CHEST MEDICINE

Essentials of Pulmonary and Critical Care Medicine

Fifth Edition

CHEST MEDICINE

Essentials of Pulmonary and Critical Care Medicine

Fifth Edition

Editors

Ronald B. George, MD
Professor of Medicine, Emeritus
Former Chairman
Department of Medicine
Louisiana State University School of Medicine
Shreveport, Louisiana

Richard W. Light, MD
Professor of Medicine
Vanderbilt University
Director of Pulmonary Disease Program
Department of Medicine
St. Thomas Hospital
Nashville, Tennessee

Michael A. Matthay, MD
Professor of Medicine and Anesthesia
Division of Pulmonary and Critical Care Medicine
Cardiovascular Research Institute
University of California, San Francisco
San Francisco, California

Richard A. Matthay, MD
Professor of Medicine and Associate Director
Section of Pulmonary and Critical Care Medicine
Department of Internal Medicine
Yale University School of Medicine
New Haven, Connecticut

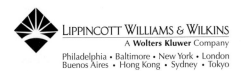

LIPPINCOTT WILLIAMS & WILKINS
A **Wolters Kluwer** Company
Philadelphia • Baltimore • New York • London
Buenos Aires • Hong Kong • Sydney • Tokyo

Acquisitions Editor: Danette Somers/Sonya Seigafuse
Developmental Editor: Joanne Bersin
Project Manager: Fran Gunning
Senior Manufacturing Manager: Ben Rivera
Marketing Manager: Kathleen Neely
Design Coordinator: Doug Smock
Production Services: Laserwords Private Limited
Printer: Edwards Brothers

5th Edition
© 2005 by LIPPINCOTT WILLIAMS & WILKINS
530 Walnut Street
Philadelphia, PA 19106
www.lww.com
4e–LWW, 2000; 1e–Churchill Livingston, 1983

Library of Congress Cataloging-in-Publication Data
Chest medicine : essentials of pulmonary and critical care medicine /
[edited by] Ronald B. George—[et al.]—5th ed.
    p. ; cm.
  Includes bibliographical references and index.
  ISBN 0-7817-5273-6
  1. Chest—Diseases. 2. Lungs—Diseases. 3. Respiratory intensive care. I. George, Ronald B.
[DNLM: 1. Lung Diseases. 2. Critical Care—methods. WF 600 C525 2005]
RC941.C5675 2005
616.2'4—dc22

                                                                        2005005876

Care has been taken to confirm the accuracy of the information presented and to describe generally accepted practices. However, the authors, editors, and publisher are not responsible for errors or omissions or for any consequences from application of the information in this book and make no warranty, expressed or implied, with respect to the currency, completeness, or accuracy of the contents of the publication. Application of this information in a particular situation remains the professional responsibility of the practitioner.

The authors, editors, and publisher have exerted every effort to ensure that drug selection and dosage set forth in this text are in accordance with current recommendations and practice at the time of publication. However, in view of ongoing research, changes in government regulations, and the constant flow of information relating to drug therapy and drug reactions, the reader is urged to check the package insert for each drug for any change in indications and dosage and for added warnings and precautions. This is particularly important when the recommended agent is a new or infrequently employed drug.

Some drugs and medical devices presented in this publication have Food and Drug Administration (FDA) clearance for limited use in restricted research settings. It is the responsibility of health care providers to ascertain the FDA status of each drug or device planned for use in their clinical practice.

The publishers have made every effort to trace copyright holders for borrowed material. If they have inadvertently overlooked any, they will be pleased to make the necessary arrangements at the first opportunity.

To purchase additional copies of this book, call our customer service department at (800) 638-3030 or fax orders to (301) 824-7390. Lippincott Williams & Wilkins customer service representatives are available from 8:30 am to 6:30 pm, EST, Monday through Friday, for telephone access. Visit Lippincott Williams & Wilkins on the Internet: http://www.lww.com.

10 9 8 7 6 5 4 3 2 1

DEDICATION

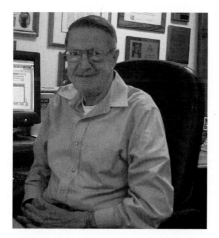

We dedicate the fifth edition of *Chest Medicine* to the esteemed clinician–educator Thomas L. Petty, M.D. Dr. Petty served as Chief of the Pulmonary Sciences Division at the University of Colorado from 1971 to 1985. Subsequently, he was Director of the Webb Waring Institute at the University of Colorado from 1983 to 1989, Director of Academic and Research Affairs at Presbyterian St. Luke's Medical Center in Denver from 1989 to 1995, and Chairman of the National Lung Health Education Program (NLHEP) from 1997 to 2004.

One of Dr. Petty's many achievements is the description of the acute respiratory distress syndrome (ARDS) with Drs. Ashbaugh, Levine, and Bigelow in *Lancet* in 1967. Along with colleagues in Denver, Dr. Petty was a major force in the introduction of oxygen therapy for chronic obstructive pulmonary disease (COPD), still the only therapy shown to improve survival in patients with COPD. Dr. Petty has also championed the early diagnosis of COPD and lung cancer.

When Dr. Petty began his career in medicine, intensive care—especially ventilator management of medical patients—was largely directed by anesthesiologists. Dr. Petty believed that internists, especially pulmonologists and critical care medicine specialists, should have a major role in the care and treatment of these patients. Perhaps more than any other person, Dr. Petty deserves credit for ensuring that pulmonologists and critical care medicine physicians have a predominant role in the care of critically ill patients in medical intensive care units throughout the United States.

As an educator in pulmonary and critical care medicine, Dr. Petty has been unsurpassed. Between 1971 and 1985, he and his colleagues in Denver trained 148 fellows. Substantially more than half of these fellows entered academic medicine, 12 became division chiefs, 2 became department chairmen of medicine, and several became hospital chiefs.

Tom Petty is one of the great academic leaders of the past century. It is with high respect and deep gratitude that we dedicate this edition of *Chest Medicine* to Thomas L. Petty.

Ronald B. George, MD
Richard W. Light, MD
Michael A. Matthay, MD
Richard A. Matthay, MD

CONTRIBUTING AUTHORS

Luis F. Angel, MD
Assistant Professor of Medicine
Department of Medicine
University of Texas Health Science Center at San Antonio
San Antonio, Texas

Alejandro C. Arroliga, MD
Professor of Medicine
Cleveland Clinic Lerner College of Medicine
Department of Pulmonary, Allergy and Critical Care Medicine
The Cleveland Clinic
Cleveland, Ohio

Kamran Atabai, MD
Post Doctoral Fellow
Lung Biology Center
Department of Medicine
University of California
San Francisco, California

John R. Balmes, MD
Professor of Medicine
Department of Medicine
University of California
Chief, Division of Occupational and Environmental Medicine
San Francisco Corner Hospital
San Francisco, California

Richard B. Berry, MD, DABSM
Professor of Medicine
Department of Medicine, Division of Pulmonary
    and Critical Care Medicine
University of Florida
Director, Sleep Laboratory
Department of Pulmonary and Critical Care Medicine
Malcolm Randall VAMC
Gainesville, Florida

Carolyn S. Calfee, MD
Fellow
Division of Pulmonary and Critical Care Medicine
Cardiovascular Research Institute
University of California
San Francisco, California

G. Douglas Campbell Sr. MD
Professor
Department of Medicine
Director
Division of Pulmonary, Critical Care
    and Sleep Medicine
University of Mississippi School of Medicine
Jackson, Mississippi

Donna L. Carden, MD
Professor of Medicine
Department of Emergency Medicine, Internal Medicine
Louisiana State University Health Sciences Center
Vice-Chair for Research
Department of Emergency Medicine
Louisiana State University Health Sciences Center
Shreveport, Louisiana

Darryl C. Carter, MD
Professor of Pathology, Emeritus
Department of Pathology
Yale University School of Medicine
New Haven, Connecticut

Brian M. Daniel, RRT, RCP
Director, Clinical Education
Respiratory Care Program
Skyline College
San Bruno, California
Clinical Specialist
Department of Respiratory Care Service
UCSF Medical Center
San Francisco, California

James F. Donohue, MD
Professor of Medicine
Department of Medicine
University of North Carolina
Chief
Department of Pulmonary
    and Critical Care Medicine
UNC Health Systems
Chapel Hill, North Carolina

Rachel H. Dotson, MD
Department of Medicine
Division of Pulmonary and Critical Care Medicine
University of California
San Francisco, California

Jane M. Eggerstedt, MD
Professor of Surgery
Department of Surgery
Louisiana State University Health Sciences Center
Shreveport, Louisiana

Mark D. Eisner, MD, MPH
Assistant Professor of Medicine
Department of Medicine
Moffitt-Long Hospital
University of California
San Francisco, California

E. Wesley Ely, MD, MPH
Associate Professor of Medicine
Department of Medicine
Vanderbilt University
Associate Director of Research
Geriatric Research Education and Clinical Center (GRECC)
Veterans Affairs Tennessee (VATN), Valley Health Care System
Nashville, Tennessee

M. Chad Foster
Attending Radiologist
Department of Diagnostic Radiology
Hospital of St. Raphael
New Haven, Connecticut

James A. Frank, MA, MD
Assistant Professor of Medicine in Residence
Division of Pulmonary and Critical Care Medicine
University of California
Director, MICU
Department of Pulmonary and Critical Care Medicine
San Francisco VA Medical Center
San Francisco, California

Ronald B. George, MD
Professor of Medicine, Emeritus
Former Chairman
Department of Medicine
Louisiana State University School of Medicine
Shreveport, Louisiana

Michael B. Gotway, MD
Assistant Professor in Residence
Director, Radiology Residency Training Program
Vice-Chair, Department of Diagnostic Radiology, Pulmonary
    and Critical Care Medicine
University of California
Interim Director, Thoracic Imaging
Department of Radiology
San Francisco General Hospital
San Francisco, California

Michael A. Gropper, MD, PHD, FCCP
Professor of Medicine
Departments of Anesthesia and Physiology
University of California
Director, Critical Care Medicine
Department of Anesthesia and Perioperative Care
Moffitt-Long Hospital
San Francisco, California

Robert J. Homer, MD, PHD
Associate Professor
Department of Pathology
Yale University School of Medicine
New Haven, Connecticut

Director of Anatomic Pathology
Pathology and Laboratory Medicine Service
VA CT Healthcare System
West Haven, Connecticut

Stephen G. Jenkinson, MD
Professor of Medicine
Director, Division of Pulmonary Diseases and Critical Care Medicine
Department of Medicine
University of Texas Health Science Center at San Antonio
San Antonio, Texas

Mani S. Kavuru, MD
Director, Pulmonary Function Lab
Department of Pulmonary, Allergy, Critical Care Medicine
Cleveland Clinic Foundation
Cleveland, Ohio

Gary T. Kinasewitz, MD
Professor and Chief, Pulmonary and Critical Care
Department of Medicine
University of Oklahoma Health Sciences Center
Oklahoma City, Oklahoma

Stephanie M. Levine, MD
Professor of Medicine
Department of Medicine, Division of Pulmonary
    and Critical Care Medicine
University of Texas Health Science Center
Co-Medical Director, Lung Transplant Program
University Hospital
San Antonio, Texas

Cari R. Levy, MD
Assistant Professor
Department of Internal Medicine
University of Colorado Health Sciences Center
Arora, Colorado
Assistant Professor
Department of Internal Medicine
University Hospital
Denver, Colorado

Richard W. Light, MD
Professor of Medicine
Vanderbilt University
Director of Pulmonary Disease Program
Department of Medicine
St. Thomas Hospital
Nashville, Tennessee

John M. Luce, MD
Professor of Medicine
Department of Medicine and Anesthesia
University of California
Member
Division of Pulmonary and Critical Care Medicine
San Francisco General Hospital
San Francisco, California

C. Kees Mahutte, MD, PHD
Professor of Medicine
University of California, Irvine
Orange, California
Chief
Department of Pulmonary and Critical Care Section
UA Long Beach HCS
Long Beach, California

Boaz A. Markewitz, MD
Assistant Professor
Department of Internal Medicine, Division of Respiratory,
    Critical Care and Occupational Pulmonary Medicine
University of Utah
University of Utah Hospital
Salt Lake City, Utah

Michael A. Matthay, MD
Professor of Medicine and Anesthesia
Division of Pulmonary
  and Critical Care Medicine
Cardiovascular Research Institute
University of California, San Francisco
San Francisco, California

Richard A. Matthay, MD
Professor of Medicine and Associate Director
Section of Pulmonary and Critical Care Medicine
Department of Internal Medicine
Yale University School of Medicine
New Haven, Connecticut

Frank M. Mele, MD
Attending Radiologist
Department of Diagnostic Radiology
Hospital of St. Raphael
New Haven, Connecticut

Shawn A. Milligan, MA, FCCP
Professor of Medicine
Department of Medicine, Division of Pulmonary
  and Clinical Care Medicine
Louisiana State University Health Sciences Center
Shreveport, Louisiana

David G. Morris, MD
Assistant Professor of Medicine
Department of Medicine, Division of Pulmonary
  and Critical Care Medicine
Yale University School of Medicine
Attending Physician
Department of Medicine, Division of Pulmonary
  and Critical Care Medicine
Yale-New Haven Hospital
New Haven, Connecticut

Michael S. Niederman, MD
Professor and Vice-Chairman
Department of Medicine
Stony Brook, New York
Chairman
Department of Medicine
Winthrop University Hospital
Minneola, New York

Paul W. Noble, MD
Professor of Medicine
Department of Internal Medicine, Division of Pulmonary
  and Critical Care
Yale University School of Medicine
Director, Interstitial Lung Disease Clinic
Yale-New Haven Hospital
New Haven, Connecticut

Michael W. Owens, MD
Associate Professor and Vice-Chairman
Department of Medicine
Louisiana State University Health Sciences Center
Chief of Medicine
Overton Brooks VAMC
Shreveport, Louisiana

D. Keith Payne, MD
Professor of Medicine
Department of Medicine, Division of Pulmonary
  and Critical Care Medicine
Louisiana State University Health Sciences Center
Chief
Department of Pulmonary
  and Critical Care Medicine
Louisiana State University Health Sciences Center
Shreveport, Louisiana

Jay I. Peters, MD
Professor of Medicine
Department of Medicine, Division of Pulmonary Diseases
  and Critical Care Medicine
University of Texas Health Science Center
San Antonio, Texas

Margaret A. Pisani, MD, MPH
Assistant Professor
Department of Internal Medicine
Yale University
New Haven, Connecticut

Carrie A. Redlich, MD, MPH
Professor of Medicine (Internal Medicine)
Department of Pulmonary and Critical Care, Occupational
  and Environmental Medicine
Yale University School of medicine
Staff Physician
Internal Medicine
Yale-New Haven Hospital
New Haven, Connecticut

Herbert Y. Reynolds, MD
Professor of Medicine
Department of Medicine
Pennsylvania State University College of Medicine
Milton S. Hershey Medical Center
Hershey, Pennsylvania
Medical Officer
Division of Lung Diseases
National Heart Lung Blood Institute
National Institute of Health
Department of Health and Human Resources
Bethesda, Maryland

R. Michael Rodriguez, MD, FCCP
Associate Professor Medicine
Department of Pulmonary Medicine
St. Thomas Hospital and Vanderbilt University
Nashville, Tennessee

Sanjay Saint, MD, MPH
Associate Professor of Medicine
Department of Internal Medicine
University of Michigan
Lansing, Michigan
Research Investigator
Health Services Research and Development
Ann Arbor VA Medical Center
Ann Arbor, Michigan

Gerardo S. San Pedro, MD
Associate Professor of Clinical Medicine
Department of Internal Medicine, Division of Pulmonary
  and Critical Care Medicine
Louisiana State University Health Sciences Center
Shreveport, Louisiana

George A. Sarosi, MD, MACP
Professor of Medicine
Chief, Medical Service
Roudebush VA Medical Center
Indianapolis, Indiana

Richard H. Savel, MD
Assistant Professor
Department of Medicine
Mt. Sinai School of Medicine
New York, New York
Associate Director
Surgical ICU
Maimonides Medical Center
Brooklyn, New York

H. Dirk Sostman, MD, FACR
Executive Vice Dean
Professor and Chair of Radiology
Weill Medical College of Cornell University
Ithaca, New York
Chief Radiologist
Weill Cornell Medical Center
NewYork - Presbyterian Hospital
New York, New York

Annette Stralovich-Romani, RD, CNSD
Adult Critical Care Nutritionist
Nutrition and Dietetics
UCSF Medical Center
San Francisco, California

Lynn T. Tanoue, MD
Associate Professor
Department of Internal Medicine, Division of Pulmonary
    and Critical Care Medicine
Yale University School of Medicine

Medical Director
Yale Lung Cancer Center
Yale New Haven Hospital
New Haven, Connecticut

Lorraine B. Ware, MD
Assistant Professor
Department of Medicine
Vanderbilt University
Attending Physician
Allergy, Pulmonary and Critical Care Medicine
Vanderbilt University Medical Center
Nashville, Tennessee

Herbert P. Wiedemann, MD
Professor of Medicine
Cleveland Clinic Lerner College of Medicine
Chairman
The Department of Pulmonary, Allergy and Critical Care Medicine
Cleveland Clinic Foundation
Cleveland, Ohio

PREFACE

It has been 25 years since the editors initiated the plans for *Chest Medicine*. The first edition appeared in 1983 after two years in development. At that time, we had a different publisher and only three editors. There was to be a fourth editor, Dr. Roger Bone, but he had to bow out and was later replaced by Dr. Michael Matthay. We feel that five editions of this textbook, appearing over a quarter of a century, qualify it as a standard in the field of pulmonary and critical care medicine.

From the start, we have tried to fill a specific need: a concise yet complete textbook for the busy physician, containing the essential knowledge in our field. We have kept the book at a "laptop" size so that it is portable and thus available to clinicians and students for studying when away from their office or home. We have also attempted to keep the price low enough for students and house staff physicians to afford. Each new edition is a complete rewrite of the previous ones, with elimination of some sections and addition of new ones, new authors, and new illustrations. At the same time, there is some overlap with previous editions; for example, many of the figures are repeated if they are still current and appropriate, and some sections like those on history taking and physical examination are similar to those in the previous editions.

We have attempted to keep up with the vast changes in our subspecialty over the years. We have greatly expanded the critical care sections so that they now comprise a major portion of the book. Considerable space has been devoted to sleep medicine, pulmonary hypertension and fibrosis, and newer diagnostic studies. We continue to discuss new procedures and new applications of old ones.

As in the past, we wish to thank our contributing authors and the many people who have worked with us in the production of this textbook, including our secretaries, our audiovisual departments, and our fellow faculty members. We thank the students, residents, and fellows who continue to question us and stimulate us to stay current. We also thank the many editorial personnel we have worked with at Lippincott Williams and Wilkins, particularly Joyce Rachel-John, Joanne Bersin, and Jolene Lehr. Finally, we wish to thank our friend, mentor and advisor, Dr. Tom Petty, to whom this edition is dedicated.

Ronald B. George, MD
Richard W. Light, MD
Michael A. Matthay, MD
Richard A. Matthay, MD

CONTENTS

SECTION 1

ANATOMY AND PHYSIOLOGY OF THE RESPIRATORY SYSTEM

SECTION 2

GATHERING THE DATABASE

SECTION 3

MANAGEMENT OF RESPIRATORY DISEASES

ANATOMY AND PHYSIOLOGY OF THE RESPIRATORY SYSTEM

Functional Anatomy of the Respiratory System

Donna L. Carden

Michael A. Matthay

Ronald B. George

The lungs perform many important functions, including the filtering of systemic venous blood prior to its entry into the left ventricle and the production and metabolism of vasoactive substances. Their most important function, however, is the exchange of carbon dioxide—a by-product of cellular metabolism—for oxygen, which is necessary for cellular activity. The respiratory system is ideally designed to perform this vital function 24 hours a day with a minimum amount of work (1).

During a lifetime of breathing, the delicate tissues of the lung periphery are constantly exposed to environmental toxins and irritants of varying potency, including viruses, bacteria, and other living organisms, as well as cigarette smoke, dust particles, and toxic chemicals. This constant exposure to a hostile environment has resulted in the development of an elaborate defense mechanism for the purpose of maintaining the integrity of the lung periphery.

Table 1-1 outlines the functional components of respiration and lung defenses and the structures involved. This chapter provides an overview of these structures as they relate to the functions for which they have been designed.

VENTILATORY PUMP

The ventilatory pump consists of the chest wall, the respiratory muscles, and the pleural space, which connects the lungs to the chest wall. The chest wall acts as a rigid cylinder within which the lungs are expanded and deflated by the action of the respiratory muscles. The diaphragm, the principal muscle of quiet breathing, moves like a piston within the cylinder, and the movement of this wide-bore piston over relatively short distances represents an efficient method of moving large volumes of air with minimum work. Air moves into and out of the lungs in a to and fro manner like the tides of the ocean; thus, it is called *tidal* flow.

CHEST WALL

The bony thorax consists of the spine, ribs, and sternum. The basic shape of the thorax is that of a truncated cone (Fig. 1-1). Both the superior and inferior ends of the cone are inclined anteriorly so that the posterior portion of the cone, the spine, is

TABLE 1-1.   Respiratory Structures as Related to Their Function

Function	Structures
Ventilatory pump	Chest wall and pleura Respiratory muscles
Distribution of ventilation	Upper respiratory tract Conducting airways Respiratory bronchioles
Distribution of blood	Pulmonary arteries and veins Pulmonary capillaries
Gas exchange	Terminal respiratory unit
Bronchial clearance	Mucociliary escalator Macrophages
Alveolar clearance and defense	Pulmonary lymphatics Alveolar macrophages Humoral mediators Inflammatory cells

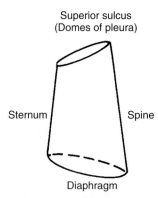

FIGURE 1-1.   Simplified diagram of the cone-shaped thorax (lateral view). There is anterior–posterior compression, so the thorax is widened laterally; the anterior wall is shorter than the posterior wall and the superior and inferior planes are inclined anteriorly.

longer than the anterior portion, the sternum. These structures are innervated and may be a source of chest pain. The ribs are hinged on the spine by ligaments and cartilage in such a way that the ribs move upward and outward during inspiration and downward and inward during expiration. This hinging movement results in a change in thoracic volume. In addition, the connective tissue components of the chest wall function as a spring, storing mechanical energy. This elastic property of the chest wall is a function both of the geometry of chest wall structures and of their composition. The extracellular matrix components that determine the mechanical properties of the chest include both the calcified bony ribs and the proteoglycans, elastin, and collagen of the cartilaginous ribs.

The expansion of the chest wall driven by respiratory muscles causes a fall in pressure of the air contained within the lungs, which in turn causes the flow of gas into the lungs. Air continues to flow into the lungs until the intrapulmonary gas pressure equals the atmospheric pressure. As the respiratory muscles relax, expiration begins and the elastic recoil of the chest wall and lungs compresses the air contained within the lungs, resulting in a pressure greater than atmospheric pressure. This causes gas to flow out of the lungs. The movement of the chest wall and lungs during inspiration and expiration is shown in Figure 1-2.

RESPIRATORY MUSCLES

The respiratory muscles are the only skeletal muscles that are essential to life; they have been called "the vital pump" by Macklem and associates (2). Clinical investigations have shown that weakness or fatigue of the respiratory muscles is a common cause of hypercapnic respiratory failure and difficulty of weaning from mechanical ventilation (3,4).

Inspiration requires active work, which is provided by the muscles of inspiration. These include the diaphragm, the inspiratory intercostal muscles, and the accessory muscles of inspiration (the scalenes and sternomastoids). Expiration under normal, quiet conditions is passive and requires no work; however, when ventilatory needs increase because of exertion or when the lungs are abnormal, as in asthma or chronic obstructive pulmonary disease (COPD), expiration often becomes an active process. The muscles of expiration include the internal intercostal muscles and the muscles of the abdominal wall (Fig. 1-3). In quadriplegic

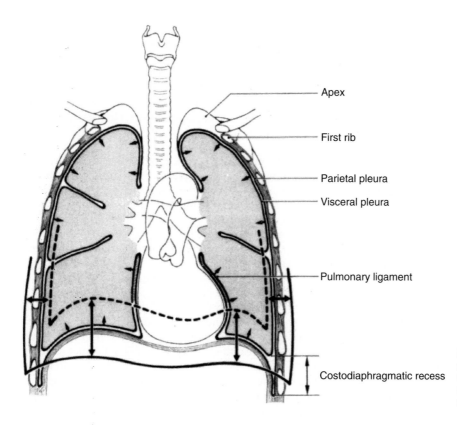

Apex

First rib

Parietal pleura

Visceral pleura

Pulmonary ligament

Costodiaphragmatic recess

FIGURE 1-2. Frontal section of chest and lung showing pleural space. *Single arrows* indicate retractive force and *double arrows* show the excursion of the lung bases and periphery between deep inspiration and expiration.

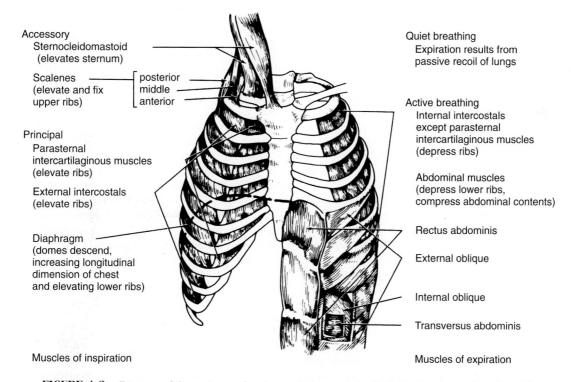

Accessory
  Sternocleidomastoid
  (elevates sternum)

Scalenes
  (elevate and fix
  upper ribs)
    [posterior
      middle
      anterior

Principal
  Parasternal
  intercartilaginous muscles
  (elevate ribs)

  External intercostals
  (elevate ribs)

  Diaphragm
  (domes descend,
  increasing longitudinal
  dimension of chest
  and elevating lower ribs)

Muscles of inspiration

Quiet breathing
  Expiration results from
  passive recoil of lungs

Active breathing
  Internal intercostals
  except parasternal
  intercartilaginous muscles
  (depress ribs)

  Abdominal muscles
  (depress lower ribs,
  compress abdominal contents)

Rectus abdominis

External oblique

Internal oblique

Transversus abdominis

Muscles of expiration

FIGURE 1-3. Diagram of the anatomy of major respiratory muscles. Left side, inspiratory muscles; right side, expiratory muscles. (Reprinted from Garrity ER, Sharp JT. Respiratory muscles: function and dysfunction. *Pulmonary and critical care update*, Vol. 2. Park Ridge, IL: American College of Chest Physicians, 1986, with permission.)

patients, the pectoralis major and serratus anterior muscles may be used during expiration (5).

Like all skeletal muscles, and unlike the smooth muscle that lines airways, the muscles of respiration have no basal tone. Release of acetylcholine at the neuromuscular junction is required to initiate the contraction process. Binding of acetylcholine to the N_2 nicotinic cholinergic receptor on the target muscle cell initiates a depolarization that in turn releases calcium from the T-tubule system into the cytoplasm. This calcium then activates the adenosine triphosphatase (ATPase) of the myosin heavy chain, which converts adenosine triphosphate (ATP) to adenosine diphosphate (ADP), causing the myosin to move along the actin fibers present within the cellular cytoplasm. This movement results in cellular shortening, and in this manner, chemical energy is converted from ATP to the mechanical energy needed to drive ventilation. The ATP, in turn, is generated by the mitochondria of the muscle cell by oxidative metabolism or, for brief intervals, by glycolysis. Repolarization of the cell membrane, resequestration of calcium, and cleavage of acetylcholine by acetylcholinesterase result in relaxation of the muscle cell and readies it for another round of contraction.

Resting tidal breathing depends on the diaphragm, which is composed of two distinct portions. The costal and crural portions of the diaphragm have separate functions and innervations. The motor innervation to the diaphragm is via the phrenic nerve, which is derived from the third, fourth, and fifth cervical nerves. Sensory nerves to the crural portion of the diaphragm are also carried by the phrenic nerve; thus, irritation of the center of the diaphragm may cause pain that is referred to the ipsilateral neck or shoulder areas, which are also innervated by the third, fourth, and fifth cervical segments. Sensory innervation of the costal portion of the diaphragm is via the intercostal nerves from the adjacent chest wall, which they also innervate, and pain from the lateral portion of the diaphragm is referred to the chest wall.

The dome of the diaphragm moves downward with contraction, displacing abdominal contents; therefore, during inspiration the abdomen normally moves outward. Because of the fulcrum effect of the relatively fixed abdominal contents, diaphragm contraction also elevates and increases the diameter of the lower rib cage (Fig. 1-2). The accessory muscles of inspiration become important only during high levels of ventilation and with hyperinflation of the thorax associated with obstructive lung disease. The accessory muscles move the cage upward so that the ribs themselves lie in a more horizontal plane, thus increasing the diameter of the thoracic cage.

Fatigue of the inspiratory muscles occurs when the energy supply is exceeded as a result of increased ventilatory demands (vigorous exercise), increased work of breathing (asthma or COPD), or inadequate energy generation by the muscles (hypoxemia or congestive heart failure). Dyspnea is the major complaint when the respiratory muscles become fatigued. The sensation of dyspnea has not been completely explained, but it may be related to a disproportion between the amount of work required and the amount of work the respiratory muscles can perform. Healthy respiratory muscles can increase minute ventilation from a normal resting level of 6 to 7 L/min to a maximum of over 100 L/min with voluntary effort. However, this maximum level of ventilation cannot be sustained over long periods, and with vigorous exercise, minute ventilation is more

often maintained at five to six times the normal resting level. The body adapts to the increased ventilatory demand by increasing the circulation to the muscles of inspiration and by increasing the extraction of oxygen from the diaphragmatic capillaries. Lactate production occurs in normal persons only as a result of breathing against a high resistance, leading to fatigue, or breathing low-oxygen mixtures. High levels of blood lactate have been found in patients during severe asthma attacks (6).

Hyperinflation, which occurs in patients with emphysema and during asthma attacks, places the diaphragm at a distinct disadvantage. With hyperinflation, the diaphragm is already low and flat; contraction neither moves the diaphragm downward nor moves the lower rib cage outward. In fact, with severe hyperinflation, diaphragm contraction may pull the lower rib cage inward *(Hoover's sign)*, causing an expiratory effect on the rib cage (7).

The clinical signs of inspiratory muscle fatigue have been summarized by Macklem's group (2,3,8). During early muscle fatigue, the ratio of high-frequency to low-frequency electrical activity of the diaphragm, as recorded on an electromyogram, decreases. This is manifested by an increased respiratory rate; rapid, shallow breathing; and an early fall in the measured arterial P_{CO_2}. As muscle fatigue increases, the diaphragm movement diminishes and the accessory muscles assume a greater role. The contraction of accessory muscles produces a negative pressure in the thorax that may actually pull the flaccid diaphragm upward, causing the abdomen to move inward during inspiration; this is called *paradoxical respiration* and indicates significant diaphragm fatigue (3). Respiration may also shift back and forth from predominantly diaphragmatic breathing to predominantly accessory muscle breathing *(respiratory alternans).* In summary, the clinical signs of inspiratory muscle fatigue include rapid, shallow respiration with an initial increase in minute ventilation; an initial fall in Pa_{CO_2}; often paradoxical respiration and respiratory alternans; and finally, a decrease in respiratory rate and minute ventilation, leading to hypoventilation and respiratory acidosis.

Tobin and associates have compared the clinical findings used to assess the state of the respiratory muscles prior to weaning from mechanical ventilation (9). The ratio of the respiratory rate to the tidal volume (f/V_T) is the most useful of the bedside measurements of respiratory muscle function. They also found that although respiratory muscle dysfunction is a primary cause of ventilatory failure in patients with neuromuscular disorders, respiratory muscle fatigue per se is not a primary cause of ventilatory failure in patients with COPD; rather, the increased demands on the respiratory muscles by airway obstruction and hyperinflation seem to be the primary factors in ventilatory failure (10).

PLEURA

As the lungs grow laterally from the mediastinum during fetal development, they grow into a part of the celomic cavity that is lined with undifferentiated mesenchyme. As the lungs extend into the cavity, they are covered by these mesenchymal cells, which become the parietal pleura. The mesenchymal cells that line the chest wall and mediastinum become the visceral pleura. The visceral and parietal pleura join one another at the lung hila. The parietal pleura contains abundant pain fibers derived from the intercostal nerves, and irritation of this membrane produces a characteristic, well-localized type of chest pain, which is exacerbated by chest wall movement *(pleuritic pain)*.

The pleural space is airtight; the two pleural surfaces, parietal and visceral, are separated only by a thin film that contains hyaluronic acid and provides lubrication during lung movement. In the intact system at rest, the lung has a natural tendency to become smaller and the chest wall has a natural tendency to become larger. They are thus pulling against each other across the pleural space and, because it is airtight, a negative pressure is produced. It is this negative pleural pressure that links the lung to the chest wall and transmits movements of the chest wall to the lung. At rest, the average negative intrapleural pressure is about 4 cm H_2O. In the upright position, this negative pressure is greater at the top of the lungs than at the lung bases because of the effects of gravity on the lungs themselves.

Fluid flows constantly through the pleural space, forming a lubricating film over the surface of the lungs. Recent studies show that approximately 100 mL of pleural fluid is formed each hour; because this fluid is rapidly absorbed, the pleural space contains a minimal amount of fluid at any given time. Previous theories proposed that pleural fluid was formed from the systemic capillaries adjacent to the parietal pleura and absorbed into the plexus of capillaries under the visceral pleura. However, recent studies suggest that the absorption of pleural fluid is more complicated than this and that the parietal pleural lymphatics play a role in the removal of liquid, protein, and other large particles from the pleural cavity (11,12). The visceral pleural capillaries drain via the pulmonary veins into the left atrium.

DISTRIBUTION OF AIR

Before atmospheric air reaches the alveolar–capillary membrane, the air must be conditioned so that it does not injure this delicate surface area. The *upper respiratory tract* is primarily designed to purify, warm, and humidify the air; it consists of the nose, paranasal sinuses, pharynx, and larynx.

NOSE

The nose contains a layer of epithelial cells overlying a rich capillary plexus, all resting on thin bony plates, the turbinates. The vascular and epithelial structures are responsive to neural and humoral mediators. Therefore, the nasal tissues can provide for rapid heat exchange, transudation of fluid, or recruitment of inflammatory cells to the nose. The nasal mucosa is normally bathed by thin, watery secretions designed to trap foreign particles and to add moisture to the inspired air. With normal, quiet breathing, inspired air is heated to body temperature and the relative humidity is increased to over 90% during passage through the nose. Resistance to airflow is higher in the nose than in the mouth because of the intricate system of baffles. This is the explanation for mouth breathing during vigorous exercise; in this case, the air-conditioning function of the nose is lost, and dry, cold air may enter the lower airways. In patients with abnormal irritability of the bronchial tree, inspiration of cold air through the mouth during exercise may initiate bronchospasm. Patients with tracheostomy and those being ventilated via endotracheal tubes also lose the function of the nose, and inspired gas must be artificially humidified and warmed to prevent drying and irritation of the lower airways.

PARANASAL SINUSES

The paranasal sinuses are lined by ciliated columnar epithelium and communicate with the nasal passages by narrow openings, which may become occluded when they are inflamed. Cilia within the sinus cavities beat in a pattern that tends to propel secretions toward the opening into the nasal cavity. The function of paranasal sinuses is not completely clear, but they add resonance to voice sounds and may insulate the cranial vault. They also provide lightness to the skull without unduly compromising its protective function. The sinuses may become inflamed and cause drainage of material into the pharynx (postnasal drip). This material may be aspirated into the lower respiratory tract, especially during sleep, and this may be a source of chronic bronchial irritation.

PHARYNX

The pharynx is divided by the soft palate into the nasopharynx and the oropharynx. The adenoids, tonsils, and eustachian tubes are located in the nasopharynx. The epiglottis, which protects the laryngeal opening during swallowing, is at the base of the tongue. In unconscious patients, the base of the tongue may fall posteriorly and obstruct the laryngeal opening. To avoid this, the head should be hyperextended and the lower jaw pulled forward. Alternatively, the patient may be placed in a position in which gravity causes the tongue to fall forward. The oropharynx is easily seen through the open mouth; it serves as an entryway to both the larynx and the esophagus.

LARYNX

The larynx has evolved from a simple valve, designed to prevent aspiration into the trachea, into a complex structure containing the vocal cords, capable of phonation (13). The larynx is also vital to the defense of the respiratory system because the vocal cords participate in coughing. Coughing is a major clearance mechanism for material that collects in the larger airways; it is initiated by irritation of nerves in the walls of the trachea and large bronchi. Coughing is produced by closure of the vocal cords combined with contraction of the respiratory and abdominal muscles, so that high pressures are created in the lower airways. Sudden opening of the vocal cords then allows a rush of air, carrying larger particles of mucus with it. Normally, the respiratory tract is free of bacteria below the level of the larynx.

One or both vocal cords may become paralyzed by surgery or injury to the nerves in the neck or thorax. The left recurrent laryngeal nerve descends into the mediastinum and around the arch of the aorta before returning to the larynx. This nerve may become disrupted by cancer involving lymph nodes adjacent to the left hilum, and hoarseness is an ominous sign in patients with carcinoma of the lung. Other diseases such as granulomas, lymphomas, and aortic aneurysms may also interrupt the left recurrent laryngeal nerve in the mediastinum. The right recurrent laryngeal nerve descends only to the level of the subclavian artery; therefore, it is affected less often.

If both vocal cords are paralyzed, they become flaccid near the midline and breathing may be hindered. Large airway

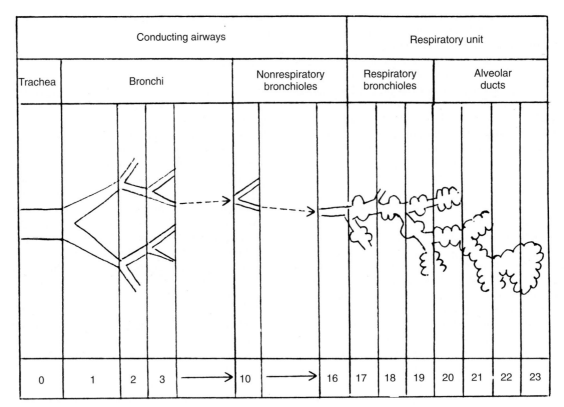

Conducting airways				Respiratory unit	
Trachea	Bronchi	Nonrespiratory bronchioles	Respiratory bronchioles	Alveolar ducts	
0	1 2 3 ⟶ 10 ⟶ 16		17 18 19	20 21 22 23	

FIGURE 1-4.   Conducting airways and terminal respiratory unit of the lung. The relative size of the respiratory unit is greatly enlarged. Figures at the bottom indicate the approximate number of generations from trachea to alveoli. (Modified from Weibel ER. *Morphometry of the human lung.* Heidelberg: Springer-Verlag, 1963, with permission.)

obstruction produces a characteristic combination of symptoms, signs, and pulmonary function abnormalities (14). Bilateral vocal cord paralysis causes a variable extrathoracic airway obstruction, which produces inspiratory stridor associated with hoarseness, dyspnea, and anxiety. Tests of ventilatory function, such as a flow-volume loop or a spirogram, may show relatively normal forced expiration; however, there is a decrease in peak airflow during inspiration. Carcinoma of the larynx also produces the combination of hoarseness and stridor. However, because this is a fixed obstruction, stridor occurs usually during both inspiration *and* expiration, and pulmonary function tests show both inspiratory and expiratory flow limitation.

The *lower respiratory tract* begins at the junction of the larynx with the trachea and includes the trachea, bronchi, bronchioles, and alveoli. The air conduction system of the lungs is a series of dichotomously branching bronchi and bronchioles, ending blindly in some 300 million alveoli, which collectively form the gas exchange surface (Fig. 1-4). There are normally about 23 generations of airways, of which the first 16 or so are conducting airways, where no gas exchange occurs, and the last 7 or so are respiratory airways, where alveoli appear in progressively larger numbers (15). The average diameter of a daughter branch is smaller than that of its parent branch, but the *total cross-sectional area* of each successive generation *increases* from trachea to alveoli; thus, the total area of the respiratory bronchioles is much greater than that of the trachea (Fig. 1-5).

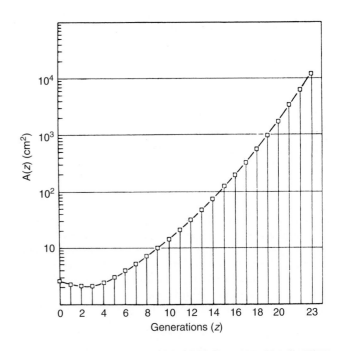

FIGURE 1-5.   Total cross section of the airways in the human lung by generation. Although each generation of airways is smaller than its parent, the *total* cross-sectional area of each generation is greater than the *total* area of the previous generation. (From Weibel ER. *Morphometry of the human lung.* Heidelberg: Springer-Verlag, 1963, with permission.)

TRACHEA

The trachea begins at the base of the neck and extends about 10 to 12 cm to its bifurcation into the right and left main bronchi. It lies immediately anterior to the esophagus and behind the aorta and often lies slightly to the right of the midline after entering the thorax. Its transverse diameter is greater than its anterior–posterior diameter, and it is held open by a series of anterior horseshoe-shaped cartilaginous rings bound posteriorly by fibrous bands. The position of the carina varies according to the position of the neck and the level of inspiration but is normally at about the level of the second anterior rib, just below the aortic arch. The angle between the right and left main bronchi is normally acute, varying from 50 to 100 degrees.

BRONCHI

The right main bronchus divides almost immediately into the upper lobe bronchus and the intermediate bronchus. The left main bronchus is considerably longer, extending across the midline approximately 5 cm before it divides into the left upper-lobe and left lower-lobe bronchi. The major bronchi contain large numbers of mucous glands; their surface is innervated by branches of both the parasympathetic and the sympathetic nervous systems. These nerves are connected to the brain via the vagus nerves. Irritant receptors in large airways initiate the cough reflex, and resultant motor stimuli through the vagi cause bronchoconstriction and mucous secretion. Airway nerves also permit axon–axonal reflexes; therefore, irritation of one site in the airway can lead to bronchoconstriction or secretion diffusely. Neuropeptides, including substance P and the neurokinins, are thought to be important mediators released by these sensory nerves in the airways (16).

The right main bronchus is larger and less deviated from the axis of the trachea than the left; it thus may be considered an extension of the trachea itself. This is an explanation for the more frequent aspiration of foreign material into the right lung. The main bronchi divide into five lobar bronchi—the upper, middle, and lower on the right and the upper and lower on the left. The left upper lobe divides into the apical-posterior and anterior segments and the lingula, which developmentally corresponds to the right middle lobe. The lobes are separated from each other by fissures, which are lined by two layers of visceral pleura.

The lobar bronchi divide into segmental bronchi, 10 on the right and 9 on the left (Fig. 1-6). Segments are usually separated by delicate connective tissue planes but not by fissures. There is some disagreement concerning the nomenclature of the bronchopulmonary segments; however, the classification of the Thoracic Society of Great Britain (shown in Fig. 1-6) is most commonly used. A thorough knowledge of the lung segments has become necessary in recent years because of the high incidence of bronchogenic carcinoma, one of the most common neoplasms. These neoplasms commonly occur in lobar and segmental bronchi and produce characteristic patterns, based on their anatomic location, on the chest x-ray film.

The epithelial cells that line the airways change in character from the proximal to the distal airways. In the trachea, the epithelium is pseudostratified with as many as four or five nuclei arranged above each other. Most of the surface area of the basement membrane, however, is covered by basal cells. These

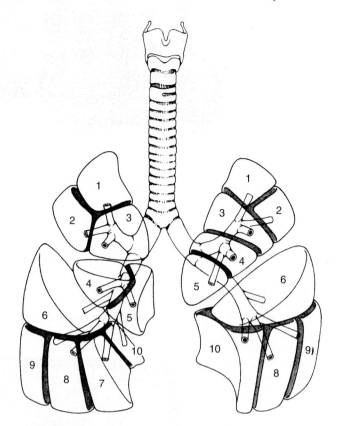

FIGURE 1-6. The bronchopulmonary segments. *Upper lobes:* (1) apical; (2) posterior; (3) anterior; (4) superior lingular; and (5) inferior lingular segments. *Middle lobe:* (4) lateral and (5) medial segments. *Lower lobes:* (6) apical (superior); (7) medial basal; (8) anterior basal; (9) lateral basal; and (10) posterior basal segments. The medial basal segment (7) is absent in the left lung. (From Weibel ER. Design and structure of the human lung. In: Fishman AP, ed. *Assessment of pulmonary function.* New York: McGraw-Hill, 1980, with permission.)

small cells with scant cytoplasm have numerous hemidesmosomes, which anchor them to the basement membrane, as well as numerous desmosomes, which provide mechanical anchors for the columnar cells of the epithelium. It is currently thought that all columnar cells extend a slender process that contacts the basement membrane and hence the designation "pseudostratified." These processes may function to regulate the differentiated phenotype of the epithelial cells.

The columnar cells consist predominantly of ciliated cells, with smaller numbers of goblet cells and brush cells. *Ciliated cells* contain motile cilia, which beat in a coordinated manner to move the mucous layer toward the mouth. *Goblet cells,* interspersed among the ciliated epithelial cells, secrete mucus. *Brush cells* contain microvilli resembling those of basal cells in the gut and may function to control fluid balance in the airway lumen. These cells may also represent immature ciliated cells. Following injury, the epithelial cellular components change, and goblet cells or squamous cells, which are usually nonkeratinizing and stratified, may replace the population of ciliated cells.

The columnar cells are connected by several types of junctions. Mechanical integrity is thought to depend on desmosomes formed with basal cells and with other columnar cells. Gap junctions between epithelial cells provide for exchange of nutrients and metabolites and may be important in permitting cell-to-cell exchange of mediators that coordinate epithelial functioning. Near the epithelial surface, the epithelial cells are linked by tight junctions. These junctions permit a fusion of the outer leaflet of the lipid bilayer cell membrane of adjacent cells. These junctions prevent exchange between the apical and basolateral membranes because they extend entirely around each cell. Tight junctions thus permit the airway epithelium to form a barrier segregating the airway lumen from the airway parenchyma. In addition, the apical cell surface is segregated from the basolateral cell surface. Many functions, particularly those involved in the regulation of secretion, depend on processes that are localized within the cell membranes.

The epithelium contains numerous glands with ducts that penetrate and empty into the airway lumen. In addition to the trachea, glands are particularly prevalent in the medium-sized bronchi but are sparse in the smaller bronchi. Glands contain two types of secretory cells: *serous cells,* which secrete a variety of peptides, including lysozyme, lactoferrin, and the secretory leukoprotease inhibitor, as well as ions and water; and *mucous cells,* which secrete mucins. Because the volume of glands is estimated to be 40-fold greater than that of the luminal goblet cells, they are thought to be the major sources of bronchial mucous secretions. Luminal secretory cells and glands, however, may be regulated differently and may make qualitatively different contributions to airway secretions. Hypertrophy of the mucous glands can occur in chronic bronchitis; the *Reid index* (a ratio of the depth of gland penetration to the thickness of the bronchial wall) is a measure of this hypertrophy.

The columnar cells are highly elongated in the proximal airways and basal cells are common (Fig. 1-7). In more peripheral airways, the columnar cells gradually become shorter and basal cells become fewer, disappearing in the terminal airways. The total height of the epithelium diminishes as its character changes from pseudostratified to columnar. Ciliated cells become less numerous and glands gradually disappear in the smaller bronchi. *Clara cells* are often seen scattered between ciliated cells and may project into the airway lumen (17). These cells contribute, along with the type II alveolar cells, to the surface lining layer of the bronchioles and alveoli. Clara cells may

also function as progenitors for ciliated cells, brush cells, and goblet cells. This may explain why there is a decrease in Clara cells with an increase in epithelial mucous cells in the bronchi of heavy smokers.

BRONCHIOLES

The segmental bronchi continue to bifurcate for about 10 generations until the nonrespiratory bronchiole is reached (Fig. 1-4). Bronchioles usually are 1 mm in diameter or smaller (18). Respiratory bronchioles, which are 0.5 mm or smaller in diameter, have alveoli in their walls and communicate directly with the alveolar ducts (Fig. 1-8). The bronchioles have a lining mucosa that contains Clara, ciliated, and basal cells. Clara cells are scattered between ciliated cells and may project into the airway lumen (17). Clara cells tend to disappear with an increase in epithelial mucous cells in the bronchi of heavy smokers. Surrounding the bronchiolar mucosal layer are a basement membrane, a lamina propria, an elastic tissue layer, a layer of smooth muscle, and an adventitial layer that is attached to the surrounding alveoli and perivascular interstitium. The total cross-sectional circumference of the terminal bronchioles in human lungs is nearly 2000 times that of the trachea (Fig. 1-5) (15). Beyond the terminal bronchiole, the airways contain progressively larger numbers of alveoli. As shown in Figure 1-4, *alveolar ducts* are found after approximately three generations of respiratory bronchioles. These are totally lined by alveolar type I cells.

Direct communications occur between bronchioles and surrounding alveoli *(canals of Lambert),* and it is through these canals that bronchiolar epithelium may grow into the alveoli in the healing phase of bronchiolitis (18). This has been called *lambertosis* or *peribronchiolar metaplasia.* Ventilation of the conducting airways ceases to be bulk flow at the level of the alveolar ducts. Farther distally, movement of gases is by gaseous diffusion. Ventilation of the gas-exchange surfaces, therefore, depends on how far the gases must travel from the alveolar duct to the alveolar wall. If small peripheral airways become partly or completely occluded, collateral ventilation of alveoli may occur via the *pores of Kohn*—holes in the alveolar walls that connect

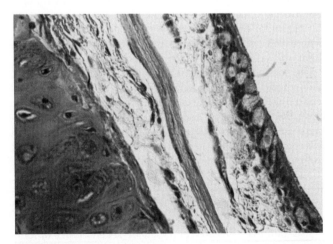

FIGURE 1-7. Section through the wall of a large bronchus (×400). The lumen (right) is lined with pseudostratified columnar epithelial cells containing tiny cilia, which propel mucus toward the trachea. The submucosa is surrounded by a thin layer of smooth muscle. To the left is a part of the cartilage that lends support to the bronchial wall. (Courtesy of Warren D. Grafton, MD.)

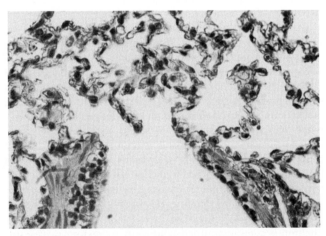

FIGURE 1-8. Section through a terminal bronchiole (×400). At the center of the picture, the terminal bronchiole is dividing into two respiratory bronchioles whose walls contain alveoli. The respiratory bronchioles end in alveolar sacs. (Courtesy of Warren D. Grafton, MD.)

alveoli directly—or via the canals of Lambert. This collateral ventilation increases the physiologic dead space and adds to the ventilation–perfusion mismatching seen in diseases that affect the small airways (19). However, it prevents lung segments distal to obstructed airways from becoming atelectatic.

METABOLIC AND SECRETORY FUNCTIONS OF THE RESPIRATORY MUCOSA

In addition to their role as conducting airways, the respiratory bronchi and bronchioles have been shown to perform everexpanding duties involving the production of secretory products and the transport of electrolytes and water. Surfactant is a highly heterogeneous mixture of phospholipid–protein aggregates. It is produced by the nonciliated cells of the bronchioles as well as the type II cells of the alveoli. In the adult lung, phosphatidylcholine and phosphatidylglycerol are the most abundant phospholipids; lesser amounts of sphingomyelin, neutral lipids, glycolipids, and other lipids are found in surfactant as well. Toward the end of fetal gestation, surfactant phospholipids increase markedly in the lungs and are secreted into the amniotic fluid. The levels of phospholipids in amniotic fluid correlate with postnatal respiratory function. Four surfactant proteins, SP-A, SP-B, SP-C, and SP-D, are produced by respiratory epithelial cells (20). They play important roles in surfactant function and host defenses. Other proteins produced by the respiratory epithelial cells include the Clara Cell Protein (CC16, CC10) and mucin-associated antigens (KL-6, 17-Q2, 17-B1). These proteins are important for host defenses (20). Beyond this, the epithelial goblet cells and the mucous glands secrete the complex mucous blanket, which serves a vital role in the defense of the lungs and the removal of foreign particles.

The respiratory epithelium also serves an important role in the movement of solutes and water, contributing to the maintenance of lung fluid balance. The epithelial cells are joined at their apical surface by tight junctions with selective permeabilities to ions, other solutes, and water (21). Furthermore, the apical membrane, which contains the epithelial sodium channel (ENaC) and the cystic fibrosis transmembrane conductance regulatory (CFTR) chloride channel, differs from the basolateral membrane, which contains the ATPase-powered sodium–potassium pump (22). These cellular pathways provide for selective ion transport (Fig. 1-9). Recent evidence suggests that active sodium transport in the distal lung epithelium is the primary mechanism that drives fluid clearance from the distal airspaces. The rate of fluid transport from the airspaces can be increased by cyclic adenosine monophosphate (cAMP) stimulation. Catecholamine-independent mechanisms including hormones, growth factors, and cytokines also contribute to epithelial fluid clearance in the lung (23).

Epithelial cells of patients with cystic fibrosis (CF) lack CFTR chloride channels. Normally, the fluid in the bronchi has a low salt concentration, with chloride levels of 80 to 90 mM. However, in patients with CF, surface fluid has higher chloride levels, in the range of 130 to 170 mM, suggesting that chloride absorption through CFTR channels tends to lower the salt concentration in the mucosal fluid. High salt concentrations in CF airway fluid may prevent bacterial killing by antibacterial factors from the epithelium and may also affect the normal hydration of mucus (24).

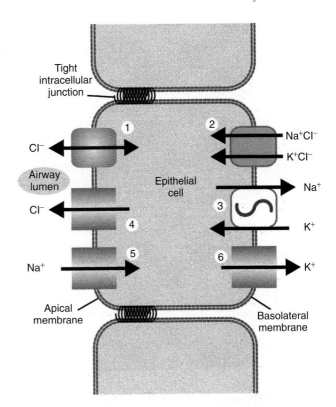

FIGURE 1-9. Mechanisms of electrolyte transport through the respiratory epithelium. Rounded boxes indicate passive pathways of ion exchange, whereas square boxes indicate active transport channels. (1) CFTR chloride channel, which is powered by cAMP; patients with cystic fibrosis lack this pathway. (2) Electrically neutral cotransport channel moves Cl^- into the cell coupled with Na^+ and K^+. (3) The ATPase-powered sodium–potassium pump maintains high intracellular K^+ levels and low intracellular Na^+ levels. (4) Chloride exits passively into the mucosa via apical membrane channels. (5) Sodium enters the cell passively via epithelial Na^+ channels (ENaC). (6) Passive K^+ exit via basolateral K^+ channels.

DISTRIBUTION OF BLOOD

The lungs contain approximately 450 mL of blood, or 12% of the body's total blood volume. Seventy to one hundred milliliters of this blood are contained within the pulmonary capillaries; the rest is equally divided between the pulmonary arteries and veins (25).

The lungs are the only organs to receive essentially the entire cardiac output, a feature that facilitates their role in gas exchange and allows them to modify the blood before it is returned to the left ventricle. The lungs receive blood from two sources: the bronchial arteries, which contain oxygenated blood; and the pulmonary arteries, which contain systemic venous blood. The bronchial arteries are part of the systemic circulation and supply the supporting tissue of the lungs, including the walls of the bronchi and bronchioles to the level of the alveoli. In contrast, the pulmonary arteries are components of the low-pressure, highly compliant pulmonary circulation that originates from the right ventricle and supplies the dense capillary network surrounding the alveolar wall. The structure of this dense vascular meshwork facilitates the critical gas exchange as well as metabolic functions of the lung.

RIGHT VENTRICLE

The pulmonary circulation begins as the main pulmonary artery leaves the right ventricle. Because the left ventricle contracts with extreme force compared to the right ventricle, it assumes a globular shape and the septum protrudes into the right heart. Because both sides of the heart pump essentially the same quantity of blood, the external wall of the right ventricle bulges outward, surrounding a large portion of the left ventricle to accommodate the blood volume (Fig. 1-10) (25). As a result of the lower pressures generated by the right side of the heart, the right ventricular muscle is only one-third as thick as that of the left ventricle (25).

PULMONARY ARTERIES AND VEINS

The main pulmonary artery, carrying mixed venous blood from the right side of the heart, extends only 5 cm beyond the apex of the right ventricle before dividing into the right and left main branches, which supply the two respective lungs. The main pulmonary artery and its subdivisions are thin-walled, distensible vessels (25). Furthermore, the subdivisions of the pulmonary artery, including the small arteries and arterioles, have much larger diameters than the corresponding systemic arteries. This anatomic feature makes the pulmonary vascular tree extremely compliant, averaging 7 mL/mm Hg, which is almost equal to that of the entire systemic arterial tree. This large compliance allows the pulmonary arteries to accommodate the stroke volume output of the right heart (25).

Like the airways, the main pulmonary artery successively branches the pulmonary arteries accompanying the bronchi through the centers of the primary lobules as far as the terminal bronchioles (26). Beyond that point, the pulmonary arterioles form a dense capillary network (Fig. 1-11) within the alveolar wall, an arrangement exceedingly efficient for gas exchange (26,27).

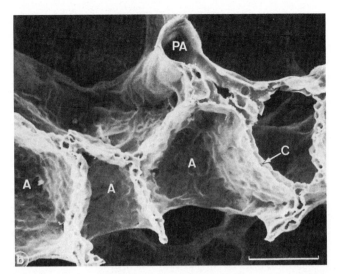

FIGURE 1-11. Blood flow in pulmonary capillaries (C) surrounds the alveoli (*A*) in a dense vascular network. PA, pulmonary arteriole; marker = 50 μm. (Reprinted with permission from Weibel ER. Design and morphometry of the pulmonary gas exchanger. In: Crystal RG, West JB, Weibel WR, et al., eds. *The lung: scientific foundations.* New York: Lippincott-Raven, 1997:1147–1159.)

Oxygenated blood leaves the pulmonary capillaries in the short, distensible, pulmonary veins that form at the periphery of the terminal respiratory unit (TRU) and that later coalesce to form the four large pulmonary veins that empty into the left atrium. In addition to the alveolar capillaries, a portion of the bronchial system also empties into the pulmonary veins. The deoxygenated blood added to the pulmonary veins by the bronchial system accounts for a significant portion of the right-to-left anatomic shunt that normally occurs in the lungs.

PULMONARY CAPILLARIES

The majority of lung vasculature consists of alveolar capillaries (28). The alveolar walls are occupied by a dense meshwork or sheet of capillaries and supporting tissue that together form a barrier to transvascular fluid exchange (Fig. 1-11). Arteriolar branches of the pulmonary artery feed at regular intervals into this dense capillary meshwork that then coalesce into venules (29). The pulmonary capillaries are surrounded by air rather than supported by tissue, as is the case in the systemic circulation. Although this arrangement facilitates gas exchange, it exposes the pulmonary capillaries to stress failure or rupture if intravascular pressure becomes excessive (30). Recent evidence suggests that injury to the pulmonary capillary can also occur as a result of excessive alveolar pressures and repeated opening and collapse of atelectatic alveoli, as occurs during mechanical ventilation (31).

The closely apposed epithelial and endothelial barriers of the alveolar–capillary membrane are both involved in the regulation of fluid and solute exchange in the lung (Fig. 1-12) (32). The alveolar capillary allows a net outward movement of fluid and small solutes from the vascular to the interstitial space. In contrast, the alveolar epithelium forms a highly restrictive barrier that limits the movement of water and ions into the alveolus. Although the vascular layer of the alveolus appears to be formed only by endothelial cells, the alveolar airspace is

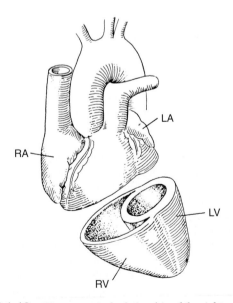

FIGURE 1-10. The anatomical relationship of the right ventricle to the left ventricle demonstrating the globular-shaped left ventricle protruding into the right heart. LA, left atrium; LV, left ventricle; RA, right atrium; RV, right ventricle. (Adapted with permission from Guyton AC. The pulmonary circulation. *Textbook of medical physiology*, 9th ed. Philadelphia: WB Saunders, 1996:491–501.)

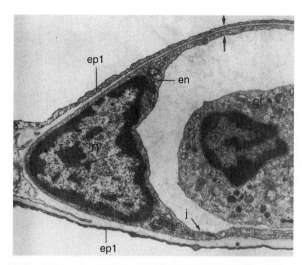

FIGURE 1-12. The alveolar–capillary membrane constitutes the primary barrier at the air–blood interface and consists of an endothelial cell (*en*) and the adjacent type I epithelial cell (*ep1*) with their fused basement membranes. (Reprinted with permission from Weibel ER. Lung cell biology. In: Fishman AP, ed. *Handbook of physiology,* Vol 1, *The respiratory system.* Baltimore: Williams & Wilkins, 1985:47–91.)

lined by at least two types of epithelial cells (Table 1-2) (33). Flat alveolar type I cells make up approximately 90% of the alveolar surface area and are easily injured. Cuboidal alveolar type II cells are involved in surfactant production, ion transport, and proliferation and differentiation into type I cells following injury (32). Interstitial cells provide support for the structures in the alveolar walls, whereas alveolar macrophages are an important component of the host defense and lung-clearance mechanisms.

ALVEOLAR–CAPILLARY BARRIER

The major site of fluid exchange in the lung is in the alveolar capillaries, although some fluid also leaks from the small arterioles and venules at the junctions of alveolar walls (34). Two separate barriers form the alveolar–capillary barrier, the

TABLE 1-2. Cells of the Alveolar Region of the Human Lung

Cells	$n \times 10^9$	Total (%)
Alveolar epithelial cells		
Type I cells	19	8.3
Type II cells	37	15.9
Endothelial cells	68	30.2
Interstitial cells	84	36.1
Macrophages	23	9.4

Reprinted with permission from Crapo JD, Barry BE, Gehr P, et al. Cell number and cell characteristics of the normal human lung. *Am Rev Respir Dis* 1982;125:740–745.

microvascular (capillary) endothelium and the alveolar epithelium (Figs. 1-12 and 1-13). The forces that govern microvascular fluid exchange are discussed in detail in Chapter 23, Acute Hypoxemic Respiratory Failure.

ALVEOLAR–EPITHELIAL BARRIER

Once thought to be composed of passive, structural cells, the alveolar epithelium is now recognized as the primary barrier against fluid movement into the alveolus. In fact, current evidence suggests that the alveolar epithelium is at least an order of magnitude less permeable than the pulmonary endothelium; hence, it is the main regulator of fluid and solute exchange across the alveolar–capillary membrane (35,36). The restrictive properties of the epithelial barrier are thought to depend on the adhesion of several specialized proteins found in the tight and adherens junctions (37–39). Moreover, the alveolar epithelium plays an active role in the reabsorption of any fluid that leaks into the alveolus (40).

CAPILLARY–ENDOTHELIAL BARRIER

The pulmonary vasculature is composed of continuous or nonfenestrated endothelium characterized by organelle-free zones that provide an exceptionally thin barrier to gas exchange (41). Most of the exchange of fluid and solute across

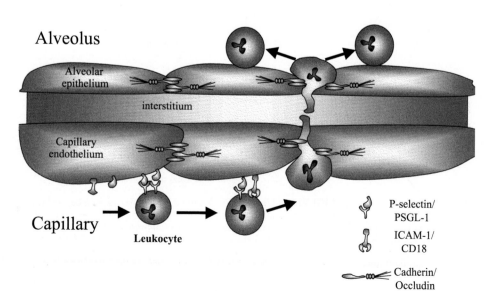

P-selectin/ PSGL-1

ICAM-1/ CD18

Cadherin/ Occludin

FIGURE 1-13. The interaction of the adhesion glycoprotein, P-selectin, on the alveolar endothelium with P-selectin glycoprotein ligand (PSGL-1) on white blood cells mediates leukocyte rolling along the vascular wall. The interaction of endothelial ICAM-1 with the leukocyte adhesive determinant, CD18, contributes to firm leukocyte adhesion and extravascular migration. These events contribute to leukocyte trafficking in the lung and alter the barrier properties of the alveolar–capillary membrane.

the vascular endothelium occurs at endothelial cell–cell junctions (Fig. 1-13) (42,43). The structural components of these junctions consist of *occludin*, a major component of tight junctions, and *cadherins*, which form the adherens junction (38,44). Alterations in these junctional proteins in response to inflammatory stimuli correlate with widening of interendothelial junctions and increased microvascular permeability (45).

Pulmonary endothelial cells express adhesion molecules that facilitate leukocyte–endothelial cell interaction and that contribute to enhanced transvascular fluid leak in response to a variety of lung insults (Fig. 1-13). The interaction of these endothelial cell adhesive proteins with specific white blood cell counter-receptors mediates leukocyte slowing, arrest, and tissue migration in response to lung injury or inflammation (46,47).

PHYSIOLOGY OF THE PULMONARY CIRCULATION

PULMONARY VASCULAR PRESSURES

Because the pulmonary circulation supplies only one organ, the right ventricle is required to generate only enough pressure in the pulmonary artery to pump blood to the top of the lung. Consequently, pressures in the pulmonary circulation are approximately 10-fold less than pressures in the systemic circulation (Fig. 1-14) (26). As a result of the remarkably low pressures in the pulmonary vasculature, the walls of the pulmonary artery and its branches are extremely thin, with little surrounding connective tissue and minimal smooth muscle.

Figure 1-14 illustrates that the pressure drop within the pulmonary vasculature is more uniform than in the systemic circulation. In addition, the capillaries are more important determinants of vascular resistance in the pulmonary circulation than in the systemic circulation, where the primary resistance vessels are the small, muscular arterioles (48).

PULMONARY VASCULAR RESISTANCE

Pulmonary vascular resistance (PVR) can be described by the following relationship:

$$\text{PVR (mm Hg/L/min)} = \frac{\Delta P \text{ (mm Hg)}}{Q \text{ (L/min)}}$$

where ΔP is the pressure gradient between the pulmonary artery and the pulmonary veins or left ventricle and Q is pulmonary blood flow. The total pressure drop from the pulmonary artery to the left ventricle is about 10 mm Hg in contrast to a pressure gradient of about 100 mm Hg in the systemic circulation (Fig. 1-14). As blood flow through the pulmonary and systemic circulations is essentially identical, PVR is only one-tenth of systemic vascular resistance.

Resistance to blood flow through the vasculature is directly related to vessel length and inversely related to vessel diameter (25). Consequently, anything that increases pulmonary capillary diameter will decrease PVR. The unique arrangement of the pulmonary capillaries in dense sheets (Fig. 1-11) over the alveolar wall provides much less resistance than flow through systemic capillaries (49).

Although the PVR is normally low, it has an extraordinary capacity to become even lower as pressure within the pulmonary vasculature rises (26,50). Figure 1-15 demonstrates that an increase in either pulmonary arterial or venous pressure causes PVR to decrease. Two mechanisms contribute to this decrease. First, as pulmonary vascular pressure rises, previously collapsed vessels begin to conduct blood, a process termed *capillary recruitment*. Recruitment is the primary mechanism responsible for the fall in PVR as pulmonary artery pressure rises. Second, as intravascular pressure rises, previously patent pulmonary capillaries become *distended*, thereby increasing their internal diameter and resulting in a decline in PVR.

Another important determinant of PVR is lung volume. As the lung expands, alveolar pressure rises and may exceed the

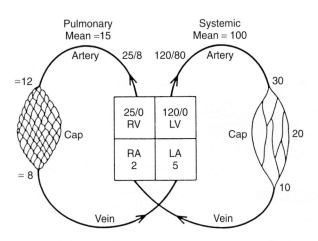

FIGURE 1-14. Comparison of pressure (in mm Hg) in the pulmonary and systemic circulations. LA, left atrium; LV, left ventricle; RA, right atrium; RV, right ventricle. (Reproduced with permission from West JB. *Respiratory physiology: the essentials*, 4th ed. Baltimore: Williams & Wilkins, 1989.)

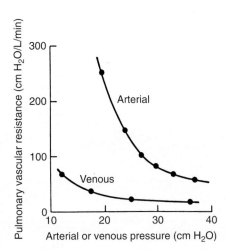

FIGURE 1-15. Fall in pulmonary vascular resistance as the pulmonary arterial or venous pressure is raised. Venous pressure is held constant at 12 cm H_2O when the arterial pressure is changed and arterial pressure is held at 37 cm H_2O when the venous pressure is changed. Data from an excised dog preparation. (Adapted with permission from West JB. *Respiratory physiology: the essentials*, 4th ed. Baltimore: Williams & Wilkins, 1989.)

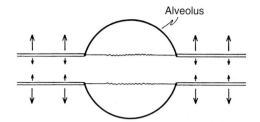

Alveolus

FIGURE 1-16. As lung volume and alveolar pressure rise, alveolar capillaries collapse causing vascular resistance in these vessels to increase. In contrast, extra-alveolar capillaries are pulled open by surrounding connective tissue as lung volume increases, resulting in a fall in vascular resistance. (Adapted with permission from Hughes JMB, Glazier JB, Maloney JE, et al. Effect of lung volume on the distribution of pulmonary blood flow in man. *Respir Physiol* 1968;4:58.)

intravascular pressure in *alveolar capillaries*. When alveolar pressure exceeds alveolar capillary intravascular pressure, these vessels collapse, resulting in an increase in their vascular resistance. In contrast, the connective tissue scaffolding surrounding *extra-alveolar capillaries* pulls them open as lung volume rises, causing vascular resistance in these vessels to fall (Fig. 1-16). Thus, changes in lung volume produce opposing effects on vascular resistance in alveolar and extra-alveolar capillaries.

DISTRIBUTION OF PULMONARY BLOOD FLOW

The distribution of blood flow throughout the pulmonary vasculature is not uniform (26). In the upright human lung, blood flow decreases from the bottom to the top of the lung, reaching lowest levels at the lung apex (26). The effect of gravity on pulmonary vascular pressures is one of the major factors causing these regional inequalities in blood flow. The pulmonary arterial system behaves as a continuous column of blood with a hydrostatic pressure difference of about 30 cm H_2O (or 23 mm Hg) in the upright lung (26). This large pressure gradient has a significant impact on the low-pressure pulmonary circulation.

The effect of hydrostatic pressure gradients on regional lung blood flow is illustrated in Figure 1-17. In zone 1, at the top of the lung, pulmonary arterial pressure may fall below alveolar pressures, causing the capillaries to collapse and blood flow to

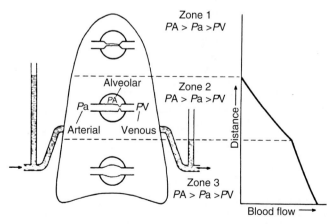

FIGURE 1-17. The zone model of regional inequalities in blood flow in the lung based on hydrostatic pressure differences affecting the capillaries. (Adapted with permission from West JB, Dollery CT, Naimark A. Distribution of blood flow in isolated lung: relation to vascular and alveolar pressure. *J Appl Physiol* 1964;19:713.)

cease. Under normal conditions, this does not occur because the pulmonary arterial pressure is sufficient to raise blood to the top of the lung. However, zone 1 conditions could occur if pulmonary arterial pressure falls (e.g., following severe hemorrhage) or if alveolar pressure is raised (e.g., during positive pressure ventilation).

Zone 2 occurs near the middle of the lung. Pulmonary arterial pressure rises in zone 2 because of the hydrostatic effect of gravity on the column of blood. In zone 2, pulmonary arterial pressure exceeds alveolar pressure. However, venous pressure remains lower than alveolar pressure because the veins in this zone may be below the level of the heart. In zone 2, the pressure gradient determining blood flow is the arterial–alveolar pressure difference, not the typical arterial–venous pressure gradient. Blood flow increases down zone 2 because the hydrostatic effect increases arterial pressure, while alveolar pressure remains unchanged. Moreover, capillary *recruitment* occurs down zone 2 (26).

Zone 3 occurs near the bottom of the lung where the hydrostatic effect causes both arterial and venous pressure to exceed alveolar pressure. Blood flow in zone 3 is determined by the usual arterial–venous pressure gradient. Blood flow also increases down zone 3 because of *distention* of patent capillaries.

Some evidence suggests that blood flow decreases again in zone 4, at the very bottom of the lung. Excessive intravascular pressure resulting in interstitial edema and collapse of alveolar capillaries has been proposed as a possible mechanism for diminished blood flow in zone 4.

REGULATION OF THE PULMONARY CIRCULATION

The pulmonary circulation is regulated by *active* factors, such as the autonomic nervous system, circulating vasoactive substances, and alveolar oxygen content. However, it is also influenced by *passive* factors, such as changes in cardiac output and left atrial pressure as well as gravitational forces. It is likely that the normally low pulmonary vascular tone is maintained by a tightly regulated balance of locally and systemically produced vasoactive substances. The lung actively participates in the synthesis, storage, or degradation of these factors.

Resting Vascular Tone

Although the pulmonary circulation is a low-resistance system, some degree of resting vascular tone is maintained by the pulmonary vasculature, as evidenced by the fact that administration of vasodilators elicits a further decline in pulmonary artery pressure and resistance (51). In normal subjects, basal pulmonary vascular tone is regulated at least in part by continuous local production of nitric oxide (52). It is likely that the sympathetic nervous system, as well as circulating catecholamines, prostaglandins, and endothelins, also contributes to basal vascular tone in the pulmonary circulation.

Autonomic Nervous System

There are both α- and β-adrenergic receptors in the pulmonary vascular bed, with a prevalence of α-receptors (53,54). Evidence suggests that although there is some degree of basal sympathetic tone in the pulmonary circulation, it is less than that in the systemic vascular bed (50).

Catecholamines and Other Vasoactive Substances

Release of substantial amounts of epinephrine or norepinephrine may elicit mild pulmonary vasoconstriction because of the prevalence of α-receptors within the pulmonary vasculature (53,55). Other vasoactive substances also produce pulmonary vasoconstriction. For example, histamine—a mediator of type I (immediate) hypersensitivity reactions—is widely distributed throughout the lung parenchyma, pulmonary mast cells, and within the pulmonary circulation (56). In contrast to its vasodilating properties in the systemic circulation, histamine causes constriction of pulmonary vessels through interaction with H_1 receptors (57).

Other substances that are metabolically altered by the lung appear to contribute to basal or stimulated pulmonary vascular tone. For example, serotonin (5-hydroxytryptamine), released from argentaffin cells in the intestine or lung or from platelets, elicits a rise in PVR by increasing both pre- and postcapillary tone (50,58). Angiotensin II, prostaglandins of the F series, and the leukotrienes are also pulmonary vasoconstrictors. In contrast, bradykinin and prostaglandins of the E series elicit pulmonary vasodilation. Prostacyclin (PGI_2), one of the major eicosanoids produced by the lung, is also a vasodilator and platelet aggregation inhibitor that may contribute not only to low PVR but also to the antithrombogenic properties of the pulmonary vasculature (59). The overall balance of vasodilating and vasoconstricting substances that are delivered to or metabolically altered by the lung probably contributes to basal as well as stimulated pulmonary vascular tone. Local alterations in the production of vasoconstrictors, such as endothelin-1 or eicosanoids, or vasodilators, such as nitric oxide or prostacyclin, may contribute to the pathogenesis of pulmonary hypertension (60).

Endothelial-Derived Vasoactive Factors

In addition to metabolizing or converting a multitude of vasoactive agents, the pulmonary vascular endothelium synthesizes substances that actively participate in the regulation of normal pulmonary vascular tone (61). These substances, such as endothelin-1 and nitric oxide, induce vasoconstriction or vasodilation, respectively (62,63).

ENDOTHELINS. Endothelin (ET)-1, ET-2, and ET-3 are members of a family of vasoconstrictor peptides that are synthesized as larger propeptides, termed *big ETs*. Following activation of big ET-1 by endothelin-converting enzyme expressed on pulmonary endothelial cells, it can bind to two major endothelin receptors: ET-A and ET-B. Low concentrations of ET-1 elicit pulmonary vasodilation possibly through interaction with ET-B receptors (64), while higher concentrations produce significant and sustained vasoconstriction mediated through ET-A receptors (65). A role for ET-1 in asthma and pulmonary hypertension has been suggested because enhanced expression of this peptide has been identified in patients with these disorders (66,67).

NITRIC OXIDE. Nitric oxide (NO) is synthesized in pulmonary endothelial cells through the action of NO synthase (NOS) on the amino acid precursor L-arginine. NO diffuses to the underlying vascular smooth muscle cell where it activates guanylate cyclase, thereby increasing intracellular concentrations of

cGMP (cyclic guanosine monophosphate) and inducing smooth muscle relaxation (68). Not only does NO appear to contribute to low basal pulmonary vascular tone, it may also contribute to pulmonary hypoxic vasoconstriction because alveolar hypoxia inhibits NOS activity, thereby reducing production of this potent vasodilator (69–71).

Hypoxic Vasoconstriction

In the systemic circulation, local hypoxia induces vasodilation that elicits increased blood flow to hypoxic regions. In contrast, hypoxia in the pulmonary circulation acts as a vasoconstrictor, diverting blood flow away from poorly ventilated, hypoxic areas of lung (72). The vasoconstriction occurs on the arterial side of the pulmonary circulation when *alveolar* oxygen tension approaches 60 mm Hg. Hypoxic pulmonary vasoconstriction is exaggerated in the presence of arterial acidosis (Fig. 1-18). In contrast to the effect of alveolar hypoxia, pulmonary arterial hypoxemia does not induce the vasoconstrictor response (53).

Pulmonary hypoxic vasoconstriction is beneficial in patients with pneumonia, pulmonary edema, or respiratory failure in that blood flow is shunted away from poorly ventilated areas, thereby reducing the degree of venous admixture and hypoxemia. However, considerable attention has been given to the deleterious effects of hypoxic pulmonary vasoconstriction in chronic conditions such as severe COPD with hypoventilation. The marked increase in PVR resulting from the hypoxic vasoconstrictor response predisposes to cor pulmonale and right heart failure (73,74). Therapy with low-flow oxygen can relieve some of the pulmonary hypertension seen in hypoxic patients with COPD and prolong life (74).

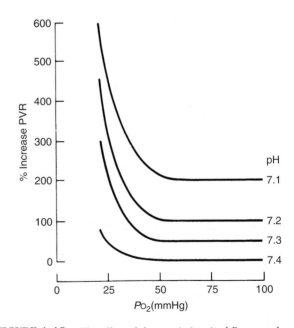

FIGURE 1-18. The effect of changes in inspired PO_2 on pulmonary vascular resistance (PVR) under conditions of different arterial blood pH in newborn calves. As inspired PO_2 is decreased, pulmonary vascular resistance increases, an effect exaggerated by acidosis. (Reproduced from Rudolph AM, Yuan S. Response of the pulmonary vasculature to hypoxia and H$^+$ ion concentration changes. *J Clin Invest* 1966;45:399–411, by copyright permission of the American Society for Clinical Investigation.)

Pulmonary hypoxic vasoconstriction appears to be an intrinsic property of pulmonary vascular smooth muscle and is dependent upon increased intracellular calcium concentrations within small pulmonary arteries and arterioles (75). Three mechanisms have been proposed to explain hypoxic vasoconstriction: (a) Hypoxia may stimulate the production of a vasoconstricting substance, (b) it may inhibit the production of a vasodilating substance, and (c) it may directly affect vascular smooth muscle (76). Although the mechanisms responsible for initiating and perpetrating pulmonary hypoxic vasoconstriction are not entirely clear, it appears that endothelial-derived NO, endothelin, and arachidonic acid derivatives modulate the response. Furthermore, there is evidence that red blood cell–NO interactions facilitate pulmonary hypoxic vasoconstriction (71). For example, chronic hypoxia-induced polycythemia appears to contribute to hemoglobin-mediated inactivation of NO and an augmented pulmonary vasoconstrictor response to hypoxia (77).

Passive Forces

As described in the preceding section, increased pulmonary arterial or venous pressure can elicit a decrease in PVR (Fig. 1-15) through capillary recruitment as well as capillary distention. In addition, the hydrostatic pressure effects on regional blood flow in the lung are significant (Fig. 1-17). Changes in cardiac output, left atrial pressure, and the effects of gravity all contribute to the regulation of the pulmonary circulation. In contrast to the effect of active factors such as vasoactive substances, passive factors change PVR or blood flow independent of changes in pulmonary vascular tone.

METABOLIC, NONRESPIRATORY FUNCTIONS OF THE LUNG

In addition to gas exchange, the lung performs a large number of metabolic functions in response to normal or inflammatory stimuli. The vast surface area of the pulmonary endothelium, strategically located to receive the entire output of the right ventricle, modifies the composition of the circulating blood before it returns to the left heart. The pulmonary microvascular endothelium has evolved elaborate systems for the synthesis, storage, degradation, or activation of inflammatory, chemical, and mechanical stimuli to accomplish these metabolic tasks.

The fate of several vasoactive substances during a single pass through the pulmonary circulation is indicated in Table 1-3. The extent of removal indicated applies only when the concentration of the substance in the pulmonary arteriolar blood is normal. In pathologic disturbances, when large amounts of compounds may be released or administered, the capacity of the lung to deal with them may be overwhelmed (50). Moreover, the efficacy of removal may be markedly altered in patients with lung disease (56,76,78).

VASOACTIVE SUBSTANCES

Biogenic Amines

Pulmonary endothelial cells possess receptors for biogenic amines; however, the metabolism of these substances is not uniform. Some amines, such as serotonin, are rapidly internalized

TABLE 1-3. Summary of the Fate of Circulating Substances during a Single Pass through the Intact Pulmonary Circulation

Substance	Fate
Amines	
Acetylcholine	Uncertain
Serotonin	Almost completely removed
Norepinephrine	Up to 40% removed
Epinephrine	Unchanged
Dopamine	Unchanged
Histamine	Unchanged
Peptides	
Bradykinin	Up to 80% inactivated
Angiotensin I	Converted to angiotensin II
Angiotensin II	Unchanged
Vasopressin	Unchanged
Arachidonic acid metabolites	
Prostaglandin E_2	Almost completely removed
Prostaglandin F_2	Almost completely removed
Prostaglandin A_2	Unchanged
Prostaglandin I_2 (prostacyclin)	Unchanged
Thromboxane	Unknown
Leukotrienes	Almost completely removed
Adenine nucleotides	
Adenosine triphosphate	Almost completely removed
Adenosine monophosphate	Almost completely removed

Reproduced with permission from Murray JF. *The normal lung.* Philadelphia: WB Saunders, 1986.

by endothelial cells and extensively degraded by monoamine oxidase (MAO) during a single pass through the lungs (79,80). Norepinephrine is also internalized and metabolized by the lungs, although less efficiently than serotonin. Biogenic amines such as propranolol are internalized and stored unchanged in lung endothelial cells, whereas others such as histamine, dopamine, and epinephrine pass through the pulmonary circulation without alteration (81). The fact that histamine is not removed from the pulmonary circulation is surprising, given its widespread pulmonary distribution and the fact that most vascular beds metabolize histamine (81).

Proteins and Peptides

Many circulating peptides and proteins exhibit potent vasoactive properties that must be modified to function appropriately. The pulmonary endothelium contains enzymes that modulate circulating peptides, proteins, or amino acids as they traverse the pulmonary circulation under normal as well as pathologic conditions. For example, bradykinin, a potent endogenous vasodilator implicated in the pathogenesis of bronchial asthma and anaphylaxis, is almost completely removed during passage through the lungs by the action of enzymes and peptidases on the endothelial cell surface (82,83). Furthermore, the pulmonary endothelial uptake of the NO precursor, L-arginine, as well as proteins required for antioxidant synthesis are increased by inflammatory stimuli or oxidant injury (84–86).

One of the best characterized enzymes on the luminal surface of the pulmonary endothelium is the angiotensin-converting enzyme (ACE). ACE is uniformly distributed along the pulmonary endothelium and plays a critical role in the control of systemic vascular pressures and volume homeostasis by regulation of the renin–angiotensin system. Angiotensin I is formed in circulation from an α-2 globulin precursor by the action of the enzyme renin. ACE converts the inactive decapeptide angiotensin I into the powerful vasoconstrictor angiotensin II in a single pass through the lung (87). No physiologically significant conversion of angiotensin I to angiotensin II has been demonstrated outside the lung (82).

Eicosanoids

Arachidonic acid (AA) is synthesized in the lung and other tissues from the cleavage of cellular membrane phospholipids (Fig. 1-19). The metabolites of AA, the *eicosanoids,* are not only synthesized by pulmonary endothelial cells but also inactivated to a large extent by the pulmonary vasculature. AA can be metabolized by either the cyclooxygenase pathway, resulting in the production of the *prostaglandins* and *thromboxanes,* or the lipoxygenase pathway, resulting in the production of the *leukotrienes* (Fig. 1-19).

Prostaglandins, specifically PGI_2 and PGE_2, are the major eicosanoids produced by the pulmonary endothelium (87). In general, prostaglandins of the F series constrict pulmonary and systemic blood vessels as well as bronchial smooth muscle, whereas prostaglandins of the E series elicit vasodilation and bronchodilation. The lungs inactivate AA and over 90% of prostaglandins of the E and F series but have little effect on prostaglandins of the A series and PGI_2 (88).

Leukotrienes induce enhanced microvascular permeability and marked bronchoconstriction and contribute to the airway inflammatory response. The leukotrienes are almost entirely removed within a single pass by the pulmonary circulation.

Nucleotides

The pulmonary microvascular endothelium contributes significantly to the regulation of adenosine, a potent vasodilator, and its nucleotide derivatives by rapidly removing them

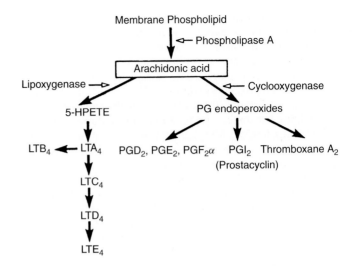

FIGURE 1-19. Pathways of arachidonic acid metabolism. Prostaglandins and thromboxane A_2 are generated by the cyclooxygenase pathway; the leukotrienes are generated by the lipoxygenase pathway. (Adapted with permission from Murray JF. *The normal lung.* Philadelphia: WB Saunders, 1986.)

from the circulation (89). In addition, pulmonary capillary endothelium has a high density of *caveolae intracellulare* that communicate with the vasculature and are the site of adenine nucleotide metabolism (Fig. 1-20) (90).

Endothelial-Derived Substances

Eighty percent of ET-1 and ET-3 are removed from the circulation by first-pass elimination by the lung (91). In contrast, there is basal production of NO that appears to contribute to normal pulmonary vascular tone. NO production in pulmonary endothelial cells is enhanced by changes in shear stress, blood flow, oxygen tension, and the binding of acetylcholine to specific endothelial receptors.

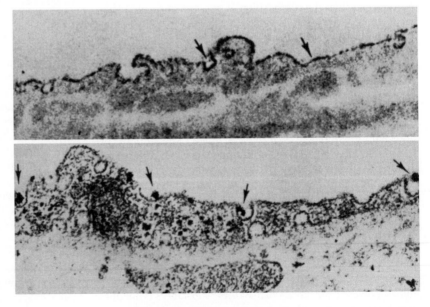

FIGURE 1-20. **A:** Section of rat pulmonary capillary endothelium demonstrating the location of angiotensin-converting enzyme. The electron-dense reaction product (*arrows*) is located on the plasma membrane and *caveolae intracellulare* facing the vascular lumen (original magnification × 76,000). (Reprinted by permission from Ryan US, Ryan JW, Whitaker C, et al. Localization of angiotensin-converting enzyme (Kinase II). II, Immunocytochemistry and immunofluorescence. *Tissue Cell* 1976;8:125–146.) **B:** Cytochemical localization of 5' nucleotidase on rat pulmonary endothelial cell (arrows) (original magnification × 95,000). (Reprinted by permission from Smith U, Ryan JW. Pinocytotic vesicles of the pulmonary endothelial cell. *Chest* 1971;59:12S–15S.)

GAS EXCHANGE AREA

TERMINAL RESPIRATORY UNIT

In the past, different authors have used various names for the smaller divisions of the lung architecture. To prevent confusion, the *terminal respiratory unit* (TRU) is herein defined as the portion of lung distal to a terminal nonrespiratory bronchiole (92,93). The TRU has been called the acinus by Lauweryns and the primary lobule by Miller (94,95). Three to five TRUs together form a *pulmonary lobule,* which is separated from its neighboring lobules by an interlobular septum containing lymphatic channels; these interlobular septa may become visible as Kerley's "B" lines on the chest x-ray film when they are distended by fluid or fibrosis (96).

A stylized version of a TRU is illustrated in Figure 1-21. The unit is designed to perform its basic function of gas exchange efficiently. The terminal bronchiole enters the center of the TRU accompanied by a branch of the pulmonary artery carrying unoxygenated blood from the body tissues. The arteriole divides into a rich network of pulmonary capillaries that cover the alveolar walls and drain into pulmonary venules, which lie in the periphery of the TRU. These venules converge into larger branches situated in the interlobular septa. This arrangement results in organized perfusion of a lobule from the center to the periphery.

LUNG CLEARANCE AND DEFENSES

The lung is in danger of injury by virtue of its direct contact with the atmosphere, which is necessary for gas exchange. Major irritants that invade the respiratory tract include organic agents (e.g., bacteria, fungal spores, and viruses) and inorganic agents (e.g., industrial exhaust, dusts, and cigarette smoke). These infectious and noninfectious agents may act together to

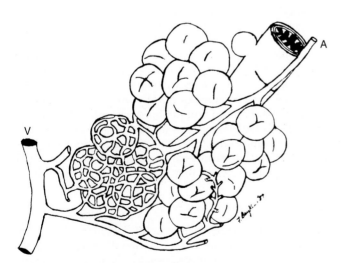

FIGURE 1-21. A terminal respiratory unit (TRU), the basic gas-exchanging unit of the lungs. The pulmonary arterial branch (*A*) enters the center of the TRU along with the terminal bronchiole. It anastomoses with the pulmonary venule in the alveolar walls, forming a dense capillary network for gas exchange. Venous drainage is to the periphery of the TRU, where the venous branches (*V*) lie. They coalesce to form the major pulmonary veins, which carry oxygenated blood.

produce acute or chronic disease. Complicated and effective defense mechanisms have evolved to protect the respiratory tract from these inhaled substances (97).

PARTICLE DEPOSITION IN THE RESPIRATORY TRACT

The deposition of particles in the lungs depends on their size and density, the distance over which they must travel, and the relative humidity. The method of breathing (i.e., mouth breathing versus nose breathing), the rate of airflow, the minute ventilation, and the depth of breathing also influence the deposition of the aerosol. Defense mechanisms vary depending on the position in the respiratory tract where particles are deposited as well as on their size and composition. In general, particles larger than 10 μm in diameter are deposited by impaction in the upper respiratory passages. Particles between 2 and 10 μm are carried in the airstream into the lower respiratory tract, where they impact in the bronchial tree. Particles between 0.5 and 3 μm are too small to impact in the airways but are deposited in the gas exchange areas of the lungs (the TRUs). Particles smaller than 0.2 μm are not efficiently deposited in the lung and may be exhaled. Modern nebulizers are capable of generating aerosols containing small particles of controlled size in high concentrations; thus, they are efficient means of depositing particles in the distal parts of the respiratory tract.

TRANSPORT SYSTEMS OF THE LUNGS

Three transport systems are available for the removal of inhaled particles from the alveoli: the mucociliary escalator, the phagocytes, and the lymphohematogenous drainage system. These systems work together, although they operate through different pathways at different rates (97).

MUCOCILIARY ESCALATOR

The mucociliary escalator functions to transport deposited particles from the level of the terminal bronchioles to the major airways, where they are coughed up and either expectorated or swallowed. The transport rate of this system is about 3 mm per minute and becomes more rapid proximally, where the streams converge. Approximately 90% of the particles directly deposited on the mucous layer are cleared within 2 hours. In the main bronchi, the mucociliary apparatus is formed by the ciliated epithelial cells, the mucus-producing goblet cells, and the mucous glands, which open directly onto the mucosa. In the smaller bronchi and bronchioles, mucus is formed from goblet cell secretions. In the smallest peripheral bronchioles, goblet cells are not normally seen, and the epithelium is lined by a thin layer of material containing surfactant that is derived from the Clara cells and the type II alveolar cells. This layer flows proximally and is continuous with the mucous layer of the mucociliary escalator.

The mucus, which is the transport medium, is a complex mucopolysaccharide arranged in a double layer on the surface of the epithelium (Fig. 1-22). The external layer is a viscous gel, which acts as a trap to catch and transport deposited particles. The mucous gel is elastic; therefore, the mechanical beating of cilia is able to propel both mucus and any entrapped particulates proximally. Loss of mucous elasticity can impair clearance. The internal sol layer is a thin liquid in which the cilia are

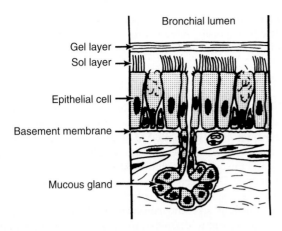

FIGURE 1-22.   The mucociliary escalator. The gel layer of mucus is propelled toward the trachea by the movement of the cilia on the surface of the cells.

able to move easily. The cilia themselves move with a characteristic biphasic rhythm. Beating within the liquid layer and striking the gel layer with their tips, they exhibit a periodic movement, forming wave bands that move the mucus up the bronchial tree toward the larynx. Efficient beating of cilia requires that the sol layer has an appropriate viscosity. In addition, the sol layer must be of the proper thickness so that cilia tips contact the mucous gel on the forward beat but release on the reverse beat. Effective clearance, therefore, requires a sol layer of appropriate composition and amount.

Many factors can alter clearance. Ciliary motion can be affected by exposure to a variety of substances. Toxic fumes and cigarette smoke, for example, may disrupt normal wave patterns or cause cilia to stop beating completely. Hereditary abnormalities of the cilia alter their movement and result in the "immotile cilia syndrome" (98). This syndrome can result from a variety of cilia defects, several of which can be recognized by electron microscopy of cilia. These hereditary diseases are associated with immotile cilia not only in the lung and upper respiratory tract but also at other sites where cilia are present, such as sperm cells and cells lining the nasal sinuses. Immotile sperm and male infertility, therefore, may be associated with the immotile cilia syndromes. Cilia in the developing embryo are responsible for pushing the developing heart to the left. With immotile cilia, localization is nearly random, and approximately half of individuals have dextrocardia or situs inversus. The triad of situs inversus associated with bronchiectasis and sinusitis, associated with immotile cilia, is termed *Kartagener's syndrome.*

Chronic bronchitis, asthma, CF, and acute respiratory infections may cause loss of cilia or abnormal ciliary function. These conditions are also associated with altered mucous secretion. Deoxyribonucleic acid (DNA) derived from inflammatory cells can increase viscosity, and proteolytic enzymes can disrupt mucous elasticity; thus, these disorders are associated with impaired clearance for a number of reasons. It is likely that increased susceptibility to infection in these disorders results, at least in part, from these clearance defects.

The alveolar surface itself is protected to some extent by the normal movement of the surface lining layer into the peripheral bronchi. However, the alveolar phagocytes and the lymphohematogenous drainage system are more important to alveolar clearance.

ALVEOLAR MACROPHAGE

The principal resident phagocyte of the alveoli is the alveolar macrophage. Some replication of these cells may take place in the lung, but they are ultimately derived from precursors in bone marrow that migrate in the peripheral blood as monocytes. Compared to mononuclear phagocytes at other sites (e.g., peritoneal macrophages), alveolar macrophages possess adaptations for the aerobic environment of the lung. Macrophages can phagocytose surfactants and are probably involved in the metabolic turnover of many of the extracellular components of the alveoli. Macrophages also phagocytose both bacteria and nonliving particulates. This process can be augmented by both specific and nonspecific opsonins, which can bind to particulates and subsequently interact with specific macrophage receptors. Bacteria may be killed and particles digested by powerful enzymes in the cellular lysosomes following phagocytosis. Organic molecules may be further detoxified by oxidases and a variety of transferases.

Macrophages are also able to release a host of cytokines. Through the release of these mediators, macrophages are able to recruit and activate other inflammatory cells. Neutrophils, recruited in response to macrophage-derived chemotactic factors such as leukotriene B_4 or interleukin-8, can greatly augment the phagocytic defenses of the lung. Cytokines derived from macrophages can also recruit and activate lymphocytes and pulmonary parenchymal cells. Macrophages are likely, therefore, to play a central role in initiating and maintaining chronic inflammatory processes in the lungs. The ability of macrophages to regulate parenchymal cells, combined with their capability to release proteases capable of degrading all components of the extracellular matrix, suggests that they may also be crucial regulators of tissue repair and remodeling.

LYMPHOHEMATOGENOUS DRAINAGE

The third transport system of the lungs is the lymphohematogenous drainage system. The alveolar septum contains connective tissue and is a space that may potentially act as a vehicle for the exit of macrophages from the alveoli. From there, macrophages may enter the pulmonary capillaries or the lymphatics of the lung periphery. Inhaled particles probably do not enter lymphatics directly unless inflammation is present but are carried within phagocytic cells. The speed of transport via the lymphatic system is variable and may take months or years. Collections of macrophages containing large amounts of foreign particles are frequently seen in the lymph nodes of the lungs, where they may remain permanently.

PULMONARY LYMPHATICS

The lungs and pleura are richly supplied with lymphatics. The purpose of the large flow of lymph from the lungs is twofold. First, it forms a natural mechanism for the removal of excess fluid that moves into the interstitial spaces from the pulmonary capillaries, thus keeping the alveoli relatively free of fluid. Second, it forms an important part of the alveolar defense mechanism by transporting macrophages containing inhaled particles from distal areas of the lungs. It is largely because of this rich lymphatic system that bronchogenic carcinoma travels out of the lungs so readily. The lymphatics in the terminal respiratory units converge in the interlobular septa. Movement of lymph is increased by respiratory movements coupled with a series of valves in the lymphatic vessels, which ensures proximal flow. Chronic increased pulmonary capillary pressure, and presumably increased production of pulmonary lymph, can be associated with increased capacity for lymphatic clearance. The lymphatics line the pulmonary arteries and veins as well as the bronchi themselves and converge at the pulmonary hila, where the hilar lymph nodes are found. From here, the thoracic duct drains the left lung and the right lymphatic duct drains the right. These vessels enter the systemic venous circulation at the junctions of the subclavian and internal jugular veins.

The bronchopulmonary lymph nodes surround the divisions of the lobar bronchi, and hilar glands are clustered at the lung roots. The hilar lymph nodes occur around the upper and lower lobe bronchi and communicate richly via the subcarinal nodes with the opposite side. Paratracheal nodes are found on either side of the trachea and are most prominent on the right. The *azygos* node is found adjacent to the azygos vein at the junction of the right upper lobe bronchus and the right main bronchus. The pulmonary lymphatic system communicates with the lower deep cervical nodes above and the abdominal lymphatics below. In addition to the hilar and mediastinal lymph nodes, there are also lymphatics along the distribution of the internal mammary arteries, near the intercostal arteries adjacent to the posterior ribs, and in the anterior and posterior mediastinum, which receive drainage primarily from the chest wall.

There is some disagreement as to the drainage of the various lobes of the lung, and indeed, drainage channels may vary among individuals. In general, the lower lobes drain into the hilar and subcarinal nodes, whereas the upper lobes more often drain directly to the paratracheal nodes. Thus, cancers arising in lower-lobe bronchi must traverse an extra set of lymph nodes, the hilar group, before reaching the paratracheal chain. The rich system of anastomoses among lymph node groups may account, at least in part, for the variation in lymphatic drainage of the lobes. Lymphocytes in intrapulmonary and regional nodes may become reactive and the nodes may enlarge in a variety of inflammatory lung diseases, both infectious (e.g., granulomas) and noninfectious (e.g., silicosis).

Lymphocytes accumulate beneath the epithelium of airways, where they are termed *bronchus-associated lymphoid tissue* (BALT). These airway lymphocytes are thought to participate in the system of mucosal immunity and to be responsible for local responses to antigen with both local and generalized production of immunoglobulin, particularly IgA. Lymphocytes are also present in the pulmonary parenchyma, and their numbers may increase significantly in disease states. Although the mechanisms responsible are not fully elucidated, lymphocytes present in the lungs are thought to be capable of migrating to regional nodes, circulating in the blood, and then relocalizing at specific tissue sites by virtue of the expression of specific "homing receptors."

Acknowledgment

This work was supported in part by a grant from the National Institutes of Health (NIDDK 2 PO1 DK 4378506).

REFERENCES

1. Staub NC, Albertine KH. The structure of the lungs relative to their principal function. In: Murray JF, Nadel JA, eds. *Textbook of respiratory medicine.* Philadelphia: WB Saunders, 1988:12–16.
2. Macklem PT. Respiratory muscles: the vital pump. *Chest* 1980;78:753–758.
3. Cohen CA, Zagelbaum G, Gross D, et al. Clinical manifestations of inspiratory muscle fatigue. *Am J Med* 1982;73:308–316.
4. Garrity ER Jr, Shart JT. Respiratory muscles: function and dysfunction. *ACCP Pulm Crit Care Update* 1986;2:lesson 10:1–4.
5. De Troyer A, Estene M, Heilporn A. Mechanisms of active expiration in tetraplegic patients. *N Engl J Med* 1986;314:740–744.
6. Roncoroni AJ, Androgue HJA, DeObrutsky CW, et al. Metabolic acidosis in status asthmaticus. *Respiration* 1976;33:85–94.
7. Minh VD, Dolan GF, Konopka RF, et al. Effect of hyperinflation on inspiratory function of the diaphragm. *J Appl Physiol* 1976;40:67–73.
8. Roussos C, Macklem PT. The respiratory muscles. *N Engl J Med* 1982;307:786–797.
9. Yang KL, Tobin MJ. A prospective study of indexes predicting the outcome of trials of weaning from mechanical ventilation. *N Engl J Med* 1991;325:1445–1450.
10. Tobin MJ. Respiratory muscles in disease. *Clin Chest Med* 1988;9:263–286.
11. Weiner-Kronish JP, Albertine KH, Licko V, et al. Protein egress and entry rates in pleural fluid and plasma in sheep. *J Appl Physiol* 1984;56:459–463.
12. Broaddus VC, Wiener-Kronesh JP, Berthiaume Y, et al. Removal of pleural liquid and protein in lymphatics in awake sheep. *J Appl Physiol* 1988;64:384–390.
13. Armstrong WB, Netterville JL. Anatomy of the larynx, trachea, and bronchi. *Otolaryngol Clin North Am* 1995;28:685–699.
14. Light RW, George RB. Upper airway obstruction (editorial). *Arch Intern Med* 1977;137:281.
15. Weibel ER. *Morphometry of the lung.* New York: Academic Press, 1963:111.
16. Barnes PJ. Airway neuropeptides: roles in fine tuning and in disease? *News Physiol Sci* 1989;4:116–120.
17. Massaro G. Nonciliated bronchiolar epithelial (Clara) cells. In: Massaro D, ed. *Lung biology in health and disease,* Vol. 41, *Lung cell biology.* New York: Marcel Dekker, 1989:81–114.
18. Colby TV. Bronchiolitis: pathological considerations. *Am J Clin Pathol* 1998;109:101–109.
19. Terry PB, Traystman RJ, Newball HH, et al. Collateral ventilation in man. *N Engl J Med* 1978;298:10.
20. Hermans C, Bernard A. Lung epithelium-specific proteins. *Am J Respir Crit Care Med* 1999;159:646–678.
21. Boucher RC. Human airway ion transport. *Am J Respir Crit Care Med* 1994;150:271–281.
22. Riordan JR. The cystic fibrosis transmembrane conductance regulator. *Annu Rev Physiol* 1993;55:609–630.
23. Matthay MA, Clerici C, Sauman G. Active fluid clearance from the distal air spaces of the lung. *J Appl Physiol* 2002;93:1533–1541.
24. Smith JJ, Travis SM, Greenberg EP, et al. Cystic fibrosis airway epithelia fail to kill bacteria because of abnormal airway surface fluid. *Cell* 1996;85:229–236.
25. Guyton AC. The pulmonary circulation. *Textbook of medical physiology,* 9th ed. Philadelphia: WB Saunders, 1996:491–501.
26. West JB. *Respiratory physiology,* 4th ed. Baltimore: Williams & Wilkins, 1990:31–49.
27. Weibel ER. Design and morphometry of the pulmonary gas exchanger. In: Crystal RG, West JB, Weibel ER et al., eds. *The lung: scientific foundations.* New York: Lippincott-Raven, 1997:1147–1159.
28. Weibel ER. Lung cell biology. In: Fishman AP, ed. *Handbook of physiology,* Vol. 1, *The respiratory system.* Baltimore: Williams & Wilkins: 1985:47–91.
29. Weibel ER, Gil J. Structure-function relationships at the alveolar level. In: West JB, ed. *Bioengineering aspects of the lung,* Vol. 3, *Lung biology health and disease series.* New York: Marcel Dekker, 1977:1–81.
30. West JB, Mathieu-Costell O. Structure, strength, failure and remodeling of the pulmonary blood-gas barrier. *Annu Rev Physiol* 1999;61:543–572.
31. Slutsky AS, Tremblay LN. Multiple system organ failure: is mechanical ventilation a contributing factor? *Am J Respir Crit Care Med* 1998;157:1721–1725.

32. Ware LB, Matthay MA. The acute respiratory distress syndrome. *N Engl J Med* 2000;342:1334–1349.

33. Crapo JD, Barry BE, Gehr P, et al. Cell number and cell characteristics of the normal human lung. *Annu Rev Respir Dis* 1982;125:740–745.

34. Matthay MA, Matthay RA. *Chest medicine: essentials of pulmonary and critical care medicine.* Baltimore: Williams & Wilkins, 1995:593–618.

35. Taylor AE, Gaar KA. Estimation of equivalent pore radii of pulmonary capillary and alveolar membranes. *Am J Physiol* 1970;218:1133–1140.

36. Normand ICS, Olver RE, Reynolds EOR, et al. Permeability of lung capillaries and alveoli to non-electrolytes in the fetal lamb. *J Physiol* 1971;219:303–330.

37. Gumbiner B, Simons K. A functional assay for proteins involved in establishing an epithelial occluding barrier: identification of a uvomorulin-like polypeptide. *J Cell Biol* 1986;102:457–468.

38. Volk T, Geiger B. A-cam: A 135-kD receptor of intercellular adherens junctions. II. Antibody-mediated modulation of junction formation. *J Cell Biol* 1986;103:1451–1464.

39. Gumbiner B, Stevenson B, Grimaldi A. The role of the cell adhesion molecule uvomorulin in the formation and maintenance of the epithelial junctional complex. *J Cell Biol* 1988;107:1575–1587.

40. Matthay MA, Landolt CC, Staub NC. Differential liquid and protein clearance from the alveoli of anesthetized sheep. *J Appl Physiol* 1982;53:96–104.

41. Simionescu M. Lung endothelium: structure-function correlates. In: Crystal RG, West JB, Weibel ER et al., eds. *The lung: scientific foundations.* New York: Lippincott-Raven, 1997:615–629.

42. Allport JR, Ding H, Collins T, et al. Endothelial dependent mechanisms regulate leukocyte transmigration: a process involving the proteasome and disruption of the vascular endothelial cadherin complex at endothelial cell to cell junctions. *J Exp Med* 1997;186:517–527.

43. Burns AR, Walker DC, Brown ES, et al. Neutrophil transendothelial migration is independent of tight junctions and occurs preferentially at tricellular corners. *J Immunol* 1997;159:2893–2903.

44. Lampugnani MF, Resnati M, Raiteri M, et al. A novel endothelial specific membrane protein is a marker of cell–cell contacts. *J Cell Biol* 1992;118:1511–1522.

45. Alexander JS, Elrod JW. Extracellular matrix, junctional integrity, and matrix metalloproteinase interactions in endothelial permeability regulation. *J Anat* 2002;200:561–574.

46. Carden DL, Alexander JS, George RB. The pathophysiology of the acute respiratory distress syndrome. *Pathophysiology* 1998;5:1–13.

47. Diamond MS, Staunton DE, Marlin SD, et al. Binding of the integrin Mac-1 (CD11b/CD18) to the third Ig-like domain of ICAM-1 (CD54) and its regulation by glycosylation. *Cell* 1991;65:961–967.

48. Guyton AC. Overview of the circulation: medical physics of pressure, flow and resistance. *Textbook of medical physiology*, 9th ed. Philadelphia: WB Saunders, 1996:493.

49. Powell FL. Structure and function of the respiratory system. In: Johnson LR, ed. *Essential medical physiology*, 2nd ed. Philadelphia: Lippincott-Raven, 1998:248–249.

50. Murray JF. *The normal lung.* Philadelphia: WB Saunders, 1986:150.

51. Bergofsky EH, Bass BG, Ferretti R, et al. Pulmonary vasoconstriction in response to precapillary hypoxemia. *J Clin Invest* 1963;4:1201–1205.

52. Cooper CJ, Landzberg MJ, Anderson TJ, et al. Role of nitric oxide in the local regulation of pulmonary vascular resistance in humans. *Circulation* 1996;93:266–271.

53. Bergofsky EH. Active control of the normal pulmonary circulation. In: Moser KM, ed. *Pulmonary vascular disease.* New York: Marcel Dekker, 1979:1–18.

54. Widdicombe JG, Sterling G. The autonomic nervous system and breathing. *Ann Intern Med* 1970;126:311.

55. Murray PA, Lodato RF, Michael JR. Neural antagonists modulate pulmonary vascular pressure-flow plots in conscious dogs. *J Appl Physiol* 1986;60:1900–1907.

56. Gillis CN, Roth JA. Pulmonary disposition of circulation vasoactive hormones. *Biochem Pharmacol* 1976;25:2547–2553.

57. Tucker A, Weir EK, Reeves JT, et al. Histamine H_1 and H_2 receptors in the pulmonary and systemic vasculature of the dog. *Am J Physiol* 1975;229:1008–1013.

58. Bhattacharya JH, Nanjo S, Staub NC. Micropuncture measurement of lung microvascular pressure during 5-HT infusion. *J Appl Physiol* 1982;52:634–637.

59. Grygkewsju RJ, Korbut R, Ocetkiewicz A. Generation of prostacyclin by lungs in vivo and its release into the arterial circulation. *Nature* 1978;273:765–767.

60. Christman BW, McPherson CD, Newman JH, et al. *N Engl J Med* 1992;327:70–75; Giaid A, Yanagisawa M, Langleben D, et al. Expression of endothelin-1 in the lungs of patients with pulmonary hypertension. *N Engl J Med* 1993;328: 1732–1739; Giaid A, Saleh D. *N Engl J Med* 1995;333:214–221.

61. Aaronson PI, Robertson TP, Ward JP. Endothelium-derived mediators and hypoxic pulmonary vasoconstriction. *Respir Physiol Neurobiol* 2002;132:107–120.

62. Moncada S, Higgs A. The L-arginine-nitric oxide pathway. *N Engl J Med* 1993;329:2002–2012.

63. Dinh-Xuan AT. Endothelial modulation of pulmonary vascular tone. *Eur Respir J* 1992;5:757–762.

64. Sato K, Oka M, Hasunuma K, et al. Effects of separate and combined ETA and ETB blockade on ET-1-induced constriction in perfused rat lungs. *Am J Physiol* 1995;269:L668–L672.

65. Bonvallet ST, Oka M, Yano M, et al. BQ123, an ET_A receptor antagonist, attenuates endothelin-1 induced vasoconstriction in rat pulmonary circulation. *J Cardiovasc Pharmacol* 1993;22:39–43.

66. Mattoli S, Soloperto M, Marini M, et al. Levels of endothelin in the bronchalveolar lavage fluid of patients with symptomatic asthma and reversible airflow obstruction. *J Allergy Clin Immunol* 1991;88:376–384.

67. Stewart DJ, Levy RD, Cernacek P, et al. Increased plasma endothelin-1 in pulmonary hypertension: marker or mediator of disease? *Ann Intern Med* 1991;114:464–469.

68. Palmer RMJ, Ashton DS, Moncada S. Vascular endothelial cells synthesize nitric oxide from L-arginine. *Nature* 1988;333:664–666.

69. Stamler JS, Loh E, Roddy MA, et al. Nitric oxide regulates basal systemic and pulmonary vascular resistance in healthy humans. *Circulation* 1994;89:2035–2040.

70. Rodman DM, Yamaguchi T, Hasunuma K, et al. Effect of hypoxia on endothelium-dependent relaxation of rat pulmonary artery. *Am J Physiol* 1990;258:L207–L214.

71. Deem, S. Nitric oxide scavenging by hemoglobin regulates hypoxic pulmonary vasoconstriction. *Free Radical Biol Med* 2004;36:698–706.

72. Naeije R, Brimioulle S. Physiology in medicine. Importance of hypoxic vasoconstriction in maintaining arterial oxygenation during acute respiratory failure. *Crit Care* 2001;5:67–71.

73. Burrows B, Kettel LJ, Niden AH, et al. Patterns of cardiovascular dysfunction in chronic obstructive pulmonary disease. *N Engl J Med* 1972;286:912–918.

74. Nocturnal Oxygen Therapy Trial Group. Continuous or nocturnal oxygen therapy in hypoxemic chronic obstructive lung disease: a clinical trial. *Ann Intern Med* 1981;93:391–398.

75. Gelband CH, Gelband H. Ca^{2+} release from intracellular stores is an initial step in hypoxic pulmonary vasoconstriction of rat pulmonary artery resistance vessels. *Circulation* 1997;96:3647–3654; Hillier SC, Graham JA, Hanger CC, et al. Hypoxic vasoconstriction in pulmonary arterioles and venules. *J Appl Physiol* 1997;82:1084–1090.

76. Fishman AP. Hypoxia on the pulmonary circulation. *Circ Res* 1976;38:221–231.

77. Defoilloy C, Teifer E, Sediame S, et al. Polycythemia impairs vasodilator response to acetylcholine in patients with chronic hypoxemic lung disease. *Am J Respir Crit Care Med* 1998;157:1452–1460.

78. Gillis CN, Catravas JD. Altered removal of vasoactive substances by the injured lung: detection by lung microvascular injury. *Ann N Y Acad Sci* 1982;384:458–474.

79. Fisher A, Block ER, Pietra G. Environmental influences on uptake of serotonin and other amines. *Environ Health Perspect* 1980;35:191–198.

80. Roth RA, Wallace KB, Alper RH, et al. Effect of paraquat treatment of rats on disposition of 5-hydroxytryptamine and angiotensin I by perfused lung. *Biochem Pharmacol* 1979;28:2349–2355.

81. Youdim MBH, Bakhle YS, Ben-Harari RR. Inactivation of monoamines by the lung. *Ciba Found Symp* 1980;78:105–128.

82. Vane JR. The release and fate of vasoactive hormones in the circulation. *Br J Pharmacol* 1969;35:202–208.

83. Baker CRF Jr, Little AD, Little GH, et al. Kinin metabolism in the perfused ventilated rat lung. I: Bradykinin metabolism in a system modeling the normal, uninjured lung. *Circ Shock* 1991;33:37–47.

84. Cendan JC, Moldawer LL, Souba WW, et al. Endotoxin-induced nitric oxide production in pulmonary artery endothelial cells is regulated by cytokines. *Arch Surg* 1994;129:1296–1300.

85. Souba WW, Salloum RM, Bode BP, et al. Cytokine modulation of glutamine transport by pulmonary artery endothelial cells. *Surgery* 1991;110:295–302.

86. Deneke SM, Baxter DF, Phelps DT, et al. Increase in endothelial cell glutathione and precursor amino acid uptake by diethyl maleate and hyperoxia. *Am J Physiol* 1989;257:L265–L271.

87. Bunning P, Budeck W, Escher R, et al. Characteristics of angiotensin converting enzyme and its role in the metabolism of angiotensin I by endothelium. *J Cardiovasc Pharmacol* 1986;8(Suppl. 10):S52–S57.

88. McGiff JC, Terragno NA, Strand JC, et al. Selective passage of prostaglandins across the lung. *Nature* 1969;216:762–766.

89. Pearson JD, Carleton JS, Hutchings A, et al. Uptake and metabolism of adenosine by pig aortic endothelial and smooth-muscle cells in culture. *Biochem J* 1978;170:265–271.

90. Smith U, Ryan JW. An electron microscopic study of the vascular endothelium as a site for bradykinin and adenosine-5′-triphosphate inactivation in rat lung. *Adv Exp Med Biol* 1979;8:249–261.

91. De Nucci G, Thomas R, D'Orleans JP, et al. Presser effects of circulating endothelin are limited by its removal in the pulmonary circulation and by the release of protacyclin and endothelium-derived relaxing factor. *Proc Natl Acad Sci U S A* 1988;85:9797–9800.

92. Von Hayek H. *The human lung* (trans. Krohl VE). New York: Hafner, 1960.

93. Staub NC. The interdependence of pulmonary structure and function. *Anesthesiology* 1963;24:831.

94. Lauweryns JM. The blood and lymphatic microcirculation of the lung. In: Sommers SC, ed. *Pathology annual 1971*. New York: Appleton-Century-Crofts, 1971.

95. Miller WS. *The lung*. Baltimore: Charles C Thomas Publisher, 1937.

96. Reid L, Simon G. The peripheral pattern in the normal bronchogram and its relation to peripheral pulmonary anatomy. *Thorax* 1958;13:103.

97. Green GM. In defense of the lung. *Am Rev Respir Dis* 1970;102:691.

98. Eliasson R, Mossberg B, Camner P, et al. The immotile cilia syndrome: a congenital ciliary abnormality as an etiologic function in chronic infection and male sterility. *N Engl J Med* 1977;297:1–6.

CHAPTER **2**

Mechanics of Respiration

Richard W. Light

**LUNG VOLUMES: THE DIMENSIONS
OF THE RESPIRATORY SYSTEM**

**VOLUME–PRESSURE RELATIONS OF THE
RESPIRATORY SYSTEM DURING RELAXATION**
Pressure–Volume Curves for the Chest Wall, Lung,
and Respiratory System

**VOLUME–PRESSURE RELATIONS OF THE
RESPIRATORY SYSTEM DURING MUSCULAR EFFORTS**
Measurement of Pleural Pressure
Pleural Pressure Gradients

Factors Holding the Lung Against the Chest Wall
Factors Influencing the Pressure–Volume Curve of the Lung

DYNAMICS OF THE RESPIRATORY SYSTEM
Airway Resistances
Pressure–Flow Relationships
Density Dependence of Maximal Airflow
Distribution of Ventilation
Work of Breathing

In this chapter, the factors that determine the volume of the lungs and hemithorax and the movement of air into and out of the lungs are described.

LUNG VOLUMES: THE DIMENSIONS OF THE RESPIRATORY SYSTEM

Figure 2-1 illustrates the subdivisions of the lungs during various respiratory maneuvers. The total lung capacity (TLC) is the total amount of air in the lungs after a maximal inspiration. The TLC is dependent on the height, age, and sex of the subject and is greater in taller, younger, and male individuals.

The vital capacity (VC) is the maximal amount of air that a subject is able to exhale after a maximal inhalation. The residual volume (RV) of the lungs is the amount of air remaining in the lungs at the end of a maximal exhalation. Normally, it is approximately 25% of the TLC. The sum of the RV and the VC equals the TLC.

The functional residual capacity (FRC) is the quantity of air in the lungs and airways at the end of a spontaneous exhalation. Therefore, it is the resting volume of the lungs. Normally, it is about 40% of the TLC.

The tidal volume (V_T) is the volume of air inhaled or exhaled during a respiratory cycle. It averages about 600 mL in normal subjects under resting conditions. The minute ventilation is the total amount of air moving into and out of the lungs per minute. It is equal to the product of the V_T and the respiratory rate.

The inspiratory capacity (IC) is the maximal volume of air that can be inspired from the resting level (FRC). The IC is approximately 60% of the TLC. The inspiratory reserve volume (IRV) is the difference between IC and V_T, or the maximal volume of air that can be inspired beyond the V_T. The expiratory reserve volume (ERV) is the maximal volume of air that can be exhaled beyond the FRC. The sum of the ERV and the IC equals the VC.

VOLUME–PRESSURE RELATIONS OF THE RESPIRATORY SYSTEM DURING RELAXATION

Everyone who has observed an autopsy realizes that when the chest is opened, the lungs collapse and the thorax enlarges. This simple observation illustrates two fundamental static properties of the respiratory system: the lungs tend to recoil inward and the chest wall tends to recoil outward.

24

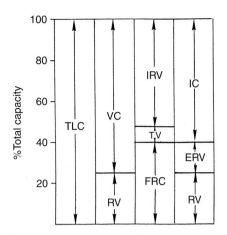

FIGURE 2-1. The subdivisions of the lung volume.

The lungs and the chest wall are distensible objects. As with any distensible object, their volumes are dependent on their elastic properties and their distending pressures. The distending pressure is the pressure difference between the inner and outer surfaces. The distending pressures for the lungs and the chest are illustrated in Figure 2-2.

The distending pressure of the lung is termed the *transpulmonary pressure* (P_L) and is the difference between alveolar pressure (P_A) and pleural pressure (P_{pl}).

$$P_L = P_A - P_{pl} \qquad (2.1)$$

The distending pressure for the chest wall (P_W) is the difference between the pleural pressure and the pressure at the body surface (P_{bs}).

$$P_W = P_{pl} - P_{bs} \qquad (2.2)$$

Note the importance of the pleural pressure in both these expressions. The distending pressure for the entire respiratory system (P_{rs}) is the sum of the distending pressures for the lung and the chest wall. Because the pleural pressures cancel out, it is the difference between alveolar pressure and the pressure at the body surface.

$$P_{rs} = P_A - P_{bs} \qquad (2.3)$$

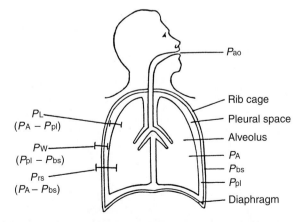

FIGURE 2-2. Respiratory pressures influencing ventilation. P_{ao}, pressure at the airway opening; P_{pl}, pressure within the pleural space; P_A, pressure within the alveoli; P_{bs}, pressure at the body surface; P_L, pressure difference across the lung; P_W, pressure difference across the chest; P_{rs}, pressure across the respiratory system.

The elastic properties of a distensible object can be defined by means of its volume–pressure diagram. To construct such a diagram, the volumes of the object at different distending pressures are determined. The relationship between changes in volume and pressure define the *compliance* of the object, which is expressed as follows:

$$\text{Compliance} = \text{change in volume/change in pressure} \qquad (2.4)$$

PRESSURE–VOLUME CURVES FOR THE CHEST WALL, LUNG, AND RESPIRATORY SYSTEM

If the respiratory muscles are completely relaxed and the heart and lungs are removed from the thorax, the elastic properties of the thorax can be studied by adding or removing air from it and observing the relationship between the distending pressure and the volume of the thorax. A pressure–volume curve obtained in this manner is depicted in Figure 2-3(A). Note that the resting volume of the chest wall—that is, the volume at which the distending pressure is zero—is about 50% of the VC.

In a similar manner, if the lungs are removed from the thorax, a pressure–volume curve for them can be obtained. Such a curve is illustrated in Figure 2-3(B). As the inflating pressure becomes higher, the volume increment with a given pressure increase becomes progressively smaller.

If the subject is relaxed, a pressure–volume curve for the respiratory system can be obtained by increasing or decreasing the alveolar pressures. A curve depicting this for the respiratory system is shown in Figure 2-3(C). It is the sum of the curves for the chest wall and the lungs. The resting volume of the respiratory system is the volume at which P_A is equal to P_{bs} and the distending pressure is zero. Note that it is the volume at which the distending pressures of the lungs and the chest wall are equal but are opposite in sign. This resting volume is the FRC.

VOLUME–PRESSURE RELATIONS OF THE RESPIRATORY SYSTEM DURING MUSCULAR EFFORTS

For the volume of the respiratory system to be different than the FRC, muscular effort must be present if the glottis is open and there is no airflow. In Figure 2-4, the alveolar pressures that can be generated at various lung volumes with maximal inspiratory ($P_{max_{insp}}$) and expiratory ($P_{max_{exp}}$) efforts are shown. Also shown are the alveolar pressures during relaxation at various lung volumes when there is no airflow. The horizontal difference between $P_{max_{insp}}$ or $P_{max_{exp}}$ and the relaxation pressure gives the net maximal pressure generated by the inspiratory or expiratory muscles, respectively. Note that the higher the lung volumes, the lower the maximal inspiratory pressure and the higher the maximal expiratory pressure. At FRC, the maximal inspiratory pressure is about -100 cm H_2O, whereas the maximal expiratory pressure is about $+150$ cm H_2O.

From Figure 2-4, it is easy to see that the TLC is the volume at which the maximal negative pressure generated by the inspiratory muscles is equal to the relaxed positive pressure of the respiratory system. Accordingly, the TLC is reduced if the lungs or the chest wall become stiffer (less compliant) or if the inspiratory muscles become weaker. Conversely, the TLC is increased if the lungs or chest wall become more compliant or if the muscles become stronger.

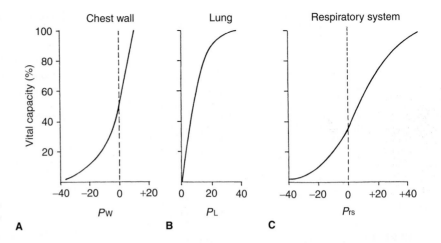

FIGURE 2-3. Static pressure–volume relationships for **(A)** the chest wall, **(B)** the lungs, and **(C)** the respiratory system.

In a similar fashion, the RV is the volume at which the maximal positive expiratory pressure is equal to the relaxed negative pressure of the respiratory system. The RV increases if there is expiratory muscle weakness or if the pressure–volume curve of the respiratory system is shifted to the left, as occurs with a noncompliant chest wall or very compliant lungs (Fig. 2-3). The RV decreases if the lower end of the pressure–volume curve for either the lungs or the chest wall is shifted to the right.

MEASUREMENT OF PLEURAL PRESSURE

Because the pleural pressure is the pressure at the inner surface of the chest wall and the outer surface of the lungs, it is an important parameter to be measured when studying either normal subjects or patients with pulmonary disease. The pleural pressure can be measured directly by inserting needles, trocars, catheters, or balloons into the pleural space. However, direct measurement of the pleural pressure is not usually performed because of the danger of producing a pneumothorax or an infection of the pleural space. At present, pleural pressures are usually measured indirectly using a fluid-filled catheter or a balloon positioned in the subject's esophagus. Because the esophagus is located between the two pleural spaces, esophageal pressure measurements provide a close approximation of the pleural pressure at the level of the device in the thorax (1). Estimation of

pleural pressure by means of an esophageal balloon is not without pitfalls (1). The volume of air within the balloon must be small so that the balloon is not stretched and the esophageal walls are not displaced; otherwise, falsely elevated pleural pressure measurements will be obtained. Moreover, the balloon must be short and must be placed in the lower part of the esophagus. If care is taken, reliable pressure–volume curves of the lungs can be obtained by measuring esophageal pressure at different lung volumes while the subject holds his or her breath with the glottis open to eliminate the effect of changes in alveolar pressure. Reliable measurements of esophageal pressures can also be made with liquid-filled catheter manometer systems (2). Use of these devices circumvents some of the problems associated with esophageal balloons.

PLEURAL PRESSURE GRADIENTS

Although estimation of the pleural pressure via an esophageal balloon gives a value, the pleural pressure is not uniform throughout the chest. There is a gradient in pleural pressure between the top and the bottom of the lung, the pleural pressure being the lowest, or most negative, at the top of the lung and the highest, or least negative, at the bottom. The main factors responsible for the pleural pressure gradient are probably gravity, mismatching of the shapes of the chest wall and lung,

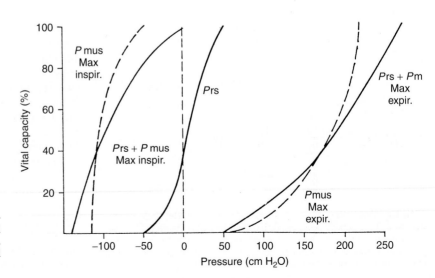

FIGURE 2-4. Schematic demonstrating the relationship between the alveolar pressures generated during maximal inspiratory and expiratory efforts. The dashed lines indicate the pressure contributed by the muscles.

and the weight of the lungs and other intrathoracic structures (3).

The magnitude of the pleural pressure gradient is on the order of 0.30 cm H_2O per centimeter of vertical distance (3). Therefore, in the upright position, the difference in the pleural pressure between the apex and the base of the lungs may be 8 cm H_2O or more. Because the alveolar pressure is constant throughout the lungs, the effect of the pleural pressure gradient is that different parts of the lungs have different distending pressures (P_L). The transpulmonary pressure is approximately 12 cm H_2O higher in the uppermost than in the lowermost portion of the lungs.

It is thought that the pressure–volume curve is the same for different regions of the lung regardless of their location. Therefore, the variation in pleural pressure results in the alveoli in the superior parts of the lung being larger than those in the inferior parts. Moreover, because separate alveoli are at different positions on the pressure–volume curves, a given change in distending pressure causes varying volume changes throughout the lung. For these reasons, at lung volumes above FRC, alveoli in the inferior parts of the lungs expand considerably more than those at the top, as illustrated in Figure 2-5. At low lung volumes, the pleural pressure may become positive in the lower regions of the lung. This positive pressure can compress airways, resulting in alveoli that are not ventilated. This phenomenon is the basis for the closing volume test, which is described in Chapter 6, Clinical Pulmonary Function Testing, Exercise Testing, and Disability Evaluation.

FACTORS HOLDING THE LUNG AGAINST THE CHEST WALL

The pleural pressure throughout most of the thorax is negative at FRC because the lungs and chest wall are, respectively, above and below their resting volumes. Why does the potential space between the lungs and chest wall (the pleural space) not become filled with either gas or liquid?

Gases move in and out of the pleural space from the capillaries in the visceral and parietal pleura. Because the sum of all the partial pressures in capillary blood ($P_{H_2O} = 47$, $P_{CO_2} = 46$, $P_{N_2} = 573$, and $P_{O_2} = 40$ mm Hg) averages 706 mm Hg, there will be a net movement of gas into the pleural space only if the pleural pressure is below 706 mm Hg, or below −54 mm Hg relative to atmospheric pressure. Because mean pleural pressures this low virtually never occur, the pleural space does not fill up with gas unless there is a communication between the pleural space and the lungs or the atmosphere or unless there are gas-forming organisms in the pleural space. It is for this same reason that air from a pneumothorax is absorbed if the communication between the alveoli and the pleural space closes.

There is normally a small amount of liquid (~8 mL) present in each pleural space (4). This liquid forms a very thin film of uniform thickness that couples the parietal and visceral pleural surfaces, enabling them to slide over one another with a minimal amount of friction. Normally, a small amount of fluid (~0.01 mL/kg/h) continuously enters the pleural space from either the visceral or parietal pleura (5). Most of the liquid in the pleural space leaves via the lymphatics in the parietal pleura. These lymphatics have the capacity to remove about 0.28 mL/kg/h (6). The movement of fluid into and out of the pleural space is more fully discussed in Chapter 17, Diseases of the Pleura, Mediastinum, Chest Wall, and Diaphragm.

FACTORS INFLUENCING THE PRESSURE–VOLUME CURVE OF THE LUNG

Elastic Recoil of the Lungs

Pressure–volume curves for the lungs from a normal individual, a patient with emphysema, and a patient with interstitial fibrosis are illustrated in Figure 2-6. As volume of the lungs increases, pressure is generated within the system because of the tendency of the elastic component of the lungs to recoil inward. As the volume is further increased, the pressure increase

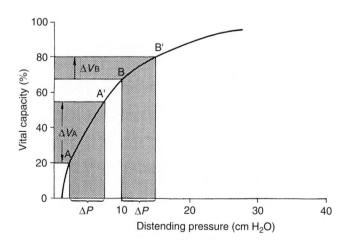

FIGURE 2-5. Pressure–volume curve of a normal lung. At functional residual capacity, the alveoli in the lower part of the lung *(A)* are at a smaller volume than those in the upper part of the lung *(B)* on account of the pleural pressure gradient. Then, when a given amount of distending pressure (ΔP) is applied to both sets of alveoli, the volume increase of those in the lower parts of the lung (ΔV_A) is much greater than that in the upper parts of the lung (ΔV_B) because of the shape of the pressure–volume curve.

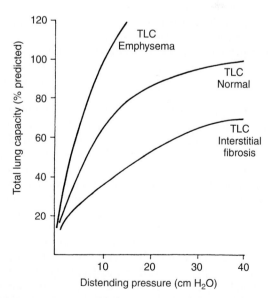

FIGURE 2-6. Representative pressure–volume curves from a normal subject, a patient with emphysema, and a patient with interstitial fibrosis.

with each volume increment becomes larger. Eventually, the pressure–volume curve becomes almost flat as the elastic elements reach their limits of distensibility. If the volume increases furthermore, the lungs are liable to rupture because of the very high transpulmonary pressure.

Under static conditions, the pressure generated by the lung is determined solely by its elastic recoil pressure $Pst(L)$. In other words, when the airways are open and there is no airflow, $Pst(L)$ is equal to PL. If the glottis is open so that the alveolar pressure is zero, the pleural pressure must be equal, but opposite in sign, to the recoil pressure.

$$Pst(L) = PL = PA - Ppl$$
$$\text{but because } PA = 0, Pst(L) = -Ppl$$

The lungs of patients with emphysema are more distensible than normal lungs because many alveolar walls have been destroyed, resulting in a loss of elastic elements. As illustrated in Figure 2-6, the pressure–volume curve of a patient with emphysema is shifted to the left. The transpulmonary pressure at any given lung volume is less than that for a normal lung. In contrast, the lungs of patients with interstitial fibrosis are less distensible than normal lungs because the retractive forces of the tissue are increased. Therefore, the pressure–volume curve of the patient with interstitial fibrosis is shifted to the right. The stiffness of the lung may also be increased when the pulmonary vessels are engorged with blood or when the interstitial spaces are filled with fluid.

Origin of Lung Elastic Recoil

The total force causing the inflated lung to recoil inward has two components: the first arises from the elastic properties of the lung tissue itself and the second arises from surface tension. In Figure 2-7, pressure–volume curves are shown for an excised lung when it is first inflated with saline and then with air. When a normal excised lung is deflated and then inflated with air, the volume increases very slowly until a pressure of 8 cm H_2O is reached. At pressures above this, the volume increases rapidly until the TLC is approached at about 30 cm H_2O. The filling of the lung is uneven, as is evident from the rapid inflation of the different areas of the lung. If the pressure is then decreased, the volume of air remaining in the lung will be much greater than that at the same pressure during inflation, and the lung will deflate evenly. Microscopic observations of subpleural air spaces show that these air spaces are recruited sequentially from largest to smallest during inflation from the gas-free state but that they tend to deflate in parallel without extensive derecruitment (7). This difference between the inflation and deflation curves and the failure of the lung to return to its original state after deformation is called *hysteresis*.

When the lungs are filled with a liquid such as isotonic saline, they begin to expand at a lower pressure, fill uniformly, and require less pressure to fill completely. When the lung empties after being filled with the liquid, very little hysteresis is noted. The differences in the pressure–volume curves with air and saline inflation are due to differences in surface tension.

Surface tension does not represent a true force but arises because any surface has the tendency to decrease to a minimum. The molecules present at the surface of an air–liquid interface are pulled toward the liquid by molecules in the liquid, and this pull is not counterbalanced because the molecules lie on

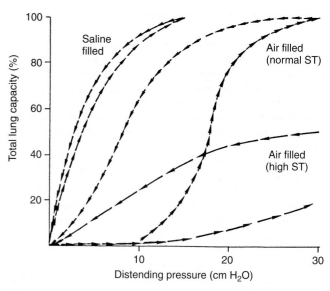

FIGURE 2-7. Pressure–volume curves of lungs filled with saline and with air with normal and high surface tension (ST). The arrows indicate whether the lung is being inflated or deflated. When the lung is filled with saline, the effects of surface forces at the air–liquid interfaces are eliminated. The differences between the curves of the saline-filled and air-filled lungs are due to surface forces. The differences between the curve of the lung with normal surface tension and that of the lung with high surface tension are due to the reduction of surface forces by surfactant.

the surface. When one considers a spherical bubble, the surface tension (T) in the wall of the bubble tends to contract the bubble and the pressure (P) owing to the gas inside the bubble tends to expand it. At equilibrium,

$$P = 2T/r \qquad (2.5)$$

where r is the radius of the bubble.

From this equation (Laplace's equation), it can be seen that the larger the bubble, the smaller the pressure inside the bubble if T is constant. The lungs are essentially two sets of millions of bubbles. Consider what would happen if T were the same throughout the lungs. At any given time, if all the alveoli were not exactly the same size, the pressure in the smaller alveoli would be greater than the pressure in the larger alveoli. Hence, air would flow from the smaller to the larger alveoli. This would exacerbate the pressure differences, and after a short period, most alveoli would be collapsed or fully distended, obviously a less than ideal situation.

However, in the normal lung, there is no such instability. The reason why the normal lung is stable is because of a substance called *surfactant* (8). Surfactant is a complex mixture composed of lipids, proteins, and carbohydrates secreted by the type II pneumocytes that are present in all alveoli. The major surface-active component of pulmonary surfactant is the phospholipid dipalmitoyl phosphatidylcholine. Surfactant has two main functions. First, when it is present, the surface tension decreases dramatically as the surface area is decreased. The result of this is that the T in Laplace's equation becomes a variable depending on the radius of the alveoli, such that

$$P = 2T'/r = \text{constant} \qquad (2.6)$$

where T' is the varying surface tension in the presence of surfactant. In this manner, surfactant promotes alveolar stability.

Its presence is partly responsible for the hysteresis observed with the inflating lung. It is difficult to open alveoli initially, but once they are inflated, the presence of surfactant allows them to empty evenly in parallel. The second characteristic of surfactant is that it markedly decreases surface tension and thereby reduces the transpulmonary pressure necessary to achieve a given lung volume. It has the lowest surface tension of any biologic substance ever measured. The presence of surfactant also increases the antibacterial capabilities of alveolar macrophages and modulates lymphocyte responsiveness (8).

The difference between the pressure–volume curves obtained with saline and with air indicate how much of the elastic recoil is due to surface tension (Fig. 2-7). On the inflation part of the curve, there is much more elastic recoil secondary to surface tension than to the elastic properties of the lung. For example, to reach a volume of 50% TLC, a total pressure of 18 cm H_2O is necessary with air inflation but only 3 cm H_2O with saline inflation, indicating that 15 of the 18 cm H_2O of the elastic recoil is due to surface tension. Alternatively, on the deflation limb of the air inflation curve, a pressure of 8 cm H_2O is necessary for a volume of 50% TLC and the elastic recoil due to surface tension is only 5 cm H_2O.

The importance of surfactant in reducing the surface tension can be appreciated by comparing the pressure–volume curves of isolated lungs with and without surfactant (Fig. 2-7). In the lung with no surfactant and therefore high surface tension, the TLC is not approached even with a distending pressure of 30 cm H_2O. Moreover, at 50% TLC, the distending pressure of the deflating lung devoid of surfactant is more than double that of the lung with normal surfactant.

Surfactant is important in several different clinical situations. The infant acute respiratory distress syndrome (ARDS) occurs in infants born prematurely, before they have developed sufficient ability to produce surfactant. As a result of the inadequate level of surfactant, their lungs are unstable and have very low compliance. This instability leads to complete atelectasis of many alveoli, producing a right-to-left shunt and profound hypoxemia. The decreased compliance and atelectatic alveoli lead to alveolar hypoventilation. Surfactant production can be augmented by the administration of corticoids to the mother prenatally, which results in a decreased incidence of the respiratory distress syndrome (9). Studies have consistently shown that the administration of exogenous surfactant therapy to premature babies with the infant respiratory distress syndrome results in improved gas exchange and lung mechanics as well as a reduced mortality rate. The administration of exogenous surfactant is now considered to be routine therapy for infants with the infant respiratory distress syndrome (8,10).

A lack of surfactant is also thought to play a role in producing the adult ARDS (Chapter 23, Acute Hypoxemic Respiratory Failure: Pulmonary Edema and Acute Lung Injury). This condition is characterized by diffuse pulmonary infiltrates and marked hypoxia refractory to high concentrations of inspired oxygen. The marked hypoxia is secondary to perfusion of atelectatic alveoli. Because of atelectasis, the lungs are very noncompliant, as would be predicted from Figure 2-7. Therapy for ARDS is primarily directed toward increasing lung volume to prevent alveoli from becoming atelectatic (Chapter 23, Acute Hypoxemic Respiratory Failure: Pulmonary Edema and Acute Lung Injury). Despite several studies evaluating the therapeutic efficacy of exogenous surfactant, none has definitively shown that surfactant replacement therapy is efficacious in the adult ARDS. Further studies are necessary before exogenous surfactant can be recommended in the treatment for this syndrome (11).

DYNAMICS OF THE RESPIRATORY SYSTEM

The dynamics of breathing are discussed in this section. First, different types of airflow and resistances to airflow are described. Next, the relationship between alveolar pressures and airflow is reviewed, including the dynamic compression of the airways by positive pleural pressure on forced exhalation. Finally, factors influencing the distribution of ventilation and the work of breathing are discussed.

AIRWAY RESISTANCES

Air moves into and out of the lungs whenever the alveolar pressure differs from the atmospheric pressure (assuming the airways are not obstructed). The airway resistance (Raw) is defined as the frictional resistance of the entire system of air passages to airflow from outside the body to within the alveoli. By definition,

$$Raw = (P_A - Pao)/\dot{V} \tag{2.7}$$

where P_A is the alveolar pressure, Pao is the pressure at the airway opening, and $\dot{V}$ is the flow rate. This system is analogous to an electrical circuit:

$$R = V/I \tag{2.8}$$

where R is the electrical resistance, V is the voltage difference, and I is the current.

Patterns of Airflow

The resistance to airflow in a tube depends on the type of flow, the dimensions of the tube, and the viscosity and density of the gas. Airflow through tubes can be either *laminar* or *turbulent* or a combination. Laminar flow is organized, and the streamlines are parallel everywhere to the sides of the tube and are capable of sliding over one another (Fig. 2-8). The streamlines at the center of the tube move faster than those closest to the walls, producing a flow profile that is parabolic. With laminar flow, the relation between pressure and flow is given by Poiseuille's equation,

$$P = 8\eta l \dot{V}/\pi r^4 = K_1 \dot{V} \tag{2.9}$$

or

$$\dot{V} = P\pi r^4/8\eta l \tag{2.10}$$

where $\dot{V}$ is the flow rate, P is the driving pressure (pressure drop between the beginning and end of the tube), r and l are the radius and the length of the tube respectively, and η is the viscosity of the gas. Because flow resistance (R) is the driving pressure divided by the flow (Eq. 2.7), the resistance with laminar flow is independent of the flow rate:

$$R = 8\eta l/\pi r^4 = K_1 \tag{2.11}$$

Note the critical importance of the tube radius—if the radius of the tube is halved, the airway resistance increases 16-fold.

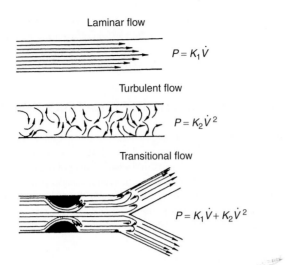

Laminar flow

$$P = K_1\dot{V}$$

Turbulent flow

$$P = K_2\dot{V}^2$$

Transitional flow

$$P = K_1\dot{V} + K_2\dot{V}^2$$

FIGURE 2-8.   Patterns of airflow in tubes.

Note also that laminar flow is dependent on the viscosity of a gas but is independent of its density.

Turbulent flow occurs at high flow rates and is characterized by a complete disorganization of the streamlines so that molecules of gas move laterally, collide with one another, and change their velocities (Fig. 2-8). Owing to this disorganization, the pressure drop across the tube is not proportionate to the flow rate, unlike laminar flow, but rather it is proportional to the square of the flow rate:

$$P = K_2\dot{V}^2 \qquad (2.12)$$

It follows from Equation 2.7 that the resistance to airflow is proportional to the flow rate

$$R = K\dot{V} \qquad (2.13)$$

in contrast with laminar flow. In addition, with turbulent flow, an increase in gas density increases the pressure drop for a given flow, but the viscosity of the gas becomes unimportant.

Whether airflow is laminar or turbulent depends to a large extent on a dimensionless quantity called the Reynolds number, *Re*, which is given by

$$Re = 2rvd/\eta \qquad (2.14)$$

where r is the radius of the tube, v is the average velocity, d is the density of the gas, and η is the viscosity of the gas. In straight, smooth, rigid tubes, turbulence occurs when *Re* exceeds 2000.

In the lung, laminar flow occurs only in the small peripheral airways, where, owing to the large overall cross-sectional area, flow through any given airway is extremely slow. Turbulent flow occurs in the trachea. In the remainder of the lung, owing in large part to the multiple branching of the tracheobronchial tree, flow is neither laminar nor turbulent but rather mixed or transitional (Fig. 2-8). With a transitional flow pattern, flow is dependent on both the viscosity and the density of the gas.

Distribution of Airway Resistance

Toward the periphery in the tracheobronchial tree, the airways become successively narrower. Therefore, from Equation 2.11, one would anticipate that the major part of the airway resistance would reside in the narrow peripheral airways. However,

direct measurements of airway resistance have shown that less than 20% of the total airway resistance is confined to airways with diameters <2 mm. The explanation for this apparent paradox is that the progressive branching of the tracheobronchial tree results in an increased average cross-sectional diameter of the peripheral airways; therefore, resistance does not increase disproportionately (12).

During nasal breathing, the resistance offered by the nose is the largest single fraction, constituting one-half to two-thirds of the total resistance at low flow rates. The nasal resistance increases disproportionately with increasing flow rates; therefore, during heavy exercise, one switches from nasal breathing to mouth breathing. During quiet breathing, the mouth, pharynx, larynx, and trachea provide 20% to 30% of the airway resistance. Most of the remainder of the airway resistance is in the bronchi with diameters >2 mm (13).

Factors Influencing Airway Resistance

Airway resistance depends on the number, length, and cross-sectional area of the conducting airways. Because resistance to airflow in a given airway changes according to the fourth power of its radius, the cross-sectional area within the tracheobronchial tree is by far the most important determinant of airway resistance. The airways, like the lung parenchyma, exhibit elasticity and are capable of being compressed or distended. Therefore, the diameter of an airway varies with the transmural pressure applied to that airway—that is, the difference between the pressure within the airway and the pressure surrounding the airway. The pressure surrounding the intrathoracic airways approximates pleural pressure.

As the lung volume increases, the traction applied to the walls of the intrathoracic airways also increases, widening the airways and decreasing their resistance to airflow. The relationship between the lung volume and airway resistance is not linear (Fig. 2-9A). However, the relationship between the reciprocal of the airway resistance, the *airway conductance* (Gaw), and lung volume is linear (Fig. 2-9B). The *specific airway conductance* (SGaw) is defined as

$$SGaw = Gaw/V_L \qquad (2.15)$$

where V_L is the volume at which Gaw is measured. As *SGaw* is nearly independent of the lung volume in a given patient, it is the index of airway resistance that should be used in the clinical situation. Furthermore, use of this index reduces the variations in resistance measurements from individual to individual owing to varying body size (14).

Contraction of the bronchial smooth muscles narrows the airways and increases airway resistance. Normally, there is a small amount of resting smooth muscle tone in the bronchial smooth muscles. Administration of inhaled bronchodilator drugs to normal subjects leads to a significant decrease in the airway resistance (15). The tone of the bronchial smooth muscle is under the control of the autonomic nervous system. Sympathetic stimulation causes bronchodilation, whereas parasympathetic stimulation causes bronchoconstriction. Stimulation of the irritant receptors in the tracheobronchial tree induces bronchoconstriction reflexly via the parasympathetic nerve fibers contained in the vagus nerve (16). In patients with lung disease, mucosal edema, hypertrophy and hyperplasia of mucous glands, increased production of mucus, and

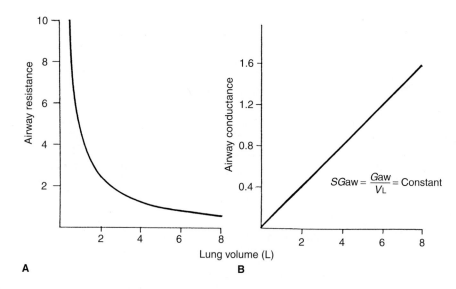

$$SGaw = \frac{Gaw}{V_L} = \text{Constant}$$

FIGURE 2-9. **A:** The relationship between airway resistance and lung volume. **B:** The relationship between airway conductance and lung volume. Note that the relationship between airway resistance and lung volume is not linear, whereas that between airway conductance and lung volume is linear.

hypertrophy of the bronchial smooth muscle all tend to decrease airway caliber and contribute to the increased airway resistance.

PRESSURE–FLOW RELATIONSHIPS

It has been recognized for a long time that there is a limit to the flow rate that can be attained during exhalation and that, once this limit is achieved, greater muscular effort does not augment flow. With both laminar flow (Eq. 2.10) and turbulent flow (Eq. 2.12), one would expect higher pressures to be associated with higher flows.

The limitation of flow at different lung volumes is best appreciated from the examination of isovolume pressure–flow curves at different lung volumes. Isovolume pressure–flow curves are constructed by simultaneously measuring the flow, volume, and pleural pressure as a subject inhales and exhales with varying amounts of effort that are reflected by changes in pleural pressure. Thus, for any given lung volume, there is a set of pleural pressures and flow rates. Because at any given lung volume the elastic recoil pressure of the lung is constant, the pleural pressures can be converted to alveolar pressures by adding the elastic recoil pressure at that particular lung volume to the pleural pressure.

Figure 2-10 depicts a family of isovolume pressure–flow curves at different lung volumes. Two main characteristics of these curves should be noted. First, for a given alveolar pressure, the higher the lung volume, the greater the flow rate during both inhalation (negative alveolar pressure) and exhalation (positive alveolar pressure). The explanation for this during inhalation is that the higher the lung volume, the lower the airway resistance. The explanation during exhalation is that, at higher lung volumes, not only is the airway resistance lower but the elastic recoil of the lung is also greater. The importance of elastic recoil in determining expiratory flow rates is discussed in the next section.

Second, as alveolar pressure increases during exhalation at all but the higher lung volumes, flow rates increase until a certain alveolar pressure is reached. Then, further increases in alveolar pressure do not result in increased flow. This flow

limitation in the face of increasing alveolar pressure is surprising because, with both laminar flow (Eq. 2.10) and turbulent flow (Eq. 2.12), one would expect higher pressures to be associated with higher flows. The explanation for this upper limit on expiratory flow is dynamic compression of the airways, which is discussed in the next section. Note that there is no similar limitation of flow on inspiration. Note also that the alveolar pressure necessary to generate the maximum flow is lower at lower lung volumes.

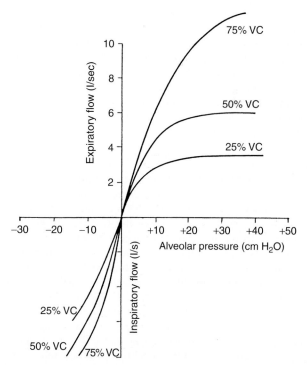

FIGURE 2-10. Isovolume pressure–flow curves at 25%, 50%, and 75% of the vital capacity (VC). Note the limitation of airflow on exhalation at alveolar pressures above 20 and 28 cm H_2O at 25% and 50% of the VC, respectively.

At volumes greater than 75% of the VC, airflow increases progressively with increasing alveolar pressure and is considered *effort dependent*. In contrast, at lung volumes below 75% of the VC, the flow rate reaches a maximum once a given alveolar pressure is reached. At these lung volumes, airflow is considered *effort independent*, but the critical alveolar pressure must be reached in order to have maximum flow.

The limitation of flow on exhalation, demonstrated in Figure 2-10, is very important to the clinician. The majority of patients with lung disease have obstructive lung disease, which means that it takes them longer than normal to get the air out of their lungs. The two main tests used to diagnose and assess the response of these patients to therapy are the *forced expiratory spirogram* and the *flow–volume loop* (Chapter 6, Clinical Pulmonary Function Testing, Exercise Testing, and Disability Evaluation). With both of these tests, the patient takes a maximal inspiration and then exhales as hard and as long as he or she is able. From Figure 2-10, it can be seen that at lung volumes below about 75% of the VC, these tests are independent of effort once the critical alveolar pressure is reached. Therefore, the tests are reproducible and are invaluable in the management of these patients. Because there is no flow limitation on inspiration, tests dependent on inspiratory flow rates are much less reproducible than are tests dependent on expiratory flow rates.

Dynamic Compression of the Airways

Limitation of flow during exhalation results from dynamic compression of the airways. To illustrate the mechanisms involved in producing flow limitation during a maximal expiratory maneuver, it is useful to consider a model of the lung in which the alveoli are represented by an elastic sac and the intrathoracic airways by a compressible tube, both of which are enclosed within a pleural space (Fig. 2-11).

At a given lung volume when there is no flow (Fig. 2-11A), the alveolar pressure is zero. The pleural pressure is subatmospheric and exactly counterbalances the elastic recoil of the lung. To generate expiratory flow, the alveolar pressure must be increased above zero, which is accomplished by increasing the pleural pressure. Because the lung volume has not changed, increase in the alveolar pressure is the same as increase in the pleural pressure.

$$P_A = P_{pl} + P_{st(L)} \qquad (2.16)$$

As one moves downstream (toward the mouth) from the alveolus, the intrabronchial pressure decreases on account of the resistance to airflow. During quiet breathing, if the pleural pressure does not become positive, the intrabronchial pressure is always greater than the pleural pressure (Fig. 2-11B). When sufficient expiratory effort is generated, however, the pleural pressure becomes positive. In this situation, the intrabronchial pressure at some point along the airways is equal to the extrabronchial pleural pressure (Fig. 2-11C). Mead and coworkers designated this point the *equal-pressure point* (EPP) (17). The EPP divides the airways into two components arranged in series: an *upstream segment* from the alveoli to the EPP, where the distending pressure of the bronchi is positive, and a *downstream segment* from the EPP to the airway opening, where the distending pressure of the bronchi is negative intrathoracically. It is these downstream segments of the airways that are dynamically compressed during forced exhalation.

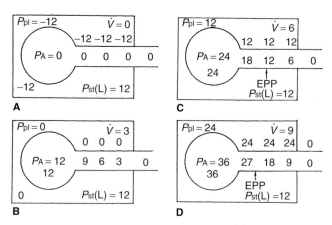

FIGURE 2-11. A schematic representation of the equal-pressure point (EPP) concept. **A:** The alveolar pressure is zero, so there is no flow. **B:** The increase in the alveolar pressure is equal to the $P_{st(L)}$, so the pleural pressure is zero. Here, the EPP is at the airway opening. **C:** The alveolar pressure has increased more, so the pleural pressure must be positive. The pressure drops from the alveolus to different points along the airway are greater because $\dot{V}$ is higher. Accordingly, the EPP moves closer to the alveolus. **D:** The P_{pl} has been increased even more and the EPP has moved farther upstream because flow has increased. When flow limitation occurs, the EPP becomes fixed, and $\dot{V}$max is determined by Equation 2.18.

Location of Equal-Pressure Point

When the pleural pressure is subatmospheric, there is no EPP (Fig. 2-11A). When the pleural pressure becomes atmospheric, the EPP is at the airway opening (Fig. 2-11B). As the pleural pressure becomes more positive, the EPP moves upstream (Fig. 2-11C, D)—but how far? When flow in the upstream segment is considered, the pressure drop from the alveolus to the EPP is the difference between alveolar pressure and the pleural pressure, which is the elastic recoil pressure of the lung. The resistance of the upstream segment is designated R_{us}. Therefore, it follows from Equation 2.7 that

$$\dot{V} = P_{st(L)}/R_{us} \qquad (2.17)$$

At a constant lung volume, $P_{st(L)}$ is constant. Therefore, the only way that $\dot{V}$ can be increased is for R_{us} to decrease, which can be accomplished only by having the EPP move upstream. With more and more effort, the EPP moves upstream (Fig. 2-11B–D) until the pleural pressure reaches a level at which further increases in it do not lead to further increases in $\dot{V}$. The $\dot{V}$ at this pleural pressure is called $\dot{V}$max and corresponds to the flat top on the isovolume pressure–flow curve (Fig. 2-10).

Note by this analysis that

$$\dot{V}max = P_{st(L)}/R_{us} \qquad (2.18)$$

and, therefore, $\dot{V}$max is dependent on two factors: (a) the resistance of the upstream segment and (b) the recoil pressure of the lung. In other words, a decreased elastic recoil of the lung is just as important in reducing $\dot{V}$max as is increased airway resistance.

Pride and coworkers (18) developed a different analysis of the mechanisms of forced exhalation. Their analysis is similar to that of Mead and coworkers but also takes into account the resistance to collapse of the intrathoracic airways. The analysis has not been publicized as much as the EPP analysis, but it better explains the mechanics of forced exhalation.

In the model of Pride and coworkers (Fig. 2-12), the airways are divided into two rigid tubes connected in series by a short segment of a collapsible tube. They divided the airways into an upstream segment, between the alveoli and the distal end of the collapsible segment, and a downstream segment, from the end of the collapsible segment to the airway opening. Moreover, they defined the *critical closing pressure of the collapsible segment* (Ptm') as the transmural pressure (Ptm) at which the segment collapsed. As with any distensible object, the transmural pressure is the difference between the pressure inside and outside the wall. Therefore, the value for Ptm' indicates the distending pressure that must be maintained to keep the collapsible segment patent. They further assumed that the short, collapsible segment was fully open whenever its distending pressure exceeded Ptm' and fully collapsed whenever Ptm fell below Ptm'.

The transmural pressure in the collapsible segment is given by the following:

$$Ptm = PA - (\dot{V} \times Rs) - Ppl \qquad (2.19)$$

where Rs is the resistance of the segment upstream from the collapsible segment. (Note the distinction from Rus, which is the resistance of the segment upstream from the EPP in the analysis of Mead et al.) Given that

$$PA = Pst(L) + Ppl \qquad (2.20)$$

then

$$Ptm = Pst(L) - (\dot{V} \times Rs) \qquad (2.21)$$

Therefore, as $\dot{V}$ increases, Ptm decreases. When $\dot{V}$ increases to a critical level ($\dot{V}max$), Ptm drops to Ptm'. This is illustrated in Figure 2-12(B), where $Ptm = 6 - 6 = 0$ and it is assumed that $Ptm' = 0$. If flow rates increase further, as illustrated in Figure 2-12(C), the Ptm would fall below Ptm' (in the illustration, $Ptm = -4$), but by our assumptions, the collapsible segment would collapse completely and there would be no flow (Fig. 2-12D). However, as soon as flow ceases, the intrabronchial pressure equals the alveolar pressure and again Ptm exceeds Ptm' and flow resumes. If the collapsible segment opens all the way, $\dot{V}$ again exceeds $\dot{V}max$, Ptm falls below Ptm', and airflow ceases. Therefore, it is postulated that the collapsible segment acts as a variable resistor, as illustrated in Figure 2-12(E) and (F). Once the pleural pressure is reached, at which dynamic compression of the airways occurs, the collapsible

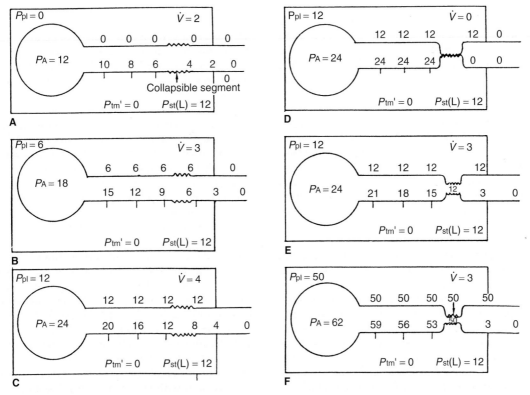

FIGURE 2-12. A schematic representation of the collapsible-segment concept. In these diagrams, the lung volume is that giving a $Pst(L)$ of 12 and it is assumed that Ptm' is zero. **A:** Pressures along the airways when Ptm still exceeds Ptm'. There is no collapse. **B:** Pressures along the airways when Ptm approaches Ptm'. Note that the flow rate increases from **A. C:** Pressures along the airways when pleural pressures are further increased. Note that Ptm at the collapsible segment is now $8 - 12 = -4$, which is below $Ptm' = 0$, so this higher flow is impossible because the collapsible segment must collapse. **D:** Pressures along the airways when there is no flow. Now, Ptm is $24 - 12 = 12$, so the airways must open. **E:** Pressure along the airways when the collapsible segment is partially collapsed such that $Ptm = Ptm'$. **F:** Pressures along the airways when the alveolar pressure is raised much higher. Note that the collapsible segment is more collapsed than in **E** and that the flows in **B**, **E**, and **F** are also identical. The airway pressures downstream from the collapsible segment in **B**, **E**, and **F** are also identical.

segment partially collapses. It collapses to the degree where the pressure drop between the alveoli and the collapsible segment is such that the Ptm is equal to the Ptm'. As pleural pressures progressively increase (Fig. 2-12F), there is a larger pressure drop across the collapsible segment. Note that by this analysis, flow and intrabronchial pressures downstream from the collapsible segment do not change once flow limitation is achieved (Fig. 2-12B, E, F). From Equation 2.21, flow limitation occurs when Ptm = Ptm'. Therefore, when Ptm is substituted for Ptm in Equation 2.21,

$$Ptm' = Pst(L) - \dot{V}max \times Rs \qquad (2.22)$$

which can be rewritten as follows:

$$\dot{V}max = (Pst(L) - Ptm')/Rs \qquad (2.23)$$

Note that this analysis of respiratory mechanics is conceptually analogous to a waterfall. The height of the waterfall (i.e., the pressure drop across the collapsible segment) does not affect flow either above or below the waterfall. The flow above the waterfall is given by Equation 2.23 regardless of the height of the waterfall. The flow below the waterfall is determined by the flow above the waterfall. As the resistance to flow below the waterfall is fixed, the pressure immediately downstream from the collapsible segment is equal to the product of $\dot{V}max$ and the resistance of the downstream segment.

When Equation 2.23 is analyzed, it is seen that $\dot{V}max$ depends on three different factors: (a) the elastic recoil of the lung (Pst(L)), (b) the tendency of the airways to collapse (Ptm'), and (c) the resistance of the upstream segment (Rs). Emphysema, chronic bronchitis, and asthma are the three main diseases that cause reduced flow rates on exhalation. Analysis of Equation 2.23 reveals that the predominant mechanism causing reduced flow rates is different with each of these three diseases. With emphysema, the main abnormality is decreased elastic recoil of the lungs (Pst(L)); with chronic bronchitis, the predominant abnormality is increased resistance of the upstream segment (Rs); with asthma, the constriction of the bronchial smooth muscles greatly increases the tendency of the airways to collapse (Ptm') and thereby reduces flow rates by this mechanism. With all three diseases, the three factors interact to some extent to produce reduced expiratory flow rates. An explanation for air trapping is also given by Equation 2.23. Air trapping occurs when the Pst(L) is less than Ptm' because when this condition is met, $\dot{V}max$ is zero. Therefore, the lungs cannot empty at lung volumes below which Ptm' exceeds Pst(L).

Experimental evidence supporting this analysis of flow limitation was provided by Smaldone and Bergofsky (19). They monitored intrabronchial pressures in excised lungs and demonstrated that the flow-limiting segment consisted of well-demarcated short lengths of the trachea at large lung volumes but lobar or segmental bronchi at low lung volumes. There was a large pressure drop across the collapsible segment, which at any given lung volume was closely related to the driving pressure. Leaver and coworkers (20) investigated the contribution of the three factors in Equation 2.23 in producing decreased expiratory flow rates in 17 patients with chronic bronchitis and emphysema. They found that all three factors contributed to reduction in maximal flow. In 3 of their 17 patients, the reduction in expiratory flow rates could be entirely accounted for by loss of lung elastic recoil and enhanced airway collapsibility.

Although dynamic compression of the airways produces limitation of flow on exhalation, it is not without value because it does improve the effectiveness of coughing. In the collapsible segment, the linear velocity of airflow is markedly increased owing to the smaller cross-sectional area. This increased linear velocity leads to a greater shearing force that serves to dislodge secretions and particles from the walls of airways. The shift of the collapsible segment from the trachea to the segmental bronchi as lung volumes get smaller increases the ease with which coughing can remove secretions from most of the larger airways.

DENSITY DEPENDENCE OF MAXIMAL AIRFLOW

In the normal lung during forced exhalation, flow in the peripheral airways is laminar, flow in the medium-sized airways is transitional, and flow in the large airways is turbulent. Only laminar flow is independent of gas *density*. Therefore, if maximal expiratory flow rates are measured with the patient breathing gases of varying densities, the flow rates should remain stable only if there is laminar flow in the flow-limiting segment. If there is either turbulent flow or transitional flow in this segment, breathing a gas with a lower density should result in increased flow rates at a given lung volume. In contrast, laminar flow is dependent on gas *viscosity*.

A mixture of 80% helium and 20% oxygen (He–O$_2$) has a viscosity very similar to that of air but a density that is approximately one-third that of air (21). Because the viscosity of He–O$_2$ is similar to that of air but the density of He–O$_2$ is much lower, one would expect higher maximal flows with the He–O$_2$ only if the flow in the flow-limiting segment were turbulent or transitional. Flow–volume loops from a normal subject obtained while breathing air and with He–O$_2$ are illustrated on the left in Figure 2-13. At all lung volumes above 15% of the VC, the maximum flow rate with He–O$_2$ is greater than that with air. At 50% of the VC, the flow rate with He–O$_2$ is 50% higher than it is with air. The percent increase in flow rates with He–O$_2$ at 50% VC is termed the $\Delta \dot{V}max_{50}$. The point at which the flow rates with He–O$_2$ and with air become identical is termed the *isoflow volume* (VisoV̇). The normal $\Delta \dot{V}max_{50}$ is 47.3 ± 27.4% (two standard deviations) and does not change with age. The normal VisoV̇ at age 40 is 16.5 ± 13.8% and increases 0.3% for each additional year (22).

In normal subjects, flow at low lung volumes is density independent because the collapsible segment is more peripheral and flow rates are lower. Owing to the much lower flow rates, the Reynolds number (Eq. 2.14) dictates that the flow will be laminar. Flow–volume loops for a smoker obtained with room air and with He–O$_2$ are illustrated on the right in Figure 2-13. Although the flow–volume loops with room air for the normal person and the smoker are virtually identical, the increases in the flow rates with He–O$_2$ are much less for the smoker. The $\Delta \dot{V}max_{50}$ for the smoker is only 15% compared with 50% for the nonsmoker, and the VisoV̇ is 30% compared with 15% for the nonsmoker.

The use of He–O$_2$ flow–volume loops has its greatest utility in detecting disease of the small peripheral airways. Because the small airways usually contribute only a minor portion to the total airway resistance, changes in these airways may not be detectable by measurements of airway resistance. Increased resistance in the small airways should reduce maximal flow, but

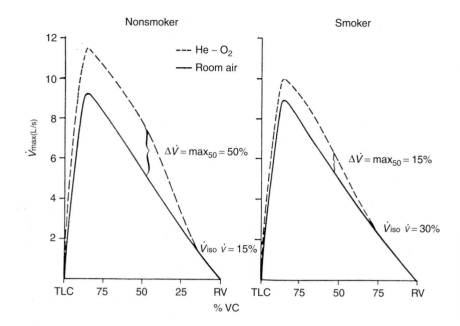

FIGURE 2-13. Flow–volume loops obtained with room air and He–O₂ on a normal non-smoker and an asymptomatic smoker. Although the flow–volume loops in room air are identical, there is a substantially greater improvement in the flow rates with He–O₂ in the normal person than in the smoking individual.

because of the great variability of flow–volume curves in normal individuals, flow may not be reduced below the normal range. However, disease in the peripheral airways should decrease the relative contribution of density-dependent flow to the total pressure drop between the alveoli and the collapsible segment.

Dosman and coworkers obtained flow–volume loops with air and He–O₂ for 66 nonsmokers and 48 smokers whose forced expiratory volume in 1 second divided by the forced vital capacity (FEV_1/FVC%) values exceeded 70% (22). With air, only 12% of the smokers had a $\dot{V}max_{50}$ and only 2% had a $\dot{V}max_{25}$ that were more than two standard deviations below those of the nonsmokers. In contrast, with He–O₂, 40% of the smokers had a $\Delta\dot{V}max_{50}$ that was more than two standard deviations below that of the nonsmokers and 52% had a $\dot{V}iso\dot{v}$ that exceeded those of the nonsmokers by more than two standard deviations. These results show that use of He–O₂ during a forced expiratory maneuver allows the detection of functional abnormalities in smokers at a stage when their $\dot{V}max$ is still within the normal range while they are breathing room air. However, the significance of these functional abnormalities in terms of the patient eventually developing chronic obstructive pulmonary disease (COPD) remains to be proved.

Despite the theoretical considerations described in the preceding section, there has not been widespread utilization of the He–O₂ flow–volume loops in clinical pulmonary disease. This is because they have proved difficult to use in healthy subjects and patients because of large intrasubject and intersubject variability and variability in interpretation of the same series of curves by different observers (23).

DISTRIBUTION OF VENTILATION

The regional distribution of ventilation depends on the distensibility of the peripheral gas exchange units and the resistance of the airways leading to them. The emptying of an elastic reservoir, such as the lung, through a resistive conduit resembles the discharge of a capacitor through a resistor. If the volume V remaining in the reservoir as a fraction of the initial volume V_0 is plotted against time t, an exponential curve is obtained for which the equation is

$$V/V_0 = e^{-t/RC} \tag{2.24}$$

where R is the resistance and C is the compliance of the system. When t is equal to RC, the exponent has a value of unity and $V/V_0 = e^{-1} = 0.37$. The product RC is the time that the system takes to reach 37% of its original volume, and this product is termed the *time constant* of the respiratory unit.

When two or more parallel units are subjected to the same inflation or deflation pressure, they each fill or empty at a rate determined by their individual time constants. If their time constants are equal, the units fill and empty uniformly. If their time constants are unequal, the units fill or empty nonuniformly. From Equation 2.24, it can be seen that an increase in either the resistance or the compliance of a respiratory unit increases the time it takes the unit to empty or fill.

Frequency Dependence of Compliance

As the time constants of the respiratory units are relatively small (0.01 second), during quiet breathing equilibration between alveolar and mouth pressures occurs both at the end of exhalation and at the end of inspiration. Therefore, the dynamic compliance of the respiratory system (the change in volume divided by the change in pleural pressure) during quiet breathing is the same as the static compliance. In the normal lung, increases in the breathing frequency up to rates of 80 breaths per minute do not affect the measured compliance. This is because the time constants are small and equilibration between alveolar and mouth pressures still occurs. However, in patients with peripheral airway disease, the time constants of at least some of the respiratory units are increased so that with more rapid breathing, equilibration between alveolar and mouth pressures does not occur at either end-inspiration or end-exhalation. Accordingly, the volume change with a given pleural pressure change falls with increasing respiratory rate, and the compliance is said to be frequency dependent (24).

In patients with relatively normal expiratory flow rates, the decrease in dynamic compliance with increasing respiratory rates may be marked. Woolcock and coworkers found that the dynamic compliance of mild asthmatics breathing at a respiratory frequency of around 80 per minute was less than 50% of the static compliance (24). A large proportion of the decrease in dynamic compliance is due to the fact that at times of zero flow at the mouth, air is flowing within the lung from one region to another *(pendelluft)*. The mechanism for this is illustrated in Figure 2-14. During inspiration, alveolus 1 fills more rapidly than alveolus 2 because of the increased airway resistance of the airways leading to alveolus 2 and, hence, its larger time constant. If the inspiratory time is short, alveolus 2 never becomes completely filled. Then, on exhalation, the pressure in alveolus 1 is higher than the pressure in alveolus 2 because of its larger volume; therefore, flow goes not only from alveolus 1 to the mouth but also from alveolus 1 to alveolus 2. The higher the frequency, the lower the tidal volume to the abnormal region.

Tests of dynamic compliance are sensitive indicators of peripheral airway disease. The time constants of the lung units distal to airways 2 mm in diameter are on the order of 0.01 second. Fourfold increases in some time constants are necessary to cause dynamic compliance to become frequency dependent. However, measurements of frequency dependence of compliance are not performed in most pulmonary function laboratories because they are time consuming, technically difficult, and require the patient to swallow an esophageal balloon.

From the preceding discussion, it can be readily appreciated that the time constants of the respiratory units markedly influence the distribution of ventilation. A second factor that is influential is the regional differences in pleural pressures, as discussed earlier in this chapter. Owing to the regional differences in pleural pressure, dependent parts of the lung are better ventilated. Other factors that influence the distribution of ventilation are the *interdependence* that exists between adjacent lung units and the presence of collateral pathways for ventilation.

INTERDEPENDENCE. The lung has a connective tissue framework containing elastic elements. Because contiguous units are attached to each other, they are not free to move independently. Rather, the behavior of one unit is influenced by the behavior of its neighbors. This dependence of one respiratory unit on the movements of its neighbors is termed *tissue interdependence*. Another factor that influences interdependence is the relationship between the lung and the adjacent chest wall. If, with an inspiratory effort, any part of the lung lags in its filling, the shape of the chest wall will be distorted. The local distortion of the chest wall will produce a local decrease in pleural pressure over the slowly filling lung. This local decrease in pleural pressure will be transmitted to the alveoli, thereby producing a greater pressure differential between the mouth and the alveoli. This in turn augments the flow to the area that was lagging and promotes uniformity of ventilation. It has been shown that this interaction between the lung and the chest wall is more important for the preservation of homogeneous ventilation than is lung tissue interdependence (25).

COLLATERAL VENTILATION. *Collateral ventilation* is ventilation of the alveolar structures through passages that bypass the normal airways (26). Without collateral ventilation, alveoli distal to obstructed airways would become atelectatic. The possible pathways for collateral ventilation include interalveolar communications (pores of Kohn), bronchiole-alveolar communications (canals of Lambert), and the interbronchiolar communications of Martin. The relative contributions of these three different types of communications to collateral ventilation is unknown. In a normal human lung, the resistance to collateral ventilation is high and ventilation via collateral channels takes a long time in relation to the time taken for inspiration. However, in patients with emphysema, the overall resistance to collateral ventilation is less than the airway resistance (26). Therefore, collateral ventilation may be very important in preserving the uniformity of ventilation in patients with emphysema and other lung diseases. In normal humans, there is very little collateral ventilation between different lobes or different segments (27). However, in patients with emphysema, there is substantial collateral ventilation between adjacent segments via the interbronchiolar communications of Martin (26).

WORK OF BREATHING

During breathing, the respiratory muscles must work to overcome the elastic, flow-resistive, and inertial forces of the lung and chest wall. In the respiratory system, work is expressed as the product of pressure and change in volume according to the following equation:

$$\text{Work} = \int P \times \Delta V \tag{2.25}$$

Therefore, to measure the mechanical work that is performed during breathing, it is necessary to obtain simultaneous measurements of both the volume change and the pressure that is exerted across the respiratory system.

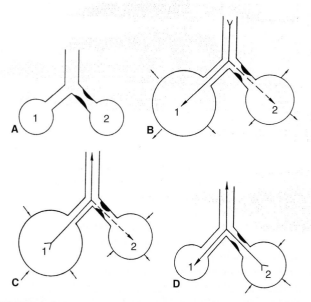

FIGURE 2-14. Effects of uneven time constants on ventilation. The airway leading to unit 2 is partially obstructed and, therefore, unit 2 has a longer time constant. **A:** After a slow exhalation, the units have the same size. **B:** With a rapid inspiration, unit 1 fills more than unit 2 because it has a faster time constant. **C:** Shortly after the start of a rapid exhalation, air moves not only from unit 1 to the airway opening but also from unit 1 to unit 2 because the pressure in unit 2 is less than the pressure in unit 1. **D:** During the latter phases of exhalation, flow moves from unit 2 to unit 1. As the respiratory rate is progressively increased, the tidal volume of the abnormal region becomes smaller and smaller.

At present, there is no method available for measuring the total amount of work being done on the lung, the respired gases, the chest wall, the diaphragm, and the abdominal contents because no technique has been developed for determination of the nonelastic resistance of the chest wall. However, the mechanical work performed on the lungs during a breathing cycle can be estimated by simultaneously measuring the changes in the intrathoracic pressures and the volume of the lungs throughout a respiratory cycle (28).

Figure 2-15 illustrates the information concerning work done on the lungs available from such measurements. In the figure, the line *ABC* is the static inflation–deflation curve of the lung. The mechanical work necessary to overcome the elastic resistance of the lung is the trapezoidal area *0ABCD*. The mechanical work required to overcome the nonelastic resistance is the area of the loop *AECF*. The portion of the loop that falls to the right of line *ABC* (*AECB*) represents the mechanical work necessary to overcome the nonelastic resistance during inspiration. The portion of the loop that falls to the left of line *ABC* (*ABCF*) represents the mechanical work required to overcome the nonelastic resistance during exhalation. Note

that in Figure 2-15(A), this area (*ABCF*) lies entirely within area *0ABCD*, which represents the elastic energy stored in the system during inspiration. The fact that the area *ABCF* lies within *0ABCD* indicates that this stored energy is sufficient to overcome the flow-resistive forces of exhalation and no work is required from the expiratory muscles.

When lung disease is present, the work of breathing can increase substantially. The mechanical work done on a lung in which the compliance is reduced by 50% is shown in Figure 2-15(B). Note that the trapezoidal area *0ABCD* is nearly doubled; hence, the work necessary to overcome the elastic resistance is nearly double that for the normal lung. The mechanical work necessary to overcome nonelastic resistance has not changed. In Figure 2-15(C), the mechanical work done on a lung in which the airway resistance is markedly increased is shown. Owing to the increased airway resistance, more negative pleural pressures must be generated to achieve the same inspiratory flow rates. Therefore, the distance between lines *ABC* and *AEC* is markedly increased and the inspiratory work (*0AECD*) is increased. Also, on account of the increased airway resistance, positive pleural pressure occurs during exhalation, indicating that muscular work is performed. The stored elastic energy is no longer sufficient. The net work during exhalation is the area *DF0*. Therefore, the total work during the respiratory cycle is the sum of the inspiratory work (*0ECD*) and the expiratory work (*DF0*), and this is increased substantially over the total work in Figure 2-15(A).

Relationship between Mechanical Work and Alveolar Ventilation

The work of breathing at any given level of alveolar ventilation is dependent on the pattern of breathing. Large tidal volumes increase the elastic work of breathing, whereas rapid breathing frequencies increase the work against flow-resistive forces (Fig. 2-16). With small tidal volumes, a higher total ventilation is required because more ventilation is wasted. Several studies have shown that both normal individuals and patients with lung disease adopt the respiratory pattern in which work is minimal (Fig. 2-16). The respiratory rate at which the minimum work occurs increases progressively with increased alveolar ventilation. Individuals with pulmonary fibrosis, which is characterized by increased elastic work of breathing, tend to breathe rapidly and shallowly. Individuals with airway obstruction, which is characterized by increased nonelastic work of breathing, usually breathe more deeply and slowly.

Oxygen Cost of Breathing

To perform the mechanical work necessary for breathing, the respiratory muscles require oxygen. The oxygen cost of breathing provides an indirect measure of the work of breathing. The oxygen cost of breathing is measured by determining the total oxygen consumption of the body at rest and at increased levels of ventilation produced by voluntary hyperventilation.

During quiet breathing, the total oxygen consumption of the body is between 200 and 300 mL/min. In normal subjects, the oxygen cost of breathing is on the order of 1.0 mL/L of ventilation. If a minute ventilation of 10 L/min is assumed, the cost of breathing accounts for approximately 5% of the total oxygen consumption. When an individual exercises, the

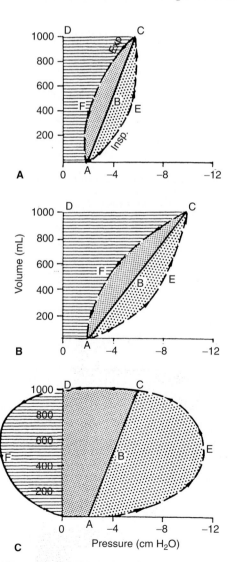

FIGURE 2-15. The mechanical work done during a respiratory cycle on **(A)** a normal lung, **(B)** a lung with reduced compliance, and **(C)** a lung with increased airway resistance. See text for explanation.

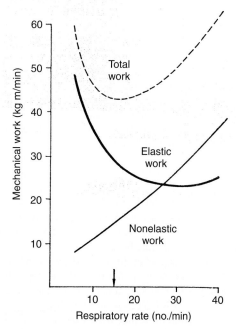

FIGURE 2-16.   The effect of respiratory rate on the elastic, nonelastic, and total mechanical work of breathing at a given level of alveolar ventilation. Subjects tend to adopt the respiratory rate at which the total work of breathing is minimal (*arrow*).

increase in the oxygen cost of breathing parallels the increase in the oxygen consumption and remains about 4% of the oxygen consumption (29). The oxygen cost of breathing is much greater in patients with lung disease. In one report, the oxygen cost of breathing in patients with COPD with a mean FEV_1 of 0.54 L was 16 mL/L of ventilation (30). In these patients, the oxygen cost of breathing accounted for more than 50% of the total oxygen uptake; these patients had a markedly increased basal metabolic index (30).

REFERENCES

1. Milic-Emili J, Mead J, Turner JM, et al. Improved technique for estimating pleural pressure from esophageal balloons. *J Appl Physiol* 1964;19:207–211.
2. Hartford CG, Rogers GG, Turner MJ. Correctly selecting a liquid-filled nasogastric infant feeding catheter to measure intraesophageal pressure. *Pediatr Pulmonol* 1997;23:362–369.
3. Lai-Fook SJ. Pleural mechanics and fluid exchange. *Physiol Rev* 2004;84:385–410.
4. Noppen M, De Waele M, Li R, et al. Volume and cellular content of normal pleural fluid in humans examined by pleural lavage. *Am J Respir Crit Care Med* 2000;162(3 pt 1):1023–1026.
5. Nahid P, Broadus VC. Liquid and protein exchange. In: Light RW, Lee YC, eds. *Textbook of pleural diseases*. London: Arnold Publishers, 2003:35-44.
6. Broaddus VC, Wiener-Kronish JP, Berthiaume Y, et al. Removal of pleural liquid and protein by lymphatics in awake sheep. *J Appl Physiol* 1988;64:384–390.
7. Radford EP Jr. Mechanical factors determining alveolar configuration. *Am Rev Respir Dis* 1960;81:743–744.
8. Ainsworth SB, Milligan DW. Surfactant therapy for respiratory distress syndrome in premature neonates: a comparative review. *Am J Respir Med*. 2002;1:417-433.
9. Elimian A, Verma U, Canterino J, et al. Effectiveness of antenatal steroids in obstetric subgroups. *Obstet Gynecol* 1999;93:174–179.
10. Jobe AH. Pulmonary surfactant therapy. *N Engl J Med* 1993;328:861–868.
11. Warren WH. Is there a role for surfactant replacement therapy in adult pulmonary dysfunction? *Crit Care Med* 1998;26:1626–1627.
12. Hogg JC, Macklem PT, Thurlbeck WM. Site and nature of airway obstruction in chronic obstructive lung disease. *N Engl J Med* 1968;278:1355–1360.
13. Ferris BG Jr, Mead J, Opie LH. Partitioning of respiratory flow resistance in man. *J Appl Physiol* 1964;19:653–658.
14. Briscoe WA, Dubois AB. The relationship between airway resistance, airway conductance and lung volume in subjects of different age and body size. *J Clin Invest* 1958;37:1279–1285.
15. Skinner C, Palmer KNV. Changes in specific airways conductance and forced expiratory volume in one second after a bronchodilator in normal subjects and patients with airways obstruction. *Thorax* 1974;29:574–577.
16. Barnes PJ. *Managing chronic obstructive pulmonary disease*, 2nd ed. London: Scientific Press Limited, 2001:42.
17. Mead J, Turner JM, Macklem PT, et al. Significance of the relationship between lung recoil and maximum expiratory flow. *J Appl Physiol* 1967;22:95–105.
18. Pride NB, Permutt S, Riley RL, et al. Determinants of maximal expiratory flow from the lungs. *J Appl Physiol* 1967;23:646–662.
19. Smaldone GC, Bergofsky EH. Delineation of flow-limiting segment and predicted airway resistance by movable catheter. *J Appl Physiol* 1976;40:943–952.
20. Leaver DG, Tattersfield AE, Pride NB. Contributions of loss of lung recoil and of enhanced airways collapsibility to the airflow obstruction of chronic bronchitis and emphysema. *J Clin Invest* 1973;52:2117–2128.
21. Drazen JM, Loring SH, Ingram RH Jr. Distribution of pulmonary resistance: effects of gas density, viscosity, and flow rate. *J Appl Physiol* 1976;41:388–395.
22. Dosman J, Bode F, Urbanetti J, et al. The use of a helium-oxygen mixture during maximum expiratory flow to demonstrate obstruction in small airways in smokers. *J Clin Invest* 1975;55:1089–1090.
23. Lam S, Abboud RT, Chan-Yeung M, et al. Use of maximal expiratory flow-volume curves with air and helium-oxygen in the detection of ventilatory abnormalities in population survey. *Am Rev Respir Dis* 1981;123:234–237.
24. Woolcock AJ, Vincent NJ, Macklem PT. Frequency dependence of compliance as a test for obstruction in the small airways. *J Clin Invest* 1969;48:1097–1106.
25. Zidulka A, Sylvester JT, Nadler S, et al. Lung interdependence and lung-chest wall interaction of sublobar and lobar units in pigs. *J Appl Physiol* 1979;46:8–13.
26. Morrell NW, Wignall BK, Biggs T, et al. Collateral ventilation and gas exchange in emphysema. *Am J Respir Crit Care Med* 1994;150:635–641.
27. Morrell NW, Roberts CM, Biggs T, et al. Collateral ventilation and gas exchange during airway occlusion in the normal human lung. *Am Rev Respir Dis* 1993;147:535–539.
28. Milic-Emili J, Orzalesi MM. Mechanical work of breathing during maximal voluntary ventilation. *J Appl Physiol* 1998;85:254–258.
29. Coast JR, Rasmussen SA, Krause KM, et al. Ventilatory work and oxygen consumption during exercise and hyperventilation. *J Appl Physiol* 1993;74:793–798.
30. Mannix ET, Manfredi F, Farber MO. Elevated O_2 cost of ventilation contributes to tissue wasting in COPD. *Chest* 1999;115:708–713.

CHAPTER **3**

Alveolar Ventilation, Gas Exchange, Oxygen Delivery, and Acid–Base Physiology

Ronald B. George
Gary T. Kinasewitz

The major function of the respiratory system is to provide gas exchange between the body and the environment. Oxygen is required for energy generation via oxidative phosphorylation, as well as for support of various metabolic processes. Carbon dioxide (CO_2) is produced as the endpoint of the metabolism of ingested food. The body is limited in its ability to store oxygen and CO_2; thus, there must be a continuous exchange of these gases with the environment to prevent hypoxemia and respiratory acidosis.

Gas exchange occurs by passive diffusion across a thin alveolar–capillary membrane, the functional unit of the lungs, which separates pulmonary capillaries from alveolar air spaces. The respiratory muscles bring in fresh air to the alveoli, creating an atmosphere of relatively high oxygen and low CO_2. The heart and pulmonary circulation deliver mixed venous blood from the tissues, which have low oxygen and relatively high CO_2 tensions. The gradients thus produced result in the passive transfer of CO_2 out of the blood and of oxygen into the blood.

One can determine if alveolar–capillary gas exchange is adequate by measuring arterial blood PO_2 and PCO_2; if these gas tensions are normal, the gas exchange apparatus is functioning adequately. However, much more can be learned about gas exchange by using a few simple formulas that allow an estimation of the efficiency of ventilation and perfusion. Information about the delivery of oxygen to the tissues where it is required can be gained by the careful use of additional tests, including the analysis of expired gas and mixed venous blood. This chapter will demonstrate how this information can be used to assess the efficiency of gas exchange in the lungs and oxygen transport from the lungs to the tissues.

NORMAL BLOOD GAS TENSIONS

In normal subjects at sea level, the arterial PCO_2 is 35 to 45 mm Hg and the arterial PO_2 is 80 to 100 mm Hg. Normal arterial pH is 7.35 to 7.45. Average normal gas pressures at sea level for alveoli, arterial blood, and mixed venous blood are shown in Table 3-1. The development of reliable convenient pulse oximetry allows for the noninvasive monitoring of arterial hemoglobin saturation (SaO_2) levels. At a normal arterial PO_2 of 80 mm Hg or above, SaO_2 should be 95% or more. The effect of the oxyhemoglobin dissociation curve on the oxygen content of the blood will be discussed in the section on oxygen transport.

In a resting adult, cardiac output, and thus pulmonary blood flow, is approximately 6 L per minute. Alveolar ventilation is normally about 4.5 L per minute, and the overall *ventilation–perfusion ratio* is approximately 0.8. Normal oxygen consumption

$(\dot{V}O_2)$ is approximately 250 to 300 mL per minute and normal CO_2 production ($\dot{V}CO_2$) is approximately 200 to 250 mL per minute; therefore, the average *respiratory exchange ratio* ($\dot{V}CO_2/\dot{V}O_2$) is also about 0.8. With a normal hemoglobin concentration of 15 g per dL, and a normal ratio of cardiac output to oxygen consumption, the mixed venous blood contains approximately 5 mL per dL less oxygen than the arterial blood under "steady state" conditions.

ALVEOLAR–ARTERIAL OXYGEN GRADIENT

In Table 3-1, note that there is a small difference between alveolar and arterial PO_2 levels. This is the result of the normal anatomic shunts, through which 1% to 3% of mixed venous blood flows directly into the systemic circulation without perfusing the alveolar capillaries. This occurs mainly through the bronchial, mediastinal, and left thebesian veins. In normal young adults, the average alveolar–arterial gradient ($PAO_2 - PaO_2$) is 5 to 10 mm Hg (1). With the normal aging process, there are gradually more and more lung units with uneven ventilation and perfusion. Thus, in a group of normal adults between 61 and 75 years old, Mellemgaard found that the average $PAO_2 - PaO_2$ was 16 mm Hg (1). The gradient may go up as high as 30 mm Hg in normal subjects over age 70.

ALVEOLAR VENTILATION

Of a resting tidal volume of 500 mL, approximately 150 mL (one-third) is required to fill the large airways in which no gas exchange occurs. Because this air is not involved in gas exchange, it is considered wasted and is a part of the *physiologic dead space*. This portion of the "wasted ventilation" is called the *anatomic dead space* and is present in all individuals. It is approximately equal to the body weight in pounds. Thus, at a resting minute ventilation of 7 L, if the tidal volume is 500 mL, the respiratory rate is 14 per minute, and the physiologic dead space is composed of only the conducting airways (150 mL), the effective alveolar ventilation per minute will be 4.9 L. In normal young subjects, the physiologic dead space is similar to the anatomic dead space; however, with aging or in the presence of disease, the physiologic dead space is greatly increased by the presence of underperfused alveoli (*alveolar dead space*).

HYPOVENTILATION

Overall hypoventilation of the lungs causes a decreased flow of inspired air relative to the venous blood perfusing the lungs. This results in a predictable fall in PO_2 and a rise in PCO_2 in alveolar gas and capillary blood. Although arterial PO_2 is dependent on several factors that affect gas exchange, arterial PCO_2 is dependent on the relationship of CO_2 production to alveolar ventilation. Thus, at a given level of CO_2 production ($\dot{V}CO_2$), the volume of alveolar ventilation ($\dot{V}A$) per minute may be calculated by using the *alveolar ventilation equation*:

$$\dot{V}A = \dot{V}CO_2 \times 0.863/PACO_2 \qquad (3.1)$$

$\dot{V}CO_2$ is the CO_2 production per minute and may be measured by collecting an expired gas sample. The factor 0.863 corrects

TABLE 3-1. Normal Gas Tensions in Alveoli and Arterial and Mixed Venous Blood at Sea Level

	Alveoli	*Arterial Blood*	*Mixed Venous Blood*
PO_2	100	95	40
PCO_2	40	40	46
PH_2O	47	47	47
PN_2	573	573	573
P TOTAL	760	755	706

for differences in measurement units and conversion from body temperature to standard temperature (BTPS to STPD). In practice, arterial pressure (P_{aCO_2}) may be substituted for alveolar pressure (P_{ACO_2}) because they are essentially equal.

The alveolar ventilation equation provides a means for relating inflow of fresh air ($\dot{V}_A$) to the rate of CO_2 production $\dot{V}_{CO_2}$. In practice, it is seldom necessary to measure expired CO_2, and for practical purposes, the equation may be simplified to express the inverse relationship between alveolar (and arterial) P_{CO_2} and alveolar ventilation:

$$P_{ACO_2} \approx 1/\dot{V}_A \tag{3.2}$$

The inverse relationship of alveolar and arterial P_{CO_2} to alveolar ventilation is shown in Figure 3-1. With a steady CO_2 output of 200 mL per minute, halving the alveolar ventilation from 5 L per minute to 2.5 L per minute doubles the P_{ACO_2} to 80 mm Hg, and doubling alveolar ventilation to 10 L per minute halves the P_{ACO_2} to 20 mm Hg. From the shape of this curve, it may be evident that relatively small increases in alveolar ventilation are associated with impressive reductions in P_{aCO_2} when the patient is hypercapnic. P_{aCO_2} can also rise quickly when alveolar ventilation changes by only a small amount in this setting. Conversely, in the setting of hypocapnia, relatively large changes are required to decrease P_{aCO_2} further. It is not uncommon to observe large fluctuations in P_{aCO_2} in hypercapnic patients responding to minor changes in ventilation. In response to metabolic acidosis, large increases in ventilation and work of breathing result in only modest changes in acid–base status. Obviously, if $\dot{V}_{CO_2}$ should change owing to increased metabolic activity, as with exercise, a new curve would be derived to the right of the one shown in Figure 3-1.

THE BOHR EQUATION

Although the arterial P_{CO_2} provides a simple method of estimating effective alveolar ventilation, it is also useful in estimating the amount of dead space, or "wasted ventilation." This tells us how efficient a patient's breathing pattern is (i.e., how much of each breath is useful and how much is "wasted"). Figure 3-2 illustrates the variables used in calculating dead space ventilation. Note that *partial pressures* are used rather than *concentrations* of gases. The total minute ventilation ($\dot{V}_E$) and expired carbon dioxide (P_{ECO_2}) are composed of the effective alveolar ventilation ($\dot{V}_A$), which contains alveolar levels of CO_2

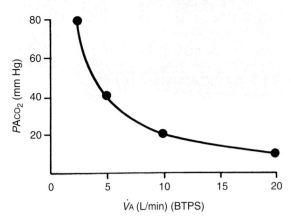

FIGURE 3-1. The relationship of alveolar ventilation ($\dot{V}_A$) to alveolar CO_2 (P_{ACO_2}) at a given CO_2 production ($\dot{V}_{CO_2}$) of 200 mL/minute. Increased CO_2 production, as with exercise, shifts the curve to the right.

(P_{ACO_2}), and the dead space ventilation ($\dot{V}_D$), which contains inspired levels of CO_2 (P_{ICO_2}). This sentence may be written in the form of an equation:

$$\dot{V}_E \times P_{ECO_2} = (\dot{V}_A \times P_{ACO_2}) + (\dot{V}_D \times P_{ICO_2}) \tag{3.3}$$

Rearranging and solving for $\dot{V}_D/\dot{V}_E$ (the portion of $\dot{V}_E$ that is wasted), we have the *Bohr equation*:

$$\dot{V}_D/\dot{V}_E = P_{ACO_2} - P_{ECO_2}/P_{ACO_2} - P_{ICO_2} \tag{3.4}$$

Furthermore, because P_{ICO_2} breathing room air is zero, this factor can be eliminated and arterial CO_2 (P_{aCO_2}) can be substituted for alveolar CO_2 as follows:

$$\dot{V}_D/\dot{V}_E = P_{aCO_2} - P_{ECO_2}/P_{aCO_2} \tag{3.5}$$

Arterial P_{CO_2} can be substituted for alveolar P_{CO_2} because they are assumed to be in complete equilibrium (and therefore identical). The CO_2 dissociation curve is relatively flat in the physiologic range (see Fig. 3-3). Furthermore, the difference between the mixed venous and arterial P_{CO_2} is only about 6 mm Hg, and although venous admixture significantly affects P_{aO_2}, it has relatively little effect on P_{aCO_2}.

If you collect expired gas for a minute or two, mix it, and determine the partial pressure of CO_2, the normal value will be approximately 25 to 30 mm Hg. With a normal arterial P_{CO_2}

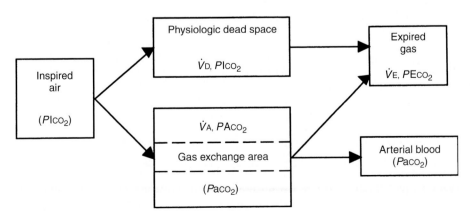

FIGURE 3-2. A gas exchange diagram, showing the variables that are measured for the Bohr equation. P_{ICO_2}, partial pressure of inspired CO_2 (normally zero); P_{ACO_2}, partial pressure of CO_2 in alveolar air (equal to arterial P_{CO_2}); P_{aCO_2}, partial pressure of CO_2 in arterial blood; P_{ECO_2}, partial pressure of CO_2 in expired gas; $\dot{V}_D$, dead space ventilation; $\dot{V}_E$, total minute ventilation; $\dot{V}_A$, effective alveolar ventilation.

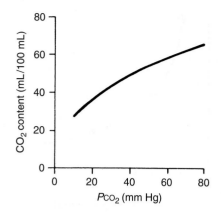

FIGURE 3-3. CO_2 dissociation curve for a subject with a normal level of saturated hemoglobin. The curve shifts to the right with polycythemia and to the left with anemia. Oxygenation shifts the curve to the right and hypoxemia shifts it to the left (Haldane effect).

of 40 and a PE_{CO_2} of 25 mm Hg, the dead space is calculated as follows:

$$\dot{V}_D/\dot{V}_E = 40 - 25/40$$
$$= 15/40$$
$$= 0.37 \text{ or } 37\%$$

In patients with lung disease, the difference between expired P_{CO_2} and arterial P_{CO_2} increases as the physiologic dead space increases. Comparison of expired P_{CO_2} with the arterial P_{CO_2} gives an estimate of the percentage of wasted ventilation (see Eq. 3.5).

THE ALVEOLAR AIR EQUATION

By comparing *arterial* blood gas values with *alveolar* values, one may estimate the impedance to gas transfer across the alveolar capillary membrane. End-expired alveolar gas may be sampled directly; however, the analysis of this expired gas sample includes both functional and nonfunctional alveoli (those that are perfused and those that are not). Although there is variation among alveoli, depending on their relative ventilation and perfusion, the *average* alveolar P_{CO_2} so nearly equals arterial P_{CO_2} that Pa_{CO_2} may substitute for PA_{CO_2} in the alveolar ventilation equation (Eq. 3.1). Thus, $PA_{CO_2} - Pa_{CO_2}$ differences are not sensitive indicators of problems with gas exchange. On the other hand, large differences exist between mean alveolar *oxygen* tension and measured arterial oxygen tension, and the *alveolar–arterial oxygen difference* ($PA_{O_2} - Pa_{O_2}$) is a practical and relatively sensitive test for assessment of gas exchange. Fortunately, mean alveolar oxygen tension can be calculated with reasonable accuracy by using the *simplified alveolar air equation*:

$$PA_{O_2} = \frac{PI_{O_2} - Pa_{CO_2}}{R} \qquad (3.6)$$

where PA_{O_2} is the calculated alveolar P_{O_2}, PI_{O_2} is the partial pressure of inspired oxygen, arterial P_{CO_2} is substituted for alveolar P_{CO_2}, and R is the respiratory exchange ratio.

This is a modification of the actual alveolar air equation. In practice, a respiratory exchange ratio (R) of 0.8 is used in Equation 3.6. Begin and Renzetti have shown that these modifications using an R of 0.8 yield calculated values of PA_{O_2} that are accurate enough for clinical purposes (2). For example, a subject breathing room air at sea level has an arterial P_{CO_2} of 40 and an arterial P_{O_2} of 90. What are his calculated alveolar P_{O_2} and alveolar–arterial oxygen difference?

We must first calculate PA_{O_2}. With the patient breathing room air (21% O_2) at sea level (barometric pressure 760 mm Hg and body temperature 37°C), water vapor pressure is 47 mm Hg. Equation 3.6 becomes

$$PA_{O_2} = 0.21 (760 - 47) - 40/0.8$$
$$= 0.21 (713) - 50$$
$$= 150 - 50$$
$$= 100 \text{ mm Hg}$$

This gives an estimate of the mean alveolar oxygen tension. The difference between alveolar and arterial oxygen tensions can then be calculated by subtracting the measured Pa_{O_2} (90 mm Hg) from the calculated PA_{O_2} (100 mm Hg) to give an alveolar–arterial oxygen difference of 10 mm Hg. The normal $PA_{O_2} - Pa_{O_2}$ in young adults averages about 8 mm Hg, and this increases gradually to a mean of 16 mm Hg in the 61 to 75 age group of healthy adults (1). Values significantly above this level indicate the presence of a lung abnormality causing a defect in gas transfer, and this may be assessed whether or not alveolar hypoventilation is present. The simplified alveolar air equation is extremely useful in clinical practice and should be committed to memory.

GAS TRANSFER (DIFFUSION)

Gas transfer across the alveolar–capillary membrane occurs by passive diffusion, which is related to the partial pressures of oxygen and carbon dioxide in the alveoli and in the pulmonary capillaries. The difference in oxygen and CO_2 tensions across the membrane represents the driving pressure for diffusion of each gas. It is impossible to measure diffusing capacity for oxygen because the capillary tension cannot be measured. In practice, carbon monoxide diffusion (D_{CO}) is measured because the trace amounts of CO inhaled do not increase the P_{CO} in capillary blood. Diffusing capacity for oxygen (D_{O_2}) is about 1.23 times the D_{CO}, or about 40 mL/minute per mm Hg (3). During exercise, D_{O_2} may increase by more than three times through pulmonary capillary recruitment and an increase in capillary blood volume.

In the normal human capillary, equilibrium between alveolar and arterial P_{O_2} occurs in less than 0.25 second. Under normal resting conditions, blood spends about 0.75 second in the capillaries. Because it takes only one-third of this time for equilibration to occur, a wide safety margin exists, and even a large decrease in diffusion fails to affect gas exchange. The D_{CO} must fall to about 10% of the predicted value before any change in arterial oxygen at rest occurs because of an isolated diffusion defect.

The diffusion process may be affected by an abnormal resistance to diffusion, as in a thickened alveolar–capillary membrane; a decrease in the partial pressure gradient for oxygen across the membrane; or a shortened time for equilibration. At least two of these must coexist before arterial oxygen is affected. Thus, diffusion may become a factor in gas exchange during exercise (shortened equilibrium time) in a patient with interstitial fibrosis (thickened membrane) or at high altitude (decreased gradient).

For practical purposes, abnormal diffusion plays only a minor role in the hypoxemia seen in patients with lung diseases. This defect can easily be corrected by small increases in the inspired oxygen.

VENTILATION–PERFUSION RELATIONSHIPS

In the ideal gas exchange unit, ventilation and perfusion are equally matched and gas exchange is optimum. In real life, however, the situation is much more complex, and a *gradation* occurs from well-ventilated but underperfused areas, to equally ventilated and perfused areas, to areas that are well perfused but underventilated. In diseases that affect the lungs, the areas of equal matching are relatively small, and areas of mismatching of ventilation and perfusion are more important.

Using radioactive xenon scans, West demonstrated that normally, in the upright position, blood flow increases progressively from the top to the bottom of the lungs, and blood flow per unit of lung area is increased approximately 10-fold from apex to base (4). Because of the movement of the diaphragm and larger pressure changes with inspiration around the lower lobe, *ventilation* also increases from top to bottom but not as much as perfusion. The bases are ventilated approximately three times as well as the apices. Thus, there is normally a gradient of both ventilation and perfusion from the top to the bottom of the lungs, in the upright position. When lying supine, these gradients occur from the anterior to the posterior portions of the lungs.

Because blood flow increases relatively more from apex to lung base than does ventilation, there is a decreasing *ratio* of ventilation to perfusion on descending from the apex to the base of the lungs. This is illustrated by the O_2–CO_2 diagram in Figure 3-4, which is taken from West monograph. Using the figures from the O_2–CO_2 diagram, West has estimated that in normal resting humans in the upright position, the $\dot{V}/\dot{Q}$ ratio in the lung apices is about 3.3, whereas near the lung bases, it is only about 0.63. For this reason, oxygen tension in the alveoli at the apex is around 130 mm Hg, whereas in those at the lung base, it is only about 90 mm Hg.

Note that according to the principles outlined in the preceding, the majority of the blood flows to the lung bases. Thus, areas at the apices, which are relatively well ventilated and have high $\dot{V}/\dot{Q}$ ratios, are poorly perfused, thus contributing relatively little to the measured Pa_{O_2} in the systemic arterial blood. The gas exchange units near the lung bases, where perfusion is relatively high and $\dot{V}/\dot{Q}$ ratios relatively low, contribute much more to the arterial blood, and because their effects predominate, arterial P_{O_2} primarily reflects areas with relatively low $\dot{V}/\dot{Q}$ relationships. This is a second reason why in normal humans arterial P_{O_2} is slightly less than alveolar P_{O_2}. The remainder of the normal $PA_{O_2} - Pa_{O_2}$ gradient is explained by the normal anatomic shunts discussed in the preceding. Note in Figure 3-4 that the P_{CO_2} also varies normally from lung apices to lung bases. Because of relative hyperventilation, the P_{CO_2} at the top of the lungs is about 30 mm Hg, whereas that at the lung bases is around 40 mm Hg.

The $\dot{V}/\dot{Q}$ mismatching discussed earlier is that which occurs normally in the upright position. Patients with abnormal lungs have much more severe mismatching of ventilation to perfusion. Moreover, at the same horizontal level, a lung lobule may contain terminal respiratory units that are adequately ventilated adjacent to underventilated terminal lung units whose bronchioles are completely occluded. Collateral ventilation may occur from a well-ventilated to a poorly ventilated pulmonary lobule, thus increasing the distance that the air must travel and increasing the dead space. The mismatching of ventilation to perfusion in disease occurs throughout the lungs and is difficult to measure with such gross tests of ventilation and perfusion as lung scans and arteriograms. In clinical practice, the amount of $\dot{V}/\dot{Q}$ mismatch is estimated from the amount of hypoxemia that remains after the effects of hypoventilation and true shunting are removed. The effects of hypoventilation are determined from the arterial P_{CO_2} (Eq. 3.1), and the effects of true shunts are estimated by measuring the Pa_{O_2} while the patient breathes 100% oxygen.

EFFECTS OF BREATHING 100% OXYGEN

The portion of venous admixture caused by true right-to-left shunts can be separated from that caused by poorly ventilated lung units by having the subject breathe 100% oxygen for at least 15 minutes and then calculating the resultant change in shunt fraction (see Eq. 3.9). It is important that the patient take deep breaths during this procedure so that even poorly ventilated alveoli receive oxygen. The principle of this maneuver is that breathing 100% oxygen ultimately replaces the nitrogen in all functional lung units, even those that are poorly ventilated. Thus, the hemoglobin in the perfusing capillaries becomes completely saturated. These poorly ventilated alveoli then function as normal lung units as far as oxygen exchange is concerned. Alveolar oxygen tension is calculated from the alveolar air equation (using a respiratory exchange ratio of 1.0), and from that, capillary oxygen content is estimated. Arterial and mixed venous oxygen tensions are measured and

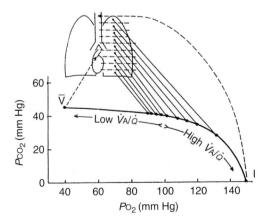

FIGURE 3-4. The O_2–CO_2 diagram showing normal ventilation-perfusion ratios in upright humans, from the top of the lungs to the bottom. The high $\dot{V}/\dot{Q}$ ratio at the apex results in a high P_{O_2} and low P_{CO_2} there. A low P_{O_2} and a high P_{CO_2} are found at the lung base. (Reprinted from West JB. *Ventilation/blood flow and gas exchange*, 4th ed. Oxford: Blackwell Scientific Publications, 1985. With permission from the author and publisher.)

oxygen contents are then calculated. Because defects in gas transfer owing to $\dot{V}/\dot{Q}$ inequality are eliminated by breathing 100% oxygen, the remaining $\dot{Q}s$ is owing solely to true right-to-left shunting. Subtracting the true shunt fraction from the total venous admixture (measured while breathing room air) yields an estimate of the contribution of $\dot{V}/\dot{Q}$ mismatching to arterial hypoxemia.

It should be noted that the alveolar–arterial oxygen tension difference normally increases as the F_{IO_2} is increased because the effects of poorly oxygenated blood from the normal right-to-left shunts on the PaO_2 become more pronounced. It is also common for the breathing of pure oxygen to cause absorption atelectasis. This phenomenon occurs when nitrogen from poorly ventilated alveoli is replaced by oxygen, which is subsequently absorbed into the pulmonary capillary blood.

OXYGEN TRANSPORT

The pulmonary venous blood leaves the pulmonary capillaries, after equilibration with the alveolar gases, as arterial or oxygenated blood. It goes to the left atrium and ventricle, and from there to the systemic arteries. Arterial blood gas levels reflect the ability of the lungs to oxygenate the blood and remove excess CO_2. The oxygenated blood is distributed to the tissues via the systemic arteries and capillaries.

CARDIAC OUTPUT

The cardiac output is the total amount of blood leaving the heart and going to the tissues. The normal resting cardiac output in an adult is about 6 L per minute. The cardiac output may be measured by several techniques, including thermodilution using a pulmonary artery catheter; dye dilution using pulmonary and systemic arterial catheters; or Doppler flow analysis. Cardiac output can be calculated using the Fick principle. The Fick principle states simply that the rate at which oxygen enters the blood during its passage through the lungs is a product of the blood flow and the difference between the oxygen content in the mixed venous blood and that of the arterial blood:

$$\dot{V}O_2 = \dot{Q}t (CaO_2 - C\bar{v}O_2) \quad (3.7)$$

where $\dot{Q}t$ is the total blood flow from the right ventricle (i.e., the cardiac output). Solving for $\dot{Q}t$, we can rewrite this equation as follows:

$$\dot{Q}t = \dot{V}O_2 / CaO_2 - C\bar{v}O_2 \quad (3.8)$$

OXYGEN CONTENT AND THE OXYHEMOGLOBIN DISSOCIATION CURVE

It should be emphasized that we are now dealing with oxygen *content* in arterial and mixed venous blood rather than with oxygen *tension*, and thus blood hemoglobin levels and the shape of the oxyhemoglobin dissociation curve must be considered. Because hemoglobin is the major oxygen carrier in the blood and because of the sigmoid shape of the oxyhemoglobin dissociation curve, we must calculate oxygen content from PaO_2 using the dissociation curve and measured levels of hemoglobin.

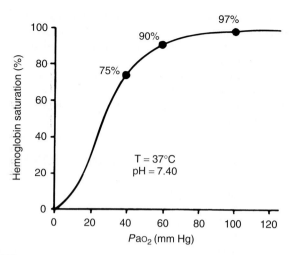

FIGURE 3-5. The normal oxyhemoglobin dissociation curve at pH 7.4 and temperature 37°C. Saturations at three key points are marked. Hyperthermia shifts the curve to the right and hypothermia shifts it to the left. Acidemia shifts it to the right and alkalemia to the left (Bohr effect).

At this point, it is reasonable to review the oxyhemoglobin dissociation curve. A few numbers are worth keeping in mind (see Fig. 3-5). At a normal pH of 7.4 and a normal PaO_2 of 100 mm Hg, the hemoglobin is approximately 97% saturated. At the shoulder of the oxyhemoglobin dissociation curve, with a PaO_2 of 60 and pH of 7.4, the hemoglobin is about 90% saturated. From here, saturation drops quickly, and at a PaO_2 of 40 (the normal mixed venous oxygen tension), the hemoglobin is only about 75% saturated.

The vast majority of the oxygen contained in blood is carried on the hemoglobin molecule. One gram of hemoglobin fully saturated carries 1.39 mL/g of oxygen (5). For example, with a hemoglobin content of 15 g per dL and a saturation of 97%, the oxygen content of arterial blood that is attached to hemoglobin is

$$15 \text{ g/dL} \times 0.97 \times 1.39 \text{ mL/g} = 19.5 \text{ mL/dL}$$

In addition to the oxygen attached to hemoglobin, a small quantity is dissolved in arterial plasma, according to the solubility of oxygen in plasma (0.003 mL per dL per mm Hg PO_2) At a normal PaO_2 of 100 mm Hg, the dissolved content is

$$100 \times 0.003 = 0.3 \text{ mL/dL}$$

The oxygen content of arterial blood for the normal patient in this example would be 19.8 (or about 20) mL per dL. In the normal range of PaO_2, the amount of dissolved oxygen is relatively minute and can be ignored; however, in situations where the F_{IO_2} is high, the amount of dissolved oxygen may become significant.

The blood normally loses about 25% of its oxygen content as it passes through the tissues. With a hemoglobin content of 15 g per dL, the arterial blood carries about 20 mL of oxygen per dL. With a normal $P\bar{v}O_2$ of 40 mm Hg and a mixed venous saturation of 75%, this same blood carries 15 mL of oxygen per dL. Thus, the normal *a-v̄ oxygen difference* is 5 mL per dL, and this difference may increase as tissue demands increase in relation to oxygen delivery. With an increase in metabolic demand, the a-$\bar{v}$ oxygen difference increases at the same time the cardiac output increases, thus increasing oxygen delivery simultaneously by two mechanisms.

If cardiac output is insufficient to meet the body's needs, there is a drop in the $P\bar{v}_{O_2}$, because more oxygen must be extracted from the same amount of hemoglobin. In certain situations (e.g., sepsis syndrome), mixed venous oxygen content may increase in the face of low oxygen delivery, owing to inability of the tissues to utilize oxygen adequately. Thus, the measurement of mixed venous oxygen (saturation or tension) by indwelling catheters must be interpreted with caution in patients with gas exchange problems. In general, serial measurements are more useful for comparison than are single measurements.

THE SHUNT EQUATION

Although calculation of the alveolar–arterial oxygen gradient ($PA_{O_2} - Pa_{O_2}$) yields an assessment of gas transfer and therefore tells us whether there is wasted perfusion, the actual *percent* of the cardiac output that is shunted through the lungs and unavailable for gas transport may be estimated by using the *shunt equation*

$$\frac{\dot{Q}s}{\dot{Q}t} = \frac{Cc'_{O_2} - Ca_{O_2}}{Cc'_{O_2} - C\bar{v}_{O_2}} \qquad (3.9)$$

where $\dot{Q}s/\dot{Q}t$ is the shunt fraction or venous admixture and Cc'_{O_2}, Ca_{O_2}, and $C\bar{v}_{O_2}$ are the oxygen contents of end-capillary, arterial, and mixed venous blood, respectively. The Cc'_{O_2} is estimated by assuming that end-capillary P_{O_2} is the same as PA_{O_2} (calculated from the alveolar air equation). Ca_{O_2} is calculated from the measured arterial P_{O_2} and the oxyhemoglobin dissociation curve. The $C\bar{v}_{O_2}$ may be estimated by assuming a normal a-$\bar{v}$ oxygen content difference of 5 mL per dL. This estimate of $C\bar{v}_{O_2}$ is not valid unless the cardiac output is adequate and stable, and tissue utilization is intact. If left ventricular function fails to meet the oxygen needs of the tissues, the a-$\bar{v}$ difference is widened; conversely, if tissue utilization is impaired, the a-$\bar{v}$ difference may be narrowed.

At a normal PA_{O_2} of 100 mm Hg and a hemoglobin of 15 g, the hemoglobin is 97% saturated and Cc'_{O_2} is 19.5 mL per dL. If the measured Pa_{O_2} is 80 mm Hg, the hemoglobin is 96% saturated and the Ca_{O_2} is 19.3 mL per dL. Assuming a normal cardiac output, and therefore an a-$\bar{v}$ oxygen content difference of 5 mL per dL, we can calculate the shunt fraction as follows:

$$\begin{aligned}
\frac{\dot{Q}s}{\dot{Q}t} &= \frac{Cc'_{O_2} - Ca_{O_2}}{Cc'_{O_2} - C\bar{v}_{O_2}} \\
&= \frac{19.5 - 19.3}{19.5 - 14.5} \qquad (3.10) \\
&= \frac{0.2}{5.0} = 0.04 \text{ or } 4\%
\end{aligned}$$

This relatively small percentage of the cardiac output that represents the normal shunting of blood in healthy people is made up of two components: blood that is perfusing relatively underventilated alveoli, and true shunts that perfuse areas that are not ventilated at all.

ARTERIAL HYPOXEMIA

The potential causes of arterial hypoxemia are listed in Table 3-2. In patients who are seen for evaluation of lung disease, arterial hypoxemia is usually the result of an increase in mismatching of ventilation to perfusion, and the causes of hypoxemia not related to $\dot{V}/\dot{Q}$ mismatch (low inspired oxygen concentration, alveolar hypoventilation, diffusion defect, and low $P\bar{v}_{O_2}$) are usually readily identifiable. This discussion addresses the differential diagnosis of arterial hypoxemia using a few simple observations and calculations to differentiate among the causes listed in Table 3-2. However, it should be noted that several causes often coexist in the same patient. For instance, the patient who is admitted with an acute exacerbation of COPD may have a combination of alveolar hypoventilation and a defect in gas transfer owing to mismatching of ventilation to perfusion. The relative contribution to the arterial hypoxemia should be determined for each of the factors when possible, as the various causes are treated differently and respond differently to an increase in inspired oxygen.

LOW INSPIRED OXYGEN CONCENTRATION

A review of the simplified alveolar air equation emphasizes the importance of F_{IO_2} and barometric pressure on the partial pressure of alveolar oxygen. In the example given in the preceding, the barometric pressure at sea level (760 mm Hg) was used; however, people frequently live at higher altitudes and are able to adapt quite well to living at altitudes as high as 2500 m (8200 ft). Nearly 30 million people live at altitudes even higher, in the Rocky Mountains of North America, the Andes of South America, the Himalayas of Asia, and elsewhere (6). At 8000 ft, barometric pressure is approximately 565 mm Hg, the inspired P_{O_2} is about 120 mm Hg, and the alveolar oxygen is approximately 80 mm Hg. In subjects with normal lungs, the Pa_{O_2} remains high enough to achieve nearly complete hemoglobin saturation so that oxygen content is not severely affected.

In people living at altitudes above 8000 ft, compensation occurs with increased hemoglobin levels and a shift in the oxygen–hemoglobin dissociation curve to the right so that oxygen is unloaded more efficiently to the tissues. Cardiac output increases in response to hypoxemia; however, this decrease in red cell transit time through the pulmonary capillaries in addition to a decrease in mixed venous P_{O_2} tends to emphasize existing $\dot{V}/\dot{Q}$ inequalities. Furthermore, pulmonary hypertension occurs at very high altitudes, and this is associated with an alteration in ventilation–perfusion relationships, which may result in further arterial hemoglobin desaturation. For a further discussion of altitude physiology and adaptation to high altitudes, the reader is referred to the work of West et al. (7).

TABLE 3-2. Potential Causes of Arterial Hypoxemia

Low F_{IO_2}
Hypoventilation
Diffusion defect
Ventilation–perfusion mismatch
Right-to-left shunt
Low mixed venous oxygen tension

Patients undergoing mechanical ventilation because of diffuse lung disease with severe defects in gas exchange (e.g., pneumonia, pulmonary edema, adult respiratory distress syndrome) may suffer rapid worsening of hypoxemia if the delivered FIO_2 falls because of ventilator malfunction or manipulation of the ventilator controls. Such patients are often maintained at the lowest FIO_2 that results in nearly complete saturation of the arterial hemoglobin. At levels of PaO_2 below 60 mm Hg, a small decrease in FIO_2 results in a severe decline in SaO_2 and arterial oxygen content, owing to the steep slope of the oxyhemoglobin dissociation curve. Constant monitoring of SaO_2 with pulse oximetry alerts the clinician to such sudden and potentially dangerous decreases in oxygen content.

HYPOVENTILATION

As noted in the preceding section, alveolar PCO_2 is inversely related to alveolar ventilation; thus, if alveolar ventilation is halved, alveolar and arterial PCO_2 values double. The hallmark of alveolar hypoventilation is an increase in $PaCO_2$. Alveolar hypoventilation decreases alveolar PO_2 because as CO_2 accumulates in the alveoli it displaces oxygen; therefore, the displaced oxygen is not available for gas exchange. If the arterial PCO_2 is normal or low, hypoxemia cannot be explained by alveolar hypoventilation.

In normal patients, alveolar ventilation ($\dot{V}A$) is a fixed proportion of minute ventilation ($\dot{V}E$) because dead space ventilation is limited mainly to the anatomic dead space (conducting airways). Thus, we can consider the $\dot{V}E$ and $PaCO_2$ to be inversely proportional (Eq. 3.2). In patients with respiratory problems, the ventilatory pattern may change so that breathing becomes rapid and shallow; thus, a greater part of each breath is composed of dead space ventilation. In such patients, $\dot{V}A$ may decrease and $PaCO_2$ may rise without a change in measured minute ventilation ($\dot{V}E$). A change to slow, deep breaths results in a decrease of $PaCO_2$ without a change in $\dot{V}E$. In patients with chronic lung disease, minute ventilation may be increased, although $PaCO_2$ is elevated, because of an increase in the alveolar dead space and $\dot{V}/\dot{Q}$ mismatching.

Hypoventilation causes hypoxemia owing to its effects on the alveolar PO_2, a relationship described in the *alveolar air equation* (Eq. 3.6). Any rise in $PaCO_2$ causes a drop in the alveolar and thus the arterial PO_2. Thus, with moderate degrees of alveolar hypoventilation, the $PAO_2 - PaO_2$ remains normal. It has been shown that marked hypercapnia reduces the increased $PAO_2 - PaO_2$ that might otherwise exist because of abnormalities in gas exchange (8).

In patients who are hypoxemic and retaining CO_2, the relative contribution to the hypoxemia of alveolar hypoventilation can be determined by calculating $PAO_2 - PaO_2$. If this is normal, one can assume that the observed hypoxemia can be corrected by achieving adequate alveolar ventilation. If, however, the $PAO_2 - PaO_2$ is elevated, there is a defect in gas transfer (usually a $\dot{V}/\dot{Q}$ mismatch) in addition to the hypoventilation. In comatose patients who have no associated lung disease, the $PAO_2 - PaO_2$ is within normal limits and the hypoxemia can be corrected completely with adequate ventilation. If, however, the $PAO_2 - PaO_2$ is elevated in the presence of a high $PaCO_2$, there is an additional defect in gas transfer, and an increased FIO_2 or the addition of positive end-expiratory pressure (PEEP) may be necessary.

DIFFUSION DEFECT

A defect in gas transfer because of diffusion limitation does not occur in normal humans at sea level because even at high cardiac outputs, the blood remains in the capillaries long enough for adequate equilibrium. However, during exercise at high altitudes, the driving pressure (PAO_2) of oxygen in the alveoli may be low enough and the transit time of blood in the capillaries so short that a limitation of diffusion of oxygen into the blood may become a factor in the development of hypoxemia (9). As noted, three factors may decrease oxygen diffusion and cause hypoxemia: (a) a defect in the lung diffusion capacity of oxygen, (b) a decrease in the oxygen gradient between alveoli and capillary blood, and (c) a decrease in equilibration time. Two or more of these abnormalities must occur for diffusion defects to become a factor in hypoxemia; however, defects in diffusion may play a minor role in patients with other problems. Diffusion defects are easily corrected by increasing the FIO_2.

VENTILATION–PERFUSION MISMATCH

Ventilation–perfusion mismatching is the most common cause of hypoxemia in patients with lung disease. Marked $\dot{V}/\dot{Q}$ mismatching is manifested by hypoxemia in the presence of a normal, low, or high $PaCO_2$. By definition, wasted ventilation ($\dot{V}D/\dot{V}T$) and wasted perfusion ($\dot{Q}s/\dot{Q}t$) are both increased. Measurement of $\dot{V}D/\dot{V}T$ yields an estimate of the amount of wasted ventilation, whereas calculating the shunt fraction indicates the amount of wasted perfusion.

The $PAO_2 - PaO_2$ is a useful index of the degree of $\dot{V}/\dot{Q}$ inequality in the lungs. Because the distribution of lung abnormalities is not uniform in the presence of disease, various units of the lungs are affected to different degrees. Thus, some areas have relatively high $\dot{V}/\dot{Q}$ ratios and others relatively low ratios. Arterial blood reflects areas with relatively high blood flow, and thus areas with relatively low $\dot{V}/\dot{Q}$ ratios. The majority of diffuse lung diseases, including those affecting the airways (e.g., chronic bronchitis and asthma) and those affecting the alveoli (e.g., emphysema and interstitial fibrosis), all result in increased $PAO_2 - PaO_2$ owing to $\dot{V}/\dot{Q}$ mismatching. Furthermore, therapeutic measures (e.g., administration of bronchodilators) may actually hinder the physiologic attenuation of perfusion to areas of localized hypoventilation, resulting in more severe shunting and a further drop in $PAO_2 - PaO_2$ (10).

The greater the degree of $\dot{V}/\dot{Q}$ inequality present, the higher the $\dot{V}E$ must be to maintain a normal or reduced $PaCO_2$. An elevated $\dot{V}E$ with a normal $PaCO_2$ is evidence for the presence of a $\dot{V}/\dot{Q}$ abnormality. This is due to an increase in the dead space ventilation. The overventilation of normal lung units required to compensate for low $\dot{V}/\dot{Q}$ units results in an increased gradient between the expired PCO_2 and the $PaCO_2$, and thus an increase in the $\dot{V}D/\dot{V}T$.

At some point, the work of increasing $\dot{V}E$ becomes too great to sustain, and any further increase in $\dot{V}/\dot{Q}$ mismatch results in a rise in $PaCO_2$. This may be slow (e.g., COPD) or rapid (e.g., acute asthma attacks). The respiratory center and the respiratory muscles determine the point at which $PaCO_2$ begins to rise. The increased $PaCO_2$ that occurs is a method of boosting the efficiency of a compromised ventilatory system. The higher the concentration of CO_2 in the alveolar gas, and thus in each expired breath, the lower the $\dot{V}E$ required to remove a specific amount of CO_2. The effect of the rise in $PaCO_2$ on blood pH and central nervous system function limits the extent of this compensatory mechanism. However, with renal compensation, chronic elevations of $PaCO_2$ are well tolerated.

During acute hypercapnic exacerbations of COPD, oxygen therapy almost always leads to a further rise in the $PaCO_2$. Although this has been thought to be caused by further depression of the respiratory drive, Aubier et al. showed that $PaCO_2$ may rise without a significant reduction in $\dot{V}E$ (11). Other investigators have disputed their findings; at any rate, other factors seem to be active in causing the further rise in $PaCO_2$ associated with oxygen administration. There is a further increase in $\dot{V}/\dot{Q}$ mismatching owing to vasodilation and increased perfusion of poorly ventilated lung units; and the hemoglobin affinity for CO_2 is reduced as oxygen saturation increases (Haldane effect). Because the increase in $PaCO_2$ is not entirely due to respiratory center depression, progressively worsening hypercapnia is not inevitable.

A moderate increase in $PaCO_2$ without mental changes requires no intervention. If hypercapnia progresses and CO_2 narcosis ensues, mechanical ventilation may be required. A common practice is to decrease the FIO_2 slightly to "stimulate the respiratory center." This is a mistake because it may result in severe hypoxemia. Progressive hypercapnia rarely kills a patient; severe hypoxemia often does. A reasonable approach is to increase the FIO_2 in small increments while monitoring with a pulse oximeter, using only the FIO_2 necessary to achieve a hemoglobin saturation of about 90%.

RIGHT-TO-LEFT SHUNT

The other potential cause of arterial hypoxemia is a true right-to-left shunt. Shunting may occur in conjunction with $\dot{V}/\dot{Q}$ mismatching or hypoventilation, in which case it adds to the severity of the hypoxemia. The contribution of shunting in patients with arterial hypoxemia may be assessed by calculating the shunt fraction with the patient breathing 100% oxygen, as outlined earlier. The $\dot{Q}s/\dot{Q}t$ that remains after breathing oxygen (correcting that portion caused by $\dot{V}/\dot{Q}$ mismatching) is the percentage of the cardiac output actually shunted through unventilated areas.

When breathing mixtures high in oxygen, the amount of oxygen dissolved in the plasma must be included in the estimation of $Cc'O_2$, CaO_2, and $C\bar{v}O_2$. This is calculated by multiplying the PaO_2 by the solubility coefficient of oxygen in plasma at body temperature, which is 0.003 mL/dL/mm Hg. On breathing 100% oxygen at sea level, about 2 mL oxygen is dissolved in each 100 mL plasma. It should also be noted that the calculation of $PAO_2 - PaO_2$ while breathing 100% oxygen does not require the usual correction for R because only oxygen and carbon dioxide are left in the alveoli, the nitrogen having been washed out.

Acute lung injuries, such as the adult respiratory distress syndrome (ARDS), cause severe hypoxemia mostly as a result of shunting. Serial changes in gas transfer cannot be determined using the $PAO_2 - PaO_2$ gradient because the increased FIO_2 required to treat the hypoxemia is associated with a variable effect on the calculated gradient. An estimate of serial changes in gas transfer can be obtained by comparing the ratio of PaO_2 to the FIO_2 (12). A PaO_2/FIO_2 of 250 or greater is indicative of a relatively mild defect in gas transfer in patients with ARDS; a ratio of 100 or less is a grave prognostic sign, indicating severe lung damage.

LOW MIXED VENOUS OXYGEN TENSION

A reduction in $P\bar{v}O_2$ may result in worsening arterial hypoxemia in patients with $\dot{V}/\dot{Q}$ mismatching, right-to-left shunts, or low hemoglobin levels (13). The drop in $P\bar{v}O_2$ may result from a decrease in cardiac output or from an increase in oxygen uptake by the tissues. The lower $P\bar{v}O_2$ increases the effects of right-to-left shunts on arterial PO_2 (depending on the intensity of hypoxemic vasoconstriction), further limiting oxygen delivery. In patients with limited cardiac output who require mechanical ventilation, factors such as fever, anxiety, and increased work of breathing may be corrected by measures such as lowering the temperature, administering sedation, or adjusting the ventilator. Decreasing oxygen uptake then results in an increased $P\bar{v}O_2$ (assuming oxygen delivery is unchanged); this in turn increases arterial oxygen.

SYSTEMIC OXYGEN DELIVERY

In a normal adult, approximately 300 mL of oxygen is used per minute at rest. During exercise, oxygen delivery is related linearly to oxygen uptake. The amount of oxygen delivered to the tissues per minute can be calculated by multiplying the arterial blood oxygen content (CaO_2) in mL per dL by the cardiac output ($\dot{Q}$) in L per minute. The arterial oxygen content depends on the concentration of functional hemoglobin in arterial blood and the saturation of that hemoglobin with oxygen. The saturation of hemoglobin is dependent on the partial pressure of oxygen in the arterial blood. Thus, systemic oxygen delivery depends on the interaction of the *circulatory system* (delivery of arterial blood), *erythropoietic system* (hemoglobin in red blood cells), and *respiratory system* (gas exchange area) according to the following equation:

$$\text{Systemic oxygen transport (mL/minute)}$$
$$= \dot{Q} \text{ (L/minute)} \times CaO_2 \text{ (mL/L)}$$
$$= \dot{Q} \times \text{(g hemoglobin} \times 1.39) \times SaO_2 \quad (3.11)$$
$$\underset{\text{system}}{\text{circulatory}} \quad \underset{\text{system}}{\text{erythropoietic}} \quad \underset{\text{system}}{\text{respiratory}}$$

where $\dot{Q}$ is the cardiac output and SaO_2 is the percent saturation of the hemoglobin. The respiratory system provides the oxygen tension in the pulmonary capillaries, which in turn determines hemoglobin saturation. The preceding equation does not include the (normally inconsequential) volume of oxygen that is dissolved in the blood.

THE CIRCULATORY SYSTEM

With a normal resting cardiac output ($\dot{Q}$) of about 6 L per minute, because each 100 mL of arterial blood contains about 20 mL oxygen, the total amount of oxygen delivered per minute to the tissues at rest is about 1200 mL. The cells use only about 300 mL of this oxygen, which means that about 900 mL remains in the mixed venous blood. The percent of oxygen remaining in the mixed venous blood represents the *average* extraction of oxygen from blood by all the tissues. It is important to understand that although the average oxygen extraction is about 25% of the oxygen present in the arterial blood, oxygen use differs markedly from one organ system to another. For instance, the heart uses essentially all the oxygen it receives, whereas the kidneys use only a small percentage. It is physiologically appropriate to have a surplus of oxygen available in case sudden changes in availability or use occur. Thus, the oxygen remaining in the mixed venous blood represents a reservoir for the tissues to call on should the normal adjustments to demand be temporarily inadequate.

The oxygen extracted from the blood during its passage through the tissues determines the *arterial-mixed venous difference* in oxygen tension ($PaO_2 - P\bar{v}O_2$). The $P\bar{v}O_2$ is normally about 40 mm Hg, so that with a normal arterial PO_2 of 90 mm Hg and an adequate delivery of blood to the tissues, the a-$\bar{v}$ oxygen difference is about 50 mm Hg. A fall in mixed venous PO_2 with an increase in the a-$\bar{v}$ oxygen tension difference occurs during exercise, and whenever the oxygen delivery system is stressed. When an abnormal a-$\bar{v}$ difference occurs in the absence of normal stress mechanisms, it is evidence for failure of the circulatory system (14–16).

THE ERYTHROPOIETIC SYSTEM

Each 100 mL of blood normally contains about 15 g of hemoglobin. It is this hemoglobin content that allows for the remarkable oxygen-carrying ability of the blood, normally about 20 mL per dL. This is possible because 1 g of hemoglobin when fully saturated carries 1.39 mL of oxygen. At a normal PaO_2 of more than 80 mm Hg, the hemoglobin molecule is almost completely saturated, whereas at a mixed venous PO_2 of 40 mm Hg, the hemoglobin is only about 75% saturated. The ability of hemoglobin to bind oxygen at normal values of arterial PO_2 and to give it up at lower values of PO_2 is described by the oxyhemoglobin dissociation curve (Fig. 3-5).

To calculate arterial oxygen content, the percent saturation of the hemoglobin (SaO_2) must be determined. The SaO_2 may be estimated from the oxyhemoglobin dissociation curve, provided the PaO_2 and pH are known and the hemoglobin is normal. This is the procedure used in most blood gas laboratories, where SaO_2 is calculated rather than measured. Alternatively, SaO_2 may be measured by using a cooximeter for *in vitro* measurement or a pulse oximeter for *in vivo* measurement. Actual measurement is necessary if the shape or position of the oxyhemoglobin dissociation curve is abnormal because of changes in the hemoglobin molecule.

Normally, the relationship of SaO_2 to PO_2 is not static but changes with differing conditions, usually to the benefit of the individual. A decrease in blood pH is associated with a shift in the curve toward the right, as shown in Figure 3-6; thus, at the higher pH levels found in the lungs, oxygen is bound more easily, whereas at lower pH levels found in the tissues, oxygen is freed more easily (the Bohr effect). Lower temperatures shift the curve to the left, whereas higher temperatures shift the curve to the right.

The binding capacity for oxygen is also affected by an increase or decrease in the 2,3-diphosphoglycerate (2,3-DPG) content of the red cells. Because the 2,3-DPG competes with oxygen for sites on the hemoglobin molecule, increased levels of 2,3-DPG shift the curve to the right and allow for improved

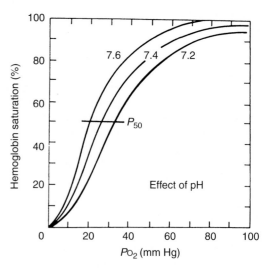

FIGURE 3-6.   The oxyhemoglobin dissociation curve. The effects of shifts in pH on the affinity of hemoglobin for oxygen (the Bohr effect) are shown. Acidosis shifts the curve toward the right and thus increases oxygen delivery at the tissue level. The affinity of hemoglobin for oxygen is expressed as the P_{50} (the PAO_2 at which the hemoglobin is 50% saturated).

oxygen delivery. Carbon monoxide (CO) binds extremely readily with hemoglobin to form carboxyhemoglobin. This decreases the ability of the hemoglobin to carry oxygen. Some inherited abnormal types of hemoglobin are associated with marked changes in the oxyhemoglobin dissociation curve, with either an increased or a decreased affinity of hemoglobin for oxygen.

Although almost all the oxygen in arterial blood is carried on the hemoglobin molecule, a small amount is also carried in the plasma as dissolved oxygen. Because the solubility of oxygen in plasma is very low, this portion of the oxygen content is insignificant except in unusual situations, such as in the breathing of high concentrations of oxygen. In patients with carbon monoxide poisoning, CO replaces oxygen on the hemoglobin molecule because its affinity for hemoglobin is greater, producing tissue hypoxia in the presence of a normal hemoglobin level and a normal PaO_2. In such cases, ventilation with high-oxygen mixtures may prevent hypoxic tissue damage and will augment the elimination of CO.

The affinity of hemoglobin for oxygen and its ability to give up oxygen at the tissue level are commonly assessed by calculating the P_{50}, the partial pressure of oxygen at which the hemoglobin is 50% saturated. The P_{50} can be calculated by equilibrating the patient's blood in a tonometer at various PO_2 levels and then measuring the saturation of the hemoglobin and plotting a dissociation curve. The normal P_{50} of human blood is about 26 mm Hg, with a fairly large variability around this level in the presence of disease. The P_{50} may be estimated from a random venous blood sample according to a formula proposed by Lichtman et al. (17). In a group of 38 healthy subjects, the mean P_{50} calculated by using their technique was 26 ± 1.3 mm Hg. It is important to note that most values of SaO_2 reported from the blood gas laboratory are calculated from a nomogram that assumes a normal hemoglobin dissociation curve. For estimation of P_{50}, saturation of the hemoglobin must be measured directly, for obvious reasons.

THE RESPIRATORY SYSTEM

The respiratory system is assessed by measurement of Pao_2 while breathing room air. If the arterial blood is not adequately oxygenated, there is a defect in gas transfer at the pulmonary capillary level. This may be due to precapillary shunting within the lungs, to mismatching of ventilation with perfusion in the gas transfer units of the lungs, or to hypoventilation. Frequently, several of these factors are abnormal in the same patient. Factors outside the lungs can also affect Pao_2. These include extrapulmonary right-to-left shunts, in which case blood never gets to the lungs to be oxygenated, and a decrease in mixed venous Po_2.

Inadequate oxygen delivery affects arterial oxygen content by decreasing the mixed venous Po_2. In patients with intrapulmonary shunts, because the mixed venous blood is added directly to the arterial blood, there is a dramatic fall in Pao_2 secondary to the decrease in $P\bar{v}o_2$ (13). Thus, when the Pao_2 deteriorates in a patient with multiple organ system failure, factors other than those directly related to abnormal gas exchange in the lungs must be considered.

NORMAL ACID–BASE BALANCE

Healthy individuals have a normal $[H^+]$ that is maintained within a narrow range between 36 and 44 nanoequivalents per liter (see Table 3-3). Clinically, the hydrogen ion activity of a fluid is expressed as its pH, that is, the negative log (base 10) of the $[H^+]$. The normal pH of arterial blood is 7.40 (range 7.36–7.44). Because pH is the negative log of the hydrogen ion activity, there is an inverse relationship between pH and $[H^+]$ (see Fig. 3-7), that is, an increasing $[H^+]$ is reflected by a fall in the pH. When the pH of arterial blood falls below 7.36 ($[H^+]$ >44 nEq per L), the patient is *acidemic*, whereas if the pH is greater than 7.44 ($[H^+]$ <36 nEq per L), the patient is *alkalemic*. The terms acidemic and alkalemic refer to the actual pH of the blood, whereas *acidosis* and *alkalosis* refer to the processes that respectively cause acid and alkali to accumulate.

Despite the curvilinear inverse relationship between pH and $[H^+]$ depicted in Figure 3-7, a relatively accurate estimate

TABLE 3-3. Normal Laboratory Values for Acid–Base Measurements

Measurement	Normal Value	Normal Range
pH	7.40	7.36–7.44
$[H^+]$	40 n Eq/L	36–44 nEq/L
Pco_2 (arterial blood)	40 mmHg	36–44 mmHg
Serum HCO_3^-	24 mEq/L	22–26 mEq/L
Total CO_2	26 mEq/L	24–28 mEq/L

of the $[H^+]$ between pH 7.2 and 7.5 can be obtained if one estimates the change in $[H^+]$ as 1 nEq per L for each 0.01 unit change in pH (18). By this method, when there is decrease in pH of 0.10 units, one would estimate the increase in $[H^+]$ as 10 nEq per L. If the initial $[H^+]$ was 40 nEq per L, the new $[H^+]$ would be 40 + 10 = 50 nEq per L. At more extreme deviations from the normal range, this "one for one" relationship does not hold. When the pH is above this range, the last two digits of total increment in pH above 7.40 is multiplied by 0.7 to yield the fall in $[H^+]$, whereas for pH below this range, the total decrement in pH is multiplied by 1.3 to indicate the magnitude of the increase in $[H^+]$. Thus, by this method, an increment in pH to 7.60 would correspond to a fall in $[H^+]$ of 14 nEq per L, whereas a decrease in pH to 7.10 would correspond to an increase in $[H^+]$ of 39 nEq per L. The accuracy of this method of estimating $[H^+]$ is illustrated in Figure 3-7.

The $[H^+]$ of plasma and the extracellular fluid is normally maintained within a narrow range by the buffering systems of the body. An acid is a substance that surrenders H^+ ion in solution, whereas a base is a substance that accepts it. This relationship may be expressed as

$$Acid \leftrightarrows Base + H^+ \qquad (3.12)$$

When additional hydrogen ions are generated, they combine with the base and drive the above reaction to the left, whereas when there is a lack of hydrogen ions, the reaction moves to the right. A buffer may be thought of as an acid–base pair that can either absorb or donate hydrogen ions when

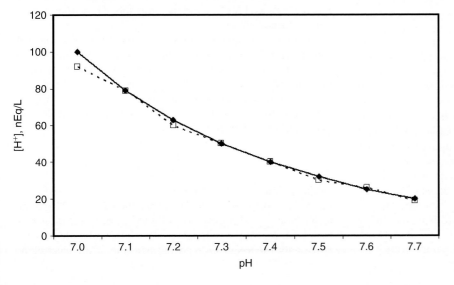

FIGURE 3-7. Inverse relationship between pH and hydrogen ion concentration, $[H^+]$. Solid line and closed diamonds indicate actual $[H^+]$; dashed line and open squares indicate the value estimated by the method described in the text.

there is a rise or fall in the $[H^+]$ of a solution, thereby blunting (but not entirely preventing) the swings in pH that would otherwise ensue. Strong acids by definition are almost completely dissociated at a physiologic pH and therefore are poor buffers. The strength of an acid (its inherent tendency to ionize) is described by its ionization constant. The stronger an acid, the higher its ionization constant or, in keeping with the concept of pH, the lower will be its pK (which is defined as the negative log [base 10] of the ionization constant). The most effective *in vivo* buffers are those weak acids that have pKs close to the physiologic pH. $H_2CO_3, H_2PO_4^-$ and many of the plasma proteins such as hemoglobin that have pKs between 6.0 and 7.0 are important buffer systems.

The importance of plasma proteins and other nonvolatile weak acids such as phosphate in determining the pH has been clearly illustrated by the physical–chemical approach to acid–base analysis described by Stewart (19). He demonstrated how the $[H^+]$ is determined by the P_{CO_2}, nonvolatile weak acids, and strong ion difference. The latter is the difference between these cations ($Na^+ + K^+ + Ca^{2+} + Mg^{2+}$) and anions ($Cl^-$) that are completely dissociated in plasma. This approach is applicable to patients with complex acid–base disturbances but its complexity requires a computer for analysis (20). A simpler approach that can be utilized at the bedside is presented in the following equation.

The isohydric principle states that all buffer pairs in a homogeneous system are in equilibrium with the same $[H^+]$, that is,

$$[H+] = K1 \frac{[Acid1]}{[Base1]} = K2 \frac{[Acid2]}{[Base2]} \qquad (3.13)$$

It should be apparent that this relationship allows the clinician to analyze disturbances in acid–base equilibrium by measuring the components of any one of the body's buffering systems. The buffer pair that is most commonly measured to determine a patient's acid–base status is the H_2CO_3/HCO_3^- system.

This system is unique among the body's buffers in that it has an open-ended ventilatory outlet. Approximately 13,000 mEq of CO_2 are generated each day by the cellular combustion of carbohydrate and fat. The CO_2 consequent to cellular respiration behaves as any other gas in solution and its concentration in plasma is proportional to its partial pressure, the P_{CO_2}. A portion of the dissolved CO_2 added by the tissues is rapidly hydrated by the ubiquitous enzyme carbonic anhydrase to form H_2CO_3 (which dissociates into H^+ and HCO_3^-). Fortunately, this reaction is reversed in the lungs, and the generated CO_2 is excreted. Thus, the respiratory system that regulates the level of P_{CO_2} in the blood in effect controls the $[H_2CO_3]$ of the body fluids.

In addition to the volatile acid (CO_2) produced as a consequence of the cellular metabolism of carbohydrate and fat, approximately 70 mEq per day of nonvolatile acids are generated via the metabolism of protein and phospholipid. If it were not for the ability of the kidneys to excrete these metabolic acids via two mechanisms, the body stores of bicarbonate would be consumed in buffering the H^+ ion liberated by these nonvolatile acids and a metabolic acidosis would ensue. Therefore, just as the lungs regulate the P_{CO_2} and $[H_2CO_3]$ of the blood, the kidneys regulate the $[HCO_3^-]$ of the body.

Classically, the relationship between the pH, H_2CO_3, and HCO_3^- is expressed by the Henderson–Hasselbalch equation:

$$pH = pK + \log \frac{[H_2CO_3]}{[HCO_3^-]} \qquad (3.14)$$

It is apparent from this relationship that the pH of the blood is determined by the ratio of HCO_3^- to H_2CO_3. However, the use of logarithms in Equation 3.14 makes it cumbersome and impractical to use in everyday clinical practice. A far more useful expression can be derived if we express the relationship between H^+, HCO_3^-, and H_2CO_3 in the original form proposed by Henderson:

$$[H^+] = K \frac{[H_2CO_3]}{[HCO_3^-]} \qquad (3.15)$$

The CO_2 determined in the routine measurement of the serum electrolytes is the total CO_2 rather than the actual bicarbonate. Total CO_2 includes the HCO_3^-, H_2CO_3, and CO_2 dissolved in the blood. The sum of the latter two components are proportionate to the P_{CO_2} and may be calculated by multiplying the P_{CO_2} by its solubility constant (0.03 mmol/L/mm Hg). At a normal P_{CO_2} of 40 mm Hg, the dissolved CO_2 and $[H_2CO_3]$ is 1.2 mEq per L (0.03×40). Thus, it should be apparent that the total CO_2 reported by the clinical laboratory is predominantly a measure of the $[HCO_3^-]$ and for practical purposes, the total CO_2 may be considered interchangeable with the $[HCO_3^-]$.

Kassirer and Bleich have taken advantage of the relationship between P_{CO_2} and $[H_2CO_3]$ and adjusted the dissociation constant of the H_2CO_3/HCO_3^- buffer system to account for the dissolved CO_2 (18). They have rewritten Equation 3.15 in the more clinically useful form:

$$[H^+] = 24 \times \frac{P_{CO_2}}{[HCO_3^-]} \qquad (3.16)$$

This expression emphasizes the interdependence of $[H^+]$, P_{CO_2}, and $[HCO_3^-]$. It is important to recognize that the $[H^+]$ is determined by the ratio of P_{CO_2} and $[HCO_3^-]$ rather than by the absolute value of either. When there are changes in the P_{CO_2} and $[HCO_3^-]$ that are proportionate, as might be seen in a patient with pneumonia and lactic acidosis who might have a P_{CO_2} of 20 mm Hg and a $[HCO_3^-]$ of 12 mEq per L, then the ratio of P_{CO_2} to $[HCO_3^-]$ and therefore the pH of arterial blood will be normal (7.40).

Equation 3.16 also provides the physician caring for critically ill patients with a useful means to verify the accuracy of the laboratory data. Once any two components of the equation are measured, the third may be readily calculated. In a healthy individual with a pH of 7.40 ($[H^+]$ of 40 nEq per L), a P_{CO_2} of 40 mm Hg, and a $[HCO_3^-]$ (or total CO_2) of 24 mEq per L, Equation 3.16 would read

$$40 = 24 \times \frac{40}{24}$$

Many times, one can be confused by apparently conflicting data. Most laboratories measure the pH and P_{CO_2} of arterial blood with highly accurate electrodes and then read the $[HCO_3^-]$ from a nomogram. This latter estimate may not agree with the total CO_2 reported with the serum electrolytes that were drawn a few hours earlier. For example, the blood gas laboratory may report a pH of 7.30, a P_{CO_2} of 40 mm Hg, and a bicarbonate of 26 mEq per L, whereas the total CO_2 reported by the clinical laboratory was 20 mEq per L. Substituting the bicarbonate value reported with the blood gases into Equation 3.16 yields

$$50 = 24 \times \frac{40}{26}$$

which is obviously incorrect. However, the total CO_2 value reported a few hours previously is consistent with the measured pH and P_{CO_2}. (Remember that, as previously discussed, the actual $[HCO_3^-]$ is slightly less than the total CO_2.) This indicates that the discrepancy between the two bicarbonate determinations is due to a misreading of the nomogram rather than an acute change in the patient's status.

DISTURBANCES IN ACID–BASE BALANCE

Conditions that initially increase or decrease the P_{CO_2} of the blood are termed *respiratory acidosis* or *alkalosis* respectively. Diseases that initially affect the plasma $[HCO_3^-]$ are termed *metabolic acidosis* or *alkalosis*. It is important to remember that the change in arterial pH (and $[H^+]$) is determined by the ratio of P_{CO_2} to HCO_3^-. Primary respiratory disturbances will initiate compensatory renal responses to blunt the change in the P_{CO_2}/HCO_3^- ratio; for example, a rise in P_{CO_2} will induce the renal generation of bicarbonate, so that the fall in pH consequent to the respiratory acidosis is partially offset. Similarly, a primary metabolic disturbance will induce compensatory changes in the level of ventilation that tend to restore the P_{CO_2}/HCO_3^- ratio toward normal. In general, these compensatory responses will not totally restore the pH to normal because to do so would remove the compensatory stimulus. The normal compensatory responses to the different types of primary acid–base disturbances can be predicted with relative certainty. It is important to understand the degree of expected compensation for each primary disturbance because deviations from the predicted response will indicate a mixed acid–base disturbance. For example, a patient with a metabolic acidosis should have a low P_{CO_2}; the presence of a "normal" P_{CO_2} indicates an inappropriate compensation and thereby defines a second primary disorder, respiratory acidosis. On the other hand, a P_{CO_2} that is lower than expected for the degree of metabolic acidosis indicates the coexistence of a second primary acid–base disorder, respiratory alkalosis. Only by understanding the normal degree of compensation for a given primary disturbance can we diagnose these second primary disorders.

RESPIRATORY ACIDOSIS

Any process that reduces the effective level of alveolar ventilation will result in an elevation of the P_{CO_2} and produce a respiratory acidosis. When alveolar ventilation decreases, there is an imbalance initially between the rates of CO_2 production and excretion, resulting in hypercapnia. Eventually, the increment in P_{CO_2} is sufficient to provide an excretory rate (which can be calculated as the product of alveolar ventilation and the

TABLE 3-4. Causes of Respiratory Acidosis

CNS depression
  Drug overdose
  Structural lesions, e.g., tumors
Neuromuscular diseases
  Neuropathies, e.g., Guillain-Barré
  Myopathies, e.g., muscular dystrophy
Impaired lung expansion
  Chest wall deformities, e.g., kyphoscoliosis
  Pneumothorax
  Abdominal distention
  Pleural effusion
Obstructive lung disease
  Upper airway, e.g., laryngospasm
  Asthma
  Chronic obstructive lung disease
Infiltrative pulmonary disease
  Pulmonary fibrosis (end-stage)
  Pulmonary edema
  Severe pneumonia
Miscellaneous, e.g., ventilator malfunction

alveolar concentration of CO_2) equal to the rate at which it is being produced and a steady state is restored. Clinical situations that can reduce the effective level of alveolar ventilation and produce an increase in P_{CO_2} are listed in Table 3-4.

The primary abnormality in a respiratory acidosis is an increase in the P_{CO_2} and $[H_2CO_3]$ of the blood. As the P_{CO_2}/HCO_3^- ratio increases and the $[H^+]$ of extracellular and intracellular fluid rises, there is a compensatory increase in the generation of HCO_3^- from nonbicarbonate buffers, which blunts the increase in the P_{CO_2}/HCO_3^- ratio. The pH returns toward but not to normal. The source and magnitude of this compensatory generation of bicarbonate depends on the duration of the respiratory acidosis.

Acutely a portion of the rise in H^+ ion is neutralized by nonbicarbonate cellular buffers. As the P_{CO_2} increases and H_2CO_3 is generated by hydration of CO_2, protons from the additional H_2CO_3 are taken up by hemoglobin and other intracellular proteins, leaving behind newly formed HCO_3^- ions. This intracellular buffering is extremely rapid, occurring within minutes, but the total amount of bicarbonate that can be generated in this manner is quite small (21,22). An acute increase in P_{CO_2} to 80 mm Hg will produce a rise in bicarbonate of <4 mEq per L (22). Thus, in a pure acute respiratory acidosis, the serum bicarbonate should not exceed 30 mEq per L (total CO_2, 32 mEq per L). There is approximately a 1 mEq per L increase in HCO_3^- for each 10 mm Hg increment in P_{CO_2} (23). The patient with an acute rise in P_{CO_2} to 70 mm Hg and a HCO_3^- level of 34 mEq per L should be recognized as having a coexisting metabolic alkalosis. Brackett et al. (22) have analyzed the acid–base response to acute rises in P_{CO_2} and determined that the relationship between the increase in $[H^+]$ ($\Delta[H^+]$) and the rise in P_{CO_2} (ΔP_{CO_2}) can be expressed as:

$$\Delta[H^+] = 0.8\,(\Delta P_{CO_2}) \tag{3.17}$$

If the P_{CO_2} increased acutely from 40 to 60 mm Hg, the corresponding rise in $[H^+]$ would be 16 nEq per L for a final $[H^+]$ of 56 nEq per L. A 20 mm Hg increase in P_{CO_2} will produce a 2 mEq per L increase in $[HCO_3^-]$, whereas the pH will fall by 0.01 unit for each 1 nEq per L rise in $[H^+]$ to 7.24 (assuming an initial pH of 7.40).

If the elevation in P_{CO_2} persists for more than a few hours, there is an increase in the renal excretion of acid, primarily in the form of NH_4Cl and a net synthesis of HCO_3^- by the kidney (24,25). Because chloride is excreted with the ammonium ion during this generation of bicarbonate, the serum electrolytes will demonstrate a fall in chloride concentration as well as the rise in bicarbonate, characteristic of the compensatory metabolic response to chronic respiratory acidosis. In addition, hypercapnia elevates the renal threshold for bicarbonate and promotes its reabsorption from the glomerular filtrate (26,27). If the elevation in P_{CO_2} is sustained for several days, the increase in bicarbonate generated via the above mechanisms will further blunt (but never entirely correct) the fall in arterial pH produced by the hypercapnia. For each 10 mm Hg increment in P_{CO_2}, the plasma $[HCO_3^-]$ can be expected to increase by 3.5 mEq per L during a chronic respiratory acidosis. The increase in $[H^+]$ per increment in P_{CO_2} during chronic hypercapnia can be calculated from the following relationship:

$$\Delta[H^+] = 0.3 \, \Delta P_{CO_2} \tag{3.18}$$

The resulting change is less than half of that produced by an acute respiratory acidosis. Indeed, it is possible that many patients who had an arterial pH in the high normal range prior to the onset of the respiratory acidosis may have a pH that, though lower than before, is still within the normal range, for example, 7.37. For mild degrees of hypercapnia ($P_{CO_2} \leq 50$ mm Hg), this is extremely likely (28,29). Of special interest to the physicians caring for patients with acute respiratory failure is the compensatory response to an acute elevation in P_{CO_2} occurring in an individual with a chronic respiratory acidosis. It would appear that the body's ability to defend pH against sudden shifts in P_{CO_2} is dependent upon its buffer stores. When the bicarbonate levels are increased above normal, the same increment in P_{CO_2} will produce a smaller increase in $[H^+]$ (30,31). This should be expected from Equation 3.16 in which the $[H^+]$ is described as a function of the P_{CO_2}/HCO_3^- ratio. Conversely, if the bicarbonate level has fallen because of a superimposed metabolic acidosis, then the same rise in P_{CO_2} will have a more pronounced effect on the P_{CO_2}/HCO_3^- ratio and therefore on the $[H^+]$.

RESPIRATORY ALKALOSIS

The changes in acid–base balance due to a simple respiratory alkalosis are in most respects the opposite of those seen during respiratory acidosis. In a respiratory alkalosis, the level of alveolar ventilation is increased so that CO_2 excretion initially exceeds CO_2 production and the arterial P_{CO_2} falls. Eventually, because of the falling alveolar CO_2 concentration, the rate of CO_2 excretion will again match that of CO_2 production and a new steady state will be established, albeit at a lower arterial P_{CO_2}. It can be seen from Table 3-5 that many of the disorders that cause a respiratory alkalosis are associated with respiratory failure.

In respiratory alkalosis, the acute decrease in P_{CO_2} evokes a rapid decrease in $[HCO_3^-]$ that occurs within minutes and is independent of any renal compensation (32). Similar to the situation in respiratory acidosis, it is hemoglobin and other

TABLE 3-5. Causes of Respiratory Alkalosis

Central hyperventilation
    CNS disorders, e.g., cerebrovascular disease
    Drug-induced, e.g., salicylate intoxication
    Hormonal, e.g., pregnancy, hyperthyroidism
Increased peripheral respiratory drive
    Hypoxia
    Hypotension
    Pain, anxiety
Infiltrative pulmonary disease
    Pulmonary edema
    Pneumonia
    Pulmonary fibrosis
    Pulmonary embolism
Obstructive pulmonary diseases
    Asthma
    Chronic obstructive lung disease
Miscellaneous
    Hepatic insufficiency
    Sepsis
    Ventilator-induced

intracellular proteins that play a major role in buffering the change in $[H^+]$ during an acute respiratory alkalosis. However, in this instance, these buffers release hydrogen ions to combine with HCO_3^- and counteract the rise in pH. The magnitude of this initial rapid decrease in HCO_3^- is small, roughly 2 mEq per L per 10 mm Hg decrease in P_{CO_2} (32). Only after several hours is it possible to demonstrate a decrease in renal acid excretion and the consumption of tissue bicarbonate stores due to the retention of the endogenously produced acid (33,34). The decrease in $[H^+]$ during an acute respiratory alkalosis is proportionate to the decrease in P_{CO_2} (32) and may be described by the following equation:

$$[H^+] = 0.8 \, \Delta P_{CO_2} \tag{3.19}$$

Note that Equations 3.17 and 3.19 are identical. In both acute respiratory alkalosis and acute respiratory acidosis, the change in $[H^+]$ will be 80% of the change in P_{CO_2}.

The chronic suppression of renal acid secretion, which may persist for a week or more, substantially lowers the plasma HCO_3^- level and restores the pH toward normal. The plasma bicarbonate level will fall by 5 mEq per L for each 10 mm Hg decrease in P_{CO_2}. Because of this remarkable ability to compensate, the decline in $[H^+]$ per mm Hg decrease in P_{CO_2} in chronic respiratory alkalosis, which may be calculated as

$$[H^+] = 0.17 \, \Delta P_{CO_2} \tag{3.20}$$

is far less than the change in the opposite direction produced by chronic respiratory acidosis (33). Indeed, most individuals with P_{CO_2}'s ≥ 20 mm Hg will have arterial pH's in the normal range. The reason for this enhanced buffering observed in chronic respiratory alkalosis is presently unknown.

METABOLIC ACIDOSIS

Metabolic acidosis is the state produced by any process that reduces the $[HCO_3^-]$. This reduction may occur either because of HCO_3^- loss from the body or via the retention of nonvolatile acids that cannot be excreted by the lungs. It is

TABLE 3-6. Causes of Metabolic Acidosis

High Anion Gap
   Renal failure
   Ketoacidosis
      Diabetic
      Alcoholic
   Lactic acidosis
   Intoxications
      Methanol
      Ethylene glycol
      Salicylate
      Paraldehyde
Normal Anion Gap
   Diarrhea
   Acetazolamide
   Chloride administration, e.g., unbuffered parenteral
      hyperalimentation
   Ureterosigmoidostomy
   Interstitial renal disease
Renal tubular acidosis

clinically convenient to classify the metabolic acidoses by first determining the anion gap (AG) (see Table 3-6).

The AG may be calculated from the serum electrolytes as the difference between the sodium concentration and the sum of the chloride and bicarbonate concentrations, as indicated below:

$$AG = Na^+ - (Cl^- + HCO_3^-) \qquad (3.21)$$

The AG represents those anions other than Cl^- and HCO_3^- that counterbalance the positive charge of Na^+. The normal anion gap of 8 to 12 mEq per L is due to the sulfates, phosphates, negatively charged plasma proteins, and other organic acids that are present in the plasma of a healthy individual. Quantitatively, albumin accounts for most of the normal AG, contributing about 2.5 mEq per L for each 1 g per dL [35,36]. With rare exception, an increase in the AG is diagnostic of the presence of a metabolic acidosis [37,38]. (The converse is not true. Some metabolic acidosis may have a normal AG.) The AG increases when there is an excess accumulation of any acid (HA), which is strong enough to dissociate and react with the $NaHCO_3$ in plasma to form H_2CO_3 and NaA. The H_2CO_3 thus formed is excreted as CO_2 by the lungs, leaving behind Na^+ and the unmeasured anion. Thus, there should be a one-to-one correspondence between the rise in unmeasured anion, for example, lactate, and the fall in plasma bicarbonate levels [37]. If the HCO_3^- level is disproportionately elevated relative to the level of circulating anion, a mixed acid–base disturbance (metabolic acidosis and metabolic alkalosis) should be suspected. In contrast, some metabolic acidoses are produced by a primary loss of bicarbonate and/or the addition of excess chloride ion. These hyperchloremic acidoses are characterized by a normal AG. Regardless of its etiology, any metabolic acidosis will stimulate respiration and thereby reduce the arterial P_{CO_2}. In contrast to the rapid acute adaptation to a primary respiratory disturbance in acid–base balance previously discussed, the respiratory compensation for a metabolic disturbance is somewhat slower and may take 24 hours or longer to be fully manifest [39]. The respiratory response to a metabolic acidosis is mediated via the chemoreceptors of the medullary respiratory center [40], and the lag in the ventilatory response is thought to be due to the slow penetration of H^+ into the cerebrospinal fluid (CSF). The delay in ionic movement across the blood brain barrier also presumably accounts for the maintained hyperventilation and low P_{CO_2} observed after a metabolic acidosis has been rapidly corrected. Despite normalization of the plasma bicarbonate, the CSF may still be acidotic [41] and the hyperventilation may persist, resulting in a respiratory alkalemia.

Once it is fully developed (i.e., after 24 hours), the respiratory response to a metabolic acidosis will produce a fall in P_{CO_2} that is proportionate to the reduction in plasma bicarbonate [42]. The expected P_{CO_2} for a measured bicarbonate level can be predicted from the relationship:

$$P_{CO_2} = 1.5\,[HCO_3^-] + 8(\pm 2) \qquad (3.22)$$

Thus, a patient with chronic renal failure and a HCO_3^- of 16 mEq per L should have a P_{CO_2} of 32($\pm$2) mm Hg. A P_{CO_2} of 24 mm Hg would indicate a coexistent respiratory alkalosis, whereas a normal P_{CO_2} of 40 mm Hg would indicate the presence of a respiratory acidosis. In general, the P_{CO_2} decreases by 1.0 to 1.3 mm Hg for each 1 mEq per L decrement in serum HCO_3^- [22,23]. It has been empirically observed that the P_{CO_2} during a chronic steady state metabolic acidosis will approximate the last two digits of the pH [23]. Thus, a patient with a pH of 7.25 due to a metabolic acidosis should have a P_{CO_2} of 25 mm Hg. It is important to remember that all of these methods for assessing the ventilatory response to a metabolic acidosis are applicable only when the acidosis has been present for 24 hours. If the predictive formulas are employed prior to this time, the P_{CO_2} may not have fallen to its steady state level and a complicating respiratory acidosis would be erroneously diagnosed.

METABOLIC ALKALOSIS

Metabolic alkalosis is the result of any process that tends to elevate the plasma $[HCO_3^-]$ (see Table 3-7). Clinically, it is useful to separate the various types of metabolic alkaloses on the basis of the amount of chloride present in the urine [43]. If, in the absence of diuretics, the urinary chloride concentration is >10 mEq per L, a chloride-resistant alkalosis should be suspected. If the urinary chloride is <10 mEq per L, the alkalosis is likely to be chloride responsive.

The classic example of a chloride-responsive alkalosis is that due to gastrointestinal chloride loss as a consequence of vomiting or nasogastric suction. The renal reabsorption of Na^+ may occur proximally in association with chloride or in the distal tubule in which Na^+ is exchanged for K^+ and H^+. When the amount of chloride present in the glomular filtrate is inadequate for the complete reabsorption of the Na^+ presented to the proximal tubule, more Na^+ is delivered to the distal tubule in which K^+ and H^+ are secreted; every mEq of H^+ added to the urine adds 1 mEq of HCO_3^- to the blood, producing the hypokalemic metabolic alkalosis characteristic of these conditions [44]. Most of the chloride-resistant alkaloses are also associated with an increased distal tubular reabsorption of Na^+. However, in these conditions, the extracellular fluid volume is usually normal or elevated. The renal response to this volume

TABLE 3-7. Causes of Metabolic Alkalosis

Chloride-responsive
    GI chloride loss
        Vomiting
        Nasogastric suction
        Chloride diarrhea
    Alkali administration
        $NaHCO_3$ (baking soda)
        Transfusions, lactated Ringer's
        Antacids
    Chloruretic diuretics
    Administration of poorly reabsorbed anions
        Carbenicillin, ticarcillin
    Posthypercapnia
Chloride-resistant
    Increased distal tubular Na^+ reabsorption
        Endogenous
            Primary hyperaldosteronism
            Cushing's syndrome
            Adrenal hyperplasia
            Bartter's syndrome
        Exogenous
            Steroid therapy
            Licorice ingestion
            Carbenoxolone
    Impaired chloride reabsorption
        Severe K^+ depletion
        Hypercalcemia and hypoparathyroidism

stimulus is appropriate and a fraction of the NaCl presented to the proximal tubule escapes reabsorption, accounting for the high chloride levels in the urine (44).

In contrast to the three simple acid–base disorders presented previously, the compensatory response to a metabolic alkalosis is highly variable (45). The alkalemia should depress the respiratory center and elevate the Pco_2 in a manner analogous to that described for metabolic acidosis. In functionally anephric patients, when a chronic metabolic alkalosis is produced by varying the alkali concentration of the dialysis bath, the following relationship was observed (46):

$$Pco_2 = 0.9\ \Delta[HCO_3^-] + 15.6 \qquad (3.23)$$

However, this sort of consistent response has not been observed clinically. Clearly, there are some individuals who will develop profound CO_2 retention in the presence of a metabolic alkalosis (47,48). However, hypoxemia that is a consequence of alveolar hypoventilation acts as a potent respiratory stimulant, which in turn may offset the respiratory depression and prevent an increase in Pco_2. Although some hypoventilation may occur in those individuals with a pronounced elevation of HCO_3^- (up to 35 mEq per L), the degree of respiratory compensation is usually mild. Any Pco_2 exceeding 55 mm Hg should suggest the coexistence of a primary respiratory acidosis rather than a true compensatory response to the metabolic alkalosis.

MIXED ACID–BASE DISTURBANCES

Thus far, we have been focusing on simple primary acid–base disorders and the expected compensation for these derangements. However, it is not unusual for two or even three of these simple acid–base disturbances to coexist in the same patient, in which case the patient is said to be suffering from a mixed acid–base disturbance. In a number of clinical situations, the two acid–base disturbances might arise simultaneously, for example, the metabolic and respiratory acidoses due to cardiac arrest. In other instances, a new, acute acid–base disturbance may be superimposed on a chronic disorder such as might be seen in a patient with renal failure who already has a chronic metabolic acidosis and then develops a respiratory alkalosis because of pneumonia. A "triple" disturbance can be diagnosed in the patient with an elevated HCO_3^- and a high AG (mixed metabolic alkalosis-metabolic acidosis) who also has a primary respiratory disturbance, either alkalosis or acidosis. To diagnose these mixed disturbances, a clear understanding of how the four simple acid–base orders alter pH, Pco_2, and HCO_3^- is required. If the extent of the expected compensation for any primary disturbance is known, then deviations from the expected response should alert the physician to the presence of a second, simultaneously occurring primary acid–base disorder. These principles are outlined in the following section.

DIAGNOSIS OF ACID–BASE DISTURBANCES

The first step in analyzing any acid–base disturbance is to review the clinical history for potential causes of a metabolic or respiratory acid–base disorder. Virtually all patients with respiratory failure will have a primary respiratory disorder, either alkalosis or acidosis, depending on the etiology of their respiratory failure. In addition to seeking information about clinical conditions such as vomiting or diabetes mellitus that could potentially induce metabolic disturbances, one should also consider the possibility of drug ingestion. A review of the order sheets may identify therapeutic maneuvers such as salt restriction or steroid administration that could produce acid–base disturbances.

The physical examination may reveal additional clues about the presence and cause of an acid–base disturbance. Fever, hypotension, cyanosis, jaundice, and even something as obvious as the presence of a nasogastric tube can indicate the etiology of the acid–base disorder. Only after these initial steps should one turn his attention to the laboratory data. Examination of the serum electrolytes can provide important clues about the type of acid–base abnormality present. Remember that the total CO_2 routinely measured in the clinical lab is primarily bicarbonate. An elevated total CO_2 should suggest the presence of either a metabolic alkalosis or respiratory acidosis. The AG should be calculated. A high AG is diagnostic of a metabolic acidosis. [Alkalemia will increase anaerobic glycolysis and slightly elevate the plasma lactate concentration by ≤ 2 mEq per L (49).] In addition, the liberation of H^+ from plasma proteins to buffer HCO_3^- will increase the amount of unmeasured anions. However, even during a severe alkalemia, the total increase in the AG will be small, 2 to 4 mEq per L.

The serum K^+ can also provide an important clue as to the type of acid–base disturbance present. Most of the buffering that takes place during an acute acid–base disturbance occurs intracellularly. As hydrogen ion shifts into cells during a metabolic acidosis, Na^+ and K^+ move in the opposite direction,

TABLE 3-8. Primary Alterations and Compensation in Simple Acid–Base Disturbances

Disorder	pH	P_{CO_2}	HCO_3^-	Expected Compensation
Respiratory acidosis—acute	$\downarrow\downarrow$ [a]	$\uparrow\uparrow$	$\downarrow$	$\Delta[H^+] = 0.8\,(\Delta P_{CO_2})$ $\Delta[HCO_3^-] = 0.1\,(\Delta P_{CO_2})$
—chronic	$\downarrow\downarrow$	$\uparrow\uparrow$	$\uparrow$	$\Delta[H^+] = 0.3\,(\Delta P_{CO_2})$ $\Delta[HCO_3^-] = 0.35\,(\Delta P_{CO_2})$
Respiratory alkalosis—acute	$\uparrow\uparrow$	$\downarrow\downarrow$	$\downarrow$	$\Delta[H^+] = 0.8\,(\Delta P_{CO_2})$ $\Delta[HCO_3^-] = 0.2\,(\Delta P_{CO_2})$
—chronic	$\uparrow\uparrow$	$\downarrow\downarrow$	$\downarrow$	$\Delta[H^+] = 0.17\,(\Delta P_{CO_2})$ $\Delta[HCO_3^-] = 0.5\,(\Delta P_{CO_2})$
Metabolic acidosis (< 24 h)	$\downarrow\downarrow$	$\downarrow$	$\downarrow\downarrow$	$P_{CO_2} = 1.5\,[HCO_3^-] + 8$
Metabolic alkalosis (< 24 h)	$\uparrow\uparrow$	$\uparrow$	$\uparrow\uparrow$	$P_{CO_2} = 0.9\,[HCO_3^-] + 15$ (Response highly variable)

[a] The symbol $\downarrow\downarrow$ or $\uparrow\uparrow$ indicates direction of primary disturbance; $\downarrow$ or $\uparrow$ direction of compensatory response (which may be within the normal range if the disturbance is not severe).

raising the plasma K^+ concentration. Conversely, during alkalosis, intracellular hydrogen ion moves into the extracellular fluid in exchange for K^+ and the serum K^+ will be low. Although K^+ tends to reflect the extracellular $[H^+]$, it cannot be substituted for the direct measurement of pH. In a severely potassium-depleted individual and in those patients whose acidosis is the result of $KHCO_3$ loss, the serum K^+ may be low despite the presence of acidemia. The acidoses produced by diarrhea, acetazolamide, and renal tubular acidosis are examples of the latter problem.

Ultimately, the precise identification of the type of acid–base disorder present in an individual patient depends on a thoughtful correlation of the blood gas results with the clinical picture and the serum electrolytes. The characteristic change in each of these parameters in simple acid–base disturbances, which has already been discussed, is summarized in Table 3-8. The presence of a mixed disturbance should be suspected when the magnitude of the compensatory response is inappropriate for the primary disturbance. These mixed acid–base disorders are easy to recognize when the effects of both disturbances on pH are additive. For example, in a mixed metabolic acidosis respiratory acidosis, the pH is lower than would be expected on the basis of either the decrease in bicarbonate or the increase in P_{CO_2} alone (see Table 3-9). Remember that in such a mixed disturbance, the "decreased" bicarbonate or "elevated" P_{CO_2} may actually lie within the normal range—the terms "elevated" and "decreased" refer to the values expected in compensation if there were only a single, simple metabolic (or respiratory) acidosis present.

When two primary acid–base disturbances that produce opposing effects on the $[H^+]$ coexist, the pH will be near or within the normal range. Such a mixed disturbance, for example, respiratory alkalosis–metabolic acidosis, is recognized when one calculates that "overcompensation" for a single simple acid–base disturbance is present. For example, a patient with acute respiratory failure might be admitted with the following room air blood gases: pH = 7.39, P_{O_2} = 42 mm Hg, P_{CO_2} = 60 mm Hg, and HCO_3^- = 35.1 mEq/L. On the basis of

these blood gases, a reasonable first guess is that the patient has a chronic respiratory acidosis. If this indeed were the case, we would expect the $[H^+]$ to be 46 nEq per L from the relationship $\Delta[H^+] = 0.3\,\Delta P_{CO_2}$ (Eq. 3.18), which describes the expected compensation for a chronic respiratory acidosis. However, the $[H^+]$ is lower than expected and the increase in HCO_3^- is greater than the 3.5 mEq per L rise predicted for each 10 mm Hg increase in P_{CO_2}, indicating that there is an additional metabolic alkalosis present.

Nomograms have been developed that enable one to plot the pH, P_{CO_2}, and HCO_3^- and determine whether a set of values lies within the confidence bands predicted for a given acid–base disturbance. The use of such a device cannot substitute for the thoughtful evaluation of the patient and his or her laboratory results (50). In the example cited above, if the pH and bicarbonate were slightly lower, the values would lie within the confidence band for a chronic respiratory acidosis. Yet if the clinical history were that of alcohol intoxication with nausea and vomiting followed by the acute onset of respiratory distress, the pH, P_{CO_2}, and HCO_3^- reported above would be more likely to represent an acute respiratory acidosis superimposed on a metabolic alkalosis due to Cl^- loss from the

TABLE 3-9. Laboratory Values in Mixed Acid–Base Disturbances

Disorder	pH	P_{CO_2}	HCO_3^-
Respiratory acidosis–metabolic alkalosis	$\pm$ [a]	$\uparrow$	$\downarrow$
Respiratory acidosis–metabolic acidosis	$\downarrow\downarrow$	$\uparrow$	$\uparrow$
Respiratory alkalosis–metabolic alkalosis	$\uparrow\uparrow$	$\downarrow$	$\uparrow$
Respiratory alkalosis–metabolic acidosis	$\pm$	$\downarrow$	$\downarrow$
Metabolic alkalosis–metabolic acidosis	$\pm$	$\pm$	$\uparrow$ [b]

[a] The symbol $\pm$ indicates the value is close to or within the normal range; the number of arrows indicates the magnitude of the deviation from normal.

[b] Anion gap increased in this disturbance.

gastrointestinal (GI) tract. Furthermore, if the AG on this patient's serum electrolytes was elevated, one would diagnose a triple acid–base disturbance such as might be observed if alcoholic ketoacidosis were superimposed on the above preceding problems.

REFERENCES

1. Mellemgaard K. The alveolar–arterial oxygen difference: its size and components in normal man. *Acta Physiol Scand* 1966;67:10–20.
2. Begin R, Renzetti AD. Alveolar–arterial oxygen pressure gradient. Comparison between an assumed and actual respiratory quotient in stable chronic pulmonary disease. *Respir Care* 1977;22: 491–500.
3. Dantzker DR. Pulmonary gas exchange. In: Bone RE, Dantzker DR, George RB et al., eds. *Pulmonary and critical care medicine.* St Louis: Mosby, 1993:B-1–B-13.
4. West JB. *Ventilation/blood flow and gas exchange,* 4th ed. Oxford: Blackwell Scientific Publications, 1985:17–29.
5. Murray JF. *The normal lung,* 2nd ed. Philadelphia: WB Saunders, 1986:201–209.
6. Baker PT. The adaptive fitness of high altitude populations. In: Baker PT, ed. *The biology of high altitude peoples.* Cambridge: Cambridge University Press, 1978:317–346.
7. West JB, Hackett PH, Maret KH, et al. Pulmonary gas exchange on the summit of Mount Everest. *J Appl Physiol* 1983;55:678–687.
8. Gray BA, Blalock JM. Interpretation of the alveolar–arterial oxygen difference in patients with hypercapnia. *Am Rev Respir Dis* 1991;143:4–8.
9. West JB, Lahiri S, Gill MB, et al. Arterial oxygen saturation during exercise at high altitude. *J Appl Physiol* 1962;17:617–621.
10. Tai E, Reid J. Response of blood gas tensions to aminophylline and isoprenaline in patients with asthma. *Thorax* 1967;22:543–549.
11. Aubier M, Marviano D, Millic-Emili J, et al. Effects of the administration of O_2 on ventilation and blood gases in patients with chronic obstructive pulmonary disease during acute respiratory failure. *Am Rev Respir Dis* 1980;122:747–754.
12. Murray JF, Matthay MA, Luce JM, et al. An expanded definition of the adult respiratory distress syndrome. *Am Rev Respir Dis* 1988;138:720–723.
13. Dantzker DR. The influence of cardiovascular function on gas exchange. *Clin Chest Med* 1983;4:149–159.
14. Kandel G, Aberman A. Mixed venous oxygen saturation. Its role in the assessment of the critically ill patient. *Arch Intern Med* 1983;143:1400–1402.
15. Kasnitz P, Druger GL, Yorra F, et al. Mixed venous oxygen tension and hyperlactatemia. *JAMA* 1976;236:570–574.
16. Bell RC, Coalson JJ, Smith JD, et al. Multiple organ system failure and infection in adult respiratory distress syndrome. *Ann Intern Med* 1983;99:293–298.
17. Lichtman MS, Murphy MS, Adamson JW. Detection of mutant hemoglobins with altered affinity for oxygen: a simplified technique. *Ann Intern Med* 1976;84:517–520.
18. Kassirer JP, Bleich HL. Rapid estimation of plasma carbon dioxide from pH and total carbon dioxide content. *N Engl J Med* 1965;272:1067.
19. Stewart PA. Modern quantitative acid-base chemistry. *Can J Physiol Pharmacol* 1983;61:1444–1461.
20. Fencl V, Leith DE. Stewart's quantitative acid-base chemistry: applications in biology and medicine. *Respir Physiol* 1993;210:1–16.
21. Cohen JJ, Brackett NC, Schwartz WB. The nature of the carbon dioxide titration curve in the normal dog. *J Clin Invest* 1964;43:777.
22. Brackett NC, Cohen JJ, Schwartz WB. Carbon dioxide titration in man. *N Engl J Med* 1965;272:6.
23. Narins RG, Emmett M. Simple and mixed acid-base disorders: a practical approach. *Medicine* 1980;59:161.
24. Polak A, Haynie GD, Hays RM. Effects of chronic hypercapnia on electrolyte and acid-base equilibrium. *J Clin Invest* 1965;44:291.
25. Schwartz WB, Brackett NC, Cohen JJ. The response of extracellular hydrogen ion concentration to graded degrees of chronic hypercapnia. The physiologic limits of defense of pH. *J Clin Invest* 1961;40:1223.
26. Engel K, Dell RB, Rahill J. Quantitative displacement of acid-base equilibrium in chronic respiratory alkalosis. *J Appl Physiol* 1968; 24:288.
27. Warren Y, Luke RB, Kashgarian M, et al. Micropuncture studies of chloride and bicarbonate reabsorption in the proximal renal tubule of the rat in respiratory acidosis and chloride depletion. *Clin Sci* 1970;38:375.
28. Van Ypersele de Strihou C, Brasseur CL, DeConinck J. The "carbon dioxide response curve" for chronic hypercapnia in man. *N Engl J Med* 1966;275:117.
29. Alfaro V, Torras R, Ibáñez J, et al. A physical-chemical analysis of the acid-base response to chronic obstructive pulmonary disease. *Can J Physiol Pharmacol* 1996;74:1229–1235.
30. Goldstein MB, Gennari FJ, Schwartz WB. Influence of graded degree of chronic hypercapnia on the acute carbon dioxide titration curve. *J Clin Invest* 1971;50:208.
31. Madias NE, Adrogue HJ. Influence of chronic metabolic acid-base disorders on the acute CO_2 titration curve. *J Appl Physiol* 1983;55: 1187.
32. Arbus GS, Herbert LA, Levesque PR. Characterization and clinical application of the "significance band" for acute respiratory alkalosis. *N Engl J Med* 1969;280:1.
33. Gennari FJ, Goldstein MB, Schwartz WB. The nature of the renal adaptation to chronic hypocapnia. *J Clin Invest* 1972;51:1722.
34. Glenhill N, Beirne GJ, Dempsey JA. Renal response to short term hypocapnia in man. *Kidney Int* 1975;8:376.
35. Figge J, Mydosh T, Fencl V. Serum proteins and acid-base equilibria: a follow-up. *J Lab Clin Med* 1992;120:713–719.
36. Jurado RL, Del Rio C, Nassar G, et al. Low anion gap. *South Med J* 1998;91:624–629.
37. Emmett M, Narins RG. Clinical use of the anion gap. *Medicine* 1977;56:38.
38. Oh MS, Carroll HJ. The anion gap. *N Engl J Med* 1977;297:814.
39. Pierce NF, Fedson DS, Brigham KL. The ventilatory response to acute base deficit in humans. Time course during development and correction of metabolic acidosis. *Ann Intern Med* 1970;72:633.
40. Fencl V, Miller TB, Pappenheimer JR. Studies on the respiratory responses to disturbances of acid-base balance, with deductions concerning the ionic composition of cerebral interstitial fluid. *Am J Physiol* 1966;210:459.
41. Posner JB, Plum F. Spinal-fluid pH and neurologic symptoms in systemic acidosis. *N Engl J Med* 1967; 277:605.
42. Albert MD, Dell RB, Winters RW. Quantitative displacement of acid-base equilibrium in metabolic alkalosis. *Ann Intern Med* 1967; 66:312.
43. Narins RG, Jones ER, Stom MD. Diagnostic strategies in disorders of fluid, electrolyte and acid-base homeostasis. *Am J Med* 1982;72:496.
44. Seldin DW, Rector FC, Jr. The generation and maintenance of metabolic alkalosis. *Kidney Int* 1972;1:306.
45. Goldring RM, Cannon PJ, Heinemann HO, et al. Respiratory adjustment to chronic metabolic alkalosis in man. *J Clin Invest* 1968;47:188.
46. Van Ypersele de Strihou C, Frans A. The respiratory response to metabolic alkalosis and acidosis in disease. *Clin Sci Mol Med* 1973;45:439.
47. Tuller MA, Mehdi F. Compensatory hypoventilation and hypercapnia in primary metabolic alkalosis. *Am J Med* 1971;50:281.
48. Lifschitz MD, Brasch R, Cuomo AJ, et al. Marked hypercapnia secondary to severe metabolic alkalosis. *Ann Intern Med* 1972;77:405.
49. Hood VL, Tannen RL. Protection of acid-base balance by pH regulation of acid production. *N Engl J Med* 1998;339:819.
50. Fulop M, Fulop M. Acid-base diagnosis: maths, myths and measurements. *Lancet* 1974;2:637.

SECTION 2

GATHERING
THE DATABASE

CHAPTER 4

The Respiratory History and Physical Examination

Ronald B. George

D. Keith Payne

OBTAINING A USEFUL HISTORY
Occupational and Exposure History

SYMPTOMS OF RESPIRATORY DISEASES
Upper Respiratory Tract Symptoms
Chest Pain
Breathlessness
Cough
Sputum Expectoration
Hemoptysis

PHYSICAL EXAMINATION
Inspection and Palpation
Percussion
Auscultation
Extrapulmonary Signs

OFFICE AND HOME TESTING OF PATIENTS WITH RESPIRATORY DISEASE

The process of obtaining a meaningful history, performing a good physical examination, and putting the information together to form an initial impression is an art that must be learned by experience. The history and physical examination should lead to a reasonable list of differential diagnoses. This list of impressions, in turn, forms the basis for a diagnostic plan, whereby the number of possible diagnoses is gradually decreased by the results of selected laboratory tests, radiographs, and specialized procedures. This chapter includes some guidelines for this important task.

OBTAINING A USEFUL HISTORY

The interview is designed to identify the important symptoms and to determine their duration. To do this without being led into blind areas of discussion is an important step toward identifying the problem. The interviewer must lead the discussion, avoiding lengthy digressions; on the other hand, the

patient must have the freedom to mention items that may prove important as the history unfolds. The patient should not be badgered but should be made to feel that the interviewer is truly interested in his or her problems. The interviewer should not yawn or act bored but should instead appear interested in the patient's story.

The chief complaint—the symptom that caused the patient to seek help—and its duration should be identified. Frequently, the patient will say that he or she was referred because of an abnormal finding on a chest film or some other laboratory test. However, it is important to determine why that test was made and, if it was part of a routine examination, what changes from previous films resulted in the referral.

Once the major complaint and its duration are identified, the development of the patient's symptoms should be investigated chronologically, beginning at the time the patient first noted a departure from feeling well. The patient should be questioned concerning current and past medications, any allergic reactions or intolerance to foods or drugs, or exposure to contagious illnesses. It is important to determine if other members of the household or co-workers have similar symptoms. It is also useful to obtain information from previous examinations or diagnostic tests. For instance, a previously negative tuberculin skin test is important if tuberculosis is suspected. Elements of the personal, occupational, and social history should be included in the present illness if they are directly pertinent to the patient's current symptoms.

A systematic review of the symptoms of respiratory illnesses and their character and duration should be reported. Nonrespiratory symptoms should also be reviewed because they may be related to the respiratory disease. Patients with carcinoma of the lung may present with complaints of headaches or seizures related to cerebral metastases; ankle swelling or a history of injury to the lower extremities is important if the patient has a suspected pulmonary embolism. Ascites and edema of the legs may be secondary to heart failure, cor pulmonale, or liver disease, all of which may cause abnormalities on the chest film, whereas joint pain may be caused by hypertrophic pulmonary osteoarthropathy. It is important to determine whether a patient's complaints are seasonal, especially in patients with hay fever, sinusitis, postnasal drip, or asthma.

Previous illnesses and operations should be recorded because they may be related to the present illness. For instance, childhood measles or pertussis may be the origin of bronchiectasis, and asthma that had occurred in childhood and had disappeared at puberty may return at a later age. Patients with reactivation tuberculosis often relate a history of household contact during their childhood years. Previous operations and biopsies may be the source of pathologic specimens that might be useful for reexamination. If previous chest films are available, they should be obtained for comparison with recent ones.

OCCUPATIONAL AND EXPOSURE HISTORY

Cigarette smoking is the most common preventable cause of death in the United States today (1). A smoking history is especially important in patients with respiratory complaints. Passive exposure to cigarette smoke in the home or workplace is an increasingly recognized cause of respiratory symptoms in children whose parents smoke, and passive smoking has been shown to increase the incidence of respiratory infections (2).

The occupational history is especially important in patients with lung problems because the lungs are constantly in contact with the environment. The patient should be encouraged to relate his or her job history in chronologic order. Occupational exposure may have occurred many years ago; exposure to asbestos may result in the development of a pleural mesothelioma 25 years or more after the exposure has ceased. It is important to ask the patient whether he or she was advised to wear a mask at work and whether his or her fellow workers did so. The type of mask worn and the air source should be identified. Construction workers who are not directly involved in hazardous activities may work in closed areas containing toxic materials; for instance, carpenters, plumbers, and welders often work in areas where sandblasting is occurring. Although the sandblaster may have extensive protection, the workers nearby may be exposed.

Some symptoms of toxic reactions are not related to the lungs. Patients working with galvanized metal (zinc fumes) may complain of nausea, vomiting, and other systemic symptoms. Allergic alveolitis due to thermophilic actinomycetes in workers exposed to moldy hay (farmer's lung) or sugar cane residue (bagassosis) is associated with fever, malaise, and headache, in addition to nonproductive cough. The patient should be questioned about particularly irritating odors or upper respiratory symptoms because toxic fumes usually affect the eyes, nose, and throat and this serves as an early sign of chemical exposure. Upper respiratory symptoms are common in toxic smoke inhalation.

Workers may not be aware of exposures to toxic materials. For instance, office workers have developed allergic alveolitis from air conditioners and humidifiers that were contaminated with fungal spores (3).

The family history is often useful. Cystic fibrosis and the immotile cilia syndromes are inherited, as are the hemoglobinopathies and α_1-antitrypsin deficiency. Patients with asthma often have a family history of allergic rhinitis, asthma, or other allergic symptoms. In addition, family members may have similar exposures. Tuberculosis is often spread by household contact, and viral respiratory diseases often affect several family members. Families may be exposed to the oxides of nitrogen (silo-filler's disease) or moldy hay while working together on a farm.

SYMPTOMS OF RESPIRATORY DISEASES

UPPER RESPIRATORY TRACT SYMPTOMS

Rhinorrhea, conjunctivitis, and sneezing are common in patients with allergic rhinitis (hay fever) who may also have asthma; the two syndromes often coincide. Postnasal drip occurs in patients with upper respiratory disease and is manifested during the daytime by frequent clearing of the throat rather than by actual coughing. A postnasal drip is often a problem at night and may produce a morning cough caused by chronic irritation of the upper airways.

Nosebleeds (epistaxis) may be a symptom of sinusitis or may be produced by trauma, foreign bodies, or tumors of the nose and nasopharynx. Systemic diseases such as hypertension, polycythemia, and bleeding disorders can also lead to bouts of epistaxis. Wegener's granulomatosis causes necrotizing granulomas of the upper respiratory tract as well as of the lungs. Blood from the nose and nasopharynx sometimes accumulates in the oropharynx and is coughed up; therefore, the patient thinks that it is coming from the lungs. A history of epistaxis and the finding of blood clots in the nose or nasopharynx are clues that the expectorated blood may be coming from the upper respiratory tract. Hoarseness may result from lesions of the recurrent laryngeal nerve (surgical trauma, mediastinal tumors, or infections) or from diseases of the larynx (tuberculosis, tumors, or allergy).

Patients who present with anaerobic infections of the lungs and pleura (lung abscess, empyema) often have upper respiratory abnormalities leading to aspiration of oral secretions. The patient should be questioned concerning recent mouth or dental surgery, anesthesia, aspiration of a foreign body, neurologic abnormalities, periods of unconsciousness, and seizures.

CHEST PAIN

Thoracic pain is an alarming symptom because most people are aware of its association with cardiac disease, lung tumors, and other serious life-threatening diseases. There are two basic types of chest pain: that which arises in the chest wall structures and is conducted through the intercostal and phrenic nerves (lateral or chest wall pain) and that which arises in the internal organs and is conducted through the afferent fibers of the vagus nerve (central or visceral pain). These two types of chest pain are discussed separately.

Visceral chest pain occurs with neoplasms of the major bronchi or mediastinum; abnormalities of the heart, aorta, and pericardium; or diseases that cause esophageal pain, especially reflux esophagitis or tumors. Pain associated with acute bronchitis is usually central and is often accentuated by coughing.

Pain in the substernal area may indicate disease of the heart, pericardium, aorta, or esophagus. Angina pectoris is usually an effort-induced pain that is relieved by rest and vasodilators. It is often referred to the neck, shoulder, or arm. Pericardial pain is sometimes relieved by sitting up or leaning forward. Pain associated with a dissecting aortic aneurysm is frequently reported as being severe and deep and may be referred to the interscapular area of the back. Esophageal pain may mimic angina pectoris and may be relieved by sublingual nitroglycerin, which relaxes esophageal spasm. It is often related to meals and relieved by antacids. Patients with significant esophageal reflux are subject to aspiration, especially at night, and may present with recurrent bouts of acute bronchospasm and cough, mimicking asthma attacks.

Chest wall pain is sharp, often well localized, and is increased by deep breathing or coughing (pleuritic pain or pleurisy). Pleuritic pain is associated with any disease that causes inflammation of the parietal pleura such as infections (pneumonia, empyema, tuberculosis), trauma (pneumothorax, hemothorax, rib fracture), or tumors (cancer, lymphoma, mesothelioma). Older patients may suffer rib fractures following minor trauma or even severe coughing bouts. These fractures may not be visible on the initial chest film, but later, callus formation around the fracture may make it apparent in retrospect. Irritation of the intercostal nerves (herpes zoster, spinal nerve root disease) may also lead to localized chest wall pain. Costochondritis of the second to fourth costosternal articulations (Tietze's syndrome) is common and may mimic the pain of myocardial ischemia or other serious diseases. The pain is clearly localized to the costal cartilage, and there is tenderness to pressure and often a palpable enlargement of the costosternal junction.

The peripheral innervation of the diaphragm is from the local intercostal nerves, and irritation of the peripheral diaphragm is referred to the adjacent chest wall. The central diaphragmatic pain fibers are conducted through the phrenic nerves, and pain in the central diaphragm is often felt in the ipsilateral trapezius region at the base of the neck and the shoulder, an area also supplied by the phrenic nerve.

BREATHLESSNESS

Breathlessness (dyspnea) is the sensation of difficulty in breathing, sometimes interpreted as the inability to take a deep breath. It is one of the most common reasons for which patients with chest diseases consult a physician. Breathlessness is difficult to quantitate because it is subjective and, in certain situations (e.g., during and following exercise and at high altitudes), it is normal. Although exercise normally produces dyspnea, a rapid increase in breathlessness or a decrease in exercise tolerance is an important symptom. Breathlessness may occur intermittently, as with attacks of asthma, or it may be persistent, as with chronic obstructive pulmonary disease (COPD). It may be influenced by position, as in patients with left heart failure who complain of orthopnea (dyspnea when lying flat). Orthopnea may also be seen in patients with asthma or chronic airway obstruction.

There are three basic causes of the sensation of breathlessness: an increased awareness of normal breathing, an increase in the work of breathing, and an abnormality of the ventilatory system itself. Increased awareness of normal breathing is usually a result of anxiety; in this situation, the common complaint is that the patient cannot take a satisfactorily deep breath. The breathing pattern is often irregular, with frequent sighs. Severe psychogenic breathlessness is associated with rapid breathing, tingling of the hands and feet, circumoral numbness, respiratory alkalosis, and, occasionally, tetanic seizures. This *hyperventilation syndrome* is diagnosed only after organic causes, both respiratory and nonrespiratory, have been excluded and the respiratory mechanics and blood oxygen level have been determined to be normal.

The second cause of breathlessness is an increase in the work of breathing. This may be due to either airway obstruction, in which case greater pressures are required to move air into and out of the lungs, or restriction of lung volumes and loss of compliance, in which case greater effort is required to expand the lungs and chest wall.

The third cause of breathlessness is an abnormality of the ventilatory apparatus. This involves dysfunction of the nerves, the respiratory muscles, or the thoracic cage itself. Neurologic abnormalities producing breathlessness include spinal cord injury, ascending polyneuritis, myasthenia gravis, amyotrophic lateral sclerosis, poliomyelitis, and exposure to paralytic agents or neurotoxins. Primary diseases of the respiratory muscles include polymyositis and muscular dystrophy, whereas examples of chest wall abnormalities include extreme obesity, kyphoscoliosis, large pleural effusions, and space-occupying lesions of the thorax.

COUGH

Cough receptors are located in the large bronchi, trachea, and larynx and respond to respiratory secretions in the large airways. Irritation of the cough receptors may occur in the absence of abnormal secretions, as with inhalation of toxic fumes or a mild asthma attack. In such cases, the nonproductive cough serves no useful purpose and may cause mechanical trauma, leading to more coughing. A nonproductive cough may also be a manifestation of anxiety. In such instances, it may be useful to suppress the cough; however, in most cases, coughing aids in airway clearance and suppression is not indicated.

A change in the character or frequency of cough is a common complaint in patients with pulmonary diseases. Most acute and self-limiting coughs are secondary to a viral respiratory infection (4), whereas chronic and persistent coughs are most often secondary to chronic bronchitis or postnasal drip. Patients who smoke cigarettes have a characteristic smoker's cough, a manifestation of chronic bronchitis, most noticeable in the morning on awaking. This cough may produce mucoid sputum and is often ignored by the chronic cigarette smoker.

Cough may be the sole complaint in patients with mild asthma (5). In such patients, the cough may be relieved by a bronchodilator or by the avoidance of inhaled allergens. If bronchospasm is not present at the time of examination, reversible airway obstruction may be demonstrated with the use of a nonspecific bronchial challenge such as methacholine (6). Cough (with or without bronchospasm) may occur as a side effect of β-adrenergic antagonists as well as angiotensin converting enzyme (ACE) inhibiting drugs (7).

SPUTUM EXPECTORATION

If the patient has a productive cough, the duration of sputum expectoration, the character of the sputum, and the presence or absence of blood should be determined. Cigarette smokers with chronic bronchitis have mucoid or occasionally purulent sputum without much change in character for months or years and without hemoptysis. The sputum is the result of chronic stimulation and hypertrophy of the bronchial glands as a defense mechanism (8).

In patients with COPD and chronic sputum production, it is important to examine thoroughly the character of an expectorated sputum sample (color, opacity, and consistency). The patient should be asked about any changes in the quantity, color, or opacity, which may indicate an acute infectious exacerbation requiring antibiotic therapy. It is useful to look at an unstained wet preparation of purulent-appearing sputum to identify neutrophils or eosinophils as the cause of the purulence because therapy is with antibiotics in the case of neutrophils and with antiinflammatory agents in the case of eosinophils (9). It is not usually necessary to obtain a Gram stain in cases of chronic bronchitis with acute exacerbation, and the results usually indicate a mixed flora with both gram-positive and gram-negative organisms. Likewise, a sputum culture and sensitivity are rarely indicated; antibiotic therapy is empiric, based on the usual causes of such exacerbations.

Viral infections of the lower respiratory tract are first associated with scant mucoid sputum, which may contain a few streaks of blood. Later, the sputum may become copious and purulent with or without bacterial superinfection. Patients recovering from influenza who begin to produce large volumes of purulent sputum associated with a febrile relapse most likely have a bacterial superinfection. Viral and mycoplasmal pneumonias are associated with relatively scant sputum production initially.

Patients with acute lower respiratory tract infections usually produce sputum containing neutrophils. A Gram stain of grossly purulent sputum may help to identify a predominant bacterial organism. In pneumococcal lobar pneumonia, the sputum produced early is usually scanty and is composed of mucus tinged with blood ("rusty"); later, sputum may become purulent. As opposed to the scant mucoid sputum in early lobar pneumonia, the sputum in patients with bronchopneumonia (frequently a complication of chronic bronchitis) is usually copious and purulent. The chronic production of purulent sputum with episodes of blood streaking is suggestive of severe bronchitis, bronchiectasis, bronchogenic tumor, or the presence of an aspirated foreign body. Suppurative lung diseases—including bronchiectasis, lung abscess, or bronchopleural fistula with empyema—are associated with expectoration of large volumes of yellow or green sputum. The color is produced by pigments released from degenerating neutrophils. Approximately 60% of patients with lung abscess have foul-smelling sputum associated with bad breath, anorexia, and weight loss (10).

Asthmatics who are recovering from an acute attack usually produce sputum that is thick and tenacious and contains bronchial mucous plugs. The sputum may be purulent but, when examined, is found to predominantly contain eosinophils rather than neutrophils. A simple wet preparation or a Wright stain allows ready determination of the predominant cell type (9).

Lung tumors and tuberculosis are associated most often with the chronic production of mucoid sputum that may be associated with blood streaking. Hemoptysis is an important symptom in such patients; it is the appearance of bloody sputum that often brings the patient to the physician.

Sputum Induction

If the patient is unable to produce sputum, inhalation of a nebulized solution of 3 or 4 mL distilled water or 10% sodium chloride results in the induction of an adequate specimen for examination in over 90% of cases. Any type of nebulizer may be used; however, ultrasonic nebulizers, which produce a concentrated mist, are preferred. The patient should be placed in a private room or an isolation booth if he or she is suspected of having a contagious disease. The patient inhales the nebulizer mist deeply and is encouraged to cough frequently, saving all material produced. Chest percussion and/or postural drainage may be used. The procedure is terminated when an adequate specimen is obtained, the nebulizer solution is exhausted, or after a maximum of 15 to 20 minutes. The procedure is most often used for patients suspected of having tuberculosis or a lung malignancy, and to search for *Pneumocystis carinii* infection in patients with acquired immunodeficiency syndrome (AIDS). Sputum induction has largely replaced gastric lavage for obtaining specimens for mycobacteria or fungi because sputum induction results in higher yield and less patient discomfort (11).

HEMOPTYSIS

The term *hemoptysis* means simply the coughing of blood; to say that a patient has hemoptysis is not enough. It is important to determine the duration of the hemoptysis and to note whether there is gross blood, blood-tinged sputum, or blood-streaked sputum. An attempt should be made to determine the amount of blood produced and to record whether it is bright red or dark and whether it contains blood clots.

Hematemesis, or vomiting of blood, may be confused with hemoptysis; however, hemoptysis tends to produce bloody sputum that is at least partly frothy, whereas hematemesis does not. Hematemesis more often produces dark red blood that is usually acidic, whereas hemoptysis produces alkaline blood. With hematemesis, blood streaking of sputum is unusual, whereas with hemoptysis it is common. Vomited blood frequently contains food particles, whereas this is rare with hemoptysis.

The more recently reported common causes of submassive and massive hemoptysis are shown in Tables 4-1 and 4-2. Massive hemoptysis is frequently defined as expectoration of blood exceeding 200 mL in a 24-hour period. Although massive hemoptysis is much less common than submassive hemoptysis, it is associated with a significant mortality and is

TABLE 4-1. Reported Causes of Submassive Hemoptysis (<200 mL/24 h) by Percent of Total Cases

Author	Hirshberg(12)	Johnston(13)	McGuiness(14)
Country	Israel	USA	USA
Number of Cases	80	102	57
Bronchitis	23	44	7
Bronchiectasis	11	0	25
Bronchogenic Carcinoma	19	24	12
Tuberculosis	0	5	16
Cardiogenic	8	2	0
Aspergilloma	0	0	12
Pneumonia	19	6	0
Other[a]	10	15	9
Unknown	10	4	19

[a]Includes pulmonary embolism, adenoma, trauma, vasculitis, pulmonary hypertension, broncholith, and Kaposi sarcoma.

TABLE 4-2. Reported Causes of Massive Hemoptysis (>200 mL/24 h) by Percent of Total Cases

Author	Hirshberg(12)	Johnston(13)	Knott-Craig(15)
Country	Israel	USA	South Africa
Number of Cases	128	22	120
Bronchitis	15	27	0
Bronchiectasis	25	4	51 (all had TB)
Bronchogenic Carcinoma	19	4	5
Tuberculosis	0	18	73
Cardiogenic	2	0	1
Aspergilloma	0	9	6
Pneumonia	14	0	3
Other[a]	18	34	4
Unknown	7	4	8

[a]Includes pulmonary embolism, adenoma, trauma, vasculitis, pulmonary hypertension, broncholith, and Kaposi sarcoma.

commonly a sign of serious underlying lung disease. The etiologies of both massive and submassive hemoptysis depend greatly on the population of patients studied (e.g., older patients usually have a higher incidence of lung cancer) and the diagnostic modalities employed to investigate the cause [the use of high resolution CT scanning of the lungs (HRCT) may demonstrate unsuspected bronchiectasis in a patient previously thought to have bronchitis]. In general, the "three Bs"—bronchitis, bronchiectasis, and bronchogenic carcinoma—along with active tuberculosis account for the majority of cases of both massive and submassive hemoptysis. Other common causes include aspergillomas, heart disease, pulmonary vascular disease, and necrotizing pneumonias. Even with an intensive investigation including bronchoscopy and HRCT, a cause may not be discovered for a significant percentage of cases.

A careful history may be very useful in guiding the physician to identify the source of hemoptysis. Bleeding may occur with tumors of the larynx; hoarseness is frequently present in this case. Problems in the nasopharynx and oropharynx are usually associated with obvious abnormalities of these areas on physical examination. Bleeding dyscrasias often cause

hemoptysis, in which case there is usually evidence of hemorrhage elsewhere (e.g., in the skin or gastrointestinal tract). Hemoptysis from pulmonary embolism may be suspected when the patient complains of dyspnea and pleuritic chest pain. The gradual onset of shortness of breath along with complaints of leg swelling, orthopnea, and paroxysmal nocturnal dyspnea may lead the examiner to implicate heart failure as a potential cause of hemoptysis. Similarly, pneumonia may be suspected when the patient complains of dyspnea with fever, chills, and purulent sputum. Smokers complaining of blood-streaked mucopurulent sputum may have bronchitis as the cause of hemoptysis, while patients with bronchiectasis may complain of expectorating large volumes of purulent secretions. Hemoptysis in male adolescents or young men, particularly with a history of repeated episodes of bronchitis or pneumonia, may be a clue to the presence of unsuspected cystic fibrosis.

PHYSICAL EXAMINATION

As in recording the medical history, it is important to develop an organized, systematic approach to examining the patient. Initially, the patient's general condition should be observed and his or her body habitus and state of nutrition noted. The presence of acute distress, such as pain, dyspnea, or mental confusion, should be recorded. Evidence of chronic illness, such as weight loss or debilitation, should also be noted. The patient's psychological attitude, awareness, and appreciation of events, handicaps, and use of prosthetic devices should be noted. If the patient is receiving oxygen, the amount and method of administration should be recorded.

INSPECTION AND PALPATION

During the inspection and palpation of the head, neck, and chest, it is useful to have the chest radiograph handy. This is true during the entire examination of the chest because it allows correlation of physical and radiographic findings. In examining the chest, it is useful to recall the normal location of the five lobes of the lungs and their areas of contact with the chest wall (see Fig. 4-1).

The nose, throat, and ears should be examined carefully because lower respiratory diseases are often associated with upper respiratory tract abnormalities. Rhinorrhea and the presence of pale, edematous nasal mucosa occur with allergic rhinitis. Nasal polyps occur with respiratory allergies and may cause epistaxis. The frontal, ethmoid, and maxillary sinuses are often tender in the presence of sinusitis, which may produce postnasal drip or bleeding. A red, edematous throat may result from infection, toxic fume exposure, or chronic postnasal drip. Patients with pneumonia often have inflamed mucous membranes caused by associated viral or bacterial upper respiratory infections. Oropharyngeal candidiasis (thrush) may be associated with inhaled steroids or antibiotic therapy and is also common in immunosuppressed patients. Tumors, strictures, or inflammation of the oropharynx can cause upper airway obstruction, leading to extreme breathlessness; sleep-related disorders of breathing may occur in the presence of lesions that obstruct the upper airway. Patients with lung abscess or empyema frequently have poor dental hygiene and foul-smelling breath and may have problems with swallowing.

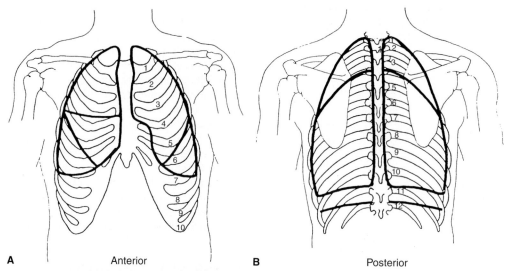

FIGURE 4-1.   **A:** Normal relationship of the lungs to the anterior chest wall. The upper part of the chest overlies the upper lobes. The middle lobe lies under the fourth and fifth interspaces to the right of the heart. The lower lateral chest wall lies over the anterior and lateral basal segments of the lower lobes. **B:** Normal relationship of the lungs to the posterior chest wall. The upper lobe areas are covered by the bones and muscles of the shoulder girdle and are therefore not readily accessible to percussion and auscultation. Most of the posterior chest wall overlies the lower lobes. Diaphragm positions at inspiration and expiration are shown. (From Prior JA, Silberstein JS, Stang JM. *Physical diagnosis, the history and examination of the patient*, 6th ed. St. Louis: CV Mosby, 1981, with permission)

Sarcoidosis may involve the salivary and lacrimal glands, with dryness of the oral mucosa and conjunctivae; involvement of the parotid gland may be associated with paralysis of the facial nerve (Bell palsy). Inflammation of the uveal tract in sarcoidosis is detected by slit lamp examination. Drying of the oral mucous membranes may be associated with anticholinergic drug therapy or with rheumatoid disease (keratoconjunctivitis sicca), which may affect the lungs also.

The position and mobility of the trachea should be determined because shift of the mediastinum is associated with shift of the trachea, whereas fixation of the mediastinum by carcinoma or mediastinal fibrosis is associated with decreased tracheal mobility. The position of the trachea is easily ascertained from the front by comparing the distance from the trachea to each clavicular head. Nodes and masses in the neck and supraclavicular areas are usually best palpated from the rear.

An examination of the neck veins is important in patients with lung diseases. Right heart failure and severe obstructive airway disease are associated with neck vein distention. With airway obstruction, the veins usually collapse during inspiration unless elevated venous pressure is also present. With obstruction of the superior vena cava, there is marked distention of neck veins, sometimes associated with edema of the neck, eyelids, and hands, and dilation of veins over the anterior chest wall.

The presence of tenderness, discoloration, bruises, or scars over the chest wall should be noted. If there is a history of recent trauma and if chest pain is present, an attempt should be made to palpate the chest wall for crepitus, indicating the presence of a rib fracture or subcutaneous emphysema. If scars from previous surgery are noted, the patient should be questioned about this. Examination of the spine for kyphoscoliosis may reveal the cause in patients with restrictive lung disease. Expansion of the chest wall should be evaluated both

by inspection and palpation. In patients with severe hyperinflation of the chest owing to COPD or asthma, the chest is rounded and barrel-shaped, and because the diaphragm is low and flat, there may be inward deflection of the lower chest with inspiration (Hoover sign). In each step of the physical examination, advantage should be taken of the fact that the chest is a bilaterally symmetrical structure and each side should be compared with the other as a control. For example, tension pneumothorax produces an ipsilateral hyperinflation of the chest, with hyperresonance and decreased breath sounds.

In patients with significant emphysema and air trapping, pneumothorax may occur spontaneously or with minor trauma, such as chest physical therapy. The presence of a pneumothorax may be difficult to detect on physical examination in such patients because the findings are similar to those of the underlying COPD (increased thoracic diameter, hyperresonance, decreased breath sounds, decreased fremitus) (16). The pneumothorax may not be evident on inspiratory chest films because of the pulmonary hyperinflation; an expiratory film is useful in such cases.

PERCUSSION

Percussion of the chest is useful because the chest contains structures of both air and fluid density; in the presence of disease, their relationships may vary. With pleural effusions, consolidation, large intrathoracic masses, or atelectasis, the chest is dull to percussion. With pneumothorax or hyperinflation, the chest is hyperresonant. The generalized hyperresonance in patients with emphysema may cause the examiner to miss a small pneumothorax; in such patients, mediastinal shift may be limited because of air trapping on the opposite side (16).

Percussion over the area of the diaphragm during maximal inspiration and expiration allows the examiner to estimate the extent of diaphragm motion. This is one of the few objective measurements for assessing diaphragm movement. The diaphragm is low and flat and movement is minimal with emphysema.

AUSCULTATION

The examiner should become familiar with the character of normal breath sounds. In the average resting person, inspiration involves approximately one-third of the respiratory cycle and expiration, the remaining two-thirds. Breath sounds vary according to the site of auscultation. Bronchial breath sounds are a normal finding over the trachea.

Transmission of voice-generated sounds to the chest wall can be evaluated by either palpation or auscultation. Again, it is important to compare the two sides while listening for the conduction of voice sounds. A localized increase in the clarity of whispered or spoken sounds is associated with bronchial breathing and occurs with consolidation around open airways. Several terms have been devised to describe this increased conduction of sound through fluid—*bronchophony*, *egophony*, and *whispered pectoriloquy*. Decreased conduction of whispered or spoken sounds occurs in the presence of obstructed bronchi, pneumothorax, or large collections of fluid or tissue between the lung and chest wall.

The terminology of adventitious sounds in the chest has been confusing in the past, and there are still differences in terminology in different countries. In an attempt to unify the terminology, a series of symposia have been held in several countries. The terminologies used in this chapter are the recommendations of the International Lung Sounds Association (17).

Discontinuous Sounds

The term *rale* was originally devised by Laennec to signify a variety of abnormal chest sounds. Because of the confusion associated with this term, Robertson and Coope introduced the term *crackles* to describe the series of tiny explosions heard over the chest wall during inspiration (18). A number of qualifying adjectives have been used, such as crepitant, subcrepitant, dry, and wet. To avoid confusion, only the terms coarse and fine should be used.

A careful analysis of chest physical findings using waveform analysis has revealed that the *timing* of crackles is important. Those that begin early in inspiration are likely to be associated with airway obstruction (see Table 4-3). Early, fine

TABLE 4-3. Clinical Conditions and Timing of Crackles

Early Crackles	Late Crackles
Chronic bronchitis	Diffuse interstitial fibrosis
Asthma	Airspace pneumonia
Emphysema	Pulmonary congestion and edema
"Atelectatic crackles"	Sarcoidosis
	Scleroderma
	Bronchopneumonia
	Rheumatoid lung
	Asbestosis

crackles are usually caused by small airway closure at end-expiration and disappear after a few deep breaths. Coarse, early inspiratory crackles are usually associated with bronchitis or bronchopneumonia. Fine, superficial crackles that occur late in inspiration ("Velcro") are usually associated with diseases that cause a restrictive ventilatory defect, such as idiopathic diffuse interstitial fibrosis, asbestosis, and sarcoidosis.

Continuous Sounds

These sounds have a longer duration than crackles, usually lasting more than 250 milliseconds. They have a musical quality that crackles do not have. Continuous breath sounds are either wheezes, which are high pitched and arise in small airways, or rhonchi, which are low pitched and occur in large airways (19). Wheezes generally occur in the presence of bronchospasm and are an important finding in asthma. Occasionally, a wheeze may begin with an audible pop as a small airway opens during inspiration. This crackle, followed by a high-pitched wheeze, has been called a *sibilant crackle* and has the same significance as a wheeze.

The term *rhonchus* means snore; rhonchi are common in severely ill patients whose secretions are collected in proximal airways. They occur in the presence of large-airway disease (stricture, foreign body, tumor, or mucous secretions), and those that clear with coughing are associated with sputum in larger airways. The presence of a localized wheeze or rhonchus that does not clear with coughing and does not change from one examination to another suggests an intrinsic defect in a large airway, such as a bronchogenic neoplasm. Because of the constricting nature of these lesions, the rhonchus usually occurs during both inspiration and expiration.

Other Adventitious Sounds

In the presence of air in the pericardium or mediastinum, a coarse, crackling sound called a *mediastinal crunch* may be heard that is synchronous with systole. This sound may be associated with a pericardial friction rub.

A pleural friction rub is a grating sound associated with breathing. Rapid tape recordings have demonstrated that pleural friction rubs are actually a series of tiny explosions, just as crackles are (19). Pleural friction rubs are generally loud and sound as if they are immediately under the stethoscope. They occur during both inspiration and expiration, generally at the end of inspiration and at the beginning of expiration. If a patient has pleuritic chest pain, it is useful to ask him or her to point to the location of the pain and to listen over that area because the rub will be loudest there. The rub often occurs simultaneously with the patient's chest pain.

Pericardial friction rubs are similar to pleural rubs except that they occur with atrial and ventricular systole and diastole. They are best heard at the left sternal border at about the third interspace. It is useful to have the patient stop breathing, at which time the pericardial friction rub should persist. Pericardial and pleural friction rubs may occur simultaneously.

EXTRAPULMONARY SIGNS

A wide variety of physical findings outside the thorax may occur in patients with pulmonary diseases. Hypoxemia is

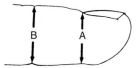

FIGURE 4-2. Clubbing of the fingers is best assessed by determining the ratio of the diameter at the base of the nail (*A*) to the diameter at the distal interphalangeal joint (*B*). This ratio is normally less than 1.

associated with cyanosis if 5 g per dL or more of reduced hemoglobin is present in the capillary blood. Central cyanosis implies involvement of gas transfer in the lungs and affects the tongue as well as the extremities. Peripheral cyanosis without central cyanosis implies a circulatory problem (e.g., vascular spasm or shock).

Clubbing of the digits may or may not be associated with cyanosis. It is seen with many chest diseases, including neoplasms, bronchiectasis, and lung abscess. It may be inherited as a familial trait or may occur with diseases of other organs (e.g., the liver). The most reliable evidence of digital clubbing is an increase in the ratio of the diameter of the digit at the base of the nail to the diameter of the distal interphalangeal joint (Fig. 4-2). This ratio is always less than unity unless clubbing is present.

Patients who have pulmonary neoplasms may have one of several paraneoplastic syndromes, which are usually related to the production of hormones by tumor cells (Chapter 14, Lung Neoplasms). Horner syndrome occurs when apical lung tumors invade outside the pleura and into the superior cervical ganglion. There is ipsilateral enophthalmos, loss of sweating, and meiosis. Invasion of the brachial plexus nerves by these tumors may produce pain, atrophy, and loss of function in the ipsilateral arm.

OFFICE AND HOME TESTING OF PATIENTS WITH RESPIRATORY DISEASE

Increasingly, the emphasis in medical care is shifting to the outpatient setting. Economic considerations and patient preference have resulted in a shift of diagnostic activity from the inpatient hospital setting to outpatient facilities, including the physician's office. This important trend has been facilitated by the development of technologically advanced, highly accurate, portable diagnostic equipment. Appropriate use of this equipment combined with a thorough history and physical examination may greatly enhance the speed and accuracy of the initial evaluation of the patient with suspected lung disease.

Office-based spirometry can be useful in several ways. Spirometry may be used to evaluate and characterize signs and symptoms of lung disease as well as to monitor disease progression (or regression) in patients with known lung disease. Therapeutic interventions by the physician may be more accurately quantitated using spirometry. Preoperative risk assessment can be facilitated with data obtained by spirometry. Prognostic information concerning the patient's disease may be obtained as well. On occasion, data obtained with spirometry may be useful in better defining occupational exposures causing or contributing to the observed pulmonary dysfunction. The degree of physical impairment based on lung function may

be quantitated, providing valuable information that may help the lung-impaired patient find appropriate employment or gain appropriate disability benefits.

It is important to select the appropriate equipment for office spirometry. Volume-displacement spirometers may be the water-seal, rolling-seal, or bellows type. The Stead–Wells water-seal type spirometer has been considered the gold standard for many years. Volume-displacement machines are highly accurate and frequently less costly than other types of spirometers; however, they tend to be bulky and less portable and require manual calculations unless they are connected to computers. Flow-sensing spirometers are highly computerized and offer the advantage of small size and portability. They are probably the instruments of choice in most office settings. The pneumotachograph is the most common type of flow-sensing spirometer. Other types include machines that operate with thermistors, turbines, or vortex-sensing devices. Several companies manufacture spirometers. Not all of these machines are equally accurate, and the American Thoracic Society has established minimal standards for spirometers used for diagnostic and monitoring purposes (20). In addition, technician training is important and should not be neglected (21).

Peak flowmeters are inexpensive and readily available. Although peak flowmeters are less accurate than spirometry, they, nonetheless, may provide useful data regarding airflow, especially in asthmatic patients. Current expert panel guidelines recommend the measurement of peak flow, particularly in asthma patients with moderate to severe disease (22). Peak flow can be utilized as a formal part of an action plan for the patient to follow during exacerbations. Out-of-office phone consultations between patient and physician may be expedited if the patient can compare his or her current peak flow to his or her personal best. Patients with asthma that is difficult to control may benefit from recording peak flow in the morning and afternoon for several weeks. During an office visit, the physician and patient can observe the variability in airflow patterns, which correlates with the degree of airway hyperresponsiveness.

Oximeters are an important addition to the office equipment of the pulmonologist. The ability to measure accurate oxygen saturation both at rest and with varying degrees of exertion is of great importance in the evaluation of lung disease. Because oxygen is the only therapeutic modality that has been demonstrated to prolong survival in COPD, it is important to identify those individuals who require supplemental oxygen. After a resting value is obtained, saturation values with exercise should also be measured. By use of a treadmill or simply by walking a known distance in the hallway, accurate oxygen saturation values with exercise may be obtained. Saturation values at rest and with exercise should be recorded in the chart for documentation purposes and for providing the basis for reimbursable oxygen prescriptions.

REFERENCES

1. U.S. Public Health Service. *The health consequences of smoking—cardiovascular disease. A report of the Surgeon General.* Washington, DC: US Government Printing Office, 1983.
2. Wall M, Brooks J, Holsclaw D, et al. Health effects of smoking on children. ATS statement. *Am Rev Respir Dis* 1985;132:1137–1138.

3. Banaszak EF, Thiede WH, Fink JN. Hypersensitivity pneumonitis due to contamination of an air conditioner. *N Engl J Med* 1970; 283:271–276.

4. Irwin RS, Rosen MJ, Braman SS. Cough, a comprehensive review. *Arch Intern Med* 1977;137:1186–1191.

5. Corrao WM, Braman SS, Irwin RS. Chronic cough as the sole presenting manifestation of bronchial asthma. *N Engl J Med* 1979;300: 633–637.

6. Pratter MR, Irwin RS. The clinical value of pharmacologic bronchoprovocation challenge. *Chest* 1984;85:260–265.

7. Bucknall CE, Neilly JB, Carter R, et al. Bronchial hyperreactivity in patients who cough after receiving angiotensin converting enzyme inhibitors. *Br Med J* 1988;296:86–88.

8. Reid L. Measurement of the bronchial mucous gland layer: a diagnostic yardstick in chronic bronchitis. *Thorax* 1960;15:132–141.

9. Epstein RL. Constituents of sputum: a simple method. *Ann Intern Med* 1972;77:259–265.

10. Bartlett JG. Anaerobic infections of the lung. *Chest* 1987;91:901–909.

11. Elliott RC, Reichel J. The efficacy of sputum specimens obtained by nebulizer versus gastric aspirates in the bacteriologic diagnosis of pulmonary tuberculosis. *Am Rev Respir Dis* 1963;88:223–227.

12. Hirshberg B, Biran I, Glazer M, et al. Hemoptysis: Etiology, evaluation, and outcome in a tertiary referral hospital. *Chest* 1997;112: 440–444.

13. Johnston H, Reisz G. Changing spectrum of hemoptysis. *Arch Intern Med* 1989;149:1666–1668.

14. McGuinness G, Beacher JR, Harkin TJ, et al. Hemoptysis: prospective high-resolution CT/bronchoscopic correlation. *Chest* 1994;105:1155–1162.

15. Knott-Craig C, Oostuizen G, Rossouw G, et al. *J Thorac Cardiovasc Surg* 1993;105:394–397.

16. George RB, Herbert SJ, Shames JM, et al. Pneumothorax complicating pulmonary emphysema. *JAMA* 1975;234:389–393.

17. Mikami R, Murao M, Cugell DW, et al. International symposium on lung sounds: synopsis of proceedings. *Chest* 1987;92: 342–345.

18. Robertson AJ, Coope R. Rales, rhonchi, and Laennec. *Lancet* 1957; 2:417–422.

19. Forgacs P. Crackles and wheezes. *Lancet* 1967;2:203–205.

20. American Thoracic Society. Standardization of spirometry: 1994 update. *Am J Respir Crit Care Med* 1995;152:1107–1136.

21. Wanger J, Irvin CG. Office spirometry: equipment selection and training of staff in the private practice setting. *J Asthma* 1997;34: 93–104.

22. National Heart, Lung, and Blood Institute. *Expert Panel Report II: Guidelines for the diagnosis and management of asthma.* Bethesda: National Institutes of Health [NIH Publication No. 97–4051], 1997.

CHAPTER 5

Chest Imaging

H. Dirk Sostman

Frank M. Mele

M. Chad Foster

Richard A. Matthay

The lungs are composed of a complex of tissues, each of which has a unique function but all of which together perform the act of respiration (1). The morphologist examines each tissue and describes its normal or abnormal characteristics. The radiologist, similarly, can assess individual components of the lungs through application of special techniques such as bronchography and angiography. The most commonly and generally used examination is the plain chest film (taken without added contrast material) (see Figs. 5-1 and 5-2). The plain radiograph is the cornerstone of chest radiographic diagnosis (1). All other radiographic procedures (e.g., fluoroscopy, tomography, and special contrast studies) are strictly ancillary. With few exceptions, establishing the presence of a disease process by plain radiography of the chest should constitute the first step; if this first examination does not show clearly the nature and extent of the lesion, additional studies can be performed to complement the plain chest radiograph.

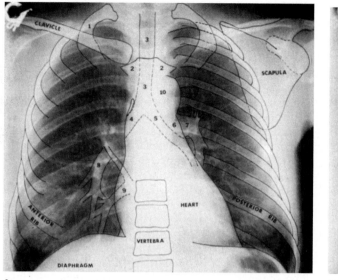
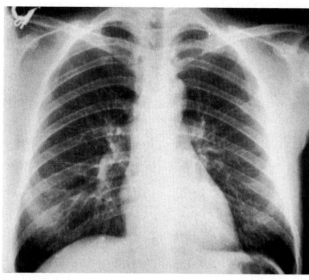

A   B

FIGURE 5-1.   **A:** Posteroanterior (PA) chest radiograph with diagrammatic overlay. Various structures are identified by labels or numbers. *1,* first rib; *2,* upper portion of manubrium; *3,* trachea; *4,* right main bronchus; *5,* left main bronchus; *6,* main pulmonary artery; *7,* left pulmonary artery; *8,* right interlobar pulmonary artery; *9,* right pulmonary vein; *10,* aortic arch. **B:** Chest radiograph of the same subject without diagrammatic overlay.

Accordingly, in this chapter the normal chest radiograph and the normal radiographic anatomy of the airways and the pulmonary vasculature are discussed first; then, special chest radiographic views, fluoroscopy, tomography, ultrasound, magnetic resonance imaging, contrast examinations, and ventilation–perfusion scans are reviewed. Radiographic manifestations of diseases of the lungs, mediastinum, diaphragm, chest wall, and pleura are discussed in subsequent chapters.

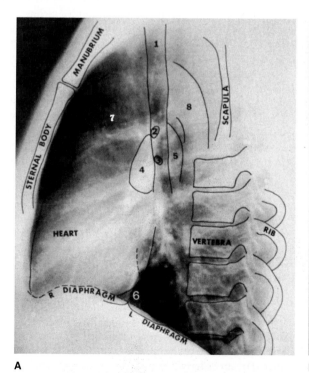
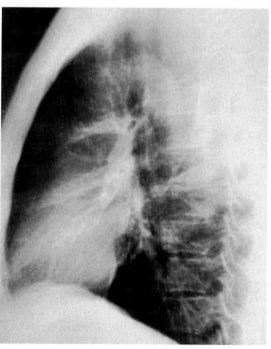

A   B

FIGURE 5-2.   **A:** Lateral chest radiograph of the same patient as in Figure 5-1, with diagrammatic overlay. Structures are identified by labels or numbers. *1,* trachea; *2,* right upper lobe bronchus; *3,* left upper lobe bronchus; *4,* right pulmonary artery; *5,* left pulmonary artery; *6,* inferior vena cava; *7,* ascending aorta; *8,* descending aorta. **B:** Lateral chest radiograph without diagrammatic overlay.

CONVENTIONAL CHEST RADIOGRAPHY

RADIOGRAPHIC TECHNIQUE

The basic principles of radiographic technique are as follows: (a) positioning must be such that the x-ray beam is properly centered, the patient's body is not rotated, and the scapulae are rotated sufficiently anteriorly to be projected free of the lungs; (b) respiration must be fully suspended, preferably at total lung capacity; (c) exposure factors should be such that the resultant radiograph permits faint visualization of the thoracic spine and the intervertebral discs so that lung markings behind the heart are clearly visible (2).

ROUTINE PROJECTIONS

The normal chest radiograph in the posteroanterior (PA) and lateral projections is shown in Figures 5-1 and 5-2. A diagrammatic overlay shows the normal anatomic structures numbered or labeled in both projections. In young persons or in asymptomatic patients, a PA projection alone is generally used as a screening procedure (3). From an analysis of over 100,000 chest radiographs of a hospital-based population, Sagel et al. concluded that routine screening examinations, obtained solely because of hospital admission or scheduled surgery, are not warranted in patients under 20 and that the lateral projection can be safely eliminated from routine screening examination in patients 20 to 39 years of age (4). A lateral film should be obtained whenever chest disease is suspected and during screening examination of patients 40 years of age or older.

For the PA film, the x-ray beam is projected from the back to the front of the patient, with the film cassette against the anterior thorax. Because the heart is in the front of the thorax, there is much less cardiac and mediastinal magnification on a PA than on an anteroposterior (AP) film (5).

The upright position is used because the diaphragms are lower, and the lungs are larger in this position because the abdominal viscera do not push the diaphragms up as they do in the supine position. If pleural fluid is present, it is more easily identified on the upright film than on a supine film because it gravitates to the dependent portion of the thorax, where small spaces (e.g., the costophrenic angles) are filled and altered in contour. Ultrasound is more sensitive than the chest radiograph for detecting small to moderate-size pleural effusions. Air-fluid levels, as seen in lung abscess and hydropneumothorax, are clearly visible on the upright chest film. If fluid must be identified and if the patient cannot stand or sit upright, a lateral decubitus film should be obtained.

It is not always possible or advisable to take films upright or in the PA projection. A very sick patient must be recumbent, and infants and young children are usually radiographed in the supine position.

The lateral view adds valuable information about certain areas that are not seen well on the PA view (3). This is particularly true of the anterior part of the lung, close to the mediastinum, which may be obscured by the overlying heart and aortic shadows, the mediastinum, and the vertebral column (Figs. 5-1 and 5-2). Moreover, a small pleural effusion is best seen, and often only seen, as blunting of a costophrenic sulcus posteriorly (3).

PORTABLE CHEST RADIOGRAPHS

Portable x-ray films that are made in the intensive care unit, operating suite, or patient's room are generally of poorer quality than the erect PA x-ray or even recumbent films made in the radiology department. Positioning is difficult in a hospital bed; consequently, the patient's true position is often unknown, which causes difficulty in assessing the pulmonary vascularity or the presence of pleural fluid. The film focal distance is short, with resultant magnification of the heart and aorta and obscuration of part of the lung fields. Further, the x-ray generator used on portable equipment is not as powerful as stationary generators available in the x-ray department. Hence, it is preferable to obtain a film in the radiology department unless the patient absolutely cannot be moved without hazard. If a portable film must be taken, an upright portable film is preferable to a supine film. The position and distance from the beam generator to the film should be recorded on the film.

Recent advances in storage phosphor technology have made it possible to significantly improve the consistency and quality of portable radiographs and to produce them in a digital format so that they may be transmitted easily to video terminals (which might be located, e.g., in the intensive care unit).

OBSERVER ERROR

As Fraser and Paré have emphasized, radiologic diagnosis of chest disease begins with identification of an abnormality on a radiograph; what is not seen cannot be appreciated (1). Many studies of the accuracy of diagnostic procedures, notably those by Garland et al., have revealed an astonishingly high incidence of both intraobserver and interobserver error among experienced radiologists (6–9). For example, in one series, the interpreters missed almost one-third of radiographically positive minifilms and overread about 1% of negative films; in another series, based only on positive radiographs, interobserver error ranged from 9% to 24% and intraobserver error from 3% to 31% (6,7). As these figures are derived from studies by competent, experienced observers, it is clear that no student of chest radiography should be lulled into a false sense of security concerning his or her competence to detect a lesion.

To minimize observer error, a radiograph can be inspected in two ways, each of which may be employed usefully in different situations. *Directed search* is a method by which a specified order of inspections is carried out (e.g., thoracic and extrathoracic scans), followed by examination of soft tissues, bony thorax, mediastinum, diaphragm, pleurae, and finally the lungs themselves (1). The lungs are usually analyzed by individual inspection and the zones of the two lungs are compared from apex to base. Such a method *must* be used by those in training because it is only through the exercise of this routine that the pattern of the normal chest can be recognized (1).

The alternative method of inspection is *free search*, in which the radiograph is scanned without a preconceived orderly pattern. This is the method employed by the majority of experienced radiologists. However, such free search must be followed by an orderly pattern of inspection to avoid overlooking less obvious abnormalities.

It is important to view every chest radiograph from a distance of at least 6 to 8 feet or through diminishing lenses (1). There are two reasons: (a) the slight nuances of density variation between similar zones of the two lungs can be better appreciated at a distance, and (b) the visibility of shadows with ill-defined margins is improved significantly by minification (10).

As a further means of reducing the frequency of "missing" lesions radiographically, the practice of double viewing has been advocated (1,6,10). In one study, dual interpretation by the same observer on two occasions or by two different observers decreased by at least one-third the number of positive films missed (6). Many physicians, particularly chest physicians and surgeons, become highly competent in radiograph interpretation as a result of many years of personal viewing; if their chest radiograph reading is done in consultation with the radiologist, the second look may reveal abnormalities missed on the first interpretation.

RADIOGRAPHIC ANATOMY OF THE AIRWAYS

THE TRACHEA AND MAIN BRONCHI

The trachea is a midline structure; however, a slight deviation to the right after entering the thorax is a normal finding and should not be misinterpreted as evidence of displacement (Fig. 5-1) (1). The walls of the trachea are parallel except on the left side just above the bifurcation, where the aorta commonly impresses a smooth indentation; rarely, the azygos vein causes a smaller indentation at the tracheobronchial angle on the right side (1).

The trachea divides into the two major bronchi at the carina. The angle of bifurcation is varied and is most acute in asthenic persons (1). The distal course of the right main bronchus is more vertical than that of the left.

The transverse diameter of the right main bronchus at total lung capacity is greater than that of the left (average 15.3 mm versus 13.0 mm in adults), although its length before the origin of the upper lobe bronchus as measured at necropsy is shorter (average 2.2 cm compared with 5 cm on the left) (see Fig. 5-3) (11–13).

The air column of the trachea, both major bronchi, and the intermediate bronchus should be visible on well-exposed standard radiographs of the chest in the frontal projection (Fig. 5-1). A thin vertical shadow is usually well visualized on lateral chest radiographs; it is formed by the posterior boundary of the tracheal air column (Fig. 5-2). This thin band is chiefly the posterior tracheal wall and is formed anteriorly by the junction of the tracheal air column and the tracheal wall and posteriorly by the junction of aerated lung in the right retrotracheal space with the external aspect of the tracheal wall and a thin layer of areolar tissue (14).

Pathologic processes within the mediastinum (e.g., carcinoma of the middle third of the esophagus) or in the medial portion of the right upper lobe can lead to deformity or obliteration of the posterior tracheal band, providing evidence for a pathologic process that might not be readily apparent otherwise (1).

THE LOBAR BRONCHIAL SEGMENTS

The anatomic distribution of the bronchial segments is illustrated in Figure 5-3. Each of the lobes divides into segments, which have been classified by the nomenclature shown in Table 5-1 (1).

Of clinical significance is the fact that several segmental bronchi are located posteriorly, which renders them frequent recipients of aspirated material and likely sites for the development of aspiration pneumonia. The dorsally located segments

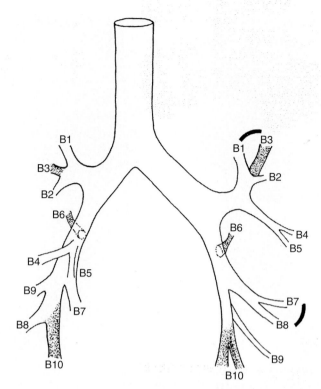

FIGURE 5-3. Diagram of the bronchopulmonary segments, following the Boyden classification. Segments that are relatively more posteriorly located are shaded; these areas are frequent sites of aspiration pneumonia. See Table 5-1 for correspondence of the Boyden system with the more frequently used Jackson–Huber classification. Note that the latter combines the segments connected with bars on the diagram into single segments.

TABLE 5-1. Nomenclature of Bronchopulmonary Anatomy

Jackson–Huber	Boyden
Right upper lobe	
Apical	B1
Anterior	B2
Posterior	B3
Right middle lobe	
Lateral	B4
Medial	B5
Right lower lobe	
Superior	B6
Medial basal	B7
Anterior basal	B8
Lateral basal	B9
Posterior basal	B10
Left upper lobe	
Upper division	
Apical-posterior	B1, B3
Anterior	B2
Lower (lingular) division	
Superior lingular	B4
Inferior lingular	B5
Left lower lobe	
Superior	B6
Anteromedial	B7, B8
Lateral basal	B9
Posterior basal	B10

From Fraser RG, Paré JAP, Paré PD et al. *Diagnosis of diseases of the chest,* Vol. 1, 3rd ed. Philadelphia: WB Saunders, 1988:37, with permission.

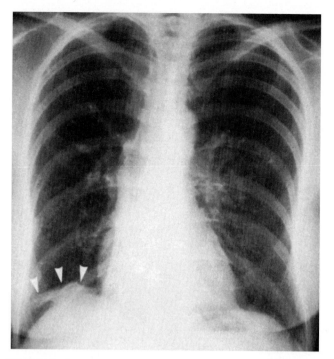

FIGURE 5-4. Posteroanterior chest radiograph showing density in the right lung base behind the right portion of the cardiac silhouette obliterating the medial silhouette of the right hemidiaphragm. This is right lower lobe atelectasis. Note the relative paucity of vascular markings in the aerated portion of the right lung due to compensatory overaeration. Immediately above the right hemidiaphragm there is an area of linear atelectasis as well (*arrowheads*).

that are frequent sites for aspiration include the posterior segment of the right upper lobe (*B3*); the posterior basal and superior segments of the right lower lobe (*B10*, *B6*); and the posterior basal and superior segments of the left lower lobe (*B10*, *B6*) (see Fig. 5-3).

Lobar consolidation of the lung is frequently associated with loss of volume (atelectasis). However, atelectasis of pulmonary segments occurs less often because collapse is prevented by collateral air drift; thus, most x-ray presentations of atelectasis are lobar (3). The patterns of atelectasis of various lobes are illustrated in Figures 5-4 to 5-8. It is important to recognize the patterns of atelectasis because it is a common manifestation of bronchial obstruction by carcinoma of the lung. Atelectasis is common in the postoperative period, when it is due in part to inadequate clearing of secretions, and it may be seen in other conditions, such as asthma, in which viscid mucus occludes bronchi. It may also occur secondary to aspiration of a foreign body.

RADIOGRAPHIC ANATOMY OF THE HILA AND PULMONARY VASCULAR SYSTEM

The major vascular structures in the thorax that are visible on the normal chest radiograph are the aorta, pulmonary arteries, and pulmonary veins (15). Each is discussed individually; first the normal hila is described.

The hila are composed of the pulmonary arteries and their main branches, the upper lobe pulmonary veins, the major bronchi, and the lymph nodes. The lower lobe pulmonary veins

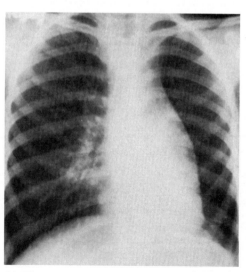

A

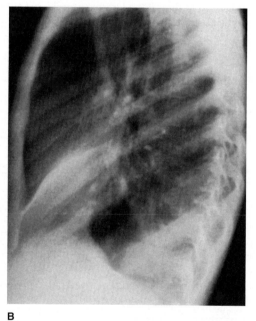

B

FIGURE 5-5. **A:** Posteroanterior chest radiograph demonstrating middle lobe and left lower lobe atelectasis. The middle lobe atelectasis is seen as a triangular density obliterating the right cardiac silhouette. The left lower lobe atelectasis is demonstrated as a triangular-shaped area of increased density behind the left cardiac silhouette. Note that the medial silhouette of the left hemidiaphragm is not visible. **B:** Lateral view of the same patient. The middle lobe atelectasis is more easily visible on this view, seen as a linear area of density overlying the heart silhouette. The left lower lobe atelectasis is seen as an area posteriorly and inferiorly, giving increased density to the vertebral bodies, which it overlies, and obliterating the silhouette of the left hemidiaphragm posteriorly.

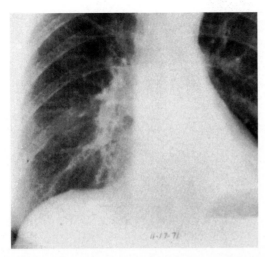

FIGURE 5-6. Posteroanterior chest radiograph of another patient with left lower lobe atelectasis. Note the similarity to Figure 5-5A.

do not cross the hila and, therefore, do not contribute to the hilar shadows (15). The bronchi account for little of the hilar opacity because they are filled with air, and normally, lymph nodes are too small to add to the size or density. Therefore, normal hilar shadows consist mostly of the large pulmonary arteries and upper lobe veins (see Figs. 5-9 and 5-10) (15).

The main pulmonary artery is 4 to 5 cm in length and about 3 cm in diameter in adults. It lies entirely within the pericardial sac, as does its bifurcation (15). The right pulmonary artery lies posterior to the aorta and the superior vena cava and anterior to the right main bronchus (Figs. 5-9 and 5-11).

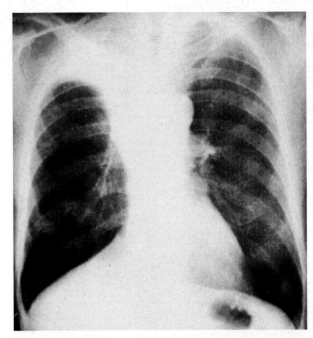

FIGURE 5-8. Right upper lobe atelectasis shown on the posteroanterior chest radiograph. Note the disparity in vascular markings between the right and left lungs. This is evidence of compensatory hyperinflation of the nonatelectatic portions of the right lung. Note that the right upper lobe collapse does not obliterate the cardiomediastinal silhouette as much as the left upper lobe collapse does. This is partly because the left upper lobe moves forward as well as upward as it collapses (see Fig. 5-7A and B), while the right upper lobe moves mostly upward, and partly because of differences in the mediastinal contour.

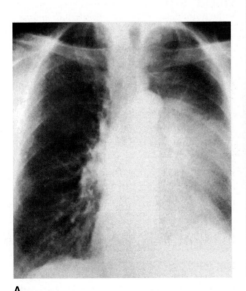

A

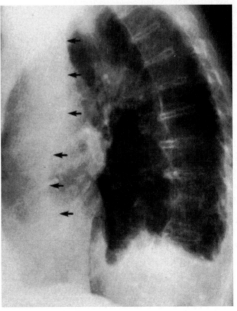

B

FIGURE 5-7. **A:** Chest radiograph of a patient with left upper lobe atelectasis. Note that the upper portion of the left heart border is not visible and there is a hazy density in the left upper lung field. There is evidence of volume loss in the left hemithorax (elevation of the left hemidiaphragm, shift of the heart and mediastinal structures to the left, and closer spacing of the left ribs than the right ribs). **B:** Lateral view of the same patient. The collapsed left upper lobe forms an anteriorly located density, which is outlined in the figure by *arrows.* This is because the left upper lobe collapses upward and forward.

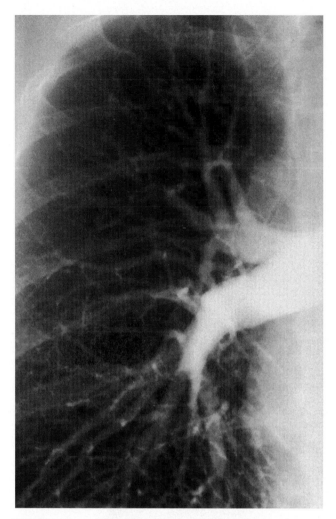

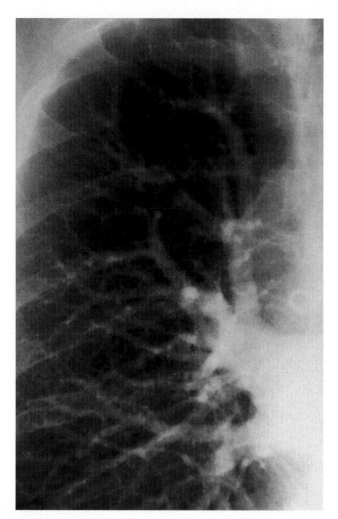

FIGURE 5-9. Normal pulmonary artery anatomy is shown on the arterial phase of a normal pulmonary arteriogram, obtained by injecting iodinated contrast material directly into the right main pulmonary artery.

FIGURE 5-10. Levophase (venous and left heart phase) of the same pulmonary arteriogram shown in Figure 5-9. Note the differing course of the pulmonary veins as related to the pulmonary arteries.

It remains within the pericardium until it gives off its first branch, and the artery continues as the descending or interlobar division to supply the middle lobe and right lower lobe. It accounts for the lower portion of the right hilum (15).

The left pulmonary artery lies within the pericardium for a short distance before entering the lung. This vessel divides within the left hilum after passing immediately anteriorly and laterally to the lower portion of the left main bronchus (Figs. 5-9 and 5-11) (1).

The component distribution pattern of pulmonary veins (Fig. 5-10) involves two large veins on each side, entering the mediastinum slightly below the pulmonary arteries and anterior to them (Figs. 5-10 and 5-11). It may be difficult to distinguish arterial and venous trunks within the lungs owing to superimposition of artery and vein, especially in the upper lobes where their course is parallel; in the lower lung fields, the veins run more horizontally than the arteries and can often be distinguished (1).

The caliber of the hilar pulmonary artery is important and should be assessed carefully. A significant sign is a change in caliber from one examination to another, particularly in relation

to the diagnosis of pulmonary hypertension (1). Radiographic measurement of a segment of the pulmonary vascular tree may provide useful information (16). The width of the right descending pulmonary artery has been measured in over 1,000 normal adult subjects (16). The upper limit in inspiration is 16 mm in men and 15 mm in women; during expiration, it is 1 to 3 mm greater. Pulmonary artery hypertension is generally associated with enlargement of the right descending pulmonary artery.

SPECIAL CHEST RADIOGRAPHIC VIEWS

OBLIQUE VIEWS

In addition to the PA and lateral views, other projections serve special purposes. Oblique views may be invaluable in delineating a pulmonary or mediastinal mass or pulmonary infiltrate from structures that overlie it in the PA and lateral view. A pleural effusion or mediastinal mass is often well demonstrated in oblique views (5). Oblique views are also useful for studying lesions that are visible in the PA view but not in the

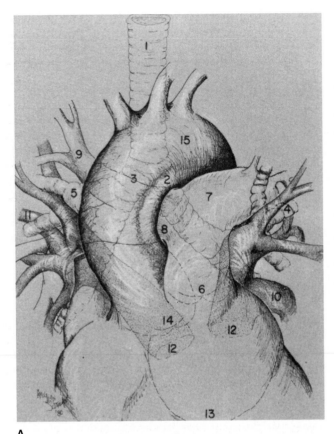

A

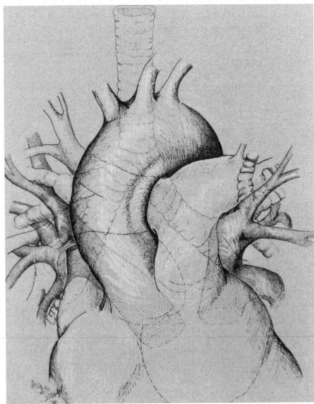

B

FIGURE 5-11. **A:** Depiction of the bronchial and vascular interrelationships in the mediastinum and hilum. Some of the individual structures are identified by numbers. *1,* trachea; *2,* left main bronchus; *3,* right main bronchus; *4,* segmental left upper lobe bronchus; *5,* right upper lobe bronchus; *6,* pulmonary valve; *7,* left main pulmonary artery; *8,* right main pulmonary artery; *9,* right upper lobe (truncus anterior) pulmonary artery; *10,* left lower lobe pulmonary vein; *11,* right upper lobe pulmonary vein; *12,* entrance of pulmonary vein to left atrium; *13,* left atrium; *14,* aortic valve; *15,* aortic arch. **B:** Depiction of the mediastinal, bronchial, and vascular structures without overlying identifying numbers.

lateral view. They may help in determining the site of origin of an intrathoracic lesion. By observing the rotation of a lesion in relation to a rib or to the heart or aorta, it may be possible to ascertain how close the lesion is to that structure and thereby infer its site and sometimes even its point of origin (5). When there are bilateral lesions on the PA view, it may be difficult to decide from the lateral view as to which shadow belongs to which side. Oblique views usually resolve this dilemma (5). Some reports have emphasized the value of oblique chest radiographs in detecting pleural plaques caused by asbestosis. They are also helpful in the differential diagnosis of cardiac and great-vessel enlargement, because the border-forming structures of the cardiomediastinal silhouette are different in oblique projections than those in the frontal and lateral views.

Oblique positions are named according to the part of the chest that is closest to the cassette: right anterior oblique (RAO) view, with the right front of the patient against the cassette, and left anterior oblique (LAO) view, with the left front of the patient against the cassette. The standard angles relative to the coronal plane are 45 degrees for the RAO and 60 degrees for the LAO (5).

As the availability of CT has become universal, oblique images are being used less frequently. The main indication at present is to determine if a low suspicion lesion may be a nipple shadow or an osseous (i.e., rib) abnormality.

LATERAL DECUBITUS VIEWS

The lateral decubitus film is useful for demonstrating a small amount of free pleural fluid or pneumothorax, the extent of a cavity or lung abscess, and the mobility of a mediastinal mass with gravity. As little as 25 to 50 mL of pleural fluid can be visualized (17). This view is particularly useful in determining if the blunting of a costophrenic sulcus is owing to pleural effusion or to pleural thickening (3). Pleural thickening is usually a scar that is formed following organization of an exudate or blood in the pleural space (3). The decubitus film may also be helpful in shifting free fluid out of the way to visualize the underlying lung (2,3,5). Bilateral decubitus films are usually necessary if the effusion is moderately sized or large.

A lateral decubitus view is taken with the patient on his or her side, the x-ray beam aimed parallel to the floor, and the area of interest positioned closest to the film. Air rises and fluid falls; therefore, when right pneumothorax is suspected, for example, the patient should be placed on the left side, with the film and x-ray beam centered over the uppermost part of the right chest. For right-sided pleural fluid, on the other hand, the patient should be lying on the right side, with the x-ray beam centering over the dependent portion of the right chest (5).

LORDOTIC VIEW

The original purpose of the lordotic view of the chest was to partially uncover the pulmonary areas from the bony grid created by the ribs and clavicles on the PA film. When the tube is angled upward, the shadows of the clavicles are projected above the thorax and the ribs become more horizontal (see Fig. 5-12) (5). The anterior part of each rib is thereby superimposed on its posterior portion, reducing the number of obscuring bony structures. Thus, the lordotic projection enables evaluation of the apical portion of the lungs by displacing shadows of the first rib and the clavicle, which may be confusing on the PA projection (3). The lordotic view is also useful for recognizing collapse of the lingula or middle lobe when these areas become very thin and cast minimal shadows on the PA film (5). Lordotic and reverse lordotic views are often good for determining if a lesion is anterior or posterior. An anterior lesion is projected upward, as are other anterior structures (such as ribs and clavicles). The opposite is true for a posterior lesion. A reverse lordotic film produces exactly the opposite changes. Like the oblique images, the computerized tomography (CT) scan has largely replaced this view.

EXPIRATION FILM

Although chest radiographs are routinely taken at full inspiration, an expiratory film may be helpful under appropriate circumstances. For example, a small pneumothorax is often difficult or impossible to be seen on a routine inspiratory PA film. On expiration, the volume of the thorax and of the lungs within it is reduced, but the amount of air in the pleural sac remains essentially unchanged. The pneumothorax then occupies a larger percentage of the area of the thorax and is more easily visible. Also, when a film is taken in expiration, the lungs appear denser because the blood-containing vessels are crowded into a smaller space. Because the blackness of the pneumothorax does not change, the density gradient between the pneumothorax and the lungs becomes larger and this also makes it easier to see the pneumothorax.

Another indication of the expiratory film is to demonstrate air trapping. The bronchi increase in diameter with each inspiration and decrease with each expiration. With a foreign body or tumor in a main bronchus, a valve action may occur, with air bypassing the obstruction on inspiration and becoming trapped on expiration. With expiration, the normal lung reduces in volume and becomes less radiolucent. The obstructed

portion of the lung retains its air, thereby retaining its radiolucency and forcing the mediastinum to shift toward the contralateral side. If a patient has a unilateral respiratory wheeze, air trapping is likely, and an expiratory film is mandatory (5).

OTHER VIEWS

The *overpenetrated grid* radiograph is useful for evaluating densities that lie behind the heart or diaphragm and are seen poorly on routine radiographs. Stereoscopic views can be helpful in localizing any pulmonary lesion and are particularly useful with apical lesions because they can separate pulmonary lesions from the overlying clavicle and first rib (3). *Magnification* radiographs are used occasionally in diffuse lung disease to clarify minute details of the pulmonary parenchyma (10). Double-exposed films in inspiration and expiration are sometimes helpful in evaluating motion of the diaphragms.

FLUOROSCOPY

Fluoroscopy of the chest is useful for examining the movement of pulmonary and cardiac structures and for localizing a pulmonary lesion that is only visible in one of the two conventional radiographic projections. It is particularly helpful for examining diaphragmatic motion (3,18). When searching for diaphragmatic paralysis, it is often best to use the lateral projection so that motion of both hemidiaphragms can be observed simultaneously (3). A paralyzed hemidiaphragm moves paradoxically. This paradoxical motion is often difficult to appreciate during quiet breathing but usually becomes readily apparent during a quick, short "sniff" (sniff test). Localized weakness in part of one hemidiaphragm (eventration) is often misinterpreted as diaphragmatic paralysis. This error can be avoided by fluoroscopy in the lateral projection; partial eventration is then manifested by paradoxical motion of one portion of the hemidiaphragm, whereas the other portion moves normally. Eventration of an entire hemidiaphragm is impossible to distinguish from paralysis because, in both instances, the entire hemidiaphragm moves paradoxically (3).

When fluoroscopy is combined with a barium swallow, lesions within the esophagus can be seen. Moreover, the pattern of displacement of the esophagus by a mass in the middle mediastinum helps to determine the nature of the mass (3,18). Respiratory maneuvers affect the size of large venous structures in the chest, which become smaller during a Valsalva maneuver and larger during a Müller maneuver. These maneuvers do not change the size of solid masses. Pulsation of a mediastinal mass suggests it is vascular. However, pulsation must be interpreted with care: masses that are adjacent to the

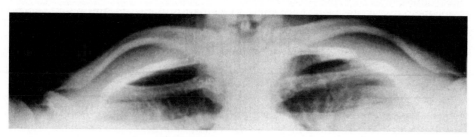

FIGURE 5-12. Normal apical lordotic view of the chest. Compare with Figure 5-1 to appreciate the difference in visualization of the lung apices.

aorta often transmit its pulsations and appear to be pulsating; in contrast, large aortic aneurysms often pulsate poorly (3).

Chest fluoroscopy also can be useful when trying to determine if a suspected pulmonary nodule on a chest radiograph (a) is real versus a superimposition of unrelated shadows, or (b) is intrapulmonary versus extrapulmonary.

In past years, fluoroscopy of the chest was used as a screening procedure for routine chest examination (2,3). This is no longer acceptable for at least three reasons: (a) the patient's exposure to x-rays is much greater during even a short fluoroscopic examination than during standard radiographs, (b) small lesions in the lung fields are overlooked at fluoroscopy, and (c) usually no permanent record of the fluoroscopic examination is available. However, fluoroscopy of the chest is warranted when specific information is being sought or when it is necessary to monitor "online" the performance of a special procedure, such as needle aspiration of a pulmonary mass or transbronchial biopsy (3).

TOMOGRAPHY

INDICATIONS FOR TOMOGRAPHY

Tomography is useful when there is a need for precise knowledge of the morphologic characteristics of lesions visible on plain radiographs whose nature is obscured by superimposed images lying superficial or deep to them (2).

CONVENTIONAL TOMOGRAPHY

If the x-ray tube and film are in motion during exposure, the resulting radiograph (called a *tomogram* or *laminagram*) will show a sharply focused plane or "cut" through the body, with adjacent planes being blurred (18). The thinness of the plane and successful blurring of the other planes are factors that can be controlled to some degree to determine the ultimate appearance of the film. As the distance of the x-ray tube from the table determines the plane in focus, the films are usually made in a series of cuts so that each level through the lung is visualized sharply, without overlying shadows (see Fig. 5-13) (18). Posterior oblique tomography at an angle of 55 degrees has been recommended for displaying a clearer outline of the anatomic components of the hila (19). Conventional tomography accurately detects calcification within pulmonary nodules and other thoracic lesions.

In most institutions, conventional tomography has been largely or completely superseded by CT in evaluating pulmonary nodules, the hila, the mediastinum, and the lung parenchyma. However, conventional tomography remains an accurate and useful technique.

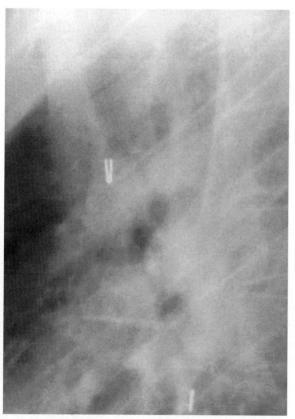

A

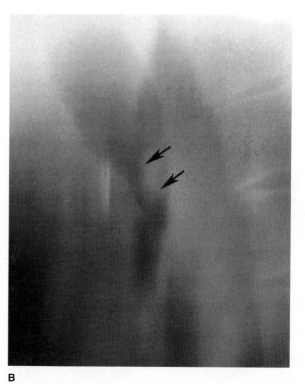

B

FIGURE 5-13. The value of plain tomography in evaluating pathology of the central airways. **A:** Lateral chest radiograph after resection of esophageal carcinoma in a patient who presented with wheezing. The lower portion of the tracheal air column is not well seen, but the presence of a lesion is not clear. **B:** Lateral tomogram through the trachea. Note that the overlying surgical clip that is seen clearly in (A) is blurred on the tomogram. This is the means by which tomography produces clearer visualization of selected planes. The tomogram clearly shows the presence of a constricting tumor recurrence narrowing the lower trachea (*arrows*).

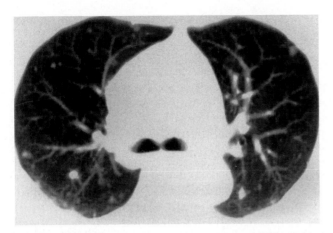

FIGURE 5-14. Computerized tomography (CT) is the method of choice for detecting pulmonary metastases (as shown here in a patient with metastatic melanoma) and other kinds of pulmonary nodules.

COMPUTED TOMOGRAPHY

The development of CT brought diagnostic medical imaging into the modern age (Figs. 5-14–5-21). It combined the basic phenomenon upon which the field of radiology was founded (differential x-ray attenuation by tissues) with the basis of subsequent developments (use of nonfilm x-ray detectors, digital computers, and video displays). Previous methods of forming x-ray images used direct geometric projection of an x-ray shadowgraph of the patient's body on a piece of film by a large-area beam of x-ray photons. CT uses a series of planar projections made by a thin beam of x-ray photons. These planar projections are mathematically recombined by the *computer* to form the patient's cross-sectional *tomographic* image that displays the attenuation values of the many small areas ("picture elements" or "pixels"). CT thus introduced into clinical practice an entirely new approach to diagnostic imaging, aspects of which have subsequently been utilized in digital

radiography, fluoroscopy, ultrasound, and magnetic resonance imaging. The diagnostic advantages of CT are owing to its transaxial tomographic (slicelike) format and its high sensitivity to differences in electron density (and thus in x-ray attenuation) between different tissues. In addition, because the x-ray attenuation measurements are stored in the computer, the image can be enhanced or manipulated mathematically. Adjustments of the computer data (windowing) allow for differences in contrasts. For example, a wider window [2200/–600 Hounsfield units (HU)] allows for better evaluation of the lung parenchyma and a narrower window (400/40 HU) is better for assessing mediastinal structures (see Figs. 5-15 and 5-16). The technique of high-resolution CT (HRCT), a valuable method of studying the lung parenchyma, combines very thin slices with mathematical filtering of the computer data to produce increased edge definition in the final image.

Thoracic CT has found widespread use in the assessment of masses and neoplasms, including primary lung cancer, hilar and mediastinal masses, and pulmonary nodules (Figs. 5-14 and 5-17) (20–33). It is now the standard of care for patients with such conditions, who require diagnostic imaging beyond the plain chest radiograph and its simple variants (e.g., fluoroscopy). HRCT of the lung parenchyma has been developed in the last few years and has been widely used for evaluating interstitial lung disease and bronchial abnormalities (see Fig. 5-18) (34–42). CT has application in vascular imaging in the thorax, most notably for suspected aortic dissection and superior vena cava obstruction (see Fig. 5-19) (43,44). In addition, CT is unsurpassed in the detection and localization of pericardial and pleural fluid collections (see Fig. 5-20) (45–48). Finally, CT may be used effectively to guide percutaneous biopsy and drainage of thoracic lesions (49,50). The patient is imaged to localize the lesion, and the skin entry site is identified with the aid of the CT scanner's positioning lights. A similar approach can be used to localize fluid collections or pneumothoraces that are not responding to blindly placed thoracostomy tubes and then to guide percutaneously placed drains into the refractory collections.

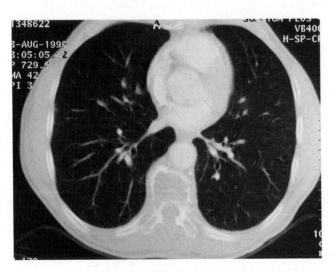

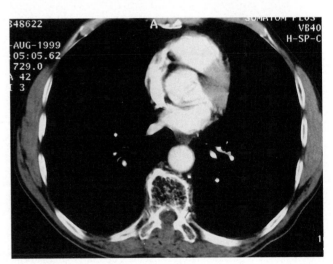

FIGURES 5-15 AND 5-16. Images obtained of the chest at the level of the heart demonstrating differences in appearance owing to computer manipulations. The lungs (Fig. 5-15) are well seen with the wider window while the heart and mediastinal structures (Fig. 5-16) are better visualized with the narrow settings.

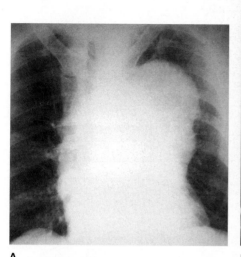 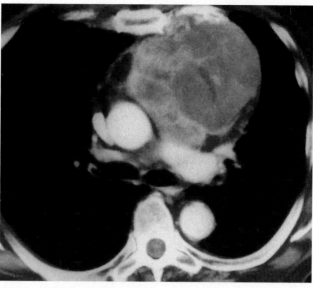

A   B

FIGURE 5-17. Computerized tomography (CT) is the method of choice for detailed evaluation of most patients with mediastinal masses. **A:** The posteroanterior chest radiograph in this patient shows a large mass. **B:** The CT scan clearly delineates the anterior mediastinal location of the mass and separates it from the mediastinal vasculature, facilitating both the differential diagnosis and the surgical planning.

Helical CT

Over the past decade, CT has benefited from advances in technology with the advent of helical scanning (51). Conventional CT obtains images one section at a time as the x-ray tubes stop and rotate around the patient at each subsequent station. Conversely, with helical acquisition, the patient continuously moves as the x-ray tube rotates, resulting in a helical (spiral) pathway. As all of the data are available from the entire acquisition, the images can be reconstructed at select levels and locations. A further benefit is the rapid speed of helical CT, which allows for acquisition during a single breath hold—an important feature in lung imaging that reduces respiratory motion artifacts.

CT pulmonary angiography utilizing helical CT is a less invasive method than conventional pulmonary angiography for evaluating patients with suspected pulmonary thromboembolism (PE) (52). In a prospective study of 75 patients, Remy-Jardin et al. found that helical CT angiography was highly sensitive (91%) and specific (78%) for detecting PE (51, 52). Direct signs of PE on the CT pulmonary angiogram include vessel cutoff and a filling defect (see Fig. 5-21). Indirect signs include low attenuation in a segmental or subsegmental distribution (oligemia) or wedge-shaped infarct. Limitations include respiratory motion artifact, observer inexperience, and inability to detect emboli in small peripheral pulmonary arteries. The CT pulmonary angiogram in the diagnostic algorithm for PE has yet to be defined, and a National Heart, Lung, and Blood Institute (NHLBI) trial is under way to study this issue.

Contrast Helical CT for Assessing Solitary Pulmonary Nodules

The solitary pulmonary nodule is frequently encountered on the chest radiograph or chest CT scan. Although the detection of

these nodules may be challenging, the diagnostic evaluation of these lesions can be even more challenging. Goals include minimizing removal of benign nodules, maximizing removal of malignant nodules at a curable stage, maximizing use of noninvasive studies, and maintaining cost effectiveness.

It has been recognized that malignant neoplasms have an abundant vascular supply (53). Applying this knowledge, Swensen et al. theorized that the degree of enhancement of a solitary pulmonary nodule on CT should be related to the amount of contrast entering that nodule, which is in turn related to the lesion's blood supply (54,55). These investigators imaged lung nodules using the helical technique with bolus IV contrast injection in 105 patients. Swensen found that malignant neoplasms enhanced significantly more than benign neoplasms (median 40 HU versus median 12 HU) and, with a threshold of 20 HU, sensitivity was 100% and specificity was 77%. No malignant nodule enhanced <20 HU; the authors concluded that the degree of enhancement is an indicator of malignancy.

Other Helical CT Applications

Other uses of helical CT include virtual bronchoscopy for evaluation of endobronchial abnormalities, three-dimensional reconstruction of mediastinal and vascular abnormalities, and coronary artery evaluation (51,56,57). Evaluation of coronary arteries for calcification by chest CT is a noninvasive method to assess hemodynamically significant stenoses and may be used as a screening study in selected populations. By acquiring thin section helical images with cardiac gaiting, image quality is markedly improved and the amount of coronary artery calcification may be quantified. Recent studies have reported sensitivities and specificities of 88% to 91% and 52%, respectively (57,58).

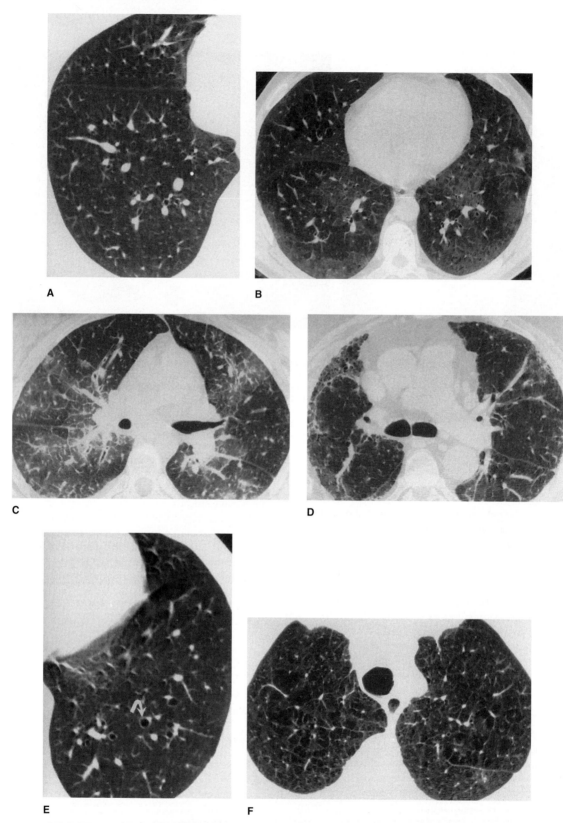

FIGURE 5-18. Examples of various common findings on high-resolution CT of the lung parenchyma. **A:** Normal lung. The vessels, bronchi, and fissures are seen clearly. **B:** Patient with alveolitis. There is multifocal faint opacification of the lungs, referred to as "ground-glass opacity." This usually, but not always, indicates the presence of an active, treatable process. **C:** Patient with lymphangitic carcinomatosis. Nodularity, bronchial wall thickening, and interlobular septal (interstitial) thickening are present. **D:** Patient with idiopathic pulmonary fibrosis. Characteristically subpleural changes of fibrosis and cyst formation ("honeycombing") are clearly visible on the HRCT image. **E:** Patient with focal bronchiectasis. Note the dilated bronchi compared with (A) and also compared with associated vessels in the same area, forming the so-called "signet-ring" (*arrow*) appearance. **F:** Patient with diffuse emphysema. Areas of destroyed lung tissue are apparent (due to their low density) as dark regions, usually without definite walls.

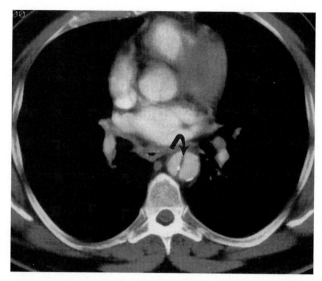

FIGURE 5-19. This contrast-enhanced CT section shows a Type B aortic dissection. The intimal flap, containing a fleck of calcium, is well seen (*arrow*).

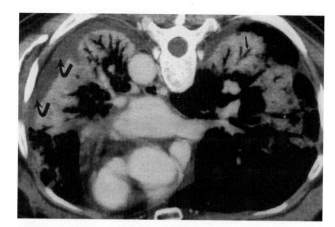

FIGURE 5-20. The left pleural effusion (*curved arrows*) is clearly visualized in this patient and easily distinguished from the adjacent lung consolidation. Note, in the consolidated areas of both left and right lungs, the presence of "air bronchograms" (one is indicated in the right lung by a small straight *arrow*).

MAGNETIC RESONANCE

Magnetic resonance imaging (MRI) is based on magnetization of the patient's tissue, generation of a weak electromagnetic signal by the application of a radiofrequency pulse, and spatially mapping that signal by manipulating its frequency and phase in a location-dependent manner using magnetic field gradients. Unlike CT, MRI does not require mechanical motions of the scanner; therefore, it can image directly in nontransaxial planes. However, like CT, it is a tomographic technique.

Although electromagnetic radiation is involved, the energy levels used in MRI are well below the levels needed to ionize molecules, and MRI appears to be remarkably free of significant bioeffects. However, the strong magnetic field is a major safety hazard because the magnetic forces near a whole-body MR imager are strong enough to cause significant projectile hazards. For example, an oxygen cylinder brought into an MR examination room will fly into the bore of the magnet with a

terminal velocity of about 45 miles per hour. The possibility of displacements or torques on metallic implants within patients must also be considered. Finally, the magnetic field can operate reed relays in cardiac pacemakers and can cause a change in the pacing mode. Accordingly, strict security around MR facilities is essential to prevent patients with certain types of metallic implants from entering the scanner and to prevent medical personnel from carrying objects that could become projectiles into the scan room.

MRI produces extremely high contrast between different types of soft tissues. This soft tissue contrast is based on intrinsic properties of the tissues and also on operator-selectable machine parameters. The tissue properties are: (a) the tissue concentration of protons available to produce an MR signal ("proton density"); (b) the presence of motion or blood flow; and (c) two tissue properties known as T1 and T2, time constants that describe how quickly an MR signal can be generated (T1) from a tissue and how quickly the MR signal, once generated, decays (T2). In general, pathologic tissues have

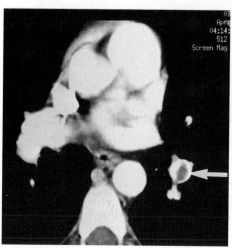

A

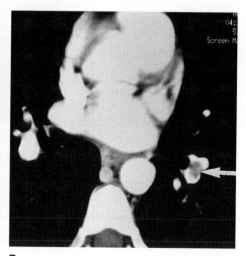

B

FIGURE 5-21. (A,B) Contrast enhanced CT scan of the mediastinum demonstrating a nonocclusive thrombus in the left lower lobar artery at its branch point consistent with an acute saddle embolus.

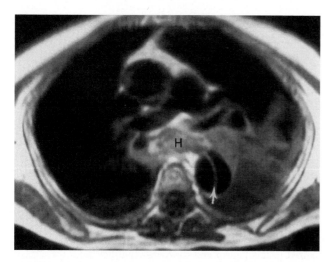

FIGURE 5-22. Magnetic resonance imaging (MRI) was done in this patient with suspected aortic dissection who had renal dysfunction and thus was a poor candidate for intravenous contrast-enhanced CT. The intimal flap of a type B dissection is visible (*arrow*), and a mediastinal hematoma (*H*) was found as well.

long T1 times and appear dark on those MR images whose appearance is conditioned primarily by T1 effects ("T1-weighted images"). Usually, pathologic tissues also have long T2 times and appear bright on T2-weighted images. Flowing blood also can appear either bright or dark on MR images, depending on the examination technique that is used.

The usefulness of MRI in thoracic diseases is more limited than that of CT; for most patients who require further imaging

beyond the plain chest radiograph, CT is the preferred initial choice because it is more effective, less expensive, and more widely available (59). In certain situations, however, MRI is useful to answer questions that remain after a CT examination has been performed. These situations include indeterminate mediastinal, chest wall, or vascular invasion by lung carcinoma and the evaluation of suspected hilar masses (20, 23,25,26,59). In still other patients, MRI is the initial procedure of choice because the patient is allergic to contrast material that may be deemed necessary for a particular CT examination (60). The most common setting in which this occurs is suspected aortic dissection, but an allergy to contrast material can mandate the use of MRI for other vascular imaging problems as well (see Fig. 5-22) (43,59,61–63). Finally, there are a few conditions in which MRI has a real diagnostic advantage over CT and should be used as the initial procedure of choice. These include upper-extremity deep venous thrombosis (DVT), brachial plexopathies and superior sulcus tumors, and cardiac and paracardiac masses (see Fig. 5-23) (64–69).

ULTRASOUND

Like CT and MRI, ultrasound is a tomographic technique. Ultrasound has limited usefulness in evaluating the lungs because the sound beam is transmitted poorly by the air-containing alveoli and airways. However, there are three situations in which ultrasound is useful for evaluating chest diseases. First, ultrasound is widely used to evaluate disorders of the heart and aortic root. Areas in which the heart and mediastinal structures touch the chest wall without lung intervening are used as "acoustic windows" for transmission of the sound beam into the mediastinum. Ultrasound is the procedure of

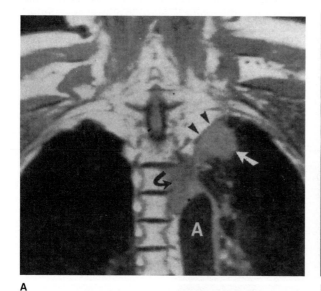

A

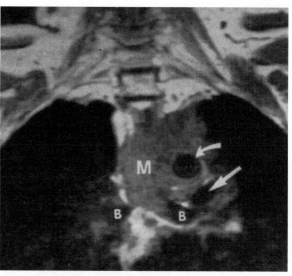

B

FIGURE 5-23. Magnetic resonance (MR) images of a 61-year-old man with a left superior sulcus (Pancoast) tumor, a squamous cell carcinoma. **A:** Coronal T1-weighted MR scan reveals a mass (*white arrow*) that is confined within the apical pleura. The subpleural fat, which has high signal intensity (*arrowheads*), is preserved. Medially, the mass is infiltrating the mediastinum (*black curved arrow*) and is contiguous with the thoracic aorta (*A*). **B:** Coronal MR scan 20 mm anterior to first image (*left*) demonstrates extension of the mass (*M*) into the mediastinum. The relationship of the mass to the aortic arch (*curved arrow*), main pulmonary artery (*straight arrow*), and bronchi (*B*) can be appreciated. (From Takasugi JE, Rapaport S, Shaw C. Superior sulcus tumors: the role of imaging. *J Thorac Imaging* 1989;4:41–48, with permission.)

choice to detect or exclude pericardial effusion. Unique information can also be obtained concerning valvular heart disease (e.g., mitral stenosis), the presence of vegetations or clots in the cardiac chambers, and global or segmental abnormalities of cardiac contraction. The second situation in which ultrasound is useful in the evaluation of chest pathology is in precisely localizing pleural effusions for aspiration or drainage (70,71). It should be emphasized that ultrasound should not be routinely used for this purpose because most effusions can be safely and easily aspirated after localization by physical examination. Finally, ultrasound may be used to assess diaphragm motion analogous to the fluoroscopic "sniff" test. This is particularly useful in ICU settings where the study can be done portably with ultrasound.

CONTRAST EXAMINATIONS

Air is the "natural" contrast material on which the diagnostic value of the plain chest film depends. Supplementary information is gained by introducing extraneous contrast material into different structural compartments of the thorax. "Positive" contrast material (e.g., barium sulfate suspension) is commonly introduced into the esophagus, whereas other suitable media are used to visualize cardiac chambers, trachea and bronchi, pulmonary vessels, aorta, bronchial and mediastinal arteries, superior vena cava, and mediastinal veins. Intravenously administered contrast material has become commonly used in many CT and MRI examinations outside of the thorax. Iodinated contrast material is used for CT, whereas metal chelates are employed for MRI. In thoracic imaging with CT and MRI, the use of contrast is more selective and contrast is administered in a minority of examinations. To achieve "negative" contrast, air or other gases can be introduced, although this is no longer done in clinical practice.

BARIUM SWALLOW

Of all the contrast examinations, the barium swallow, which is usually performed under fluoroscopic guidance, is the simplest to perform. The esophageal lumen is outlined by radiopaque barium sulfate. Abnormalities of the esophagus itself, such as tumor or achalasia, can be seen (3). Formerly used to assess mediastinal masses and cardiac enlargement, the barium swallow has been replaced for these purposes by more specific tests (e.g., CT, MRI, and ultrasound).

BRONCHOGRAPHY

The trachea and bronchi can be better defined by instillation of radiopaque contrast medium into the lumina of the trachea and bronchial tree (bronchography). It is mostly used for diagnosing bronchiectasis and for mapping its location before surgical resection. In the past, prior to development of the flexible bronchoscope, bronchography was used to demonstrate an obstructing lesion that was inaccessible to the rigid bronchoscope. Today, bronchography is rarely performed. Bronchiectasis is infrequent and seldom requires surgical treatment (5). When present, it can be visualized accurately with the less hazardous CT examination. The advent of fiberoptic bronchoscopy has rendered fewer lesions inaccessible to direct vision, and bronchoscopic brush or forceps biopsy and transthoracic needle puncture are more precise methods of diagnosing a pulmonary lesion than bronchography is. If bronchography is performed, it should be done in conjunction with fiber-optic bronchoscopy.

PULMONARY ANGIOGRAPHY

Pulmonary angiography involves the rapid injection of a radiopaque dye into the pulmonary circulation via a catheter into the superior vena cava, right atrium, right ventricle, or main pulmonary artery; or by selective injection into the right or left pulmonary artery or branches of these (Figs. 5-9 and 5-10) (2,3). Direct injection into the pulmonary artery branches invariably produces the clearest opacification of the pulmonary vascular tree; this superior visualization usually outweighs any disadvantage inherent in the catheterization procedure (2).

Angiography is principally useful for investigating pulmonary thromboembolic disease. In recent years, the popularization of ventilation and perfusion scans of the lung ($\dot{V}/\dot{Q}$) using radioactive isotopes has relegated pulmonary angiography to a secondary role in most cases. The accuracy of $\dot{V}/\dot{Q}$ scans for diagnosing pulmonary thromboemboli has recently been assessed and has been shown to be definitive in some circumstances but inaccurate in others (72). Angiography is almost always indicated when massive pulmonary embolus is suspected as the basis for circulatory collapse and when immediate surgical intervention is contemplated. If surgical interruption of the inferior vena cava is planned because of failure of medical therapy or if thrombolytic therapy is planned, pulmonary angiography should usually be performed. Angiography is commonly used in a clinical setting in which anticoagulation is considered dangerous or in patients whose $\dot{V}/\dot{Q}$ scan results are equivocal or the clinical and lung scan evaluations lead to markedly different conclusions.

Less common indications for angiography include: (a) suspected congenital abnormalities of the arterial system, such as agenesis or hypoplasia of a pulmonary artery; (b) suspected congenital abnormalities of the pulmonary venous circulation, such as anomalous pulmonary venous drainage and pulmonary varix; and (c) suspected pulmonary AV malformations. In some instances, noninvasive techniques such as CT, ultrasound, and MRI provide diagnostic information in these settings.

The decision to perform pulmonary angiography should be made carefully because the procedure is associated with slight morbidity and rare mortality. However, these risks are not great in experienced hands (73).

Before injection of contrast material into the pulmonary artery, the pulmonary artery pressure should always be measured because it is dangerous to perform angiography in a patient with severe pulmonary arterial hypertension. If physiologic measurements such as wedge pressure or oxygen saturations are needed, they should be obtained before contrast material is injected because contrast material has numerous physiologic effects that may alter these parameters.

VENTILATION–PERFUSION LUNG SCANNING

There has been a rapid evolution of imaging devices and radiopharmaceuticals for the study of regional pulmonary function by inhalation and perfusion scintigraphy. Although the number of indications for lung scanning has increased, the major clinical application is in the evaluation for pulmonary thromboembolism and the performance of preoperative lung function studies (72,74–78). It is beyond the scope of this chapter to describe in detail the imaging techniques and methods of interpretation of lung scans. They are only summarized here, and the interested reader is referred to reviews of this subject (74–76).

Lung scans are obtained by measuring gamma radiation emitted from the chest after radiopharmaceuticals are injected into the bloodstream or are inhaled into the air spaces. Ventilation–perfusion scintigraphy is performed with gamma cameras, which permit viewing a large area at once.

Interfacing the gamma camera with a computer allows quantification of pulmonary $\dot{V}/\dot{Q}$ scans and measurement of regional ventilation and perfusion ratios. Thus, prior to lung resection, the surgeon can determine the contribution to overall pulmonary function of the region of lung to be resected. Perfusion lung scans can be obtained for either particulate or gaseous radionuclides. For the particulate type, a standard quantity of particles (usually macroaggregates of human serum albumin) with a size of 10 to 60 mm is injected into a peripheral vein. Because the particles are larger than capillaries, they lodge in the first capillary bed encountered (74). Techniques for assessing pulmonary ventilation involve the inhalation of a radioactive gas or a nebulized aerosol of a radioactive material (such as albumin labeled with Technetium-99). For the latter, the particles must be small enough (<1 mm in diameter) to reach the alveoli.

As stressed previously, the major indication for lung scanning is the investigation of pulmonary thromboembolism. Perfusion studies are diagnostically valuable only when the scan image is normal or comparable with a current chest radiograph and ventilation scan. The absence of perfusion in an area of lung is nonspecific. It can be due to thromboembolic disease or to primary pulmonary vascular disease such as arteritis; it can be secondary to airway obstruction or other abnormalities of ventilation; or it can result from destruction of lung parenchyma, as in bullous emphysema. Only when the areas of perfusion abnormality correspond to pulmonary segments or subsegments (indicating a distribution comparable with the distribution of the pulmonary arteries) and when ventilation in the analogous area is normal can pulmonary vascular disease be diagnosed with confidence. Pulmonary vascular disease is most commonly owing to pulmonary embolism, and thus the assumption is made that areas of normal ventilation and abnormal perfusion are owing to pulmonary embolism. The diagnostic scheme for evaluating perfusion defects with and without ventilation and chest x-ray abnormalities is presented in detailed reviews (74–77). A normal lung scan excludes pulmonary embolism for all practical purposes (see Fig. 5-24). Multiple perfusion defects in areas of normal ventilation are characteristic of pulmonary embolism (see Fig. 5-25A, B). Intermediate patterns are more difficult to interpret. In many of

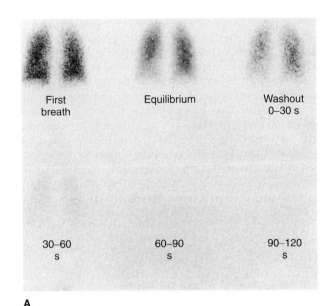

A

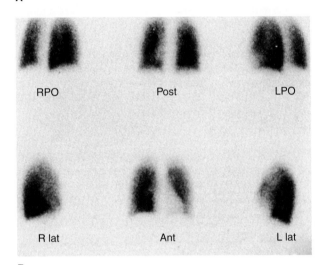

B

FIGURE 5-24. **A:** Ventilation phase of a ventilation–perfusion scan. Note that in the "first-breath" and in "equilibrium" images there is homogeneous distribution of the radioactivity in both lungs. Note that in the "wash-out" phase (which is performed by serial imaging when the patient is no longer breathing in radioactive gas, so that the gas already in the lungs is imaged as it exits from the lungs), there is no evidence of abnormal retention of radioactive gas. **B:** Perfusion images of the same patient. It is important to obtain at least six views of the lungs. In this patient, the perfusion is normal, with no focal defects seen in the images. The radioactive particles are injected with the patient lying supine. Note on the right and left lateral views that there is more perfusion in the posterior (dependent) portions of the lungs. This is a graphic demonstration of the effect of gravity on the pulmonary perfusion gradient.

those cases, a pulmonary angiogram must be performed to make the diagnosis accurate (Fig. 5-25C). Alternatively, evaluation of the deep venous system with ultrasound may be used as an ancillary study. If the ultrasound is diagnostic of clots in the deep venous system, pulmonary angiography may be avoided.

An additional use of lung scanning has been in the preoperative evaluation of patients potentially undergoing lung

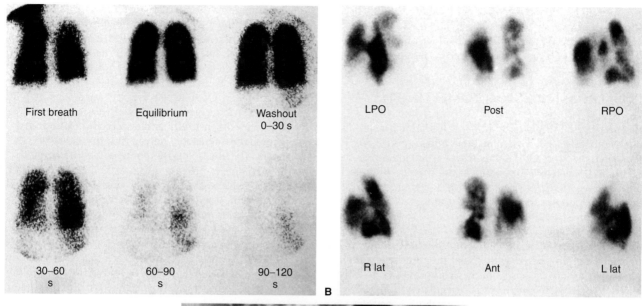

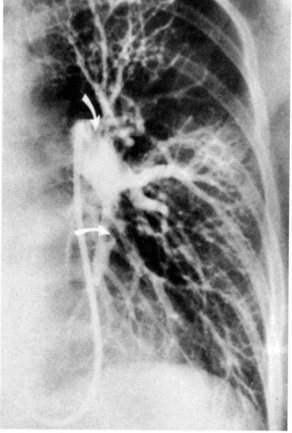

FIGURE 5-25. **A:** Ventilation scan in a patient with pulmonary embolism. There is no significant abnormality in ventilation. Focal activity in the later images is due to concentration of xenon in the liver. **B:** Perfusion scan in the same patient. Multiple perfusion defects that are wedge-shaped and bilateral are seen in the perfusion images. This is a classic appearance for pulmonary embolism. **C:** Selective pulmonary arteriogram on the same patient. Multiple filling defects in pulmonary arteries are demonstrated (*arrows*). This is angiographic proof of pulmonary embolism.

resection (e.g., lobectomy or pneumonectomy) (78). By obtaining quantitative lung measurements of lung perfusion and ventilation, an estimation of the percentage of function that each lobe or lung contributes can be assessed.

POSITRON-EMISSION TOMOGRAPHY

Positron-emission tomography, or PET, scanning is an imaging technique based on annihilation of positrons (79,80). Photons from positron annihilation travel 180 degrees from each other, and when these photons strike the crystal detectors around the patient, the origin of the annihilation can be calculated. Only photons that strike the detectors 180 degrees apart within a very short interval are accepted for imaging, improving sensitivity, and resolution.

PET uses physiologically and metabolically active radiopharmaceuticals labeled with positron emitters, resulting in data that produce an image on the basis of metabolic activity and not anatomy. Owing to their deregulated growth properties, most malignant tumors utilize metabolic substrates such as glucose more readily than normal tissue does. The glucose analog fluorine-18 fluorodeoxyglucose (FDG) is currently used in the diagnosis and staging of cancers such as nonsmall and small cell lung cancer (NSCLC), lymphoma, breast and colon cancer, and melanoma.

However, glucose metabolism is affected in many disease states and is not specific for neoplastic processes. This can potentially result in false-positive FDG PET studies in inflammatory or other nonneoplastic conditions such as hamartomas, granulomas, tuberculosis, some fungal infection, and Wegener granulomatosis (see Fig. 5-26). Benign pulmonary nodules show only very low or no FDG uptake (81). With multiple possibilities for false-positive results, PET data need to be incorporated with clinical and radiographic findings to best assess any given abnormality and to guide appropriate management.

In an attempt to reduce false-positive results, PET images are compared side by side or are fused with CT images for anatomic correlation. With PET/CT detectors, a whole-body low-dose CT scan is acquired separately from the PET but during the same examination, for attenuation correction. Some authors advocate performing the CT acquisition for fully diagnostic CT data with intravenous and oral contrast agents in all patients. Still other authors state that low radiation, "nondiagnostic" data are sufficient for attenuation correction and anatomic correlation (82,83).

The PET and CT data sets are generated separately by the system but can be fused. PET/CT fusion has proven to provide increased sensitivity and specificity for findings versus each modality alone or viewed side by side (84). PET/CT scanners allow for acquisition of both the PET and CT scan in one study, thus improving interpretation of the data. PET/CT is currently the most accurate imaging modality for staging in NSCLC, with sensitivity and specificity near 90% for each. This data fusion improves lesion localization, which is difficult, if not impossible, by PET alone; the resolution of most units is approximately 6 to 8 mm.

Applications of PET in lung cancer currently include mediastinal staging, evaluation of indeterminate pulmonary nodules, assessment of distant metastases, and restaging for response to treatment and recurrence after treatment with chemotherapy and radiation (85). Use of PET has also shown to help target radiation therapy fields (82,85) and to guide biopsies. PET has also had an impact on patient management when subclinical distant disease is detected, halting unnecessary thoracotomies. Multiple studies have demonstrated the utility of FDG PET for pulmonary nodule evaluation (81,86). With the advent of low-dose screening for lung cancer, more and more asymptomatic pulmonary nodules are being discovered (81,87). While the long-term outcome of this has yet to be determined, PET imaging is now and will likely continue to be an important part of the algorithm.

One of the more promising applications of PET/CT is staging of mediastinal lymph nodes in the tumor, node, and metastasis (TNM) staging system. In the current TNM staging system, pathologic staging, via mediastinoscopy, is considered more accurate than clinical or radiographic staging (88). Although anatomic radiographic staging alone frequently underestimates the extent of disease, PET/CT may offer additional advantages of demarcation of the primary tumor,

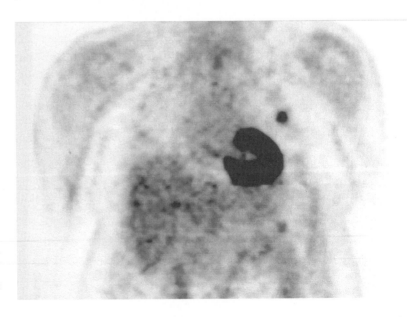

FIGURE 5-26. Positron-emission tomography scan shows focal nodule in the left lung (SUV 4.6) suspicious for malignancy. Biopsy has proven granuloma. Note physiologic uptake of FDG in liver. Physiologic cardiac uptake can vary.

precise localization of mediastinal lymph node metastases, and classification and localization of extrathoracic lesions (see Fig 5-27). This offers more precise surgical management, mediastinal staging, and radiation therapy.

Today, PET/CT represents an important advance in the staging of lung cancer. When using PET in evaluating lung cancer and, particularly, in staging the mediastinum, one must take into account the need for anatomic correlation (CT) and the significance of false-positive and false-negative results. A positive PET may not represent malignant disease, as mentioned above, but may reflect potential benign or inflammatory processes. PET/CT may be used in this setting to guide biopsies, especially if initial biopsy results are unexpectedly negative (89). A negative PET/CT scan result has a negative predictive value reported near 88.3% (88,90). Patients with negative PET mediastinal results may not require mediastinoscopy before exploration for resection and mediastinal lymph node dissection (89). Nevertheless, mediastinoscopy currently remains the standard in staging the mediastinum in patients with lung cancer, especially in patients with high pretest probability for cancer (81). PET/CT has demonstrated economic advantages with exclusion of unnecessary examinations for unclear findings, avoidance of ineffective surgery and radiation therapy, and for the assessment of tumor recurrence and scar. As a complimentary modality to other imaging and surgical methods, PET improves the overall accuracy, clinical evaluation, and staging of lung cancer.

REFERENCES

1. Fraser RG, Paré JAP, Paré PD, et al. The normal chest. In: Fraser RG, Paré JAP, Paré PD et al., eds. *Diagnosis of diseases of the chest,* 3rd ed. Philadelphia: WB Saunders, 1988:1–291.
2. Fraser RG, Paré JAP, Paré PD, et al. Methods of roentgenologic and pathologic investigation. In: Fraser RG, Paré JAP, Paré PD et al., eds. *Diagnosis of diseases of the chest,* 3rd ed. Philadelphia: WB Saunders, 1988:315–387.
3. Miller TW. Radiographic evaluation of the chest. In: Fishman AP, ed. *Pulmonary diseases and disorders,* 2nd ed. New York: McGraw-Hill, 1988:479–528.
4. Sagel SS, Evans RG, Forrest JV, et al. Efficiency of routine screening and lateral chest radiographs in a hospital based population. *N Engl J Med* 1974;291:1001–1004.
5. Felson B. The chest roentgenologic work up. *Basics R D* 1980; 81:1–4.
6. Garland LH. Studies on the accuracy of diagnostic procedures. *Am J Roentgenol* 1959;82:25–38.
7. Garland LH. On the scientific evaluation of diagnostic procedures. *Radiology* 1949;52:309–327.
8. Garland LH, Cochrane AL. Results of international test in chest roentgenogram interpretation. *JAMA* 1952;149:631–634.
9. Felson B, Morgan W, Bristol VC, et al. Observations on the results of multiple readings of chest films on coal miners pneumoconiosis. *Radiology* 1973;109:19–23.
10. Tuddenham WJ. Problems of perception in chest roentgenology: facts and fallacies. *Radiol Clin North Am* 1963;1:277–289.
11. Fraser RG. Measurements of the caliber of human bronchi in three phases of respiration by cinebronchography. *J Can Assoc Radiol* 1961;12:102–112.
12. Merendino KA, Kirilak LB. Human measurements involved in tracheobronchial resection and reconstruction procedures: report of case of bronchial adenoma. *Surgery* 1954;35:590–597.
13. Jesseph JE, Merendino KA. The dimensional interrelationships of the major components of the human tracheobronchial tree. *Surg Gynecol Obstet* 1957;105:210–214.
14. Bachman AL, Teixidor HS. The posterior tracheal band: a reflector of local superior mediastinal abnormality. *Br J Radiol* 1975;48:352–359.
15. Felson B. *Chest roentgenology.* Philadelphia: WB Saunders, 1973.
16. Chang CH. The normal roentgenographic measurements of the right descending pulmonary artery in 1,085 cases. *Am J Roentgenol* 1962;87:929–935.
17. Hesser I. Roentgen examination of pleural fluid. A study of the localization of free effusions, the potentialities of diagnosing minimal quantities of fluid and its existence under physiological conditions. *Acta Radiol Suppl (Stockh)* 1951;86:1–80.
18. Scanlon GT. Use of radiology in the diagnosis of lung disease. In: Baum GL, ed. *Textbook of pulmonary diseases,* 2nd ed. Boston: Little, Brown and Company, 1974:85–102.
19. Favez G, Willa C, Heinzer F. Posterior oblique tomography at an angle of 55 degrees in chest roentgenology. *Am J Roentgenol* 1974; 120:907–915.
20. Webb WR, Gatsonis C, Zerhouni EA, et al. CT and MR imaging in staging non-small cell bronchogenic carcinoma: report of the Radiologic Diagnostic Oncology Group. *Radiology* 1991;178:705–713.
21. Patterson GA, Ginsberg RJ, Poon PY, et al. A prospective evaluation of magnetic resonance imaging, computed tomography, and mediastinoscopy in the preoperative assessment of mediastinal node status in bronchogenic carcinoma. *J Thorac Cardiovasc Surg* 1987;94:679–684.

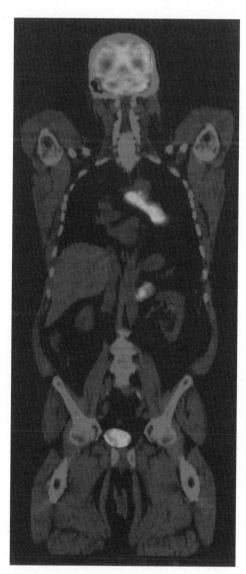

FIGURE 5-27. Fused PT/CT coronal slice of a patient with a hypermetabolic lung mass. Left adrenal mass consistent with metastasis.

22. Friedman PJ. Lung cancer staging: efficacy of CT. *Radiology* 1992;182:307–309.
23. Heelan RT, Demas BE, Caravelli JF, et al. Superior sulcus tumors: CT and MR imaging. *Radiology* 1989;170:637–641.
24. McLoud TC, Bourgouin PM, Greenberg RW, et al. Bronchogenic carcinoma: analysis of staging in the mediastinum with CT by correlative lymph node mapping and sampling. *Radiology* 1992;182:319–323.
25. Levitt RG, Glazer HS, Roper CL, et al. Magnetic resonance imaging of mediastinal and hilar masses: comparison with CT. *Am J Roentgenol* 1985;145:9–14.
26. Glazer GM, Gross BH, Aisen AM, et al. Imaging of the pulmonary hilum: a prospective comparative study in patients with lung cancer. *Am J Roentgenol* 1985;145:245–248.
27. Khan A, Herman PG, Vorwerk P, et al. Solitary pulmonary nodules: comparison of classification with standard, thin-section and reference phantom CT. *Radiology* 1991;179:477–481.
28. Zwirewich CV, Vedal S, Miller RR, et al. Solitary pulmonary nodule: high resolution CT and radiologic-pathologic correlation. *Radiology* 1991;179:469–476.
29. Davis SD. CT evaluation for pulmonary metastases in patients with extrathoracic malignancy. *Radiology* 1991;180:1–12.
30. Chang AE, Schaner EG, Conkle DM, et al. Evaluation of computed tomography in the detection of pulmonary metastases: a prospective study. *Cancer* 1979;43:913–916.
31. Robertson PL, Boldt DW, DeCampo JF. Paediatric pulmonary nodules: a comparison of computed tomography, thoracotomy findings and histology. *Clin Radiol* 1988;39:607–610.
32. Costello P, Anderson W, Blume D. Pulmonary nodule: evaluation with spiral volumetric CT. *Radiology* 1991;179:875–876.
33. Feuerstein IM, Jicha DL, Pass HI, et al. Pulmonary metastases: MR imaging with surgical correlation—a prospective study. *Radiology* 1992;182:123–129.
34. Remy-Jardin M, Remy J, Deffontaines C, et al. Assessment of diffuse infiltrative lung disease: comparison of conventional CT and high-resolution CT. *Radiology* 1991;181:157–162.
35. Munk PL, Müller NL, Miller RR, et al. Pulmonary lymphangitic carcinomatosis: CT and pathologic findings. *Radiology* 1988;166:705–709.
36. Mathieson JR, Mayo JR, Staples CA, et al. Chronic diffuse infiltrative lung disease: comparison of diagnostic accuracy of CT and chest radiography. *Radiology* 1989;171:111–116.
37. Lee JS, Im J-G, Ahn JM, et al. Fibrosing alveolitis: prognostic implication of ground-glass attenuation at high-resolution CT. *Radiology* 1992;184:451–454.
38. Aberle DR, Gamsu G, Ray CS, et al. Asbestos-related pleural and parenchymal fibrosis: detection with high-resolution CT. *Radiology* 1988;166:729–734.
39. Munro NC, Cooke JC, Currie DC, et al. Comparison of thin section computed tomography with bronchography for identifying bronchiectatic segments in patients with chronic sputum production. *Thorax* 1990;45:135–139.
40. Silverman PM, Godwin JD. CT/bronchographic correlations in bronchiectasis. *J Comput Assist Tomogr* 1987;11:52–56.
41. Grenier P, Maurice F, Musset D, et al. Bronchiectasis: assessment by thin-section CT. *Radiology* 1986;161:95–99.
42. Naidich DP, Funt S, Ettenger NA, et al. Hemoptysis: CT-bronchoscopic correlations in 58 cases. *Radiology* 1990;177:357–362.
43. Petasnick JP. Radiologic evaluation of aortic dissection. *Radiology* 1991;180:297–305.
44. Godwin JD. Conventional CT of the aorta. *J Thorac Imaging* 1990;5(4):18–31.
45. McLoud TC, Flower CDR: Imaging the pleura: sonography, CT, and MR imaging. *Am J Roentgenol* 1991;156:1145–1153.
46. Waite RJ, Carbonneau RJ, Balikian JP, et al. Parietal pleural changes in empyema: appearances at CT. *Radiology* 1990;175:145–150.
47. Aberle DR, Balmes JR. Computed tomography of asbestos-related pulmonary parenchymal and pleural diseases. *Clin Chest Med* 1991;12:115–131.
48. Friedman AC, Fiel SB, Fisher MS, et al. Asbestos-related pleural disease and asbestosis: a comparison of CT and chest radiography. *Am J Roentgenol* 1988;150:268–275.
49. Fink I, Gamsu G, Harter LP. CT-guided aspiration biopsy of the thorax. *J Comput Assist Tomogr* 1982;6:958–962.
50. Lee KS, Im J-G, Kim YH, et al. Treatment of multiloculated empyemas with intracavitary urokinase: a prospective study. *Radiology* 1991;179:771–775.
51. Zeman RK, Baron RL, Jeffrey RB, et al. Helical body CT: evolution of scanning protocols. *Am J Roentgenol* 1998;170:1427–1438.
52. Remy-Jardin M, Remy J, Deschildre F, et al. Diagnosis of pulmonary embolism with spiral CT: comparison with pulmonary angiography and scintigraphy. *Radiology* 1996;200:699–706.
53. Viamonte M. Angiographic evaluation of lung neoplasms. *Radiol Clin North Am* 1965;3:529–542.
54. Swensen SJ, Brown LR, Colby TV, et al. Pulmonary nodules: CT evaluation of enhancement with iodinated contrast material. *Radiology* 1995;194:393–398.
55. Swensen SJ, Brown LR, Colby TV, et al. Lung nodule enhancement at CT: prospective findings. *Radiology* 1996;201:447–455.
56. Nardich DP, Graden JF, McGuiness G, et al. Volumetric (helical spiral) CT (VCT) of the airways. *J Thorac Imaging* 1997;12:11–28.
57. Broderick LS, Shemesh J, Wilensky RL, et al. Measurement of coronary artery calcium with duel-slice helical CT compared with coronary angiography: evaluation of CT scoring methods, interobserver variations and reproducibility. *Am J Roentgenol* 1996;167:439–444.
58. Shemesh J, Apter S, Rosenman J, et al. Calcification of coronary arteries: detection and quantification with double-helix CT. *Radiology* 1995;197:779–783.
59. Webb WR, Sostman HD. MR imaging of thoracic disease: clinical uses. *Radiology* 1992;182:621–630.
60. Katayama H, Yamaguchi K, Kozuka T, et al. Adverse reactions to ionic and nonionic contrast media. *Radiology* 1990;175:621–628.
61. White RD, Dooms GC, Higgins CB. Advances in imaging thoracic aortic disease. *Invest Radiol* 1986;21:761–778.
62. Solomon SL, Brown JJ, Glazer HS, et al. Thoracic aortic dissection: pitfalls and artifacts in MR imaging. *Radiology* 1990;177:223–228.
63. Kersting-Sommerhoff BA, Higgins CB, White RD, et al. Aortic dissection: sensitivity and specificity of MR imaging. *Radiology* 1988;166:651–655.
64. Hansen ME, Spritzer CE, Sostman HD. Assessing the patency of mediastinal and thoracic inlet veins: value of MR imaging. *Am J Roentgenol* 1990;155:1177–1182.
65. Rapoport S, Blair DN, McCarthy SM, et al. Brachial plexus: correlation of MR imaging with CT and pathologic findings. *Radiology* 1988;167:161–165.
66. Castagno AA, Shuman WP. MR imaging in clinically suspected brachial plexus tumor. *Am J Roentgenol* 1987;149:1219–1222.
67. Gupta RK, Mehta VS, Banerji AK, et al. MR evaluation of brachial plexus injuries. *Neuroradiology* 1989;31:377–381.
68. Freedberg RS, Krozon I, Runnancik WM, et al. The contribution of magnetic resonance imaging to the evaluation of intracardiac tumors diagnosed by echo-cardiography. *Circulation* 1988;77:96–103.
69. Barakos JA, Brown JJ, Higgins CB. MR imaging of secondary cardiac and paracardiac lesions. *Am J Roentgenol* 1989;153:47–50.
70. Yan PC, Luh KT, Shen JC, et al. Ultrasonography and ultrasound guided aspiration biopsy. *Radiology* 1985;155:451–456.
71. Ammann AM, Brewer WH, Maull KI, et al. Traumatic rupture of the hemidiaphragm: real-time sonographic diagnosis. *Am J Roentgenol* 1983;140:915–916.
72. The PIOPED Investigators. Value of the ventilation-perfusion scan in acute pulmonary embolism: results of the prospective investigation of pulmonary embolism diagnosis. *JAMA* 1990;263:2753–2759.
73. Nicod P, Peterson K, Levine M, et al. Pulmonary angiography in severe chronic pulmonary hypertension. *Ann Intern Med* 1987;107:565–568.
74. Anderson PO, Martin EC. Pulmonary embolism: diagnosis with multiple imaging modalities. *Radiology* 1987;164:297–312.
75. Gottschalk A, Juni J, Sostman HD, et al. Ventilation-perfusion scintigraphy in the PIOPED study. Part I: data collection and tabulation. *J Nucl Med* 1993;34:1109–1118.
76. Gottschalk A, Sostman HD, Juni J, et al. Ventilation-perfusion scintigraphy in the PIOPED study. Part II: evaluation of criteria and interpretations. *J Nucl Med* 1993;34:1119–1126.
77. Wernly JA, DeMeester TR, Kirchner PT, et al. Clinical value of quantitative ventilation-perfusion lung scans in the surgical

management of bronchogenic carcinoma. *J Thorac Cardiovasc Surg* 1980;80:535–543.

78. Boysen PG, Block AJ, Olsen GN, et al. Prospective evaluation for pneumonectomy using the 99m-technetium quantitative perfusion lung scan. *Chest* 1977;72:422–425.

79. Scott WJ, Dewan NA. Use of positron emission tomograph to diagnose end stage lung cancer. *Clin Pulm Med* 1999;6:198–204.

80. Som P, Atkins HL, Bandoypadhyay D, et al. A fluorinated glucose analogue, 2-fluoro-2-deoxy-D-glucose (F-18): nontoxic tracer for rapid tumor detection. *J Nucl Med* 1980;21:670–675.

81. Fletcher J. PET scanning and the solitary pulmonary nodule. *Semin Thorac Cardiovasc Surg* 2002;14:268–274.

82. Goerres GW, Gustav K, von Schulthess K, et al. Why most PET of lung and head-and-neck cancer will be PET/CT. *J Nucl Med* 2004;45:66S–71S.

83. Kinahan PE, Townsend DW, Beyer T, et al. Attenuation correction for a combined 3D PET-CT scanner. *Med Phys* 1998;25:2046–2053.

84. Antoch G, Stattaus J, Nemat AT, et al. Non-small cell lung cancer: Dual modality PET/CT in preoperative staging. *Radiology* 2003; 229:526–533.

85. Dezendorf EV, Baumert BG, von Schulthess GK, et al. Impact of whole-body 18F-FDG PET on staging and managing patients for radiation therapy. *J Nucl Med* 2003;44:24–29.

86. Gupta NC, Frank AR, Dewan NA, et al. Solitary pulmonary nodules: Detection of malignancy with PET with 2-F18-fluoro-2deoxy glucose. *Radiology* 2000;184:441–444.

87. Henschke C. Early lung cancer action project overall design and findings from baseline screening. *Cancer* 2000;89:2474–2482.

88. Gonzalez-Stawinski G, Lemaire A, Merchant F. A comparative analysis of positron emission tomography and mediastinoscopy in staging non-small cell lung cancer. *J Thorac Cardiovasc Surg* 2003;126:1900–1905.

89. Kalff V, Hicks RJ, MacManus MP, et al. Clinical impact of (18) F fluorodeoxyglucose positron emission tomography in patients with nonsmall cell lung cancer: a prospective study. *J Clin Oncol* 2001;19:111–118.

90. Kernstine K. Positron emission tomography with 2-F18 fluoro-2-deoxy-D-glucose: Can it be used to accurately stage the mediastinum in non-small cell lung cancer as an alternative to mediastinoscopy? *J Thorac Cardiovasc Surg* 2003;126:1700–1703.

CHAPTER 6

Clinical Pulmonary Function Testing, Exercise Testing, and Disability Evaluation

Richard W. Light

MEASUREMENTS OF VENTILATORY FUNCTION
Measurement of Expiratory Flow Rates
Measurement of Airway Hyperresponsiveness
Measurement of Lung Volumes
Airway and Pulmonary Tissue
    Mechanics
Distribution of Ventilation
Gas Transfer and Exchange

EXERCISE AND EXERCISE TESTING
Exercise Physiology and Pathophysiology
Measures of Work Capacity
Determinants of Work Capacity ($\dot{V}o_2max$)
Training
Aging and Exercise Performance
Performance of Exercise Testing
Use of Pulmonary Function and Exercise Tests

Pulmonary function testing consists of the performance of a set of maneuvers to detect and quantitate disorders of pulmonary ventilation and gas exchange. These tests provide objective evidence of the presence, type, and degree of abnormality. They allow for assessment of the course of a disease state over time, evaluation of the effectiveness of a therapeutic intervention, and determination of the risk of pulmonary complications of surgical procedures. In general, testing of the pulmonary system is minimally invasive and has low risk, enabling one to undergo repeated studies over relatively short intervals.

This chapter provides an overview of clinical pulmonary function testing as it exists today. The tests commonly performed in well-equipped clinical laboratories are discussed. The objective is not to detail the techniques but, rather, to emphasize the fundamental concepts.

The field of pulmonary function testing has acquired a system of nomenclature that may appear confusing to the student but has an underlying structure that is easily mastered. The American College of Chest Physicians (ACCP) and the American Thoracic Society (ATS) Joint Committee on Pulmonary Nomenclature

have provided a set of recommendations that are followed in this chapter (1). Where older terminology is commonplace, it is given as well.

MEASUREMENTS OF VENTILATORY FUNCTION

MEASUREMENT OF EXPIRATORY FLOW RATES

Measurements of flow rates and cumulative exhaled volumes are the backbone of pulmonary function testing. The reader is referred to a monograph by the American Thoracic Society for guidance in the selection and calibration of equipment for this testing (2).

Simple Spirometry

With this test, the subject inhales maximally to total lung capacity (TLC) and then exhales as rapidly and forcefully as possible. The cumulative exhaled volume is recorded on the *y*-axis

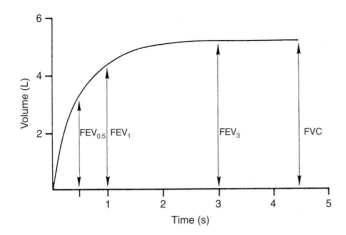

FIGURE 6-1. A typical forced expiratory spirogram showing the timed volumes obtained from the graph. $FEV_{0.5}$, FEV_1, and FEV_3 represent the forced expired volume at 0.5, 1, and 3 seconds, respectively. The forced vital capacity (FVC) is the maximum volume that can be forcefully exhaled.

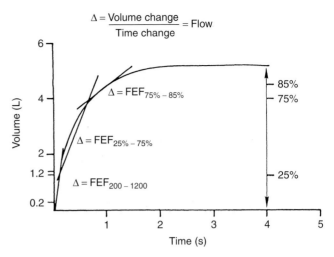

FIGURE 6-2. A typical forced expiratory spirogram showing the averaged flows obtained from the graph. The flow between 200 and 1200 mL of expired air ($FEF_{200-1200}$) is taken at high lung volume near TLC. The average flow between 25% and 75% of the expired vital capacity ($FEF_{25\%-75\%}$) measures flow in the midportion of the expired volume. The average flow between 75% and 85% of the expired vital capacity ($FEF_{75\%-85\%}$) measures flow at low lung volumes.

and time on the *x*-axis (see Fig. 6-1). From the curve, a series of timed volumes and flows are measured. The forced vital capacity (FVC) is the total volume exhaled. The $FEV_{0.5}$, FEV_1, and FEV_3 are the cumulative volumes exhaled after 0.5, 1.0, and 3.0 seconds, respectively. Although the $FEV_{0.5}$, FEV_1, and FEV_3 are volume measurements, they convey information on obstruction to flow because they are measured over a known period of time. They may be decreased by any process that inhibits expiratory flow, by a decrease in the TLC, or by lack of effort by the subject.

A more sensitive means of evaluating obstruction is to express the forced expiratory volumes (FEVs) as a percentage of the vital capacity, abbreviated as FEV_t/FVC, with *t* representing time of measurement. The ratio is relatively independent of the patient's size. The FEV_1/FVC is a specific measure of airway obstruction with or without associated restriction of lung volumes. Normally, it is 75% or greater. The FEV_3/FVC includes flows at relatively low lung volumes when flow rates are decreased relatively early in disease; thus, it may be abnormal in early airway obstruction. It is normally 95% or greater in adults.

Average flows can be graphically measured from the spirogram. Because flow is the change in volume with time, these forced expiratory flows (FEFs) may be determined graphically by dividing the volume change by the time required to make the change. Typically, the average flow between 25% and 75% of the vital capacity ($FEF_{25\%-75\%}$)—formerly called the maximal midexpiratory flow rate (MMF)—is recorded (see Fig. 6-2). Other flows that are frequently reported include the flow between 75% and 85% of the vital capacity ($FEF_{75\%-85\%}$) and between 200 and 1200 mL of expired air ($FEF_{200-1200}$). These three average flow rates demonstrate marked variability in normal subjects (3). Accordingly, the 95% confidence limits for their normal values are so wide that they are of limited value in detecting disease in an individual subject.

Measurements obtained from the FVC maneuver, whether recorded as spirograms or flow–volume loops, require the cooperation of the patient. It is recommended that a minimum of three acceptable FVC maneuvers be performed. If a subject

has large variability between expiratory maneuvers, reproducibility criteria may require that up to eight acceptable maneuvers be performed. For the test results to be considered valid, the largest FVC and the second-largest FVC should not vary by more than 5% or 100 mL, whichever is greater. In addition, the largest FEV_1 and the second-largest FEV_1 should meet the same criteria. These reproducibility criteria are used as a guide to determine whether more than three FVC maneuvers are needed. The largest FVC and the largest FEV_1 should be recorded (2).

Flow–Volume Studies

The development of sophisticated electronic pulmonary function testing equipment has led to the popularity of the flow–volume curve. For this test, the subject makes a forced exhalation from TLC, as with the forced expiratory spirogram, followed by a forced inspiration. The recording device plots volume on the horizontal axis and flow on the vertical axis. Values of FEF are taken at volumes representing 25%, 50%, and 75% of the exhaled vital capacity and are recorded as $FEF_{x\%}$ ($\dot{V}max_{x\%}$), with *x* representing the exhaled fraction of the vital capacity (VC).

The flow–volume curve during forced exhalation has a characteristic appearance. The curve shows a rapid ascent to peak flow and a subsequently slow linear descent proportional to volume (see Fig. 6-3). The initial portion of the curve depends, at least in part, on the effort of the patient. As a subject exerts increasing effort during exhalation, higher flow rates are generated. However, the latter two-thirds of the curve is relatively effort independent. For each point on the volume curve, a maximal flow exists that cannot be exceeded regardless of the effort of the patient (see discussion of isovolume pressure–flow curves in Chapter 2, Mechanics of Respiration). However, it must be emphasized that the maximal flow at a given lung

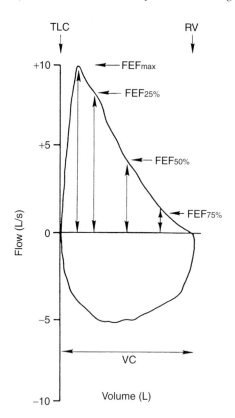

FIGURE 6-3. A typical flow–volume loop from a normal subject showing both expiratory (upper) and inspiratory (lower) portions. Instantaneous flows may be measured after 25% ($FEF_{25\%}$), 50% ($FEF_{50\%}$), and 75% ($FEF_{75\%}$) of the vital capacity has been exhaled. The peak flow is easily measured as the value of the peak of the graph.

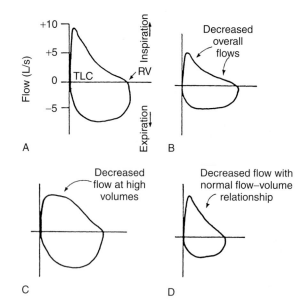

FIGURE 6-4. Common examples of abnormal flow–volume loops. **A:** Mild obstructive airway disease characterized by decreased flow at low lung volume when elastic support is reduced. **B:** Significant obstructive airway disease characterized by decreased overall flows, with a further decrease at low lung volumes. **C:** Variable intrathoracic large airway obstruction in which peak flow is decreased at higher lung volumes, with preservation of normal flow–volume relationship at lower lung volumes. **D:** Restrictive pulmonary disease with decreased vital capacity and flows but with preservation of normal flow–volume relationships.

volume will be achieved only if the patient generates sufficient intrathoracic pressure to reach flow limitation.

The flow–volume loop carries a great deal of information (4). Early in the development of obstructive airway disease, expiratory flow at low lung volumes is decreased but the volume exhaled is normal. This results in an expiratory curve that declines rapidly until the lung volume gets low and then persists at a low flow rate until the residual volume (RV) is reached (see Fig. 6-4A). More severe obstructive disease results in an accentuation of upward concavity with a greatly decreased maximal flow (Fig. 6-4B) (5). Intrathoracic large airway obstruction, as in the trachea, results in decreased flows at larger lung volumes, whereas the flows at low volumes are relatively unaffected. The result is a flattening of the flow–volume loop (Fig. 6-4C). The curve for patients with restrictive lung disease has a decreased volume and peak flow but a normal relationship between the two (Fig. 6-4D).

There have been many studies comparing the flow–volume curves obtained when the subject is breathing air and breathing low-density gas mixtures such as 80% helium and 20% oxygen. The clinical usefulness of these tests remains to be proved (6). The reader is referred to Chapter 2, Mechanics of Respiration, for further discussion of these tests.

Peak Expiratory Flow Rate

The peak expiratory flow (PEF) is the highest flow rate that occurs during a forced exhalation from TLC. The PEF occurs very early in exhalation when the flow rates are effort dependent. A

low value can result from a submaximal effort as well as from airway obstruction. In general, a relatively accurate prediction of the FEV_1 can be obtained from the PEF by multiplying the PEF (in liters per minute) by 9 to get the FEV_1 in milliliters (7).

The most common situation in which the PEF is used clinically is home monitoring. The availability of inexpensive, small, portable devices allows patients to objectively measure their degree of airway obstruction on an ambulatory basis. Essentially, all published asthma practice guidelines recommend the use of PEF monitoring as an adjunct to asthma education in selected groups of patients (8,9). Groups most likely to benefit from home PEF monitoring are those who have labile asthma and those who require repeated burst prednisone therapy, emergency room visits, and hospital admissions (9).

Maximal Voluntary Ventilation

The maximal voluntary ventilation (MVV) is the volume of air a subject can ventilate with maximal effort over a brief period. In this test, subjects are instructed to breathe rapidly and deeply for 12 to 15 seconds and the cumulative expired volume is recorded. The results of the test are heavily dependent on subject cooperation and effort. As the MVV can be predicted relatively accurately ($r = 0.94$) from the FEV_1 by multiplying the FEV_1 by 35 to 40, routine performance of this test is not recommended (10).

MEASUREMENT OF AIRWAY HYPERRESPONSIVENESS

Individuals with asthma have, by definition, hyperresponsive airways. At times when they are evaluated in the pulmonary function laboratory, their spirometry may be within normal limits. The diagnosis of asthma can still be established by demonstrating bronchial hyperreactivity to the inhalation of various agents. The two agents most commonly used to provoke bronchial responses are histamine and methacholine. Additional challenges that are used at times include distilled water, cold air, and exercise. In the typical procedure, the inhaled dose of the provocative agent is plotted on a logarithmic scale against the change in lung function, expressed as a percentage change from the normal value measured after an initial test dose of normal saline. The dose that produces a 20% fall in the FEV_1 is then determined. Hyperresponsiveness is said to be present when the dose of histamine or methacholine that causes a 20% fall in the FEV_1 is 8.0 µmol or less. The lower the dose that induces the 20% decrease in FEV_1, the more hyperresponsive the individual is. The primary uses of these tests are to establish the diagnosis of asthma in patients whose spirometry is normal and to quantitate the degree of hyperresponsiveness in known asthmatics (11).

One of the primary uses of bronchoprovocation tests is to exclude the diagnosis of asthma in patients with asthma-type symptoms or cough (11). A positive test in this situation is suggestive that the patient has asthma, but it should be remembered that 3% to 35% of asymptomatic individuals have airway hyperresponsiveness (11). Asymptomatic hyperresponsiveness is more frequently observed in subjects with atopy, in members of families with asthma, and in those individuals exposed to tobacco smoke (11). It is associated with airway inflammation and remodeling (11).

A second use is to diagnose and follow subjects with occupational asthma. A third use is to document the severity of asthma and to assess the response to treatment (11). It should be noted that there is a high incidence of airway hyperresponsiveness in smokers with obstructive airway disease. In a recent study of 3700 male and 2200 female smokers with FEV_1/FVC less than 70%, 63% of the men and 87% of the women had a positive response to methacholine (12). It has also been shown that the presence of increased airway responsiveness is a significant predictor of subsequent accelerated decline in pulmonary function in adults (13).

MEASUREMENT OF LUNG VOLUMES

Spirometric Volume Determinations

The spirometric volume determinations are relatively simple to perform. The typical testing procedure consists of having a subject breathe several times with a normal, resting tidal pattern while continuously recording the volume. The subject is then instructed to inspire maximally, then exhale slowly and as completely as possible, and then return to tidal breathing. A forceful exhalation may induce air trapping, resulting in a lower volume measurement. A typical graph is given in Figure 6-5, from which the following measurements can be made:

Tidal volume (VT): The average of the normal resting ventilatory excursions.

Inspiratory reserve volume (IRV): The maximum volume that may be inhaled beyond a normal tidal breath.

Expiratory reserve volume (ERV): The maximum volume that may be exhaled from a resting ventilatory level after a normal tidal exhalation.

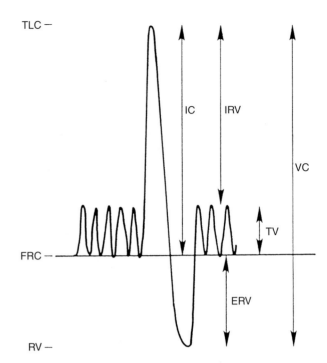

FIGURE 6-5. Volume tracing of a spirometer, showing the lung volumes and compartments measured from the tracing. The tracing is obtained by having the patient breathe quietly for a period of time, followed by a deep inspiration, and then a slow, complete exhalation. The patient then returns to tidal breathing. The total lung capacity (*TLC*), functional residual capacity (*FRC*), and residual volume (*RV*) are shown for orientation. The measurements include the tidal volume (*TV*), inspiratory reserve volume (*IRV*), expiratory reserve volume (*ERV*), inspiratory capacity (*IC*), and vital capacity (*VC*).

Vital capacity (slow) (VC): The total volume of air that may be moved into or out of the lungs, which is equal to the sum of IRV, VT, and ERV.

Inspiratory capacity (IC): The maximum volume of air that may be inhaled from a resting level, which is equal to the sum of the VT and the IRV.

The main problem with the spirometrically determined lung volumes is that they do not provide any indication of the volume of air remaining after a maximal exhalation, which is the RV. Therefore, alternative methods must be used if one desires to measure the TLC, which is the sum of the RV and VC. These alternative methods include gas dilution methods and body plethysmography.

Gas Dilution

The closed-circuit helium dilution method is performed by having the subject rebreathe a known volume of gas in a closed-circuit spirometer containing helium as a tracer (see Fig. 6-6) (14). Helium is inert and does not readily diffuse across the alveolar–capillary membrane. The helium equilibrates throughout the volume of the entire patient–spirometer system. The carbon dioxide generated is removed and the oxygen lost is replenished with 100% oxygen to maintain a constant volume in the system. If the patient begins and ends the test at the end of a normal exhalation, the functional residual capacity (FRC) is determined. The residual volume is then obtained by subtracting the measured ERV from the calculated FRC.

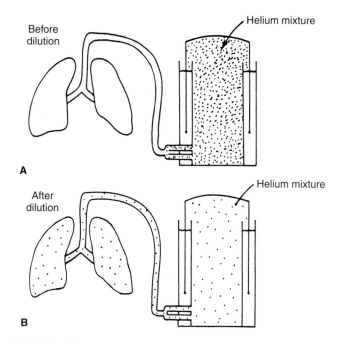

FIGURE 6-6. Diagram of the closed-circuit helium method for determination of the functional residual capacity. **A:** Prior to equilibration, the helium tracer is distributed in the spirometer circuit only. **B:** After equilibration with the patient's lungs by having him or her rebreathe the gas mixture, the helium is diluted and distributed throughout the lungs and spirometer. Measurement of the spirometer gas volume and the amount of dilution of the helium tracer enables calculation of the total system volume. The FRC is calculated by subtracting the spirometer volume from the system volume.

This method is sensitive to errors from leakage of gas and also fails to measure the volume of gas in lung bullae.

A second method is the open circuit, or multibreath, nitrogen washout technique (see Fig. 6-7) (15). The nitrogen normally present in the lungs is used as the tracer gas. The subject begins breathing 100% oxygen at the end of a normal exhalation (FRC). As the nitrogen is "washed out," the exhaled gas is collected and the concentration of nitrogen is continuously monitored. When the concentration in the expirate falls to a low level, the FRC may be determined by measuring the volume of gas exhaled, and the nitrogen concentration of this gas may be determined in a manner similar to that used in the helium dilution method. This method has the advantage of permitting a simultaneous assessment of intrapulmonary gas mixing. This method is also sensitive to errors from gas leakage and does not measure the volume of gas in poorly communicating air spaces such as bullae.

Two other measurements of lung volume can be obtained from the dilution of gases used in standard tests of pulmonary function. One involves the measurement of the mean concentration of nitrogen in the air exhaled after an inspiration of 100% oxygen in the single-breath nitrogen washout test. The other involves measuring the change in concentration of helium used as the inert tracer gas in the single-breath measurement of the diffusing capacity. However, because the time for dilution of the tracer gas is relatively short for both of these methods, the TLC is underestimated in patients with moderate or severe maldistribution of ventilation (16).

The measurements obtained by spirometry with either of the gas dilution methods allow determination of all of the lung volumes. Any of the three techniques can give faulty results if the

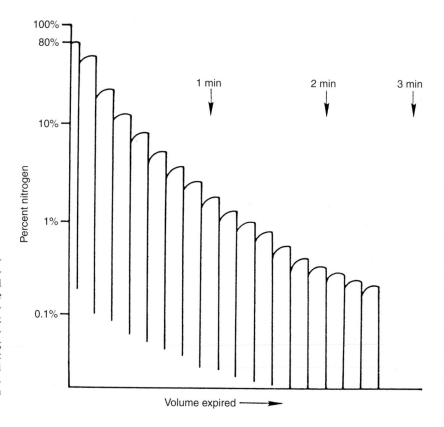

FIGURE 6-7. Graph of log nitrogen concentration versus volume exhaled in the multibreath nitrogen washout test used for determination of FRC and intrapulmonary gas mixing. The peak of the curve for each breath represents the end-tidal N_2 concentration. Analysis of the curve generated by the peak concentrations enables assessment of the homogeneity of gas distribution. On the log scale, mixing in the presence of ideal gas distribution would result in a curve that is nearly a straight line, with a rapid decrease in the concentration of N_2 to below 2.5%. By monitoring the volume exchanged, along with the N_2 concentration, the FRC may be calculated.

test begins and ends at a volume different from that to be measured, which is either the FRC or the RV. In the helium dilution method, gas leaks in the system can cause an overestimation of helium dilution and thus yield falsely elevated values.

Plethysmographic Volume Determinations

The technique of plethysmography is an alternate method used to measure the volume of the lungs (17). It is important to note that the results of these tests may differ from the results obtained by using gas dilution or washout methods. The gas dilution methods measure communicating FRC or RV, whereas the plethysmographic techniques measure both the communicating and noncommunicating compartments. Noncommunicating or poorly communicating air spaces are often present as a result of disease in which "air trapping" occurs. A pneumothorax is another example of a noncommunicating space. These gas compartments are compressible and, therefore, are included in the plethysmographic measurement but are not reflected in the gas dilution determination. The gas volume measured by a plethysmograph is known as the *thoracic gas volume* (V_{TG}) and in disease states is frequently higher than the value measured by gas dilution.

The measurement of V_{TG} via plethysmography is based on Boyle's law, which states that the product of the pressure and the volume of the gas in the thorax is constant if the temperature is unchanged. The subject is seated comfortably in the airtight plethysmograph and temperature equilibration is allowed to occur (see Fig. 6-8). With the airway occluded, the subject makes inspiratory and expiratory efforts against the occluded airway. Because changes in the volume of the thorax are reflected by changes in the pressure in the airtight box and because changes in the thoracic pressure are reflected

by changes in the pressure recorded at the mouth, the lung volume can be calculated.

The procedure described above is usually initiated at the end of a normal exhalation, so the V_{TG} is equivalent to FRC. By combining this measurement with spirometric measurements, one can determine all the lung volume compartments, as in the gas dilution methods. The volumes determined by plethysmography are subject to error if the test is performed at an inappropriate starting volume. The measurement reflects the actual volume in the thorax at the start and at the end of the test.

AIRWAY AND PULMONARY TISSUE MECHANICS

The tests discussed so far are affected by such extrapulmonary factors as thoracic and abdominal muscle function and the properties of the thoracic cage. It is possible to assess the mechanical properties of the lungs themselves by using tests that require more sophisticated equipment. These tests are discussed briefly in the paragraphs that follow.

Airway Resistance

Airway resistance (Raw) must be measured during airflow. By definition, the airway resistance is the driving pressure divided by the flow that results from the pressure differential. Resistance to flow in the airways may be measured with a body plethysmography (18). In measuring total airway resistance, the pressure differential is that between the alveoli and the atmosphere. It is not possible to measure alveolar pressure directly when air is flowing, but it can be measured indirectly with a body plethysmograph. The flow at the mouth may be measured simultaneously to enable calculation of airway resistance. It is important to measure Raw at low flow rates (less than 0.5 L per second) so that the measurement does not reflect dynamic compression of the airways (see Chapter 2, Mechanics of Respiration).

Airway resistance changes with lung volume, so the Raw determination is made at a known volume, usually the FRC. The relationship is inverse; thus, an increase in lung volume results in a decreased resistance (see Fig. 2-9A). The reciprocal of airway resistance is *airway conductance* (Gaw = 1/Raw). The relationship between the airway conductance and the lung volume is nearly linear (Fig. 2-9B). The specific airway conductance (Gaw/V_L or SGaw) is therefore independent of the lung volume. It is the measurement that should be used to evaluate changes in airway resistance with time in an individual patient or in comparing measures of airway resistance in a given patient to normal values.

Lung Compliance

The distensibility of the lungs is assessed by measuring lung compliance, which is determined from the relationship between changes in *transpulmonary pressure* and changes in lung volume (see Chapter 2, Mechanics of Respiration).

The measurement of static compliance is performed with a spirometer to measure volume change and with pressure transducers to measure pressures in the airway and esophagus. The pleural pressure is estimated from the pressure within a balloon placed in the esophagus. The subject inspires to TLC

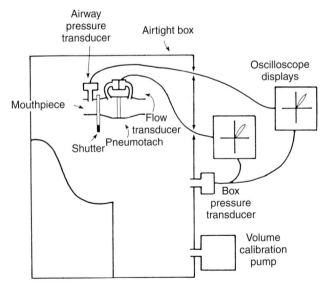

FIGURE 6-8. Body plethysmograph for the measurement of thoracic gas volume and airway resistance. The type shown is a pressure plethysmograph, which uses pressure changes in the box to estimate lung volume changes. Pressure transducers are used to monitor the box and mouth pressures. A flow transducer allows simultaneous recording of flow at the mouth. From these measurements, the thoracic gas volume and the airway resistance may be calculated using the techniques outlined in the text.

and begins a slow exhalation. The airflow at the mouth is interrupted at small volume decrements of approximately 500 mL, during which time the volume and pressures are recorded. As the airway pressure during occlusion of the airway is identical to alveolar pressure, the transpulmonary pressure is calculated as the difference between airway and esophageal pressures. The lung volumes and corresponding transpulmonary pressures are plotted to give a static lung compliance curve (see Fig. 6-9). The slope of the curve ($\Delta V/\Delta P$) at any given volume represents the *static lung compliance* (C_{Lst}) at that volume. The portion of the curve 500 to 1000 mL above the FRC is usually chosen for the measurement because, at higher lung volumes, the relationship becomes highly nonlinear. The static compliance is often normalized to the absolute lung volume at which the measurement is made and is termed *specific compliance* (C_{Lst}/V_L). The reason for this is that compliance is directly related to absolute lung volume.

Static lung compliance reflects the elasticity of the lung parenchyma. It increases slightly with advancing age owing to changes in the elastic fibers of the lungs. It also increases in emphysema. A decreased compliance suggests interstitial disease or a disease associated with alveolar filling such as pulmonary edema.

During the measurement of static lung compliance, the transthoracic pressure (alveolar minus atmospheric) may be recorded in addition to the transpulmonary pressure to permit calculation of *total lung compliance* (C_{Tst}). This measurement includes pulmonary and chest wall factors. The difference between the transthoracic and transpulmonary pressures may be used to calculate the *chest wall compliance* (C_{wst}).

DISTRIBUTION OF VENTILATION

Tests of gas distribution are used to give a measure of the homogeneity of the distribution of inspired gas to the alveoli. In the normal lung, gas is transported along all airways and is distributed relatively equally to all areas of the lung, with more distribution to the lower regions of the lung in the upright subject. This is because alveoli in the upper zones are more distended than in the lower zones at FRC and are less able to expand. In certain disease states, especially those with destruction of pulmonary tissue, there is a variable degree of inhomogeneity that alters the intrapulmonary distribution of gas within each region. Several tests are available to detect this type of abnormality.

Single-Breath Nitrogen Elimination Test

The single-breath nitrogen (N_2) test may be used to assess the homogeneity of gas distribution (19). The results of the test give an index that reflects the overall mixing ability of the lungs, but no anatomic indication of areas of poor distribution is possible.

The test is performed with the subject seated after normal breathing of room air for a few moments. The subject exhales to residual volume and then slowly inhales a breath of 100% oxygen to total lung capacity. During a slow exhalation (under 1 L per second), the concentration of nitrogen in the exhaled air is recorded continuously as a function of the volume exhaled. The resulting curve consists of four phases, which are depicted in Figure 6-10.

The shape of the curve can be explained on the basis of the underlying physiology. At RV, the alveoli in the upper portions of the lungs are larger than those in the lower portions because of the more negative pleural pressure in the top part of the lung. At TLC, all the alveoli are approximately the same size. Therefore, when an individual takes a breath of 100% O_2 from RV, the nitrogen concentration in the alveoli in the upper portion of the lungs will be greater at TLC than that in the lower portion of the lungs. On exhalation, the dead space gas (100% oxygen) is exhaled first and is noted as phase *I*, in which the nitrogen concentration is zero. The nitrogen concentration rises abruptly (phase *II*) when alveolar gas with nitrogen begins to be exhaled. Phase *III* represents alveolar gas exhalation. If gas distribution were perfectly homogeneous, all alveoli would empty at an approximately equal rate and the phase *III* line would be horizontal. Nonhomogeneous

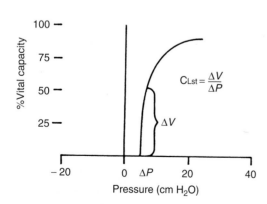

FIGURE 6-9. Volume–pressure graph obtained by measuring the pressure during static conditions at various lung volumes with the glottis closed. The test is usually performed by interrupting flow intermittently during an exhalation from TLC while recording transpulmonary pressure and volume above FRC. The transpulmonary pressure is the alveolar pressure measured at the mouth minus the pleural pressure measured with an esophageal balloon. The pressure and volume points are plotted as a curve. The static compliance is measured as the slope of the curve at a given point, usually just above FRC.

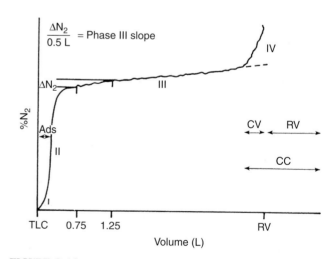

FIGURE 6-10. Graph of nitrogen concentration versus volume exhaled in the single-breath nitrogen test. Measurement of ΔN_2 is the change in nitrogen concentration over the curve from 750 to 1250 mL. The *phase III slope* is the slope of the line over an initial portion of the curve, equal to the change in N_2 concentration over a 1-L portion of the curve. Measurements of closing volume and anatomic dead space are made directly from the graph.

emptying of the lungs results in different rates of nitrogen exhalation, and there is normally a slight rise of the phase *III* line. In conditions of abnormal intrapulmonary mixing, the beginning of phase *IV* occurs when the small airways in the bases of the lungs begin to close, leaving only the upper zones, which have higher N_2 concentration, to empty, causing the abrupt increase in slope (20).

From the curve, the following measurements are made:

Anatomic dead space (V_{Danat}): The volume of phase *I* and approximately half of phase *II*.

Phase III slope: The change in nitrogen concentration over 1 L of the initial portion of phase *III*.

Closing volume (CV): The volume above the RV, at which phase *IV* begins to occur, reported as percent of VC.

Closing capacity (CC): The sum of the CV and the RV, reported as percent of TLC.

The phase *III* slope is an index of uniformity of gas distribution. Normally, there is less than a 2% change in nitrogen concentration per liter during phase *III*. Increases in its value reflect relatively greater inhomogeneity than normal. Indeed, in one large study of over 2,500 adults, the slope of phase *III* was more strongly associated with mortality than was the FEV_1 (21). At one time, the CV was proposed as a sensitive indicator of small airway disease and was thought to hold promise as a predictive test for the development of chronic obstructive pulmonary disease (COPD) (22). However, subsequent studies designed to prove this contention were disappointing (23). At the present time, this test is rarely used in the clinical situation.

Multibreath Nitrogen Washout

The use of this test to measure the FRC was described in a previous section (Fig. 6-7). It may also be used to assess the homogeneity of ventilation. The nitrogen concentration after 7 minutes is used as an index of the homogeneity of ventilation. Normally, it is less than 2.5%. If uneven gas distribution exists owing to slower emptying of some lung compartments, the washout is prolonged and the nitrogen concentration after 7 minutes is greater than 2.5%. Occasionally, the multibreath nitrogen washout test may be abnormal when the single-breath nitrogen test is normal. This has been attributed to the exchange of gas with bullae or similar compartments, which is too slow to affect the single-breath test but is detectable by the washout method owing to the prolonged tidal breathing.

Radioactive Xenon Distribution

The two tests of distribution described in the preceding section provide an index, giving some overall indication of the degree of inhomogeneity. Visualization of the distribution of gas may be performed in the radioactive xenon test, in which the subject breathes a gas mixture containing ^{133}Xe while his or her chest is scanned with a gamma camera. The ^{133}Xe isotope may also be dissolved in saline and injected intravenously. Because the gas is poorly soluble in blood, it is almost completely eliminated in one passage through the lungs. Scanning over the chest wall immediately after injection yields an estimate of relative perfusion to various areas, and the rate of clearance from these areas indicates their relative ventilation.

GAS TRANSFER AND EXCHANGE

The ability of gases to transfer across the alveolar–capillary membrane is assessed by analyzing the concentration of respiratory gases on both sides of the membrane or by assessing the ease with which a foreign gas transfers from the alveoli to the blood. There are several factors that affect the process of gas exchange, including the total surface area available for gas exchange, the diffusion characteristics of the alveolar–capillary membrane, the perfusion of the capillaries with blood, and the matching of ventilation to perfusion. These tests, however, give an overall index of diffusion and do not allow an assessment of each of the factors involved.

Blood Gas and Acid–Base Analysis

The measurement of the pH and partial pressures of oxygen and carbon dioxide in the arterial and venous blood is fundamental to the diagnosis and management of patients with pulmonary disorders. These measurements are not only valuable in the management of critically ill patients but also enable one to determine a number of clinically useful indexes of cardiopulmonary function, including venous admixture (physiologic shunt fraction) and physiologic dead space fraction. They reflect the overall function of the cardiopulmonary system with respect to gas exchange. Detailed information on the use and interpretation of these measurements is presented in Chapter 3, Alveolar Ventilation, Gas Exchange, Oxygen Delivery, and Acid–Base Physiology.

Carbon Monoxide Diffusing Capacity

The diffusing capacity of the lungs (D_L) is a measure of the ability of gases to diffuse from the alveoli into the pulmonary capillary blood. Carbon monoxide is the usual test gas because it is not normally present in the lungs or blood and because it is much more soluble in blood than in lung tissues. When the diffusing capacity is measured with carbon monoxide, it is called the carbon monoxide diffusing capacity (D_{LCO}).

To determine D_{LCO}, the amount of CO transferred per unit time and the average partial pressure difference of the gas across the alveolar–capillary membrane must be measured. The following equation represents this basic principle:

$$D_{LCO} = \dot{V}_{CO}/(P_{ACO} - P_{cCO}) \tag{6.1}$$

where $\dot{V}_{CO}$ is the uptake of carbon monoxide and P_{ACO} and P_{cCO} are the partial pressures of carbon monoxide in the alveolar gas and capillary blood, respectively. The final result for D_{LCO} is expressed as milliliters of carbon monoxide transferred per minute per millimeter of mercury pressure gradient. As the D_{LCO} is directly related to the alveolar volume, it is frequently normalized to this value (D_L/V_A), which allows for its interpretation in the presence of abnormal lung volumes.

Techniques

The most common manner by which the diffusing capacity is measured is the single-breath carbon monoxide test ($D_{LCO_{SB}}$) (24). With this method, the subject exhales to RV and then inhales a full breath of a gas mixture containing a low concentration of CO and a known concentration of an insoluble tracer gas, which is most commonly helium. The subject holds

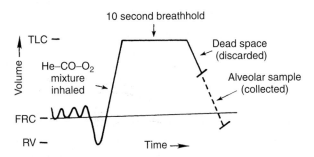

FIGURE 6-11. Kymograph tracing during the single-breath D_{LCO} maneuver. The patient first exhales to residual volume, then takes a full breath of a known mixture of oxygen, helium, and carbon monoxide. The breath is held at full inspiration for 10 seconds to allow gas transfer, then the subject exhales. After the initial dead space is exhaled, a sample of alveolar gas is collected and analyzed. The difference in gas concentration between the inhaled gas and the alveolar gas sample allows for calculation of the transfer of carbon monoxide from the lungs.

his or her breath for 10 seconds and then exhales completely (see Fig. 6-11). The initial alveolar volume and alveolar concentration of carbon monoxide are derived from measurements of the concentration of the tracer gas in the inhaled and exhaled air and the carbon monoxide concentration in the inspired gas. The final P_{ACO} is assumed to be the end-expiratory partial pressure of carbon monoxide. It is assumed that the P_{ACO} declines exponentially and that the capillary partial pressure is negligible. The D_{LCO} can then be easily computed from the following equation:

$$D_{LCO} = (V_A \times 60/(Pbar - 47) \times t) \times (\ln P_{ACO_i}/P_{ACO_t}) \quad (6.2)$$

where V_A is the original lung volume, $Pbar$ is the barometric pressure, t is the time of breath holding, and P_{ACO_i} and P_{ACO_t} are the initial and final partial alveolar pressures of carbon monoxide, respectively (2). Recommendations for the standard technique for this measurement have been published (24). In smokers, the level of carbon monoxide in the blood due to smoking is usually not taken into consideration and, accordingly, the measured D_{LCO} is less than the actual D_{LCO} (25).

A second technique is the steady state method ($D_{LCO\,SS}$), of which there are several variations. In these methods, the subject rebreathes a gas with a known CO concentration until CO uptake reaches a steady state, at which point several measurements are made for the calculation of the entities in Equation 6.1. The various methods differ in the way in which the mean P_{ACO} and the capillary P_{CCO} are calculated (26).

A less commonly used technique is the rebreathing method ($D_{LCO\,RB}$), in which a subject rebreathes a CO–He mixture for approximately one minute (27). The gas mixture, the measurement, and calculations are nearly identical to those for the single-breath technique.

The choice of the technique used depends on several factors. The single-breath technique is most widely used because it is simple and quick to perform. It is possible, however, that this technique does not give truly physiologic results because breath holding does not provide proper conditions for complete gas distribution. It is also the method that is most sensitive to ventilation–perfusion abnormalities and cannot be used for measurements during exercise. The steady state and rebreathing methods can be applied to exercise testing and are less affected by ventilation–perfusion abnormalities but are more difficult and time consuming to perform.

Factors Influencing the Diffusing Capacity

The resistance to the diffusion of carbon monoxide from the alveoli to the blood is determined primarily by two factors: the state of the alveolar–capillary membrane and the amount of hemoglobin in the pulmonary capillaries available for uptake of carbon monoxide (28). Mathematically, the following formula expresses this relationship:

$$1/D_L = 1/D_M + 1/\theta V_c \quad (6.3)$$

where D_L is the diffusing capacity of the lung, D_M represents the membrane component, V_c is the capillary blood volume, and the coefficient θ is the rate at which CO binds to intracellular oxyhemoglobin. Normally, the two components on the right side of Equation 6.3 contribute approximately equally to the measured D_{LCO} (29).

Both quantitative and qualitative abnormalities in the alveolar–capillary membrane may alter the measured D_{LCO}. The measured D_{LCO} depends on the total surface area available for gas exchange. Therefore, large individuals will have a higher D_{LCO} than small individuals. Also, the removal of a portion of the lung will reduce the D_{LCO}. In areas of the lung that are poorly ventilated, carbon monoxide will not be transferred and a reduced diffusing capacity will result. In a given patient, a higher D_{LCO} will be obtained with a higher lung volume (30).

The D_{LCO} may also be reduced if there is increased resistance to diffusion across the alveolar membrane. Historically, qualitative abnormalities in the alveolar–capillary membrane have been considered to be due primarily to an increased membrane thickness. However, the relative contribution of a "thick" membrane to a decrease in the D_{LCO} appears to have been overestimated. In diseases with interstitial thickening, other factors such as alterations in the alveolar architecture with loss of surface area for gas exchange appear to play a greater role in producing a decreased D_{LCO} (28).

The second major factor that influences the diffusing capacity, represented by the last term in Equation 6.3, is the ability of the blood to accept and bind carbon monoxide. Fundamentally, this is dependent on two factors: the pulmonary capillary blood volume and the level of hemoglobin in this capillary blood. The pulmonary capillary blood volume is obviously reduced in areas of the lung that are not perfused. Changes in position and alterations in intrathoracic pressure at the time of measurement can each alter pulmonary capillary blood volume.

Diffusing capacity measurements are usually made to determine the status of the lung. As anemia can result in a decreased diffusing capacity in the presence of a normal lung, it is recommended that diffusing capacity measurements be corrected for the level of hemoglobin in the blood by using the following equations (31):
In men,

$$\text{Adjusted } D_{LCO} = \text{observed } D_{LCO} + 1.40 (14.6 - [Hb]) \quad (6.4)$$

In women,

$$\text{Adjusted } D_{LCO} = \text{observed } D_{LCO} + 1.40 (13.4 - [Hb]) \quad (6.5)$$

EXERCISE AND EXERCISE TESTING

In recent years, exercise pathophysiology and exercise testing have received increased attention. This is because an individual's capacity to function on a daily basis is more closely related to the maximal performance of his or her pulmonary and cardiovascular systems than to the performance of these organ systems at rest. If an individual is perfectly comfortable at rest but becomes very dyspneic with minimal exercise, he or she will be miserable. Life is a series of exercises that range from grooming oneself to feeding oneself to generating an income through work. Under normal conditions, the ability to perform exercise depends on the capacity of the circulatory and respiratory systems to increase the transport of oxygen to exercising muscles and the status of the local factors that determine whether the increased quantity of oxygen reaches the cell interior, where it is used to produce energy for muscle fiber contraction. If a certain activity requires a greater oxygen consumption than can be generated by the individual, then that activity is closed to that individual.

In addition, it has been shown that the exercise capacity of patients is a more powerful predictor of mortality than other established risk factors for cardiovascular disease (32). In one study of 6213 men consecutively referred for treadmill exercise testing for clinical reasons, each one unit increase in metabolic equivalents (METS) conferred a 12% improvement in survival (32). In patients with COPD, the $\dot{V}O_2$max is a better predictor of mortality than is spirometry (33).

There are at least nine reasons to study individuals while they exercise. First, an exercise test can quantitate the degree of functional impairment. The maximal workload tolerated by the individual or the oxygen consumption during maximal exercise ($\dot{V}O_2$max) can be measured and compared with those predicted for individuals of the same age, size, and sex. Second, analysis of the results of the exercise test can help indicate whether the limiting factor is pulmonary, cardiac, a lack of conditioning, or poor effort. Third, responses to various therapeutic interventions (e.g., vasodilator therapy for intractable heart failure) can be assessed with serial exercise tests. Fourth, results of exercise tests can provide the basis for the development of a rational reconditioning program. Fifth, the results of exercise testing are sometimes useful in the preoperative assessment of patients with bronchogenic carcinoma (34). Sixth, exercise test results are sometimes used to select patients for lung or heart transplantation. Seventh, exercise tests can be used to diagnose exercise-induced asthma (35). Eighth, they can be used to monitor disease progress, especially early interstitial lung disease. Ninth, exercise test results are the best predictors of mortality in normal individuals (32) and in patients with COPD (33) and cardiovascular disease (32).

This section briefly considers alterations that occur in the respiratory and circulatory systems during exercise. Excellent reviews are available that discuss the actual performance of exercise testing and the physiologic responses to exercise and training in more depth (35–39). In addition, the use of exercise testing in the differential diagnosis of work intolerance and disability evaluation is discussed.

EXERCISE PHYSIOLOGY AND PATHOPHYSIOLOGY

To exercise, an individual must generate more energy. Adenosine triphosphate (ATP) is the obligatory energetic intermediary in the transduction of ingested food energy into the mechanical energy for muscle contraction and work. ATP is generated primarily through the oxidation of carbohydrate and fat. When insufficient oxygen is present, ATP can also be generated via the anaerobic metabolism of carbohydrates to lactic acid. However, anaerobic metabolism is much less efficient than aerobic metabolism. To generate the same amount of energy with anaerobic as with aerobic metabolism, approximately 18 times as much glucose must be used. Accordingly, to all intents and purposes, an individual's ability to exercise is limited by his or her capacity to deliver oxygen to the exercising muscles and by the ability of exercising muscles to use the delivered oxygen (40).

The oxygen required to perform various tasks is shown in Table 6-1. Note that the oxygen requirements vary more than 15-fold, from 200 mL/minute at rest to more than 3,200 mL/minute for carrying loads up stairs. Note also that eating and conversing require relatively low levels of oxygen consumption. Therefore, it becomes evident that if a patient is breathless during an interview or during eating, it will be very difficult for that patient to dress himself or herself, take a shower, drive a car, or do any housekeeping. The fact that propulsion of a wheelchair takes much less oxygen than does walking at 2.5 miles per hour suggests that more people with severe exercise limitation might benefit from this device. If physicians keep in mind the oxygen requirements for the activities listed in Table 6-1, they can counsel their patients more rationally in what they should and should not do.

MEASURES OF WORK CAPACITY

As mentioned earlier, an individual's ability to perform muscular work is dependent on his or her capacity to transport

TABLE 6-1. Energy Requirements for an Average-Sized Adult during Various Activities

Activity	O_2 Consumption (mL/min)
Rest, supine	200
Sitting	240
Standing relaxed	280
Eating	280
Conversation	280
Typing	360
Dressing, undressing	460
Propulsion, wheelchair	480
Driving car	560
Peeling potatoes	580
Walking 2.5 mph	720
Making beds	780
Bricklaying	800
Showering	840
Swimming 20 yd/min	1,000
Golfing	1,000
Walking 3.75 mph	1,120
Tennis	1,420
Ambulation, braces, and crutches	1,600
Shoveling snow	1,700
Ascending stairs, 22-lb load, 54 ft/min	3,240

From Gordon EE. Energy costs of activities in health and disease. *Arch Intern Med* 1958;101:702. Reproduced with permission of the author and publisher.

oxygen from the atmosphere to the mitochondria of the cells in the exercising muscles. The best metabolic index of the work capacity in a given individual is the maximum O_2 consumption per unit time ($\dot{V}O_2max$) of the individual. As the oxygen requirement to perform a given task depends on the weight of the individual, the best indication of an individual's exercise capacity is the $\dot{V}O_2max/kg$. Prediction equations for the $\dot{V}O_2max$ are given later in this chapter (see Eqs. 6.9–6.16). The $\dot{V}O_2max$ is determined by measuring oxygen consumption ($\dot{V}O_2$) at progressively higher workloads (37). Eventually, a point is reached where higher workloads do not result in higher $\dot{V}O_2$, and, by definition, the highest $\dot{V}O_2$ value attained is $\dot{V}O_2max$. The leveling off of $\dot{V}O_2$ provides objective evidence that the subject has attained maximal aerobic power. However, it is notable that one cannot demonstrate such a plateau in most individuals undergoing exercise testing, and the $\dot{V}O_2max$ is taken as the highest $\dot{V}O_2$ attained by the patient (41). As the energy for the additional work is provided by anaerobic metabolism, a demonstration that the blood lactate levels are substantial (8 mmol/L or greater) also indicates that the subject has attained maximal aerobic power.

Because maximum exercise is at times uncomfortable for the subject, many exercise laboratories attempt to derive the $\dot{V}O_2max$ from a $\dot{V}O_2$ measured at a submaximal load. This can be done because, in most individuals, there is a linear relationship between heart rate and $\dot{V}O_2$ after the $\dot{V}O_2$ reaches a certain level. The maximum heart rate for an individual can be estimated by subtracting the patient's age from 220. Therefore, if $\dot{V}O_2$ is measured at two submaximum exercise levels, the $\dot{V}O_2max$ can be estimated as demonstrated in Figure 6-12. This method of determining the $\dot{V}O_2max$ by derivation from submaximal load is relatively accurate for normal subjects, deconditioned patients, and most patients with heart disease. However, it is usually not applicable to patients with moderate to severe pulmonary disease because their exercise is limited by their ventilatory abilities; thus, they do not achieve

their predicted maximum heart rate. It is also not applicable for patients who are taking β-blockers, which reduce the patient's maximal heart rate. Many patients with left ventricular failure also fall far short of reaching their predicted maximal heart rate (42).

Other indices of work capacity frequently used are watts, kilopound meters (kpm) per minute, and multiples of resting O_2 consumption (METS). The relationship between these indices of work capacity and the $\dot{V}O_2$ is shown in Table 6-2. Most bicycle ergometers are calibrated in watts or in kpm per minute. Therefore, a reasonable estimate of the $\dot{V}O_2$ for bicycle ergometer exercise can be obtained from Table 6-2. When exercise is performed on a treadmill, the $\dot{V}O_2$ is dependent on the patient's weight, the speed of the treadmill, and the inclination of the treadmill. Nomograms are available for the prediction of an individual's $\dot{V}O_2$ from his or her weight and from the speed and inclination of the treadmill (43). Therefore, relatively accurate estimates of $\dot{V}O_2$ can be obtained without the collection of exhaled gases. Such estimates do not take into consideration the contribution of anaerobic metabolism to the work performed. Moreover, with repeated testing, individuals tend to become more efficient on both the treadmill and the bicycle ergometer. Hence, these indirect estimates of the $\dot{V}O_2max$ tend to overestimate actual improvements in the $\dot{V}O_2max$.

DETERMINANTS OF WORK CAPACITY ($\dot{V}O_2max$)

The oxygen consumption ($\dot{V}O_2$) of an individual is given by the following equation:

$$\dot{V}O_2 = \dot{Q} \times (CaO_2 - C\bar{v}O_2) \qquad (6.6)$$

where $\dot{Q}$ is the cardiac output, CaO_2 the oxygen content of arterial blood, and $C\bar{v}O_2$ the oxygen content of mixed venous blood. As almost all the oxygen in the blood is bound to hemoglobin, Equation 6.6 can be rewritten as follows:

$$\dot{V}O_2 = \dot{Q} \times [Hb] \times (SaO_2 - S\bar{v}O_2) \times 1.34 \qquad (6.7)$$

where Hb is the concentration of hemoglobin in the blood, SaO_2 is the hemoglobin saturation in arterial blood, $S\bar{v}O_2$ is the hemoglobin saturation of mixed venous blood, and 1.34 is the amount of oxygen it takes to fully saturate 1 g of hemoglobin. From Equation 6.7, one can readily appreciate that the $\dot{V}O_2max$ is dependent on the cardiac output, the hemoglobin concentration, the arterial oxygen saturation, and the ability

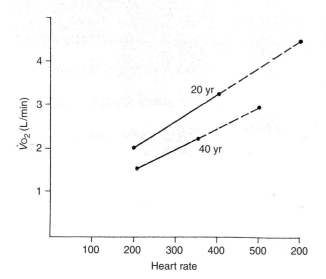

FIGURE 6-12. Predicting the $\dot{V}O_2max$ from submaximal exercise levels. The top line represents the $\dot{V}O_2$ of a 20-year-old; $\dot{V}O_2$ is 2,100 at a heart rate of 120 and is 3,250 at a heart rate of 160. By extrapolating to a heart rate of 200 (220 − 20), we find an estimated $\dot{V}O_2max$ of 4,500. In an analogous manner, the 40-year-old represented by the bottom line was found to have an estimated. $\dot{V}O_2max$ of 3,000 mL/minute.

TABLE 6-2. Relationship between O_2 Consumption and Other Measures of Work

O_2 Consumption (mL/min)	kpm/min	W	METS
225	0	0	1
900	300	50	4
1,500	600	100	7
2,100	900	150	10
2,800	1,200	200	13
3,500	1,500	250	16
4,200	1,800	300	19
5,000	2,100	350	22

of the exercising muscles to extract oxygen from blood during maximum exercise, as reflected by the $S\bar{v}O_2$. We will discuss exercise physiology by examining the factors that influence the different terms in Equation 6.7.

Cardiac Output

The cardiac output is the limiting factor for $\dot{V}O_2$max in normal subjects (37). Attempts to go beyond maximal work capacity are associated with a further increase in ventilation but no further increase in the cardiac output or $\dot{V}O_2$max. The cardiac output during exercise increases linearly with increasing $\dot{V}O_2$. Although an increase in cardiac output can result from an increase in either heart rate or stroke volume or both, most of the increase in cardiac output during exercise is related to increases in the heart rate, and the increases in stroke volume are proportionately smaller.

The cardiac output at a given $\dot{V}O_2$ is essentially identical in trained and untrained subjects during arm and leg exercise and during running, bicycling, and swimming. Therefore, the $\dot{V}O_2$ provides an indirect measure of the cardiac output. The cardiac output is approximately 5 L plus the $\dot{V}O_2$ times 5. Therefore, the cardiac output with a $\dot{V}O_2$ of 1 L/minute is approximately 10 L/minute, whereas the cardiac output with a $\dot{V}O_2$ of 3 L/minute is approximately 20 L/minute.

The work capacity of patients with heart disease is also limited by their cardiac output. In general, cardiac patients generate the same maximal heart rates as do normal subjects. However, because they have much lower stroke volumes than normal individuals, the cardiac output at a given heart rate is reduced in proportion to the reduction in the stroke volume. In these patients, the cardiac output can be improved by surgical correction of valvular defects, by improvement in the perfusion of the myocardium by rehabilitative training or surgery, or by administration of inotropic agents such as digitalis (42).

Hemoglobin Concentration

From Equation 6.7, it is obvious that hemoglobin (Hb) is a critical factor in determining $\dot{V}O_2$max. An abnormally high or a low Hb may be associated with a decreased work capacity. The explanation for the decrease in work capacity with a low Hb is obvious. Support for the relationship between the Hb and exercise tolerance is provided by a study of patients with kidney disease receiving chronic dialysis. When these patients were given erythropoietin such that their Hb increased from 7.3 to 10.8 g/dL, their exercise capacity increased from 108 to 130 W (44).

The detrimental effects of a very high Hb on $\dot{V}O_2$max is not immediately apparent from Equation 6.6. Nevertheless, too high a hematocrit and Hb can result in increased viscosity of the blood, which in turn can decrease the maximum cardiac output. If the reduction in cardiac output is proportionately greater than the increase in Hb, $\dot{V}O_2$max is reduced. This appears to be the case for both the experimental animal and the COPD patient with polycythemia. In dogs, the systemic oxygen transport during exercise is reduced when the animals are made polycythemic (45). In COPD patients, reduction of the hematocrit from above 60% to below 55% results in a marked improvement in exercise tolerance, which indicates that the increase in cardiac output is proportionately greater than the decrease in Hb (46).

In recent years, athletes have attempted to increase their performance by the administration of erythropoietin or transfusions; the practice is popularly called "blood doping." It appears that such practices do indeed result in a significant increase in the $\dot{V}O_2$max. One report summarized the results from 30 subjects who participated in four different investigations (47). These individuals exercised before and within 72 hours of reinfusing two 450-mL blood units. Overall, erythrocyte reinfusion led to a mean increase in the $\dot{V}O_2$max of 0.357 L/min. In general, for every 1% increase in Hb, there was a 1% increase in the $\dot{V}O_2$max, but there was marked interindividual variability in this relationship. At the present time, the policing of blood doping via transfusion or the administration of erythropoietin is a major problem for sporting organizations (48).

Smoking can affect work capacity by transforming normal hemoglobin into carboxyhemoglobin (CO–Hb), which has no value in terms of O_2 transport. Smokers generally have CO–Hb values around 4% to 7%. In normal subjects, it has been shown that $\dot{V}O_2$max decreases proportionately to the level of CO–Hb. A CO–Hb of 10% is associated with an approximately 10% decrease in the $\dot{V}O_2$max (49).

Peripheral O_2 Extraction ($S\bar{v}O_2$)

During exercise, there is increased O_2 extraction by the exercising muscles, which results in a lowered mixed venous saturation ($S\bar{v}O_2$). The contribution of the decreased $S\bar{v}O_2$ to $\dot{V}O_2$ is obvious from Equation 6.7. Mixed venous blood is a mixture of the venous blood returning to the right heart from exercising muscles and from the remainder of the body. Blood returning from heavily exercising muscles is quite desaturated, with a $P\bar{v}O_2$ of 10 to 15 mm Hg and an $S\bar{v}O_2$ of less than 10% (50). In superbly conditioned subjects at exhaustion, the mixed venous saturation averages about 10% (50).

Some authors have proposed that exercise is limited by the diffusion of oxygen from the capillaries to the mitochondria in the exercising muscles (40). In particular, there seems to be a "bottleneck" in the diffusion of oxygen from the capillary to the mitochondria as the oxygen enters the muscle cell before it combines with myoglobin (40). However, most maintain that the oxygen delivery to the muscles is the factor that limits exercise because the hemoglobin is less than 10% saturated in the blood emanating from a highly trained muscle.

During exercise, the distribution of the systemic vascular resistance is altered such that a higher percentage of blood is distributed to the exercising muscles. In unfit people, this vasoregulation during exercise is suboptimal. They fail to adjust their regional peripheral vascular resistance; thus, their exercising muscles receive less of the cardiac output. Therefore, their $S\bar{v}O_2$ at exhaustion is considerably higher than 25%. It follows from Equation 6.7 that their $\dot{V}O_2$ at a given level of cardiac output is lower than it is in the conditioned individual because the $SaO_2 - S\bar{v}O_2$ is smaller (38). Other dysfunctions of the peripheral circulation can also result in a suboptimal distribution of cardiac output and a high $S\bar{v}O_2$ at maximal exercise.

Arterial Oxygen Saturation (SaO_2)

The SaO_2 depends on the alveolar O_2 tension (PAO_2) and the alveolar–arterial O_2 gradient ($PAO_2 - PaO_2$). The PaO_2, in turn, is dependent on the partial pressure of the inspired O_2 (PIO_2), the $PaCO_2$, and the respiratory exchange ratio (R), as shown by the alveolar air equation:

$$PAO_2 = PIO_2 - PaCO_2 \times [FIO_2 + (1 - FIO_2)/R] \qquad (6.8)$$

where FIO_2 is the fractional concentration of O_2 in inspired gas. Note that an elevation of the $PaCO_2$ will decrease the PAO_2. In normal subjects, the $PaCO_2$ tends to remain constant or decrease with increasing levels of exercise to maintain a constant pH (51). Therefore, the PAO_2 remains constant or increases. However, in some patients with COPD, the ventilatory reserve is insufficient to eliminate the additional CO_2 produced with exercise. Accordingly, the $PaCO_2$ increases and the PAO_2 decreases (52). For a given level of pulmonary dysfunction, patients whose $PaCO_2$ increases during exercise will have higher exercise tolerance because they do not have to breathe as much to get rid of the same amount of CO_2 (52).

The alveolar–arterial oxygen gradient ($PAO_2 - PaO_2$) results from venous admixture ($\dot{Q}va/\dot{Q}t$), which is the fraction of the cardiac output that reaches arterial blood and acts as though it had not been exposed to alveolar gas. Venous admixture has three components: (a) that which results from the perfusion of units with low $\dot{V}/\dot{Q}$ ratios, (b) that which results from the failure of the capillary PO_2 and the alveolar PO_2 in reaching equilibrium, and (c) that which results from true right-to-left shunts. In patients with lung disease, the majority of the $PAO_2 - PaO_2$ gradient is due to inadequate ventilation of perfused alveoli. The amount of ventilation required to fully oxygenate the blood in a given alveolus is dependent on both the amount of perfusion and the degree of venous desaturation. West has shown that in a lung unit with a ventilation–perfusion ratio ($\dot{V}/\dot{Q}$) of 1, the PaO_2 will fall from 100 to 42 mm Hg as $P\bar{v}O_2$ falls from 100 to 10 mm Hg (53).

The best way to understand this phenomenon is to consider a numerical example. Table 6-3 lists the oxygen requirements to achieve full saturation of 100 mL blood at different $S\bar{v}O_2$ levels and the corresponding PAO_2 if this much oxygen is extracted from 100 mL of ventilated air. When the $S\bar{v}O_2$ falls below 55%, the resulting PAO_2 falls drastically and, accordingly, the PaO_2 must fall. In the same example, if the $\dot{V}/\dot{Q}$ ratio increases to 3, the PAO_2 would still be over 100 mm Hg when the $S\bar{v}O_2$ is 25%.

The preceding example illustrates that a $\dot{V}/\dot{Q}$ ratio of 1 is not ideal during exercise. If the $S\bar{v}O_2$ is substantially decreased, the $\dot{V}/\dot{Q}$ ratio must increase above 1, or arterial desaturation will result. The cardiac output of a normal subject at rest is about 5 L/minute and increases fourfold to a level of 20 L/minute on maximal exercise. The minute ventilation increases from 5 L/minute at rest to 80 L/minute during maximal exercise. Thus, the overall $\dot{V}/\dot{Q}$ ratio increases from 1 at rest to 4 during maximal exercise, and arterial desaturation does not normally result from the above mechanism.

Another factor that can increase the $PAO_2 - PaO_2$ is a reduced diffusing capacity of the lungs. If, at the end of the capillary, the PO_2 of the blood has not reached that of the alveolus, the $PAO_2 - PaO_2$ will be increased. Such an increase is said to be due to a diffusion abnormality. It is generally accepted that in normal individuals, complete equilibrium occurs between alveolar and capillary blood at most levels of exercise except when the individual is breathing low levels of oxygen. However, the SaO_2 is decreased in nearly 50% of elite cyclists and runners when they are performing maximally. A diffusion limitation is the most likely explanation for the desaturation in these athletes, but ventilation–perfusion imbalances could play a role (54).

It is thought that a reduced diffusing capacity does not contribute to the $PAO_2 - PaO_2$ at rest, even in patients with lung disease and markedly reduced diffusing capacities. However, when a patient with a reduced diffusing capacity exercises, equilibrium between the alveolar and capillary PO_2 may not occur because the venous blood is more desaturated and the capillary transit time is shorter during exercise. Shepard, in a theoretical analysis, demonstrated that a reduced diffusing capacity can cause a substantial reduction in SaO_2 during exercise (55). Moreover, once the $PAO_2 - PaO_2$ is increased due to diffusion limitations, slight increases in $\dot{V}O_2$ lead to dramatic reductions in SaO_2. For example, if the diffusing capacity is 16, the SaO_2 will start to fall when the $\dot{V}O_2$ reaches 1,600 mL/minute and will fall to less than 70% when the $\dot{V}O_2$ reaches 1,800 mL/minute, assuming that the $S\bar{v}O_2$ was 50%. In general, the higher the cardiac output, the more rapid the transit of blood in the pulmonary capillaries. Once the level is reached at which equilibrium between the alveoli and capillaries does not occur, further increases in the velocity of flow or decreases in $S\bar{v}O_2$ lead to large decreases in SaO_2.

The reduction in SaO_2 due to a given fractional shunt ($\dot{Q}s/\dot{Q}t$) depends on the $S\bar{v}O_2$. For example, if the $\dot{Q}s/\dot{Q}t$ is 25%, the SaO_2 will be 94% if $S\bar{v}O_2$ is 75%, but will decrease to 81% if $S\bar{v}O_2$ is 25%. In view of the marked reduction in the $S\bar{v}O_2$ during strenuous exercise, one might expect that the SaO_2 would decrease substantially in many individuals during heavy exercise and that this reduction would limit their exercise capabilities. However, SaO_2 does not change in normal subjects even during exhaustive physical work. Most patients with lung disease have an increased $PAO_2 - PaO_2$ at rest, and the majority of this increase is due to perfusion of units with low $\dot{V}/\dot{Q}$ ratios. As mentioned previously, patients with COPD increase their ventilation more than their cardiac output during exercise so that their PAO_2 does not decrease. This increase in total ventilation tends to improve the ventilation of units with low $\dot{V}/\dot{Q}$ ratios and decreases the fraction of the ($\dot{Q}s/\dot{Q}t$) that is due to perfusion of poorly ventilated alveoli. The net effect of exercise on SaO_2 depends on whether the ($\dot{Q}s/\dot{Q}t$) decreases enough to compensate for the decreased $S\bar{v}O_2$.

Ventilatory Limitation

As mentioned earlier, the cardiac output is the factor limiting exercise in normal subjects. At maximal exercise, they have

TABLE 6-3.   Influence of $S\bar{v}O_2$ on PAO_2, Assuming R Is 0.8 and Hb 15 g/100 mL

$S\bar{v}O_2$ %	O_2 Required for $SaO_2 = 100\%$ mL	PAO_2 if $SaO_2 = 100\%$	
		$\dot{V}/\dot{Q} = 1$	$\dot{V}/\dot{Q} = 3$
75	5	115	138
65	7	101	134
55	9	87	129
45	11	73	124
35	13	58	120
25	15	44	115

ventilatory reserve, as manifested by their ability to increase their ventilation voluntarily. However, the exercise capacity of most individuals with moderate or severe lung disease is limited by their ventilatory abilities. Normal individuals are unable to maintain minute ventilations above 60% of their MVV. Patients with lung disease are also unable to sustain minute ventilations much above 60% of their MVV without developing dyspnea (56). Therefore, their exercise capabilities are limited by their ventilation even though their arterial blood gases frequently remain unchanged at exhaustion.

In addition to their reduced ventilatory reserves, patients with lung disease have increased ventilatory requirements for a given level of exercise. The ventilatory requirement is determined by the CO_2 production ($\dot{V}CO_2$), the $PaCO_2$, and the wasted ventilation fraction of each breath (V_D/V_T). In patients with lung disease, the V_D/V_T is much higher at rest (mean 0.45) than it is in normal individuals (mean 0.28). Moreover, during exercise, the V_D/V_T on an average does not change in patients with COPD, whereas it falls below 0.20 in normal individuals (52,57).

Therefore, the patient with lung disease needs more ventilation for a given workload. The ventilatory equivalent for CO_2 ($\dot{V}E/\dot{V}CO_2$) is a measure of the efficiency with which additional CO_2 is eliminated. The normal $\dot{V}E/\dot{V}CO_2$ is about 30, but with COPD, it can exceed 50 (58).

Anaerobic Metabolism

Exercise requires an increase in the O_2 flow to the mitochondria of the exercising muscles. If the increase in O_2 flow is insufficient to generate the required ATP, anaerobic metabolism must be used to generate the ATP. The anaerobic threshold is the highest level of work that can be done without inducing a sustained metabolic acidosis. The anaerobic threshold normally occurs between 50% and 60% of the $\dot{V}O_2max$.

Lactic acid is the end product of anaerobic metabolism. The metabolic acidosis that results from its accumulation produces the subjective feeling of fatigue that precludes extensive periods of anaerobic exercise. When lactic acid is produced, it is immediately buffered, predominantly by the bicarbonate system:

$$H^+ lactate^- + Na^+HCO_3^- \rightarrow Na^+lactate^- + CO_2 + H_2O$$

The above reaction causes a reduction in the bicarbonate levels and an increase in the production of carbon dioxide gas. Until the anaerobic threshold is reached, the relationship between the workload or the $\dot{V}O_2$ and the $\dot{V}E$ is linear with progressive workloads. Above the anaerobic threshold, $\dot{V}E$ increases proportionately more than $\dot{V}O_2$ for two reasons: (a) the increased carbon dioxide produced by the buffering of lactate must be eliminated, and (b) the metabolic acidosis produced by the buffering process acts as a respiratory stimulant such that $\dot{V}E$ increases proportionately more than the $\dot{V}CO_2$, and the $PaCO_2$ falls. In general, normal individuals and patients with cardiovascular or pulmonary disease attempt to regulate their ventilation such that the arterial pH remains stable at rest and during exercise levels of varying intensities (59).

The anaerobic threshold is best documented by demonstrating an increase in the blood lactate concentration. This is usually accompanied by a decrease in the plasma bicarbonate concentration. One can also try to identify the anaerobic

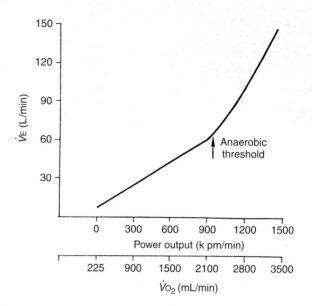

FIGURE 6-13. Determination of anaerobic threshold from plot of $\dot{V}E$ versus workload or $\dot{V}O_2$. The anaerobic threshold is identified as the workload at which the $\dot{V}E$ starts to increase out of proportion to the $\dot{V}O_2$ or the work load.

threshold by examining the results of the exhaled gas analysis. One method is to plot $\dot{V}E$ versus the workload. The anaerobic threshold occurs when $\dot{V}E$ increases disproportionately to the workload (see Fig. 6-13). A second method examines plots of the $\dot{V}E/\dot{V}O_2$ and the $\dot{V}E/\dot{V}CO_2$ versus the workload. The anaerobic threshold is the point where $\dot{V}E/\dot{V}O_2$ rises, whereas $\dot{V}E/\dot{V}CO_2$ remains stable, when plotted against work rate. A third method examines the relationship between the $\dot{V}O_2$ and the $\dot{V}CO_2$ and identifies the anaerobic threshold as the point where the $\dot{V}CO_2$ increases disproportionately to the $\dot{V}O_2$ (60). In general, noninvasive methods are relatively inaccurate in identifying the anaerobic threshold in patients with COPD (61). Moreover, the majority of patients with severe lung disease do not reach their anaerobic threshold (61).

TRAINING

It is widely recognized that it is possible to increase the maximum amount of exercise a subject can perform by a period of physical training. By the same token, periods of inactivity will decrease the maximum amount of exercise an individual can perform. In one study, $\dot{V}O_2max$ was measured in a group of elite Swedish swimmers at the height of their competitive swimming careers and, then, 4, 6, and 8 years after they had stopped swimming competitively (62). In these individuals, the $\dot{V}O_2max$ decreased much more rapidly than would be expected from aging alone, and the rapid decrease persisted even between the sixth and eighth years. In another study, five adult males with varying degrees of physical fitness were studied before and after 21 days of bed rest and, then, periodically during 60 days of intensive reconditioning (see Fig. 6-14) (63). During the 21 days of bed rest, $\dot{V}O_2max$ fell by over 25% in each of the five individuals. During the reconditioning period, $\dot{V}O_2max$ initially increased rapidly, then increased at a slower rate, and then appeared to level off after a

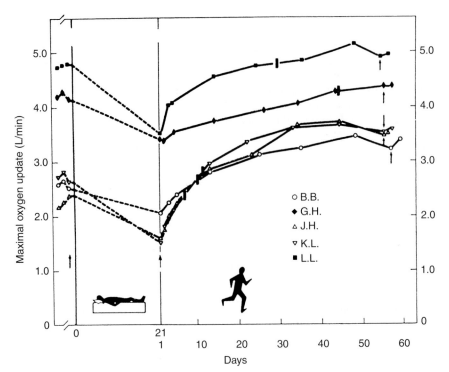

FIGURE 6-14. Changes in $\dot{V}O_2max$ with bed rest and training. *Heavy bars* mark the time during the training period at which the maximal oxygen uptake had returned to the control value obtained before bed rest. Originally, the top two patients were well conditioned, whereas the bottom three patients were poorly conditioned. [From Saltin B, Blomqvist G, Mitchell JH, et al. Response to exercise after bed rest and after training. A longitudinal study of adaptive changes in oxygen transport and body composition. *Circulation* 1968;38(Suppl. 7):1. By permission of the American Heart Association, Inc.]

mean of about 45 days. The $\dot{V}O_2max$ at the end of the training period had increased substantially more in the unfit than in the fit individuals.

In general, there are three different factors that should be considered in conditioning programs, namely, the intensity, the duration, and the frequency of the exercise (64). Of the three, the intensity is the most important. To increase $\dot{V}O_2max$, the oxygen transport system must be challenged with exercise, demanding at least 50% of the person's $\dot{V}O_2max$. Moreover, above 50% of $\dot{V}O_2max$, the higher the intensity of the exercise, the more rapid the improvement in $\dot{V}O_2max$ and the greater the eventual change will be. However, training should not be performed much above the anaerobic threshold. One can use the pulse to guide the intensity of exercise in that the anaerobic threshold is usually exceeded when the pulse is greater than 77% of the predicted maximal pulse (65). The exercise program should be performed at least twice a week, but every other day is preferable. The minimal duration of each training session should be 15 minutes, with 45 minutes being optimal. The degree of improvement in $\dot{V}O_2max$ after 2 months of training is dependent on the initial level of fitness and on the intensity of the exercise, as outlined in Table 6-4 (64).

TABLE 6-4. Expected Improvement in $\dot{V}O_2max$ after Training Three Times a Week for 45 Minutes for 2 Months

Initial Status		Expected Improvement (%)		
Level of Fitness	$\dot{V}O_2$ max mL/kg/min	Exercise at 50%–70% $\dot{V}O_2max$	Exercise at 70%–90% $\dot{V}O_2max$	Exercise at 90%–100% $\dot{V}O_2max$
Low	30	10	25	40
Medium	45	3	8	20
Excellent	60	0	0	5

The improvement in physical performance capacity that results from regularly performed vigorous exercise involves multiple adaptive reactions occurring primarily in the circulatory system. The maximum cardiac output increases via an increase in the maximum stroke volume arising from two factors. First, the myocardial function improves such that, with a given peripheral vascular resistance, the maximum cardiac output is increased. Second, local adaptive processes in the exercising muscle decrease the vascular resistance of the exercising muscles such that a higher fraction of the cardiac output is distributed to the exercising muscles. With conditioning, the improved myocardial function is a generalized process so that if unconditioned muscles are exercised, the maximum cardiac output will still be increased. In contrast, the redistribution of the cardiac output is specific in that if unconditioned muscles are exercised, the distribution of the cardiac output to them will not be facilitated.

An important by-product of the redistribution of the cardiac output to the exercising muscles is its effect on $S\overline{v}O_2$. When a larger fraction of the cardiac output goes to the exercising muscles, the $S\overline{v}O_2$ decreases because of the very low $S\overline{v}O_2$ of the larger fraction of the cardiac output returning from the exercising muscles. From Equation 6.7, it can be readily appreciated that this decrease in $S\overline{v}O_2$ will increase $\dot{V}O_2max$ substantially.

Training also leads to changes in muscle that has undergone training such that it can take up more oxygen (39). In particular, there is an increase in the oxidative capacity owing to an increase in mitochondrial volume and an enhancement of the enzyme systems that promote the use of free fatty acids. These changes lead to a lower SaO_2 at the end of the capillary. In addition, an increase in the vascular conductance owing to an increase in the capillary density leads to an increase in oxygen extraction by enlarging the surface area for oxygen movement.

It should be noted that the expected improvements outlined in Table 6-4 are those for healthy individuals. Even though patients with COPD frequently have a very low $\dot{V}O_2$max at the start of a physical training program, their $\dot{V}O_2$max does not increase by as much as normal individuals because their ventilatory capabilities, which limit their exercise performance, do not increase significantly during a training program (66,67). In recent years, there has been much interest in training the respiratory muscles of patients with lung disease. However, a meta-analysis of the results of respiratory muscle training concluded there was little evidence that patients with COPD clinically benefited from respiratory muscle training (68).

AGING AND EXERCISE PERFORMANCE

As an individual ages, his or her capacity to exercise decreases. In untrained individuals, there is approximately a 10% decrease per decade in the $\dot{V}O_2$max, starting at the age of 25 (38). In trained individuals, the decrease in the $\dot{V}O_2$max is approximately 6% per decade (38). The initial $\dot{V}O_2$max is approximately 50% higher in the trained individual; however, the absolute decrease in the $\dot{V}O_2$max is less in the trained individual. In the sedentary individual, most of the decline (72%) in the $\dot{V}O_2$max is due to a decreased cardiac output, whereas the remaining 28% is due to reduced peripheral oxygen extraction (38). Decreases in the stroke volume are more important than decreases in the maximal heart rate in producing the decrease in the $\dot{V}O_2$max (38). Interestingly, sedentary individuals above the age of 60 who embark on a vigorous training program can improve their $\dot{V}O_2$max by approximately 25% (69). However, their exercise capabilities still remain far below those of individuals who have remained trained throughout their lives (38,69).

PERFORMANCE OF EXERCISE TESTING

The reader is referred to a comprehensive ATS/ACCP statement of cardiopulmonary exercise testing for technical details regarding testing (70). Although the exercise test must, in general, be tailored to the individual patient, this author believes that most exercise tests should be conducted along the following guidelines: The patient should be studied on a treadmill or bicycle ergometer at increasing workloads. The test should be performed with continuous cardiac monitoring, with a physician at least in the vicinity. Resuscitation equipment, including a defibrillator, should be immediately at hand. The workload should be increased until the patient becomes physically exhausted.

However, it should be noted that the progressive ergometer test has little relevance to normal activities and may give no insight into the patient's difficulties in coping with daily living. Therefore, self-paced walking tests such as the 6-minute walk (71) or the shuttle walk (72) have been developed. These tests have the advantage of being a more natural test of exercise capacity and are reproducible and simple. However, they give information only on overall exercise tolerance and allow no physiologic measurements during exercise.

In the 6-minute walk, the distance that a patient walks during a self paced 6-minute period is recorded. The ATS has recently issued guidelines on the performance of this test (73). In the shuttle walk, the patient walks in an oval whose largest diameter is 10 m. The patient starts out walking slowly, and each minute, the walking speed is increased by 0.17 m per second

until the patient cannot keep up or is too short of breath to continue (72). As this is a progressive test, its results correlate better with progressive exercise tests than do those of the 6-minute walk test. However, results from the 6-minute walk test are better correlated with the patient's activities of daily living.

The data collected during ergometer or treadmill exercise tests depend on the information desired from the test. In general, there are four stages of exercise testing (43). In stage 1 exercise testing, the patient is exercised at increasing workloads until exhaustion, with the heart rate and ventilation being monitored. An estimate of the $\dot{V}O_2$ can be obtained from nomograms that relate the power output or the treadmill grade and speed to the $\dot{V}O_2$ (43). Cardiovascular dysfunction is suggested by a stage-1 test demonstrating a heart rate that is high relative to the workload and an early onset of the anaerobic threshold, as evidenced by nonlinear increases in ventilation. A ventilatory limitation is suggested when the maximum ventilation reaches 35 times the FEV_1 and when the anaerobic threshold and the maximum predicted heart rates are not achieved.

In stage 2 exercise testing, mixed expired gases are also collected and analyzed. The additional information provided includes the $\dot{V}O_2$, $\dot{V}CO_2$, $\dot{V}E/\dot{V}O_2$, and $\dot{V}E/\dot{V}CO_2$. Therefore, the aerobic capacity ($\dot{V}O_2$max) can be accurately determined. In addition, cardiac outputs and stroke volumes can be estimated if a rebreathing procedure is used to obtain the mixed venous PCO_2. These measurements are useful in further defining the factors limiting exercise but are unnecessary if the exercise capacity is normal. With stage 2 exercise testing, the end-tidal PCO_2 and PO_2 are usually also recorded. However, during exercise, there is no close correlation between the changes in the end-tidal PCO_2 and the arterial PCO_2 (74).

In stage 3 exercise testing, arterial blood gases are also collected. The additional data permit detection of hypoxemia, hypercapnia, and respiratory or metabolic acidosis during exercise. In addition, the VD/VT can be calculated. If the only reason for the measurement of arterial blood gases is to detect hypoxemia, a pulse oximeter is a possible noninvasive alternative. One study revealed that when the SaO_2 from pulse oximetry was compared to SaO_2 as determined by cooximetry, the mean difference was 1.7% and the standard deviation of the difference was 2.9% (75).

In stage 4 exercise testing, a Swan-Ganz catheter is inserted into the pulmonary artery. The additional information provided includes the pressures in the lesser circulation, the mixed venous blood gases, and the cardiac output as calculated by the Fick method.

Predicted Values for $\dot{V}O_2$max

The following equations provide predicted values for the $\dot{V}O_2$max (76,77).
In men,

$$\dot{V}O_2\text{max (L/minute)} = 4.2 - 0.032 \times \text{age (SD} \pm 0.4) \quad (6.9)$$

$$\dot{V}O_2\text{max (mL/kg/minute)} = 60 - 0.55 \times \text{age (SD} \pm 7.5) \quad (6.10)$$

Over the age of 55,

$$\dot{V}O_2\text{max (L/minute)} = 2.43 \text{ (SD} \pm 0.44) \quad (6.11)$$

$$\text{Workload (W)} = 179 \text{ (SD} \pm 36) \quad (6.12)$$

In women,

$$\dot{V}O_2\text{max (L/minute)} = 2.6 - 0.014 \times \text{age (SD} \pm 0.4) \quad (6.13)$$

$$\dot{V}O_2\text{max (mL/kg/minute)} = 48 - 0.37 \times \text{age (SD} \pm 7.0) \quad (6.14)$$

Over the age of 55,

$$\dot{V}O_2\text{max (L/minute)} = 1.49 \text{ (SD} \pm 0.31) \quad (6.15)$$

$$\text{Workload (W)} = 104 \text{ (SD} \pm 25) \quad (6.16)$$

USE OF PULMONARY FUNCTION AND EXERCISE TESTS

Pulmonary function tests and exercise tests can be used to answer many questions. This section is organized according to the various questions that might be asked.

Does My Patient Have Lung Disease?

This is the question most frequently asked. The answer to this question is obtained primarily by comparing the results from a given individual to those obtained from a normal population. The predicted value of a test for a given patient represents the mean value of a group of normal individuals with similar characteristics. The characteristics involved depend on the test but usually include height, age, and sex. The predicted value is calculated from a prediction equation, usually an algebraic equation derived from multiple linear regression. Associated with each predicted value is a range representing the expected variation in the group of normal individuals. Conventionally, this range has been defined as a somewhat arbitrary percentage of the predicted value. A better approach, which is gaining acceptance, is to use a range on the basis of the standard error of the estimate obtained in the analysis of the normal group. In this manner, the range that includes 95% of the normal individuals can be calculated. A test result is labeled as abnormal only if it falls outside the range into which 95% of normal individuals fall. This method takes into account intersubject variability. For specific equations, a number of references are available (78–85).

When a patient is initially evaluated, it is recommended that only spirometry be obtained. If the FEV_1, FVC, and FEV_1/FVC are all within normal limits, one can assume that the patient does not have significant obstructive or restrictive ventilatory dysfunction (86). At times, a diffusing capacity is obtained in addition to the spirometry because patients with lung disease, especially pulmonary vascular disease, may have normal spirometry but an abnormal diffusing capacity. Usually, there is no reason to obtain lung volume measurements or spirometry after the administration of bronchodilators in patients who have normal spirometry.

At times, inhalational challenge tests are useful in patients with normal spirometry. Asthma is an episodic disease, and many patients have normal spirometry at least part of the time. Inhalational challenge tests can demonstrate airway hyperresponsiveness in such patients and can suggest the diagnosis. In a similar manner, in some patients, cough is due to airway hyperresponsiveness, and an inhalational challenge test may be necessary to demonstrate the airway hyperresponsiveness if the spirometry is within normal limits (11). It should be remembered that 3% to 6% of asymptomatic individuals have airway hyperresponsiveness.

It should also be pointed out that the maximal exercise test is sometimes abnormal in patients with mild lung disease when the spirometry and diffusing capacity are normal. In one study of 30 patients with sarcoidosis, results from the maximal exercise tests were more sensitive than spirometry or the diffusing capacity were in identifying abnormalities. Excess ventilation and an increased V_D/V_T during exercise were the most common abnormalities (87).

What Type of Lung Disease Does My Patient Have?

Once a patient has been found to have abnormal pulmonary function, an effort to determine the type and degree of dysfunction should be made. In general, abnormalities in pulmonary function can be classified as obstructive ventilatory dysfunction, restrictive ventilatory dysfunction, and mixed ventilatory dysfunction.

OBSTRUCTIVE VENTILATORY DYSFUNCTION. By definition, obstructive ventilatory dysfunction occurs when there are reduced expiratory flow rates with maximal effort owing to increased expiratory resistance. As discussed in Chapter 2, Mechanics of Respiration, the increased expiratory resistance can be due to either increased airway resistance or decreased elastic recoil of the lung.

In determining whether airway obstruction is present, one should look at the FEV_1/FVC and the FEV_3/FVC. In general, if the FEV_1/FVC is above 0.75 and the FEV_3/FVC is above 0.95, the patient does not have significant obstructive ventilatory dysfunction. The forced vital capacity is often reduced with moderate to severe airway obstruction as a result of air trapping. The PEF and the FEF at different lung volumes are also reduced.

The degree of obstructive ventilatory dysfunction can be quantified as outlined in Table 6-5. The absolute value of the FEV_1 should be used only if the patient does not have restrictive ventilatory dysfunction also. The patient is classified according to the most severe criterion that he or she meets. For example, if the FEV_1/FVC is 0.35 and the FEV_1 is 1800 mL, the individual is classified as having severe obstructive ventilatory dysfunction.

RESTRICTIVE VENTILATORY DYSFUNCTION. By definition, restrictive pulmonary dysfunction indicates that the TLC is reduced. Most volume compartments are affected, resulting in decreases in VC, RV, and FRC, as well as the total lung capacity. Frequently, the residual volume is not reduced by as great a percentage as the other lung volumes. A diagnosis of restrictive impairment is made when the vital capacity falls below the predicted normal range and is associated with reductions in the other volume compartments. If the FVC is

TABLE 6-5. Criteria for Quantitating Degree of Obstruction

Grade	FEV_1/FVC	FEV_1 (mL)
Very severe	<0.30	<600
Severe	0.3–0.4	600–1,000
Moderate	0.4–0.6	1,000–2,000
Mild	0.6–0.7	2,000–3,000
Very mild	0.7–pred. value	>3,000

within normal limits, it is unlikely that the TLC is abnormal and lung volume measurements are usually not indicated (86). If the patient has no obstructive ventilatory dysfunction, restrictive ventilatory dysfunction can be established from spirometry. However, if the patient has obstructive ventilatory dysfunction, the FVC can be reduced due to the obstruction. Therefore, the diagnosis of restrictive ventilatory dysfunction can only be established if lung volumes, including RV, are measured. In one study of 206 patients with obstructive ventilatory dysfunction and a reduced FVC, only 40 (19%) had restrictive pulmonary dysfunction when lung volume measurements were obtained (88). When both the FEV_1 and the FVC are reduced with spirometry, one can get some idea as to whether the individual has predominantly obstructive or restrictive ventilatory dysfunction by comparing the value for the FEV_1 and the FVC expressed as a percentage of the predicted value. If the individual has predominantly restrictive dysfunction, the FVC will be reduced proportionately more than the FEV_1. Alternatively, if the individual has predominantly obstructive dysfunction, the FEV_1 will be reduced proportionately more than the FVC.

The degree of restrictive ventilatory dysfunction can be quantified as outlined in Table 6-6. Results of other ventilatory function tests—such as time-forced expiratory volumes, expiratory flows, and MVV—are either normal or slightly reduced with restrictive impairment. Although the FEV_1 and FEV_3 expressed as a percentage of the predicted value are reduced in individuals with restrictive ventilatory dysfunction, the FEV_1/FVC and the FEV_3/FVC are normal or greater than predicted, indicating an absence of airway obstruction.

MIXED VENTILATORY DYSFUNCTION. Some patients have concomitant obstructive and restrictive ventilatory dysfunction. Lung volume measurements, including a determination of the residual volume, are necessary in these individuals to quantify the degree of dysfunction. As the FEV_1 is reduced from the restrictive dysfunction, only the FEV_1/FVC should be used in quantifying the obstruction.

Does My Patient Have Predominantly Asthma, Chronic Bronchitis, or Emphysema?

The three main diseases that produce obstructive ventilatory dysfunction are asthma, chronic bronchitis, and emphysema. Some indication as to the pathogenesis of the obstruction can be obtained from the pulmonary function laboratory. However, it must be noted that, in the older smoker, the obstructive ventilatory dysfunction is usually due to a combination of all three diseases.

Measures of airway resistance are useful in separating the three entities. With pure emphysema, airway resistance is normal and the expiratory flow limitation is due to loss of lung

TABLE 6-6. Criteria for Quantitating Degree of Restriction

Grade	VC % Predicted	TLC % Predicted
Very mild	>80	>90
Mild	60–80	70–90
Moderate	30–60	50–70
Severe	<30	<50

elastic recoil. Therefore, an increased airway resistance indicates that the airways are abnormal and that the patient has a component of asthma or bronchitis. Emphysema results in destruction of pulmonary parenchyma and, therefore, loss of surface area for gas exchange. Accordingly, the DLCO is reduced with emphysema, whereas it is normal in asthma and chronic bronchitis.

BRONCHODILATOR TESTING. By definition, the obstructive ventilatory dysfunction with asthma is reversible. Therefore, many laboratories perform spirometry before and after administration of bronchodilators to distinguish asthma from chronic bronchitis and emphysema. A positive response is said to be present if the FEV_1 improves by at least 12% and 200 mL above baseline. However, it should be noted that most patients who appear to have chronic bronchitis or emphysema may periodically have an improvement of 15% or more in their FEV_1 if they are repeatedly tested (89). Although one might hypothesize that an acute response to a bronchodilator would predict chronic improvement in pulmonary function with bronchodilator therapy, this does not appear to be the case (90,91).

LARGE AIRWAY OBSTRUCTION. A relatively uncommon cause of obstructive ventilatory dysfunction is upper or large airway obstruction. However, it is important not to overlook this possibility because its presence can be life threatening. Upper airway obstruction is manifested by reduced flows early in exhalation and by normal flows during the latter part of exhalation (Fig. 6-4C). If the obstruction in the large airway is variable, its site inside or outside the thoracic inlet determines its effects on flow rates. Variable intrathoracic obstruction primarily affects FEF because positive pleural pressures cause further decrease in the size of the large airway. Variable extrathoracic obstruction affects forced inspiration because the negative intratracheal pressure on inspiration tends to make the trachea more collapsible. These changes are best demonstrated with the flow–volume loop, as described earlier in this chapter. The ratio of the FEV_1 to the $FEV_{0.5}$ is almost always greater than 1.5 except when obstruction of the large airways is present (92).

Is My Patient Going to Develop Lung Disease?

In the natural history of COPD, disease first develops in the small peripheral airways. As these airways contain only 10% to 20% of the total airway resistance, the usual tests for obstructive ventilatory dysfunction, such as the FEV_1/FVC, are normal when significant disease is present (93). Accordingly, many different tests have been proposed, including the closing volume, the slope of phase *III* on the single-breath nitrogen washout test, comparison of flow–volume loops obtained with room air and a mixture of helium and oxygen, and sophisticated analyses of the forced expiratory spirogram. However, none of these has been shown to be very useful in predicting the development of significant COPD and are not recommended (23). A more cost-effective alternative is to ask the patient if he or she smokes. If he or she does smoke, efforts directed toward smoking cessation should be undertaken.

Is My Patient Responding to Therapy?

Once the diagnosis of pulmonary dysfunction is confirmed and therapy is undertaken, how should the response of the patient to therapy be monitored? The simplest way is to ask the patient how he or she feels. However, patients with lung disease are notoriously poor at assessing their pulmonary function. In one study of 82 asthmatics, more than 20% had an FEV_1 less than 70% of the predicted value when they reported no symptoms, and many did not become symptomatic when the FEV_1 fell to less than 50% of the predicted value, after the inhalation of methacholine (94). Likewise, the physical examination of patients with COPD is less than ideal in quantifying the response to therapy. It has been shown that there is a very poor correlation between the auscultatory findings and the pulmonary function test results in patients with COPD (95).

Therefore, to evaluate the response to therapy, serial tests of pulmonary function should be obtained. Usually, spirometry is sufficient, and it is recommended that spirometry be performed each time a patient with pulmonary dysfunction is seen. The best indices for following patients with obstructive lung disease are the absolute values of the FEV_1 and the FVC and not the FEV_1/FVC ratio because the latter is dependent on the duration of exhalation. It should be noted that spirometry is not perfect for assessing the response to therapy. For the patient, the most important consideration is whether his or her functional capabilities improve. Significant improvements in spirometric results are not necessarily associated with increased exercise tolerance (96). Nevertheless, it is impractical to perform repeated exercise tests on most patients with pulmonary dysfunction.

Recent theories concerning the pathogenesis of chronic airway obstruction have focused on airway inflammation and airway hyperresponsiveness (11). Accordingly, serial inhalational challenge tests are being used with increasing frequency to assess a patient's response to a therapeutic regimen. For example, one study documented that when aerosolized steroids were given to 16 mild asthmatics for 1 year, the hyperresponsiveness improved in 15 of the 16 and the methacholine test became normal in 5 individuals (97). Although, at present, such tests are used primarily in research situations, their use in the clinical setting will probably become more widespread in the future.

Why Is My Patient Short of Breath on Exertion?

Many patients complain of exercise intolerance. An explanation for the exercise intolerance is frequently lacking even after a careful history, physical examination, chest roentgenogram, electrocardiogram, and routine tests of pulmonary function. The performance of an exercise test frequently permits identification of the factor producing limitation in an individual patient. The characteristic profiles of exercise tests in patients limited by obstructive ventilatory dysfunction, exercise-induced asthma, restrictive ventilatory dysfunction, pulmonary hypertension, cardiovascular dysfunction, poor physical condition, and poor effort are described in the following sections.

OBSTRUCTIVE VENTILATORY DYSFUNCTION. The exercise capacity of most patients with COPD is limited by their respiratory system. In general, this limitation is due to their reduced ventilatory capacity in conjunction with their increased ventilatory requirement for a given workload because their wasted ventilation (V_D/V_T) is increased. The cardiovascular response to exercise in patients with COPD appears to be

relatively normal because the cardiac output for a given $\dot{V}O_2$ is normal (98).

The typical results of an exercise test of a patient with ventilatory limitation are as follows: (a) the patient stops exercising because of shortness of breath rather than leg fatigue (although, even among those with FEV_1 below 40% of predicted, a sizable percentage stop because of leg fatigue) (99); (b) the $\dot{V}O_2$max is reduced, and $\dot{V}E$ at exhaustion is at least 35 times the FEV_1 or 70% of the MVV (99); (c) the V_D/V_T at rest is usually elevated and does not decrease with exercise, and the $\dot{V}CO_2/\dot{V}E$ is above 30; (d) for a given $\dot{V}O_2$, the heart rate is higher than normal, but the maximum heart rate is reduced because the $\dot{V}O_2$max is so low (36); (e) the anaerobic threshold is frequently not reached due to the ventilatory limitation; and (f) arterial blood gases during exercise may be unchanged from rest or may reveal an increased $PaCO_2$ or a decreased PaO_2.

EXERCISE-INDUCED ASTHMA. Exercise can precipitate bronchospasm in some individuals. If exercise-induced asthma is suspected, spirometry should be obtained before the exercise test and at 5-minute intervals after completion of the exercise test. The duration of the exercise should be for at least 6 to 8 minutes at an intensity sufficient to reach 85% to 90% of the predicted maximal heart rate. The diagnosis is established if the FEV_1 falls more than 10% after performance of the exercise test (100).

RESTRICTIVE VENTILATORY DYSFUNCTION. Restrictive lung disease encompasses a large and diverse group of disorders characterized by diminished lung volumes. In general, the functional disability in these patients is often out of proportion to the impairment in lung function, and there is only a weak (r ~ 0.5) correlation between any resting measure of lung function and exercise tolerance (101,102). Abnormal gas exchange is a major factor limiting exercise in patients with significant pulmonary interstitial disease. This is manifested during exercise by a decline in arterial oxygen saturation, a widened alveolar–arterial oxygen gradient, and an elevated V_D/V_T (101). The reduced FVC results in a relatively low maximal tidal volume (V_T), necessitating a high respiratory rate. This limitation, coupled with a decreased efficiency of gas exchange (increased V_D/V_T), leads to decreased exercise tolerance. Arterial blood gases during exercise usually reveal hypoxemia, and endurance exercise can be prolonged with supplemental oxygen (103).

PULMONARY HYPERTENSION. The exercise tolerance as reflected by the $\dot{V}O_2$max of patients with primary pulmonary hypertension is markedly reduced. The exercise capacity of these patients appears to be limited by a low cardiac output because of a decrease in the functional pulmonary vascular bed. The anaerobic threshold occurs at a relatively low workload, and the oxygen pulse is much lower than normal. The PaO_2 also tends to decrease in these patients with exercise. Although the ventilation at any given workload is higher in these patients than in normal individuals because of the increased V_D/V_T and the early onset of anaerobic metabolism, there is no evidence that these patients have ventilatory limitations (104). Exercise testing in patients with pulmonary hypertension carries a significant mortality risk and should not be performed when there is a history of arrhythmias, syncope, or clinical signs of right heart failure (35, 70).

CARDIOVASCULAR DYSFUNCTION. The exercise capacity of patients with cardiovascular dysfunction as well as of normal individuals is limited by their cardiac output. The main abnormality in these patients is a decreased stroke volume. Accordingly, their cardiac output at a given heart rate is less than normal. The maximum heart rate is also often reduced (42,105). Interestingly, there is a poor correlation between the left ventricular ejection fraction and the $\dot{V}O_2$max (105). The $\dot{V}O_2$max has been used to select patients for cardiac transplantation because a $\dot{V}O_2$max of <12 mL/kg identifies patients with a poor 1-year prognosis (105). When patients with cardiac dysfunction undergo maximal exercise tests, about 50% of them stop because of fatigue and 50% stop because of dyspnea. The patients who stop because of dyspnea do not appear to have less ventilatory reserve than those who stop because of fatigue (106).

The typical results of an exercise test in a patient with cardiac dysfunction are as follows (58): (a) the $\dot{V}O_2$max is reduced, but the $\dot{V}E$ is less than 35 times the FEV_1 and less than 70% of the MVV; (b) the VD/VT is near normal and the $\dot{V}CO_2/\dot{V}E$ is below 30; (c) the heart rate is elevated relative to the $\dot{V}O_2$ secondary to the low stroke volume, and the anaerobic threshold is reached at a low $\dot{V}O_2$; (d) arterial blood gases reveal a normal PaO_2 but a reduced $PaCO_2$ and metabolic acidosis.

LACK OF FITNESS. The results of an exercise test in an unfit individual are similar to those in a patient with cardiovascular disease (70). The anaerobic threshold will be reached at a low $\dot{V}O_2$ because of the poor distribution of the cardiac output. The maximum heart rate is normal and the $\dot{V}E$ is below 35 times the FEV_1. Arterial blood gases are similar to those of patients with cardiovascular dysfunction.

MALINGERING. Some individuals complain of exercise intolerance when their initial evaluation reveals no abnormalities that can explain such intolerance. Frequently, the question arises as to whether they are actually impaired, particularly when litigation or disability compensation is involved. When subjected to a maximal exercise test, such individuals may not give maximum effort. Therefore, they have a decreased $\dot{V}O_2$max. However, aside from this decrease, there is no evidence that they are limited by any of the above mechanisms. More specifically, their $\dot{V}E$ is less than 35 times their FEV_1; their maximal heart rate is reduced, but the $\dot{V}O_2$ for a given heart rate is normal; they fail to reach their anaerobic threshold and their blood lactate levels are <8 mmol/L; and arterial blood gases do not demonstrate hypercapnia, hypoxia, or metabolic acidosis.

If an individual appears to not give a maximal effort, a good approximation of their actual $\dot{V}O_2$max can be obtained by extrapolating the results of their exercise test to the maximal predicted heart rate, as shown in Figure 6-12. If their ventilatory reserve at exhaustion is less than their cardiac reserve percentagewise, then the extrapolation should be made using ventilation rather than heart rate.

Is My Patient Physically Impaired from His or Her Lung Disease?

New and revised social legislation entitles an increasing number of Americans to compensation for disability. As a result,

physicians are being asked with increasing frequency to quantify impairment of health. The term *impairment* implies a physiologic, anatomic, or mental functional deficit, whereas the term *disability* implies an inability to perform or a limitation in the performance of tasks within a social environment. Rating of impairment falls within the sphere of the physician's expertise. In contrast, adjudication of disability requires consideration of additional factors, such as educational or cultural level and availability of suitable work, and is generally an administrative function outside the realm of the physician's practice (107). The following discussion addresses only quantifying the degree of impairment. The recommendations are those of the American Thoracic Society (108,109).

TESTS OF PULMONARY FUNCTION. In the evaluation of respiratory impairment, the first step is to obtain pulmonary function tests. It is recommended that this initial testing include both forced spirometric measurements and the single-breath diffusing capacity. The results of these tests allow the majority of subjects to be appropriately categorized as to their degree of impairment as follows:

Normal: FVC $\geq$ 80% of predicted *and* FEV_1 $\geq$ 80% of predicted *and* FEV_1/FVC $\geq$ 0.75 *and* $DLCO$ $\geq$ 80% of predicted.

Mildly impaired (usually not correlated with diminished ability to perform most jobs): FVC 60% to 79% of predicted *or* FEV_1 60% to 79% of predicted *or* FEV_1/FVC 0.60 to 0.74 *or* $DLCO$ 60% to 79% of predicted.

Moderately impaired (progressively lower levels of lung function, correlated with diminishing ability to meet the physical demands of many jobs): FVC 51% to 59% of predicted *or* FEV_1 41% to 59% of predicted *or* FEV_1/FVC 0.41 to 0.59 *or* $DLCO$ 41% to 59% of predicted.

Severely impaired (unable to meet the physical demands of most jobs, including traveling to work): FVC 50% or less of predicted *or* FEV_1 40% or less of predicted *or* FEV_1/FVC <0.40 *or* $DLCO$ 40% or less of predicted.

EXERCISE TESTING. Subjects found to have no impairment or mild impairment on the basis of their pulmonary function tests are usually able to perform all but the most physically demanding of jobs. Patients with severe impairment are usually unable to perform almost all jobs, if for no other reason than that they are frequently unable to travel back and forth to their place of employment.

Patients with mild or moderate impairment who complain of shortness of breath while working should be considered as possible candidates for exercise testing. Exercise testing is useful because there is no close relationship between tests of pulmonary function and $\dot{V}O_2$max (see Fig. 6-15). In such cases, the exercise testing is performed for two reasons: first, to determine whether an individual is significantly impaired and, second, to determine whether the impairment is due to pulmonary dysfunction or some other cause. At a minimum, the testing should include measurement of ventilation ($\dot{V}E$), VT, respiratory rate, and heart rate. Most testing should be done in laboratories that can also measure the composition of exhaled gas and arterial oxygen saturation.

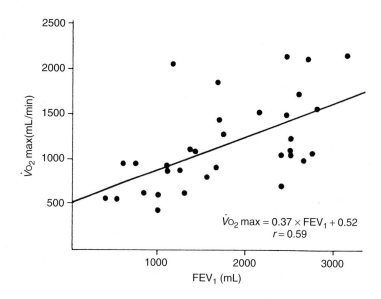

FIGURE 6-15. Relationship between the $\dot{V}O_2max$ and the FEV_1. Note how poorly the $\dot{V}O_2max$ correlates with the FEV_1. (Data courtesy VD Minh.)

The following rating of impairment is recommended:

1. If the $\dot{V}O_2max$ is >25 mL/kg/minute, the subject will be capable of continuous heavy exertion throughout an 8-hour shift for all but the most physically demanding jobs.
2. If the $\dot{V}O_2$ is between 15 and 25 mL/kg/minute and if 40% of the observed $\dot{V}O_2max$ is greater than the average metabolic work requirement of the subject's job, the subject should be able to perform that job comfortably.
3. If the $\dot{V}O_2$ max is <15 mL/kg/minute, the subject will be unable to perform most jobs because he or she will be uncomfortable in traveling back and forth to the place of employment.

IMPAIRMENT WITH ASTHMA. The determination of impairment in patients with asthma differs from that with other respiratory diseases because of the following factors: (a) in asthmatics, the condition is much more variable; (b) the condition is associated with hyperresponsiveness to various agents such as dusts, fumes, and gases that the patient may encounter while working; and (c) environmental or occupational exposures may increase airway inflammation, which on repeated exposures can become chronic and irreversible.

The American Thoracic Society has also developed guidelines for the evaluation of impairment in patients with asthma (109). In summary, these guidelines suggest that the following three factors be considered in determining the level of impairment: (a) the postbronchodilator FEV_1, (b) the reversibility of the FEV_1 or the degree of airway hyperresponsiveness, and (c) the minimal amount of medication required by the patient. An asthmatic is severely impaired if the FEV_1 is less than 50% of predicted while taking at least 20 mg prednisone orally. The reader is referred to the recent ATS statement for further details regarding impairment in the asthmatic (109).

REFERENCES

1. Pulmonary terms and symbols: a report of the ACCP-ATS Joint Committee on Pulmonary Nomenclature. *Chest* 1975;67:583–593.
2. Official Statement of the American Thoracic Society. Standardization of spirometry—1994 update. *Am J Respir Crit Care Med* 1995; 152:1107–1136.
3. Cochrane GM, Prieto F, Clark TJ. Intrasubject variability of maximal expiratory flow volume curve. *Thorax* 1977;32:171–176.
4. Hyatt RE, Black LF. The flow volume curve: a current perspective. *Am Rev Respir Dis* 1973;107:191–199.
5. Kapp MC, Schachter EN, Beck GJ, et al. The shape of the maximum expiratory flow volume curve. *Chest* 1988;94:799–806.
6. Meadows JA III, Rodarte JR, Hyatt RE. Density dependence of maximal expiratory flow in chronic obstructive pulmonary disease. *Am Rev Respir Dis* 1980;121:47–53.
7. Heaf PJD, Gillam PMS. Peak flow rates in normal and asthmatic children. *Br Med J* 1962;1:1595–1596.
8. National Heart, Lung, and Blood Institute. *National Asthma Education Program: expert panel report 2: guidelines for the diagnosis and treatment of asthma.* Bethesda: National Institutes of Health, May 1997 (NIH Publication No. 97-4051).
9. Jain P, Kavuru MS, Emerman CL, et al. Utility of peak expiratory flow monitoring. *Chest* 1998;114:861–876.
10. ATS/ACCP statement on cardiopulmonary exercise testing. *Am J Respir Crit Care Med* 2003;167:21–277.
11. Boulet LP. Asymptomatic airway hyperresponsiveness. A curiosity or an opportunity to prevent asthma? *Am J Respir Crit Care Med* 2003;167:371–378.
12. Buist AS, Connett JE, Miller RD, et al. Chronic obstructive pulmonary disease early intervention trial (Lung Health Study). Baseline characteristics of randomized participants. *Chest* 1993;103:1 863–1872.
13. O'Connor GT, Sparrow D, Weiss ST. A prospective longitudinal study of methacholine airway responsiveness as a predictor of pulmonary function decline: the normative aging study. *Am J Respir Crit Care Med* 1995;152:87–92.
14. Meneely GR, Ball CO, Kory RC, et al. A simplified closed circuit helium dilution method for the determination of the residual volume of the lungs. *Am J Med* 1960;28:824–831.
15. Darling RC, Cournand A, Richards DW. Studies on the intrapulmonary mixing of gases. II. An open circuit method for measuring residual air. *J Clin Invest* 1940;19:609–618.
16. Burns CB, Scheinhorn DJ. Evaluation of single-breath helium dilution total lung capacity in obstructive lung disease. *Am Rev Respir Dis* 1984;130:580–583.
17. Dubois AB, Botelho SY, Bedell GN, et al. A rapid plethysmographic method for measuring thoracic gas volume: a comparison with a nitrogen washout method for measuring functional residual capacity in normal subjects. *J Clin Invest* 1956;35:322–326.
18. Dubois AB, Botelho SY, Comroe JH Jr. A new method for measuring airway resistance in man using a body plethysmograph: values in normal subjects and in patients with respiratory disease. *J Clin Invest* 1956;35:327–335.
19. Comroe JH, Fowler WS. Lung function studies. IV. Detection of uneven alveolar ventilation during a single breath of oxygen: a new test of pulmonary disease. *Am J Med* 1951;10:408–413.

20. Buist AS, Ross BR. Quantitative analysis of the alveolar plateau in the diagnosis of early airway obstruction. *Am Rev Respir Dis* 1973;108:1078–1087.

21. Menkes HA, Beaty TH, Cohen BH, et al. Nitrogen washout and mortality. *Am Rev Respir Dis* 1985;132:115–119.

22. McCarthy DS, Spencer R, Greene R, et al. Measurements of "closing volume" as a simple and sensitive test for early detection of small airway disease. *Am J Med* 1972;52:747–753.

23. Buist AS, Vollmer WM, Johnson LR, et al. Does the single-breath N_2 test identify the smoker who will develop chronic airflow limitation? *Am Rev Respir Dis* 1988;127:293–301.

24. Crapo RO, Hankinson JL, Irvin C, et al. Single-breath carbon monoxide diffusing capacity (transfer factor). Recommendations for a standard Technique—1995 update. *Am J Respir Crit Care Med* 1995;152:2185–2198.

25. Graham BL, Mink JT, Cotton DJ. Effects of increasing carboxyhemoglobin on the single breath carbon monoxide diffusing capacity. *Am J Respir Crit Care Med* 2002;165:1504–1510.

26. Lewis BM, Lin TH, Noe FE, et al. The measurement of pulmonary diffusing capacity for carbon monoxide by a rebreathing method. *J Clin Invest* 1959;38:2073–2086.

27. Official statement of the American Thoracic Society. Single breath carbon monoxide diffusing capacity (transfer factor). Recommendations for a standard technique. *Am Rev Respir Dis* 1987;136: 1299–1307.

28. Weinberger SE, Johnson TS, Weiss ST. Use and interpretation of the single breath diffusing capacity. *Chest* 1980;78:483–488.

29. Bates DV, Varvis CJ, Donevan RE, et al. Variations in the pulmonary capillary blood volume and membrane diffusion component in health and disease. *J Clin Invest* 1960;39:1401–1412.

30. Ferris BG, ed. Epidemiology standardization project: recommended standardized procedures for pulmonary function testing. *Am Rev Respir Dis* 1978;118(pt 2):62–72.

31. Marrades RM, Diaz O, Roca J, et al. Adjustment of DLCO for hemoglobin concentration. *Am J Respir Crit Care Med* 1997;155: 236–241.

32. Myers M, Prakash M, Froelicher V, et al. Exercise capacity and mortality among men referred for exercise testing. *N Engl J Med* 2002;346:793 – 801.

33. Oga T, Nishimura K, Tsukino M, et al. Analysis of the factors related to mortality in chronic obstructive pulmonary disease. *Am J Respir Crit Care Med* 2003;167:544–549.

34. Larsen KR, Svendsen UG, Milman N, et al. Exercise testing in the preoperative evaluation of patients with bronchogenic carcinoma. *Eur Respir J* 1997;10:1559–1565.

35. Roca J, Whipp BJ, Agusti AGN, et al. Clinical exercise testing with reference to lung diseases: indications, standardization and interpretation strategies. *Eur Respir J* 1997;10:2662–2689.

36. Wasserman K, Hansen JE, Sue DY, et al. *Principles of exercise testing and interpretation: including pathophysiology and clinical applications*, 3rd ed. Philadelphia: Lippincott Williams & Wilkins, 1999.

37. Jones NL, Killian KJ. Exercise limitation in health and disease. *N Engl J Med* 2000;343:632–641.

38. Ogawa T, Spina RJ, Martin WH III, et al. Effects of aging, sex and physical training on cardiovascular responses to exercise. *Circulation* 1992;86:494–503.

39. Crawford MH. Physiologic consequences of systematic training. *Cardiol Clin* 1992;10:209–221.

40. Honig CR, Connett RJ, Gayeski TEJ. O_2 transport and its interaction with metabolism: a systems view of aerobic capacity. *Med Sci Sports Exerc* 1992;24:47–53.

41. Myers J, Walsh D, Buchanan N, et al. Can maximal cardiopulmonary capacity be recognized by a plateau in oxygen uptake? *Chest* 1989;96:1312–1316.

42. Arnold SB, Byrd RC, Meister W, et al. Long-term digitalis therapy improves left ventricular function in heart failure. *N Engl J Med* 1980;303:1443–1448.

43. Jones NL, Campbell EJM. *Clinical exercise testing*, 2nd ed. Philadelphia: WB Saunders, 1981.

44. Barany P, Freyschuss U, Pettersson E, et al. Treatment of anaemia in haemodialysis patients with erythropoietin: long-term effects on exercise capacity. *Clin Sci* 1993;84:441–447.

45. Weiss AB, Calton FM, Kuida H, et al. Hemodynamic effects of normovolemic polycythemia in dogs at rest and during exercise. *Am J Physiol* 1964;207:1361–1366.

46. Chetty KG, Light RW, Stansbury DW, et al. Exercise performance of polycythemic chronic obstructive pulmonary disease patients. Effect of phlebotomies. *Chest* 1990;98:1073–1077.

47. Sawka MN, Young AJ, Muza SR, et al. Erythrocytes reinfusion and maximal aerobic power. *JAMA* 1987;257:1496–1499.

48. Leigh-Smith S. Blood boosting. *Br J Sports Med* 2004;38:99–101.

49. Horvath SM, Raven PB, Dahms TE, et al. Maximal aerobic capacity at different levels of carboxyhemoglobin. *J Appl Physiol* 1975; 38:300–303.

50. Astrand PO, Rodahl K. *Textbook of work physiology*, 2nd ed. New York: McGraw-Hill, 1977.

51. Oren A, Wasserman K, Davis JA, et al. Effect of CO_2 set point on ventilatory response to exercise. *J Appl Physiol* 1981;51:185–189.

52. Light RW, Mahutte CK, Brown SE. Etiology of CO_2 retention at rest and during exercise in chronic airflow obstruction. *Chest* 1988;94:61–67.

53. West JB. Ventilation-perfusion relationships. *Am Rev Respir Dis* 1977;116:919–943.

54. Powers SK, Martin D, Dodd S. Exercise-induced hypoxaemia in elite endurance athletes. Incidence, causes and impact on $\dot{V}_{O_2}$max. *Sports Med* 1993;16:14–22.

55. Shepard RH. Effect of pulmonary diffusion capacity on exercise tolerance. *J Appl Physiol* 1958;12:487–488.

56. Belman MJ, Mittman C. Ventilatory muscle training improves exercise capacity in chronic obstructive pulmonary disease patients. *Am Rev Respir Dis* 1981;121:273–280.

57. Jones NL. Normal values for pulmonary gas exchange during exercise. *Am Rev Respir Dis* 1984;129(Suppl. 2 pt 2):S44–S46.

58. Brown HV, Wasserman K. Exercise performance in chronic obstructive pulmonary diseases. *Med Clin North Am* 1981;65:525–547.

59. Koike A, Hiroe M, Taniguchi K, et al. Respiratory control during exercise in patients with cardiovascular disease. *Am Rev Respir Dis* 1993;147:425–429.

60. Beaver WL, Wasserman K, Whipp BJ. A new method for detecting anaerobic threshold by gas exchange. *J Appl Physiol* 1986;60: 2020–2027.

61. Belman MJ, Epstein LJ, Doornbos D, et al. Noninvasive determinations of the anaerobic threshold. Reliability and validity in patients with COPD. *Chest* 1992;102:1028–1034.

62. Eriksson BO, Engstrom I, Karlberg P, et al. A physiological analysis of former girl swimmers. *Acta Paediatr Scand* 1971;217(Suppl.): 68–72.

63. Saltin B, Blomqvist G, Mitchell JH, et al. Response to exercise after bed rest and after training. A longitudinal study of adaptive changes in oxygen transport and body composition. *Circulation* 1968;38(Suppl. 7):1–78.

64. Knuttgen HG. Development of muscular strength and endurance. In: Knuttgen HG, ed. *Neuromuscular mechanisms for therapeutic and conditioning exercise*. Baltimore: University Park Press, 1976:97.

65. Goldberg L, Elliot DL, Kuehl KS. Assessment of exercise intensity formulas by use of ventilatory threshold. *Chest* 1988;94:95–98.

66. Holle RHO, Williams DV, Vandree JC, et al. Increased muscle efficiency and sustained benefits in an outpatient community hospital-based pulmonary rehabilitation program. *Chest* 1988;94: 1161–1168.

67. Sala E, Roca J, Marrades RM, et al. Effects of endurance training on skeletal muscle bioenergetics in chronic obstructive pulmonary disease. *Am J Respir Crit Care Med* 1999;159:1726–1734.

68. Smith K, Cook D, Guyatt GH, et al. Respiratory muscle training in chronic airflow limitation: a meta-analysis. *Am Rev Respir Dis* 1992;145:533–539.

69. Kohrt WM, Malley MT, Coggan AR, et al. Effects of gender, age, and fitness level on response of VO$_2$max to training in 60 to 71 year olds. *J Appl Physiol* 1991;71:2004–2011.

70. Weisman IM, Beck KC, Casaburi R, et al. ATS/ACCS statement on cardiopulmonary exercise testing. *Am J Respir Crit Care Med* 2003;167:211-277.

71. Enright PL. The six-minute walk test. *Respir Care* 2003;48:783-785.

72. Singh SJ, Morgan M, Scott S, et al. Development of a shuttle walking test of disability in patients with chronic airway obstruction. *Thorax* 1992;47:1019–1024.

73. ATS Committee on Proficiency Standards for Clinical Pulmonary Function Laboratories. ATS statement: guidelines for the six-minute walk test. *Am J Crit Care Med* 2002;166:111–117.

74. Liu Z, Vargas FS, Stansbury DW, et al. Comparison of the end-tidal arterial PCO_2 gradient during exercise in normal subjects and in patients with severe COPD. *Chest* 1995;107:1218–1224.

75. McGovern J, Sasse SA, Stansbury DW, et al. Comparison of oxygen saturation by pulse oximetry and co-oximetry during exercise testing in patients with COPD. *Chest* 1996;109:1151–1155.

76. Blackie SP, Fairbarn MS, McElvaney GN, et al. Prediction of maximal oxygen uptake and power during cycle ergometry in subjects older than 55 years of age. *Am Rev Respir Dis* 1989;139: 1424–1429.

77. Jones NL, Makrides L, Hitchcock C, et al. Normal standards for an incremental progressive cycle ergometer test. *Am Rev Respir Dis* 1985;131:700–708.

78. American Thoracic Society. Lung function testing: selection of reference values and interpretative strategies. *Am Rev Respir Dis* 1999;144:1202–1218.

79. Morris AH, Kanner RE, Crapo RO, et al. *Clinical pulmonary function testing: a manual of uniform laboratory procedures*, 2nd ed. Salt Lake City: Intermountain Thoracic Society, 1984.

80. Clausen JL, Zarins LP, eds. *Pulmonary function testing—guidelines and controversies.* New York: Academic Press, 1982.

81. Knudson RJ, Lebowitz MD, Holberg CJ, et al. Changes in the normal maximal expiratory flow-volume curve with growth and aging. *Am Rev Respir Dis* 1983;127:725–734.

82. Morris JF, Koski A, Temple WP, et al. Fifteen-year interval spirometric evaluation of the Oregon predictive equations. *Chest* 1988; 92:123–127.

83. Withers RT, Bourdon PC, Crockett A. Lung volume standards for healthy male lifetime nonsmokers. *Chest* 1988;92:91–97.

84. Crapo RO, Morris AH. Standardized single breath normal values for carbon monoxide diffusing capacity. *Am Rev Respir Dis* 1981; 123:185–189.

85. Knudson RJ, Kaltenborn WT, Knudson DE, et al. The single-breath carbon monoxide diffusing capacity. Reference equations derived from a healthy nonsmoking population and effects of hematocrit. *Am Rev Respir Dis* 1987;135:805–811.

86. Glady CA, Aaron SD, Lunau M, et al. A spirometry-based algorithm to direct lung function testing in the pulmonary function laboratory. *Chest* 2003;123:1939–1946.

87. Miller A, Brown LK, Sloane MF, et al. Cardiorespiratory responses to incremental exercise in sarcoidosis patients with normal spirometry. *Chest* 1995;107:323–329.

88. Aaron SD, Dales RE, Cardinal P. How accurate is spirometry at predicting restrictive pulmonary impairment? *Chest* 1999;115: 869–873.

89. Curtis JK, Liska AP, Rasmussen HK, et al. The bronchospastic component in patients with chronic bronchitis and emphysema. *JAMA* 1966;197:693–696.

90. Tashkin D, Kesten S. Long-term treatment benefits with tiotropium in COPD patients with and without short-term bronchodilator responses. *Chest* 2003;123:1441-1449.

91. Guyatt GH, Townsend M, Nogradi S, et al. Acute response to bronchodilator. An imperfect guide for bronchodilator therapy in chronic airflow limitation. *Arch Intern Med* 1988;148:1949–1952.

92. Rotman HH, Liss HP, Weg JG. Diagnosis of upper airway obstruction by pulmonary function testing. *Chest* 1975;68:796–799.

93. Wright JL, Lawson LM, Pare PD, et al. The detection of small airways disease. *Am Rev Respir Dis* 1984;129:989–994.

94. Rubenfeld AR, Pain MC. Perception of asthma. *Lancet* 1976;1: 882–884.

95. Marini JJ, Pierson JD, Hudson LD, et al. The significance of wheezing in chronic airflow obstruction. *Am Rev Respir Dis* 1979;120:1069–1072.

96. Tobin JM, Hughes JA, Hutchison DC. Effects of ipratropium bromide and fenoterol aerosols on exercise tolerance. *Eur J Respir Dis* 1984;65:441–446.

97. Juniper EF, Kline PA, Vanzieleghem MA, et al. Effect on long-term treatment with an inhaled corticosteroid (budesonide) on airway hyperresponsiveness and clinical asthma in nonsteroid-dependent asthmatics. *Am Rev Respir Dis* 1990;142:832–836.

98. Light RW, Mintz HM, Linden GS, et al. Hemodynamics of patients with severe chronic obstructive pulmonary disease (COPD) during progressive upright exercise. *Am Rev Respir Dis* 1984;130:391–395.

99. Killian KJ, Leblanc P, Martin DH, et al. Exercise capacity and ventilatory, circulatory, and symptom limitation in patients with chronic airflow limitation. *Am Rev Respir Dis* 1992;146:935–940.

100. Mahler DA. Exercise-induced asthma. *Med Sci Sports Exerc* 1993;25: 554–561.

101. Hsia CCW. Cardiopulmonary limitations to exercise in restrictive lung disease. *Med Sci Sports Exerc* 1999;31:S28–S32.

102. LoRusso TJ, Belman MJ, Elashoff JD, et al. Prediction of maximal exercise capacity in obstructive and restrictive pulmonary disease. *Chest* 1993;104:1748–1754.

103. Bye PB, Anderson SD, Woolcock AJ, et al. Bicycle endurance performance of patients with interstitial lung disease breathing air and oxygen. *Am Rev Respir Dis* 1982;126:1005–1012.

104. D'Alonzo GE, Gianotti LA, Pohil RL, et al. Comparison of progressive exercise performance of normal subjects and patients with primary pulmonary hypertension. *Chest* 1987;92:57–62.

105. Piña IL, Fitzpatrick JT. Exercise and heart failure. A review. *Chest* 1996;110:1317–1327.

106. Russell SD, McNeer FR, Higginbotham MB. Exertional dyspnea in heart failure: a symptom unrelated to pulmonary function at rest or during exercise. *Am Heart J* 1998;135:398–405.

107. Taiwo OA, Cain HC. Pulmonary impairment and disability. *Clin Chest Med* 2002;23:841-851.

108. Medical Section of the American Lung Association. Evaluation of impairment/disability secondary to respiratory disease. *Am Rev Respir Dis* 1986;133:1205–1209.

109. Medical Section of the American Lung Association. Guidelines for the evaluation of impairment/disability in patients with asthma. *Am Rev Respir Dis* 1993;147:1056–1061.

CHAPTER **7**

Invasive Diagnostic Procedures

Richard W. Light
R. Michael Rodriguez

The majority of chest diseases can be diagnosed on the basis of the history, physical findings, pulmonary function tests, and chest imaging, including computed tomography (CT) scans. When these basic procedures are not adequate to define a patient's illness, additional studies are available that allow the physician to define lung abnormalities with precision. These invasive tests, including the various biopsy procedures, not only carry increased risks but also are costly. In this time of fiscal responsibility, the clinician must choose those tests most likely to yield the desired results, minimizing the risk and cost to the patient. This chapter discusses some of these specialized techniques: thoracentesis, pleural biopsy, bronchoscopy with specialized procedures including bronchoalveolar lavage (BAL), protected specimen brushing and transbronchial needle aspiration (TBNA), transthoracic needle aspiration (TTNA) and biopsy, thoracoscopy, mediastinoscopy, and open-lung biopsy. Other tests, such as arterial blood gases and oximetry, capnography, metabolic and nutritional evaluation, and various invasive and non-invasive tests for venous thrombosis, are discussed in the chapters devoted to the diseases for which they are most often used.

THORACENTESIS AND PLEURAL FLUID EXAMINATION

Pleural involvement often accompanies diseases of the lung parenchyma and is usually associated with abnormal amounts of fluid in the pleural space. The volume of pleural fluid present can be semiquantitated by obtaining a lateral decubitus chest radiograph, with the suspected side down, and measuring the thickness of the fluid between the inner border of the ribs and the lower part of the lung (see Fig. 7-1). If the thickness of the fluid is >10 mm, a sample of fluid can usually be obtained for diagnostic purposes.

THORACENTESIS

The site for insertion of the needle should be determined with care. It is best to make the insertion in the posterior thorax, where the ribs are easily palpable and to where the fluid gravitates. With the patient in an upright seated position, the level is identified at which tactile fremitus is lost and the percussion note becomes dull. Thoracentesis should be attempted first in the interspace below this level. In recent years, thoracenteses have increasingly been performed by interventional radiologists, which is fast and safe (1).

The handling of the pleural fluid for the different tests is outlined in Table 7-1. For bacterial cultures, 5 mL of pleural fluid should be put into each aerobic and anaerobic culture medium. For determination of pleural fluid pH, the sample should be sent to the laboratory on ice in the original syringe and then analyzed with a blood gas machine. The specimen sent for cell count and differential should be placed in an anticoagulation tube to prevent cells from clumping, which can result in inaccurate cell counts (2).

PLEURAL FLUID APPEARANCE

The gross appearance of pleural fluid yields useful diagnostic information. Therefore, the color, turbidity, viscosity, and odor

TABLE 7-1.   Distribution of Pleural Fluid Obtained with Diagnostic Thoracentesis

Laboratory	Amount (mL)	Tests Ordered
Bacteriology	10	Aerobic and anaerobic cultures Gram stain
Tuberculosis and mycology	5	Tuberculosis and fungal cultures
Cytology	10	Cytology
Hematology	5	Red-cell count White-cell count Wright stain
Chemistry	5	Glucose Amylase Lactic dehydrogenase Protein Marker for tuberculosis
Blood gas	5	pH

of the pleural fluid should be recorded (3). Most transudative and many exudative effusions are clear, straw-colored, nonviscid, and odorless. A white milky appearance indicates chylothorax, a chyliform pleural effusion, or empyema. Pus in the pleural fluid can be distinguished from chylothorax and chyliform effusion, as after centrifugation, there is a clear, yellowish, supernatant fluid in purulent effusions, whereas the fluid with a chylous or chyliform effusion remains cloudy after centrifugation. If the pleural fluid smells foul, the patient likely has an anaerobic pleuropulmonary infection.

Only 5,000 to 10,000 red blood cells per cubic millimeter are required to impart a red color to a pleural effusion. Thus, 1 mL of blood in a moderately sized effusion will result in blood-tinged pleural fluid. The diagnostic value of blood-tinged fluid

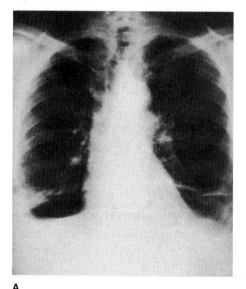

A

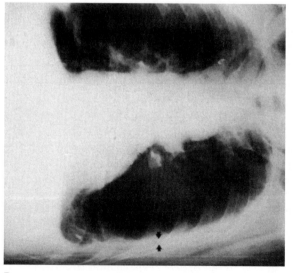

B

FIGURE 7-1.   Lateral decubitus radiograph demonstrating pleural effusion. On the erect posteroanterior radiograph **(A)**, both costophrenic angles are blunted. In the left lateral decubitus position **(B)**, there is a definite fluid line between the outer part of the lung and the inside of the chest wall. Because the distance between the *arrows* was >10 mm, a diagnostic thoracentesis was performed.

is limited because more than 15% of transudates and more than 40% of exudates are blood-tinged(3). Grossly bloody effusions have red-cell counts above 100,000 per mm^3 or a hematocrit above 1%. This finding is suggestive of one of three disease processes: trauma, malignancy (including malignant mesothelioma and metastatic neoplasms), or, less commonly, pulmonary embolism (4). A hematocrit should be obtained on grossly bloody pleural fluid to determine whether a hemothorax is present. A hemothorax is present if the pleural fluid hematocrit is more than 50% that of the peripheral blood (see Chapter 17, Diseases of the Pleura, Mediastinum, Chest Wall, and Diaphragm).

SEPARATION OF TRANSUDATES FROM EXUDATES

The first question that must be answered when a pleural effusion is discovered is whether the effusion is a transudate or an exudate. Transudates, by definition, are pleural effusions that result from imbalances of the hydrostatic and oncotic forces in the pulmonary or systemic circulation. Exudates are pleural effusions that result from increased permeability of the pulmonary or systemic circulation (5). If the effusion is a transudate, no additional diagnostic procedures are necessary, and therapy is directed toward the underlying congestive heart failure, cirrhosis, or nephrosis. Alternatively, if the effusion proves to be an exudate, more extensive diagnostic procedures are needed to delineate the cause of the pleural disease.

Exudative pleural effusions can be separated effectively from transudative pleural effusions with the simultaneous use of protein and lactic acid dehydrogenase (LDH) levels in the pleural fluid and serum (Light's criteria). Exudates meet at least *one* of the following three criteria, whereas transudates meet *none* (6).

1. The pleural fluid protein divided by the serum protein is greater than 0.5.
2. The pleural fluid LDH divided by the serum LDH is greater than 0.6.
3. The pleural fluid LDH is greater than two-thirds of the upper limit of normal for the serum LDH.

The problem with Light criteria is that although they correctly identify essentially all exudates, they incorrectly identify 20% to 25% of transudates as exudates. This is particularly likely to occur in patients with congestive heart failure who are on diuretics (7). If a patient is thought clinically to have a transudative effusion, but the pleural fluid meets Light's exudative criteria by just a small margin, the difference between the protein levels in the serum and the pleural fluid should be calculated. If this is more than 3.1 gm per dL, the patient most likely has a transudative effusion (7).

PLEURAL FLUID CELL COUNT AND DIFFERENTIAL

The pleural fluid white blood cell count (WBC) is of limited value in the differential diagnosis of pleural effusions. In general, a WBC above 1000 per mm^3 suggests an exudate. Pleural fluid WBCs above 10,000 per mm^3 are most commonly seen with parapneumonic effusions, however, pleural fluid WBCs above 10,000 are also seen with pancreatitis, pulmonary infarction, collagen vascular diseases, malignancy, and tuberculosis (3,4).

The differential WBC should be obtained on all exudative pleural effusions. The cells in the pleural fluid can include neutrophils, small lymphocytes, mesothelial cells, other mononuclear cells, and eosinophils. The presence of neutrophils suggests an acute inflammatory response. Pleural fluid neutrophilia is seen in effusions associated with pneumonia, pancreatitis, pulmonary embolism, and peritonitis. Occasionally, very early tuberculous effusions will have a predominance of neutrophils.

If the pleural fluid contains more than 50% lymphocytes, the patient probably has malignancy, tuberculosis, or a pleural effusion secondary to coronary artery bypass surgery (8). Mesothelial cells normally line the pleural cavity and are rarely present in the pleural fluid associated with tuberculous pleuritis or other processes in which the pleural surfaces are diffusely involved. Most effusions with eosinophil counts greater than 10% are either bloody or associated with a pneumothorax. If there is no air or blood in the pleural space, no etiology is found for the effusion in about 40% (9). The next most common cause of eosinophilic pleural effusion is malignancy (9). Other etiologies for eosinophilic effusions include a drug reaction, paragonimiasis, asbestos exposure, the Churg–Strauss syndrome, or a resolving parapneumonic effusion.

PLEURAL FLUID CHEMISTRIES

It is recommended that all exudative pleural effusions be analyzed for protein, LDH, and glucose. As discussed above, the protein and LDH are used to separate transudative from exudative pleural effusions. The pleural fluid LDH should be measured each time a thoracentesis is performed because it serves as an index of the degree of pleural inflammation (3). If the pleural fluid LDH increases with serial thoracenteses, the process responsible for the effusion is worsening and one should be more active in pursuing a diagnosis.

Pleural Fluid Glucose

Measurement of the pleural fluid glucose level is useful because a low pleural fluid glucose level (<60 mg per dL) indicates that the patient probably has one of four disorders, namely, a complicated parapneumonic effusion, a malignant pleural effusion, tuberculous pleuritis, or a rheumatoid effusion. Other rare causes of a low glucose pleural effusion include paragonimiasis, hemothorax, the Churg–Strauss syndrome, and occasionally lupus pleuritis (3).

Pleural Fluid Amylase

An elevated pleural fluid amylase (above the upper limit of normal for serum) indicates that the pleural effusion is due to pancreatic disease, esophageal rupture, or pleural malignancy. The main reason to measure the pleural fluid amylase is to screen for pancreatic disease and esophageal rupture. Pleural fluid amylase measurements are indicated if either of these diseases is suspected. Because only a small percentage of pleural effusions is due to these entities, it is not cost effective to routinely obtain amylase measurements on pleural fluid (10). The elevated amylase with esophageal rupture is due to saliva, with its high amylase content, entering the pleural space. The pleural fluid amylase level is elevated in approximately 10% of patients with malignant pleural effusions, and the primary tumor is usually not in the pancreas (11).

Because the pleural fluid amylase with malignancy is the salivary type, determination of the pleural fluid amylase isoenzyme pattern can differentiate malignancy from pancreatic disease (11).

Pleural Fluid pH

The determination of pleural fluid pH is most useful in patients with parapneumonic effusions because the lower the pH, the worse the prognosis. A pleural fluid pH below 7.00 suggests that the patient will require invasive procedures directed toward the effusion (12) (see Chapter 17, Diseases of the Pleura, Mediastinum, Chest Wall, and Diaphragm). The pleural fluid pH determination must be made with a blood gas machine because pH meters and pH indicator strips are not sufficiently accurate for clinical decision making (13). Other types of effusions that may have a pleural fluid pH below 7.20 are malignant pleural effusions, tuberculous pleural effusions, and any other types of pleural effusions that have a low pleural fluid glucose (3).

PLEURAL FLUID BACTERIOLOGY

When a diagnostic thoracentesis is performed on a patient with an exudative effusion, the fluid should be cultured for both aerobic and anaerobic organisms. A Gram stain of the fluid should be examined for the presence of bacteria. Mycobacterial and fungal cultures should also be obtained if there is a possibility of tuberculosis or fungal infection.

PLEURAL FLUID TESTS FOR MALIGNANCY

Pleural Fluid Cytology

If a patient has malignancy, cytologic examination of the pleural fluid is a fast, efficient, and minimally invasive means by which to establish the diagnosis. The percentage of malignant pleural effusions that are diagnosed with cytology has been reported to be anywhere between 40% and 87% (3). There are several factors that influence the diagnostic yield with cytology. If the patient has a malignancy but the pleural effusion has another etiology such as heart failure, pulmonary emboli, pneumonia, lymphatic obstruction, or hypoproteinemia, the cytology will be negative. The frequency of positive cytology also depends on the tumor type. Almost all adenocarcinomas will be diagnosed with cytology, but the yield is less with squamous cell carcinomas, Hodgkin disease, and sarcomas. Obviously, the yield is also dependent on the skill of the cytologist. Overall, if three separate pleural fluid specimens are submitted to an experienced cytologist, a positive diagnosis should be expected in about 70% to 80% of patients.

Flow Cytometry

Flow cytometry provides a rapid quantification of the nuclear DNA. The majority of malignancies are aneuploid and, consequently, have abnormal DNA levels. In contrast, the majority of benign effusions are diploid with normal DNA levels. However, because some benign effusions have abnormal DNA levels and some malignancies have normal DNA levels, the diagnosis of malignancy cannot be ruled either in or out with this test (14). The routine use of flow cytometry, therefore, is not recommended. Flow cytometry is useful in patients with lymphoma for demonstrating the homogeneity of a population of cells (15).

Immunohistochemical Testing

Immunohistochemical stains of malignant cells are used to confirm a diagnosis and to specify tumor types (16). The most common application of immunocytochemistry is to distinguish adenocarcinoma from mesothelioma. Thus, adenocarcinoma can be identified and separated from mesothelioma or reactive mesothelial cells by its positive staining with a panel of antibodies to epithelial markers, B72.3, Ber-EP4, or Leu-M1, whereas mesothelioma will stain with antibodies to calretinin (a calcium-binding protein), mesothelin (a glycoprotein identified on the surface of mesothelial cells), or specific cytokeratins (cytokeratin 5/6) (16). Immunohistochemical staining is not useful for distinguishing malignant mesothelioma cells from benign mesothelial cells.

Tumor Markers in the Pleural Fluid

There have been many publications evaluating the utility of tumor markers, such as CEA, AFP, CA 15–3, CA 19–9, and enolase, in the diagnosis of pleural malignancy. In general, the results with all have been disappointing because of the number of false positives. Because of the poor prognosis associated with malignant pleural effusions, it is important not to make the diagnosis mistakenly. One possible use of tumor markers is to select those patients with higher marker levels for additional invasive tests.

PLEURAL FLUID MARKERS FOR TUBERCULOSIS

Pleural Fluid Adenosine Deaminase Levels

Measurement of the adenosine deaminase (ADA) level in pleural fluid is diagnostically useful because ADA levels tend to be higher in tuberculous pleural effusions than in other lymphocytic exudates. In one study, the ADA was above 47 U per L in 253 of 254 patients with tuberculous pleuritis (17). In a second report of 100 nontuberculous pleural effusions that contained more than 50% lymphocytes, the pleural fluid ADA level exceeded 40 U per L in only 3 (18).

Pleural Fluid γ Interferon Levels

Pleural fluid γ interferon levels are also elevated with tuberculous pleuritis. Pleural fluid γ interferon levels are very efficient at separating tuberculous from nontuberculous pleural effusion. Using a cutoff level of 3.7 U per mL, Villena et al. demonstrated that the specificity and sensitivity of γ interferon were both 0.98 in a series of 595 patients, including 82 patients with tuberculous pleuritis (19).

Pleural Fluid Polymerase Chain Reaction Tests

With polymerase chain reaction (PCR), one can demonstrate the presence of DNA from *Mycobacterium tuberculosis* in the pleural fluid, which should be diagnostic of tuberculous pleuritis. Querol et al. (20) performed PCR on the basis of detecting a

123-bp DNA segment specific for *M. tuberculosis*. In their series of 21 patients with pleural tuberculosis and 86 controls, the sensitivity and specificity of PCR were very similar to those of ADA (20). Other series, however, have reported much poorer results with PCR (21). Because PCR testing is more expensive and more technically difficult than either ADA or γ interferon, testing it is not recommended.

PLEURAL BIOPSY

The primary use of needle biopsy of the pleura over the past 40 years has been to diagnose tuberculous pleuritis. However, as outlined above, markers for tuberculosis obtained from the pleural fluid are very efficient at establishing this diagnosis. In recent years, with the emergence of multidrug-resistant tuberculosis, cultures for *M. tuberculosis* have become important in guiding the therapy of tuberculosis. Some have advocated performing a needle biopsy of the pleura so that a specimen of the pleura can be cultured. However, only about 33% of patients with tuberculous pleuritis will have a positive pleural biopsy culture and a negative pleural fluid culture (22). In addition, to our knowledge, no patient has developed disseminated multidrug-resistant tuberculosis after presenting with a pleural effusion and receiving a standard course of antituberculous drugs. In view of the above, pleural biopsy is usually not indicated for the diagnosis of tuberculous pleuritis.

Pleural biopsy can also establish the diagnosis of malignant pleural disease. However, in most series, pleural fluid cytology is much more sensitive in establishing the diagnosis. If the fluid cytology is negative, the pleural biopsy is usually nondiagnostic. In one series, the pleural biopsy was positive in only 20 of 118 (17%) patients with pleural malignancy and negative cytology (23). Because thoracoscopy is diagnostic in more than 90% of patients with pleural malignancy and negative cytology, it is the preferred diagnostic procedure in the patient with a cytology negative pleural effusion who is suspected of having malignancy.

BRONCHOSCOPY

Bronchoscopy is the invasive procedure most commonly used in the diagnosis of pulmonary disease. The role of the rigid and flexible bronchoscope has broadened as innovations in technology have developed. These applications include the diagnosis, treatment, and monitoring of chest disease. Directly visualized endobronchial biopsies (EBB), transbronchial biopsies (TBB), and bronchial washings are considered standard procedures with flexible bronchoscopy. Moreover, the diagnostic capabilities of flexible bronchoscopy have been markedly increased because of the development of an ultrathin bronchoscope and, most recently, a bronchovideoscope (24,25). Additional procedures that can be performed through a rigid or flexible bronchoscope include electrocautery, brachytherapy, laser therapy, balloon dilatation, and stenting (26–28). Although these procedures are available to the pulmonologist, a recent survey suggests that, other than brachytherapy, these therapeutic modalities are being used infrequently (29). In the following sections, we will discuss the role of rigid and flexible bronchoscopy in the diagnosis and management of pulmonary diseases.

RIGID BRONCHOSCOPY

Rigid bronchoscopy was first performed during the latter part of the 19th century and early 20th century (30). Foreign body and large airway endobronchial tumor removal accounted for its earliest use. The development of the flexible bronchoscope led to a period in which the use of the rigid bronchoscope waned. The renewed interest in the use of this instrument relates directly to the surge in therapeutic technology, such as laser phototherapy, cryotherapy, electrocautery, balloon dilatation, and stent placement in the patient with central airway obstruction from benign or malignant disease (31–34). The rigid bronchoscope allows control of the airway in these critically ill patients who may be candidates for one of several therapeutic strategies to relieve obstructive endobronchial lesions. This instrument, therefore, remains invaluable in the management of critically ill patients with high-grade endobronchial obstruction as well as patients with massive hemoptysis.

TRANSBRONCHIAL BIOPSY

The role of TBB has evolved from its original use to diagnose unexplained infiltrates, masses, or nodules to the diagnosis of transplant rejection in patients following lung transplantation (35–38). In addition, transbronchial biopsy has been used to evaluate small airway inflammation in asthma (39). The procedure was first described in 1974 (40). With TBB, a biopsy forceps is passed through the channel of the flexible bronchoscope and out into the lung parenchyma, usually under fluoroscopic guidance. In this manner, pieces of tissue of an average diameter of 3 mm can be obtained. Several imaging modalities may be used to assist the bronchcoscopist in obtaining adequate tissue samples. Lesions that are not easily accessed using simple fluoroscopy may be localized using CT or ultrasound. Hooper et al. have used virtual CT bronchoscopy to improve their yield from biopsy (41). Schwarz et al. recently described a new technique utilizing electromagnetic navigation for difficult-to-localize lesions (42).

Complications occur with TBB in approximately 6% of patients (43,44). Pneumothorax and hemorrhage are the most common complications. In a recent study, the ingestion of aspirin did not increase the risk of severe hemorrhage (45). The severity of bleeding after TBB in patients who have undergone lung transplantation appears not to be influenced by the type of transplant, creatinine level, infection, postoperative day, number of biopsies, or gender (46). TBB remains one of the mainstays in the diagnosis of pulmonary disease and should be performed in the majority of patients with unexplained pulmonary disease unless contraindications exist.

BRONCHOALVEOLAR LAVAGE

Bronchoalveolar lavage (BAL) is a relatively safe procedure used in the diagnosis and management of infectious and noninfectious pulmonary disease (38,47,48). The basic assumption underlying BAL is that the cells, inflammatory mediators, and infectious agents involved in pulmonary diseases may be recovered from the alveoli. BAL is performed prior to bronchial brushing or biopsy to avoid cellular contamination of the samples (49). BAL is distinct from bronchial washing. With bronchial washing, small amounts of saline are injected into the bronchi to obtain cells from the bronchi. BAL requires that the bronchoscope be advanced into a peripheral fourth- or fifth-order bronchus that conforms to the area of abnormality (49). Once the bronchoscope is wedged into the bronchus, a total volume of 150 to 400 mL of saline at room temperature or warmed to 37°C is infused in 30 to 50 mL aliquots. Hand suction or gravity drainage may then be used to withdraw the fluid. Overzealous suctioning may cause airway collapse or cellular injury. Normally, approximately 40% to 60% of the instilled fluid is recovered. The first 20 to 30 mL returned with BAL is usually discarded because it may be contaminated with bronchial cells. The recovered fluid may then be sent to the lab for cytologic analysis (including cell count and differential), microbiologic, and biochemical analysis. Guidelines to reduce variability in the BAL procedure have been developed by the European Respiratory Society (50).

The most common complication of BAL is hypoxemia; therefore patients at risk of desaturation should be monitored carefully. The incidence of fever ranges between 2% and 50%, and this appears to depend on the volume of the infusate and the number of lobes lavaged (51). In addition, patients may develop bronchospasm or, rarely, bleeding. Bleeding occurs in less than 0.7% of patients even in the presence of thrombocytopenia. BAL may be performed in patients with local anesthesia or in patients requiring mechanical ventilation. Relative contraindications include an uncooperative patient, hypercapnia, and cardiac instability (52).

TRANSBRONCHIAL NEEDLE ASPIRATION

Transbronchial needle aspiration (TBNA) is a procedure in which a needle is inserted through a bronchial wall to sample a lesion that is not visible endobronchially. It is a valuable tool for establishing the diagnosis of mediastinal or hilar adenopathy (53,54), peripheral nodules, extrinsic compression of the airway by a peribronchial process, necrotic endobronchial lesions (55), and staging of lung cancer (56–58). Selcux and Firat (59) have also used TBNA to evaluate the etiology of patients presenting with the superior vena cava syndrome. They noted no major complications from its use in this patient population (59). Experience, improved imaging techniques, and on-site cytologic evaluation increase the diagnostic yield with TBNA (60). In a study to determine the optimal number of TBNAs necessary to stage or establish a diagnosis of lung cancer, Chin et al. (61) prospectively evaluated 79 patients with suspected or diagnosed carcinoma of the lung. Aspirates were obtained without the use of CT or endobronchial ultrasound guidance. A diagnosis was established in the majority of patients with no more than seven aspirates in patients with carcinoma of the lung and mediastinal adenopathy (61). Although this procedure is minimally invasive and is complimentary to the usual diagnostic procedures performed during bronchoscopy, it remains underutilized (62). A survey of pulmonary fellows noted their lack of exposure to this procedure during training. They sensed that TBNA was not stressed during fellowship training for several reasons: philosophic beliefs regarding the value of TBNA, suboptimal bronchoscopic technique, and poor cytopathology support (62). The reason for underutilization of this procedure is probably multifactorial, not the least of which is the lack of training. As with any procedure, proper education and experience is paramount to its success (60,62). TBNA is a

useful adjunct to bronchoscopy, and its use should be encouraged during training. Efforts should also be made to educate those in practice.

The complication rate of TBNA is low (56,63,64). Pneumothorax occurs in approximately 0.5% of patients. Significant bleeding is uncommon even if pulmonary or systemic blood vessels are inadvertently aspirated. Pneumomediastinum and mediastinitis are rare complications.

ENDOBRONCHIAL ULTRASONOGRAPHY

Use of endobronchial ultrasonography (EBUS) was first described in 1990 (65). Its use was limited by air in the lungs, which distorts the ultrasonic image. With advances in technology, this limitation has essentially been resolved and interest in using this modality in the diagnosis of pulmonary disease has been renewed. Normally, the view of the bronchoscopist is limited to the visualization of the lumen and the inner surface of the airways. With EBUS, one can assess the depth of infiltration of a tumor into the bronchial wall, guide therapeutic interventions (66), biopsy abnormal lymph nodes with greater accuracy, and stage patients with carcinoma of the lung (67,68). EBUS can also be used to guide TBNA (69) and direct sampling during transbronchial biopsy (65). It is anticipated that the use of EBUS will increase as bronchoscopists become more familiar with its use and the technology improves.

COMPLICATIONS OF BRONCHOSCOPY

Flexible fiberoptic bronchoscopy is generally a well-tolerated procedure with few adverse effects. The commonly recognized complications include hypoxemia, bleeding, fever, cardiac arrhythmias, bronchospasm, pneumonia, and pneumothorax. The mortality rate is in the range of 0.01% and the rate of major complications is less than 1%. With bronchoscopy, the mean PaO_2 decreases by 15 to 20 mm Hg (70). Therefore, the oxygenation status of patients undergoing bronchoscopy should be monitored continuously with supplemental oxygen administered as required.

Bleeding is one of the most distressing and difficult management problems for the bronchoscopist. Minimal bleeding is defined as 50 mL of blood or less intermixed with saline lavage and is not considered hazardous. The incidence of clinically significant bleeding varied from a low of 0.5% to a high of 1.3% in one study and appeared to be related to the types of procedures performed during bronchoscopy, including brushing and transbronchial biopsy (71). Risk factors associated with increased bleeding include an immunosuppressed host, platelet dysfunction, coagulopathies, drugs, organ failure, chest malignancy, and uremia (71). Uremia creates a major hazard of bleeding because of platelet dysfunction, and approximately 45% of uremic patients have significant hemorrhage after transbronchial biopsy. Pulmonary hypertension is also associated with a high incidence of bleeding and is frequently considered a contraindication to transbronchial biopsy.

Fever is another common complication of bronchoscopy and has been reported in as many as 16% of patients (72). Pereira et al. (72) reported pneumonia in 6% and death from rapidly progressive pneumonia in another 1%. Bacteremia following this procedure has not been demonstrated. An outbreak of *Pseudomonas aeruginosa* and *Serratia marcescens* from contaminated bronchoscopes was reported by Kirschke et al (73). In another recent report, BAL specimens were contaminated with several types of bacteria (74). Careful disinfection, cleaning, and sterilization of equipment are mandatory to prevent these complications (75).

Laryngospasm and bronchospasm are common airway complications, and patients with asthma are at especially high risk. The most severe airway obstruction occurs in patients with chronic obstructive pulmonary disease. In these patients, who may have borderline respiratory failure, endotracheal intubation and mechanical ventilation may be necessary during or after the procedure.

Myocardial ischemia may occur following bronchoscopy. ST-segment changes and bundle branch block have been observed (76). Bronchosocopy has been performed safely in the peri-infarct period in patients without active ischemia (77). However, deferring bronchoscopy for at least six weeks following infarction has been recommended by the British Thoracic Society (78).

INDICATIONS FOR BRONCHOSCOPY

Suspected Lung Cancer

Approximately 170,000 new cases of lung cancer occur annually. Bronchoscopy is the procedure used most commonly to diagnose lung cancer. Lung cancer may present as an endobronchial lesion, as a peripheral lesion, or as a hilar mass. Bronchoscopy is useful in establishing the diagnosis in each of these instances.

ENDOBRONCHIAL LESIONS. The flexible bronchoscope is invaluable in examining the central airways to localize and diagnose endobronchial lesions. The appearance of an endobronchial tumor varies from an exophytic mass to subtle submucosal abnormalities. The diagnostic yield varies with the size and location of the tumor (79,80). Bronchial washings, bronchial brushings, and EBB have been employed in various combinations to establish a diagnosis of malignant disease (81,82). If an endobronchial lesion is *visible*, bronchoscopy with bronchial brushing and EBB will be diagnostic in more than 90% of cases (83–85). With endobronchially visible lesions, three to five biopsies are usually sufficient (84,86). The diagnostic yield is increased when bronchial brushing is combined with biopsy (87,88). It is controversial as to whether the addition of bronchial washing to bronchial biopsy and bronchial brushing increases the yield with endobronchially visible lesions (89). Dasgupta and Govert reported their results on the value of TBNA in conjunction with bronchial washings, bronchial brushings, and EBB in the diagnosis of endobronchial disease. They found that the addition of TBNA to routine bronchoscopic sampling increased the diagnosis of endobronchial malignancy (79,90). TBNA is also useful in the diagnosis of submucosal tumors that may present as erythema, loss of bronchial markings, or a thickening of the mucosa. TBNA may also be useful in tumors that extrinsically compress the bronchial lumen (91).

PERIPHERAL LUNG MALIGNANCIES. Some lung carcinomas are located in the parenchyma of the lung and are not visible endoscopically. The diagnostic approach to these lesions involves the use of each of the sampling methods available to the bronchcoscopist: bronchial washing, bronchial brushing, transbronchial biopsy, TBNA, and BAL. The diagnostic sensitivity for these masses and nodules ranges from 37% (92) to 80% (93). Use of multiple sampling methods increases the diagnostic yield for these lesions (94,95). Multiple factors influence the broad range in the results of these studies, including the size and distance from the hilum (96), sampling methods, and means used to localize the lesion. For example, Gracia et al. (97) evaluated the value of BAL in patients with suspected peripheral lung carcinoma without the use of fluoroscopic guidance. They found a 50% yield in the diagnosis of lung cancer in these patients using BAL. TBNA has also been used successfully to increase the diagnostic yield in these peripheral lesions (98). As with TBB, the successful retrieval of diagnostic material using TBNA depends on the size of the mass. The yield for lesions <2 cm or >2 cm in size is approximately 33% and 76%, respectively. Location of the lesion in the upper or lower lobes does not seem to influence the diagnostic yield, but the use of fluoroscopy or other imaging modalities is necessary when attempts are made to biopsy these lesions. Wagner et al. reported on their experience in nine patients using CT to guide TBB in patients with peripheral lesions. Despite the small number of patients, they found this approach for localization of the lesion to be possible with no increased discomfort to the patient (99). In an effort to diagnose lesions <2 cm in diameter, Shinagawa et al. used an ultrathin bronchoscope with virtual bronchoscopy to localize these lesions. In their study, the average size of the lesions was 1.32 cm. Adequate tissue samples were obtained in 17 of 26 lesions (65%). In the remainder, six lesions had insufficient samples and three were not accessible (100). They concluded that the use of an ultrathin bronchoscope with virtual bronchoscopy navigation was useful in the diagnosis of small peripheral lesions. Improvement in the diagnostic yield from bronchoscopy in patients with peripheral lesions will depend on further improvements in technology designed to guide the bronchoscopist to the desired site.

SOLITARY PULMONARY NODULES. Solitary pulmonary nodules (SPN) are defined as discrete lesions <3 cm in diameter surrounded by aerated lung without associated lymphadenopathy, atelectasis, or pneumonitis (101). The physician's goal is to determine with the least morbidity whether the nodule is benign or malignant. Features that suggest malignancy are size >3 cm, older age, prior tobacco use, growth on serial chest radiographs, lack of calcification, and a previous history of malignancy. Evaluation should include appropriate clinical history, review of previous radiographs (when available), routine laboratory data, and CT of the chest. High-resolution chest CT provides more information regarding the characteristics of the nodule than does conventional CT (102). The role of low-dose spiral CT to screen patients who were at high risk of developing carcinoma of the lung was evaluated by Swensen et al. They studied 1520 patients who were at least 50 years old and had at least a 20 pack-year history of smoking. They found that they could identify early-stage cancerous pulmonary nodules. Despite these findings, they suggest further studies are necessary to determine whether screening high-risk patients is a lifesaving and cost-effective endeavor (103). Positron emission tomography (PET) is being used in the evaluation of the solitary pulmonary nodule. Its sensitivity and specificity in identifying a malignant nodule are 96.8% and 77.8%, respectively (104).

The role of bronchoscopy in the management of SPN is limited (102). In general, if it is likely that the patient has a malignancy, it is best to proceed directly to thoracotomy since a nondiagnostic bronchoscopy does not rule out malignancy. Bronchoscopy in this situation is performed for two reasons: to rule out synchronous endobronchial disease and to establish a histologic diagnosis. In stage I disease, the likelihood of finding endobronchial disease is low. The size of the nodule is critical in determining the diagnostic yield from bronchoscopy. Nodules <2 cm in size and located in the outer third of the lung are especially difficult to diagnose. The diagnostic yield in the peripheral lesions is 14% compared to 31% for those more centrally located (105). The yield increases to 40% to 69% if the nodules are larger than 2 cm. When a "bronchus sign" is seen on a CT scan, there is an 80% chance of accurate diagnosis by transbronchial biopsy. This sign is defined as the finding of a bronchus leading directly to a peripheral pulmonary mass. In one recent study, bronchoscopy with bronchial washing, brushing, TBNA, and TBB established the diagnosis in 40 of 49 patients (82%) with the CT bronchus sign and only 19 of 43 patients (44%) without the bronchus sign (106). TBNA improves the diagnostic yield of patients undergoing bronchoscopy for the evaluation of a peripheral lesion (56). TBNA should be included in the routine bronchoscopic diagnosis of a peripheral lesion.

STAGING. Once the diagnosis of lung cancer is established, staging of the disease becomes crucial, not only to predict resectability but also to avoid unnecessary surgery and provide the patient with prognostic information. One aspect of staging is to evaluate whether or not the mediastinum is involved. In general, histologic confirmation is necessary if imaging studies suggest mediastinal involvement by tumor. Sampling of the mediastinal nodes for the purpose of staging can be accomplished using TBNA (54), cervical mediastinoscopy, anterior mediastinoscopy, CT fluoroscopic-guided TBNA (63), or endobronchial ultrasound-guided fine-needle aspiration (FNA)(107). Of these procedures, TBNA is the least invasive because it involves sampling of mediastinal nodes by aspirating through the tracheal wall at the time of bronchoscopy. This procedure is most useful in sampling paratracheal, hilar, and subcarinal nodes (108). The procedure has a reported yield of approximately 40% in patients with positive imaging studies of the mediastinum and a yield of approximately 10% in individuals with negative imaging studies (108). The yield can be increased if CT guidance is utilized to ascertain that the tip of the needle is exactly inside the node (109). False-positive results have been obtained with this procedure, but these are most likely due to faulty technique, with contamination of the sample with malignant cells from the airway (110). The addition of EBUS to guide TBNA has been shown to improve the diagnostic yield of TBNA in all stations except the subcarinal nodes (111).

Hemoptysis

Hemoptysis may be divided into two broad categories, massive and minimal, on the basis of the volume of blood expectorated and/or the physiologic effects related to the loss of blood. In general, if the patient expectorates more than 150 mL in 24 hours, the hemoptysis should be considered massive because with this amount of hemoptysis, the patient is in danger of drowning in his own blood. All patients with massive hemoptysis should undergo bronchoscopy, using a scope with a large suction channel; many prefer to use a rigid bronchoscope. If the hemoptysis is life-threatening, treatment options at the time of bronchoscopy include topical epinephrine, balloon tamponade, iced saline lavage, and insertion of a double-lumen endotracheal tube (112). Recently, *n*-butyl cyanoacrylate has been used to seal bleeding bronchial segments (113). The timing of bronchoscopy to localize the bleeding is controversial (114). Most clinicians, however, favor early bronchoscopy to localize the site in the event surgery is necessary.

The four primary causes of minimal hemoptysis are bronchiectasis, carcinoma of the lung, bronchitis, and infection (115). The primary reason to perform bronchoscopy in patients with minimal hemoptysis is to rule out endobronchial malignancy. There are certain clinical factors that should influence the decision whether to perform bronchoscopy. Patients who are less than 40 years of age, have a normal chest radiograph, have a bleeding duration of less than one week, have smoked less than 40 pack-years, or who expectorate <30 mL of blood daily are unlikely to have endobronchial carcinoma (116). The prognosis for patients with hemoptysis of undetermined origin (cryptogenic) with a negative bronchoscopy is generally good, usually with resolution of bleeding within six months of evaluation (117).

Diagnosis of Pulmonary Infections

The microbiologic diagnosis of pulmonary infections can be made using specimens collected noninvasively or invasively. The bronchoscope allows direct access to the bronchi and pulmonary parenchyma. Transbronchial biopsy, BAL, and protected brush may be used independently or in combination in the diagnosis of pulmonary infections (38,49,87). When considering indications for bronchoscopy for the diagnosis of pulmonary infections, patients are generally subdivided into those with normal immune function and those who are immunocompromised.

IMMUNOCOMPROMISED PATIENTS. With the advent of acquired immunodeficiency syndrome (AIDS), organ transplantation, and intensive chemotherapeutic regimens, the population of immunocompromised patients is increasing. Lung involvement by infectious and noninfectious agents is common in those who are immunocompromised (see Chapter 18, Pulmonary Complications in the Immunosuppressed Patient). Jain et al. reported their experience using flexible bronchoscopy to diagnose the etiology of pulmonary infiltrates in 104 non–human immunodeficiency virus (HIV) immunocompromised patients (38). The diagnostic yield using flexible bronchoscopy was 56.2%. The diagnostic yield of BAL was similar to transbronchial biopsy. The combination of BAL and TBB was superior to BAL alone in establishing a diagnosis. In this study, a diagnosis was more likely to be established if the infiltrate was due to an infectious agent (38). In patients with AIDS, the most common infectious agent was *Pneumocystis jiroveci*; however, fungal, viral, and mycobacterial organisms may be identified. In addition, HIV-positive patients may develop pulmonary lymphoma or Kaposi sarcoma (118). *P. jiroveci* may be diagnosed by inducing sputum production, but in most centers, the sensitivity with this procedure is low. Flexible bronchoscopy with the use of transbronchial biopsy, BAL, and protected brush specimen is the diagnostic procedure of choice in HIV patients with undiagnosed pulmonary infiltrates (119).

The ability to safely obtain samples from infected alveoli using BAL has led to the widespread use of this modality in the immunocompromised host. The presence of certain organisms found in the recovered fluid is diagnostic of infection, for instance, *P. jiroveci, Strongyloides, Histoplasma, Toxoplasma gondii, M. tuberculosis,* and *Mycoplasma* (52). Uses of semiquantitative cultures are necessary when infectious pathogens known to colonize the airway are recovered. At least 10^3 colony-forming units (cfu) should be present on a culture of a BAL specimen in order to consider the positive culture representative of the offending organism (120).

IMMUNE-COMPETENT PATIENTS. Bronchoscopy is also useful in identifying infectious agents in the immune-competent host. Bronchoscopy is particularly useful at identifying chronic pulmonary infections, such as fungal infections, actinomycosis, nocardiosis, and tuberculosis. When a chronic infection is suspected, BAL should be performed in conjunction with bronchoscopy. BAL is also useful in patients with community-acquired pneumonia in which the clinical course suggests progression of the infection despite appropriate antibiotic coverage (121). Furthermore, BAL may be a useful tool in the diagnosis of ventilator-associated pneumonia (122).

PROTECTED SPECIMEN BRUSHING. As the bronchoscope passes from the upper airway to the lower airways, it may become contaminated with nasal or endobronchial secretions, resulting in false-positive cultures. Protected specimen brushings (PSB) are intended to avoid false-positive cultures. These catheters are designed with a plug over the distal end to avoid contact with the secretions encountered as the bronchoscope traverses the airways. When the catheter is advanced, the plug is extruded and the brush is allowed to come in contact with the infectious site. Then, material for cultures is obtained. A positive diagnosis is made if there are more than 10^3 cfu. PSB, along with BAL, is used most commonly in patients on ventilators who develop infiltrates and in patients with community- or hospital-acquired pneumonia who are not responding to therapy (122,123).

Interstitial Lung Disease

There are numerous diseases that may result in the radiographic pattern of interstitial lung disease (ILD) (see Chapter 12, Diffuse Parenchymal and Alveolar Lung Diseases). These include malignant, infectious, immunologic, occupational, and drug-induced diseases. Some authors have advocated bronchoscopy with TBB and BAL for most patients with ILD. In general, however, the only two common diagnoses that are easily established with TBB are lymphangitic carcinomatosis and sarcoidosis. The specimens obtained with TBB are usually too small to make the diagnosis of usual interstitial pneumonia or desquamative interstitial pneumonia. This does not mean that bronchoscopy should not be performed in patients when considering one of these diagnoses. Not infrequently, bronchoscopy may yield a completely unexpected finding, avoiding the need for further invasive testing. BAL may also be a valuable tool in the diagnosis and management of patients with ILD (47). BAL fluid findings that are of diagnostic value in patients with ILD include malignant cells in patients with lymphangitic spread of carcinoma, fat globules in patients with lipoid pneumonia, or hemosiderin-laden macrophages in patients with diffuse alveolar hemorrhage (124).

Cough

Chronic cough is a frequent presenting symptom in the outpatient setting. Cough is usually due to environmental exposure (especially cigarettes), postnasal drainage syndrome (PNDS), gastroesophageal reflux disease (GERD), asthma, or medications (ACE inhibitors). Cough may also be the result of more serious pathology such as malignancy, tuberculosis, ILD, congestive heart failure, aspiration, bronchiectasis, or other disorders affecting the upper or lower airway. The American College of Chest Physicians guidelines for the evaluation of chronic cough suggest a very limited role for bronchoscopy. The initial evaluation of patients with cough should include a history and physical, chest radiograph and, in certain instances, pulmonary function testing, sinus films, and evaluation for GERD (125). Bronchoscopy is indicated only in patients with radiographic abnormalities, suggesting an underlying malignancy or other primary pulmonary process not explained by the initial noninvasive evaluation.

Undiagnosed Pleural Effusion

Bronchoscopy is useful in the diagnosis of pleural effusion only if one or more of the following three conditions are present (126): (a) There is a pulmonary infiltrate on the chest radiograph or the chest CT scan. In this situation, particular attention should be paid to the area that contains the infiltrate. (b) Hemoptysis is present. Hemoptysis in the presence of a pleural effusion is very suggestive of an endobronchial lesion. (c) The pleural effusion is massive, that is, it occupies more than three-fourths of the hemithorax. In patients with pleural effusions with positive cytology, but no hemoptysis or parenchymal infiltrates, bronchoscopy will not identify the primary tumor (127).

Bronchoscopy in the Intensive Care Unit

Bronchoscopy is invaluable as a diagnostic and therapeutic tool in the intensive care unit (128). Bronchoscopy has been used to facilitate intubation, evaluate the airway, change endotracheal tubes, and evaluate causes of stridor in the immediate postextubation period. Bronchoscopy may also be used for diagnostic purposes in patients with persistent infiltrates or hemoptysis (129). Recent cardiac events are only a relative contraindication to bronchoscopy (130).

Virtual Bronchoscopy

Conventional CT and bronchoscopy are routinely used to evaluate patients with suspected endobronchial or peripheral pulmonary disease. Conventional CT is limited in detecting central airway lesions (131). Currently, it is the preferred method of evaluating endobronchial disease. However, bronchoscopy provides minimal information about areas distal to the endobronchial abnormality in patients with high-grade obstruction. Clinically, virtual bronchoscopy is a noninvasive method to evaluate intra- and extraluminal central airway lesions. Virtual bronchoscopy has evolved from advances in computer technology that have allowed the information from CT images to be processed into three-dimensional images of the central airways (132). Virtual bronchoscopy has been used in preprocedure planning (133), the evaluation of bronchial anastomoses, and airway stenoses (134). As technology improves, the clinical applications of virtual bronchoscopy will continue to evolve.

TRANSTHORACIC NEEDLE ASPIRATION

Percutaneous transthoracic needle aspiration is used most commonly to obtain tissue from patients who are suspected of having lung tumors, but it can also be used to establish the etiology of infections. Percutaneous needle aspiration is relatively good at establishing the diagnosis of lung malignancy, but it is not very good at establishing specific benign diagnoses. In one series of 130 patients who had undergone TTNA, TTNA had a sensitivity of 74% for the detection of malignancy but established the diagnosis in only two of 28 patients (8%) with benign disease (135). TTNA is more sensitive when the lesion is larger (135). In patients who are suspected of having lung cancer and who are operative candidates, TTNA should be performed only if the results of the aspiration will influence whether or not surgery will be performed. For example, if it is decided beforehand that surgery will be performed only if the aspiration is positive, TTNA should be performed. Also, if surgery will not be performed only if the TTNA is negative, then TTNA should be performed. Visualization of the lesion for guidance of the procedure may be obtained with CT scanning, ultrasonography, or fluoroscopy (136).

TTNA is also useful in sampling mediastinal nodes in patients with lung cancer. In one recent series, Zwischenberger et al. performed CT-guided fine-needle aspiration with or without core biopsy in 89 patients with mediastinal lymphadenopathy >1.5 cm in diameter. Mediastinal TTNA was diagnostic in 69 of the 89 patients (78%) (137). They concluded that mediastinal TTNA should be performed before mediastinoscopy in the staging of lung cancer or the workup of mediastinal masses (138).

The most common complication of TTNA is pneumothorax, which occurs in approximately 35% of patients undergoing the procedure (3). Indeed, TTNA is the most common cause of iatrogenic pneumothorax (3). Approximately 10% of the patients who develop a pneumothorax are treated with tube thoracostomy. Another complication is transient hemoptysis, occurring in about 10% of patients. Other rare complications include bacterial contamination of the pleural space, allergic anesthetic reactions, vasovagal reactions, soft-tissue infection, cancer seeding at the insertion site, and air embolism (<0.1%) (136). Contraindications to the procedure include a bleeding diathesis, bullous lung disease in the area of the biopsy, local cutaneous lesions (e.g., pyoderma or herpes zoster), pulmonary hypertension, or a lesion abutting the mediastinum or hilum.

THORACOSCOPY

Although thoracoscopy has been a part of thoracic surgical practice for many years, the advent of video-assisted techniques has greatly expanded the indications and uses of this procedure. Whereas thoracoscopy was previously performed mainly for diagnostic purposes (137), video-assisted thoracic surgery (VATS) has now assumed a major role in the diagnosis and therapy of chest diseases. Indeed, in some institutions, it is now the most commonly used operative approach for some general thoracic surgical procedures (139). The primary advantage of VATS is that it is associated with less morbidity and mortality and shorter hospitalization times than is thoracotomy (140). The overall mortality with thoracoscopy is about 1%, 1.5% in patients more than 70 years old, and 2.1% in patients with an FEV$_1$ <1 L (140).

Two different techniques have emerged: VATS and medical thoracoscopy. In actuality, there is a continuous spectrum between these two procedures. The former is usually performed in an operating room by a thoracic surgeon under general anesthesia, with the patient selectively intubated to allow for single-lung ventilation. Multiple puncture sites are made in the chest wall through which the thoracoscope and surgical instruments are introduced. Medical thoracoscopy (141) differs from VATS in that the patient may not be intubated and usually breathes spontaneously. The procedure is usually performed by a pulmonologist with conscious sedation and local anesthesia. Medical thoracoscopy primarily serves as a diagnostic tool rather than being used for intervention. Medical thoracoscopy is usually performed by pulmonologists, whereas VATS is performed by thoracic surgeons (141). For diagnostic purposes, either VATS or medical thoracoscopy is appropriate, and the choice of procedure depends primarily upon its institutional availability.

PLEURAL EFFUSIONS

In the diagnosis of pleural disease, thoracoscopic procedures should be used only when the less-invasive diagnostic methods, such as thoracentesis with cytology and markers for tuberculosis, have not yielded a diagnosis. In one series of 620 patients with pleural effusions, only 48 (8%) remained without a diagnosis and were subjected to thoracoscopy (142). If the patient has malignancy, thoracoscopy will establish the diagnosis more than 90% of the time. The diagnosis of mesothelioma is probably best made with thoracoscopy. In patients with undiagnosed pleural effusions, Ferrer et al. demonstrated that predictors of malignancy included a symptomatic period of over one month, absence of fever, serosanguineous pleural fluid, and chest CT suggestion of malignancy (143). Thoracoscopy also establishes the diagnosis of tuberculous pleuritis in more than 95% of cases (144). An advantage to thoracoscopy in the diagnosis of pleural disease is that pleurodesis can also be performed at the time of the procedure. It should be emphasized, however, that thoracoscopy rarely establishes the diagnosis of benign diseases other than tuberculosis (143).

INTERSTITIAL LUNG DISEASE

VATS procedures appear to be particularly useful for obtaining lung biopsies in patients with diffuse ILD (145) and can be done as outpatient procedures (146). Lung biopsy via VATS should not be attempted if the patient requires mechanical ventilation because he or she probably will not be able to tolerate one-lung ventilation. Patients with coagulation disorders or pulmonary hypertension should have an open-lung biopsy rather than a VATS procedure. With VATS, the visualization of the lung is better than it is with a limited thoracotomy, and more areas of the lung can be sampled. However, a recent randomized controlled study showed that there was no clinical difference in outcomes for thoracoscopic versus open-lung biopsy in patients with ILD (147).

PULMONARY NODULES

Pulmonary nodules may be safely removed via VATS procedures (148). If the nodule is benign, then no additional procedures need be done. If the patient is a good surgical candidate and has a primary lung cancer, then a lobectomy should probably be performed (148). If the patient is a poor surgical candidate, this wedge resection can serve as the definitive treatment. The primary advantages of using VATS are that for patients with benign disease, it is the definitive procedure, is associated with less discomfort, and requires a shorter period of hospitalization. One problem with VATS for the removal of pulmonary nodules is that it is sometimes difficult to find the nodule. In one series, the nodule could not be localized in 46% of 92 patients (149). Nodules <10 mm in diameter and more than 10 mm deep to the pleura are particularly difficult to identify during VATS. However, if the nodule is localized immediately preoperatively with a CT-guided hookwire, the nodule can be identified more than 90% of the time even if it is <10 mm in diameter and >15 mm deep to the pleura (150).

MEDIASTINAL DISEASE

The role of thoracoscopy in the diagnosis of mediastinal masses is still controversial. Some surgeons recommend thoracoscopy only for lesions that are not within the reach of the mediastinoscope because the length of hospital stay and the complication rates are less with mediastinoscopy (151). In contrast, some surgeons now prefer VATS procedures to anterior mediastinotomy to approach mediastinal adenopathy located in the aortopulmonary window or the low periazygos area. The visibility of the entire mediastinal compartment afforded through the VATS approach is far superior to exploration through an anterior mediastinotomy (152). VATS procedures can also be used to resect benign posterior mediastinal neoplasms and carefully selected cases of early-stage thymoma (139).

MISCELLANEOUS CONDITIONS

VATS procedures have also been used for many other thoracic surgical procedures, including ligation of the thoracic duct, creation of a pericardial window, Zenker diverticulum, lobectomy, lung volume reduction surgery, treatment of spontaneous pneumothorax with stapling of blebs and pleural abrasion, thoracic sympathectomy, benign esophageal tumors, removal of chest wall tumors, and removal of clotted blood with a hemothorax.

COMPLICATIONS OF THORACOSCOPY

Although morbidity and mortality are less from VATS procedures than from thoracotomy, there are, nonetheless, significant complications. Kaiser and Bavaria (153) reviewed the complications of VATS encountered at the Hospital of the University of Pennsylvania between December 1991 and December 1992. They reported that 10% of VATS procedures were associated with complications. The most common complication was prolonged (longer than seven days) air leak (3.7%), followed by superficial wound infection (1.9%), and bleeding significant enough to require either transfusion or reoperation (1.9%). In 4.1% of patients, they were unable to successfully complete the intended procedure thoracoscopically and converted to an open procedure (153).

MEDIASTINOSCOPY

This endoscopic procedure is used to explore the mediastinum and to obtain biopsies of lymph nodes and other masses. However, some advocate mediastinoscopy only if CT-guided mediastinal transthoracic needle aspiration is nondiagnostic (137). General anesthesia is usually required, although a local anesthetic may be used safely in selected patients in a day-surgery setting. All paratracheal nodes, nodes in the tracheobronchial angle, and nodes situated proximally along the main bronchi are evaluable, as are the nodes in the anterior compartment of the subcarinal space. Lymph nodes in the aortopulmonary window and the left anterior mediastinum (usually along the phrenic nerve) cannot be reached by conventional mediastinoscopy, nor can the inferior posterior lymph nodes. In addition, nodes along the esophagus and in the inferior pulmonary ligament are not accessible (154). A modified procedure involves extension of the conventional cervical mediastinoscopy incision using a parasternal approach as an alternative to left anterior mediastinotomy (155). This can aid in the evaluation of lymph nodes in the left hilar or left upper lobe areas.

Complications from mediastinoscopy are uncommon. In one series of over 1,000 patients from the Toronto General Hospital, the complication rate was 2.3% and included hemorrhage, pneumothorax, wound infection, and recurrent laryngeal nerve palsy (156). There were no operative deaths (156).

Mediastinoscopy is recommended in patients with T2 or T3 primary cancerous lesions, as well as those with T1 lesions in whom the cell type is adenocarcinoma or large-cell carcinoma, even when the CT studies are negative. If nodes are identified, then cervical mediastinoscopy is performed. Patients with T2 or T3 lesions in the left upper lobe should undergo cervical mediastinoscopy with frozen section; if the other biopsy specimens are negative, a left anterior mediastinotomy through the second intercostal space should be performed (155). These procedures can be performed on an outpatient basis. One report of ambulatory mediastinoscopy and anterior mediastinotomy revealed that these procedures permitted a diagnosis to be made in 47 of 158 patients and confirmed unresectable malignant disease in 29 patients, thus eliminating admission to the hospital in 48% of the patients (157). Mediastinoscopy may be omitted in patients with T1 squamous cell carcinoma and negative findings on CT.

Mediastinoscopy is also used for the diagnosis of other masses in the middle or anterior mediastinum. In one series of

21 such cases (158), definitive diagnoses were obtained in 67%. Because several of these patients had diseases for which the treatment of choice was not surgery, the procedure saved the patient from more extensive exploration. Carlens (159) reported that mediastinoscopy was positive in 96% of 123 cases of sarcoidosis. However, usually the diagnosis of sarcoidosis can be established by less-invasive means, such as peripheral lymph node biopsy or TBB.

ENDOSCOPIC ULTRASOUND-GUIDED FINE-NEEDLE ASPIRATION

Staging patients with nonsmall cell carcinoma of the lung with mediastinal involvement is essential prior to surgical resection. Chest CT and PET scans have been used to noninvasively evaluate the mediastinum and adjacent structures (107,160), but a tissue diagnosis is vital in the staging process. Exploration of the mediastinum normally requires surgical intervention such as mediastinoscopy to establish a tissue diagnosis. Endoscopic ultrasound with fine-needle aspiration (EUS-FNA) offers an alternative to surgical exploration in selected patients (107,161). With this procedure, an echoendoscope is placed in the esophagus, and the lesion is localized. Lesions <1 cm in size can be detected with this method (162). Once the lesion is localized, a needle is advanced through the esophageal wall incrementally under real-time EUS guidance until the needle tip is visualized within the lesion. Material is aspirated from the lesion, smeared onto a glass slide, and sent to cytopathology (163). Fritscher–Ravens et al. recently reported their results comparing three imaging modalities to evaluate the mediastinum in patients with carcinoma of the lung who were being considered for surgical resection. They compared CT, PET scans, and EUS with or without FNA in these patients. In their hands, EUS with FNA proved to be the most useful technique to evaluate for mediastinal involvement by carcinoma (163). The authors also found that CT and PET scanning were useful in identifying other local and distant disease sites (163). It is expected that additional experience with this procedure will result in its more widespread use to evaluate mediastinal disease.

OPEN-LUNG BIOPSY

To a large extent, thoracoscopic lung biopsy has replaced open-lung biopsy, but there are no large randomized studies that compare the diagnostic efficacy, the morbidity and the cost effectiveness of thoracoscopic lung biopsy, and limited thoracotomy. One small randomized study comparing the two methods concluded that there were no clinically significant differences (147). The indications for either thoracoscopic lung biopsy or open-lung biopsy are as follows: (a) the patient with diffuse pulmonary infiltrates and progressive disease whose diagnosis is not apparent after a careful history, physical examination, sputum analysis, radiologic studies, and bronchoscopy with transbronchial biopsy; (b) the patient with a progressive localized pulmonary infiltrate whose diagnosis is not apparent after a careful evaluation as described above, including bronchoscopy and TBB; (c) the immunocompromised host with pulmonary infiltrates but no specific diagnosis after bronchoscopy with TBB or percutaneous needle aspiration; and

(d) the patient suspected of having pulmonary malignancy in whom the sputum cytologic examination, bronchoscopy, TBB, and needle aspiration are nondiagnostic.

Open-lung biopsy via limited thoracotomy is a relatively safe procedure with little morbidity (19%) and approximately 0.5% to 0.6% mortality (164,165). Biopsy specimens should be taken from at least two sites (an upper-lobe and a lower-lobe site) and should include both abnormal- and normal-appearing areas. Obtaining small subpleural samples (especially if pleuritis is present) in dependent segments of the right middle lobe or lingula may yield nonspecific findings. When the procedure is performed and the diagnosis of interstitial infiltrates with suspected fibrosis is found, the pathologist should quantitate both the extent and the severity of the inflammatory or exudative—as well as the fibrotic or reparative—tissue responses (164,165).

In patients with diffuse pulmonary infiltrates and acute respiratory failure, open-lung biopsy often reveals an unsuspected diagnosis (164,166). Open-lung biopsy provided a specific etiologic diagnosis in 66% of 80 patients in one series (164). Diagnosis influenced therapy in 70%; however, only 30% of the patients survived to hospital discharge, and only 12% of patients survived for more than one year. This study suggested that open-lung biopsy is helpful in yielding an etiologic diagnosis; however, the usefulness of establishing a diagnosis is limited by current shortcomings of therapy (164). Open-lung biopsy is also worthwhile in immunocompromised patients with pulmonary infiltrates. Cheson et al. (167) reviewed their results in 87 such patients and reported that a specific histologic diagnosis was obtained in 62 patients (71%), 33 of whom had infections. Specific therapy was available for 52 patients, and in 33 cases, a change in therapy was necessary for appropriate treatment. Forty-one patients received an adequate course of therapy, and 27 (66%) improved clinically, including those with infection, malignancies, and vasculitis. This report suggests that in immunocompromised patients in the pre-AIDS era (from 1971 to 1982), open-lung biopsy was safe and accurate in diagnosis, with clinical improvement following biopsy-directed patient management (167).

In contrast, in patients with AIDS, open-lung biopsy appears to have a limited role. In 42 patients reported by Fitzgerald et al. (168), 29 had a preceding nondiagnostic bronchoscopic procedure and 9 had open-lung biopsy because of progressive deterioration despite treatment for diseases diagnosed bronchoscopically. Diagnoses of treatable diseases such as cryptococcosis, tuberculosis, and *Pneumocystis carinii* pneumonia were made in only 5 of the 42 patients subjected to open-lung biopsy in this study, and one of the results was a false negative. On the basis of this and other studies, many investigators suggest that open-lung biopsy in patients with AIDS should be reserved for highly selected patients and that a second bronchoscopic procedure or thoracoscopy should be considered because of the morbidity associated with open-lung biopsy (169).

REFERENCES

1. Jones PW, Moyers JP, Rogers JT, et al. Ultrasound-guided thoracentesis. Is it a safer method? *Chest* 2003;123:418–423.
2. Conner BD, Lee YC (Gary), Branca P, et al. Variations in pleural fluid WBC count and differential counts with different sample containers and different methods. *Chest* 2003;123:1181–1187.

3. Light RW. *Pleural diseases*, 4th ed. Baltimore: Lippincott Williams & Wilkins, 2001.

4. Light RW, Erozan YC, Ball WC Jr. Cells in pleural fluid: their value in differential diagnosis. *Arch Intern Med* 1973;132:854–860.

5. Broaddus VC, Light RW. What is the origin of pleural transudates and exudates? [Editorial]. *Chest* 1992;102:658.

6. Light RW, MacGregor MI, Luchsinger PC, et al. Pleural effusions: the diagnostic separation of transudates and exudates. *Ann Intern Med* 1972;77:507–513.

7. Romero-Candeira S, Fernandez C, Martin C, et al. Influence of diuretics on the concentration of proteins and other components of pleural transudates in patients with heart failure. *Am J Med* 2001;110:681–686.

8. Sadikot RT, Rogers JT, Cheng D-S, et al. Pleural fluid characteristics of patients with symptomatic pleural effusion after coronary artery bypass graft surgery. *Arch Intern Med* 2000;160:2665–2668.

9. Kalomenidis I, Light RW. Eosinophilic pleural effusions. *Curr Opin Pulm Med* 2003;9:254–260.

10. Branca P, Rodriguez RM, Rogers JT, et al. Routine measurement of pleural fluid amylase is not indicated. *Arch Intern Med* 2001;161:228–232.

11. Kramer MR, Ceperao RJ, Pitchenik AE. High amylase in neoplasm-related pleural effusion. *Ann Intern Med* 1989;110:567–569.

12. Light RW, Girard WM, Jenkinson SG, et al. Parapneumonic effusions. *Am J Med* 1980;69:507–512.

13. Cheng DS, Rodriguez RM, Rogers J, et al. Comparison of pleural fluid pH values obtained using blood gas machine, pH meter, and pH indicator strip. *Chest* 1998;114:1368–1372.

14. Rodriguez de Castro F, Molero T, Acosta O, et al. Value of DNA analysis in addition to cytological testing in the diagnosis of malignant pleural effusions. *Thorax* 1994;49:692–694.

15. Moriarty AT, Wiersema L, Snyder W, et al. Immunophenotyping of cytologic specimens by flow cytometry. *Diagn Cytopathol* 1993; 9:252–258.

16. Ordonez NG. The immunohistochemical diagnosis of mesothelioma: a comparative study of epithelioid and lung adenocarcinoma. *Am J Surg Pathol* 2003;27:1031–1051.

17. Valdes L, Alvarez D, San Jose E, et al. Tuberculous pleurisy: a study of 254 patients. *Arch Intern Med* 1998;158:2017–2021.

18. Lee YCG, Rogers JT, Rodriguez RM, et al. Adenosine deaminase levels in nontuberculous lymphocytic pleural effusions. *Chest* 2001;120:356–361.

19. Villena V, Lopez-Encuentra A, Pozo F, et al. Interferon gamma levels in pleural fluid for the diagnosis of tuberculosis. *Am J Med* 2003;115:365–370.

20. Querol JM, Minguez J, Garcia-Sanchez E, et al. Rapid diagnosis of pleural tuberculosis by polymerase chain reaction. *Am J Respir Crit Care Med* 1995;152:1977–1981.

21. Villena V, Rebollo MJ, Aguado JM, et al. Polymerase chain reaction for the diagnosis of pleural tuberculosis in immunocompromised and immunocompetent patients. *Clin Infect Dis* 1998;26:212–214.

22. Light RW. Closed needle biopsy of the pleura is a valuable diagnostic procedure. *J Bronchol* 1999;5:332–336.

23. Prakash URS, Reiman HM. Comparison of needle biopsy with cytologic analysis for the evaluation of pleural effusion: analysis of 414 cases. *Mayo Clin Proc* 1985;60:158–164.

24. Tanaka H, Yamada G, Saiki T, et al. Increased airway vascularity in newly diagnosed asthma using a high-magnification bronchovideoscope. *Am J Respir Crit Care Med* 2003;168:1495–1499.

25. Schuurmans MM, Michaud GC, Diacon AH, et al. Use of an ultra thin bronchoscope in the assessment of central airway obstruction. *Chest* 2003;124:735–739.

26. Helmers RA, Sanderson DR. Rigid Bronchoscopy: the forgotten art. *Clin Chest Med* 1995;16:393–399.

27. Miyasawa T, Yamakido M, Ikeda S, et al. Implantation of Ultraflex nitinol stents in malignant tracheobronchial stenoses. *Chest* 2000;118:959–965.

28. Saad CP, Murthy S, Krizmanich G, et al. Self-expandable metallic airway stents and flexible bronchoscopy. *Chest* 2003;124:1993–1999.

29. Colt HG, Udaya B, Prakrash S, et al. Bronchoscopy in North America. *J Bronchol* 2000;7:8–25.

30. Jackson C. Bronchoscopy: past, present and future. *N Engl J Med* 1928;199:758.

31. Beamis JF. Modern use of rigid bronchoscopy. In: Bollinger CT, Mathur, PN, eds. *Interventional bronchoscopy*. Basil: Karger, 2000: 22–30.

32. Ayers ML, Beamis JF. Rigid bronchoscopy in the twenty-first century. *Clin Chest Med* 2001;22:355–364.

33. Cavalierre S, Venuta F, Foccoli P, et al. Endoscopic treatment of malignant airway obstructions in 2,008 patients. *Chest* 1996;110:1536–1542.

34. Herth F, Becker HD, LoCicero J, et al. Successful bronchoscopic placement of tracheobronchial stents without fluoroscopy. *Chest* 2001;119:1910–1912.

35. Aboyoun CL, Tamm M, Chhajed PN, et al. Diagnostic value of follow-up transbronchial biopsy after lung rejection. *Am J Respir Crit Care Med* 2001;164:460–463.

36. Soubani AO, Quershi MA, Baynes RD. Flexible bronchoscopy in the diagnosis of pulmonary infiltrates following autologous peripheral stem cell transplantation for advanced breast cancer. *Bone Marrow Transplant* 2001;28:981–985.

37. Hopkins PM, Aboyoun CL, Chhajed PN. Prospective analysis of 1,235 transbronchial lung biopsies in lung transplant recipients. *J Heart Lung Transplant* 2002;21:1062–1067.

38. Jain P, Sandur S, Meli Y, et al. Role of flexible bronchoscopy in immunocompromised patients with lung infiltrates. *Chest* 2004;125:712–722.

39. Balzar S, Wenzel SE, Chu HW. Transbronchial biopsy as a tool to evaluate small airways in asthma. *Eur Respir J* 2002;20:254–259.

40. Levin DC, Wicks AB, Ellis JH. Transbronchial lung biopsy via the fiberoptic bronchoscope. *Am Rev Respir Dis* 1974;110:4–12.

41. Hopper KD, Lucas TA, Gleeson K, et al. Transbronchial biopsy with virtual CT bronchoscopy and nodal highlighting. *Radiology* 2001;221:531–536.

42. Schwarz Y, Mehta AC, Ernst A, et al. Electromagnetic navigation during flexible bronchoscopy. *Respiration* 2003;70:516–522.

43. Milan N, Faurschou P, Munch EP. Transbronchial lung biopsy through the fiberoptic bronchoscope. Results and complications in 452 examinations. *Respir Med* 1994;88:749–753.

44. Descombes E, Gardiol D, Leunberger P. Transbronchial lung biopsy: an analysis of 530 cases with reference to the number of samples. *Monaldi Arch Chest Dis* 1997;52:324–329.

45. Herth FJ, Becker HD, Ernst A. Aspirin does not increase bleeding complications after transbronchial biopsy. *Chest* 2002;122: 1461–1464.

46. Chhajed PN, Aboyoun C, Malouf MA, et al. Risk factors and management of bleeding associated with transbronchial lung biopsy in lung transplant recipients. *J Heart Lung Transplant* 2003;195–197.

47. Baughman RP, Drent M. Role of broncholaveolar lavage in interstitial lung disease. *Clin Chest Med* 2001;22:331–341.

48. Huang L, Hecht FM, Stansell JD, et al. Suspected pneumocystis carinii pneumonia with a negative induced sputum examination. *Am J Respir Crit Care Med* 1995;151:1866–1871.

49. Reynolds HY. Bronchoalveolar lavage. *Am Rev Respir Dis* 1987; 135:250–263.

50. Klech H, Hutter C, Costabel U. Clinical guidelines and indications for bronchoalveolar lavage (BAL). *Eur Respir Rev* 1992;2:47–127.

51. Strumpf IJ, Feld MK, Cornelius MJ, et al. Safety of fiberoptic bronchoalveolar lavage in evaluation of interstitial lung disease. *Chest* 1981;80:268–271.

52. Goldstein RA, Rohatgi PK, Bergofsky EH, et al. Clinical role of bronchoalveolar lavage in adults with pulmonary disease. *Am Rev Respir Dis* 1990;142:481–486.

53. Cetinkaya E, Yildiz P, Altin S, et al. Diagnostic value of transbronchial needle aspiration by Wang 22-gauge cytology needle in intrathoracic lymphadenopathy. *Chest* 2004;125:527–531.

54. Sharafkhaneh A, Baaklini W, Gorin AB, et al. Yield of transbronchial needle aspiration in diagnosis of mediastinal lesions. *Chest* 2003;124:2131–2135.

55. Bilaceroglu S, Guel O, Cagirici U, et al. Comparison of endobronchial needle aspiration with forceps and brush biopsies in the diagnosis of endobronchial cancer. *Monaldi Arch Chest Dis* 1997;52:13–17.

56. Reichenberger MD, Weber J, Tamm M, et al. The value of transbronchial needle aspiration in the diagnosis of peripheral pulmonary lesions. *Chest* 1999;116:704–708.

57. Herth FJ, Becker HJ, Ernst A. Ultrasound-guided transbronchial needle aspiration. *Chest* 2003;123:604–607.

58. Harrow EM, Abi-Saleh W, Blum J, et al. The utility of transbronchial needle aspiration in the staging of bronchogenic carcinoma. *Am J Respir Crit Care Med* 2000;161:601–607.

59. Selcuk ZT, Firat P. The diagnostic yield of transbronchial needle aspiration in superior vena cava syndrome. *Lung Cancer* 2003;42:183–188.

60. Hsu LH, Liu CC, Ko JS. Education and experience improve the performance of transbronchial needle aspiration: a learning curve at a cancer center. *Chest* 2004;25:532–540.

61. Chin R, McCain TW, Lucia MA, et al. Transbronchial needle aspiration in diagnosing and staging lung cancer: how many aspirates are needed? *Am J Respir Crit Care Med* 2002;166:377–381.

62. Haponik EF, Cappellari JO, Chin R, et al. Education and experience improve transbronchial needle aspiration performance. *Am J Respir Crit Care Med* 1995;151:1998–2002.

63. Grapestad E, Goldberg SN, Herth F, et al. CT fluoroscopy guidance for transbronchial needle aspiration. *Chest* 2001;119:329–332.

64. Khoo KL, Chua GS, Mukhopadhyay A, et al. Transbronchial needle aspiration: initial experience in routine diagnostic bronchoscopy. *Respir Med* 2003;97:1200–1204.

65. Steiner RM, Liu JB, Goldberg BB, et al. The value of ultrasound-guided fiberoptic bronchoscopy. *Clin Chest Med* 1995;16:519–534.

66. Herth F, Becker HD. Endobronchial ultrasound of the airways and the mediastinum. *Monaldi Arch Chest Dis* 2000;551:36–44.

67. Falcone F, Fois F, Grosso D. Endobronchial ultrasound. *Respiration* 2003;70:179–194.

68. Kurimoto N, Murayama M, Yoshioka S, et al. Assessment of usefulness of endobronchial ultrasonography in determination of depth of tracheobronchial tumor invasion. *Chest* 1999;115:1500–1506.

69. Shannon JJ, Bude RO, Orens JB, et al. Endobronchial ultrasound-guided needle aspiration of mediastinal adenopathy. *Am J Respir Crit Care Med* 1996;153:1424–1430.

70. Ghows MB, Rosen MJ, Chuang MT, et al. Transcutaneous oxygen monitoring during fiberoptic bronchoscopy. *Chest* 1986;89:543–544.

71. Cordasco EM Jr, Mehta AC, Ahmed M. Bronchoscopically induced bleeding. *Chest* 1991;100:1141–1147.

72. Pereira W, Kovnat DM, Kahn MA, et al. Fever and pneumonia after flexible fiberoptic bronchoscopy. *Am Rev Respir Dis* 1975;112:59–64.

73. Kirschke DL, Jones TF, Craig AS, et al. Pseudomonas aeruginosa and Serratia marcescens contamination associated with a manufacturing defect in bronchoscopes. *N Engl J Med* 2003;348:214–220.

74. Cetre JC, Salord H, Vanhems P. Outbreaks of infection associated with bronchoscopes. *N Engl J Med* 2003;348:2039–2040.

75. Prakash UBS. Does the bronchoscope propagate infection? *Chest* 1993;104:552–559.

76. Davies L, Mister R, Spence DPS, et al. Cardiovascular consequences of fiberoptic bronchoscopy. *Eur Respir J* 1997;10:695–698.

77. Dweik RA, Mehta AC, Meeker DP et al. Analysis of the safety of bronchoscopy after recent acute myocardial infarction. *Chest* 1996;110:825–828.

78. British Thoracic Society guidelines on diagnostic flexible bronchoscopy. *Thorax* 2001;56(Suppl. 1):i1–i21.

79. Dasgupta A, Jain P, Minai OA, et al. Utility of transbronchial needle aspiration in the diagnosis of endobronchial lesions. *Chest* 1999;115:1237–1241.

80. Mazzone P, Jain P, Arroliga A, et al. Bronchoscopy and needle biopsy techniques for diagnosis and staging of lung cancer. *Clin Chest Med* 2002;23:137–151.

81. Kvale PA, Bode FR, Kini S. Diagnostic accuracy in lung cancer: comparison of techniques used in association with flexible bronchoscopy. *Chest* 1976;69:752–757.

82. Max VHF, Johnston IDA, Hetzel MR, et al. Value of washing and brushing with fiberoptic bronchoscopy in the diagnosis of lung cancer. *Thorax* 1990;45:373–376.

83. Lundgren R, Bergman F, Angstrom T. Comparison of transbronchial needle aspiration biopsy, aspiration of bronchial secretion, bronchial washing, brush biopsy and forceps biopsy in the diagnosis of lung cancer. *Eur J Respir Dis* 1983;64:378–385.

84. Popovich J Jr, Kvale PA, Eichenhorn MS, et al. Diagnostic accuracy of multiple biopsies from flexible fiberoptic bronchoscopy: a comparison of central versus peripheral carcinoma. *Am Rev Respir Dis* 1982;125:521–523.

85. Dreisin RB, Albert RK, Talley PA, et al. Flexible fiberoptic bronchoscopy in the teaching hospital: yield and complications. *Chest* 1978;74:144–149.

86. Gellert AR, Rudd RM, Sinha G, et al. Fiberoptic bronchoscopy: effect of multiple bronchial biopsies on diagnostic yield in bronchial carcinoma. *Thorax* 1982;37:684–687.

87. Kavale PA. Bronchoscopic biopsies and bronchoalveolar lavage. *Chest Surg Clin N Am* 1996;6:205–222.

88. Man V, Johnston ID, Hassle MR, et al. Value of washings and brushings at fiberoptic bronchoscopy in the diagnosis of lung cancer. *Thorax* 1990;45:373–376.

89. Butcher G, Barbaric P, Delphian MS. Diagnostic, morphologic, and histopathologic correlates in bronchogenic carcinoma. A review of 1,045 bronchoscopic examinations. *Chest* 1991;99:809–814.

90. Govert JA, Dodd LG, Kussin PS, et al. A prospective comparison of fiberoptic transbronchial needle aspiration and bronchial biopsy for bronchoscopically visible lung carcinoma. *Cancer Cytopathol* 1999;87:129–134.

91. Witte MC, Opal SM, Gilbert JG, et al. Incidence of fever and bacteremia following transbronchial needle aspiration. *Chest* 1986;89:85–87.

92. Clark RA, Grech P, Robinson A, et al. Limitation of fiberoptic bronchoscopy under fluoroscopy in the investigation of peripheral lung lesions. *Br J Radiol* 1978;432–436.

93. Chechani V. Bronchoscopic diagnosis of solitary pulmonary nodules and lung masses in the absence of endobronchial abnormality. *Chest* 1996;109:620–625.

94. Mori K, Yanase N, Kaneko M, et al. Diagnosis of peripheral lung cancer in cases of tumor 2 cm or less in size. *Chest* 1989;95:304–308.

95. Garaparini S, Ferrelti M, Bichi S, et al. Integration of transbronchial and percutaneous approach in the diagnosis of peripheral pulmonary nodules or masses: experience with 1,027 consecutive cases. *Chest* 1995;108:131–137.

96. Cortese DA, McDougal JC. Biopsy and brushing of peripheral lung cancer with fluorescence guidance. *Chest* 1979;75:141–145.

97. Gracia JD, Bravo C, Miravitilles M, et al. Diagnostic value of bronchoalveolar lavage in peripheral lung cancer. *Am Rev Resp Dis* 1993;147:649–652.

98. Wang KP, Britt EJ. Needle brush in the diagnosis of lung masses or nodules through flexible bronchoscopy. *Chest* 1991;100:1148–1150.

99. Wagner U, Walthers EM, Wolfgang G, et al. Computer-tomographically guided fiberbronchoscopic transbronchial biopsy of small pulmonary lesions: a feasibility study. *Respiration* 1996;63:181–186.

100. Shinagawa N, Yamazaki K, Onodera Y, et al. CT-guided transbronchial biopsy using an ultra thin bronchoscope with virtual bronchoscopic navigation. *Chest* 2004;125:1138–1143.

101. Ost D, Fein AM, Feinsilver SH. The solitary pulmonary nodule. *N Engl J Med* 2003;348:2535–2542.

102. Lillington GA, Caskey CI. Evaluation and management of solitary and multiple pulmonary nodules. *Clin Chest Med* 1993;14:111–119.

103. Swensen SJ, Jett JR, Sloan JA, et al. Screening for lung cancer with low-dose spiral computed tomography. *Am J Respir Crit Care Med* 2002;165:508–503.

104. Gould MK, Maclean CC, Kuschner NG, et al. Accuracy of positron emission tomography for diagnosis of pulmonary nodules and mass lesions: a meta-analysis. *JAMA* 2001;285:914–924.

105. Baaklini WA, Reinoso MA, Gorin AB, et al. Diagnostic yield of fiberoptic bronchoscopy in evaluating solitary pulmonary nodules. *Chest* 2000;117:1049–1054.

106. Bilaceroglu S, Kumcuoglu Z, Alper H, et al. CT bronchus sign-guided bronchoscopic multiple diagnostic procedures in carcinomatous solitary pulmonary nodules and masses. *Respiration* 1998;65:49–55.

107. Gress FG, Savides TJ, Sandler A, et al. Endoscopic ultrasonography, fine-needle aspiration biopsy guided by endoscopic ultrasonography, and computed tomography in the preoperative staging of non-small-cell lung cancer: comparison study. *Ann Intern Med* 1997;127:604–612.

108. Dasgupta A, Mehta AT. Transbronchial needle aspiration: an underused diagnostic technique. *Clin Chest Med* 1999;20:39–51.

109. Rong F, Cui B. CT scan directed transbronchial needle aspiration biopsy for mediastinal nodes. *Chest* 1998;114:36–39.

110. Schenk DA, Bryan CL, Bower JH et al. Transbronchial needle aspiration in the diagnosis of bronchogenic carcinoma. *Chest* 1987;92:83–85.

111. Herth F, Becker HD, Ernst A. Conventional vs endobronchial ultrasound-guided transbronchial needle aspiration: a randomized trial. *Chest* 2004;125:322–325.

112. Knott-Craig CJ, Oostuizen JG, Rossouw G, et al. Management and prognosis of massive hemoptysis. Recent experience with 120 patients. *J Thorac Cardiovasc Surg* 1993;105:394–397.

113. Bhattacharyya P, Dutta A, Samanta AN, et al. New procedure: bronchoscopic endobronchial sealing—a new mode of managing hemoptysis. *Chest* 2002;121:2066–2069.

114. Dweik RA, Stoller JK. Role of bronchoscopy in massive hemoptysis. *Clin Chest Med* 1999;20:89–105.

115. Hirshberg B, Biran I, Glazer M, et al. Hemoptysis: etiology, evaluation, and outcome in a tertiary referral hospital. *Chest* 1997;112:440–444.

116. Haponik EF, Chin R. Hemoptysis: clinicians' perspectives. *Chest* 1990;97:469–475.

117. Adelman M, Haponik EF, Bleecker ER, et al. Cryptogenic hemoptysis. *Ann Intern Med* 1985;102:829–834.

118. Narayanswami G, Salzman SH. Bronchoscopy in the human immunodeficiency virus-infected patient. *Semin Respir Infect* 2003;18:80–86.

119. Huang L, Hecht FM, Stansell JD, et al. Suspected pneumocystis carinii pneumonia with a negative induced sputum examination. *Am J Respir Crit Care Med* 1995;151:1866–1871.

120. Marrie TJ. Community-acquired pneumonia: epidemiology, etiology, treatment. *Infect Dis Clin North Am* 1998;12:723–740.

121. Souweine B, Veber B, Bedos JP, et al. Diagnostic accuracy of protected specimen brush and bronchoalveolar lavage in nosocomial pneumonia: impact of previous antimicrobial treatments. *Crit Care Med* 1998;26:236–244.

122. Fagon JY, Chastre J, Wolf M, et al. Invasive and noninvasive strategies for management of suspected ventilator-associated pneumonia. *Ann Intern Med* 2000;132:621–630.

123. Torres A, Fabregas N, Ewig S, et al. Sampling methods for ventilator-associated pneumonia: Validation using different histologic and microbiologic references. *Crit Care Med* 2000;28:2799–2804.

124. Grebski E, Hess T, Hold G, et al. Diagnostic value of hemosiderin-containing macrophages in bronchoalveolar lavage. *Chest* 1992;102:1794–1799.

125. Irwin RS, Boudet LP, Cloutier MM, et al. Managing cough as a defense mechanism and as a symptom. A consensus panel report of the American College of Chest Physicians. *Chest* 1998;114(Suppl. 2):133S–181S.

126. Chang SC, Perng RP. The role of fiberoptic bronchoscopy in evaluating the causes of pleural effusions. *Arch Intern Med* 1989;149:855–857.

127. Feinsilver SH, Barrows AA, Braman SS. Fiberoptic bronchoscopy and pleural effusion of unknown origin. *Chest* 1986;90:514–515.

128. Raoof S, Sandeep M, Prakash UB. Role of bronchoscopy in modern medical intensive care unit. *Clin Chest Med* 2001;2:241–261.

129. Ovassapian A, Randel GI. The role of the fiberscope in the critically ill patient. *Crit Care Clin* 1995;11:29–51.

130. Dunagan DP, Baker AM, Hurd DD, et al. Bronchoscopic evaluation of pulmonary infiltrates following bone marrow transplantation. *Chest* 1997;111:135–141.

131. Haponik EF, Aquino SL, Vinning DJ. Virtual bronchoscopy. *Clin Chest Med* 1999;20:201–207.

132. Bosielle PM, Ernst A. Recent advances in central airway imaging. *Chest* 2002;121:1651–1660.

133. Ferretti GR, Thony F, Bosson JL, et al. Benign abnormalities and carcinoid tumors of the central airways: diagnostic impact of CT bronchography. *Am J Roentgenol* 2000;174:1307–1313.

134. Grenier PA, Beigleman-Aubry C, Fetita C, et al. New frontiers in CT imaging of airway disease. *Eur Radiol* 2002;12:1022–1044.

135. Larscheid RC, Thorpe PE, Scott WJ. A percutaneous transthoracic needle aspiration biopsy. A comprehensive review of its current role in the diagnosis and treatment of lung tumors. *Chest* 1998;114:704–709.

136. Sokolowski JW, Burgher LW, Jones FL Jr, et al. American Thoracic Society guidelines for percutaneous transthoracic needle biopsy. *Am Rev Respir Dis* 1989;140:255–256.

137. Loddenkemper R. Thoracoscopy—state of the art. *Eur Respir J* 1998;11:213–221.

138. Zwischenberger JB, Savage C, Alpard SK, et al. Mediastinal transthoracic needle and core lymph node biopsy. Should it replace mediastinoscopy? *Chest* 2002;121:1165–1170.

139. Landreneau RJ, Mack MJ, Hazelrigg SR, et al. The role of thoracoscopy in the management of intrathoracic neoplastic processes. *Semin Thorac Cardiovasc Surg* 1993;5:219–228.

140. DeCamp MM Jr, Jaklitsch MT, Mentzer SJ, et al. The safety and versatility of video-thoracoscopy: a prospective analysis of 895 consecutive cases. *J Am Coll Surg* 1995;181:113–120.

141. Loddenkemper R. Medical thoracoscopy. In: Light RW, Lee YC, eds. *Textbook of pleural diseases.* London: Arnold Publishers, 2003:498–512.

142. Kendall SW, Bryan AJ, Large SR, et al. Pleural effusions: is thoracoscopy a reliable investigation? A retrospective review. *Respir Med* 1992;86:437–440.

143. Ferrer J, Roldan J, Teixidor J, et al. Predictors of pleural malignancy in patients with pleural effusion undergoing thoracoscopy. *Chest* 2004 (*in press*).

144. Diacon AH, Van de Wal BW, Wyser C, et al. Diagnostic tools in tuberculous pleurisy: a direct comparative study. *Eur Respir J* 2003;22:589–591.

145. Zegdi R, Azorin J, Tremblay B, et al. Videothoracoscopic lung biopsy in diffuse infiltrative lung diseases: A 5-year surgical experience. *Ann Thorac Surg* 1998;66:1170–1173.

146. Chang AC, Yee J, Orringer MB, et al. Diagnostic thoracoscopic lung biopsy: an outpatient experience. *Ann Thorac Surg* 2002;74:1942–1947.

147. Miller JD, Urschel JD, Cox G, et al. A randomized, controlled trial comparing thoracoscopy and limited thoracotomy for lung biopsy in interstitial lung disease. *Ann Thorac Surg* 2000;70:1647–1650.

148. Cardillo G, Regal M, Sera F, et al. Video thoracoscopic management of the solitary pulmonary nodule: a single-institution study on 429 cases. *Ann Thorac Surg* 2003;75:1607–1611.

149. Suzuki K, Nagai K, Yoshida J, et al. Video-assisted thoracoscopic surgery for small indeterminate pulmonary nodules. *Chest* 1999;115:563–568.

150. Ciriaco P, Negri G, Puglisi A, et al. Video-assisted thoracoscopic surgery for pulmonary nodules: rationale for preoperative computed tomography-guided hookwire localization. *Eur J Cardiothorac Surg* 2004;3:429–433.

151. Gossot D, Toledo L, Fritsch S, et al. Mediastinoscopy vs thoracoscopy for mediastinal biopsy. *Chest* 1996;110:1328–1331.

152. Massone PPB, Lequaglie C, Magnani B, et al. The real impact and usefulness of video-assisted thoracoscopic surgery in the diagnosis and therapy of clinical lymphadenopathies of the mediastinum. *Ann Thorac Surg* 2003;10:1197–1202.

153. Kaiser OR, Bavaria JE. Complications of thoracoscopy. *Ann Thorac Surg* 1993;56:796–798.

154. Pearson FG. Staging the mediastinum: role of mediastinoscopy and computed tomography. *Chest* 1993;103:346S–348S.

155. Ginsberg RJ, Rice TO, Goldbert M, et al. Extended cervical mediastinoscopy. *J Thorac Cardiovasc Surg* 1987;94:673–678.

156. Luke WP, Todd TRJ, Cooper SD. Prospective evaluation of mediastinoscopy for assessment of carcinoma of the lung. *J Thorac Cardiovasc Surg* 1986;91:53–56.

157. Vallieres E, Page A, Verdent A. Ambulatory mediastinoscopy and anterior mediastinotomy. *Ann Thorac Surg* 1991;52:1122–1126.

158. Widstrom A, Schnurer L. The value of mediastinoscopy—experience of 374 cases. *J Otolaryngol* 1978;7:103–109.

159. Carlens E. Mediastinoscopy. *Ann Otol Rhinol Laryngol* 1965;74:1102–1112.

160. Lardonis D, Weder W, Hany TF, et al. Staging of non-small-cell lung cancer with integrated positron-emission tomography and computed tomography. *N Engl J Med* 2003;348:2500–2507.

161. Serna DL, Aryan HE, Chang KJ, et al. An early comparison between endoscopic ultrasound-guided fine-needle aspiration and mediastinoscopy for diagnosis of mediastinal malignancy. *Am Surg* 1998;64:1014–1018.

162. Vilmann P. Endoscopic ultrasonography-guided-fine-needle aspiration biopsy of lymph nodes. *Gastrointest Endosc* 1996;43:24–29.

163. Fritscher-Ravens A, Bohuslavizki MD, Brandt L. Mediastinal lymph node involvement in potentially resectable lung cancer. *Chest* 2003;123:442–451.
164. Warner DO, Warner MA, Divertie MB. Open lung biopsy in patients with diffuse pulmonary infiltrates and acute respiratory failure. *Am Rev Respir Dis* 1988;137:90–94.
165. Gaensler EA, Carrington CB. Open lung biopsy for chronic diffuse infiltrative lung disease: clinical, roentgenographic, and physiological correlations in 502 patients. *Ann Thorac Surg* 1980; 30:411–426.
166. Patel SR, Karmpaliotis D, Ayas NT, et al. The role of open-lung biopsy in ARDS. *Chest* 2004;125:197–202.
167. Cheson BD, Samlowski WE, Tang TT, et al. Value of open-lung biopsy in 87 immunocompromised patients with pulmonary infiltrates. *Cancer* 1985;55:453–459.
168. Fitzgerald W, Bevelagua FA, Garay SM, et al. The role of open lung biopsy in patients with acquired immunodeficiency syndrome. *Chest* 1987;91:659–661.
169. Vander Els NJ, Stover DE. Approach to the patient with pulmonary disease. *Clin Chest Med* 1996;17:767–785.

SECTION 3

MANAGEMENT OF RESPIRATORY DISEASES

Asthma

Mani S. Kavuru

Herbert P. Wiedemann

Bronchial asthma affects 3% to 5% of the population of the United States (approximately 14 to 15 million people), making it a frequently encountered clinical problem in both the pediatric and adult population. It is a major cause of morbidity in the United States and around the world. Asthma is a heterogeneous disease, and multiple mechanisms are likely involved in the pathogenesis, rather than a single unifying mechanism. The development of specific antagonists to the various mediators is accelerating our understanding of this disease. In addition, there is a burgeoning field of pharmacogenetics to help establish that genetic variation plays a role in the clinical response to various therapies. As a product of this understanding, it is to be hoped that additional therapeutic agents will emerge for subgroups of asthmatics. This chapter reviews recent trends in epidemiology, pathogenesis, and management principles of bronchial asthma.

DEFINITION AND CLASSIFICATION

Despite a number of formal attempts, a universally accepted definition of asthma is unavailable (1,2). It is likely that asthma is not a specific disease but a syndrome that derives from multiple precipitating mechanisms and results in a common clinical complex involving reversible airflow obstruction. Important features of this syndrome include episodic occurrence of dyspnea and wheezing, airflow obstruction with a bronchodilator-reversible component, bronchial hyperresponsiveness to a variety of nonspecific and specific stimuli, and airway inflammation. All of these features need not be present. During the past 15 years, as a result of investigative bronchoscopic studies involving mild asthmatics, airway inflammation has become integral to the definition of asthma. Although there is some overlap in features between asthma and other chronic obstructive airflow disorders such as chronic bronchitis, emphysema, and cystic fibrosis, it is essential to make this distinction. Asthma typically occurs in younger individuals who are nonsmokers. In general, the baseline level of functioning, exercise tolerance, and spirometric parameters in asthmatics are much better preserved between acute exacerbations than in individuals with emphysema or chronic bronchitis. Patients with asthma exhibit a tremendous heterogeneity in the clinical features and in the severity of disease. Asthma can range from being very mild, occurring perhaps only in relation to specific triggers such as pollen or exercise, to being a severe, unrelenting, and occasionally fatal disease without a definable external cause.

Asthma has traditionally been classified as either extrinsic or intrinsic. Patients with extrinsic asthma tend to have childhood onset, positive skin-test reactions to many allergens (atopy), a strong family history of atopy and asthma, and often a predictable seasonal variation of their asthma. Intrinsic asthma is not associated with any known immunologic reactions to external allergens, usually begins in adulthood, and exhibits little seasonal variation. However, this classification system is not particularly useful to the clinical management of most asthmatic patients, especially adults. Rather, current research to help further classify and characterize the asthma syndrome is focused on a variety of biologic markers of inflammation, including oxidation products, exhaled nitric oxide, bronchoalveolar lavage cellular and cytokine profiles, urinary leukotriene products, and various genetic markers. However, current knowledge does not permit these parameters to be used in the diagnosis, assessment of disease severity, prognosis, or likelihood of responding to specific therapies.

EPIDEMIOLOGY

INCIDENCE, PREVALENCE, AND MORTALITY

The true prevalence of asthma is difficult to ascertain because of the lack of a standard definition and the variations in epidemiologic methodology that have been used. In most surveys, asthma is found to be more common in children than in adults and slightly more frequent in men than in women. In the United States, a national survey by the Public Health Service in 1970 estimated that 3% of the population had asthma (3,4). In a smaller study using better clinical documentation, performed in the Michigan town of Tecumseh, the 12-month prevalence of asthma was 4.0% in men and 3.4% in women (4,5). National Health and Nutritional Examination Surveys conducted five years apart, in 1975 and 1980, reported a significant increase in the prevalence of asthma from 4.8% to 7.6% among 6- to 11-year-old children (6). The overall annual age-adjusted hospital-discharge rate for asthma as the primary diagnosis decreased slightly from 18.4 per 10,000 population in 1982 to 17.9 per 10,000 in 1992 (7,8). From 1982 through 1992, the overall annual age-adjusted prevalence rate of self-reported asthma increased by 42%, from 34.7 per thousand to 49.4 per thousand. For persons aged 5 to 34 years, the rate increased by 52%, from 34.6 to 52.6 per thousand. The rate for women increased by 82%, from 29.4 to 53.6 per thousand.

Skobeloff et al. conducted a retrospective review of all asthma admissions from southeastern Pennsylvania to define the role of age and sex as risk factors for asthma hospital admission (9). There were 33,269 patients admitted for asthma treatment over a 4-year period that included 67 hospitals in five counties. In the 0- to 10-year-old age group, boys were admitted nearly twice as often as age-identical girls. In the 11- to 20-year-old age group, admissions for male and female patients were nearly identical. Between 20 and 50 years of age, the female-to-male ratio was nearly 3:1. Length of stay increased proportionally as the patient's age increased, and the length of stay was greater for women than for men. Overall, the authors concluded that women are more severely affected by asthma than men.

Data from the National Center for Health Statistics disclosed gradual decreases in the number of deaths from asthma each year in the United States to a low of 1674 in 1977 (7). From 1982 through 1991, however, the annual age-adjusted death rate for asthma as the underlying cause of death increased by 40% from 13.4 per million population (3154 deaths) to 18.8 per million (5106 deaths). During this period, the death rate increased by 59% for women (from 1.3 to 2.0 per 100,000) and by 34% for men (from 1.3 to 1.6 per 100,000) (7). The annual asthma death rate was consistently higher for African Americans than for whites during this period. For African Americans, the rate increased by 52% (from 2.5 to 3.8 per 100,000) compared with a 45% increase (from 1.1 to 1.6 per 100,000) for whites. The increase in the death rate for black and white women was similar; however, the increase in the death rate for black men was more than twice that for white men, and the mortality rate was three times the rate for whites. The increase in mortality rates has been even more dramatic in other countries, including Australia, England and Wales, West Germany, Japan, and Canada (10,11). The increase in asthma mortality appeared to be due to false-positive reporting in a revision in the International Classification of Disease (ICD-9) coding (12–14). However, the trend for increasing asthma-associated morbidity and mortality reported between 1980 and 1995 did not continue between 1995 and 1999 (15). The annual rates of patients reporting asthma attacks during 1997 to 1999 were lower than previously reported rates. Since 1995, the rate of outpatient visits for asthma has increased, whereas the rates of hospital admissions have decreased (from 19.5 per 10,000 population in 1995 to 15.7 in 1998). Importantly, annual rates of asthma mortality, which increased during the 1980s, plateaued and decreased slightly in the 1990s. Although it is too early to be certain, these trends are reassuring and indicate that, perhaps, the aggressive strategies of asthma management finally seem to be reaching fruition. However, African Americans continue to have higher rates of asthma, emergency department visits, hospitalizations, and deaths than whites do.

Asthma deaths are of two types: type 1, slow onset—late arrival; and type 2, sudden onset (16–19). Risk factors for type 1 fatal asthma include serious asthma requiring prior emergency-room visits or mechanical ventilation. Other factors include inadequate use of pulmonary function to objectively assess the severity of asthma. Inadequate treatment with either inhaled or systemic corticosteroids is also a frequently described finding. Factors that may interfere with compliance and access to medical care include socioeconomic factors, certain psychological features, and racial/cultural factors. Therefore, underestimation of asthma severity and undertreatment are important contributing factors in type 1 asthma-related fatalities (20). A relatively small subset of patients with status asthmaticus have a predominantly hyperacute, bronchospastic component (21). Whether the fundamental mechanism in this type 2 subset is based on bronchospasm, smooth-muscle contraction, neural mechanisms, or yet-unknown inflammatory mechanisms remains to be established (22).

In 1990, the cost of illness related to asthma was estimated to be $6.2 billion, or nearly 1% of all US health care cost (23). Inpatient hospital services represented the largest single direct medical expenditure for asthma, approaching $1.6 billion. Forty-three percent of the economic impact of asthma was associated with emergency-room use and hospitalization. Nearly two-thirds of the visits for ambulatory care were to physicians in primary care specialties, including pediatrics, family medicine, general practice, and internal medicine.

THE β-AGONIST CONTROVERSY

There has been much controversy surrounding the potential role of β-agonist preparations in asthma mortality (24). The hypothesis is that excessive or regular use of β-adrenergic bronchodilators can actually worsen asthma, perhaps contributing to morbidity and mortality. A variety of epidemiologic studies have found conflicting findings. Several studies from New Zealand suggested that the use of inhaled β-agonists increases the risk of death in severe asthma (11,25,26). Spitzer et al. conducted a matched, case-controlled study using a health insurance database from Saskatchewan, Canada, of a cohort of 12,301 patients for whom asthma medications had been prescribed (27). Data were based on matching 129 case patients who had fatal or nearly fatal asthma with 655 controls. The use of β-agonist administered by a metered-dose inhaler (MDI) was associated with an increased risk of death from asthma, with an odds ratio of 5.4 per canister of fenoterol, 2.4 per canister of albuterol, and 1.0 for background risk (i.e., no fenoterol or albuterol). The primary limitation of this study, and indeed case-controlled studies in general, is the concern regarding the comparability of the two groups in terms of the severity of the underlying disease (28).

A large, placebo-controlled trial of salmeterol, a long-acting β2-receptor agonist, was recently stopped prematurely because of concerns with interim analysis that suggested that salmeterol may be associated with excess mortality due to life-threatening asthma (29). This Salmeterol Multiple-Center Asthma Research Trial (SMART) was a 28-week safety study comparing salmeterol 42 μg MDI twice a day with placebo, in addition to other asthma therapies. Of over 26,000 patients randomized, a higher number of asthma-related deaths or life-threatening experiences (36 vs 23) and a higher number of asthma-related deaths (13 vs 4) occurred in the patients treated with salmeterol. Although there was no statistically significant difference for this primary end point for the total population, a subset analysis indicated that asthma-related deaths or life-threatening episodes were higher in African Americans using salmeterol. Interestingly, 50% of white and 38% African American patients were using concurrent inhaled corticosteroid at baseline. Among the patients using inhaled corticosteroids, there was no significant difference between the two groups.

Sears et al. conducted a placebo-controlled, crossover study in patients with mild stable asthma to evaluate the effects of regular versus on-demand inhaled fenoterol therapy for 24 weeks (26). In the 57 patients who did better with one of the two regimens, only 30% had better asthma control when receiving regularly administered bronchodilators, whereas 70% had better asthma control when they employed the bronchodilators only as needed. More recently, a study by Drazen et al. randomly assigned 255 patients with mild asthma to inhaled albuterol either on a regular basis (two puffs four times per day) or only on an as-needed basis for 16 weeks (30). There were no significant differences between the two groups in a variety of outcomes, including morning peak expiratory flow, diurnal peak flow variability, forced expiratory volume in one second, number of puffs of supplemental as-needed albuterol, asthma symptoms, or airway reactivity to methacholine. As neither benefit nor harm was seen, it was concluded that inhaled albuterol should be prescribed for patients with mild asthma on an as-needed basis. A recent meta-analysis of pooled results from 22 randomized, placebo-controlled trials that studied at least 1 week of regularly administered β2-agonist in patients with asthma compared to a placebo group (that did not permit "as-needed" β2-agonist use) concluded that regular use results in tolerance to the drug's bronchodilator and nonbronchodilator effects and may be associated with poorer disease control compared to placebo (31). However, there was no decline in the mean FEV$_1$ after regular treatment with β2-agonists.

PHARMACOGENETICS

Polymorphisms of the gene for the β2-adrenergic receptor (AR) may be important in determining the clinical response to β-agonists (30,32–35). For the β2-AR gene, single nucleotide polymorphisms (SNPs) have been defined at codons 16 and 27. The normal or "wild-type" pattern is Arg-16-Gly and Gln-27-Glu, but SNPs have been described with homozygous pairing (i.e., Gly-16-Gly, Arg-16-Arg, Glu-27-Glu, and Gln-27-Gln). Importantly, the frequency of these polymorphisms is the same in the normal population as in a population of asthmatics. Also, the presence of a gene variant itself does not appear to influence baseline lung function. However, in the presence of a polymorphism, the acute bronchodilator response to a β-agonist, or protection from a bronchoconstrictor, is affected. Studies indicate that in patients with Arg-16-Arg variant, the resulting β2-AR is resistant to endogenous circulating catecholamines (i.e., receptor density and integrity are preserved), with a subsequent ability to produce an acute bronchodilator response to an agonist. In patients with Gly-16-Gly, the β2-AR is down-regulated by endogenous catecholamines; therefore, the acute bronchodilator response is reduced or blunted. In relation to prolonged β-agonist therapy (i.e., >2 weeks), it appears that only patients who are homozygous for Arg16 and who were receiving regularly scheduled β-agonist aerosol had a persistent decrease in lung function over time (i.e., tachyphylaxis) (30). These same individuals, when switched to as-needed albuterol, had no decrease in lung function, as is the case for homozygous Gly16. Polymorphisms at the 27 loci are of unclear significance. Also, the impact of haplotypes (i.e., variant genes linked at ≥2 loci) is presently unclear.

A recent study with transgenic mouse models using β2-AR knockout as well as overexpression of β2-AR has suggested an alternative molecular mechanism for the effects of chronic exposure to β-agonists and for the effects on airway bronchodilator response (34). Interestingly and unexpectedly, the mice with absent β_2-AR had markedly reduced bronchoconstrictive response to methacholine. The overexpressors of β_2-AR who had continuous β_2-AR signaling activity demonstrated an enhanced constrictive response. In addition, the overexpressors showed increased expression of a phospholipase C β_1 enzyme, which is thought to mediate the contractile response to methacholine. Overall, this study provides a new molecular mechanism to understand the effects of chronic β-agonist therapy on attenuated bronchodilator response (i.e., tachyphylaxis).

To date, there is limited data on mutations involving the leukotriene cascade or corticosteroid metabolism (35). Polymorphisms of the 5-lipoxygenase (5-LO) promoter gene and the leukotriene C_4 (LTC$_4$) synthase gene have been described. Asthmatics with the "wild-type" genotype at 5-LO have a greater response with 5-LO inhibitor therapy compared to asthmatics with a mutant gene. However, mutations of the 5-LO promoter occur only in about 5 % of the asthmatic patients, so it is unlikely to play an important role in most patients. An SNP in the LTC$_4$ synthase promoter gene (A-444C) is associated with increased leukotriene production and has a lower response to leukotriene modifying agents. Far less is known about genetic variability in the corticosteroid pathway. Polymorphisms in the glucocorticoid receptor (GR) gene have been identified, which appear to affect steroid binding and downstream pathways in various *in vitro* studies. However, polymorphisms in the glucocorticoid pathways have not been associated with the asthma phenotype or clinical steroid resistance.

NATURAL HISTORY

The natural history of asthma is complex. In general, childhood asthma is frequently self-limited and carries a better prognosis than adult-onset asthma (4). In one large study, one half of 449 children with onset of asthma before the age of 13 became symptom-free during 20-year follow-up (5,36). Another one-fourth had only minimal symptoms, which could be prevented by avoiding specific exacerbating factors such as dust or animals. The severity of asthma in childhood correlates with the persistence of asthma into adulthood and with the severity of adult asthma in the childhood-onset group (37,38). There is increasing evidence to suggest that asthma alone can cause irreversible airflow obstruction (39,40). Recent studies indicate that the bulk of the "irreversible" loss of lung function may occur in the interval prior to the start of antiinflammatory therapy (41,42). Data from Bronnimann and Burrows suggest that after the second decade, asthmatic subjects show a low rate of remission (43). Adults with a history of childhood asthma have a significant risk of future active asthma. In general, atopy is not useful in predicting remissions or relapses. Despite common belief, allergic rhinitis is not a harbinger of subsequent asthma. Although allergic rhinitis and asthma frequently coexist, if asthma does not occur within 1 year of the onset of allergic rhinitis, then there is only a 5% to 10% risk of asthma developing later (44). About 20% of asthmatics develop disease after the age of 65.

PATHOLOGY AND PATHOGENESIS

Early pathologic observations have been made in patients who have succumbed to a severe exacerbation of asthma (45,46), although some information is available from asthmatic patients who died of other causes (46) and from patients with symptom-free asthma (47). The pathologic findings in fatal asthma include (a) infiltration with eosinophils, (b) thickening of the basement membrane, (c) hypertrophy of the airway smooth muscle, (d) desquamation of the epithelium, (e) mucosal edema, and (f) mucous plugs containing shed epithelial cells and proteinaceous and cellular components of the inflammatory reaction.

Information from experimentally induced asthma as well as studies involving bronchoalveolar lavage (BAL) and endobronchial biopsy of milder, chronic, human asthma have contributed to the hypothesis that airway inflammation is a fundamental aspect of asthma (48–52). This concept underlies the growing clinical and investigational interest in the use of various antiinflammatory agents in the treatment of asthma. The relationship between airway inflammation and bronchial hyperreactivity remains unclear (53).

There are several well-described human models of experimentally induced asthma that form the basis of our current understanding of the pathogenesis of asthma (54). A well-known model involves an allergic asthmatic challenged with an inhaled allergen to which he or she is sensitive (55,56). This challenge results in a biphasic decline in respiratory function, an early asthmatic response (EAR) that occurs within minutes and resolves by 2 hours and a late asthmatic response (LAR) that usually occurs within 6 to 8 hours and may last 24 to 96 hours or longer (see Fig. 8-1). The LAR, which appears to occur in 50% of adult asthmatics (57), is associated with increased airway reactivity to nonspecific stimuli (such as methacholine or histamine) and a cellular influx into airway lavage fluid. Pretreatment with β-agonists blocks only the EAR, whereas corticosteroids block only the LAR, and cromolyn sodium and nedocromil block both phases. In human studies, exposure to ozone results in LAR and in influx of polymorphonuclear neutrophils in BAL (53). In the allergen and western

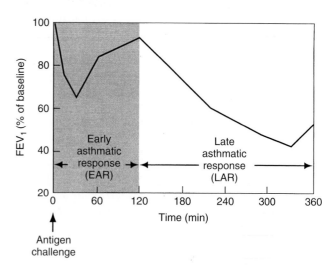

FIGURE 8-1. Biphasic decline in lung function as measured by forced expiratory volume in one second (FEV$_1$) in an allergic asthmatic after inhalation of an allergen (see text for details).

red cedar (plicatic acid) model of asthma, there again appears a LAR, but the lavage fluid has an influx of both polymorphonuclear cells and eosinophils. These and other studies suggest that the specificity of the stimulus affects the nature of the inflammatory process after exposure.

These observations in experimentally induced asthma have been extended to chronic stable asthma. Beasley et al. studied eight atopic stable asthmatics and four controls (52). Endobronchial biopsies of stable asthmatics showed extensive mucosal inflammation characterized by epithelial sloughing, eosinophil infiltration of the submucosa, and basement membrane thickening. Also, BAL studies in these stable asthmatics showed the presence of a fivefold increase in the shed epithelial cells and mast cells. These studies suggest that airway inflammation plays a significant role in both experimentally induced asthma and stable chronic human asthma. Numerous studies have suggested that the inflammation in asthma differs significantly from the inflammatory response seen in other airway or pulmonary parenchymal diseases by the distinct absence of bronchiolitis, fibrosis, and granulation tissue. The reasons for this remain unclear (49).

Numerous studies have recently advanced the notion that the T lymphocyte plays a pivotal role in the regulation and expression of local eosinophilia and in IgE production in both asthma and allergic disease (58,59). Lavage fluid from patients with atopic asthma reveals expression of CD4 positive T helper cells. It appears that T helper cells can be further categorized as T_{H1} or T_{H2} cells on the basis of the profile of cytokines these cells are capable of releasing (60). The T_{H1} cell produces interleukins 2 and 3 (IL-2, IL-3), granulocyte-macrophage colony-stimulating factor (GM-CSF), and interferon-γ (INF-γ), which leads to delayed hypersensitivity-type inflammatory response. On the other hand, T_{H2} lymphocytes mediate allergic inflammation in atopic asthmatics by a cytokine profile that involves interleukin-4 (which directs B lymphocytes to synthesize IgE), interleukin-5 (which is essential for the maturation of eosinophils), interleukin-3, and GM-CSF. Therefore, preliminary evidence suggests that atopic asthma is regulated by activation of a T_{H2}-like T-cell population (61). The so-called "hygiene hypothesis" of asthma postulates a polarization to a T_{H2}-like airway inflammation (which suppresses the T_{H1} pattern) by lack of childhood respiratory infections in the western world (62).

Lipid mediators are products of arachidonic acid metabolism. They have been implicated in the airway inflammation of asthma and, therefore, have been the target for pharmacologic antagonism by a specific class of agents: antileukotrienes (63–69). The prostaglandins are generated by the cyclooxygenation of arachidonic acid, whereas leukotrienes are generated by the lipoxygenation of arachidonic acid. The proinflammatory prostaglandins (PGD_2, PGF_2, TXB_2) cause bronchoconstriction, whereas other prostaglandins are considered protective and may elicit bronchodilation (PGE_2 and PGI_2 or prostacyclin). The cysteinyl leukotrienes (LTC_4, LTD_4, and LTE_4), formerly known as the *slow-reacting substance of anaphylaxis* (SRS-A), are formed by the lipoxygenation of arachidonic acid by the enzyme 5-lipoxygenase. These compounds, released by mast cells, eosinophils, and airway macrophages and epithelial cells, have a variety of potent effects, including bronchoconstriction, increased vascular permeability, and enhanced airway reactivity. Leukotrienes can be recovered from nasal secretions, bronchoalveolar lavage,

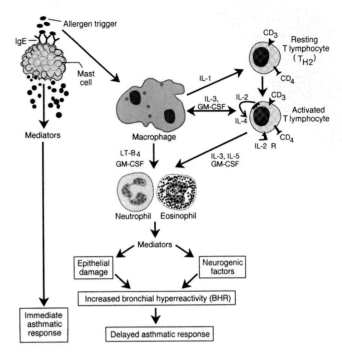

FIGURE 8-2. Asthma inflammatory cascade: summary of proposed mechanisms.

and urine of patients with asthma at much higher levels than normal individuals. Leukotriene antagonists inhibit the asthmatic responses to a variety of triggers, including allergen; exercise; cold, dry air; and aspirin (67,68).

The paradigm of the asthma inflammatory cascade involves a complex interaction of resident airway cells, recruited inflammatory cells, a variety of cytokines, and a variety of proinflammatory chemical and neurogenic mediators (see Fig. 8-2). The critical and rate-limiting steps in this process remain incompletely understood.

CLINICAL EVALUATION AND ASSESSMENT OF SEVERITY

The history and physical examination are important for several reasons: (a) to confirm a diagnosis of bronchial asthma and to exclude asthma "mimics" such as upper-airway obstruction (UAO), congestive heart failure, and so on; (b) to assess the severity of airflow obstruction and the need for hospitalization; (c) to identify factors that might place a patient at particular risk for poor outcome, including death; and (d) to identify comorbid diseases that may complicate the management of bronchial asthma, such as allergy to avoidable external triggers, sinusitis, or gastroesophageal reflux.

DIAGNOSIS

In most instances, the diagnosis of asthma is not difficult. The typical patient exhibits dyspnea, and wheezes can be heard throughout the lung fields. It is essential to inquire specifically about nocturnal symptoms because these are often missed (70). Some individuals with symptomatic airway hyperresponsiveness exhibit a bothersome nonproductive cough rather than wheezing (71–73). Identification of the "cough variant" asthma syndrome may require the use of a bronchoprovocation test to document the presence of airway hyperreactivity. Such patients may achieve symptomatic relief with the use of inhaled bronchodilator medication. However, 29% of Irwin's patients in whom reactive airway disease was diagnosed as a cause of cough required prednisone to resolve their cough (73). No trials have compared the effectiveness of inhaled β-agonists with theophylline or inhaled corticosteroids.

The most important asthma mimic is upper-airway obstruction (UAO). Such obstruction can be caused by tumors, laryngeal spasm, aspirated foreign bodies, and tracheal stenosis, to name just a few potential causes. Patients with UAO may present with dyspnea and "wheezing" (stridor) that might be very difficult to distinguish from asthma on clinical inspection alone (although careful auscultation should reveal that the "wheeze" is located over the superior aspect of the thorax or neck). Some patients with chronic UAO have been misdiagnosed and treated for months or even years as having "refractory" asthma. Failure to diagnose and treat acute life-threatening UAO can have obvious consequences as well. UAO can be detected through analysis of the flow–volume loops (expiratory and inspiratory) and can be confirmed by bronchoscopy.

The shape of the flow–volume loop may provide insight into the nature and location of airway obstruction. Figure 8-3 depicts several characteristic patterns of the loop that help localize the site of obstruction and help distinguish asthma from asthma mimics such as UAO. Both asthma and emphysema are examples of typical obstructive airway disorders characterized by a concavity of the expiratory limb of the flow–volume loop, with a fairly well-preserved inspiratory limb. With UAO,

the shape of the loop is related to the level of the obstruction (above or below the thoracic inlet) and to the net effect of pressures acting on the extrathoracic or intrathoracic airway, which include the atmospheric pressure, intraluminal pressure, and intrapleural pressure. The flow–volume loop shows flattening of the inspiratory limb with variable extrathoracic UAO, likely due to a lesion involving the glottic or subglottic area. On the other hand, flattening limited to the expiratory limb of the flow–volume loop occurs with variable intrathoracic UAO, usually on the basis of an obstructing lesion of the mid or distal trachea. "Boxlike" flattening of both the inspiratory and expiratory limbs of the flow–volume loop occurs with a fixed UAO due to any etiology.

Over the past decade, several reports have described patients with functional vocal cord disorders that mimic attacks of bronchial asthma ("factitious asthma") (74–76). The typical history involves episodes of wheezing and dyspnea that are refractory to standard therapy for asthma. These individuals may have wheezing that is often loudest over the neck, but the wheezing is often transmitted over both lung fields and may be misdiagnosed as bronchial asthma. During acute episodes, the flow–volume loop is consistent with variable extrathoracic UAO. The pathophysiology of factitious asthma, as noted by laryngoscopy, appears to be adduction of the true and false vocal cords throughout the respiratory cycle, including the inspiratory phase. During asymptomatic periods, both the flow–volume loop and the laryngoscopic examination are normal. Methacholine or histamine provocation testing is usually negative for airway hyperreactivity. Christopher et al. described a variety of personality styles and psychiatric diagnoses in these individuals and suggested that factitious asthma

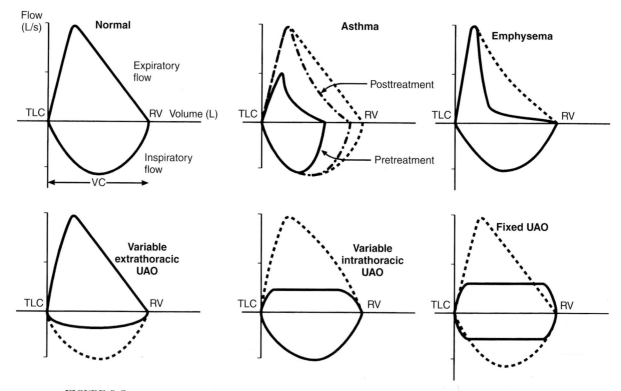

FIGURE 8-3. Representative flow–volume loops (see text for details). *RV*, residual volume; *TLC*, total lung capacity; *VC*, vital capacity; *UAO*, upper-airway obstruction.

is a form of conversion reaction (74). They reported a dramatic response to speech therapy and psychotherapy in these patients. In general, factitious asthma should be included in the differential diagnosis of difficult-to-control asthma.

More recently, McFadden et al. described vocal cord dysfunction in elite athletes that presents as "choking" during exercise (77). This entity may be distinguished from typical exercise-induced asthma by several features—symptoms are maximal during, rather than after, exercise; absence of nocturnal symptoms; UAO pattern on flow–volume loops.

ASSESSING ASTHMA SEVERITY

Assessing the severity of an asthmatic episode is important in determining the therapeutic approach. Although the magnitude of wheezing bears some relationship to the severity of airflow obstruction, use of auscultation alone is unreliable (78). In particular, wheezing may become weak or inaudible as airflow becomes significantly reduced. An early study by McFadden et al. evaluated the relationship between clinical and physiologic manifestations of acute bronchial asthma serially during initial therapy in the emergency room (79). Regardless of the initial presentation of the patients, when they became asymptomatic, the overall mechanical function of the lungs was only about 40% to 50% of predicted normal values. When they were without signs of asthma on examination, lung function was only 60% to 70% of predicted values. This study reinforces the need for objective measurement of airflow obstruction during acute asthma.

Patients may have a poor ability to perceive the presence and severity of airflow obstruction until it becomes quite severe (79–83). Some patients have remained asymptomatic even with an FEV_1 of 50% of predicted (84). Despite this, patients often have a better appreciation of the severity of airflow limitation than their physician, who is relying on the history and physical examination (85). It is true that physical findings such as pulsus paradoxus (inspiratory decline in systolic blood pressure >12 mm Hg), accessory muscle use including sternocleidomastoid muscle retraction, respiratory rate greater than 30, and heart rate greater than 130 are generally associated with more severe airflow obstruction (86,87).

However, none of these signs alone or in combination are specific or sensitive (88,89).

The importance of directly and objectively measuring airflow is underscored by the relative insensitivity of either arterial blood gases or subjective assessments for detecting anything less than severe obstruction. The measurements most frequently used for assessing airflow are the forced expiratory volume in one second (FEV_1) and peak expiratory flow (PEF). Both the FEV_1 and the PEF yield comparable results (90–93). Severe airflow obstruction is indicated by a peak flow <120 L per minute or by an FEV_1 <1 L.

Several attempts have been made to formulate a scoring index for the purpose of grading the severity of acute asthma and for predicting the need for hospitalization (see Table 8-1) (94–100). Fischl et al. described an index predicting relapse and the need for hospitalization in 205 patients with acute bronchial asthma (100). Of the 205 patients, 120 were successfully treated and discharged from the emergency room, 45 were hospitalized, and 40 were treated and discharged from the emergency room but had relapses within 10 days. A predictive index was developed on the basis of awarding one point for each of a combination of seven factors on initial presentation, including tachycardia (heart rate above 120 per minute), tachypnea (respiratory rate above 30 per minute), pulsus paradoxus (18 mm Hg or above), and PEF (120 L/minute or less). Presence of four or more of the seven factors upon presentation to the emergency room (prior to therapy) was 95% accurate in predicting the risk of relapse and 96% accurate in predicting the need for hospitalization. Another early study indicated that the response to initial therapy could be a useful guide (88). Patients whose FEV_1 improved by more than 400 mL had an early relapse rate of only 29%, whereas those who failed to demonstrate such an improvement in FEV_1 had a 67% relapse rate (101,102).

The chest roentgenogram may be helpful in excluding other pathologic conditions (pneumonia, pneumothorax) but does not provide useful information to grade the severity of asthma. In fact, hyperinflation is the most common finding on the chest roentgenogram in patients with acute asthma. Clinical judgment should be used to decide which patients receive a chest roentgenogram (103).

TABLE 8-1. Proposed Spirometric Criteria for Admission

Basis	Indications for Admission	Reference
Initial presentation	• Fischl index	100
	• Inability to perform spirometry	95,96
	• FEV_1 <0.61	96
Initial flow rate and response to first treatment	• Unresponsive to epinephrine, and PEF <60 L/min	95,97
	• Unresponsive to bronchodilators, and <16% change in initial PEF value	95,97
	• <0.15 L increase in FEV_1 after subcutaneous administration of bronchodilator	96
	• PEF <100 L/min initially and <60 L/min after 0.25 mg terbutaline	98
	• FEV1 <30% of predicted value; not improving to >40% of predicted value; >4 h therapy needed	99
Initial flow rate and response to full treatment	• PEF <100 L/min and <300 L/min after full treatment	98
	• FEV1 <0.61 L and <1.6 L after full treatment	96
	• Change in FEV1 <400 mL after bronchodilator administration	88
Other	• Deterioration of PEF by 15% after initial good response to bronchodilator therapy	97

From Brenner AS. The acute asthmatic in the emergency department: the decision to admit or discharge. *Am J Emerg Med* 1985;3:74–77, with permission.

Although life-threatening and severe hypoxemia can occur in asthma, it is relatively uncommon. Hypoxemia is secondary to ventilation–perfusion mismatch and readily responds to supplemental oxygen. Perhaps of more concern is the evaluation and correct interpretation of the arterial carbon dioxide tension ($PaCO_2$) (104,105). Mild and moderate degrees of airflow obstruction in asthma are usually accompanied by a hyperventilation response and a low $PaCO_2$. As airflow obstruction becomes more severe, $PaCO_2$ rises to about 40 mm Hg. The onset of hypercapnia usually begins when the FEV_1 declines below 750 mL or 25% of the predicted value (see Fig. 8-4) (104). Thus, the finding of a normal $PaCO_2$ in a patient with active asthma should be viewed with some concern, and increases in $PaCO_2$ above 40 mm Hg should be viewed with proportionately increasing alarm because this heralds severe airflow obstruction and respiratory muscle fatigue. Nowak et al. prospectively compared arterial blood gas and pulmonary function measurements in 102 episodes of acute bronchial asthma initially seen in the emergency room (105). The PaO_2, $PaCO_2$, and pH were unable to distinguish patients requiring admission from those who could be discharged. All patients with $PaCO_2$ >42 mm Hg and/or severe hypoxemia (PaO_2 <60 mm Hg) had a PEF <200 L per minute or an FEV_1 <1 L. In general, in patients with an acute asthma exacerbation, arterial blood gas determination can be limited to patients who have evidence of severe airflow obstruction by a screening airflow measurement.

In the absence of completely reliable objective indicators, clinical judgment is necessary to help decide which patients with acute asthma require hospitalization.

COMORBID CONDITIONS

Gastroesophageal Reflux

There is substantial literature that suggests a relationship between gastroesophageal reflux disease (GERD) and bronchial asthma (106). There are several possible associations between asthma and GERD: (a) these are two common diseases that coexist independently in some patients, (b) GERD either exacerbates or is causally related to the pathogenesis of asthma, or (c) bronchial asthma and/or antiasthma medications exacerbate or induce gastroesophageal disease. It is likely that all three of these possibilities occur in subsets of patients with bronchial asthma. Some degree of reflux appears to be normal or "physiologic," especially for several hours in the postprandial period. The probable mechanisms for GERD-induced asthma are: (a) acid stimulation of sensory nerve fibers in the lower esophagus, with reflex vagal bronchoconstriction; and (b) microaspiration of acid into the trachea.

Drug-induced Asthma

A variety of over-the-counter and prescription medications may contribute to acute bronchospasm, either as an isolated response or as part of a generalized systemic anaphylaxis. The overall magnitude of drug-induced bronchospasm in the United States remains unknown (107). Nonsteroidal antiinflammatory drugs (NSAIDs) are by far the most common cause of drug-induced asthma. Reports indicate that 5% to 20% of adults with asthma will experience exacerbation of bronchoconstriction after ingestion of aspirin or other NSAIDs. An adverse reaction to aspirin or NSAIDs may occur at any time, often following many years of employing these drugs without difficulty. These reactions are not prevented by pretreatment with antihistamines, theophylline, or cromolyn sodium. Corticosteriods do not prevent the bronchospasm unless given for an extended number of days. Other agents that have received a lot of attention in the literature include sulfites, β-adrenergic blocking agents, angiotensin converting enzyme (ACE) inhibitors, tartrazine, and a variety of miscellaneous agents (108–110). Drug-induced asthma should be suspected in all patients with difficult-to-control or steroid-dependent asthma. Careful history of all prescribed and over-the-counter medications should be obtained for all patients with asthma.

Allergic Bronchopulmonary Aspergillosis

The clinical course of an occasional patient with bronchial asthma may be complicated by pulmonary parenchymal infiltrates on the chest radiograph. The differential diagnosis for an infiltrate is extensive. However, specific entities to consider in an asthmatic include: (a) typical and atypical infections, (b) allergic bronchopulmonary aspergillosis (ABPA), (c) chronic eosinophilic pneumonia and other pulmonary infiltrate and eosinophilia (PIE) syndromes, and (d) allergic granulomatosis with angiitis (Churg–Strauss disease).

ABPA can be regarded as a complicated or special form of asthma in which immunologic reactions to *Aspergillus* species, usually *Aspergillus fumigatus*, play an important pathogenic role. Clinical syndromes analogous to ABPA have also been described in which noninvasive fungi other than *Aspergillus* appear to be the culprit. These related syndromes have been grouped under the term allergic bronchopulmonary fungoses (ABPF) (111–115).

The classic patient with ABPA has asthma, recurrent or fixed pulmonary infiltrates on the chest roentgenogram, proximal bronchiectasis, dual (immediate and late) skin-test response to *A. fumigatus*, elevated total serum IgE level (above 1,000 ng per mL), peripheral blood eosinophilia (above

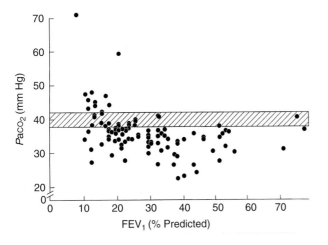

FIGURE 8-4. Correlation of the severity of acute airway obstruction with the arterial carbon dioxide tension in asthma. (From McFadden ER, Lyons HA. Arterial blood gas tension in asthma, *N Engl J Med* 1968;278:1027–1032, with permission.)

1,000 per mm^3), and serum precipitins (specific IgG) to *A. fumigatus* (112,113). *Aspergillus* species can frequently be identified or cultured from respiratory secretions.

Prednisone is the drug of choice for treatment of ABPA. Patients who receive other therapy for asthma (cromolyn, inhaled bronchodilators, inhaled corticosteroids) without systemic corticosteroids appear to have an increased number of exacerbations and a greater likelihood of a progressive deterioration of lung function. When exacerbations of ABPA are treated with prednisone, it seems that most patients will maintain stable long-term lung function (114,115).

The suggested dosage of prednisone is 0.5 mg per kg daily for 2 weeks (or longer if lung infiltrates are slow to improve), followed by conversion to alternate-day therapy for another 3 months (111). Such therapy usually clears the patient's symptoms and chest roentgenogram. The total serum IgE is usually significantly reduced as well but may not return to the normal level.

During the first year of therapy, serum IgE measurements should be obtained frequently (perhaps every 4 to 6 weeks) to determine the patient's baseline value and to detect subsequent relapse. Once a patient's baseline is determined, a subsequent 100% rise in total IgE suggests a relapse. In many cases, the chest roentgenogram will indicate a new infiltrate. According to current concepts, even asymptomatic relapses of ABPA should be treated with a reinstitution of prednisone therapy.

GENERAL MANAGEMENT

The National Asthma Education Prevention Program (NAEPP) Expert Panel Report-2 (EPR-2) provides an excellent algorithmic framework for the management of bronchial asthma (1). The general goals of asthma therapy include the following: (a) maintain normal activity levels, including exercise, (b) maintain nearly "normal" pulmonary function, (c) prevent chronic and troublesome symptoms and recurrent exacerbations of asthma, (d) avoid adverse effects from asthma medications, and (e) meet patients' and family's expectation of care. Overall, asthma therapy has four key components according to EPR-2: (a) patient education; (b) lung function measurement, both initially and during periodic evaluation, including home PEF monitoring; (c) environmental control with avoidance of asthma triggers; and (d) pharmacologic therapy. Much effort has been expended to develop and disseminate asthma guidelines. Although the various guidelines represent the best collective experience and literature review by a group of experts, many of the recommendations are not based on rigorous prospective clinical trials (e.g., utility of PEF monitoring in chronic asthma), largely due to lack of head-to-head comparisons. Studies have shown that physician understanding and/or implementation of the guidelines is poor, even among specialists (116). The overall impact of NAEPP/EPR-2 remains largely unknown. It is best to view the guidelines as a dynamic process with the aim of improving outcomes.

PATIENT EDUCATION

Nonadherence or noncompliance with therapy is a major problem in the management of asthma. A recent study of patients with chronic asthma in a general practice setting found that only one in three patients used at least half of the prescribed amount of medication daily (117). Similarly, a number of studies have documented improper MDI technique in the majority of patients (118,119). Several studies have shown that only 40% of physicians correctly performed four or more of the seven steps in the recommended MDI inhalation maneuver (120–123). Reasons for nonadherence are complex and include patient-related factors (e.g., denial of disease, cultural perception of the use of medications, socioeconomic and educational status) as well as the complexity of care (e.g., need for regular maintenance therapy, use of MDIs with spacer rather than pills, etc.). Asthma education programs that are targeted (e.g., low income, ethnic minorities) may improve overall outcomes (124).

Several studies have highlighted the beneficial effects as well as the limitations of adult asthma education and self-management in clinical practice (125,126). At Bellevue Hospital, a randomized crossover trial was conducted to evaluate an outpatient educational program involving 104 adult asthmatics previously requiring multiple hospitalizations for asthma attacks (127). The program involved a combination of widely accepted modalities, including vigorous education about self-management skills, a written crisis plan, easy access to a nurse practitioner, home PEF monitoring, and proper MDI technique. The program enrollment resulted in a threefold reduction in readmission rate and a twofold reduction in hospital days. Notably, this study excluded patients with psychiatric disease, who have increased risk of asthma morbidity and mortality (127). Wilson et al. conducted a randomized controlled trial with 1-year follow-up in a group of 323 adults with moderate-to-severe bronchial asthma (requiring three or more physician visits for asthma during a screening year) at Kaiser Health Plan Center (128). Patients were assigned to one of four treatment groups (small-group education, individual education, information workbook control group, or usual control group with no supplemental education). Both the small-group and individual asthma education programs improved patient understanding, control of asthma symptoms, and MDI technique. The small group was somewhat more effective. Additional controlled studies involving formal asthma education programs have documented their effectiveness in reducing the use of health services (129,130). Other studies have documented the cost effectiveness of an adult asthma education program (131). However, attendance rates for formal asthma education programs have ranged from 31% to 66% (132,133). Yoon et al. reported that attendees at an asthma education program were more likely to be women, nonsmokers, and patients from a higher socioeconomic status (134). The EPR-2 recommends that patients, especially those with moderate-to-severe persistent asthma or with a history of severe exacerbations, be given a written action plan based on signs and symptoms and/or PEF.

PEF monitoring has been advocated as an objective measure of airflow obstruction in patients with chronic asthma. All published asthma practice guidelines uniformly recommend the use of PEF monitoring as an adjunct to asthma education in selected groups of patients. Unfortunately, even after nearly four decades of use, many aspects of PEF monitoring remain unclear. An important and largely unanswered question is whether PEF monitoring adds anything to a well-constructed, individualized asthma education program with management based on symptoms alone. Despite a sound theoretical rationale for PEF monitoring, evaluating the usefulness of PEF monitoring in ambulatory asthma patients shows conflicting results. Over the past decade, six out of 10 randomized trials failed to show an advantage for the addition of PEF monitoring above and beyond symptom-based intervention for the control group (92).

Although PEF monitoring is not an adequate substitute for office spirometry in the initial diagnosis, currently available inexpensive devices are acceptable for serial monitoring of airflow obstruction. Regular PEF monitoring allows early detection of worsening airflow obstruction, which may be of particular value in "poor perceivers." Even though additional benefits above a well-constructed, symptom-based management plan have not been shown in patients with mild asthma, available data appear to support its role in moderate-to-severe asthma. PEF monitoring has some value in risk stratification in patients with asthma. Excessive diurnal variation and morning dip of PEF imply poor control and the need for careful reevaluation of the management plan. PEF alone is never appropriate; rather, PEF should be part of a comprehensive patient education program. Future studies to evaluate the usefulness of PEF should target patients who are at a higher risk for asthma-related morbidity and mortality. These are patients who are suspected to be poor perceivers. Future studies also need to identify the cutoff points or "action points" of high discriminatory value that can be easily applied by both patients and physicians in the primary care setting.

Aerosol delivery of the β-agonists can be achieved through the use of a handheld MDI in most patients. In the MDI technique, proper instruction is important to ensure effective use (118). It has been shown that increased deposition in the lung occurs when the actuator is held 2 to 4 cm from an open mouth position (135). Likewise, beginning inhalation at the end of normal expiration (functional residual capacity) is likely to optimize distribution of the inhaled aerosol (135). Optimal use of an MDI delivers only about 10% of the medication dose to the lung, whereas as much as 85% is deposited in the oropharynx (135). The use of a volume reservoir or spacer device is advantageous, especially in patients who are unable to learn or perform the unassisted MDI technique (136). Use of the volume reservoir may improve lung deposition to 15% of the dose and reduce oropharyngeal deposition to 5%, thereby potentially decreasing side effects as well (remaining 80% stays in the spacer device). Powered nebulizers have traditionally been used in patients with significant bronchospasm and in most hospital inpatients. However, recent studies suggest that properly supervised MDI aerosol delivery is as efficacious as powered nebulizer delivery, even in patients with acute or severe airflow obstruction (137–139). Data from non-ICU hospitalized patients suggest that use of MDIs rather than nebulizers results in substantial savings in direct costs (i.e., therapist's time) (140).

ALLERGEN AVOIDANCE: ENVIRONMENTAL CONTROL MEASURES

A variety of population and clinical studies have strongly suggested that exposure to aeroallergens in a susceptible host is associated with allergic sensitization in a subset of patients with both acute and chronic asthma (141,142). It is generally accepted that environmental control measures to reduce exposure to allergens should be considered in most asthmatics, and

immunotherapy should be reserved for selected patients only (143,144). Broadly speaking, aeroallergens can be divided into outdoor allergens (pollen and molds) and indoor allergens (house dust mites, animal allergens, cockroach allergen, and indoor molds). Exposure to outdoor allergens is best reduced during the peak pollen season by remaining indoors as much as possible in an air-conditioned environment with the windows closed.

Much attention in the literature has recently focused on the composition of house dust and indoor allergens (145). It appears that house dust itself is not an allergen, but there are allergic components within house dust. Fecal pellets from two house dust mites, *Dermatophagoides farinae* and *Dermatophagoides pteronyssinus,* contain several well-characterized allergens (Der f I, Der f II, Der p I, and Der p II) (146). Similarly, allergens from cat dander (Fel d I) and cockroaches (Bla g I, Bla g II) have been well described. Data suggest that certain environmental conditions such as high temperature, high humidity, and, perhaps, closed urban surroundings can increase allergen burden from these sources. A variety of studies have quantitatively measured these allergens and have recommended "safe" levels (147). Specific recommendations have been published to help reduce indoor allergen burden (148). Overall, it seems clear that indoor allergens contribute to some morbidity related to asthma and that strategies to minimize allergen exposure are warranted in most patients with asthma.

PHARMACOTHERAPY FOR CHRONIC ASTHMA

Table 8-2 depicts the overview of therapy, as outlined in the 1997 EPR-2 (1). The pharmacotherapy for asthma can be classified as symptomatic therapy with "relievers"/bronchodilators (β-agonists, theophylline) or "disease-modifying" therapy with "controllers"/antiinflammatory agents (corticosteroids, cromolyn, nedocromil, antileukotrienes, and anti-IgE therapy). Medications commonly used in the treatment of asthma, along with possible routes and schedules of administration, are listed in Table 8-3. The ERP-2 guidelines target therapy on the basis of the severity of asthma as assessed by frequency of symptoms or peak flow measurements (see Table 8-4). The ERP-2 defines intermittent mild asthma as brief (<1 hour) wheezing, cough, dyspnea up to two times weekly, absence of symptoms between exacerbations, and nocturnal symptoms less than two times a month. Also, the FEV_1 or PEF are greater than 80% of the patient's personal best. For mild asthma as defined in this fashion, the guidelines recommend as-needed use of one to two puffs of a β_2-agonist and/or cromolyn prior to exposure to various triggers. Persistent asthma is classified as mild persistent, moderate persistent, or severe persistent. For persistent asthma, the guidelines recommend daily controller therapy (most often, inhaled corticosteroids, alternatively, cromolyn/nedocromil or antileukotrienes). For breakthrough symptoms or nocturnal symptoms, additional therapy with salmeterol or sustained-release theophylline and/or higher doses of inhaled steroids are recommended. According to the EPR-2, severe asthma should be treated with a burst of oral corticosteroids at 40 mg a day for 1 week and then tapered for 1 week, in addition to the inhaled corticosteroids and as-needed inhaled β_2-agonists.

TABLE 8-2. Management of Chronic Asthma: Overview of Therapy

Severity	Therapy	Outcome/Goals
Mild intermittent • Symptoms ≤2 × wk • Asymptomatic, normal PEF between exacerbations	• Inhaled β-MDI as required • No daily medication	• Control symptoms • Maintain normal activity levels • Prevent exacerbations
Mild persistent • Symptoms ≤2 × wk <1 × d • May affect activity	• One daily medication: — Low-dose inhaled corticosteroid or cromolyn/nedocromil — Sustained-release theophylline or antileukotriene • Inhaled β-MDI as required	• Normalize pulmonary function • Optimize pharmacotherapy with minimal side effects • Meet patient/family expectations of care
Moderate persistent • Daily symptoms • Exacerbations ≥2 × wk • Daily use of β-MDI	• Daily medication • Medium-dose inhaled corticosteroid ± long-acting β-agonist	
Severe persistent • Continual symptoms • Limited physical activity • Frequent exacerbations	• Daily medication — High-dose inhaled corticosteroid + long-acting β-agonist — ? Prednisone — Consider anti-IgE	

PEF, peak expiratory flow; MDI, metered-dose inhaler.

From National Heart, Lung, and Blood Institute. National Asthma Education and Prevention Program. Expert Panel Report 2. *Guidelines for the diagnosis and management of asthma*. Bethesda, MD: National Institutes of Health; 1997. Publication No. 97–4051, with permission.

TABLE 8-3. Pharmacologic Agents for the Treatment of Asthma

Class	Generic Name	Brand Name (Manufacturer)	Delivery Route/Device	Suggested Dosage (Adults)	Comment
Anticholinergics	Atropine sulfate	Many	Solution 0.2% (1 mg/0.5 mL) 0.5% (2.5 mg/0.5 mL) (1.25 mg)	0.025 mg/kg diluted with 3–5 mL NS q 6–8 h	Minimal side effects with ipratropium
	Ipratropium bromide	Atrovent (Boehringer)	MDI (18 μg/puff) Solution 0.02% unit dose vial	2–4 puffs qid; max = 12 puffs/d 500 μg/tid, 1 puff per d	Approved for COPD
	Tiotropium	Spiriva (Boehringer)	DPI (HandiHaler) 18 μg/capsule		
β-Adrenergic agents	Albuterol sulfate	Airet (Medeva) Albuterol (various generic) Proventil (Schering)	Solution (0.83%) Solution (0.83%, 0.5%) MDI (90 μg/puff) Solution for nebulizer Tablets (2, 4 mg)	2.5–10 mg q 6–8 h 2.5–10 mg q 6–8 h mL (0.5 mL) Acute: 2–4 puffs q 4–6 h; max 16–20 puffs/d Prophylaxis: 2 puffs 15 min before exercise 2.5–10 mg a 6–8 h (0.083%) (3 mL) or (0.5%) (0.5 mL) 2–4 mg q 6–8 h; max: 32 mg/d	Inhaled agents have fewer systemic side effects; β₂-selective agents are albuterol, bitolterol, metaproterenol, pirbuterol, salmeterol, terbutaline
		Proventil-HFA (Schering)	MDI (90 μg/puff) Repetabs (sustained-release tablets), 4 mg	2–4 puffs q 4–6 h 4 mg q 12 h	
		Ventolin (Glaxo)	MDI (90 μg/puff) Rotohaler (200 μg/Rotacap)	Max: 16–30 puffs/d (200 puffs) 200–400 μg q 6–8 h; max dose = 2.4 mg/d	

(Continued)

TABLE 8-3.   *(Continued)*

Class	Generic Name	Brand Name (Manufacturer)	Delivery Route/Device	Suggested Dosage (Adults)	Comment
			Solution for nebulizer (0.083% μg/mL, 0.5% 20 mL)	2.5–10 mg q 6–8 h	
			Tablets (2, 4 mg)	4–8 mg qid (up to 32 mg/d)	
		Volmax (Muro)	Sustained-release tablets (4, 8 mg)	4–8 mg q 12 h	
	Bitolterol mesylate	Tornalate (Sanofi Winthrop)	MDI (370 μg /puff)	2 puffs q 6 h	
	Epinephrine	Medihaler-Epi (3M Pharm)	MDI (300 μg /puff)	2 puffs qid	
		Many	Solution for inhalation (15 mL)	Nebulized q 2–3 h	
		Adrenalin chloride (Parke-Davis)	SC injection 1:1000 (1 mg/mL)	0.2–0.5 mg SC (0.2–0.5 mL SC) q 20 min	
	Formoterol	Foradil (Novartis)	DPI (Aerolizer) 12 μg/capsule	1 puff bid	
	Isoetharine HCl	Bronkometer (Sanofi Winthrop)	MDI (340 μg /puff)	1–2 puffs q 4 h	
		Many	Solutions for inhalation	0.25–1 mL nebulized with NS	
	Isoproterenol HCl	Medihaler-150 (3M Pharm)	MDI (800 μg /puff)	1–2 puff qid	
		Isuprel Mistometer (Sanofi Winthrop)	MDI (131 μg /puff) Solution (0.5%, 1%, 5%) Tablets (glossets 10, 15 mg)	1–2 puffs qid 0.5 mL in 2.5 mL NS q 3–4 h 10–20 mg q 4 h	
	Levalbuterol	Xopenex	Solution for nebulizer (Sepracor)	0.63 mg q 6–8 h (0.63 mg)	
	Metaproterenol	Alupent (Boehringer)	MDI (650 μg /puff)	2–3 puffs q 3–4 h max = 12 puff/d	
			Solution (0.4%, 0.6%)	0.3 mL in 2.5 mL NS q 4–6 h	
			Tablets (10, 20 mg)	10 mg q 6–8 h up to 20 mg	
		Metaprel (Sandoz)	MDI (650 μg /puff) Solution (0.5%)	2–3 puffs q 3–4 h; max = 12 0.3 mL in 2.5 mL NS q 4–6 h	
			Tablet (10, 20 mg)	10 mg q 6–8 h up to 20 mg	
	Pirbuterol acetate	Maxair (3M Pharm)	MDI (200 μg /puff)	1–2 puffs q 4–6 h; max = 12 puffs/d	
			AutoHaler (200 μg /puff)	2 puffs q 6 h	
	Salmeterol	Serevent (Glaxo)	Diskus (DPI 50 μg /puff)	2 puffs q 12 h	
	Terbutaline sulfate	Brethaire (Geigy)	MDI (200 μg /puff) Solution for SC injection or nebulizer (1 mg/mL)	1–2 puffs q 4–6 h 0.25 mg SC q 15–30 min; max = 0.50 mg/4 h, 0.75–2.5 mg nebulized with NS	
			Tablet (2.5, 5 mg)	2.5–5 mg tid; max = 15 mg/24 h	
		Bricanyl (Marion Merrell Dow)	MDI (200 μg /puff) Tablets (2.5, 5 mg)	1–2 puffs q 4–6 h 2.4–5 mg tid; max = 15 mg/24 h	

(Continued)

TABLE 8-3.   *(Continued)*

Class	Generic Name	Brand Name (Manufacturer)	Delivery Route/Device	Suggested Dosage (Adults)	Comment
Cromoglycates	Cromolyn sodium	Intal (Fisons)	MDI (800 μg /puff) Solution (20 mg/2 mL ampule)	2–4 puffs qid 1 ampule qid	Contraindication in acute asthma
	Nedocromil sodium	Tilade (Fisons)	MDI (1.75 mg/puff)	2 puffs bid, tid, qid	
Inhaled corticosteroids	Beclomethasone dipropionate	Beclovent (Allen & Hanburys)	MDI (42 μg /puff)	2 puffs tid—qid; max = 20 puffs/d	Need more than 400 μg /d to maintain off oral steroids, no adrenal suppression if <800–1200 μg /d
		Qvar (HFA-BDP) (3M)	MDI (40 or 80 μg /puff)	2–8 puffs bid	
		Vanceril (Schering)	MDI (42 μg /puff)	2 puffs tid–qid; max = 20 puffs/d	
		Vanceril DS	MDI (84 μg /puff)	2 puffs tid–qid; max = 20 puffs/d	
	Budesonide	Pulmicort (AstraZeneca)	Turbuhaler (200 μg /puff)	400–1600 μg in divided doses bid–qid	Approved for 12 mo–8 yrs; only approved steroid for nebulization
		Pulmicort Respules (AstraZeneca)	Solution (0.25 mg/2 mL or 0.50 mg/2 mL)	0.25–1 mg qd–bid	
	Flunisolide	AeroBid (Forest)	MDI (250 μg /puff)	2 puffs bid; max = 8 puffs/d	
	Fluticasone propionate	Flovent (Glaxo)	MDI (44, 110, 220, μg / puff)		
			Diskus powder inhaler (50, 100, 250 μg /puff)	100–800 μg /d	
	Mometasone furoate (investigational in US)	Asmanex (Schering)	DPI (Twisthaler) 200 or 400 μg/puff	1 puff bid	
	Triamcinolone acetonide	Azmacort (Rhone-Poulenc Rorer)	MDI (100 μg /puff)	2–4 puffs qid; max = 16 puffs/d	
Combination products	Albuterol/ ipratropium	Combivent (Boehringer-Ingelheim)	MDI (18 μg ipratropium/103 μg albuterol per puff)	2 puffs qid	
	Salmeterol/ fluticasone	Advair (Glaxo)	Diskus (DPI)	50/100, 50/250, 50/500 (1 puff bid)	
	Formoterol/ budesonide (investigational in US)	Symbicort (AstraZeneca)	Turbuhaler (100 or 200 μg /puff)	1 puff bid	
Antileukotrienes	Montelukast	Singulair (Merck)	Tablet (5, 10 mg)	10 mg qd in the evening	Churg–Strauss
	Zafirlukast	Accolate (Zeneca)	Tablets (20 mg)	20 mg bid	Take on empty stomach; drug interactions
	Zileuton	Zyflo (Abbott)	Tablets (600 mg)	600 mg qid	Need to follow LFTs, drug interactions
Methylxanthines	Aminophylline	Various	IV	Load: If not on theophylline at home, 5–6 mg/kg over 20 min; if on theophylline, level pending, 3 mg/kg over 20 min; a bolus of 0.5 mg/kg will increase level by 2 in the average adult. Maintenance 0.5–0.9 mg/kg/h; 200–400 mg bid	Decreased clearance with cirrhosis, CHF, erythromycin, cimetidine, troleandomycin; increased clearance with smoking, young age, and phenobarbital. Need to follow serum levels

(Continued)

TABLE 8-3. *(Continued)*

Class	Generic Name	Brand Name (Manufacturer)	Delivery Route/Device	Suggested Dosage (Adults)	Comment
	Theophylline	Anhydrous, immediate release (Slophyllin, Theolair, Quibron, Elixophyllin, etc.)	PO	qid	Normal dose range for an average adult is 300–1200 mg/d; immediate release preparation; dose should be given every 6–8 h; sustained-release preparations: dose may be given every 12–24 h; this dose range is an approximate starting point; however, whenever possible, serum levels should be monitored, that is, 8 h after a dose after 5 to 6 consecutive doses
Systemic corticosteroids	Prednisone	Many	Tablets (1, 5, 10, 20, 50 mg)	10–50 mg/d	Long-term systemic side effects: cataracts, osteopenia, Cushingoid features, immune suppression, hypertension
	Methylpredni-sone sodium succinate	Medrol (Upjohn)	Tablets (2, 4, 8, 16, 24, 32 mg)	4–48 mg/d	
		Solu-Medrol (Upjohn)	IV (40, 125, 500, 1000 mg)	1–2 mg/kg q 4–6 h	
	Hydrocortisone sodium succinate	Solu-Cortef (Upjohn)	IV (100, 250, 500, 1000 mg)	4 mg/kg q 4–6 h	
Anti-IgE	Omalizumab	Xolair (Genentech/ Novartis)	Subcutaneous	0.016 mg × body wt (kg) × IgE level (IU/ml); also see nomogram	See text for details; urticaria 2%–3%; anaphylaxis 0.01%–0.1%

HFA, hydrofluoroalkane-134a; DPI, dry powder inhaler; MDI, pressurized metered-dose inhaler; BDP, beclomethasone dipropionate; SC, subcutaneous; LFT, liver function tests; CHF, congestive heart failure; NS, normal saline; PO, per oral.

TABLE 8-4. Classification of Asthma Severity by the National Asthma Education and Prevention Program: Expert Panel Report 2

Classification	Clinical Features before Treatment[a]		
	Symptoms[b]	Nighttime Symptoms	Lung Function
Mild intermittent	• Symptoms ≤2 times/wk • Asymptomatic and normal PEF between exacerbations • Exacerbations brief (from a few hours to a few days); intensity may vary	≤2 times/mo	• FEV$_1$ or PEF ≥80% predicted • PEF variability 20%
Mild persistent	• Symptoms >2 times/wk but <1 time/d • Exacerbations may affect activity	≤2 times/mo	• FEV$_1$ or PEF ≥80% predicted • PEF variability 20%–30%
Moderate persistent	• Daily symptoms • Daily use of inhaled short-acting β_2-agonist • Exacerbations affect activity • Exacerbations ≥2 times/wk; may last days	>1 time/wk	• FEV$_1$ or PEF ≥60% to 80% predicted • PEF variability >30%
Severe persistent	• Continual symptoms • Limited physical activity • Frequent exacerbations	Frequent	• FEV$_1$ or PEF ≥60% predicted • PEF variability >30%

PEF, peak expiratory flow; FEV$_1$, forced expiratory volume in 1 second.

[a] The presence of one of the features of severity is sufficient to place a patient in that category. An individual should be assigned to the most severe grade in which any feature occurs. The characteristics noted in this table are general and may overlap because asthma is highly variable. Furthermore, an individual's classification may change over time.

[b] Patients at any level of severity can have mild, moderate, or severe exacerbations. Some patients with intermittent asthma experience severe and life-threatening exacerbations separated by long periods of normal lung function and no symptoms.

From National Heart, Lung, and Blood Institute. National Asthma Education and Prevention Program. Expert Panel Report 2. *Guidelines for the diagnosis and management of asthma.* Bethesda, MD: National Institutes of Health, 1997. Publication No. 97–4051, with permission.

BRONCHODILATORS

β-Adrenergic Agents

The β-adrenergic agonist drugs have structural similarities by virtue of a common catechol nucleus. The catecholamines (isoproterenol or isoetharine) are rapid acting, potent, and relatively nonselective β_1-agonists (148,149). Resorcinols (metaproterenol, terbutaline, and fenoterol) and saligenins (albuterol and salmeterol) represent a modification of the central catechol nucleus, with resultant longer duration of action and greater β_2-airway selectivity. Stimulation of the β-receptors activates adenyl cyclase, causing formation of intracellular cyclic adenosine monophosphate (AMP). This, in turn, provides energy for compartmental shifts in calcium, which results in bronchial smooth-muscle relaxation. The major therapeutic actions of β-stimulation in the treatment of asthma include bronchodilation, facilitation of mucociliary clearance, and inhibition of acute mediator release from mast cells. β-Agonists do not have an effect on cellular inflammation or on the LAR.

For several reasons, the use of oral β-adrenergic agonists has fallen into disfavor (1). Oral bioavailability of these agents is significantly confounded by patient-to-patient variability in bowel absorption and by first-pass hepatic metabolism (1). Aerosol delivery provides a more rapid onset of action, a comparable sustained response, and a significantly decreased incidence of side effects (150). Aerosols have traditionally been administered through MDIs or dry powder inhalers (DPIs) for ambulatory care, while small-volume wet nebulizers have been used in emergency departments, on hospital wards and intensive care units, and for young children (151). Despite the fact that a large number of studies have found comparable bronchodilation for β-agonists administered by MDI or wet nebulization in patients with acute asthma (137–139), EPR-2 recommends delivery of aerosolized bronchodilators by wet nebulization for management of acute asthma in the emergency room (1). Nebulizer therapy continues to be widely prescribed for a number of reasons: (a) it is widely believed that acutely tachypneic patients are unable to use MDIs optimally, even with a spacer device; (b) patients are usually on MDI therapy at home, and an acute episode requiring emergency care typically represents a failure of home therapy; therefore, patients expect alternative therapy; and (c) there is a widespread belief that nebulizer therapy is more effective than MDI usage in treating acute exacerbations of airway obstruction (152).

The environmental impact of chlorofluorocarbons (CFCs) used in pressurized MDIs has received much recent attention (153–155). Most currently used MDIs contain a blend of CFC propellants including CFC-12 (primary propellant), CFC-11 (primary solvent), and CFC-114 (moderates pressure and density). The CFCs (or Freons) used in MDIs represent 0.5% of the annual worldwide production of these compounds. CFCs are ideal propellants because of their stability and clinical safety. Several international conferences have been held that have resulted in an agreement to ban the use of CFCs after 1998 to 1999, including medical use (156). A number of pharmaceutical companies have responded to this challenge by developing new inhalers that do not use CFCs. One strategy is to utilize a non-CFC propellant such as hydrofluorocarbon-134a. CFC-free preparations are available for β-agonists as well as inhaled steroids. A second strategy is to use breath-actuated DPIs. Examples of DPIs currently available (or under

development) are the Spinhaler (Fisons), Rotahaler (Allen and Hanbury), Diskhaler (Allen and Hanbury), Turbuhaler (Astra), multidisk powder inhaler (Glaxo), and Aerolizer (Novartis). In addition to being environmentally safe, the breath-actuated powder devices do not require the exact patient coordination and synchronization typically necessary for MDI use (157, 158). Also, the powder preparations can be inhaled without the need for a spacer extension device. However, these devices do require a minimum inspiratory flow rate from a spontaneously breathing patient, and their use may sometimes cause throat irritation.

Salmeterol xinafoate and formoterol are long-acting β_2-agonists (duration of action 8 to 17 hours). They are available as a DPI. Formoterol has a more rapid onset of action than salmeterol. *In vitro* studies suggest that salmeterol is more potent than albuterol and has a slower onset (159). Short-term clinical trials have shown salmeterol to be more effective than albuterol (either with regular or on-demand doses), with a similar incidence of adverse reactions (160). The EPR-2 recommends that antiinflammatory therapy be initiated prior to long-acting β-agonists in patients with chronic asthma and does not recommend monotherapy with salmeterol. Numerous recent studies in mild-to-moderate asthmatics with inadequate symptom control despite low-to-moderate doses of inhaled steroids have found greater benefits from adding a long-acting β-agonist than from increasing the inhaled steroid dose (161–163). Salmeterol or formoterol are best suited for the following clinical situations: (a) predominantly nocturnal asthma symptoms; (b) exercise-induced asthma in patients who exercise regularly (may be preferred over short-acting β-agonists) (164); (c) as adjunctive therapy in patients with suboptimal asthma control while on low-to-moderate doses of inhaled steroids (as an alternative to increasing the dose of inhaled steroids).

It is important to educate patients that salmeterol is not to be used for short-term relief of acute asthma symptoms. All patients with symptomatic asthma should be prescribed and instructed on the proper use of a short-acting β-agonist. Several studies have confirmed the overall safety of daily use of salmeterol 100 μg twice a day (total four puffs per day), when used in addition to inhaled steroids (161–163,165). Studies have also shown no tolerance to the bronchodilator effects of daily salmeterol therapy for months (166). Experimental studies do show a decrease in the bronchoprotective effect over time; the magnitude and significance of this finding remains unclear (167). Side effects of salmeterol may be additive with those of short-acting β-agonists.

β_2-Adrenergic agonists are derivatives of adrenaline and have been commercially available as racemates or as a racemic mixture of two enantiomers, levo-(R) and dextro-(S)-rotatory isomers (168). The R-isomer confers pharmacologic bronchodilating activity on the racemate, whereas the S-isomer is largely inactive, although it may be associated with inducing airway hyperreactivity in some models. Albuterol is a racemic mixture with a 1:1 ratio of the isomers R-albuterol (levalbuterol) and S-albuterol. Levalbuterol is available as a nebulized solution for prevention and treatment of bronchospasm in asthmatics over the age of 12 (169). Although the early animal data on the use of pure S-enantiomer aerosols was suggestive of an adverse effect, this has not been convincingly demonstrated in human clinical trials. A recent double-blind crossover study in mild-to-moderate asthmatics

($N = 17$) indicated that there was no adverse effect by s-albuterol compared with placebo (170). With the current data, there appears to be no advantage for levalbuterol compared to the widely used racemic albuterol (169).

Several mechanisms have been advanced to describe potential side effects related to regular administration of β-agonists. These include paradoxical bronchoconstriction, downregulation of β_2-agonist receptors, tachyphylaxis as a result of depletion of norepinephrine stores, decreased protection against various stimuli, and an increase in bronchial hyperreactivity (171–173). Several mechanisms have been postulated for paradoxical bronchoconstriction, including hypotonicity and acidity of the solution (174,175); and preservatives such as benzalkonium chloride (176), sorbitan, oleic acid, edetate disodium, sulfites (177–179), and alcohol. As discussed previously, polymorphisms in the β_2-AR gene may also play a role. Overall, paradoxical bronchoconstriction is likely quite rare.

Methylxanthines

With the development of long-acting and potent inhaled β_2-agonists and inhaled corticosteroids, the use of theophylline now has a less central role in the chronic maintenance therapy of asthma (180). The reasons for this include the fact that theophylline has weak bronchodilating properties, has modest and unclear antiinflammatory properties, and has the potential for side effects (numerous drug interactions, need to monitor serum levels, and a low therapeutic-to-toxicity ratio). However, although this medication is generally less effective as a single agent than aerosol β-agonists, at least some patients will achieve an enhanced benefit from combination therapy (181). Maintenance therapy with oral theophylline may be beneficial in steroid-dependent asthmatics. In a placebo-controlled, randomized, and double-blind trial of steroid-dependent asthmatics, theophylline reduced the daily corticosteroid requirement (182). The availability of sustained-release formulations provides theophylline with a role in the treatment of nocturnal asthma (183). Particularly useful in this regard are the "once-a-day" formulations (e.g., Theo-24 and Uniphyl) (184,185).

The potentially serious toxicity of theophylline mandates that the clinician be aware of certain pharmacokinetic features of the drug and the implication for dosing regimens. A recent retrospective chart audit evaluated 40 adult inpatients with theophylline toxicity (levels >25 mg per L) to identify preventable factors (186). The study found that two-thirds (27 of 40 patients) of the inpatients became toxic because of inpatient or emergency department theophylline administration. A set of recurring management errors included a delay in taking action from the time toxic blood levels were drawn, inappropriately high dosing of patients with congestive heart failure, failure to recognize obvious symptoms of toxicity, emergency department treatment of already toxic patients, and overlapping of intravenous and oral therapy. The clearance of theophylline is affected by many different factors and exhibits significant variation among adults.

Anticholinergic Agents

For more than two centuries, naturally occurring anticholinergic substances (stramonium, found in the Datura plant, and atropine) have been used in the treatment of asthma. In general, these agents are less effective than β-agonists, and the systemic side effects after inhalation are considerable. However, the duration of action of the anticholinergic medications is often considerably longer than that of the β-agonists (187). However, the availability of a quaternary derivative of atropine, ipratropium bromide (Atrovent), which is topically active but poorly absorbed (and therefore has minimal side effects), stimulated renewed interest in using anticholinergic agents for both asthma and chronic obstructive pulmonary disease. Ipratropium bromide is available either in solution for use in a nebulizer or in an MDI. When administered via MDI, the recommended dose is two puffs (40 μg) four times daily. Interestingly, ipratropium bromide, in contrast to atropine, does not reduce mucociliary clearance in normal subjects or in patients with airway disease (188,189). An unpleasant, bitter taste appears to be the only significant unwanted feature of inhaled ipratropium.

The role of anticholinergic agents such as ipratropium or tiotropium in the treatment of stable asthma is not yet clearly defined. When used as a single agent, ipratropium has been shown in some studies to be almost as effective as isoproterenol (190), albuterol, terbutaline (191), and metaproterenol (192). However, other clinical trials have indicated ipratropium to be less effective than either metaproterenol (193) or fenoterol (194). The discrepancy regarding the efficacy of ipratropium may be explained by patient selection; it is probable that there are "responders" and "nonresponders" to ipratropium (192). It is difficult to predict which patients might respond to ipratropium, but patients with a "psychogenic" component to their asthma (in which vagal tone may play an important role) constitute a group that might be relatively responsive (195). Several studies indicate that combining ipratropium with a β-adrenergic agent is more effective in the treatment of chronic asthma than either drug alone (196).

ANTIINFLAMMATORY AGENTS

Corticosteroids

The central role of airway inflammation in the pathogenesis of both acute and chronic asthma (both mild and severe) has been reviewed in detail. It is safe to say that there is a consensus that antiinflammatory treatment should represent a primary therapeutic approach for acute severe asthma in the emergency-room setting (by use of parenteral or oral corticosteroids), in addition to repetitive dosing of inhaled β-agonists. For long-term maintenance therapy of patients with chronic asthma, treatment focus has shifted away from use of bronchodilator therapy alone and toward earlier use of inhaled antiinflammatory therapy.

Potential mechanisms of corticosteroid action include effects on leukocytes (T lymphocytes, polymorphonuclear neutrophils), synthesis of regulator proteins, catecholamine receptors or function, eicosanoid synthesis and function, and vascular endothelial integrity. Although the precise mechanism of action of glucocorticoids is not known, recent advances in understanding the molecular mechanisms of the GR, steroid-responsive target-gene elements, and cytokine biology have provided insights (see Fig. 8-5) (197–209). There is a single GR that is localized to the cytoplasm of target cells in

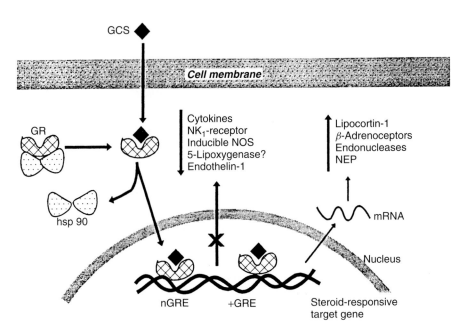

FIGURE 8-5. Molecular mechanism of glucocorticosteroid (*GCS*) action. *GCS* binds to a cytosolic glucocorticoid receptor (*GR*) that is normally bound to two molecules of heat shock protein (*hsp 90*). The activated *GR* translocates to the *nucleus*, where it binds to specific glucocorticoid receptor elements (*GREs*) in the upstream regulatory region of genes, which either inhibit (*nGRE*) or stimulate (+*GRE*) transcription of steroid-responsive target genes (of which many are likely to be relevant in asthma therapy). (From Barnes PJ, Pedersen S. Efficacy and safety of inhaled corticosteroids in asthma. *Am Rev Respir Dis* 1993;148:S2, with permission.)

airway epithelium and in endothelium of bronchial vessels. After a glucocorticoid binds to a cytosolic GR, this complex translocates to the nucleus, where it binds to specific glucocorticoid response elements of genes, which either inhibit or stimulate transcription in steroid-responsive target genes. Steroids inhibit the transcription of several cytokines, including interleukin-1 (IL-1), tumor necrosis factor-α (TNF-α), granulocyte-macrophage colony-stimulating factor (GM-CSF), and interleukins-3, -4, -5, -6, and -8. The well-known eosinopenic effect of corticosteroids is believed to be due to the inhibitory effects on circulating IL-5 and GM-CSF (200). Steroids also increase the synthesis of lipocortin-1, which has an inhibitory effect on phospholipase A_2 and, therefore, inhibits the production of lipid mediators such as leukotrienes, prostaglandins, and platelet-activating factor. Additional effects include inhibiting mucous secretion in airways and increasing the expression of β-receptors by increasing gene transcription.

A variety of studies using bronchoscopy with lavage or biopsy have been performed in asthmatics of varying severity to assess the antiinflammatory effect of inhaled and systemic steroid therapy (49,201–204). These studies suggest that inhaled corticosteroids bring about a variety of antiinflammatory effects in the airway inflammation. There are conflicting data as to whether long-term therapy with inhaled corticosteroids reduces basement membrane thickening and substantially affects airway remodeling.

Numerous studies have shown that inhaled steroid therapy provides effective symptomatic control of chronic asthma and reduces the need for oral steroids (210–218). Inhaled corticosteroids have assumed the role of first line therapy for most patients with persistent asthma. Over the past 5 to 10 years, there have been several important trends in the way these agents have been used in clinical trials as well as in practice. One trend has been the use of higher doses of inhaled steroids, especially for the more severe asthmatics. This is predicated on the hypothesis that there is a dose-response effect for these agents (219). Although quite a number of studies support

this hypothesis, there is continued debate (214–217). It is well documented that higher doses of corticosteroids facilitate a reduction in systemic corticosteroids in severe steroid-dependent asthma (217). A second trend has been the use of inhaled corticosteroids at an earlier stage of asthma (210,212). Data suggest that this might improve the long-term forced expiratory volume in one second (FEV$_1$) by preventing subepithelial fibrosis, although this hypothesis is not universally accepted (220). Several studies with follow-up over 10 years indicate that inhaled steroids do not cure asthma, and cessation of therapy often results in prompt relapse (204). A third trend is less frequent dosing, such as bid or qid, which may be equally effective. Less frequent dosing has benefits in terms of improved compliance (221). Inhaled steroids are cost effective in management of asthma with an incremental cost-effectiveness ratio for a symptom-free day of approximately $5.00 to $6.00 (213,222,223). Regular use of inhaled steroids can prevent asthmatic exacerbation, increases in bronchial hyperresponsiveness, and accelerated loss of lung function (207,210,212). Finally, a large retrospective case-control study from Canada associated regular use of inhaled steroids with a statistically significant reduction in mortality rate (224,225). Currently, there are five specific inhaled corticosteroids that are approved for maintenance therapy for asthma in the United States. Mometasone is undergoing late phase-III clinical trials (226). The EPR-2 provides a table of inhaled steroids with comparative doses to achieve a similar clinical effect.

A recent development in chronic asthma maintenance therapy is the concept of combination therapy to produce either additive or synergistic effects (1,227). A variety of studies seem to indicate that groups of mild-to-moderate asthmatics who remain symptomatic on low-to-intermediate doses of inhaled corticosteroids experience greater benefit from a long-acting inhaled bronchodilator taken in combination with inhaled steroid compared with doubling the dose of inhaled steroid. A natural extension of this concept has been the development of new inhaled products that combine both steroids and bronchodilators into a single device. This has recently become available as a diskus device with the medication, packaged as a nonchlorofluorocarbon dry–powder preparation. Several pivotal studies indicate that the combination product is superior to the individual components in patients with mild and moderately severe chronic asthma (227).

Several studies have examined the utility of inhaled steroids taken in combination with other agents such as theophylline and leukotriene antagonists (228–230). The benefits of combination therapy, as measured by symptom scores, need for rescue β-agonists, lung function, and exacerbation rates, with these other agents are, however, not as dramatic as with the addition of the long-acting inhaled bronchodilator. A study from the asthma clinical research network of the National Heart, Lung, and Blood Institute (NHLBI) found that monotherapy with salmeterol is not an adequate replacement therapy for patients controlled on an inhaled steroid 400 μg twice per day (231). The exact molecular mechanism whereby the combination of inhaled steroids and long-acting β-agonists synergistically improve asthma control is not fully known. Preliminary data indicate that long-acting β-agonists may facilitate the steroid effect, whereas the steroids upregulate the β-agonist receptors.

As discussed earlier, the conventional CFC-based MDIs are currently being reformulated with alternative propellants such as hydrofluoroalkanes (HFAs). Reformulation of beclomethasone with HFA-134a results in a solution that delivers an aerosol of extrafine particles with a mass median aerodynamic diameter (MMAD) of 1 μm, compared with the CFC-based beclomethasone dipropionate (BDP), which has a MMAD of 4 to 5 μm. In patients with moderate asthma, 400 μg HFA-134a BDP appears to produce clinical effects equivalent to an 800 μg dose of CFC-BDP in patients who had not been adequately controlled with 0 to 400 μg per day of inhaled corticosteroids (156). There was no significant difference in the morning serum cortisol level. This preliminary study indicates that the extrafine particles may deposit more peripherally in the lower airways and may be a more efficient method for delivery of steroid aerosols. Theoretically, this would mean increased clinical effectiveness with lower systemic absorption from more peripheral deposition using HFA-134a BDP.

Both the binding affinity to GR and the skin-blanching test are *in vitro* parameters that are often used to compare relative potency of inhaled glucocorticoids (198,199,219) (see Table 8-5). However, the pharmacokinetics of inhaled steroids and the subsequent clearance of these agents also determine both the efficacy and the side effects (see Table 8-6 and Fig. 8-6). Long-term comparative clinical studies are needed before the clinician can rationally choose between the currently available inhaled glucocorticoids (199).

TABLE 8-5.   Relative Binding Affinity for Human Lung Glucocorticoid Receptor and Topical Blanching Potency in Human Skin

Glucocorticosteroid	Binding Affinity	Blanching Potency
Dexamethasone	1.0	1
BDP/BMP	0.4/13.5	600/450
Budesonide	9.4	980
Flunisolide	1.8	330
Triamcinolone acetonide	3.6	330
Fluticasone propionate	18.0	1,200
	(Rat tissue)	

BDP, beclomethasone dipropionate; BMP, beclomethasone monopropionate.

From Barnes PJ, Pedersen S. Efficacy and safety of inhaled corticosteroids in asthma. *Am Rev Respir Dis* 1993;148:57, with permission.

The concept of "resistance" to corticosteroids has received a lot of attention, although the exact molecular mechanisms remain poorly understood. There is likely only one type of human GR; however, polymorphisms of the human steroid receptor have been established with unclear clinical significance. Two discrete types of relative steroid resistance have been described. Type 1 steroid resistance is a relative lack of steroid responsiveness in the airways, although there is evidence for steroid effect in other tissues of the body, usually manifested as clinical steroid side effects (i.e., Cushingoid effects). Type 1 steroid resistance is acquired and more common. On the other hand, type 2 steroid resistance is due to a generalized lack of steroid responsiveness in the airways and other organ systems. Patients with type 2 resistance have poor asthma control despite systemic corticosteroid therapy and no systemic steroid side effects. Type 2 steroid resistance is rare. The relative contribution of this concept of steroid resistance in suboptimal asthma control and in poor outcomes remains unknown. Patients with such a molecular basis for steroid resistance may be a subset who would benefit from alternative antiinflammatory approaches.

Carmichael et al. described 58 patients with chronic asthma who were clinically resistant to treatment with prednisolone (defined as absence of a 15% increase in FEV_1 after a 7-day course of at least 20 mg of prednisolone daily) (232). Dykewicz et al. studied the natural history of 40 randomly selected adult asthmatic patients refractory to inhaled beclomethasone and β-agonists and dependent on long-term prednisone therapy

TABLE 8-6.   Pharmacokinetics of Inhaled Glucocorticosteroids

	Plasma Half-Life (h)	Volume of Distribution (L/kg)	Clearance (L/min)	First-Pass (%)
Triamcinolone acetonide	1.5	2.1	1.2	—
Beclomethasone dipropionate	—	—	—	—
Flunisolide	1.6	1.8	1.0	20
Budesonide	2.8	4.3	1.0	10
Fluticasone dipropionate	3.1	3.7[a]	0.87	—

[a]Assuming a mean body weight of 70 kg

From Barnes PJ, Pedersen S. Efficacy and safety of inhaled corticosteroids in asthma. *Am Rev Respir Dis* 1993;148:S7, with permission.

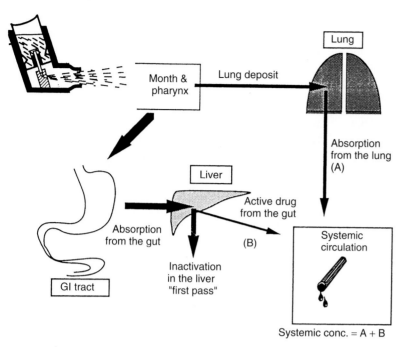

FIGURE 8-6. The fate of inhaled steroids. The amount of an inhaled glucocorticosteroid reaching the systemic circulation is the sum of the pulmonary and orally bioavailable fraction. The fraction deposited in the mouth is swallowed, and the systemic availability is determined by absorption from the gastrointestinal tract and by the degree of first-pass metabolism. The fraction deposited in the intrapulmonary airways is likely to be more or less completely absorbed in active form to the systemic circulation as there is no evidence for any degree of metabolic inactivation in currently used inhaled steroids. The systemic concentration will be reduced by continuous recirculation and inactivation in the liver. (From Barnes PJ, Pedersen S. Efficacy and safety of inhaled corticosteroids in asthma. *Am Rev Respir Dis* 1993;148:S9, with permission.)

(mean duration 6.2 ± 5 years) (233). Over a 3- to 5-year period, 24 patients (60%) had unchanged long-term prednisone requirement, 13 patients (32.5%) improved with a reduction in prednisone requirement, and 3 patients (7.5%) deteriorated with increased prednisone requirement. Unfortunately, this study did not report the maintenance dose of beclomethasone. Corrigan et al. evaluated the possible mechanism of glucocorticoid resistance in chronic asthma (234). Patients were defined as having glucocorticoid resistance if there was less than a 30% increase in FEV_1 after 2 weeks of daily prednisone, 20 mg for the first week and 40 mg for the second week. Glucocorticoid pharmacokinetics, receptor characteristics, and inhibition of peripheral blood T-cell proliferation by glucocorticoid were assayed. Overall, the investigators noted a relative insensitivity of T lymphocytes to glucocorticoid in patients with clinical glucocorticoid resistance compared with matched glucocorticoid-sensitive asthmatics. They noted that the resistance does not reflect abnormal glucocorticoid clearance. Additional studies by this group suggested that activated T lymphocytes may be the target, and, perhaps, an anti–T lymphocyte drug such as cyclosporine may be particularly useful in glucocorticoid-resistant asthmatic patients. Overall, the clinical relevance of glucocorticoid resistance in patients with chronic steroid-dependent asthma remains speculative and poorly understood (235).

Side effects of inhaled corticosteroids are being increasingly recognized as a potential problem (236,237). The factors that may contribute to toxicity include the total dose, the dosing schedule, whether a spacer device is used, whether mouth rinsing is used, and the sensitivity of the parameter used to assess systemic toxicity (199,219). The adverse effects of inhaled corticosteroids can be broadly classified as topical or systemic. The three main topical side effects are cough, oral candidiasis, and dysphonia. Slow inhalation, use of a spacer device, and gargling reduce the incidence of these side effects (238). The systemic side effects may include suppression of the HPA axis; adverse effects on bone metabolism including osteoporosis, slowing of

growth in children and adolescents; cataract formation; bruising and dermal thinning; and psychological changes (199,239,240). Many studies have suggested that doses of inhaled corticosteroids in excess of 800 μg per day in adults or 400 μg per day in children appear to result in dose-related suppression of the HPA axis, with substantial interindividual variability and response (237). Some studies suggest that beclomethasone may have a somewhat greater propensity to produce adrenal suppression in comparison with budesonide at higher doses, although the relevance of this is not clear. Inhaled corticosteroids with doses as low as 400 μg per day have been associated with the development of osteoporosis (241,242).

Studies have shown biochemical abnormalities with higher doses of inhaled steroids (199). These abnormalities may be viewed as markers for the absorption and systemic effects (toxicity) of the inhaled steroids. Parameters have included morning serum cortisol and 24-hour urinary-free cortisol excretion for HPA-axis suppression; serum osteocalcin, bone-specific serum alkaline phosphatase, urinary hydroxyproline/calcium excretion, and bone densitometry for bone metabolism (bone formation and bone resorption); and slit lamp examination for cataract formation. The clinical significance of these subtle and sensitive markers of systemic effect and how they translate into clinical toxicity such as reduced bone growth, osteoporosis, or bone fractures remain poorly established. A variety of strategies may reduce the likelihood of systemic absorption and systemic side effects from inhaled steroids. These include: (a) use the lowest dose that is clinically necessary to achieve good asthma control (e.g., step down the number of puffs per day as control is achieved); (b) routinely use a spacer device with an MDI or use a DPI; (c) routinely use mouth rinsing; (d) twice-a-day dosing or dosing once a day at 4:00 PM; (e) for patients requiring higher doses of inhaled steroids, consider options for "inhaled steroid-sparing effect" with agents such as salmeterol, antileukotrienes, nedocromil, or theophylline.

One landmark study randomized 1,041 children from ages 5 to 12 with mild-to-moderate asthma for a study duration of 4 to 6 years into 3 groups (200 μg budesonide bid, 8 mg of nedocromil bid, or placebo) (243). Asthma clinical outcomes improved the most for the budesonide group (fewer hospitalizations, fewer urgent care visits, and decreased airway hyperresponsiveness to methacholine). However, there was no significant difference in the degree of change in FEV$_1$ after bronchodilator therapy between any of the three groups. Long-term therapy with budesonide was well tolerated; even though there was a 1.1-cm smaller increase in height compared with the placebo group during the first year, this reduction in linear growth velocity was absent by the second year, and the projected height in the budesonide-treated group was no different than in the nedocromil or placebo groups. Also, there were no significant differences in bone density or in the incidence of cataracts between the three groups. Although a number of other short-term studies have noted a reduction in height and in linear growth velocity over 6 to 12 months with inhaled steroids, longer-term studies have consistently noted that the final adult height is not influenced by inhaled corticosteroids.

Cromolyn Sodium and Nedocromil Sodium

Cromolyn sodium has been available in the United States since 1973. This medication is poorly absorbed orally and, therefore, is effective only when inhaled. Initially, cromolyn was available only as a 20-mg capsule containing finely powdered cromolyn and lactose particles delivered by a turbo inhaler (Spinhaler). Its usefulness in this form was limited by oral pharyngeal irritation and cough. Subsequently, cromolyn was introduced as a nebulizer solution in 1982 and in a pressurized MDI in 1986.

Cromolyn sodium administered prior to allergen exposure blocks both the EAR and LAR following antigen inhalation (244). Cromolyn has not demonstrated smooth-muscle relaxant properties and, therefore, is not a bronchodilator. It has long been held that the primary mechanism of action appears to be inhibition of mediator release from mast cells. Although the exact mechanism by which cromolyn inhibits mast-cell mediator release is not known, it is believed to inhibit calcium influx by phosphorylation of a membrane protein. Other mechanisms of action of cromolyn include suppression of nonmyelinated vagal sensory nerve endings, inhibition of inflammatory cells other than mast cells, and reduction of airway permeability.

Cromolyn has protective effects against provocative stimuli such as allergen, cold air, SO$_2$, and exercise (244) and is most effective when administered before challenge. The protective effects against nonspecific agents such as methacholine and histamine have been less established. Studies in which cromolyn was administered for longer than 6 weeks suggest an improvement in airway reactivity. Despite initial notions that cromolyn would be more effective in extrinsic than in intrinsic asthma, most carefully designed studies do not support this concept. About 60% to 79% of asthmatics show a response to cromolyn. Studies comparing cromolyn and theophylline in the short-term management of chronic asthma suggest that both of these agents are equally effective, with perhaps greater side effects with theophylline. There are some data to show that there is an additive effect between these two agents. Toogood et al. did not find any advantage in adding cromolyn to an established regimen of beclomethasone (245).

Nedocromil sodium (Tilade) is structurally different from cromolyn, but it has very similar pharmacologic activities. Nedocromil was approved for use in the United States in MDIs in 1992. The mechanism of action of nedocromil appears to be quite similar to cromolyn. A number of *in vitro* and *in vivo* studies suggest that nedocromil blocks both the EAR and LAR (246,247). Nedocromil has antiinflammatory properties on a number of cells. There is some suggestion that nedocromil may be more potent in inhibiting bronchial C-fiber nerve endings.

A recent meta-analysis concluded that nedocromil is more effective than placebo in treating asthma and is of most benefit to patients who are receiving monotherapy with bronchodilators (247–249). The aggregate data suggested that nedocromil is less potent than inhaled corticosteroids, although some inhaled corticosteroid-sparing effects were noted. Nedocromil represents an alternative to cromolyn, although there is no clear advantage for nedocromil over inhaled steroids and the costs are higher (244).

Overall, inhaled corticosteroids are preferred in the majority of patients for chronic asthma because of proven efficacy, greater potency than cromolyn or nedocromil, and effectiveness when administered twice a day as opposed to four times a day (199). Also, there are more data supporting improvement of inflammation as assessed by BAL and endobronchial biopsy in patients treated with inhaled corticosteroids (201–204).

ANTILEUKOTRIENES

Several lines of evidence indicate that leukotrienes play an important role in asthma (243,244). First, leukotrienes stimulate airway smooth-muscle contraction, produce mucosal edema and mucous secretions, and attract a variety of cells including eosinophils and neutrophils. Second, administering aerosolized leukotrienes can produce the typical physiologic and symptomatic changes characteristic of asthma. Third, antileukotrienes inhibit asthmatic responses to a variety of stimuli, including allergen, exercise, aspirin, and cold, dry air (63–68,250). Fourth, cysteinyl leukotrienes can be recovered from nasal secretions, bronchoalveolar lavage fluid, and urine of patients with asthma in increased concentrations compared with normal individuals. Finally, clinical trials have shown that leukotriene blockade has beneficial effects on chronic, spontaneously occurring asthma (i.e., without experimental provocation or challenge) in both adults and children (251–257).

Three antileukotriene agents have been approved in the United States for maintenance therapy for persistent asthma: zileuton, zafirlukast, and montelukast (69). These agents have different mechanisms of action: zileuton blocks a critical step in leukotriene production involving 5-lipoxygenase enzyme, whereas zafirlukast and montelukast prevent leukotrienes from binding to the common leukotriene receptor. There are no published studies comparing the leukotriene synthesis inhibitors with the receptor antagonists, and the relative differences in efficacy remain unknown.

A number of randomized, placebo-controlled phase-III clinical trials have been conducted in patients with mild-to-moderate chronic asthma with each of the three oral antileukotrienes and have demonstrated significant improvement compared to placebo in numerous parameters including symptoms, FEV$_1$, morning PEF, and need for rescue β-agonist use (251,253,257). These studies have varied in length from 4 weeks to 6 months, and improvements in symptoms and FEV$_1$ were seen as quickly as the first or second day, with peak responses by 2 weeks. These three agents are available as pills, requiring dosing of once a day for montelukast, twice a day for zafirlukast, and four times a day for zileuton. Montelukast is the only agent that is approved down to the age of 6, whereas the other two agents have approval for children over the age of 12. Zafirlukast needs to be taken on an empty stomach (1 hour before or 2 hours after meals) because food decreases absorption by as much as 40%. Studies suggest that there is a 5% incidence of liver function abnormalities with zileuton, and it is recommended that baseline alanine aminotransferase (ALT) be measured as well as monitored approximately seven times during the first year. Many patients with liver function abnormalities may continue to take the drug. With 20 mg of zafirlukast twice a day, the risk of liver function abnormalities appears to be quite low and routine monitoring is unnecessary. However, there have been isolated reports of liver function abnormalities at the higher dose of 80 mg per day. There are no published reports of liver function abnormalities with montelukast. Both zafirlukast and zileuton have several drug interactions, especially agents that are metabolized with the cytochrome P-450 system. Clearance is reduced for coumadin, theophylline, phenytoin, and carbamazepine.

In the initial postmarketing experience with the antileukotrienes, a report described eight patients with steroid-dependent asthma who developed a Churg–Strauss vasculitis syndrome (allergic granulomatosis angitis) while taking zafirlukast (258). All but one of these patients were receiving corticosteroids, and this syndrome occurred with tapering or discontinuation of systemic steroid therapy. Additional cases of Churg–Strauss syndrome have been reported with zafirlukast and, more recently, with montelukast as well (259). Whether this complication is directly drug-related to montelukast (either as an idiosyncratic drug reaction or by a class effect of cysteinyl leukotriene receptor blockade) or to tapering of systemic steroids and unmasking a *forme fruste* of Churg–Strauss syndrome remains unknown.

The exact place for antileukotrienes in the chronic maintenance therapy for asthma remains to be established (69,260, 261). EPR-2 indicates a possible role for these agents in the initial therapy for mild-persistent asthma as an alternative to inhaled corticosteroids, cromolyn, or nedocromil. Also, EPR-2 indicates a possible role for these agents as adjunctive therapy (in addition to inhaled steroids) for added asthma control at any level of severity for persistent asthma. These agents have effects on early and delayed asthma response; therefore, they act as a bronchodilator within 1 to 3 hours after administration as well as an antiinflammatory agent with a response over 2 to 4 weeks. The magnitude of increase in FEV_1 at 4 weeks is about 14% above the placebo (253). Data suggest that inhaled steroids have more potent effects compared with the antileukotrienes, but once- or twice-a-day oral therapy with the antileukotrienes offers a significant compliance advantage that may be important for some patients. Montelukast represents a significant advance for pediatric patients, being approved as a 5-mg chewable tablet for use once a day for ages 6 to 14 (256). The antileukotrienes do facilitate a reduction in the need for β-agonist and inhaled steroids, thereby minimizing well-known side effects. Currently, the indications for antileukotrienes could be summarized as: (a) patients on moderate-to-high doses of inhaled steroids with breakthrough symptoms, as an alternative to increasing the dose of inhaled steroids and/or as an alternative or adjunct to inhaled salmeterol; (b) maintenance therapy for aspirin-sensitive asthmatics; (c) initial therapy for mild- or moderate-persistent chronic asthma in settings where there is a particular problem with adherence (as an alternative to inhaled steroid therapy); (d) alternative therapy to salmeterol or short-acting β-agonist for children with exercise-induced asthma.

ANTI-IgE

Omalizumab (Xolair), a monoclonal antibody that binds to IgE, was approved in June 2003 by the FDA as maintenance therapy for the prevention of asthma exacerbations and for the control of symptoms in adults and adolescents (12 years or older) with moderate-to-severe persistent allergic asthma that is inadequately controlled despite the use of inhaled corticosteroids (262–265). Additional criteria include a serum total IgE level between 30 and 700 IU/mL and a positive result on skin-prick testing or radioallergosorbent testing with at least one perennial (i.e., always present) allergen.

Omalizumab binds human IgE and prevents it from binding to mast cells. When given in sufficient dose, omalizumab can reduce free IgE levels by up to 98% (262,264). As a result of omalizumab therapy, fewer mast cells degranulate in response to allergen exposure.

Omalizumab is given subcutaneously, either monthly or every 2 weeks, depending on the dose. The dose is determined by the patient's body weight and serum IgE level (see Table 8-7). The maximum dose per injection site is 150 mg; if

TABLE 8-7. Omalizumab Doses for Asthma (Milligrams Administered Every 2 or 4 Weeks)

Pretreatment Serum IgE (IU/mL)	Body Weight (kg)			
	30–60	>60–70	>70–90	>90–150
≥30–100	150 q 4 wks	150 q 4 wks	150 q 4 wks	300 q 4 wks
>100–200	300 q 4 wks	300 q 4 wks	300 q 4 wks	225 q 2 wks
>200–300	300 q 4 wks	225 q 2 wks	225 q 2 wks	300 q 2 wks
>300–400	225 q 2 wks	225 q 2 wks	225 q 2 wks	300 q 2 wks
>400–500	300 q 2 wks	300 q 2 wks	375 q 2 wks	DO NOT USE
>500–600	300 q 2 wks	375 q 2 wks	DO NOT USE	
>600–700	375 q 2 wks	DO NOT USE		

q = every
From Omalizumab package insert. 1 DNA Way, San Francisco, CA: Genetech Inc.; June 2003, with permission.

a greater monthly dose is required, it can be split and administered at more than one site. If a monthly dose of 450 mg or more is required, the medication should be given every 2 weeks. At the current time, omalizumab is not FDA-approved at doses above 750 mg per month; therefore, some patients are ineligible for therapy because of high body weight and/or very elevated IgE levels. The current average wholesale price for a 150-mg vial is $540. Depending on the dose regimen, the cost for 1 year of treatment would range from $10,000 to $32,000.

Several aspects regarding the use or potential use of omalizumab remain to be clarified including the efficacy and safety of long-term use, its efficacy in nonatopic asthma, its ability to prevent airway remodeling, its role in patients receiving immunotherapy, its benefit in patients with severe, corticosteroid-dependent asthma (these patients have yet to be studied in large numbers), and its role in other disorders in which IgE is mechanistically involved (e.g., allergic bronchopulmonary aspergillosis).

ACUTE ASTHMA

There are about 500,000 hospitalizations for acute asthma per year in the United States, of which 65% occur in patients over 18 years of age (15,266). Acute asthma represents 4% of all emergency-room (ER) visits involving about 1.8 million people. Between 15% and 25% of ER visits result in hospital admission. About 20% to 30% of patients initially managed and discharged from the ER have a relapse (267). The average length of stay for patients admitted to the hospital is about 5 days (23). Of all hospital admissions, about 4% require intensive care and, of these, 1% to 30% require mechanical ventilation (268–271). Patients typically come to the ER and/or hospital for acute asthma when the episode is severe and when the tempo of illness is progressive and/or unresponsive to initial therapy. Acute asthma exacerbation often represents failure of outpatient maintenance therapy for several possible reasons: (a) lack of access to longitudinal medical care; (b) lack of objective monitoring of asthma, including home peak flow monitoring; (c) poor self-management skills, including patient nonadherence; and (d) inadequate pharmacotherapy prescription by the physician, most often, lack of inhaled corticosteroid maintenance therapy. For some patients, acute asthma exacerbation may be complicated by comorbid illness such as psychiatric illness, which makes outpatient management difficult (267a).

The initial management of an acute asthmatic in any setting should include administration of an aerosolized selective β_2-agonist on a repeated basis. β-Agonist may be administered by MDI with a spacer device, intermittent bolus nebulization, or continuous nebulization (138,272). Comparable clinical effects can be achieved with all three delivery methods. The potency ratio of a nebulizer to a MDI with spacer device is 7:1; therefore, one nebulization with 2.5 mg of albuterol is roughly equivalent to 4 to 12 puffs of albuterol MDI, delivering 90 μg per puff (equivalent dose range for the MDI is 0.36 to 1.08 mg). In an average adult, only 10% of the MDI dose reaches the lower airway; in patients with airflow obstruction, about 6% reaches the lower airway, with 3% to the most distal airways (135). Use of a spacer device roughly doubles this amount.

Patients with acute airflow obstruction refractory to intermittent, frequently aerosolized β-agonist therapy may be candidates for continuously nebulized bronchodilator therapy until the effects of antiinflammatory therapy are achieved (273–275). Recommended regimens are albuterol, 2.5 to 15 mg per hour, or terbutaline, 2 to 8 mg per hour. A variety of delivery methods for continuous nebulization have been described. Patients should receive continuous nebulization until they have improved enough to tolerate intermittent aerosol treatment every 4 hours. Extensive experience in children and the two reports in adults suggest that this approach is safe, although further studies in adults with underlying coronary artery disease are required.

Subcutaneous injection of β-agonist is used in the emergency treatment of acute asthma (276) when very severe airflow obstruction is present, limiting aerosol penetration into the bronchial tree. Although epinephrine (0.3 to 0.5 mL of 1:1000 aqueous solution) has long been used, terbutaline is available for subcutaneous administration as well. However, despite theoretical expectations, subcutaneous terbutaline is not associated with a decreased incidence of cardiac side effects in comparison with subcutaneous epinephrine (276,277).

Intravenous administration of β-agonist has been used in the treatment of severe acute bronchospasm (266,278). The theoretical rationale for this approach is to overcome problems related to decreased drug penetration and decreased β-adrenergic receptor responsiveness and thereby expose β-receptors to continuous and saturating levels of drug (279). Most of the experience with this therapy comes from Europe. In the United States, albuterol is not available for intravenous delivery. Albuterol might be preferable to isoproterenol because the chronotropic effect is far less. However, it is not clear in which patients, if any, intravenous delivery is preferable over aerosol or subcutaneous administration. Available comparisons between intravenous albuterol and aerosol albuterol for the treatment of acute asthma provide conflicting conclusions (278–281).

The role of aminophylline in the treatment of acute, severe asthma remains controversial (180,282–284). Early studies suggested that the addition of aminophylline to maximal therapy with inhaled β-agonists in the ER had little effect on pulmonary function parameters during 3 hours of observation (285–287). In 1988, a meta-analysis of 13 controlled trials compared aminophylline therapy with a control regimen consisting of albuterol, epinephrine, or other sympathomimetic bronchodilators (288). Overall, the pooled data found no difference between the aminophylline-treated group and the control groups, with three studies favoring aminophylline, three favoring the control regimen, and seven showing no difference between the two.

More recently, several studies have evaluated the role of aminophylline in the treatment of acute exacerbation of asthma when used in addition to inhaled β-agonists and intravenous corticosteroids, both in the emergency room and in the hospital for both adults and children (289–294). In a prospective study of 133 adult patients (290) maximally treated with intravenous corticosteroids and inhaled β-agonists, administration of aminophylline resulted in a threefold decrease in the hospital admission rate for patients treated with aminophylline (6%) compared with placebo recipients (21%). Surprisingly, the reduction in admissions occurred despite an absence of improvement in pulmonary function, as measured by spirometry. The admission decision was made by noninvestigator house staff by use of preexisting guidelines for admission. Huang et al., in a placebo-controlled randomized trial of aminophylline infusion in addition to inhaled albuterol and intravenous methylprednisolone, found that the improvement in FEV_1 at 3 hours was greater in the aminophylline group ($29\% \pm 23\%$ compared with $10\% \pm 10\%$) and that the aminophylline-treated patients required fewer nebulizations of albuterol (292). A concern with this study is whether the patients received maximal inhaled β-agonist therapy. Also, it is unclear how the decision to administer "as-needed" albuterol therapy was made because this was one of the endpoints of the study. In contrast, two recent studies in children did not find that intravenous theophylline added to the management of hospitalized pediatric asthmatics maximally treated with nebulized albuterol and intravenous corticosteroids (293,294). However, both EPR-2 and the British Thoracic Society recommend the use of intravenous theophylline in patients admitted to the hospital for an acute exacerbation of asthma (1,284).

The role of inhaled anticholinergic agents in the management of acute asthma is limited. The usefulness of atropine is limited by systemic side effects (295). Ipratropium is generally inferior to the β-agonists as sole therapy for acute asthma (296–299). Several studies have shown that the combination of high-dose ipratropium (500 μg) and the β-adrenergic agent is more effective than either drug used alone (300–302).

The efficacy of systemic corticosteroids (oral or intravenous) in acute severe asthma is quite well established in 15 clinical trials of acute asthma in adults (303). Fanta et al. demonstrated that in patients with acute severe episodes of asthma refractory to 8 hours of conventional bronchodilator therapy, those who were given intravenous corticosteroids had significantly greater resolution of airflow obstruction by the end of 24 hours (304). Littenberg and Gluck demonstrated that the prompt use of glucocorticoids in the emergency treatment of severe asthma can prevent significant morbidity, reduce the number of hospitalizations, and effect substantial savings in health care costs (305). In contrast, Stein and Cole, in a placebo-controlled trial of 81 adults with acute asthma in the ER, failed to show that early administration of intravenous corticosteroids reduces the hospital admission rate (18% for the steroid group and 13% for the control group) (306). However, the admitted patients did begin with lower PEFs and, at 2 hours, responded less to inhaled bronchodilators. It is likely that the severity of underlying airflow obstruction and inflammation on initial presentation is what determines the need for admission (303). It is clear that the onset of action is delayed at least 6 to 12 hours following systemic administration of corticosteroids (307).

As bioavailability after oral therapy is quite high for prednisone, some have recommended "noninvasive" therapy by the use of oral steroids in acute asthma exacerbation (308). Although the optimal dosage for systemic steroids has not been established, McFadden's review of the available studies suggest that hydrocortisone equivalent to 14 mg per kg per 24 hours is effective therapy for acutely ill asthmatic adults (307–313). It is common practice to administer 120 to 180 mg of methylprednisolone per day intravenously in divided doses. As an alternative, oral therapy may be given in divided doses (e.g., 150 to 225 mg of prednisone) (307). Likewise, the optimal schedule of steroid withdrawal following an acute exacerbation is not well established. In one study, Lederle et al. suggested that the relapse rate was not different between a steroid taper of 1 week compared with 7 weeks, although the relapse rate was quite high in both groups (311).

Therefore, the conventional therapy for acute severe asthma exacerbation would include repeated aerosolized β-agonist, oxygen, and systemic corticosteroids. Forced hydration and antibiotics are usually not required. Reassessment at frequent intervals by physical examination and by peak flow meter should be performed to determine whether the patient is improving, staying about the same, or deteriorating. Response to therapy is probably the single most important factor that helps in determining the need for hospital admission. It is true that patients showing improvements on this therapy and being discharged home with oral corticosteroids do well without significant relapse. A practical duration of treatment in a typical ER setting is about 4 hours (180). If a patient requires further therapy after 4 hours, then the next decision is whether to admit the patient for prolonged inpatient care or to continue therapy in the setting of an ER-based observation unit or holding room, when these facilities are available. There are conflicting data on whether these observation units (typically consisting of care for 12 to 24 hours) lessen the need for hospital admission, reduce the total length of stay, or are cost effective (314). For patients who are admitted to the hospital, the next decision is whether to manage them on a regular nursing floor or in the intensive care unit. Patients with severe airflow obstruction who are deteriorating despite conventional therapy (based on evidence of respiratory muscle fatigue and/or respiratory depression) should be managed in a closely monitored intensive care setting to assess serially the need for airway support and mechanical ventilation (278,315). For all other patients, therapy could be continued on a regular floor with frequent "every 2 to 4 hours" administration of aerosolized β-agonist and serial peak flow measurements.

For the subset of patients with a delayed or inadequate response to initial therapy, a variety of unconventional therapies may be considered. These include the use of intravenous magnesium, inhalation of helium–oxygen gas, and noninvasive positive pressure ventilation (316–320). Although there are published reports in support of each of these therapies, they should be considered experimental and be reserved for patients who are not improving despite maximal conventional therapy. The rationale for the use of intravenous magnesium is based on the fact that magnesium inhibits calcium channels, reduces the acetylcholine release, and may improve respiratory function. In addition, serum level of magnesium may be low in 50% of patients with acute asthma exacerbation. Although there are several uncontrolled studies that have shown beneficial effects with intravenous magnesium, at least two recent randomized clinical trials have not shown a benefit compared to placebo (316,317). Heliox is a blend of helium and oxygen. When inhaled by an asthmatic, turbulent flow in narrowed airways may become laminar, thereby reducing the resistive work of breathing. Several prospective, uncontrolled studies have shown improvement in peak flows, respiratory muscle fatigue, and reversal of hypercapnia (318,319). It is important to recognize that the heliox mixture typically uses 50% to 80% helium; therefore, patients who are severely hypoxemic are not appropriate candidates. Noninvasive positive pressure ventilation has been used for patients with acute asthma with an inadequate initial response to therapy. Several uncontrolled small series and case reports suggest that continuous positive airway pressure therapy with 5 to 7.5 cm H_2O can help unload the inspiratory muscles and avoid intubation (320). The use of this modality is labor intensive and should be reserved for a small number of carefully selected patients in the intensive care unit.

A small subset of patients may have such severe airflow obstruction and airway inflammation so as not to be able to maintain spontaneous ventilation despite aggressive initial therapy (278,315). These patients require intubation and mechanical ventilation. Good sedating agents to facilitate intubation include midazolam (a short-acting benzodiazepam), ketamine, or propofol (321–323). It is best to avoid morphine at the time of intubation because it can produce hypotension, induce nausea and emesis, and contribute to bronchospasm by histamine release. Ketamine, a phencyclidine that inhibits the reuptake of catecholamines, is commonly used as an induction agent prior to administration of general anesthetics. It has a rapid onset, is short acting, and has the advantage of being a bronchodilator, a vagolytic agent, and, perhaps, an antiinflammatory agent (321).

Early studies of the use of mechanical ventilation in patients with status asthmaticus in the 1970s indicated significant mortality ranging from 9% to 39% as well as significant iatrogenic complications (268). However, over the past 20 years, the prognosis for ventilated acute asthmatics has improved dramatically (324). The key principle that has evolved for mechanical ventilation of patients with status asthmaticus is controlled hypoventilation to avoid iatrogenic complications related to high airway pressures and/or auto-positive end expiratory pressure (auto-peep) (325). Specific ventilatory strategies to minimize airway pressure and auto-peep in this setting include reducing the minute ventilation by reducing the rate or tidal volume or both. This may require acceptance of hypercapnia and respiratory acidosis (a pH as low as 7.2 appears safe; supplementation with intravenous bicarbonate can be considered if the pH goes lower), a strategy referred to as "permissive hypercapnia." Patients who are mechanically ventilated by this strategy will usually require heavy sedation with benzodiazepines or narcotics, but every effort should be made to avoid neuromuscular blockade. Patients with status asthmaticus are typically treated with systemic corticosteroids, and the combination of neuromuscular blockers and corticosteroids seems to be a significant risk factor for the development of prolonged paralysis (326).

ALTERNATIVE ANTIINFLAMMATORY THERAPY

About 5% to 20% of patients continue to have troublesome asthma symptoms with frequent exacerbations, requiring hospitalization despite maximal conventional therapy (1). The reversible factors that contribute to this subset of "steroid-dependent" asthma include patient noncompliance, poor self-management skills, inadequate control of allergen burden at home, inadequate inhaler technique, and suboptimal pharmacotherapy prescription by the physician. Data from the placebo arm of a number of studies have clearly shown that a compulsory conventional management plan, with frequent follow-up, perhaps in an asthma center, can reduce the need for oral steroids by 16% to 40% in "steroid-dependent" asthmatics (327,328).

Several alternative antiinflammatory therapies with a putative steroid-sparing effect in asthma (329–336) have been evaluated. A meta-analysis reviewed the results of 11 published trials of methotrexate for steroid-dependent asthma (335). Overall, six of 11 studies concluded that methotrexate did not have a steroid-sparing effect, but subgroup analysis showed potential steroid-sparing effects with methotrexate therapy for greater than 6 months, low long-term steroid therapy ($\leq$20 mg per day), and a study design incorporating a run-in period. In summary, on the basis of the available studies, it is difficult to recommend therapy with methotrexate outside the setting of a clinical trial.

Both oral and parenteral gold preparations have been used in the therapy of steroid-dependent asthma (337–341). These studies have generally found that the addition of gold can decrease corticosteroid requirement, can improve symptoms, and, perhaps, can improve bronchial hyperreactivity as well. In addition to a number of methodologic limitations with these studies, overall patient tolerance has been poor and the incidence of side effects has been as high as 37%, including diarrhea, skin eruptions, and proteinuria. There are no data on long-term side effects or patient compliance with gold therapy for patients with bronchial asthma.

Another steroid-sparing approach in the treatment of chronic asthma has been the use of troleandomycin, a macrolide antibiotic (342–347). However, the principal effect of troleandomycin appears to be the prolongation of the plasma half-life of corticosteroids through the inhibition of their elimination, and its use does not reduce long-term steroid-induced side effects (347). There appears to be no basis to recommend the use of troleandomycin.

Cyclosporine inhibits mediator release from mast cells and basophils, as well as the synthesis of lymphokines, with resulting downregulation of CD4-positive T lymphocytes. Although CsA therapy can achieve a significant reduction in prednisone dosage in some patients (348–350), the side effects (hypertension, hypertrichosis, neurologic disturbances, and nephrotoxicity) are potentially severe. On balance, the use of cyclosporine for asthma remains investigational.

EXPERIMENTAL OR EMERGING THERAPIES

As previously discussed, T_{H2} cells and their derived cytokines IL-4, IL-5, and IL-13 play a critical role in orchestrating eosinophilia and asthmatic airway inflammation in various models of asthma. Over the past few years, there have been several early phase human studies with pharmacologic approaches to antagonize these pathways, with mixed results (351–353). Although the animal studies had been very promising, an important study using intravenous humanized monoclonal antibody to IL-5 was disappointing in a double-blind, placebo-controlled trial using an inhaled allergen-challenge model (351). Even though a single intravenous dose of anti-IL-5 decreased blood eosinophilia for 16 weeks and sputum eosinophilia for 4 weeks, there was no significant effect on the LAR or on the airway hyperresponsiveness to allergen challenge. This study raises serious questions about the relative importance of the eosinophil in mediating human asthma. Studies with inhaled soluble IL-4 receptor antagonist, altrakincept (Nuvance), found modest benefit, but further development was discontinued by the manufacturer. In a placebo-controlled, parallel-group study of 62 moderate-persistent asthmatics dependent on moderate doses of inhaled corticosteroids, IL-4R by once-weekly nebulization for 12 weeks produced modest improvements in symptom scores and in FEV_1 in the highest dose group, but the asthma exacerbation rate was not affected (352). IL-13 antagonists have shown promise in a primate model of asthma and early clinical studies are being initiated in patients.

Steroids are exquisitely active and effective in asthma, but concern for toxicity even with topical steroids has limited their wider use. A variety of approaches are being pursued to maximize local activity within the airways and, at the same time, to minimize systemic absorption and toxicity (353). These approaches include the following: (a) development of "onsite-activated steroids" such as ciclesonide, which is a nonhalogenated inhaled steroid prodrug that requires endogenous cleavage by esterases for activity; (b) development of "soft steroids" that have improved local, topical selectivity and have much less steroid effect outside the target areas (e.g., lactone–glucocorticosteroid conjugate, which may be inactivated by esterases or other enzymes); and (c) "dissociated steroids" or agents that favor monomeric glucocorticosteriod receptor complexes (produce "transrepression") and avoid dimerization or "transactivation," which is undesirable in asthma. Agents from each of these categories are undergoing clinical trials.

SUMMARY

Asthma causes significant morbidity in the United States. In response to this need, several detailed practice guidelines have been put forth by expert panels and have been disseminated widely. A major challenge is the implementation of basic asthma management principles widely at the community level. Key issues include education of primary health care providers; establishment of programs for asthma education; use of longitudinal, outpatient, follow-up care with "easy access" to providers; and emphasis on chronic maintenance anti-inflammatory therapy rather than acute episodic care.

Asthma is being aggressively targeted by a variety of research efforts. Whether asthma is a single disorder with a unique cause or a syndrome of multiple disorders with several etiologic mechanisms remains unclear. The critical and rate-limiting steps in the asthma inflammatory cascade remain to be established. The natural history of the disease is not well understood and the significance of airway hyperreactivity in asymptomatic individuals is unknown. The contribution of genetic factors, atopic status, environmental factors, and viral infections is not well understood. Future therapeutic strategies will in part be dependent on the answers to some of these unresolved issues.

REFERENCES

1. National Heart, Lung and Blood Institute. National Asthma Education and Prevention Program. Expert Panel Report 2. *Guidelines for the diagnosis and management of asthma*. Bethesda National Institutes of Health, 1997, Publication No. 97–4051.
2. National Heart, Lung and Blood Institute, National Institutes of Health. International consensus report on diagnosis and management of asthma. *Eur Respir J* 1992;5:601–641.
3. U.S. Department of Health. Prevalence of selected chronic respiratory conditions—United States, 1970. *U.S. Department of Health, Education, and Welfare Series* 10, No. 84, 1973.
4. Bonner JR. The epidemiology and natural history of asthma. *Clin Chest Med* 1984;5:557–565.
5. Broder I, Higgins MW, Mathews KD, et al. Epidemiology of asthma and allergic rhinitis in a total community, Tecumseh, Michigan. *J Allergy Clin Immunol* 1974;53:127–138.
6. Gergen PJ, Mullally DI, Evans R. National survey of prevalence of asthma among children in the U.S., 1976–1980. *Pediatrics* 1988;81:1–7.
7. Asthma mortality and hospitalization among children and young adults—United States, 1980–1993. *MMWR* 1996;45:350–353.
8. Mannino DM, Homa DM, Pertowski LA, et al. Surveillance for asthma—United States,1960–1995. *MMWR* 1998;47:1–27.
9. Skobeloff EM, Spivey WH, St. Clair SS, et al. The influence of age and sex on asthma admissions. *JAMA* 1992;268:3437–3440.
10. Jackson RT, Beaglehole R, Rea HH, et al. Mortality from asthma: a new epidemic in New Zealand. *Br Med J* 1982;285:771–774.
11. Sears MR, Rea HH, Beaglehole R. Asthma mortality: a review of recent experience in New Zealand. *J Allergy Clin Immunol* 1987;80:319–325.
12. Sears MR. Epidemiological trends in bronchial asthma. In: Kaliner MA, Barnes PJ, Persson CGA, eds. *Asthma, its pathology and treatment*. New York: Marcel Dekker Inc, 1991:1–49.
13. Buist AS, Sears MR, Reid LM, et al. Asthma mortality: trends and determinants. *Am Rev Respir Dis* 1987;135:1037–1039.
14. Sly RM. Mortality from asthma. *J Allergy Clin Immunol* 1989;84:421–434.
15. Mannino DM, Homa DM, Akinbami LJ, et al. Surveillance for asthma – United States, 1980-1999. *MMWR* 2002;51:1–13.
16. Rea HH, Sears MR, Beaglehole R, et al. Lessons from the national asthma mortality study: circumstances surrounding death. *N Z Med J* 1987;100:10–13.
17. Benatar SR. Fatal asthma. *N Engl J Med* 1986;314:423–429.
18. Rea HH, Seragg R, Jackson R, et al. A case-control study of deaths from asthma. *Thorax* 1986;41:833–839.
19. Strunk RC. Death due to asthma. *Am Rev Respir Dis* 1993;148:550–552.
20. Weiss KB, Wagener DK. Changing patterns of asthma mortality: identifying target populations at high risk. *JAMA* 1990;264:1683–1687.
21. Molfino NA, Nannini LJ, Rebuck AS, et al. The fatality-prone asthmatic patient. *Chest* 1992;101:621–623.
22. Reid LM. The presence or absence of bronchial mucous in fatal asthma. *J Allergy Clin Immunol* 1987;80:415–416.
23. Smith DH, Malone D, Lawson KA, et al. A national estimate of the economic costs of asthma. *Am J Respir Crit Care Med* 1997;156:787–793.
24. Nelson HS, Szeffler SJ, Martin RJ. Regular inhaled beta-adrenergic agonists in the treatment of bronchial asthma: beneficial or detrimental. *Am Rev Respir Dis* 1991;144:249–250.
25. Grainger J, Woodsman K, Pearce N, et al. Prescribed fenoterol and death from asthma in New Zealand, 1981-7: a further case-control study. *Thorax* 1991;46:105–111.
26. Sears MR, Taylor DR, Pring CG, et al. Regular inhaled beta-agonist treatment in bronchial asthma. *Lancet* 1990;336:1391–1396.
27. Spitzer WO, Suissa S, Ernst P, et al. The use of β-agonists and the risk of death and near death from asthma. *N Engl J Med* 1992;326:501–506.
28. Ernst P, Habbick B, Suissa S, et al. Is the association between inhaled beta-agonist use and life-threatening asthma because of confounding by severity? *Am Rev Respir Dis* 1993;148:75–79.

29. Vastag B. Health agencies update: asthma safety study stopped. *JAMA* 2003;289(7):833.
30. Drazen JM, Israel E, Boushey HA, et al. Comparison of regularly scheduled with as-needed use of albuterol in mild asthma. Asthma clinical research network. *N Engl J Med* 1996;335:841–847.
31. Salpeter SR, Ormiston TM, Salpeter EE. Meta-analysis: respiratory tolerance to regular beta2-agonist use in patients with asthma. *Ann Intern Med.* 2004 May 18;140(10):802–813.
32. Larj MJ, Bleecker ER. Effects of beta2-agonists on airway tone and bronchial responsiveness. *J Allergy Clin Immunol.* 2002;110(6 Suppl.):S304–S312.
33. Silverman EK, Kwiatkowski DJ, Sylvia JS, et al. Family-based association analysis of beta2-adrenergic receptor polymorphisms in the childhood asthma management program. *J Allergy Clin Immunol* 2003;112(5):870–876.
34. McGraw DW, Almoosa KF, Paul RJ, et al. Antithetic regulation by beta-adrenergic receptors of Gq receptor signaling via phospholipase C underlies the airway beta-agonist paradox. *J Clin Invest.* 2003;112(4):619–626.
35. Palmer LJ, Silverman ES, Weiss ST, et al. Pharmacogenetics of asthma. *Am J Respir Crit Care Med* 2002;165:861–866.
36. Rackemann FM, Edwards MC. Asthma in children. *N Engl J Med* 1952;246:858–863.
37. Blair H. Natural history of childhood asthma. *Arch Dis Child* 1977;52:613–619.
38. Martin AJ, McLennan LA, Landau LI, et al. The natural history of childhood asthma to adult life. *Br Med J* 1980;1:1397–1400.
39. Brown PJ, Greville HW, Finvcane KE. Asthma and irreversible airflow obstruction. *Thorax* 1984;39:131–136.
40. Braman SS, Kaemmerlen JT, Davis SM. Asthma in the elderly: a comparison between patients with recently acquired and long-standing disease. *Am Rev Respir Dis* 1991;143:336–340.
41. Backman KS, Greenberger PA, Patterson R. Airways obstruction in patients with long-term asthma consistent with "irreversible asthma." *Chest* 1997;112:1234–1240.
42. Selroos O, Pietinalho A, Lofroos AB, et al. Effect of early vs late intervention with inhaled corticosteroids in asthma. *Chest* 1995;108:1228–1234.
43. Bronnimann S, Burrows B. A prospective study of the natural history of asthma. *Chest* 1986;90:480–484.
44. Broder I, Barlow PP, Horton RJM. The epidemiology of asthma and hay fever in a total community, Tecumseh, Michigan. *J Allergy* 1962;33:524–531.
45. Hogg JC. The pathology of asthma. *Clin Chest Med* 1984;5:567–571.
46. MacDonald JB, MacDonald ET, Seaton A, et al. Asthma deaths in Cardiff 1963–74: fifty-three deaths in hospital. *Br Med J* 1976;2:721–723.
47. Laitinen LA, Heino M, Laitinen A, et al. Damage of the airway epithelium and bronchial reactivity in patients with asthma. *Am Rev Respir Dis* 1985;131:599–606.
48. Elias JA, Lee CG, Zheng T, et al. New insights into the pathogenesis of asthma. *J Clin Invest.* 2003;111(3):291–297.
49. Kavuru MS, Dweik RA, Thomassen MJ. Role of bronchoscopy in asthma research. *Clin Chest Med* 1999;10(1):153–189.
50. Smith DL, Deshazo RD. State of the art: bronchoalveolar lavage in asthma: an update and perspective. *Am Rev Respir Dis* 1993;148:523–532.
51. Djukanovic R, Roche WR, Wilson JW, et al. Mucosal inflammation in asthma. *Am Rev Respir Dis* 1990;142:434–457.
52. Beasley R, Roche WR, Roberts JA, et al. Cellular events in the bronchi in mild asthma and after bronchial provocation. *Am Rev Respir Dis* 1989;139:806–817.
53. Sheppard D. Airway hyperresponsiveness: mechanisms in experimental models. *Chest* 1989;96:1165–1168.
54. Bigby TD, Nadel JA. Asthma. In: Gallin JI, Goldstein IM, Snyderman R, eds. *Inflammation: basic principles and clinical correlates,* 2nd ed. New York: Raven Press, 1992:889–906.
55. Herxheimer H. The late bronchial reaction in induced asthma. *Intl Arch Allergy Appl Immunol* 1952;3:323–328.
56. Cartier A, Thomson NC, Frith PA, et al. Allergen-induced increase in bronchial responsiveness to histamine: relationship to the late asthmatic response and change in airway caliber. *J Allergy Clin Immunol* 1982;70:170–177.
57. Booij-Noord H, De Vries K, Sluiter HJ, et al. Late bronchial obstructive reaction to experimental inhalation of house dust extract. *Clin Allergy* 1972;2:43–61.
58. Robinson DS, Hamid Q, Ying S, et al. Predominant T_{H2}-like bronchoalveolar T-lymphocyte population in atopic asthma. *N Engl J Med* 1992;326:298–304.
59. Kay AB. Helper (CD4) T cells and eosinophils in allergy and asthma. *Am Rev Respir Dis* 1992;14:S22–S26.
60. Kay AB. Origin of type 2 helper T cells. *N Engl J Med* 1994;330:567–568.
61. Wilson JW, Djukanovic R, Howarth PH, et al. Lymphocyte activation in bronchoalveolar lavage and peripheral blood in atopic asthma. *Am Rev Respir Dis* 1992;145:958–960.
62. Weiss ST, Eat dirt – The hygiene hypothesis and allergic diseases. *N Engl J Med* 2002;347:930–931.
63. Samuelsson B, Dahlen SE, Lindgren JA, et al. Leukotrienes and lipoxins: structures, biosynthesis, and biological effects. *Science* 1987;237:1171–1176.
64. Drazen JM, Austen KF. Leukotrienes and airway responses. *Am Rev Respir Dis* 1987;136:985–998.
65. Drazen JM. Inhalation challenge with sulfidopeptide leukotrienes in human subjects. *Chest* 1986;89:414–419.
66. Taylor IK, O'Shaughnessy KM, Fuller Rw, et al. Effect of cysteinyl-leukotriene receptor antagonist ICI 204.219 on allergen-induced bronchoconstriction and airway hyperreactivity in atopic subjects. *Lancet* 1991;337:690–694.
67. Israel E, Dermarkarian R, Rosenberg M, et al. The effects of 5-lipoxygenase inhibitor on asthma induced by cold, dry air. *N Engl J Med* 1990;323:1740–1744.
68. Dahlen B, Kumlin M, Margolskee DJ, et al. The leukotriene-receptor antagonist MK-0679 blocks airway obstruction induced by inhaled lysine-aspirin in aspirin-sensitive asthmatics. *Eur Respir J* 1993;6:1018–1026.
69. Kavuru MS, Subramony R, Vann AR. Antileukotrienes and asthma; alternative or adjunct to inhaled steroids? *Cleve Clin J Med* 1998;65:519–523.
70. Turner-Warwick M. Epidemiology of nocturnal asthma. *Am J Med* 1998;85:6–8.
71. McFadden ER. Exertional dyspnea and cough as preludes to acute attacks of bronchial asthma. *N Engl J Med* 1975;292:555–559.
72. Corrao WM, Braman SS, Irwin RS. Chronic cough as the sole manifestation of bronchial asthma. *N Engl J Med* 1979;300:633–637.
73. Irwin RS, Corrao WM, Pratter MR. Chronic persistent cough in the adult: the spectrum and frequency of causes and successful outcome of specific therapy. *Am Rev Respir Dis* 1981;123:413–417.
74. Christopher KL, Wood RP, Eckert RC, et al. Vocal-cord dysfunction presenting as asthma. *N Engl J Med* 1983;308:1566–1570.
75. Downing ET, Braman SS, Fox MJ, et al. Factitious asthma: physiological approach to diagnosis. *JAMA* 1982;248:2878–2881.
76. Miller RD, Hyatt RE. Evaluation of obstructing lesions of the trachea and larynx by flow-volume loops. *Am Rev Respir Dis* 1973;108:475–481.
77. McFadden ER Jr, Zawadski DK. Vocal cord dysfunction masquerading as exercise-induced asthma: a physiologic cause for "choking" during athletic activities. *Am J Respir Crit Care Med* 1996;153:942–947.
78. Shim CS, Williams MH Jr. Relationship of wheezing to the severity of obstruction in asthma. *Arch Intern Med* 1983;143:890–893.
79. McFadden ER, Kiser R, DeGroot WJ. Acute bronchial asthma: relations between clinical and physiologic manifestations. *N Engl J Med* 1973;288:221–225.
80. Veen J, Smits H, Ravensberg A, et al. Impaired perception of dyspnea in patients with severe asthma. *Am J Respir Crit Care Med* 1998;158:1134–1141.
81. Guidelines for the evaluation of impairment/disability in patients with asthma. *Am Rev Respir Dis* 1993;147:1056–1061.
82. Toren K, Brisman J, Jarvholm B. Asthma and asthma-like symptoms in adults assessed by questionnaires: a literature review. *Chest* 1993;104:600–608.
83. Juniper EF, Guyatt GH, Ferrie PJ, et al. Measuring quality of life in asthma. *Am Rev Respir Dis* 1993;147:832–838.
84. McFadden ER Jr. Clinical-physiologic correlates in asthma. *J Allergy Clin Immunol* 1986;77:1–5.

85. Shim CS, William MH. Evaluation of the severity of asthma: patients versus physicians. *Am J Med* 1980;68:11–13.
86. Knowles GK, Clark TJH. Pulsus paradoxus as a valuable sign indicating severity of asthma. *Lancet* 1973;11:1356–1359.
87. Rebuck AS, Pergelly LD. Development of pulsus paradoxus in the presence of airways obstruction. *N Engl J Med* 1973;288:66–69.
88. Kelsen SG, Kelsen DP, Fleegler BF, et al. Emergency room assessment and treatment of patients with acute asthma: adequacy of the conventional approach. *Am J Med* 1978;64:622–628.
89. Carden DL, Nowak RM, Sarkar D, et al. Vital signs including pulsus paradoxus in the assessment of acute bronchial asthma. *Ann Emerg Med* 1983;12:80–83.
90. Wright BM, McKerrow CB. Maximum forced expiratory flow rate as a measure of ventilatory capacity: with a description of a new portable instrument for measuring it. *Br Med J* 1959;2:1041–1047.
91. Berube D, Cartier A, L'Archeveque J, et al. Comparison of peak expiratory flow rate and FEV$_1$ in assessing bronchomotor tone after challenges with occupational sensitizers. *Chest* 1991;99:831–836.
92. Jain P, Kavuru MS, Emerman CL, et al. Utility of peak expiratory monitoring. *Chest* 1998;114:861–876.
93. Clark NM, Evans D, Mellins RB. Patient use of peak flow monitoring. *Am Rev Respir Dis* 1992;145:722–725.
94. Brenner BE. The acute asthmatic in the emergency department: the decision to admit or discharge. *Am J Emerg Med* 1985;3:74–77.
95. Banner AS, Shah RS, Addington WW. Rapid prediction of need for hospitalization in acute asthma. *JAMA* 1976;235:1337–1338.
96. Nowak RM, Gordon KR, Wroblewski DA, et al. Spirometric evaluation of acute bronchial asthma. *JACEP* 1979;8:9–12.
97. Lulla S, Newcomb RW. Emergency management of asthma in children. *Pediatrics* 1980;97:346–350.
98. Nowak RM, Pensier MI, Sarkar DD, et al. Comparison of peak expiratory flow and FEV$_1$ admission criteria for acute bronchial asthma. *Ann Emerg Med* 1982;11:64–69.
99. Fanta CH, Rossing TH, McFadden ER Jr. Emergency room treatment of acute asthma: relationships among therapeutic combinations, severity of obstruction, and time course of response. *Am J Med* 1982;72:416–422.
100. Fischl MA, Pitchenik A, Gardner LB. An index predicting relapse and need for hospitalization in patients with acute bronchial asthma. *N Engl J Med* 1981;305:783–789.
101. Rose CC, Murphy JG, Schwartz JS. Performance of an index predicting the response of patients with acute bronchial asthma to intensive emergency department treatment. *N Engl J Med* 1984;310:573–576.
102. Centor RM, Yarbrough B, Wood JP. Inability to predict relapse in acute asthma. *N Engl J Med* 1984;310:577–580.
103. Gershel JC, Goldman HS, Stein REK, et al. The usefulness of chest radiographs in first asthma attacks. *N Engl J Med* 1983;309:336–339.
104. McFadden ER Jr., Lyons HA. Arterial blood gas tension in asthma. *N Engl J Med* 1968;278:1027–1032.
105. Nowak RM, Tomlanovich MC, Sarkar DD, et al. Arterial blood gases and pulmonary function testing in acute bronchial asthma. *JAMA* 1983;249:2043–2046.
106. Kavuru MS, Richter JE. Medical treatment of gastroesophageal reflux disease and airway disease. In: Stein MR, ed. *GERD and airway disease*. Lung Biology in Health and Disease Series. New York: Marcell Dekker Inc, 1999:179–207.
107. Meeker DP, Wiedemann HP. Drug-induced bronchospasm. *Clin Chest Med* 1990;11(1):163–175.
108. Hannaway PJ, Hopper GDK. Severe anaphylaxis and drug-induced beta-blockade. *N Engl J Med* 1983;308:1536.
109. Lois M, Honig EG. β-blockade post-MI: safe for patients with asthma or COPD. *J Respir Dis* 1997;18:568–591.
110. Moser M. Angiotensin-converting enzyme inhibitors, angiotensin II receptor antagonists and calcium channel blocking agents: a review of potential benefits and possible adverse reactions. *J Am Coll Cardiol* 1997;29:1414–1421.
111. Greenberger PA. Allergic bronchopulmonary aspergillosis and fungoses. *Clin Chest Med* 1988;9:599–608.
112. Safirstein BH, D'Souza MF, Simon G, et al. Five-year follow-up of allergic bronchopulmonary aspergillosis. *Am Rev Respir Dis* 1973;108:450–460.
113. Nichols D, Dopico GA, Braun S, et al. Acute and chronic pulmonary function changes in allergic bronchopulmonary aspergillosis. *Am J Med* 1979;67:631–637.
114. Patterson R, Greenberger PA, Halwig JM, et al. Allergic bronchopulmonary aspergillosis: natural history and classification of early disease by serologic and radiologic studies. *Arch Intern Med* 1986;146:916–918.
115. Patterson R, Greenberger PA, Lee TM, et al. Prolonged evaluation of patients with corticosteroid-dependent asthma stage of bronchopulmonary aspergillosis. *J Allergy Clin Immunol* 1987;80: 663–668.
116. Doershug KC, Peterson MW, Dayton CS, et al. Asthma guidelines: an assessment of physician understanding and practice. *Am J Respir Crit Care Med* 1999;159:824–828.
117. Dekker FW, Dieleman FE, Kaptein AA, et al. Compliance with pulmonary medication in general practice. *Eur Respir J* 1993;6: 886–890.
118. Shim C, Williams MH Jr. The adequacy of inhalation of aerosol from canister nebulizer. *Am J Med* 1980;69:891–894.
119. Epstein SW, Manning CPR, Ashley MK, et al. Survey of the clinical use of pressurized aerosol inhalers. *Can Med Assoc J* 1979;120: 813–816.
120. Kelling JS, Strohl KP, Smith RL, et al. Physician knowledge in the use of canister nebulizers. *Chest* 1983;4:612–614.
121. Guidry CG, Brown WD, Stogner SW, et al. Incorrect use of metered dose inhalers by medical personnel. *Chest* 1992;101:31–33.
122. Hanania NA, Wittman R, Kesten S, et al. Medical personnel's knowledge of and ability to use inhaling devices. *Chest* 1994;105: 111–116.
123. Tashkin DP, Rand C, Nides M, et al. A nebulizer chronolog to monitor compliance with inhaler use. *Am J Med* 1991;91(Suppl. 4A): 33S–36S.
124. Blixen CE, Havstad S, Tilley BC, et al. A comparison of asthma-related healthcare use between African-Americans and Caucasians belonging to a health maintenance organization (HMO). *J Asthma* 1999;36:199–204.
125. Clark NM. Asthma self-management education: research and implications for clinical practice. *Chest* 1989;95:1110–1113.
126. Parker SR, Mellins RB, Sogn DD. Asthma education: a national strategy. *Am Rev Respir Dis* 1989;140:848–853.
127. Mayo PH, Richman J, Harris W. Results of a program to reduce admissions for adult asthma. *Ann Intern Med* 1990;112:864–871.
128. Wilson SR, Scamagas P, German DF, et al. A controlled trial of the two forms of self-management education for adults with asthma. *Am J Med* 1993;94:564–576.
129. Tougaard L, Krone T, Sorknaes A, et al. Economic benefits of teaching patients with chronic obstructive pulmonary disease about their illness. *Lancet* 1992;339:1617–1520.
130. Bailey WC, Richards JM, Brooks M, et al. A randomized trial to improve self-management practices of adults with asthma. *Arch Intern Med* 1990;150:1664–1668.
131. Bolton MB, Tilley BC, Kuder J, et al. The cost and effectiveness of an education program for adults who have asthma. *J Gen Intern Med* 1991;6:401–407.
132. Clark NM, Feldman CH, Evans D, et al. The impact of health education on frequency and cost of health care use by low income children with asthma. *J Allergy Clin Immunol* 1986;78:108–115.
133. Hilton S, Sibbald B, Anderson HR, et al. Controlled evaluation of the effects of patient education on asthma morbidity in general practice. *Lancet* 1986;1:26–29.
134. Yoon R, McKenzie DM, Miles DA, et al. Characteristics of attenders and non-attenders at an asthma education program. *Thorax* 1991;46:886–890.
135. Dolovich M, Ruffin RE, Roberts R, et al. Optimal delivery of aerosols from metered dose inhalers. *Chest* 1981;80(Suppl.): 911–915.
136. Sackner MA, Kim CS. Auxillary MDI aerosol delivery systems. *Chest* 1985;99(Suppl.):161S–170S.
137. Shim CS, Williams MH Jr. Effect of bronchodilator administered by canister versus jet nebulizer. *J Allergy Clin Immunol* 1984;73: 387–390.
138. Turner JR, Corkery KJ, Eckman D, et al. Equivalence of continuous flow nebulizer and metered dose inhaler with reservoir bag for treatment of acute air flow obstruction. *Chest* 1988;93:476–481.
139. Colacone A, Afilado M, Wolkove N, et al. A comparison of albuterol administered by metered dose inhaler (and holding chamber) or wet nebulizer in acute asthma. *Chest* 1993;104:835–841.

140. Orens DK, Kester L, Fergus LC, et al. Cost impact of metered dose inhalers vs small volume nebulizers in hospitalized patients: the Cleveland clinic experience. *Respir Care* 1991;36:1099–1104.

141. Sporik R, Holgate ST, Platts-Mills TAE, et al. Exposure to house-dust mite allergen (Der pI) and the development of asthma in childhood. *N Engl J Med* 1990;323:502–507.

142. Call RS, Smith TF, Morris E, et al. Risk factors for asthma in inner city children. *J Pediatr* 1992;121:862–866.

143. Creticos PS. Immunotherapy with allergens. *JAMA* 1992;268:2834–2839.

144. Platts-Mills TAE. Allergen-specific treatment for asthma. *Am Rev Respir Dis* 1993;148:553–555.

145. Platts-Mills TAE, de Week AL. Dust mite allergens and asthma—a worldwide problem. *J Allergy Clin Immunol* 1989;83:416–427.

146. Platts-Mills TAE, Pollart SM, Chapman MD, et al. Role of allergens in asthma and airway hyperresponsiveness: relevance to immunotherapy and allergen avoidance. In: Kaliner MA, Barnes PJ, Persson CGA, eds. *Asthma: its pathology and treatment.* New York: Marcel Dekker Inc, 1991:595–631.

147. Hamilton RG, Chapman MD, Platts-Mills TAE, et al. House dust aeroallergen measurements in clinical practice: a guide to allergen-free home and work environments. *Immunol Allergy Pract* 1992;14:96–112.

148. Kaliner M, Lemanske R. Rhinitis and asthma. *JAMA* 1992;268:2807–2829.

149. Lands AM, Arnold A, McAuliff JP, et al. Differentiation of receptor systems activated by sympathomimetic amines. *Nature* 1967;214:597–598.

150. Popa VT. Clinical pharmacology of adrenergic drugs. *J Asthma* 1984;21:183–207.

151. Newhouse MT. Emergency department management of life-threatening asthma. *Chest* 1993;103:661–663.

152. Aerosol consensus statement. *Chest* 1991;100:1106–1109.

153. Newman SP. Metered dose pressurized aerosols and the ozone layer. *Eur Respir J* 1990;3:495–497.

154. Fisher DA, Hales CH, Wang WC, et al. Model calculations of the relative effects of CFCs and their replacement on global warming. *Nature* 1990;344:513–516.

155. Molina MJ, Rowland FS. Stratospheric risk for chlorofluoromethanes: chlorine atom-catalysed destruction of ozone. *Nature* 1974;249:810–812.

156. Gross G, Thompson PJ, Chervinsky P, et al. Hydrofluoroalkane-134a beclomethasone dipropionate, 400 μg, is as effective as chlorofluorocarbon beclomethasone dipropionate, 800 μg, for the treatment of moderate asthma. *Chest* 1999;115:343–351.

157. Brown PH, Lenny J, Armstrong S, et al. Breath-actuated inhalers in chronic asthma: comparison of Diskhaler and Turbohaler for delivery of beta-agonists. *Eur Respir J* 1992;5:1143–1145.

158. Newman SP, Weisz AWB, Talaee N, et al. Improvement of drug delivery with a breath activated pressurized aerosol for patients with poor inhaler technique. *Thorax* 1991;46:712–716.

159. Johnson M. The beta-adrenoceptor. *Am J Respir Crit Care Med* 1998;158(5 Pt 3):S146–S153.

160. Verberne AA. An overview of nine clinical trials of salmeterol in an asthmatic population. *Respir Med* 1998;92(5):777–782.

161. Greening AP, Ind PW, Northfield M, et al. Added salmeterol versus higher-dose corticosteroid in asthma patients with symptoms on existing inhaled corticosteroid. *Lancet* 1994;344:219–224.

162. Woolcock A, Lundbash B, Ringdal OL, et al. Comparison of addition of salmeterol to inhaled steroids with doubling of the dose of inhaled steroids. *Am J Respir Crit Care Med* 1996;153:1481–1488.

163. Verberne AA, The Dutch Asthma Study Group. Addition of salmeterol versus doubling the dose of beclomethasone in children with asthma. *Am J Respir Crit Care Med* 1998;158:213–219.

164. Leff JA, Busse WW, Pearlman D, et al. Montelukast, a leukotriene receptor antagonist, for the treatment of mild asthma and exercise bronchoconstriction. *N Engl J Med* 1998;339:147–152.

165. Giannini D. Inhaled beclomethasone dipropionate reverts tolerance to the protective effect of salmeterol on allergen challenge. *Chest* 1999;115:629–634.

166. Boulet LP. Tolerance to the protective effects of salmeterol on methacholine-induced bronchoconstriction: influence of inhaled corticosteroids. *Eur Respir J* 1998;11:1091–1097.

167. January B. Salmeterol-induced desensitization, internalization and phosphorylation of the human β_2-adrenoceptor. *Br J Pharmacol* 1998;123:701–711.

168. Waldeck B. Enantiomers of bronchodilating β_2-adrenoceptor agonist: is there a cause for concern? *J Allergy Clin Immunol* 1999;103:742–748.

169. Levalbuterol for asthma. *Med Lett Drugs Ther* 1999;41(1054):51–53.

170. Ramsey CM, Cowan JO, Flannery EM, et al. Broncho-protective and bronchodilator effects of single dose of the enantiomers of salbutamol [Abstract]. *Eur Respir J* 1998;12(Suppl. 28):324S.

171. Cheung D, Timmers MC, Zwinderman AH, et al. Long-term effects of a long-acting β_2-adrenoceptor agonist, salmeterol, on airway hyperresponsiveness in patients with mild asthma. *N Engl J Med* 1992;327:1198–1203.

172. Pearlman DS, Chervinsky P, LaForce C, et al. A comparison of salmeterol with albuterol in the treatment of mild-to-moderate asthma. *N Engl J Med* 1992;327:1420–1425.

173. van Schayck CP, Graafsma SJ, Visch MB, et al. Increased bronchial hyperresponsiveness after inhaling salbutamol during one year is not caused by subsensitization to salbutamol. *J Allergy Clin Immunol* 1990;86:793–800.

174. O'Callaghan C, Milner AD, Swarbrick A. Paradoxical deterioration in lung function after nebulized salbutamol in wheezy infants. *Lancet* 1986;2:1424–1425.

175. Beasley R, Rafferty P, Holgate S. Paradoxical response to nebulized salbutamol in wheezy infants [Letter]. *Thorax* 1987;42:702.

176. Zhang G, Wright WJ, Tam WK, et al. Effect of inhaled preservatives on asthmatic subjects: benzalkonium chloride. *Am Rev Respir Dis* 1990;141:1405–1408.

177. Koepke JW, Selner JC, Dunhill AL. Presence of sulfur dioxide in commonly used bronchodilator solutions. *J Allergy Clin Immunol* 1983;72:504–508.

178. Koepke JW, Christopher KL, Chai H, et al. Dose-dependent bronchospasm from sulfites in isoetharine. *JAMA* 1983;251:2982–2983.

179. Finnerty JP, Howarth PH. Paradoxical bronchoconstriction with nebulized albuterol but not with terbutaline. *Am Rev Respir Dis* 1993;148:512–513.

180. Barnes PJ. Theophylline: new perspectives for an old drug. *Am J Respir Crit Care Med.* 2003;167(6):813–818.

181. Wolfe JD, Tashkin CP, Calvarese B, et al. Bronchodilator effects of terbutaline and aminophylline alone and in combination of asthmatic patients. *N Engl J Med* 1978;298:363–367.

182. Nassif EG, Weinberger M, Thompson R, et al. The value of maintenance theophylline in steroid-dependent asthma. *N Engl J Med* 1981;304:71–75.

183. Barnes PJ, Greening AP, Neville L, et al. Single-dose slow-release aminophylline at night prevents nocturnal asthma. *Lancet* 1982;1:299–301.

184. Arkinstall WW, Atkins ME, Harison D, et al. Once-daily sustained-release theophylline reduces diurnal variation in spirometry and symptomatology in adult asthmatics. *Am Rev Respir Dis* 1987;135:316–321.

185. Tilles DS, Hales CA. Comparison of 12-hour and 24-hour sustained-release theophylline in outpatient management of asthma. *Chest* 1987;91:370–375.

186. Schiff GD, Hegde HK, LaCloche L, et al. Inpatient theophylline toxicity: preventable factors. *Ann Intern Med* 1991;114:748–753.

187. Mann JS, Geroge CF. Anticholinergic drugs in the treatment of airways disease. *Br J Dis Chest* 1985;79:209–228.

188. Yeates DB, Aspin N, Levison H, et al. Mucociliary tracheal transport rates in man. *J Appl Physiol* 1975;39:487–495.

189. Pavia D, Bateman JRM, Sheahan NF, et al. Effects of ipratropium bromide on mucociliary clearance and pulmonary function in reversible airways obstruction. *Thorax* 1979;34:501–507.

190. Schleuter DP, Neumann JL. Double blind comparison of bronchial and ventilation perfusion changes to Atrovent and isoproterenol. *Chest* 1978;73:982–983.

191. Jindal SR, Malif SR. Clinical experience with terbutaline sulfate and ipratropium bromide in bronchial asthma. *Indian J Chest Dis Allied Sci* 1979;21:130–133.

192. Storms WW, Bodman SF, Nathan RA, et al. Use of ipratropium bromide in asthma: results of a multi-clinic study. *Am J Med* 1986;81(Suppl. 5A):61–66.

193. Bruderman I, Cohen-Aronovski R, Smorzik J. A comparative study of various combinations of ipratropium bromide and metaproterenol in allergic asthmatic patients. *Chest* 1983;83:208–210.

194. Ruffin RE, McIntyre E, Crockett AJ, et al. Combination bronchodilator therapy in asthma. *J Allergy Clin Immunol* 1982;69:60–65.

195. Neild JE, Cameron IR. Bronchoconstriction in response to suggestion: its prevention by an inhaled anticholinergic agent. *Br Med J* 1985;290:674.

196. Rebuck AS, Gent M, Chapman KR. Anticholinergic and sympathomimetic combination therapy of asthma. *J Allergy Clin Immunol* 1983;71:317–323.

197. Morris HG. Pharmacology of corticosteroids in asthma. In: Middelton E, Reed CE, Ellis EF, eds. *Allergy: principles and practice.* St. Louis: Mosby, 1978.

198. Corticosteroids: their biologic mechanisms and application to the treatment of asthma. *Am Rev Respir Dis* 1990;141(Suppl.):1–96.

199. Barnes PJ, Pedersen S. Efficacy and safety of inhaled corticosteroids in asthma. *Am Rev Respir Dis* 1993;148:S1–S26.

200. Robinson D, Hamid Q, Ying S, et al. Prednisolone treatment in asthma is associated with modulation of bronchoalveolar lavage cell interleukin-4, interleukin-5, and interferon-γ cytokine expression. *Am Rev Respir Dis* 1993;148:401–406.

201. Laitinen LA, Laitinen A, Haahtela T. A comparative study of the effects of inhaled corticosteroid, budesonide, and a β_2-agonist, terbutaline, on the airway inflammation in newly diagnosed asthma: a randomized double-blind, parallel-group controlled trial. *J Allergy Clin Immunol* 1992;90:32–42.

202. Djukanovic R, Wilson JW, Britten YM, et al. Effect of an inhaled corticosteroid on airway inflammation and symptoms of asthma. *Am Rev Respir Dis* 1992;145:699.

203. Jeffery PK, Godfrey RW, Adelroth E, et al. Effect of treatment on airway inflammation and thickening of basement membrane reticular collagen in asthma. *Am Rev Respir Dis* 1992;145:890–899.

204. Lungren R, Soderberg M, Horstedt P, et al. Morphological studies on bronchial mucosal biopsies from asthmatics before and after ten years treatment with inhaled steroids. *Eur Respir J* 1988;1:883–889.

205. Wenzel SE, Szefler SJ, Leung DYM, et al. Bronchoscopic evaluation of severe asthma. Persistent inflammation associated with high-dose glucocorticoids. *Am J Respir Crit Care Med* 1997;156:737–743.

206. Juniper EF, Kline AP, van Zieleshem MA, et al. Effect of long-term treatment with an inhaled corticosteroid (budesonide) on airway hyperresponsiveness and clinical asthma in non-steroid dependent asthmatics. *Am Rev Respir Dis* 1990;142:832–836.

207. Juniper EF, Kline PA, van Zieleshem MA, et al. Long-term effects of budesonide on airway responsiveness and clinical asthma severity in inhaled steroid-dependent asthmatics. *Eur Respir J* 1990;3:122–127.

208. Li JTC, Reed CE. Proper use of aerosol corticosteroids to control asthma. *Mayo Clin Proc* 1989;64:205–210.

209. Gedes DM. Inhaled corticosteroids: benefits and risks. *Thorax* 1992;47:404–407.

210. Haahtela T, Jarvinen M, Kava T, et al. Comparison of a β-agonist, terbutaline, with an inhaled corticosteroid, budesonide, in newly detected asthma. *N Engl J Med* 1991;325:388–392.

211. Kertjens HAM, Brand PLP, Hughes MD, et al. A comparison of bronchodilator therapy with or without inhaled corticosteroid therapy for obstructive airways disease. *N Engl J Med* 1992;327:1413–1419.

212. Dompeling E, van Schayck CP, van Grunsven PM, et al. Slowing the deterioration of asthma and chronic obstructive pulmonary disease observed during bronchodilator therapy by adding inhaled corticosteroids. *Ann Intern Med* 1993;188:770–778.

213. Rutten-van Molken MP, Feenstra TL. The burden of asthma and chronic obstructive pulmonary disease: data from the Netherlands. *Pharmacoeconomics* 2001;19(Suppl. 2):1–6.

214. Smith MJ, Hodson ME. High-dose beclomethasone inhaler in the treatment of asthma. *Lancet* 1983;1:265–269.

215. Toogood JH. High-dose inhaled steroid therapy for asthma. *J Allergy Clin Immunol* 1989;83:528–536.

216. Laursen LC, Taudorf E, Weeke B. High-dose inhaled budesonide in treatment of severe steroid-dependent asthma. *Eur J Respir Dis* 1986;68:19–28.

217. Noonan M, Chervinsky P, Busse WW, et al. Fluticasone propionate reduces oral prednisone use while it improves asthma control and quality of life. *Am J Respir Crit Care Med* 1995;152:1467–1473.

218. Pauwels RA, Lofdahl CG, Postma DS, et al. Effect of inhaled formoterol and budesonide on exacerbations of asthma. *N Engl J Med* 1997;337:1407–1411.

219. Lipworth BJ. Clinical pharmacology of corticosteroids in bronchial asthma. *Pharmacol Ther* 1993;58:173–209.

220. Bousquet J, Jeffery PK, Busse WW, et al. Asthma: From bronchoconstriction to airways inflammation and remodeling. *Am J Respir Crit Care Med.* 2000;161:1720–1745.

221. Holt S, Masoli M, Beasley R. Increasing compliance with inhaled corticosteroids through the use of combination therapy. *J Allergy Clin Immunol* 2004;113(2):219–220.

222. McFadden ER, Casale TB, Edwards TB, et al. Administration of budesonide once daily by means of Turbuhaler to subjects with stable asthma. *J Allergy Clin Immunol* 1999;104:46–52.

223. Weiner P, Weiner M, Azgad Y. Long-term clinical comparison of single versus twice daily administration of inhaled budesonide in moderate asthma. *Thorax* 1995;50:1270–1273.

224. Suissa S, Ernst P, Benayoun S, et al. Low-dose inhaled corticosteroids and the prevention of death from asthma. *N Engl J Med* 2000;343:332–336.

225. Blais L, Ernest P, Boivin JF, et al. Inhaled corticosteroids and prevention of readmission to the hospital for asthma. *Am J Respir Crit Care Med* 1998;158:126–132.

226. Onrust SV, Lamb HM. Mometasone furoate: a review of its intranasal use in allergic rhinitis. *Drugs* 1998;56(4):725–745.

227. Kavuru M, Melamed J, Gross G, et al. Salmeterol and fluticasone propionate combined in a new powder inhalation device for the treatment of asthma: a randomized, double-blind, placebo-controlled trial. *J Allergy Clin Immunol* 2000;105:1108–1116.

228. Evans DJ, Taylor DA, Zetterstrom O, et al. A comparison of low-dose inhaled budesonide plus theophylline and high-dose inhaled budesonide for moderate asthma. *N Engl J Med* 1997;337:1412–1418.

229. Busse W, Nelson H, Wolfe J, et al. Comparison of inhaled salmeterol and oral zafirlukast in patients with asthma. *J Allergy Clin Immunol* 1999;103:1075–1080.

230. Schwartz HJ, Petty T, Dube LM, et al. A randomized controlled trial comparing zileuton with theophylline in moderate asthma. *Arch Intern Med* 1998;158:141–148.

231. Lazarus SC, Boushey HA, Fahy JV, et al. Long-acting beta 2-agonist monotherapy vs. continued therapy with inhaled corticosteroids in patients with persistent asthma: a randomized controlled trial. *JAMA* 2001;285:2583–2593.

232. Carmichael J, Paterson IC, Diaz P, et al. Corticosteroid resistance in chronic asthma. *Br Med J* 1981;282:1419–1422.

233. Dykewicz MS, Greenberger PA, Patterson R, et al. Natural history of asthma in patients requiring long-term systemic corticosteroids. *Arch Intern Med* 1986;146:2369–2372.

234. Corrigan CJ, Brown PH, Barnes NC, et al. Glucocorticoid resistance in chronic asthma. *Am Rev Respir Dis* 1991;144:1016–1032.

235. NIH Conference. Syndromes of glucocorticoid resistance. Moderator: Chrousos GP. *Ann Intern Med* 1994;119:1113–1124.

236. Toogood JH. Complications of topical steroid therapy for asthma. *Am Rev Respir Dis* 1990;141:S89–S96.

237. Lipworth BJ. Systemic adverse effects of inhaled corticosteroid therapy: a systemic review and meta-analysis. *Arch Intern Med* 1999;159:941–955.

238. Newman SP, Moren F, Pavia D, et al. Deposition of pressurized suspension aerosols inhaled through extension devices. *Am Rev Respir Dis* 1981;124:317–320.

239. Allen DB, Mullen M, Mullen B. A meta-analysis of the effect of oral and inhaled corticosteroids on growth. *J Allergy Clin Immunol* 1994;93:967–976.

240. Allen MB, Ray SG, Leitch AG, et al. Steroid aerosols and cataract formation. *Br Med J* 1989;299:432–433.

241. Silverstein MD, Yunginger JW, Reed CE, et al. Attained adult height after childhood asthma; effect of glucocorticoid therapy. *J Allergy Clin Immunol* 1997;99:466–474.

242. Luengo M, Picado C, Del Rio L, et al. Vertebral fractures in steroid dependent asthma and involutional osteoporosis: a comparative study. *Thorax* 1991;46:803–806.

243. Szefler S, Weiss S, Tonascia J et al., The CAMP Research Group. Long-term effects of budesonide or nedocromil in children with asthma. *N Engl J Med.* 2000;343:1054–1063.
244. Geddes DM, Turner-Warwick M, Brewis RAL, et al. Nedocromil sodium workshop. *Respir Med* 1989;83:265–267.
245. Toogood JH, Jennings B, Lefcol NM. A clinical trial of combined cromolyn/beclomethasone treatment for chronic asthma. *J Pediatr* 1981;67:317–324.
246. Edwards AM, Stevens MT. The clinical efficacy of inhaled nedocromil sodium (Tilade) in the treatment of asthma. *Eur Respir J* 1993;6:35–41.
247. Callaghan B, Teo NC, Clancy L. Effects of the addition of nedocromil sodium to maintenance bronchodilator therapy in the management of chronic asthma. *Chest* 1992;101:787–792.
248. North American Tilade Study Group. A double-blind multicenter group comparative study of the efficacy and safety of nedocromil sodium in the management of asthma. *Chest* 1990;97:1299–1306.
249. De Jong JW, Deengs JP, Postma DS, et al. Nedocromil sodium versus albuterol in the management of allergic asthma. *Am J Respir Crit Care Med* 1994;149:91–97.
250. Pearlman DS, Ostrom NK, Bronsky EA, et al. The leukotriene D$_4$ receptor antagonist zafirlukast attenuates exercise-induced bronchoconstriction in children. *J Pediatr* 1999;134:273–279.
251. Israel E, Rubin P, Kemp JB, et al. The effect of inhibition of 5-lipoxygenase by zileuton in mild-to-moderate asthma. *Ann Intern Med* 1993;119:1059–1066.
252. Lofdahl C, Reiss TF, Leff JA, et al. Randomized, placebo controlled trial of the effect of leukotriene receptor antagonist, montelukast, on tapering inhaled corticosteroids in asthmatic patients. *Br Med J* 1999;319:87–90.
253. Malmstrom K, Rodriguez-Gomez G, Guerra J, et al. Oral montelukast, inhaled beclomethasone and placebo for chronic asthma: a randomized controlled trial. *Ann Intern Med* 1999;130:487–495.
254. Kemp JP, Minkwitz MC, Bonuccelli CM, et al. Therapeutic effects of zafirlukast as monotherapy in steroid-naïve patients with severe persistent asthma. *Chest* 1999;115:336–342.
255. Lipworth BJ. Systemic adverse effects of inhaled salmeterol and oral zafirlukast in patients with asthma. *J Allergy Clin Immunol* 1999;103:1075–1080.
256. Knorr B, Matz J, Bernstein JA et al., The Pediatric Montelukast Study Group. Montelukast for chronic asthma in 6- to 14-year old children. *JAMA* 1998;3279:1181–1186.
257. Suissa S, Dennis R, Ernst P, et al. Effectiveness of the leukotriene receptor antagonist zafirlukast for mild-to-moderate asthma: a randomized double-blind placebo-controlled trial. *Ann Intern Med* 1997;126:177–183.
258. Wechsler ME, Garperstad E, Flier SR, et al. Pulmonary infiltrates, eosinophilia and cardiomyopathy following corticosteroid withdrawal in patients with asthma receiving zafirlukast. *JAMA* 1998;279:455–457.
259. Jamgleddine G, Diab K, Tabbazah Z, et al. Leukotriene antagonists and the churg-strauss syndrome. *Semin Arthritis Rheum* 2002;31:218–227.
260. Drazen JM, Israel E, O'Bryne PM. Treatment of asthma with drugs modifying the leukotriene pathway. *N Engl J Med* 1999;40:197–206.
261. Lipworth BJ. The emerging role of leukotriene antagonists in asthma therapy. *Chest* 1999;115:313–316.
262. Rambasek TE, Lang DM, Kavuru MS. Omalizumab: where does it fit into current asthma management? *Cleve Clin J Med* 2004;71:251–261.
263. Milgrom H, Fick RB, Su JQ, et al. Treatment of allergic asthma with monoclonal anti-IgE antibody. *N Engl J Med* 1999;341:1966–1973.
264. Busse W, Corren J, Lanier BQ, et al. Omalizumab, anti-IgE recombinant humanized monoclonal antibody, for the treatment of severe allergic asthma. *J Allergy Clin Immunol* 2001;108:184–190.
265. Soler M, Matz J, Townley R, et al. The anti-IgE antibody omalizumab reduces exacerbations and steroid requirement in allergic asthmatics. *Eur Respir J* 2001;18:254–261.
266. McFadden ER Jr. Acute severe asthma. *Am J Respir Crit Care Med* 2003;168(7):740–759.
267. Emerman CL, Woodruff PG, Cydulka RK et al., MARC investigators. Multicenter Asthma Research Collaboration. Prospective multicenter study of relapse following treatment for acute asthma among adults presenting to the emergency department. *Chest* 1999;115:919–927.
267a. American Thoracic Society. Proceedings of the ATS workshop on refractory asthma: current understanding, recommendations, and unanswered questions. *Am J Respir Crit Care Med* 2000;162(6):2341–2351.
268. Braman SS, Kaemmerlen JT. Intensive care of status asthmaticus. A 10-year experience. *JAMA* 1990;264:366–368.
269. Brenner BE. The acute asthmatic in the emergency department: the decision to admit or discharge. *Am J Emerg Med* 1985;3:74–77.
270. Corbridge TC, Hall JB. The assessment and management of adults with status asthmaticus. *Am J Respir Crit Care Med* 1995;151:1296–1316.
271. Reed CE, Hung LW. The emergency visit and management of asthma. *Ann Intern Med* 1990;112:801–802.
272. Kavuru MS. Beta-agonist for acute asthma: which way to deliver? *J Respir Dis* 1994;15:312–314.
273. Colacone A, Wolkove N, Stern E, et al. Continuous nebulization of albuterol (salbutamol) in acute asthma. *Chest* 1990;97:693–697.
274. Olshaker J, Jerrard D, Barish RA, et al. The efficacy and safety of a continuous albuterol protocol for the treatment of acute adult asthma attacks. *Am J Emerg Med* 1993;11:131–133.
275. Portnoy J, Nadel G, Amado M, et al. Continuous nebulization for status asthmaticus. *Ann Allergy* 1992;69:71–79.
276. Shim C. Adrenergic agonist and bronchodilator aerosol therapy in asthma. *Clin Chest Med* 1984;5:659–668.
277. Amory DW, Burham SC, Cheney FW Jr. Comparison of the cardiopulmonary effects of subcutaneously administered epinephrine and terbutaline in patients with reversible airway obstruction. *Chest* 1975;67:279–286.
278. Jederlinic RJ, Irwin RS. Status asthmaticus. *Intensive Care Med* 1989;4:166–184.
279. Parry WH, Martorano F, Colton EK. Management of life-threatening asthma with intravenous isoproterenol infusion. *Am J Dis Child* 1976;130:39–42.
280. Lawford P, Jones BJM, Milledge JS. Comparison of intravenous and nebulized salbutamol in initial treatment of severe asthma. *Br Med J* 1978;1:84.
281. Williams S, Seaton A. Intravenous or inhaled salbutamol in severe acute asthma? *Thorax* 1977;32:555–558.
282. Lam A, Newhouse MT. Management of asthma and chronic airflow limitation: are methylxanthines obsolete? *Chest* 1990;98:44–52.
283. Milgrom H, Bender B. Current issues in the use of theophylline. *Am Rev Respir Dis* 1993;147:533–539.
284. British Thoracic Society. Guidelines for management of asthma in adults. *Br Med J* 1990;301:651–653.
285. Rossing TH, Fanta CH, Goldstein DH, et al. Emergency therapy of asthma: comparison of the acute effects of parenteral and inhaled sympathomimetics and infused aminophylline. *Am Rev Respir Dis* 1980;122:365–371.
286. Siegel D, Sheppard D, Gelb A, et al. Aminophylline increases the toxicity but not the efficacy of an inhaled β-adrenergic agonist in the treatment of acute exacerbations of asthma. *Am Rev Respir Dis* 1985;132:283–286.
287. Fanta CH, Rossing TH, McFadden ER Jr. Treatment of acute asthma—is combination therapy with sympathomimetics and methylxanthines indicated? *Am J Med* 1986;80:5–10.
288. Littenberg, B. Aminophylline treatment in severe, acute asthma: a meta-analysis. *JAMA* 1988;259:1678–1684.
289. Self TH, Abou-Shala N, Burns R, et al. Inhaler albuterol and oral prednisone therapy in hospitalized adult asthmatics. Does aminophylline add any benefit? *Chest* 1990;98:1317–1321.
290. Wrenn K, Solvis CM, Murphy F, et al. Aminophylline therapy for acute bronchospastic disease in the emergency room. *Ann Intern Med* 1991;115:241–247.
291. McFadden ER. Methylxanthines in treatment of asthma: the rise, the fall, and the possible rise again [Editorial]. *Ann Intern Med* 1991;115:323–324.
292. Huang D, O'Brien RG, Harman E, et al. Does aminophylline benefit adults admitted to the hospital for an acute exacerbation of asthma? *Ann Intern Med* 1993;119:1155–1160.
293. DiGiulio GA, Kercsmar CM, Krug SE, et al. Hospital treatment of asthma: lack of benefit from theophylline given in addition to

nebulized albuterol and intravenously administered cortico-steroid. *J Pediatr* 1993;122:470–476.

294. Carter E, Cruz M, Chesrown S, et al. Efficacy of intravenously administered theophylline in children hospitalized with severe asthma. *J Pediatr* 1993;122:470–476.

295. Karpel JP, Appel D, Briedbart D, et al. A comparison of atropine sulfate and metaproterenol sulfate in the emergency treatment of asthma. *Am Rev Respir Dis* 1986;133:727–729.

296. McFadden ER Jr, Elsanadi N, Strauss L, et al. The influence of parasympatholytic on the resolution of acute attacks of asthma. *Am J Med* 1997;102:7–13.

297. Qureshi F, Prestian J, Davis P, et al. Effect of nebulized ipratropium on the hospitalization rates for children with asthma. *N Engl J Med* 1998;339:1030–1035.

298. Bryant DH. Nebulized ipratropium bromide in the treatment of acute asthma. *Chest* 1985;88:24–29.

299. Ward MJ, McFarlane JT, Davies D, et al. A place for ipratropium bromide in the treatment of severe acute asthma. *Br J Dis Chest* 1985;79:374.

300. Lanes SF, Garrett JE, Wentworth CE, et al. The effect of adding ipratropium bromide to salbutamol in the treatment of acute asthma: a pooled analysis of three trials. *Chest* 1998;114:365–372.

301. Rebuck AS, Chapman KR, Abboud R, et al. Nebulized anticholinergic and sympathomimetic treatment of asthma and chronic obstructive airways disease in the emergency room. *Am J Med* 1987;82:59–64.

302. Weber EJ, Levitt MA, Covington JK, et al. Effect of continuously nebulized ipratropium bromide plus albuterol on emergency department length of stay and hospital admission rates in patients with acute bronchospasm: a randomized, controlled trial. *Chest* 1999;115:937–944.

303. McFadden ER. Dosages of corticosteroids in asthma. *Am Rev Respir Dis* 1993;147:1306–1310.

304. Fanta CH, Rossing TH, McFadden ER. Glucocorticoid in acute asthma: a critical controlled trial. *Am J Med* 1983;74:845–851.

305. Littenberg B, Gluck EH. A controlled trial of methylprednisolone in the emergency treatment of acute asthma. *N Engl J Med* 1986;314:150–152.

306. Stein LM, Cole RP. Early administration of corticosteroids in emergency room treatment of acute asthma. *Ann Intern Med* 1990;112:822–827.

307. McFadden ER, Kiser R, deGroot WJ, et al. A controlled study of the effects of single doses of hydrocortisone on the resolution of acute attacks of asthma. *Am J Med* 1976;60:52–59.

308. Aelony Y. Non-invasive oral treatment of asthma in the emergency room. *Am J Med* 1985;78:929–936.

309. Ogirala RG, Aldrich TK, Prezant DF, et al. High-dose intramuscular triamcinolone in severe, chronic life-threatening asthma. *N Engl J Med* 1991;324:585–589.

310. Haskell RJ, Wong BM, Hansen JE. A double-blind, randomized clinical trial of methylprednisolone in status asthmaticus. *Arch Intern Med* 1983;143:1324–1327.

311. Lederle FA, Pluhar RE, Joseph AM, et al. Tapering of corticosteroid therapy following exacerbations of asthma. *Arch Intern Med* 1987;147:2201–2203.

312. Cydulka RK, Emerman CL. A pilot study of steroid therapy after emergency department treatment of acute asthma: is a taper needed? *J Emerg Med* 1998;16:15–19.

313. Vichyanond P, Irvin CG, Larsen GL, et al. Penetration of corticosteroids into the lung: evidence for a difference between methylprednisolone and prednisolone. *J Allergy Clin Immunol* 1989;84:867–873.

314. McFadden ER Jr., Elsanadi N, Dixon L, et al. Protocol therapy for acute asthma: therapeutic benefits and cost savings. *Am J Med* 1995;99:651–661.

315. Manthous CA. Management of severe exacerbations of asthma. *Am J Med* 1995;99:298–308.

316. Tiffany R, Berk WA, Todd K, et al. Magnesium bolus or infusion fails to improve expiratory flow in acute asthma exacerbations. *Chest* 1993;104:831–834.

317. Green SM, Rothrock SG. Intravenous magnesium for acute asthma: failure to decrease emergency treatment duration or need for hospitalization. *Ann Emerg Med* 1992;21:260–265.

318. Gluck EH, Onorato DJ, Castriotta R. Helium-oxygen mixtures in intubated patients with status asthmaticus and respiratory acidosis. *Chest* 1990;98:693–698.

319. Kudukis TM, Manthous CA, Schmidt GA, et al. Inhaled helium-oxygen revisited: effect of inhaled helium-oxygen during the treatment of status asthmaticus in children. *J Pediatr* 1997;130:217–224.

320. Shivaram U, Miro AM, Cash ME, et al. Cardiopulmonary responses to continuous positive airway pressure in acute asthma. *J Crit Care* 1993;8:87–92.

321. Howton JC, Rose J, Duffy S, et al. Randomized, double-blind, placebo-controlled trial of intravenous ketamine in acute asthma. *Ann Emerg Med* 1996;27:170–175.

322. Schwartz SH. Treatment of status asthmaticus with halothane. *JAMA* 1984;251:2688–2689.

323. Roy TM, Pruitt VL, Garner PA, et al. The potential role of anesthesia in status asthmaticus. *J Asthma* 1992;29:73–77.

324. Marquette CH, Saulnier F, Leroy O, et al. Long-term prognosis of near-fatal asthma. A 6-year follow-up study of 145 asthmatic patients who underwent mechanical ventilation for a near-fatal attack of asthma. *Am Rev Respir Dis* 1992;146:76–81.

325. Tuxen DV. Detrimental effects of positive end-expiratory pressure during controlled mechanical ventilation of patients with severe airflow obstruction. *Am Rev Respir Dis* 1989;140:5–9.

326. Segredo V, Caldwell JE, Matthay MA, et al. Persistent paralysis in critically ill patients after long-term administration of vecuronium. *N Engl J Med* 1992;327:524–528.

327. Mullarkey MF, Blumenstein BA, Andrade WP, et al. Methotrexate in the treatment of corticosteroid dependent asthma. A double-blind crossover study. *N Engl J Med* 1988;318:603–606.

328. Erzurum SC, Leff JA, Cochran JE, et al. Lack of benefit of methotrexate in severe steroid dependent asthma. *Ann Intern Med* 1991;114:353–360.

329. Lane DJ, Lane TV. Alternative and complementary medicine for asthma. *Thorax* 1991;46:787–797.

330. Schwartz YA, Kinity S, Ilfeld DN, et al. A clinical and immunologic study of colchicine in asthma. *J Allergy Clin Immunol* 1990;85:578–582.

331. Mazer BD, Gelfand EW. An open-label study of high-dose intravenous immunoglobulin in severe childhood asthma. *J Allergy Clin Immunol* 1991;87:976–983.

332. Mullarkey MF, Lammert JK, Blumenstein BA. Long-term methotrexate treatment in steroid dependent asthma. *Ann Intern Med* 1990;112:577–581.

333. Dyer P, Vaughan T, Weber R. Methotrexate in the treatment of steroid-dependent asthma. *J Allergy Clin Immunol* 1991;88:208–212.

334. Shiner RJ, Nunn AJ, Chung KF, et al. Randomised, double-blind, placebo controlled trial of methotrexate in steroid dependent asthma. *Lancet* 1990;336:137–140.

335. Coffey MJ, Sanders G, Eschenbacher WL, et al. The role of methotrexate in the management of steroid-dependent asthma. *Chest* 1994;105:117–121.

336. Marin MG. Low-dose methotrexate spares steroid usage in steroid-dependent asthmatic patients: a meta-analysis. *Chest* 1997;112:29–32.

337. Bernstein DI, Bernstein IL, Bodenheimer SS, et al. An open study of auranofin in the treatment of steroid dependent asthma. *J Allergy Clin Immunol* 1988;81:6–16.

338. Nierop G, Gijzel WP, Bel EH, et al. Auranofin in the treatment of steroid dependent asthma; a double-blind study. *Thorax* 1992;47:349–354.

339. Muranaka M, Myamoto T, Shida T, et al. Gold salts in the treatment of bronchial asthma; a double-blind study. *Ann Allergy* 1978;40:132–137.

340. Klaustermyer WB, Noritake DT, Kwong FK. Chrysotherapy in the treatment of corticosteroid dependent asthma. *J Allergy Clin Immunol* 1987;79:720–725.

341. Bernstein IL, Bernstein DI, Dubb JW, et al. A placebo-controlled multicenter study of auranofin in the treatment of patients with corticosteroid-dependent asthma. Auranofin multicenter drug trial. *J Allergy Clin Immunol* 1996;98:317–324.

342. Spector SL, Katz, FH, Farr RS. Troleandomycin: effectiveness in steroid dependent asthma. *J Allergy Clin Immunol* 1974;54:367–379.

343. Szefler SJ, Rose JQ, Elliott EF, et al. The effect of troleandomycin on methylprednisolone elimination. *J Allergy Clin Immunol* 1980;66:447–451.

344. Zeiger RS, Schatz M, Sperling W, et al. Efficacy of troleandomycin in outpatients with severe, corticosteroid-dependent asthma. *J Allergy Clin Immunol* 1988;66:438–446.
345. Wald JA, Friedman BF, Farr RS. An improved protocol for the use of troleandomycin in the treatment of steroid-requiring asthma. *J Allergy Clin Immunol* 1986;78:36–43.
346. Kamada AK, Hill MR, Ikhe DN, et al. Efficacy and safety of low-dose troleandomycin therapy in children with severe, steroid-requiring asthma. *J Allergy Clin Immunol* 1993;91: 873–882.
347. Nelson HS, Hamilos DL, Corsello PR, et al. A double-blind study of troleandomycin and methylprednisolone in asthmatic subjects who require daily corticosteroids. *Am Rev Respir Dis* 1993;147: 398–404.
348. Calderon E, Lockey RF, Bukantz SC, et al. Is there a role for cyclosporine in asthma? *J Allergy Clin Immunol* 1992;89:629–636.
349. Alexander AG, Barnes NC, Kay AB. Trial of cyclosporin in corticosteroid dependent chronic severe asthma. *Lancet* 1992;339:324–327.
350. Lock SH, Kay AB, Barnes NC. Double-blind, placebo-controlled study of cyclosporin A as a corticosteroid-sparing agent in corticosteroid-dependent asthma. *Am J Respir Crit Care Med* 1996;153: 509–519.
351. Leckie MJ, ten Brinkei A Kahn J, et al. Effects of an interleukin-5 blocking monoclonal antibody on eosinophils, airway hyperresponsiveness, and the late asthmatic response. *Lancet* 2000;356: 2144–2148.
352. Borish LC, Nelson HS, Corren J, et al. Efficacy of soluble IL-4 receptor for the treatment of adults with asthma. *J Allergy Clin Immunol* 2001;107:963–970.
353. Dahl R, Nielsen LP. Steriods: an overview. In: Hansel TT, Barnes PJ, eds. *New drugs for asthma, allergy, and COPD*. Basel: Karger, 2001:86–90.

CHAPTER 9

Chronic Obstructive Pulmonary Disease

James F. Donohue
Gerardo S. San Pedro

INTRODUCTION

Chronic obstructive pulmonary disease (COPD) is the fourth leading cause of chronic morbidity and mortality in the United States, affecting 5% of the adult population. In most of the world, COPD prevalence and mortality are still increasing in response to increase in smoking by women and adolescents. The morbidity data greatly underestimates the total burden of COPD because the disease is usually not diagnosed until it is clinically apparent and moderately advanced. Also, differing definitions of COPD could change estimates of its prevalence. COPD is a heterogeneous disorder that includes emphysema, chronic bronchitis, obliterative bronchiolitis, and asthmatic bronchitis. Resources directed at smoking cessation and prevention, COPD education, early detection, and improved therapy will be of benefit in the continuing efforts to control this important disease (1).

DEFINITIONS

Two recent updates of guidelines issued by expert panels representing the American Thoracic Society/European Respiratory Society (ATS/ERS) and the Global Obstructive Lung Disease (GOLD) Initiative have been published (2,3). According to the GOLD Guidelines, COPD is "a disease state characterized by airflow limitation that is not fully reversible. The airflow limitation is usually both progressive and associated with an abnormal inflammatory response of the lungs to noxious particles or gases." The ATS/ERS definition emphasizes that COPD is a preventable and treatable disease state and adds that the "noxious particles or gases are primarily caused by cigarette smoking." Although COPD affects the lungs, it also produces significant systemic consequences. *Chronic bronchitis* is defined clinically as chronic productive cough on most days for 3 months in each of 2 consecutive years in a patient in whom other causes of chronic sputum have been excluded.

Emphysema is defined pathologically as the presence of abnormal permanent enlargement of the airspaces distal to the terminal bronchioles, accompanied by destruction of their walls and without obvious fibrosis. In patients with COPD, either of these conditions may be present.

Although there is some overlap with *asthma*, substantial differences in pathogenesis and therapeutic response result in COPD being usually considered a different clinical entity. Some patients with asthma do have an irreversible component to their airflow obstruction and the two entities frequently coexist in the same patient. A 20-year longitudinal study from Tucson found that physician-diagnosed asthma was associated with an increased risk of chronic bronchitis, emphysema, and COPD (4). The presence or absence of reversibility was once thought to be the major distinction between these two entities, with reversibility of airflow obstruction being the hallmark of asthma and mainly irreversible obstruction being the hallmark of COPD. Partial reversibility is the norm for most patients with COPD, whereas asthmatics have greater reversibility to therapy. Newer definitions of both asthma and COPD acknowledge the overlap between these conditions and highlight their similarities and differences. Chronic inflammation underlies both conditions, but the nature of the inflammation differs, as does the response to different classes of medications.

Asthma is defined as a chronic inflammatory disorder of the airways, in which many cells and cellular elements play a role. Chronic inflammation causes an associated increase in airway hyperresponsiveness (AHR) that leads to recurrent episodes of wheezing, breathlessness, chest tightness, and coughing, particularly at night or early in the morning. The episodes are usually associated with widespread but variable airflow obstruction that is often reversible, either spontaneously or with treatment. International guidelines have different recommendations for bronchodilator use in asthma and COPD. Whereas β_2-agonist bronchodilators are used "as needed" in asthma management, regular bronchodilator therapy with an anticholinergic drug or β_2-agonist is the usual first-line approach in COPD.

EPIDEMIOLOGY

COPD is a leading cause of morbidity and mortality worldwide and results in an economic and social burden that is both substantial and increasing. Most of the information available on epidemiology of COPD comes from developed countries. The best prevalence data come from the third National Health and Nutrition Examination Survey (NHANES), a large national survey conducted in the United States between 1988 and 1994. In the United States, for those aged 25 to 75, the estimated prevalence of mild COPD (FEV_1/FVC 0.7 and FEV_1 >80%) is 6.9% and that of moderate COPD (FEV_1/FVC <0.7 and FEV <80% predicted) is 6.6%. The prevalence is greater in men than in women, in whites than in blacks, and it increases with age (5). COPD mortality in women has more than doubled over the last 20 years, and according to the last survey, more women have died of COPD than men have. *The Global Burden of Disease* study conducted by the World Health Organization and the World Bank estimated that the worldwide prevalence was 9.34 per thousand in men and 7.3 per thousand in women (6).

The death rates are increasing, and although they are very low among people under 45 years of age, they increase with age in older individuals. COPD was estimated to be the twelfth leading cause of morbidity and the sixth leading cause of mortality worldwide in 1990 (7). However, COPD is one of the fastest increasing conditions, and by 2020, it will be the fifth leading cause of disability and the third leading cause of death (8). A recent report from NHANES III indicates that COPD is markedly underdiagnosed. During the year 2000, an estimated 10 million Americans reported physician-diagnosed COPD (5). However, 24 million have evidence of impaired lung function (5). During the year 2000, COPD was responsible for 8 million office visits and hospital outpatient visits, 1.5 million emergency department (ED) visits, 726,000 hospitalizations, and 119,000 deaths (5). Of the estimated 225,400 adults who died because of COPD (primary or contributing cause) in 1993, 16.7% had never smoked. Those dying with COPD are more likely to be current smokers or former smokers, have a history of asthma, be underweight, and be white, as compared to those dying without COPD. Some of these observations may provide an opportunity for intervention (9).

ECONOMIC AND SOCIAL BURDEN OF CHRONIC OBSTRUCTIVE PULMONARY DISEASE. Estimates of disability attributed to major diseases use a yardstick called *Disability Adjusted Life Years* (DALYS). COPD was the fifth leading cause of DALYS loss worldwide in 2002, whereas in 1990 it ranked twelfth. The data from NHANES III indicated that COPD had a substantial effect on work loss ($9.9 billion) in 1994 and that many with severe diseases no longer participated in the labor force (10).

RISK FACTORS. Risk factors for COPD of course include both host factors and environmental exposures, with a complex interaction between the two (see Table 9-1). Genetic host factors that have been best documented are the hereditary deficiency of α-1-antitrypsin (AAT). Other candidate genes identified in the pathogenesis of COPD have included those involved in detoxification of cigarette smoke products such as microsomal epoxide hydrolase and glutathione-S-transferase. However, studies of these genetic variants have proven to be inconsistent and controversial. The genetics of COPD has been recently reviewed (11).

TABLE 9-1. Risk Factors for Chronic Obstructive Pulmonary Disease (COPD) Include Both Host Factors and Environmental Exposures

Risk Factors for COPD
Host factors
• Genetic (e.g., α-1-antitrypsin deficiency)
• Airway hyperresponsiveness
• Lung growth
Exposures
• Tobacco smoke
• Occupational dusts and chemicals
• Indoor and outdoor air pollution
• Infections
• Socioeconomic status

From GOLD Workshop Report (Updated 2004) (*www.goldcopd.org*), with permission.

Familial clustering both in patients with AAT deficiency and in those without this deficiency are described. In the population at large, PiMZ heterozygosity may account for a small number of COPD cases. An increased rate of decline in lung function is seen in PiMZ COPD patients with a family history, suggesting that other genes are involved (12). Patients with rapid FEV_1 decline may have polymorphisms in the mixed metalloprotein genes MMP1 and MMP12. Linkage of FEV_1 and/or FEV_1/FVC with different loci in the genome has been reported (chromosomes 1, 2q, 4, 6, 8, 12p, 17, 18, 19, and 21). Tumor necrosis factor-α (TNF-α) alleles are associated with smoking-related COPD, as are IL-13 promoter polymorphisms and tissue inhibitors of mixed metalloprotein (TIMP-2) polymorphisms. The relationship between the chronic bronchitis phenotype and cystic fibrosis transmembrane regulator (CFTR) mutations remain uncertain.

Environmental exposures are better understood. These include tobacco smoke; heavy exposure to occupational dust and chemicals such as vapors, irritants, and fumes; and indoor and outdoor air pollution.

Cigarette smoking is the most important etiologic factor that is significantly affected by age of onset, dose, and duration of smoking. Smoking leads to an inflammatory response, oxidative stress, lung destruction, and interference with lung repair. Smoking cessation is proven to slow the accelerated decline in FEV_1 related to COPD and to reduce all the causes of mortality rates by 27%, driven primarily by significant reduction in concurrent cardiovascular mortality. "Low-grade systemic inflammation" was present (higher C-reactive protein, fibrinogen level) in those participants in NHANES III with moderate to severe airflow obstruction (13).

The *role of gender* in COPD is controversial. Earlier studies showed men at greater risk than women, but more recent studies from developed countries show that the prevalence is equal and some studies have in fact suggested that women are more susceptible to the effects of tobacco smoke than men are. In the year 2000, for the first time, more women died of COPD than men did (59,936:59,118). The COPD death rate rose from 20.1/100,000 in 1980 to 56.7/100,000 in 2,000 in women, whereas the increase in men was a more modest 73 to 82.6/100,000 (5). Data from 1968 to 1999 are more alarming; the death rate increased by 382% in women versus 27% in men, whereas the lung cancer rate increased by 266% in women versus 15% in men. Clearly, better prevention strategies need to be targeted toward women (14).

Airway hyperresponsiveness affects 60% to 80% of patients with COPD (15). AHR is another factor that may develop after exposure to tobacco smoke or other environmental insults. This can be measured by challenging patients with low doses of histamine or methacholine, which constrict smooth muscle while lowering the FEV_1. Asthma is also characterized by increased AHR. However, in asthma, AHR correlates better with inflammation, whereas in COPD, AHR correlates with airway narrowing. Once again, women seem to be more hyperresponsive on the basis of data from the Lung Health Study. AHR has been identified as a risk factor that contributes to an accelerated loss of lung function and to the development of COPD (16–18).

Developmental risk factors like perinatal events and childhood illness also have a profound effect on lung growth. Other influences include processes occurring during gestation, low birth weight, and exposures during the first year of life. Viral infections may be important in altering lung growth, and there is some evidence that viral genomes from adenoviruses can be incorporated and expressed in airway cells, predisposing them to inflammation and injury later in life. Reduced lung function in childhood may identify individuals who are at increased risk for development of COPD. Teenage cigarette smoking, especially in girls, may be associated with less-than-projected lung development and function. Therefore, less than maximal attainable lung function during development is associated with rapid loss of function later in life and with COPD.

High levels of *urban air pollution* are harmful to people with existing lung disease. The precise role in causing COPD is unclear, but it is not as important as cigarette smoke. Exacerbations can be increased at times of ozone alerts and increased air levels of particulates and irritants. Indoor air pollution from biomass fuel burned for cooking and heating is also a risk factor, especially in Eastern Europe and in the developing world.

As mentioned above, severe childhood respiratory infections also are associated with reduced lung function and increased respiratory symptoms in adulthood. There is also evidence that the risk of developing COPD is inversely related to socioeconomic status. The role of recurrent infection in adults is controversial but many do not completely recover lung function and health status after a serious infection. *Malnutrition* can worsen COPD, it can be accelerated by infections, and it correlates with end-stage disease. This is often a contributory factor in diaphragm weakness.

NATURAL HISTORY. COPD has a variable natural history in that not all individuals follow the same path. However, the often-quoted statistic that 15% to 20% of smokers develop clinically significant COPD may be misleading and may greatly underestimate the toll of COPD. COPD may have its roots decades before the onset of symptoms. There may be impaired functional development of the lungs during childhood and adolescence, caused by recurrent infections or tobacco smoking, which lead to lower maximally attained lung function in early adulthood. As shown in the diagram from the classic study of Fletcher (see Fig. 9-1), an accelerated decline in lung function is still the single most important feature of COPD. If tobacco smoking continues, the loss of lung function progresses. If the exposure is stopped, the disease may still progress but, often, there is some improvement in lung function and a slowing, or even stabilizing, of the progression of the disease. From the NIH Lung Health Study, men who quit smoking during the first year showed an FEV_1 decline of 30 mL per year and women who quit showed a decline of 21.5 mL, whereas men who continued to smoke throughout the 11 years of the study showed a decline of 66 mL per year and women, 54.2 mL per year (19). Thus, there is a great advantage to sustained quitting (20).

PATHOLOGY, PATHOGENESIS, AND PATHOPHYSIOLOGY

Chronic obstructive pulmonary disease comprises pathologic changes in four different compartments of the lung (central airways, peripheral airways, lung parenchyma, and pulmonary vasculature), which are variably present in individuals with the disease (2).

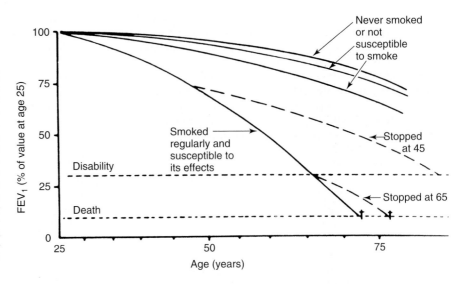

FIGURE 9-1. The effects of smoking and smoking cessation on the forced expiratory volume in one second (FEV_1) in men aged 25 years and older. The lower solid line represents a typical course in a smoker who is susceptible to developing chronic obstructive pulmonary disease (COPD). Crosses indicate death due to respiratory failure. Disability usually occurs at about age 65 years, when airflow is already markedly decreased. At that time, smoking cessation will prolong life by a few years, but disability will persist. In order to effect a major improvement in life expectancy, smoking cessation must occur at an earlier age. (From Fletcher C, Peto R. The natural history of chronic airflow obstruction. *Br. Med J* 1977;1:1645–1648, with permission.)

CENTRAL AIRWAYS (CARTILAGINOUS AIRWAYS GREATER THAN 2 MM OF INTERNAL DIAMETER). Major changes may be seen in the bronchi. The chronic hypersecretion of mucus results from changes in the central airways. Bronchial gland hypertrophy and goblet cell metaplasia result from smoking. In smokers, goblet cells are increased in number and these extend peripherally. This results in excessive mucous production that is characteristic of chronic bronchitis. Cellular infiltrates also occur in the bronchial glands. The airway wall changes include squamous metaplasia of the airway epithelium, loss of cilia and ciliary dysfunction, and increased smooth muscle and connective tissue. Different inflammatory cells predominate in the different compartments of the central airways. In the airways wall, there are lymphocytes; usually the CD8+ type predominates rather than the CD4+ helper subset (21,22). As the disease progresses, neutrophils also become prominent, while neutrophils and macrophages can also be identified. Neutrophil chemotactic factors including interleukin-8 (IL-8), leukotriene B4, and others are present in abundance.

PERIPHERAL AIRWAYS (NONCARTILAGINOUS AIRWAYS LESS THAN 2 MM INTERNAL DIAMETER). Recently, the nature of small airway obstruction in COPD was assessed in surgically resected lung tissue from 159 patients with COPD (23). The progress of COPD was strongly associated with an increase in the volume of tissue in the wall and with the accumulation of inflammatory mucous exudates in the lumen (see Fig. 9-2). Inflammation seems to persist even many years after smoking is stopped. Lymphoid follicles are often noted in the peripheral airways of people with COPD. Inflammation or bronchiolitis is present in the peripheral airways at an early stage of the disease, often when smokers are asymptomatic and when tests of lung function are still normal. There is pathologic extension of goblet cells and squamous metaplasia in the peripheral airways. The inflammatory cells in the airway wall and airspaces are similar to those in the larger airways, including the predominance of CD8+ lymphocytes and increased CD8:CD4 ratio (24). As the disease progresses, there is fibrosis and increased deposition of collagen in the airway wall.

LUNG PARENCHYMA (RESPIRATORY BRONCHIOLES, ALVEOLI, AND CAPILLARIES). Emphysema is defined in structural and pathologic terms as an abnormal enlargement of air spaces distal to the terminal bronchioles. In emphysema, there is significant loss of alveolar attachments and loss of elasticity, which contributes to small airway collapse during expiration. There are two major types of emphysema according to the distribution within the acinus: (a) centrilobular, which involves dilation and destruction of the respiratory bronchioles, the type typically seen with cigarette smoking; and (b) panlobular emphysema, which involves destruction of the whole acinus that is seen with AAT deficiency (25). In addition, irregular or scar emphysema includes enlarged airspaces around a scar unrelated to the acinus. Unilateral emphysema or McLeod syndrome is a complication of a severe childhood infection. Bullae are localized areas of emphysema that are overdistended and are classified according to their size and position (2).

In the early stages of emphysema, there are microscopic lesions. During the course of the disease, they may progress into macroscopic lesions or bullae defined as emphysematous space >1 cm in diameter (26). Bullous disease can also occur in the absence of COPD. The inflammatory cell profile in the alveolar walls and the airspaces is similar to that described in the airways and persists throughout the course of the disease. As with changes in bronchitis, there is some evidence suggesting the persistence of inflammation in the proximal and distal airspaces after smoking cessation.

PULMONARY VASCULAR CHANGES. The "blue bloater" phenotype with swollen ankles, enlarged liver, and engorged neck veins is seen in end-stage COPD. This occurs because of remodeling of the pulmonary arteries as a consequence of alveolar hypoxia in some patients with COPD. The earliest changes are seen as thickening of the intima, increase in smooth muscle, and infiltration of inflammatory cells into the vascular wall. With progression, more smooth muscle and collagen, as well as proteoglycans, thicken the vessel walls. Later in the progression, right ventricular hypertrophy and secondary pulmonary hypertension are found in those with chronic hypoxemia. The vascular changes can be aggravated by coexistent obstructive sleep apnea.

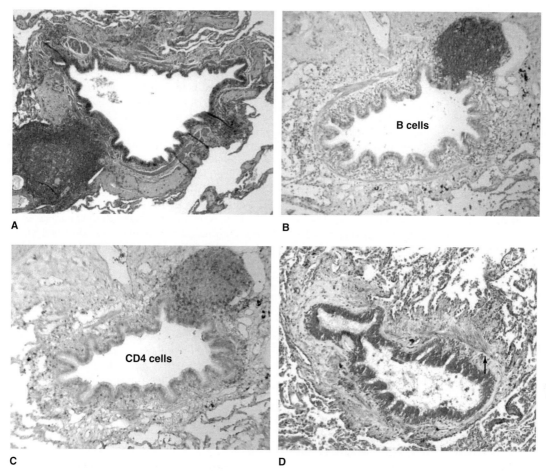

FIGURE 9-2. Pathologic findings in patients with COPD. **A:** A collection of bronchial lymphoid tissue with a lymphoid follicle containing a germinal center (*GC*) surrounded by a rim of darker staining lymphocytes that extend to the epithelium of both the small airway and the alveolar surface (Movat's stain, ×6). **B:** Another follicle in which the GC stains strongly for *B cells* (×6). **C:** A serial section of the same airway stained for *CD4 cells*, which are scattered around the edge of the follicle and in the airway wall (×6.5). **D:** An airway that has been extensively remodeled by connective-tissue deposition in the subepithelial and adventitial compartments of the airway wall. The arrow points to the smooth muscle that separates the subepithelial from the adventitial compartments (Movat's stain, ×6).

PATHOGENESIS

Tobacco smoking is the main risk factor for COPD, although other inhaled noxious particles and gases may contribute. This causes an inflammatory response in the lungs, which is exaggerated in some smokers, and leads to characteristic pathologic lesions of COPD. In addition to inflammation, imbalance of proteinases and antiproteinases in the lung, oxidative stresses, and inhibition of repair processes are also important in the pathogenesis of COPD.

INFLAMMATION. COPD is characterized by an increase in neutrophils, macrophages, and T lymphocytes, specifically $CD8^+$, in various parts of the lungs, which relate to the degree of airflow limitation. There may be an increase in eosinophils in some patients, particularly during exacerbations, which explains why corticosteroids are useful in this setting (27). These inflammatory cells are capable of releasing a variety of cytokines and inflammatory mediators, most notably leukotriene B4, interleukin-8, and TNF-α. This inflammatory pattern is markedly different from that seen in asthma. Inflammatory

changes can persist after quitting smoking. The mechanisms explaining the perpetuation of this inflammatory response in the absence of the inciting events are unknown.

PROTEINASES AND ANTIPROTEINASES IMBALANCE. The imbalance theory has been prominent for decades but cannot explain the entire pathophysiologic complex of COPD. This may occur in COPD because of increased production or activity of proteinases and reduced production or inactivity of antiproteinases. Cigarette smoke and possibly other COPD risk factors as well as inflammation itself can produce oxidative stress that, on one hand, primes several inflammatory cells (macrophages, neutrophils) to release a combination of proteinases and, on the other hand, decreases or inactivates several antiproteinases by oxidation (28). The major proteinases involved in the pathogenesis of COPD include those produced by neutrophils (elastase, cathepsin G, and proteinase-3) and macrophages (cathepsins B, L, and S), and various mixed metalloproteinases (MMPs). The major antiproteinases involved in the pathogenesis of COPD include AAT, secretory leukoproteinase inhibitor, and tissue inhibitors of MMPs.

Neutrophil elastase not only contributes to parenchymal destruction but it is also a potent inducer of mucous secretion and mucous gland hyperplasia. Therefore, long-term studies of medications such as macrolide antibiotics, which reduce neutrophil elastase, are ongoing in patients with frequent exacerbations and excessive mucous production.

OXIDATIVE STRESS. Patients with end-stage disease are cachetic and have severe exercise limitation and muscle wasting due, in part, to oxidative stress. Different markers of oxidative stress, including hydrogen peroxide, nitric oxide, and lipid peroxidation products, are found in increased amounts in the lungs, in the exhaled air breath condensate, and in the urine of smokers and patients with COPD (29). Perhaps, the oxidative stress contributes to some of the systemic manifestations of the disease. Oxidative stress can contribute to COPD by oxidizing a variety of biologic molecules that can lead to dysfunctioning of the cell or death, damaging the extracellular matrix, inactivating key antioxidant defenses, activating proteinases, or enhancing gene expression either by activating transcription factors such as nuclear factor-kB or by promoting histone acetylation (30).

PATHOPHYSIOLOGY

Pathologic changes in the lung lead to corresponding physiologic changes characteristic of the disease, including mucous hypersecretion, ciliary dysfunction, airflow limitation, pulmonary hyperinflation, gas exchange abnormalities, pulmonary hypertension, and cor pulmonale. Mucous hypersecretion and ciliary dysfunction are related to the cough and sputum production and may often be the earliest manifestation of the disease. Some patients have cough and mucus without airflow limitation. The presence of expiratory airflow limitation is the key to the diagnosis of this disease. It is due to both fixed airway obstruction and the reversibility component, leading to an increase in airways resistance. In advanced COPD, peripheral airways obstruction, parenchymal destruction, and pulmonary vascular abnormalities reduce the lung's capacity for gas exchange, producing secondary arterial hypoxemia, hypercapnia, and cor pulmonale.

CLASSIFICATION OF SEVERITY

The diagnosis of COPD is confirmed by spirometry. The presence of a postbronchodilator FEV_1 <80% of the predicted value in combination with an FEV_1/FVC ratio of <70% confirms the presence of airflow limitation. It is accepted that a single measurement of FEV_1 incompletely represents the complex clinical consequences of COPD because (a) many patients are practically asymptomatic; (b) persistent cough and sputum production often precedes the development of airflow limitation, and in others, the first symptom may be the development of dyspnea with previously tolerated activities; and (c) in the clinical course of the disease, systemic consequences such as weight loss and peripheral muscle wasting and dysfunction may develop.

The spirometric classification based on FEV_1 includes the "at risk," with the postbronchodilator FEV_1/FVC >0.7, and an FEV_1, as percent predicted, >80% (2). Usually, these are patients who smoke or have exposure to pollutants, have cough, sputum or dyspnea, or have a family history of respiratory disease.

Mild COPD is defined as an FEV_1/FVC <0.7 and an FEV_1, as percent predicted, >80%; in moderate COPD, FEV_1, as percent predicted, is 50% to 80%; in severe, it is 30% to 50%; and in very severe, FEV_1 is <30% (see Fig. 9-3). A similar classification is used in the GOLD Guidelines as stage 0 to stage 4 (3).

The body mass index, airflow obstruction, dyspnea, and the 6-minute walk distance for exercise tolerance have been combined in an index (BODE) that has recently been proposed as a 4-dimensional grading system for grading severity (31). Unlike spirometry, BODE seems to correlate well with survival. The FEV_1 is included along with the distance walked in 6 minutes. Dyspnea is measured on the Modified Medical Research Council (MMRC) scale, and the body mass index is stratified to more than or less than 21 kg per metered square. Functional dyspnea can be assessed by the Medical Research Counsel Dyspnea Scale: 0—not troubled with breathlessness except with strenuous exercise, 1—troubled by shortness of breath when walking up a slight hill, 2—walks slower than people of the same age because of breathlessness or has to stop for breath when walking at own pace on level, 3—stops for breath after walking 100 m or after a few minutes on the level, 4—too breathless to leave the house or breathless when dressing or undressing, 5—breathless at rest (31).

MANAGEMENT

There are four components of COPD management outlined by the GOLD Guidelines. These include (a) assessing and monitoring the disease, (b) reducing risk factors, (c) managing stable COPD, and (d) managing exacerbation (3).

The goals of effective COPD management are to prevent disease progression, relieve symptoms, improve exercise tolerance, improve health status, prevent and treat complications, prevent and treat exacerbations, and reduce mortality. The goals should be reached with minimal side effects from treatment. Two recent comprehensive, evidence-based reviews of COPD management are available (32,33).

ASSESS AND MONITOR THE DISEASE

Medical History

A diagnosis of COPD should be considered in any patient who has cough, sputum production or dyspnea, and/or a history of exposure to risk factors for the disease. A chronic cough is usually present either intermittently or every day. It is often present throughout the day and is seldom nocturnal. Any pattern of current sputum production may indicate COPD. Many patients produce small quantities of tenacious sputum after rather intense coughing bouts. Most patients seek medical attention because of dyspnea, which is a major cause of disability and anxiety in the disease. The dyspnea progressively worsens, is persistent, is usually present every day, and is described by the patient as "increased effort to breathe, heaviness, air hunger, or gasping." Dyspnea is worse after exercise and during respiratory infections.

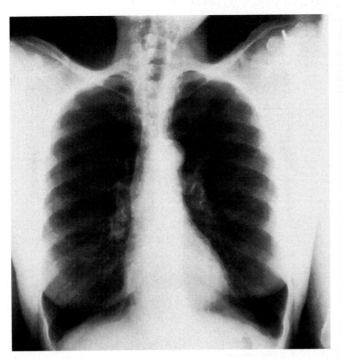 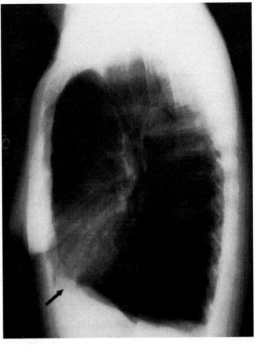

A **B**

FIGURE 9-3. Chest radiograph [posteroanterior (**A**) and lateral (**B**) views] of a 62-year-old black female smoker with emphysema (FEV_1 = 0.70 L) and a normal α1-antitrypsin (AAT) level. Vascular attenuation, hyperlucency in the upper lung zones, and diaphragm flattening [flattened costophrenic angles and an oblique sternocostal angle (*arrow*)] are demonstrated.

Past Medical History

Exposure to the risk factors and past medical history including asthma, allergy, sinusitis or nasal polyps, respiratory infections in childhood, and other respiratory disease should alert the physician that the patient may have COPD (see Table 9-2). Similarly, a family history of COPD or other chronic respiratory disease is important. The pattern of symptom development from mild cough to progressive dyspnea is noted. A history of exacerbations or previous hospitalizations for respiratory disorder may be important. The presence of comorbidity such as heart disease and rheumatoid disease can also restrict activity. It is important to assess the impact of COPD on the patient's life including limitations of activity, missed work and economic impact, effect on family routines, and feelings of depression and anxiety. The social and family support available to the patient as well as the possibilities for reducing risk factors, especially smoking cessation, should be assessed.

Physical Examination

The impressive findings on physical examination such as the "pink puffer and the blue bloater" phenotypes are seen in end-stage disease. The physical examination has low sensitivity and specificity. As lung function deteriorates, wheezing may be noted, although the physical examination is rarely diagnostic in COPD. Usually, signs of airflow limitation (e.g., prolonged expiratory phase of respiration) are present only when significant impairment in lung function has occurred.

Later in the disease, particularly with emphysema, signs of hyperinflation predominate. For example, there may be cachexia with marked weakness, fatigue, and poor muscle function. The patient may be thin and barrel chested without cyanosis or edema until the terminal stage of the disease. Some with far advanced disease have chronic alveolar hypoxia with secondary pulmonary hypertension, the so-called "blue bloater" with cyanosis, ankle edema, and cardiomegaly. Many have mixed findings.

MEASUREMENT OF LUNG FUNCTION. As mentioned earlier, spirometry should be performed for patients who have risk factors for COPD, such as smoking, symptoms of dyspnea, cough, or sputum production. Screening usually should occur in those about 50 years of age. The staging and assessment of severity is based on spirometric data although this may be less useful than the BODE Index. The hallmark of obstruction is a FEV_1/FVC <0.7 and the FEV_1 is <80% predicted.

REVERSIBILITY TO BRONCHODILATORS. Bronchodilator reversibility testing is performed once at the time of diagnosis to help rule out the diagnosis of asthma. If completely reversible, it can be used to establish the patient's best attainable lung function and to gauge the patients' prognosis. However, it has been shown over and over again that patients who do not show a significant FEV_1 response to a short-acting bronchodilator on one test may benefit symptomatically from long-term bronchodilator treatment or may be "reversible" on a subsequent testing visit.

TABLE 9-2.   Differential Diagnoses of Chronic Obstructive Pulmonary Disease (COPD)

COPD	Onset in midlife
	Symptoms are slowly progressive
	Long smoking history
	Dyspnea during exercise
	Largely irreversible airflow limitation
Asthma	Onset early in life (often childhood)
	Symptoms vary from day to day
	Symptoms at night or early morning
	Allergy, rhinitis, and/or eczema are also present
	Family history of asthma
	Largely reversible airflow limitation
Congestive heart failure	Fine basilar crackles on auscultation
	Chest x-ray shows dilated heart and pulmonary edema
	Pulmonary function tests indicate volume restriction, not airflow limitation
Bronchiectasis	Large volumes of purulent sputum
	Commonly associated with bacterial infection
	Coarse crackles on auscultation
	Chest x-ray or CT scan shows bronchial dilation and bronchial wall thickening
Tuberculosis	Onset in all ages
	Chest x-ray shows lung infiltrate
	Microbiological confirmation
	High local prevalence of tuberculosis
Obliterative bronchiolitis	Onset in younger age and nonsmokers
	Might have history of rheumatoid arthritis or fume exposure
	CT scan on expiration shows hypodense areas
Diffuse panbronchiolitis	Most patients are men and nonsmokers
	Almost all have chronic sinusitis
	Chest x-ray and HRCT scan show diffuse small centrilobular nodular opacities and hyperinflation

COPD, chronic obstructive pulmonary disease; CT, computed tomography; HRCT, high-resolution computed tomography

From GOLD Workshop Report (Updated 2004) (*www.goldcopd.org*), with permission.

Reversibility to albuterol (i.e., improvement in FEV_1 of 12% or 200 mL) may not discriminate between asthma and COPD. The bronchodilator effect is greater in peak FEV_1 and in FEV_1 area under the curve in asthma. However, many patients with COPD have reversibility to albuterol. Dorinsky et al. reviewed more than 1,000 patients and found that more than 75% had some reversibility, particularly when albuterol and ipratropium were combined (34). Donohue et al. found that approximately 73% of patients had reversibility and increased their FEV_1 12% or 200 mL following bronchodilators in the pivotal salmeterol studies of 813 patients with COPD (35). Prior to randomization, patients were tested by inhaling 2 to 4 puffs of albuterol and 2 to 4 puffs of ipratropium. Eleven percent reversed to ipratropium alone, whereas 27% reversed to albuterol alone. Thirty-five percent reversed to both agents. Mahler et al. found that 56% of patients in the trial of the combination of fluticasone and salmeterol had reversibility to albuterol at baseline (36). Calverley et al. performed bronchodilator testing at baseline in poorly

reversible COPD patients and, using ATS criteria, found that 52% changed their responder/nonresponder status between visits (37). The authors concluded that bronchodilator responsiveness in COPD is a continuous variable and classifying patients as responders or nonresponders on the basis of one observation can be misleading.

Additional evidence that many patients do not show acute bronchodilator reversal on day 1 but respond on subsequent visits can be seen in an earlier NIH sponsored multicenter–multiyear trial. Anthonisen, in a 1986 report, found that 50% of patients increased their FEV_1 15% on day 1 after breathing isoproterenol. Throughout the subsequent 9 visits over 2 years, an additional group had a 15% increase in FEV_1 on at least one visit, so that about 65% of patients had at least one visit with 15% reversibility to isoproterenol (38). Therefore, therapeutic decisions about bronchodilator use in COPD should not be based on one study of reversibility.

Lastly, Kesten and Rebuck also tried to answer the question of whether the short-term response to an inhaled β-agonist is a sensitive or specific means for distinguishing between asthma and COPD. They found that the mean change in FEV_1 in patients assessed to have asthma was different from that found in COPD patients, 16.4% versus 10.6%, respectively. However, the change in FVC in the two conditions was similar, 9.8% versus 10.3%. Nevertheless, the sensitivities and specificities of postbronchodilator changes in FEV_1 were not generally sufficient to diagnose or exclude asthma reliably. The authors concluded that the acute responses of FEV_1 and FVC following a standard dose of inhaled bronchodilator are neither sensitive nor sufficiently specific to differentiate asthma from COPD (39).

LUNG VOLUMES. Patients with COPD are hyperinflated with increased anteroposterior diameter. Static lung volumes such as total lung capacity, residual volume, and functional residual capacity, measured by either helium dilution method or by body plethysmography, can provide additional information on gas trapping and overdistention due to loss of elastic recoil. During exercise, dynamic hyperinflation occurs with reduction of inspiratory capacity or of the volume available for breathing and correlates best with dyspnea measured by the Borg scale, a visual analog scale of 0 to 10 grading from no to maximal breathlessness (40,41).

DIFFUSING CAPACITY OF CARBON MONOXIDE. Gas transfer in the lungs can be assessed by measurement of D_{LCO}. The single breath uptake of carbon monoxide over a 10-second breathhold is commonly used. The D_{LCO} tends to be low in emphysema and normal in asthma. However, many factors have influence on this test such as anemia, pulmonary vascular disease, heavy smoking, and concurrent fibrosis and atelectasis.

CHEST X-RAY. Chest x-rays are rarely diagnostic but may be valuable in excluding alternative diagnosis or in monitoring patients whose clinical status is changing (Fig. 9-3). Hyperinflation of the lungs results in (a) a low flattened diaphragm, (b) an increased retrosternal airspace (4.5 cm) on lateral film, and (c) a greater than 90-degree angle of the sternum and diaphragm. Vascular changes include (a) a reduction in the number and size of pulmonary arteries with little peripheral markings, (b) distortion of the vasculature, and (c) increased

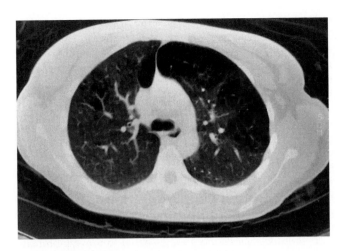

FIGURE 9-4. Computed tomographic section demonstrating extensive areas of lung destruction bilaterally consistent with the diagnosis of emphysema.

translucency. Although computerized tomography (CT) is not routinely recommended, a CT scan might help in differential diagnosis to detect and quantify emphysema and to detect bullae. CT scans are necessary if a surgical procedure such as a bullectomy or a lung volume reduction surgery (LVRS) is contemplated (see Fig. 9-4).

ARTERIAL BLOOD GASES. Secondary hypoxemia and hypercapnia are typical of end-stage COPD. Therefore, in advanced COPD such as stages 3 or 4 or in the elderly or during acute exacerbations, arterial blood gases (ABG) should be measured. While oxygen saturation is readily available, the ABG provides essential information on ventilatory status and acid–base balance. Useful situations for measuring ABG include patients with moderate to severe COPD with an FEV_1 <40% or with clinical signs suggesting respiratory failure, right heart failure, or sleep apnea. Respiratory failure is noted by a PaO_2 of <60 mm Hg with a $PaCO_2$ >55 mm Hg while breathing room air at sea level.

Exercise Testing

Direct observation of symptomatic COPD patients when challenged with the stress of exercise provides valuable insights into the severity of exertional dyspnea and the resultant functional disability (42). Simple self-paced tests such as the distanced walked over 6 minutes with measurements of oxygen saturation may provide useful information in those with moderate to severe disease; most walk 500 to 600 m. Clinical improvement after rehabilitation usually correlates with an increase in 50-m distance. Progressive symptom-limited exercise on a treadmill or bicycle is used to distinguish cardiac from respiratory causes of dyspnea.

Alpha-1-antitrypsin deficiency screening should be done in all those with early onset of COPD, often in the third or fourth decade, or in those with a strong family history of lung or liver disease. AAT is a glycoprotein produced in the liver and secreted into the blood, where it acts as a circulating serine proteinase inhibitor with neutrophil elastase, its principal substrate.

AAT is one of the serine protease inhibitors (Serpin), and its alleles can be divided into normal (M1, M2, M3), moderate deficient (S, V, F, I), and severely deficient (Z) according to their isoelectric points, concentration in the plasma, and protease inhibitory (PI) capacity. The two most frequent deficient alleles are PIS, which expresses about 50% to 60% of AAT activity, and PIZ, which expresses 10% to 20% of AAT (43). Although AAT deficiency is thought to occur predominantly in whites of Northern European heritage, it can affect all major racial groups worldwide (44).

DIFFERENTIAL DIAGNOSIS. The differential diagnosis of COPD is quite extensive (Table 9-2). The major disease to differentiate is asthma, which differs by its onset early in life, often in childhood, and by the more variable symptoms. The symptoms are more prominent at night and early morning. There may be concurrent allergic rhinitis and/or eczema, a strong family history of asthma, and a characteristic reversible airflow limitation. In contrast, COPD has an onset in midlife, the symptoms are slowly progressive, there is a long smoking history, dyspnea occurs during exercise, and there is largely irreversible airflow limitation.

Additional entities in the differential diagnosis include bronchiectasis, with large volumes of purulent sputum usually associated with infection, along with coarse crackles and clubbing on physical exam; and chest x-ray and CT scan reveal bronchodilation and bronchial wall thickening.

Tuberculosis is also an entity in the differential diagnosis but patients differ in the period of symptoms, presence of night sweats, and low-grade fever and can be diagnosed by chest x-ray with microbiologic confirmation.

Obliterative bronchiolitis has an onset in younger age and affects nonsmokers who often have a history of rheumatoid arthritis or some toxic fume exposure. CT scan on expiration shows hypodense areas. Diffuse panbronchiolitis primarily occurs in men who are nonsmokers, and all have chronic sinusitis. A chest x-ray and HRCT show diffuse small centrilobular, nodular opacities and hyperinflation.

MANAGEMENT

COMPONENT TO REDUCE RISK FACTORS. Smoking cessation is the single most effective and inexpensive intervention to reduce the risk of developing COPD and to stop its progression. A randomized double-blind placebo-controlled study of 409 patients with GOLD stage I or II COPD who smoked 15 cigarettes qd received buproprion SR 180 mg twice daily with smoking cessation and counseling for 6 months. At 5 weeks, 30% versus 15% stopped smoking; at 6 months, it was 20% versus 10% (45). Short-term tobacco dependence treatment is effective, and every tobacco user should be offered counseling and nicotine replacement (patch, gum, inhaler, and nasal spray) at every visit to the health care provider. Counseling is especially effective if it is practical and tailored to the individual. Counseling should include establishing a quit date, emphasizing abstinence, using other family members for support, and avoiding alcohol and other drugs. Several effective pharmacotherapies for tobacco dependency are available and at least one of these medications should be added to counseling. Data from the NIH Lung Health Study revealed that more participants in the Smoking Intervention Group quit compared to usual and customary therapy (in year 1, 34.4 versus 9.0; at year 5, 37.4 versus 21.9). The annual rate of decline in FEV_1 over 4 years for quitters was half that observed for smokers (31 versus 62 mL per year for 1 year). There were several additional findings: (a) women who quit had a larger improvement in first year compared with men; (b) women who continued to smoke had a greater loss of function than men with a comparative smoking rate did; and (c) heavy smokers benefit more from quitting than lighter smokers do (46). Strategies to help the patients willing to quit smoking include the 5 A's of physician interventions outlined in Table 9-3, and the 5 R's for the smoker include: (a) relevance, (b) risks, (c) rewards, (d) roadblocks, and (e) repetition.

INHALED PARTICLE AND GASES. Progression of many occupation-induced respiratory disorders can be reduced or controlled through a variety of strategies aimed at reducing the burden of inhaled particle and gases. Some may have to change employment from the so-called dusty trades or ensure that all precautions are taken. Patients with COPD should not exercise outdoors during the afternoon on "red alert" or on days when the ozone and air-pollution index are high.

MANAGEMENT OF STABLE COPD

Pharmacologic Therapy

The medications for COPD currently available can reduce or abolish symptoms, increase exercise capacity, reduce the number and severity of exacerbations, and improve health status.

Only smoking cessation and O_2 therapy can improve survival. At present, no pharmacologic treatment is shown to modify the rate of decline in lung function. The change in lung function after a brief treatment with any drug does not help in predicting other clinically relevant outcomes. In principle, the inhaled route is preferred and changes in FEV_1 following bronchodilator therapy can be small but are often accompanied by larger changes in lung volumes, which contribute to a reduction in perceived breathlessness. Another principle is that combining different agents produces a greater change in spirometry and symptoms than single agents alone can produce. As effective medication for COPD is available, all patients who are symptomatic merit a trial of bronchodilator treatment. The overall approach to managing stable COPD should be characterized by a stepwise increase in treatment (see Table 9-4).

Bronchodilator medications are essential to the symptomatic management of COPD because airflow obstruction is present in most. In the early phase of the disease, short-acting β_2-agonists or anticholinergic bronchodilators are given on an "as-needed" basis, but later on, they are given on a regular basis to prevent and relieve symptoms and to improve exercise tolerance. The inhaled route is preferred when both inhaled and oral formulations are available. Smaller doses of active treatment can be delivered directly with equal or greater efficacy and with fewer side effects when administered by inhalation. Patients must be educated in the correct use of whatever inhalation devices are employed, for a large number use metered-dose inhalers (MDIs) incorrectly (47). Furthermore, inhalation devices are changing because of regulatory actions such as the phase-out of Freon propellants that deplete ozone from the atmosphere.

TABLE 9-3. Brief Intervention Strategies to Help the Patient Willing to Quit Smoking: The Five A's

Step	Goal	Action
Ask	Systematically identify all tobacco users at every visit	Implement an office-wide system that ensures that, for EVERY patient at EVERY clinic visit, tobacco-use status is queried and documented
Advise	Strongly urge all tobacco users to quit	In a clear, strong, and personalized manner, urge every tobacco user to quit
Assess	Determine willingness to make a quit attempt	Ask every tobacco user if he or she is willing to make a quit attempt this time (e.g., within the next 30 days)
Assist	Aid the patient in quitting	Help the patient with a quit plan, provide practical counseling, provide intratreatment social support, help the patient obtain extratreatment social support, recommend use of approved pharmacotherapy except in special circumstances, and provide supplementary materials
Arrange	Schedule follow-up contact	Schedule follow-up contact, either in person or via telephone

From GOLD Workshop Report (Updated 2004) (www.goldcopd.org); and Celli BR, MacNee W. Standards for the diagnosis and treatment of patients with COPD: a summary of the ATS/ERS position paper. Eur Respir J 2004; 23(6):932-946, with permission.
http://www.thoracic.org/COPD/5/cessation_brief_intervention.asp

TABLE 9-4. The Overall Approach to Management of Stable Chronic Obstructive Pulmonary Disease (COPD) Is Characterized by a Stepwise Increase in Treatment

	0: At Risk	*I: Mild*	*II: Moderate*	*III: Severe*	*IV: Very Severe*
Characteristics	• Chronic symptoms • Exposure to risk factors • Normal spirometry	• FEV_1/FVC <70% • FEV_1 >80% • With or without symptoms	• FEV_1/FVC <70% • 50% < FEV_1 <80% • With or without symptoms	• FEV_1/FVC <70% • 30% < FEV_1 <50% • With or without symptoms	• FEV_1/FVC <70% • FEV_1 <30% or FEV_1 <50% of predicted AND chronic respiratory failure
			Avoidance of risk factor(s) and influenza vaccination		
			Add short-acting bronchodilator when needed		
			Add regular treatment with one or more long-acting bronchodilators		
			Add rehabilitation		
				Add inhaled glucocorticoids in case of repeated exacerbations	
					Add long-term oxygen in case of chronic respiratory failure
					Consider surgical treatments

From: GOLD Workshop Report (Updated 2004) (*www.goldcopd.org*), with permission.

A significant number of patients cannot effectively coordinate their breathing with an MDI but can use the breath-activated inhaler, a dry powder inhaler, or an MDI with spacer chamber. Spacers do reduce oropharyngeal deposition and subsequent local side effects. A new generation of low-volume nebulizers that use a mesh or multiple aperture plate will potentially be more efficient in delivering bronchodilators, antibiotics, proteins, and genes to the lung. These devices use a small volume, have better lung deposition characteristics, and waste less in that there is very little residual (48). Compliance with treatment in COPD is highly variable, but when assessed in large clinical trials, it was determined that at least 85% of patients take 70% of the prescribed dose, probably reflecting the fact that COPD patients are constantly symptomatic. Adherence to treatment is aided by a clear explanation of the purposes and the probable outcome of therapy, together with reinforcement and continued review of these aspects of management. As mentioned earlier, characterizing treatment responses by whether the patient is reversible or irreversible by using spirometric criteria is not useful because several studies have demonstrated worthwhile clinical benefits in groups classified initially as having irreversible disease.

BRONCHODILATORS. Three types of bronchodilators are commonly used either individually or in combination: β-agonists, anticholinergics, and methylxanthines. Bronchodilators are essential to the symptomatic management of COPD. Side effects are pharmacologically predictable in dose-dependent fashion. Adverse effects are less likely and resolve more rapidly after treatment withdrawal with the inhaled route than with oral treatment. Bronchodilators appear to work by airway smooth muscle relaxation, with improved lung emptying during tidal breathing, by causing changes in lung volume with a reduction in residual volume, and/or by delaying the onset of dynamic hyperinflation during exercises (49,50). These changes contribute to a reduction in perceived breathlessness. In general, the more advanced the COPD, the more important the changes in lung volume become relative to those in FEV_1(43).

Classes of Bronchodilator

Short-acting β₂-adrenergic bronchodilators. This type of bronchodilator, such as albuterol, pirbuterol, and terbutaline, is available as an MDI; albuterol is also available as a nebulized solution. These agents relax smooth muscle, reduce airway edema, and enhance mucociliary clearance. These agents act within a few minutes and last approximately 4 to 6 hours. They are given on an as-needed basis for relief of persistent or worsening symptoms. These agents can also increase exercise tolerance. Concerns about regular use leading to increased tolerance appear to be less of an issue in COPD than in asthma. Sestini et al. reviewed 13 studies of inhaled short-acting β₂-adrenergic bronchodilators (SABAs) in COPD. The average postbronchodilator increase in FEV_1 was 0.14 L [Weighted Mean

Difference (WMD)]. The increase in morning peak flow was 29.2 mL (WMD) and the increase in evening peak flow was 36.8 mL (WMD) (51). The author concluded that the use of SABAs administered via MDI on a regular basis modestly improves lung function and breathlessness. There is no evidence of long-term side effects.

As multiple mechanisms underlie airflow obstruction, SABAs can be added to anticholinergics to produce a very useful combination that works both peripherally and on the central airways. In three trials of 1,399 patients with advanced COPD over 3 months, combination therapy with a SABA and an anticholinergic resulted in 32% less exacerbations than monotherapy with a SABA (33) but not less than monotherapy with an anticholinergic. There are very few side effects with this combination; however, it has to be given every 4 to 6 hours (52). Recommendations in published guidelines differ for the use of SABAs: only intermittent use is recommended in asthma, whereas regular use is allowed in COPD.

Long-acting β_2-agonists (LABAs). Long-acting β_2-agonists including salmeterol 50 μg and formoterol 4.5 to 12 μg were introduced to achieve sustained and more predictable improvement in lung function than a SABA does. These agents are given every 12 hours and are particularly useful in COPD. Nine placebo-controlled clinical trials of 4,198 patients over 3 or more months demonstrated a 21% reduction in exacerbation rate (33). These agents improved health status, certainly when compared to placebo and possibly to a greater degree than regular ipratropium. Additionally, these drugs reduced symptoms and the need for rescue medication and increased the time interval between exacerbations when compared with placebo. Regular treatments with long-acting bronchodilators are more effective and convenient than treatment with short-acting bronchodilators but are more expensive. Long-acting β-agonists (LABAs), including salmeterol and formoterol, are approved for use in both asthma and COPD, but in asthma, LABAs should be combined with an antiinflammatory controller medication. In contrast, in COPD, salmeterol and formoterol can be used on a regular basis as monotherapy. As in asthma, they can be combined with agents from other bronchodilator classes and inhaled corticosteroids (ICSs) for better symptom control.

In two trials that evaluated changes in FEV₁ over 1 year, LABA improved the trough by 82 mL compared to placebo. In contrast, a systematic review by Appleton et al. performed in poorly reversible COPD identified 33 trials in their abstracts as being potentially relevant (53) but only included 4 randomized controlled trials in the review. The mean increases in FEV₁ here were 0.1 L (WMD) in the 50-μg salmeterol group and 0.12 L (WMD) in the 100-μg salmeterol group. In two crossover studies of 4 weeks' treatment, salmeterol did not produce a significant increase in FEV₁ (WMD 0.04 L). The reviewer's conclusion was that treatment of patients with COPD using LABAs produced only small increases in FEV₁, small reductions in breathlessness, and a clinically significant improvement in quality of life, which, however, was not consistent across all studies.

In contrast to formoterol, there is no dose-response effect with salmeterol. In a 16-week study, quality of life showed a significant improvement after treatment with 50 μg salmeterol but not after 100 μg (54). General health status as reflected on the Medical Outcome Short Form (SF-36) did not improve nor was there any difference in the mean change from baseline in the 6-minute walk distance.

Salmeterol has been compared with theophylline in mild to moderate COPD. In one study of 178 patients, the increase in FEV₁ was 0.13 L greater with salmeterol than with theophylline (55). Adverse event rates were fairly comparable between the two agents. Both improved quality of life, but salmeterol achieved greater improvement.

Formoterol does have a dose response, is as rapid in onset as albuterol, and is potent but is difficult to formulate. Thus, it is only available in a dry powder inhaler single dose device. The LABA salmeterol was compared with formoterol in patients with COPD (56). Formoterol had a faster onset of bronchodilator action (FEV₁ increase 0.2 L at 10 minutes); however, both agents were effective at 20 minutes (salmeterol 0.20 L, formoterol 0.25 L). The peak bronchodilator effects were the same (salmeterol 0.40 L, formoterol 0.39 L) at 60 to 120 minutes, and the duration of action was the same. Thus, both agents are comparable in COPD in efficacy and side effects.

LABAs are frequently combined with ICSs. This combination is associated with a marked increase in lung function, improvement in trough FEV₁, improvement in quality of life, and reduction in exacerbations, and may have a survival advantage.

LABAs have a good safety record in COPD. Ferguson et al. (57) reviewed 17 studies including 1,443 patients and found no increase in cardiovascular adverse effects compared with placebo. Holter monitor data revealed no significant differences from placebo in arrhythmias, QT intervals, or other parameters; usually tolerance to LABA is not seen especially in COPD. One exception was the 6-month trial of salmeterol and tiotropium where tolerance was noted (58). The recent salmeterol (SMART) study of more than 23,000 asthmatic patients was terminated early because of a slight increase in deaths, especially in African Americans. It is unknown if these findings can be extended to COPD (59).

Anticholinergics. Cholinergic mechanisms contribute to obstruction, especially in severe COPD. Anticholinergics are available as short-acting inhaled agents such as ipratropium and the long-acting agent tiotropium, which are rapidly establishing themselves as a once-a-day–preferred bronchodilators in the treatment of stable outpatients with COPD. Ipratropium bromide and tiotropium bromide are structural analogs of atropine with little systemic absorption following inhalation because their quaternary ammonia structure is lipophobic. Cholinergic nerve fibers arise in the nucleus ambiguus and in the dorsal motor nucleus of the vagus nerve. Impulses travel down the vagus nerve to parasympathetic ganglia within the walls of airways. From these ganglia, postganglionic fibers innervate airway smooth muscle, the submucosal glands, and the lung. Activation of these nerves releases acetylcholine at the neural effector junctions, where it binds to postsynaptic receptors, resulting in bronchoconstriction and increased secretion.

The effects of vagal stimulation in the lung are mediated via muscarinic receptors, of which there are several types and subtypes. The subtypes of muscarinic receptors on airway smooth muscle are M1, M2, and M3. M2 subreceptors are called *autoreceptors*; their activation inhibits further release of acetylcholine. Tiotropium selectively blocks the M3 muscarinic receptor.

The receptor half-life is 36 hours, whereas the receptor-binding half-life of ipratropium is 3 hours. Large-scale clinical trials comparing tiotropium to ipratropium and other studies against placebo for up to 1 year show the superiority of this agent (60). There is no tolerance to the bronchodilating effects of tiotropium bromide (58). Anticholinergics are more effective in COPD than in asthma. In usual doses, they are more potent than SABAs in COPD, yielding greater increases in FEV_1 area under the curve (AUC) but with similar effects on peak increase in FEV_1 and on number of responders. Calverley et al. first studied the acute response to inhaled salbutamol at one visit, and then, the response to ipratropium at another, and finally combined the two on a third visit (37). The increases in FEV_1 were similar, with a slight advantage to ipratropium. One possible advantage of ipratropium bromide is that there is a dose response in COPD whereby increasing doses of anticholinergics is associated with increasing improvement in FEV_1 (61). Because this agent is poorly absorbed, the dosage may be increased with little change in side effects. In head-to-head comparisons, short-acting anticholinergics (SACs) like ipratropium are less potent than LABAs such as formoterol and salmeterol and long-acting anticholinergics such as tiotropium (62–64). In COPD, anticholinergics are especially useful when combined with SABAs, LABAs, and/or theophyllines. Anticholinergics, particularly when administered by nebulized solution or by MDI and spacer in higher doses such as 4 puffs every 4 hours, are useful in acute exacerbations of asthma and COPD. The longer-acting agents such as tiotropium are effective in stable patients with COPD for up to 24 hours and should not be combined with SACs. Regular use of anticholinergic bronchodilators do not protect against a decline in lung function if patients continue to smoke. This was amply demonstrated in the Lung Health study.

There has been a great deal of interest in whether bronchodilator responses to ipratropium or albuterol distinguish asthma from COPD. Taube et al. found that in asthma, the increase in FEV_1 was 618 mL with the SABA fenoterol and 482 mL with the anticholinergic oxitropium. In COPD, the increase was 221 mL after fenoterol and 235 mL after oxitropium (65). Thus, it appears that there is substantial overlap. In asthma, SABAs are superior to anticholinergics, whereas in COPD the number of responders is approximately equal.

Unfortunately, ipratropium has a short duration of action, requiring administration every 6 hours. Such a regimen decreases adherence to drug therapy. Therefore, the 24-hour tiotropium was developed. Dry mouth is much more common with tiotropium than with ipratropium. The safety profiles of these drugs appear to be otherwise similar.

Van Noord et al. performed a single-center, double-blind, controlled study to characterize the onset of the pharmacodynamic steady state of tiotropium. Trough FEV_1 following 8 days of tiotropium therapy was 0.19 L, 18% above baseline. Approximately 90% of this increase (0.17 L, 16% above baseline) was achieved within 24 hours of the first dose. The trough FVC increased by 0.67 L (27%) on test day 8. Approximately 70% of the improvement (0.47 L, 19%) was observed after two tiotropium doses. Achievement of an FVC steady state was delayed compared with the FEV_1 steady state (66). Thus, it appears that FEV_1 steady state is reached within 48 hours, while an FVC increase can be expected during the first week of therapy.

Casaburi et al. found that tiotropium was a safe and effective once-daily anticholinergic agent when compared with placebo (67). The FEV_1 and FVC were 12% above baseline on day 8. These improvements were maintained at days 50 and 92. The average postdose FEV_1 was 16% higher than baseline on day 1 and 20% higher than baseline on day 92. FVC was 17% higher than baseline on day 1 and 19% higher on day 92.

Tiotropium improves health status and reduces exacerbations and hospitalizations when compared to both placebo and regular ipratropium; it appears to be superior to salmeterol over 6 months. In two 6-month trials of tiotropium versus salmeterol and placebo, in 1,207 patients, tiotropium improved health status, decreased hospital admissions, decreased dyspnea, and decreased exacerbations (68,69). Tiotropium was superior to salmeterol by 37mL in trough FEV_1, which tended to increase with time. Tiotropium has recently been shown to improve oxygen saturation during sleep, without affecting sleep quality (70). Tiotropium is associated with reduction of lung hyperinflation at rest and during exercise (71). Resultant increase in inspiratory capacity permitted greater expansion of tidal volume and improvement in dyspnea and exercise endurance. Five clinical trials of tiotropium involving 3,574 patients have uniformly shown a beneficial effect in reducing exacerbation rate when compared to either placebo [RR (relative risk), 0.74] or ipratropium bromide (RR, 0.78) but not LABAs (RR, 0.93) (33). The current trials are too short to evaluate survival effects but long-term studies are ongoing.

Theophylline. Theophylline remains one of the most widely prescribed drugs for the treatment of airways disease worldwide because it is inexpensive. However, theophylline has become a third-line agent in industrialized countries because of the frequency of side effects and its relative low efficacy. A recent study by van Andel et al. found that in 10 trials of bronchodilators in COPD from 1987 to 1995, inhaled steroid use increased from 13% to 41%, whereas theophylline use declined from 63% to 29% (72).

Theophylline is useful in both asthma and COPD and is often used as an adjunct to aerosol bronchodilators and inhaled steroids. Patients with COPD may benefit from an empiric trial over 1 to 2 months. Recommended doses today are lower than those used in the past. Lower doses have both anti-inflammatory and immunomodulatory effects in both COPD and asthma. Sustained-release theophylline is useful in controlling nocturnal symptoms.

Theophylline was initially used as a bronchodilator, and an early dose-response effect was demonstrated with increases in FEV_1 when the plasma level was increased from 10 to 20 μg per dL. More recent guidelines have recommended lower doses such as 8 to 12 μg per dL because of the narrow therapeutic window and concern about toxicity. The molecular mechanism of bronchodilation is partially explained by phosphodiesterase (PDE) inhibition, resulting in an increase in cyclic adenosine monophosphate by inhibition of PDE_3 and PDE_4 and in cyclic guanosine-3,5-monophosphate by inhibition of PDE_5. Theophylline is also an adenosine-receptor antagonist. It inhibits intracellular calcium release and increases histone deacetylase activity, possibly resulting in an increase in the efficacy of corticosteroids when the two classes are combined (73).

Theophylline has been compared with other therapies in COPD. Rossi et al. compared the efficacy of oral slow-release theophylline with formoterol in 854 patients with COPD. Both agents improved lung function (area under the FEV_1 12-hour curve). Formoterol was more effective in reducing symptoms being used as a rescue medication and in preventing falls in peak expiratory flow. More treatment-related side effects and withdrawals were seen with theophylline (74). Cazzola et al. found that salbuterol combined with titrated theophylline increased the FEV_1 by 0.157 L over baseline at 3 months. This was less than salbuterol combined with fluticasone 250 μg (0.188 L) or salbuterol with fluticasone 500 μg (0.239 L) but similar to salbuterol alone (0.163 L) (75). ZuWallack et al., in a study of 943 patients, found salmeterol to be better than theophylline in improving lung function and in producing fewer side effects. However, therapy with both agents combined was more effective and resulted in no increase in side effects compared with either agent alone (76).

Sustained-release theophylline must be monitored very carefully, particularly when used in elderly patients with asthma and COPD. The steady state pharmacokinetics of a sustained-release formulation of theophylline is altered in the elderly. Interpatient variability and peak/trough fluctuations with this formulation are higher in the elderly than those described in healthy volunteers. Therefore, the importance of theophylline monitoring is emphasized. In older patients, toxicity is usually due to drug interactions (macrolides, fluroquinolones) or due to a change in metabolism because of a concomitant condition such as pneumonia or congestive heart failure or change in health status.

Other Pharmacologic Treatment

INHALED CORTICOSTEROIDS. The use of inhaled corticosteroids in COPD remains contentious. Although COPD is an inflammatory disease, the effects of ICS on inflammatory cells and mediators in BAL, induced sputum, and endobronchial biopsy are inconsistent. Some studies show a reduced number of cells on serial studies when patients take ICS; others show higher numbers of neutrophils due to reduced neutrophil apoptosis. Regular use of ICSs does not have a substantial effect on the decline in lung function. Two recent meta-analyses including four large multiyear studies show the WMD with regular use of inhaled steroids versus placebo to be in the range of only 5.7 mL to 9.9 mL per year (77,78). However, data from the Isolde study shows that regular use of ICSs is associated with a reduction in the rate of exacerbations from 1.3 to 0.9 per year. Furthermore, those that have frequent exacerbations and more severe COPD benefit most (79). In six placebo-controlled trials in 1,741 patients, ICSs reduced exacerbations by 24% over 6 months (33). Hence, the recommendations from the GOLD Guidelines call for a consideration of inhaled corticosteroids in those whose lung function is less than 50% and in those who have exacerbations (3). The average increase in predose FEV_1 in COPD with regular use of ICSs is below 50 mL in six large trials. In addition, recent studies of the combination of an inhaled steroid such as fluticasone or budesonide versus the combination of an inhaled steroid and a LABA showed that the monotherapy arm with steroids yields an FEV_1 <100 mL (36,80–83). Surprisingly, the oft-quoted statement that a 2-week trial with oral steroids such as prednisone 40 mg daily or Medrol 32 mg is useful in predicting the response

to inhaled steroids has been proven to be false (84). A 2-week burst of inhaled steroids did not predict those who would respond to inhaled steroids over the course of the Isole study. Hence, this practice probably should be abandoned.

Patients with COPD are frequently at high risk of osteoporosis and cataracts. The question is whether inhaled steroids will accelerate the development of these degenerative conditions. Certainly, if inhaled steroids can be shown to reduce the number of bursts of oral steroids, the risk to benefit ratio will be improved. All patients with COPD, especially female smokers who are sedentary, are at risk for osteoporosis. Hence, attention to bone health should be given to every patient with this condition and replacement with calcium, vitamin D, and bisphosphonates is often appropriate. Also, patients with COPD are at risk for cataracts, and patients on ICS must be monitored yearly. The risk of osteopenia and cataracts are much less than with oral corticosteroids.

The effect of ICS on mortality is uncertain and is widely debated in the literature. A trend was observed toward reduced mortality in patients randomized to ICS (RR, 0.75) (33), and retrospective observational data is suggestive of an advantage. Inhaled corticosteroids seem to decelerate the decline in health status.

COMBINATION OF INHALED CORTICOSTEROIDS AND LONG-ACTING β-AGONIST. As in asthma, the combination of an inhaled steroid and a long-acting β-agonist has proven to be highly effective and safe in COPD. Two combinations are presently available, budesonide plus formoterol (B/F) and fluticasone plus salmeterol (F/S). At the present time, the approved dose in the United States is 250/50 μg per dL (83). The combination produced superior improvement in lung function compared to the individual components as well as the placebo in a 6-month study, with no augmented risk of side effects. The F/S at 500/50 combination is also highly effective and is the approved dose in Europe. This combination has been studied for 1 year in the Tristan study and also for 6 months in the United States (36,81). In the Trial of Inhaled Steroids and Long-Acting β_2-Agonists (TRISTAN), 1,465 patients received S/FP, S, F, or placebo. There was a significantly reduced decline in quality of life/health status and a 25% reduction in acute exacerbations in the combination group. An even greater reduction was seen in those with FEV_1 50% predicted. In the 6-month study, greater improvement in dyspnea, lung function, and health status was seen with the combination. Surprisingly, the improvement in lung function is the same with S/F at 250/50 as with 500/50, indicating that there does not appear to be a dose response to ICS in COPD (36,83). Three clinical trials of 2,951 patients demonstrated that the combination is associated with lower exacerbation rates compared to monotherapy with a LABA or placebo but not with ICS monotherapy (33). The effects of the combination on mortality are uncertain but prospective studies are ongoing.

In a short 8-week study, F/S 250/50 has proven superior to the combination of ipratropium and albuterol for a number of important outcomes including lung function, symptoms, and dyspnea, as reflected in the TDI scale. The number of responders with a significant improvement in dyspnea was 65%, which is higher than in previous studies (85).

The combination of B/F also has been highly effective in patients regardless of their bronchodilator reversibility (80,82). In these two 1-year studies with nearly 2,000 patients enrolled, the combination significantly reduced severe exacerbations and decline in health status. Obviously, further studies are needed to assess these combination agents in COPD. Furthermore, LABA and ICSs are being combined in clinical practices with long-acting agents such as tiotropium. More studies comparing the various agents alone or in combinations are ongoing. Individual empirical trials of these agents for 2 to 3 months in patients with COPD are necessary.

ORAL CORTICOSTEROIDS. Oral corticosteroids are not recommended for regular use in a long-term maintenance program because there has been no consistent evidence of efficacy nor superiority over other agents, while the adverse event profile is unpleasant. Nonetheless, many severely ill patients with few options do receive these agents and frequently have skin ecchymosis, painful compression fractures, and cataracts as a consequence, along with myopathy, which further limits exercise.

VACCINES. Influenza vaccine can reduce serious illness and death in COPD patients by about 50%. Concerns over the safety of influenza vaccination in COPD have led to suboptimal use. A population-based cohort of 12,000 patients with asthma or COPD had no adverse outcomes on the day of vaccination and over the next 2 weeks, suggesting the vaccine is safe (86). Vaccines should be given in autumn of each year. Pneumococcal vaccine containing 23 virulent serotypes probably should be used, although sufficient data to support its general use in COPD have not yet been established. However, it has been demonstrated that in the elderly population, these two vaccines reduce all-cause pneumonia and cardiac hospitalizations by 30% to 40% (87,88).

ALPHA-1-ANTITRYPSIN AUGMENTATION THERAPY. AAT is presently administered by intravenous infusion of the purified protein weekly, which can sustain circulating AAT serum levels and can have a biologic protective effect. However, it is extremely expensive, and to date, no randomized controlled trial has showed an improvement in the decline in lung function. However, the observational cohort in the United States Alpha-1 Registry has provided data suggesting that the rate of decline in lung function is less in those treated with replacement therapy than in those who did not receive therapy (89). A European trial has suggested that disease progression as shown by computerized axial tomography (CAT) scan is slower than in patients not receiving replacement therapy (90). Presently, the US market has three AAT replacement products that differ in filtering techniques used in plasma separation but are comparable in activity and in blood levels. Periodic shortfalls in availability are a constant problem with using these agents. Intravenous therapies are highly expensive and inconvenient to use. A recent ATS consensus statement provides guidance for use of these replacement products (91).

ANTIBIOTICS. These are essential to the treatment of exacerbations. In general, they are not recommended for regular use in COPD. There are some studies evaluating macrolide antibiotics for their effects on neutrophil elastase, which is important in producing mucous hypersecretion associated with infection, but these studies are investigational. Sometimes, in those with frequent infections, an HRCT will reveal concurrent bronchiectasis.

MUCOLYTIC THERAPY. There are marked differences between countries in habits for prescribing mucolytic therapy. A review of 23 trials of oral mucolytics showed a reduction in exacerbation rate of 29% per year and a reduction in DALYS (92). Mucolytic therapy, such as ambroxol and iodinating glycerol, has not been adequately evaluated in a sufficient number of studies. It has little effect on lung function. The antioxidant *N*-acetylcysteine, a drug with both mucolytic and antioxidant action, may reduce the number of exacerbations of COPD, but a three-year prospective trial in Europe will soon be reported.

The regular use of antitussives is contraindicated in stable COPD because cough has a significant airway protective effect.

LEUKOTRIENE MODIFIERS. These are not recommended in COPD unless the patient has concurrent rhinitis or asthma because they block the C4, D4, and E4 leukotriene receptor, whereas the relevant receptor in COPD is the leukotriene B4. Many studies have evaluated leukotriene modifiers in COPD, but the improvement in lung function and symptoms are modest at best.

Nonpharmacologic Treatment

CONTROLLED OXYGEN THERAPY. The long-term administration of oxygen for more than 15 hours per day to patients with COPD does increase survival. It can also have a beneficial impact on hemodynamics, hematologic characteristics, exercise capacity, lung mechanics, and mental status. Long-term oxygen therapy is generally introduced in Stage III or IV; in very severe patients with COPD who have a PaO_2 below 55 mm Hg or an SaO_2 at or below 88%, with or without hypercapnia; or a PaO_2 between 55 mm Hg and 60 mm Hg or a saturation of oxygen of 89% if there is evidence of pulmonary hypertension or peripheral edema, suggesting congestive heart failure, or polycythemia with a hematocrit >55%. The goal of long-term oxygen therapy is to increase the baseline PaO_2 to at least 60 mm Hg at sea level and at rest, and/or to produce saturation of oxygen above 90%, which will ensure adequate delivery of oxygen. As oxygen saturation may deteriorate during sleep or exercise, it may be useful to perform an overnight study to detect desaturation and/or an exercise study in patients with COPD.

PULMONARY REHABILITATION. Pulmonary rehabilitation is a multidisciplinary program of care for patients with COPD that improves exercise tolerance and health status in those whose FEV_1 is below 1.5 L. Rehabilitation is individually tailored and designed to optimize physical and social performance and autonomy (ATS definition). The primary goals of pulmonary rehabilitation are to reduce symptoms, improve quality of life, decrease disability, and increase physical and emotional participation in everyday activities by anxiety management, relaxation, identifying and changing beliefs about exercise and health related issues, as well as by exercise management. Pulmonary rehabilitation covers a range of nonpulmonary problems including exercise deconditioning, relative social isolation, altered mood states, muscle wasting, and weight loss. Patients benefit with respect to both exercise tolerance and symptoms of dyspnea and fatigue. The minimum length of an effective rehabilitation program is 2 months, but the longer the program continues, the more effective the results are. Therefore, a maintenance rehabilitation program is necessary (92). There seems to be no definite effect on survival, and data on reduction in hospitalization rates are inconsistent. Comprehensive rehabilitation includes exercise training, nutrition counseling, and education.

Surgical Treatments for Chronic Obstuctive Pulmonary Disease

Surgical treatments for COPD include bullectomy, LVRS, and lung transplantation. Pneumothorax is a common complication of COPD that might require surgical intervention.

BULLECTOMY. Bullectomy is indicated in carefully selected patients to reduce dyspnea and to improve lung function. The procedure is based on a thoracic CT scan showing a bulla with significant compression of adjoining lung, a large bulla occupying substantial part of the thorax, or respiratory embarrassment due to an enlarging bulla. Surgical candidates are carefully selected and the operative approach is based on patient factors and on the extent of disease. Often, a video-assisted thorascopy (VATS) approach is selected.

LUNG VOLUME REDUCTION SURGERY. The National Emphysema Therapeutic Trial (NETT) of LVRS failed to demonstrate that surgery improved survival but exercise tolerance did seem to improve in those individuals with upper lobe disease and poor exercise tolerance. For those with very low lung function (FEV_1 <20%), low diffusing capacity (<20%), and diffuse disease, the mortality was greater than in the controlled population treated medically. Functional benefits were noted in patients with predominant upper lobe emphysema and a high baseline exercise tolerance and in patients with non–upper lobe disease and a low baseline exercise capacity (93). Individual outcomes do vary. The NETT included a prospective economic analysis and they concluded that LVRS was costly per patient relative to medical therapy at least in the short run. The procedure may be cost effective if the benefits are sustained over time. The effect on national health care expenditures will depend on whether an estimated 2 million patients with severe emphysema will meet the criteria for surgery (94). Functional benefits were also noted in some patients with predominant upper lobe emphysema and a high baseline exercise tolerance and in patients with non–upper lobe disease and a low baseline exercise capacity.

LUNG TRANSPLANTATION. In appropriately selected patients with advanced COPD, lung transplantation may improve quality of life and functional capacity. Usually, these candidates are selected at FEV_1 less than 35%, PaO_2 of 55 to 60 mm Hg, and $PaCO_2$ above 50. Single lung transplants were offered previously, but more recently, double lung transplantation is becoming more popular. Patient with prior LVRS can successfully undergo transplantation.

MANAGING EXACERBATIONS

Many have defined an acute exacerbation of COPD as a subjective increase from baseline of some combination of dyspnea, sputum production, and sputum volume over a 2-day period. Many grading systems are used—some based on number of symptoms and type of intervention (e.g., more bronchodilator, antibiotics, corticosteroids) and others on the location of health care utilization (e.g., phone call, urgent care or ED, or hospital).

Exacerbations are often the defining clinical events in the life of a patient with COPD. There are multiple causes of exacerbation including infection, air pollution, exposure to allergens, and ozone. Usually, symptoms deteriorate. The most common symptom is increased breathlessness. This is accompanied by wheezing, chest tightness, increased cough and sputum, change in the color and/or the tenacity of sputum, and fever. There may also be nonspecific systemic complaints, such as malaise, insomnia, fatigue, depression, and confusion. There is exercise intolerance. The outcome of an exacerbation is influenced greatly by the patient's underlying severity of COPD, previous exposure to antibiotics that can change the flora, or recent use of oral corticosteroids. ABG measurements and O_2 saturations are useful in assessing the severity of an exacerbation. Simple lung function studies would be useful but are often very hard to perform. In the hospital setting, ABGs are very useful to guide O_2 therapy and to prevent sedation in a patient with impending respiratory failure. Similarly, a chest x-ray can exclude pneumonia or congestive heart failure and an electrocardiogram may rule out acute ischemic changes or arrhythmia. There is a differential diagnosis for an acute exacerbation including congestive heart failure, pneumothorax, pleural effusion, pulmonary embolism, arrhythmia, and more. These for the most part can be excluded by clinical assessment, chest x-ray, EKG, spiral CT scan, and so on.

The presence of increased cough or purulent sputum is sufficient evidence to warrant antibiotic therapy. The most common pathogens are *Streptococcus pneumoniae*, *Haemophilus influenzae*, and *Moraxella catarrhalis*. More severely affected patients (e.g., stage 4) may have gram-negative rods such as *Klebsiella* or *Pseudomonas*, which typically cause more severe infection. Rarely, atypical bacteria such as *Mycoplasma* and *Chlamydia pneumoniae* or *Legionella* can be involved. Many exacerbations are due to viruses (30%) but the findings cannot be distinguished from those due to bacteria. Similarly, air pollution due to ozone or particulates causes exacerbations that are indistinguishable from those caused by bacteria.

Management

HOME MANAGEMENT. Most exacerbations are treated at home, following a phone call or walk-in visit. An escalation in the use of β-agonist bronchodilators by increasing the dose and frequency can be done if no contraindication exists. If not being used already, an anticholinergic can be added. If the patient is only on MDIs, perhaps a high-dose nebulized therapy can be given. Antibiotics and oral glucocorticosteroids are also used (see Table 9-5).

SYSTEMIC GLUCORTICOSTEROIDS. Several recent randomized double-blind placebo-controlled studies have produced strong evidence that patients with acute exacerbation benefit

TABLE 9-5. Home Treatment of Acute Chronic Obstructive Pulmonary Disease (COPD) Exacerbation

Patient Education
>   Check inhalation technique
>   Consider use of spacer devices

Bronchodilators
>   Short-acting β_2-agonist and/or ipratropium MDI with spacer or hand-held nebulizer as needed
>   Consider adding long-acting bronchodilator

Systemic Corticosteroids
>   Prednisone, 30–40 mg, qd for 10 d
>   Consider using an inhaled corticosteroid

Antibiotics
>   May be initiated in patients with altered sputum characteristics (increased sputum volume and increased sputum purulence)
>   Choice should be based on local bacterial resistance patterns
>   Agents used successfully in clinical trials include amoxicillin/ampicillin, cephalosporins, doxycycline, and macrolides
>   If the patient has failed prior antibiotic therapy, consider amoxicillin/clavulanate and respiratory fluoroquinolones

MDI: metered-dose inhaler

From Celli BR, MacNee W. Standards for the diagnosis and treatment of patients with COPD: a summary of the ATS/ERS position paper. *Eur Respir J* 2004; 23(6):932-946, with permission.
http://www.thoracic.org/COPD/13/outpatient.asp

from systemic CS with fewer symptoms and improved lung function. For patients with modest COPD, most controlled clinical trials have shown short-term systemic CS in combination with other effective therapies lead to small but clinical significant improvement and fewer treatment failures. The usual starting dose is approximately 30 to 40 mg of prednisone given for periods of 5 to 10 days with or without a taper in dose.

ANTIBIOTICS. Sputum cultures are not usually necessary. The choice of antibiotics is based on the community patterns of bacterial resistance to antibiotics plus patient factors such as stage of disease and recent exposure to antibiotics and systemic corticosteroids. Antibiotics directed at common pathogens are used. Second- and third-generation cephalosporins, newer macrolides, amoxicillin/clavulanate, or fluroquinolones may be necessary for those who do not respond to simple oral antibiotics or for the known presence of β-lactamase–producing organisms in the sputum.

INDICATION FOR HOSPITALIZATION. The indications for a hospital assessment or admission for exacerbations of COPD are multifactorial but include insufficient home support, older age, diagnostic uncertainty, newly occurring arrhythmias, significant comorbidities, failure of an exacerbation to respond to initial medical management, onset of new physical signs such as peripheral edema or cyanosis, severe background COPD level 3 or 4, and marked increase in the intensity of symptoms, such as sudden development of resting dyspnea.

TREATMENT IN THE HOSPITAL. Adherence of ED management of COPD acute exacerbations to that recommended in treatment guidelines is poor. In a study of 224 patients with an average age of 70 years in the ED, half were admitted but 42% had a relapse at the 2-week follow-up (95). The first treatment when a patient reaches the hospital is to provide controlled oxygen therapy if necessary, with adequate levels of oxygenation as defined by a PaO_2 of 60 mm Hg and a saturation above

90%. Once oxygen therapy is started, ABG should be checked 30 minutes later to make sure there is adequate oxygenation without both CO_2 retention and acidosis.

BRONCHODILATOR THERAPY. Short-acting inhaled β_2-agonists and anticholinergics by nebulizer are usually the preferred bronchodilators for the in-hospital treatment of exacerbations of COPD. A recent systematic review of bronchodilators showed no difference in FEV_1 at 90 minutes with either SABA or SAC. When SAC was added to SABA, little advantage was noted over SABA alone (96), but the combination is widely used. The role of theophylline in treatment of COPD exacerbations remains controversial. The conclusion from four trials with 169 patients was that methylxanthine did not change FEV_1 at 2 hours, but slightly improved FEV_1 at 3 days. Nonsignificant reductions in admission rate and decreased hospital length of stay were offset by increased relapse and increase in tremor, palpitations, and arrhythmias (97).

GLUCOCORTICOSTEROIDS. Oral or intravenous glucocorticosteroids are recommended as an addition to bronchodilator therapy, although the specific dose is not known (98). Higher doses do have a higher side-effect profile. One dosing regime that was used in the Systemic Corticosteroids in Chronic Obstructive Pulmonary Disease Exacubations (SCCOPE) trial was 125 mg of intravenous methylprednisolone every 6 hours for 3 days, followed by oral prednisone tapered over 2 weeks (60 mg on days 4–7, 40 mg on days 8–11, and 20 mg on days 12–15) (99). Corticosteroids do lead to a greater improvement in lung function, reduced hospital stay, and decreased relapse rate and treatment failure.

ANTIBIOTICS. Antibiotics are always used in the hospital for exacerbations of COPD. Because of the possibility of bacterial resistance and pneumonia, a more intense regimen of broad-spectrum antibiotics directed at the common bacteria and the gram-negative bacteria is begun. The oral or intravenous route is chosen depending on the patient's status and on the likelihood of infection with *Pseudomonas*, which would require two agents.

VENTILATORY SUPPORT. Noninvasive intermittent positive pressure ventilation (NPPV) has been studied in an acute respiratory failure due to COPD, and in most randomized studies it shows a consistently positive effect. The addition of NPPV to standard care in patients with acute exacerbation of COPD decreased the rate of endotracheal intubation (RR 28%), length of hospital stay (4.57 days), and in-hospital mortality rate (10%). These reductions occur only in those with more severe exacerbations—not mild ones (100).

Selection criteria for noninvasive ventilation include moderate to severe dyspnea with the use of accessory muscles and paradoxical abdominal motion, moderate to severe acidosis with a pH <7.35, and hypercapnia with a $Paco_2$ >45 and a respiratory frequency of >25 breaths per minute. Exclusion criteria include respiratory arrest, cardiovascular instability, somnolence, impaired mental status, uncooperative patient, high aspiration risk, recent facial or gastrointestinal surgery, craniofacial trauma, and extreme obesity. Monitoring such patients closely in a high intensity unit is necessary to evaluate treatment response and facilitate intubation if NPPV fails.

Conventional invasive mechanical ventilation is indicated for those with severe dyspnea; hemodynamic instability; impending respiratory arrest with respiratory frequency >35 breaths per minute; those with life-threatening hypoxemia with a Pao_2 <40, with severe acidosis with a pH <7.25, and hypercapnia at 60 mm Hg; actual respiratory arrest; somnolence; impaired mental status; cardiovascular complications; and other complications such as sepsis, pneumonia, pulmonary embolism, and NPPV failure.

Weaning from or discontinuing mechanical ventilation can be particularly difficult and hazardous in patients with COPD. Many end-stage patients require prolonged ICU care. Therefore, the patient's preference for intervention and intense care should be determined prior to the acute event.

Hospital Discharge and Follow-up

Patients discharged from either the ED or inpatient service should be prescribed oral corticosteroids. In a prospective study of 147 patients seen in the ED with an exacerbation of COPD, the overall rate of relapse at 30 days was 43% on placebo versus 27% for those on 10 days of 40 mg of prednisone. Additional benefits versus placebo were modest improvement in FEV_1, dyspnea, and health status (101). Another prospective cohort study of 140 patients from 29 North American EDs found that one fifth of the patients discharged with an acute exacerbation of COPD have a relapse requiring urgent care within 2 weeks. Also, both chronic factors such as a history of prior ED visit in the past year and acute factors (e.g., respiratory rate at ED presentation and activity limitation over last 24 hours) are associated with an increased risk of relapse (102). The role of ICS in preventing relapse after hospitalization looks encouraging (103).

Discharge criteria following acute exacerbations of COPD vary but include: (a) the frequency of inhaled β_2-agonist is no more than every 4 hours; (b) the patient is able to walk across the room; (c) he or she is able to eat and sleep without frequent awakening by dyspnea; (d) the patient has been clinically stable

for 24 hours, including ABG; (e) the patient and home caregiver fully understand the correct use of inhalers; (f) follow-up and home-care arrangements have been completed; and (g) the patient and family physician are confident that the patient can manage successfully. The evidence is accumulating that both bronchodilators and ICS are effective in reducing exacerbation rates. The role of ICS combined with long-acting bronchodilators following an acute exacerbation is being prospectively studied. Some, but not all, observational retrospective studies suggest improved survival and reduced relapse rate when these agents are used over the year following hospitalization. Careful follow-up is imperative either by a phone call in the week following discharge or by scheduling an early clinic visit within 30 days (104).

REFERENCES

1. Mannino DM. Chronic obstructive pulmonary disease: definition and epidemiology. *Respir Care* 2003;48:1185–1191.
2. Celli BR, committee members. Standards for the diagnosis and treatment of patients with COPD: a summary of the ATS/ERS position paper. *Eur Respir J* 2004;23:932–946.
3. Fabbri L, Pauwels RA, Jurd S. Global strategy for the diagnosis, management, and prevention of chronic obstructive pulmonary disease: GOLD executive summary updated 2003. *Chronic Obstruct Pulm Dis* 2004;1:105–141.
4. Silva GE, Sherrill DL, Guerra S, et al. Asthma as a risk factor for COPD in a longitudinal study. *Chest* 2004;126:59–65.
5. Mannino DM, Homa DM, Akinbami LJ, et al. Chronic obstructive pulmonary disease surveillance—United States, 1971–2000. *MMWR* 2002;51(SS06):1–16.
6. Murray CJ, Lopez AD. Evidence-based health policy—lessons from the Global Burden of Disease study. *Science* 1996;274:740–743.
7. Murray CJ, Lopez AD, eds. *The global burden of disease: a comprehensive assessment of mortality and disability from diseases, injuries and risk factors in 1990 projected to 2020.* Cambridge, MA: Harvard University Press, 1996.
8. National Heart, Lung, and Blood Institute. Morbidity and Mortality: chart look on cardiovascular, lung, and blood disease. Bethesda: U.S. Department of Health and Human Services, Public Health Service, NIH 1198. Available from URL: *www.nhlbi.nih/gov/nhlbi/.*
9. Meyer PA, Mannino DM, Redd SC, et al. Characteristics of adults dying with COPD. *Chest* 2002;122(6):2003–2008.
10. Sin DD, Stafinski T, Ng YC, et al. The impact of chronic obstructive pulmonary disease on work loss in the United States. *Am J Respir Crit Care Med* 2002;165(5): 704–707.
11. Molfino NA. Impact of basic research on tomorrow's medicine. Genetics of COPD. *Chest* 2004;125:1929–1904.
12. Dahl M, Tybjaerg-Hansen A, Lange P, et al. Change in lung function and morbidity from chronic obstructive pulmonary disease in alpha1-antitrypsin MZ heterozygotes: a longitudinal study of the general population. *Ann Intern Med* 2002;136(4):270–279.
13. Sinn DD, Man SF. Why are patients with COPD at increased risk of cardiovascular disease? The potential role of systemic inflammation in COPD. *Circulation* 2003;107(11):1514–1519.
14. Kazerouni N, Alverson CJ, Redd SC, et al. Sex differences in COPD and lung cancer mortality trends—United States, 1968–1999. *J Womens Health* 2004;13(1):17–23.
15. Tashkin DP, Altose MD, Bleecker ER, et al. The Lung Health Study: airway responsiveness to inhaled methacholine in smokers with mild to moderate airflow limitation 1992. *Am Rev Respir Dis* 1992;145:301–310.
16. Tashkin DP, Altose MD, Connett RE, et al. Methacholine reactivity predicts change in lung function over time in smokers with early COPD. *Am J Respir Crit Care Med* 1996;153:1807–1811.
17. Connett JE, Murray RP, Buist AS, et al. Change in smoking status affect women more than men: results of the lung health. *Am J Epidemiol* 2003;157:973–979.

18. Wise RA, Kanner RE, Lindsner P, et al. The effect of smoking intervention and an inhaler bronchodilator on airway reactivity in COPD: the lung health study. *Chest* 2003;124:449–458.

19. Scanlon PD, Connett JE, Waller LA, et al. Smoking cessation and lung function in mild-to-moderate chronic obstructive pulmonary disease. The lung health study. *Am J Respir Crit Care Med* 2002;162:381–390.

20. Fletcher C, Peto N, Tinker C, et al. *The natural history of chronic bronchitis and emphysema: an eight-year study of early COPD in working men in London.* New York: Oxford University Press, 1976:1–272.

21. Saetta M, Turato U, Mastrelli P, et al. Cellular and structural bases of COPD. *Am J Respir Crit Care Med* 2001;163:1304–1309.

22. Turato U, Zuir R, Miniati M, et al. Airway inflammation in severe COPD: relationship with lung function and radiologic emphysema. *Am J Respir Crit Care Med* 2002;166:105–110.

23. Hogg JC, Chu F, Utokaparch S, et al. The nature of small-airway obstruction in chronic obstructive pulmonary disease. *N Engl J Med* 2004;350:2645–2653.

24. O'Shaughnessy TC, Ansair TW, Barnes RC. Inflammation in bronchial biopsies of subjects with chronic bronchitis: increase rates of CD8+ T lymphocytes with FEV$_1$. *Am J Respir Crit Care Med* 1997;155:852–857.

25. American Thoracic Society/European Respiratory Society. Statement: standards for the for the diagnosis and management of individuals with Alpha 1 antitrypsin deficiency. *Am J Res Crit Care Med* 2003;168(7):818–900.

26. CIBA Guest Symposium Report. Terminology, definitions, and classifications of chronic pulmonary emphysema. *Thorax* 1959;14:286.

27. Saetta M, DiStephrano A, Maestrelli P. Airway eosinophilia in chronic bronchitis during exacerbation. *Am J Respir Crit Care Med* 1994;150:1646–1652.

28. Barnes PJ, Shapiro SD, Pauwels RA. Chronic obstructive lung disease: molecular and cellular mechanisms. *Eur Respir J* 2003;22:672–688.

29. Neprine JE, Bast A, Lankhorst I. Oxidative Stress Study Group. Oxidative stress in COPD. *Am J Respir Crit Care Med* 1997;156:341–157.

30. Ito K, Lim S, Caramori G, et al. A molecular mechanism of action of theophylline: induction of histone deacytylase activity to decrease inflammatory gene expression. *Proc Natl Acad Sci USA* 2002;49:8921–8926.

31. Celli RB, Cote CG, Martin JM, et al. The body-mass index, airflow obstruction, dyspnea, and exercise capacity index in chronic obstructive pulmonary disease. *N Engl J Med* 2004;350:1005–1012.

32. Sutherland ER, Cherniack RM. Management of chronic obstructive pulmonary disease. *N Engl J Med* 2004;350:2689–2697.

33. Sin DD, McAlister FA, Man SF, et al. Contemporary management of chronic obstructive pulmonary disease. Scientific review. *JAMA* 2003;290:2301–2316.

34. Dorinsky PM, Reisner C, Ferguson GT, et al. The combination of ipratropium and albuterol optimizes pulmonary function reversibility testing in patients with COPD. *Chest* 1999;115:966–971.

35. Donohue JF, et al. Demographics and bronchoreversibility of salmeterol and ipratropium in a large population of patients with mild-to-moderate COPD [abstract]. *Am J Respir Crit Care Med* 1997;155:A227.

36. Mahler DA, Wire P, Horstman D, et al. Effectiveness of fluticasone propionate and salmeterol combination delivered via the Diskus device in the treatment of chronic obstructive pulmonary disease. *Am J Respir Crit Care Med* 2002;166:1084–1091.

37. Calverley PM, Burge PS, Spencer S, et al. Bronchodilator reversibility testing in chronic obstructive pulmonary disease. *Thorax* 2003;58:659–664.

38. Anthonisen NR, Wright EC, IPPB Trial Group. Bronchodilator response in chronic obstructive pulmonary disease. *Am Rev Respir Dis* 1986;133:814–819.

39. Kesten S, Rebuck AS. Is the short-term response to inhaled β-adrenergic agonist sensitive or specific for distinguishing between asthma and COPD? *Chest* 1994;105:1042–1045.

40. Boy G. Psychophysical basis of perceived exertion. *Med Sci Sport Exerc* 1982;84:372–381.

41. O'Donnell DE, Lam M, Webb KA. Measurement of symptoms, lung hyperinflation and endurance during exercise in COPD. *Am J Respir Crit Care Med* 1998;158:1984–1990.

42. O'Donnell DE. Assessment and management of dyspnea in COPD. In: Similowski T, Whitelaw WA, Derenne J-P, eds. *Clinical management of COPD.* New York: Marcel Dekker, 2002:113–1730.

43. Alpha 1 – reference is the ATS/ERS statement

44. de Serres FJ. Worldwide racial and ethnic distribution of alpha 1-antitrypsin deficiency: summary of an analysis of published genetic epidemiologic surveys. *Chest* 2002;122:1818–1829.

45. Tashkin D, Kanner R, Bailey W, et al. Smoking cessation in patients with chronic obstructive pulmonary disease: a double-blind, placebo-controlled, randomized trial. *Lancet* 2001;357:1571–1575.

46. Connett JE, Murray RP, Buist AS, et al. Changes in smoking status affect women more than men: results of the lung health study. *Am J Epidemiol* 2003;157:973–979.

47. Gray S, Wiiliams D, Putnam C, et al. Characteristics predicting incorrect metered dose inhaler techniques in older subjects. *Arch Intern Med* 1996;156:984–988.

48. Dhand R. New frontiers in aerosol delivery during mechanical ventilation. *Respir Care* 2004;49:666–676.

49. O'Donnell DE, Flute T, Gerker F, et al. Effects of tiotropium on lung hyperinflation, dyspnea and exercise tolerance in COPD. *Eur Respir J* 2004 23(6);832–840.

50. Celli C, ZuWallack RL, Wang S, et al. Improvement in testing inspiratory capacity and hyperinflation with tiotropium in patients with increased status lung volumes. *Chest* 2003;124(5):1743–1748.

51. Sestini P, Renzoni E, Robinson S, et al. Short-acting β2 -agonists for stable chronic obstructive pulmonary disease (Cochrane review). *The Cochrane Library*, Issue 2, 2003. File reference CD001495. Oxford: Update Software, Accessed July 20, 2003.

52. COMBIVENT Inhalation Aerosol Study Group. In chronic obstructive pulmonary disease, a combination of ipratropium and albuterol is more effective than either agent alone: an 85-day multicenter trial. *Chest* 1994;105:1411–1419.

53. Appleton S, Poole P, Smith B, et al. Long-acting β2-agonists for chronic obstructive pulmonary disease patients with poorly reversible airflow limitation (Cochran review). *The Cochrane Library*, Issue 2, 2003. File reference CD001104. Oxford: Update Software, Accessed July 10, 2003.

54. Jones PW, Bosh TK, An International Study Group. Quality of life changes in COPD patients treated with salmeterol. *Am J Respir Crit Care Med* 1997;155:1283–1289.

55. Di Lorenzo G, Morici G, Drago A et al., SLMT02 Italian Study Group. Efficacy, tolerability, and effects on quality of life of inhaled salmeterol and oral theophylline in patients with mild-to-moderate chronic obstructive pulmonary disease. *Clin Ther* 1998;20:1130–1148.

56. Çelik G, Kayacan O, Beder S, et al. Formoterol and salmeterol in partially reversible chronic obstructive pulmonary disease: a crossover, placebo-controlled comparison of onset and duration of action. *Respiration* 1999;66:434–439.

57. Ferguson GT, Funck-Brentano C, Fischer T, et al. Cardiovascular safety of salmeterol in COPD. *Chest* 2003;123:1817–1824.

58. Donohue JF, Menjoge S, Kesten S. Tolerance to bronchodilating effects of salmeterol in COPD. *Respir Med* 2003;97(9):1014–1020.

59. Knobil K, Yancey S, Kral K, et al. Salmeterol muticenter asthma research trial (SMART): results from an interim analysis. *Chest* 2003;124:335S.

60. Casaburi R, Mahler DA, Jones PW, et al. A long-term evaluation of once-daily inhaled tiotropium in chronic obstructive pulmonary disease. *Eur Respir J* 2002;19:217–224.

61. Gross NJ, Petty TL, Friedman M, et al. Dose response to ipratropium as a nebulized solution in patients with chronic obstructive pulmonary disease: a three-center study. *Am Rev Respir Dis* 1989;139:1188–1191.

62. Mahler DA, Donohue JF, Barbee RA, et al. Efficacy of salmeterol xinafoate in the treatment of COPD. *Chest* 1999;115:957–965.

63. Dahl R, Greefhorst LA, Nowak D, et al. Inhaled formoterol dry powder versus ipratropium bromide in chronic obstructive pulmonary disease. *Am J Respir Crit Care Med* 2001;164:778–784.

64. Vincken W, van Hoord JA, Greefhorst AP, et al. Improved health outcomes in patients with COPD during 1 yr's treatment with tiotropium. *Eur Respir J* 2002;19:209–216.

65. Taube C, Kannies F, Groke L, et al. Reproductivity of forced inspiratory and expiratory volumes after bronchodilation in patients with COPD or asthma. *Respir Med* 2003;97:568–577.

66. van Noord JA, Smeets JJ, Custers FLJ, et al. Pharmacodynamic steady state of tiotropium in patients with chronic obstructive pulmonary disease. *Eur Respir J* 2002;19:639–644.
67. Casaburi R, Briggs DD Jr, Donohue JF et al., US Tiotropium Study Group. The spirometric efficacy of once-daily dosing with tiotropium in stable COPD: a 13-week multicenter trial. *Chest* 2000;118:1294–1302.
68. Donohue JF, van Noord JA, Bateman ED, et al. A 6-month placebo-controlled study comparing lung function and health status changes in COPD patients treated with tiotropium or salmeterol. *Chest* 2002;122:47–55.
69. Brusasco V, Hodder R, Miravitlles M, et al. Health outcomes following treatment for six months with once daily tiotropium compared with twice daily salmeterol in patients with COPD. *Thorax* 2003;58:399–404.
70. McNicholas WT, Calverley PMA, Lee A, et al. Long-acting inhaled anticholinergic therapy improves sleeping oxygen saturation in COPD. *Eur Respir J* 2004;23:825–831.
71. O'Donnell DE, Fluge T, Gerken F, et al. Effects of tiotropium on lung hyperinflation, dyspnea and exercise tolerance in COPD. *Eur Respir J* 2004;23:832–804.
72. van Andel AE, Reisner C, Menjoge SS, et al. Analysis of inhaled corticosteroid and oral theophylline use among patients with stable COPD from 1987 to 1995. *Chest* 1999;115:703–707.
73. Barnes PJ. Theophylline: new perspectives for an old drug. *Am J Respir Crit Care Med* 2003;167:813–818.
74. Rossi A, Kristufek P, Levine BE et al., Formoterol in Chronic Obstructive Pulmonary Disease (FICOPD) II Study Group. Comparison of the efficacy, tolerability, and safety of formoterol dry powder and oral, slow-release theophylline in the treatment of COPD. *Chest* 2002;121:1058–1069.
75. Cazzola M, Di Lorenzo G, Di Perna F, et al. Additive effects of salmeterol and fluticasone or theophylline in COPD. *Chest* 2000; 118:1576–1581.
76. ZuWallack RL, Mahler DA, Reilly D, et al. Salmeterol plus theophylline combination therapy in the treatment of COPD. *Chest* 2001;119:1661–1670.
77. Highland KB, Strange C, Heffner JE. Long-term effects of inhaled corticosteroids on FEV_1 in patients with chronic obstructive pulmonary disease: a meta-analysis. *Ann Intern Med* 2003;138: 969–973.
78. Sutherland ER, Allmers H, Ayas NT, et al. Inhaled corticosteroids reduce the progression of airflow limitation in chronic obstructive pulmonary disease: a meta-analysis. *Thorax* 2003;58(11): 937–941.
79. Burge PS, Calverley PMA, Jones PW et al., ISOLDE Study Investigators. Randomised, double blind, placebo controlled study of fluticasone propionate in patients with moderate to severe chronic obstructive pulmonary disease: the ISOLDE trial. *Br Med J* 2000;320:1297–1305.
80. Calverley PM, Boonsawat W, Cseke Z, et al. Maintenance therapy with budesonide and formoterol in chronic obstructive pulmonary disease. *Eur Respir J*. 2003;22:912–919.
81. Calverley P, Pauwels R, Vestbo J et al., TRISTAN (Trial of Inhaled Steroids and Long-Acting β_2 Agonists) Study Group. Combined salmeterol and fluticasone in the treatment of chronic obstructive pulmonary disease: a randomized controlled trial. *Lancet* 2003;361:449–456. Erratum in *Lancet* 2003;361:1660.
82. Szafranski W, Cukier A, Ramirez A, et al. Efficacy and safety of budesonide/formoterol in the management of COPD. *Eur Respir J* 2003;21:74–81.
83. Hanania NA, Darken P, Horstman D, et al. The efficacy and safety of fluticasone propionate (250 microg)/salmeterol (50 microg) combined in the Diskus inhaler for the treatment of COPD. *Chest* 2003 ;124(3):834–843.
84. Burge PS, Calverley PMA, Jones PW et al., ISOLDE Study Group. Prednisolone response in patients with chronic obstructive pulmonary disease: results from the ISOLDE study. *Thorax* 2003;58: 654–658.
85. Donohue JF, Kalberg C, Emmett A, et al. A short-term comparison of fluticasone propionate/salmeterol with ipratropium bromide/albuterol for the treatment of COPD. *Treat Respir Med* 2004; 3(3):173–181.
86. Tata K. West J, Harrison T, et al. Does influenza vaccination increase consultations, corticosteroid prescriptions, or exacerbations in subjects with asthma or chronic obstructive pulmonary disease? *Thorax* 2003;58:835–839.
87. Govaent TM, This CT, Masurel N, et al. The efficacy of influenza in elderly individuals: a randomized double-blind placebo controlled trial. *JAMA* 1194;272:1661–1665.
88. Nichol KL, Nordin J, Mullooly J. Influenza vaccination and reduction in hospitalizations for cardiac disease and stroke in the elderly. *N Engl J Med* 2003;348:1322–1332.
89. The Alpha 1-Antitrypsin Deficiency Registry Study Group. Survival and FEV_1 decline in individuals with severe deficiency of alpha 1-antitrypsin. *Am J Respir Crit Care Med* 1998;158:49–59.
90. ATS Documents. American Thoracic Society/European Respiratory Society Statement: standards for the diagnosis and management of individuals with alpha-1 antitrypsin deficiency. *Am J Respir Crit Care Med*. 2003;168:818–900.
91. Dirksen A, Dijkman JH, Madsen F, et al. A randomized clinical trial of alpha-1 antitrypsin augmentation therapy. *Am J Respir Crit Care Med* 1999;160:1468–1472.
92. Poole PJ, Black PN. Mucolytic agents for chronic bronchitis or chronic obstructive pulmonary disease. *Cochrane Database Syst Rev* 2003;(2):CD001287.
93. National Emphysema Treatment Trial Research Group. A randomized trial comparing lung-volume – reduction surgery with medical therapy for severe emphysema. *N Engl J Med*. 2003;348: 2059–2073.
94. Ramsey SD, Berry B, Etzioni R, et al. Cost effectiveness of lung-volume–reduction surgery for patients with severe emphysema. *N Engl J Med* 2003;348:2092–2102.
95. Cydulka RK, Rowe BH, Clark S, et al. Emergency department management of acute exacerbations of chronic obstructive pulmonary disease in the elderly: the Multicenter Airway Research Collaboration. *J Am Geriatr Soc*. 2003;51(7):908–916.
96. McCrory DC, Brown CD. Anti-cholinergic bronchodilators versus beta2-sympathomimetic agents for acute exacerbation of chronic obstructive pulmonary disease. *Cochrane Database Syst Rev* 2002;(4):CD003900.
97. Barr RG, Rowe BH, Camargo CA Jr. Methylxanthines for exacerbations of chronic obstructive pulmonary disease: meta-analysis of randomized trials. *Br Med J* 2003;327(7416):643.
98. McCrory DC, Brown C, Gelfand SE, et al. Management of acute exacerbations of COPD: a summary and appraisal of published evidence. *Chest* 2001;119:1190–1209.
99. Niewoehner DE, Collins D, Erbland ML. Relation of FEV_1 to clinical outcomes during exacerbations of chronic obstructive pulmonary disease. Department of Veterans Affairs Cooperative Study Group. *Am J Respir Crit Care Med* 2000;161:1201–1205.
100. Keena SP, Sinuff T, Cook DJ, et al. Which patients with acute exacerbation of chronic obstructive pulmonary disease benefit from noninvasive positive-pressure ventilation? *Ann Intern Med* 2003;138:861–870.
101. Aaron SD, Vandemheen KL, Herbert P, et al. Outpatient oral prednisone after emergency treatment of chronic obstructive pulmonary disease. *N Engl J Med* 2003;348:2618–2625.
102. Kim S, Emerman CL, Cydulka RK, et al. Prospective multicenter study of relapse following emergency department treatment of COPD exacerbations. *Chest* 2004 ;125(2):473–481.
103. Sin DD, Tu JV. Inhaled corticosteroids and the risk of mortality and readmission in elderly patients with chronic obstructive pulmonary disease. *Am J Respir Crit Care Med*. 2001;164(4):580–584.
104. Sin DD, Bell NR, Svenson LW, et al. The impact of follow-up physician visits on emergency readmissions for patients with asthma and chronic obstructive pulmonary disease: a population-based study. *Am J Med*. 2002;112(2):120–125.

CHAPTER 10

Lung Transplantation and Lung Volume Reduction Surgery

Stephanie M. Levine

Luis F. Angel

Jay I. Peters

Stephen G. Jenkinson

For the past two decades, lung transplantation (LT) has become an accepted therapeutic option for patients with end-stage pulmonary parenchymal or vascular disease. Prior to this, the procedure was infrequently performed and was fraught with problems. The first human lung transplant was performed by Hardy in 1963, but the patient survived only 18 days (1). From 1963 until 1980, nearly 40 more lung transplants were attempted; however, the longest survival was only 10 months (2,3). Early attempts at LT were unsuccessful because of the development of rejection or infection in the transplant recipients (2,3).

Since that time, research has led to improved surgical techniques; markedly improved immunosuppressive therapy, initially with the discovery of cyclosporine A (4); and improved standardization of selection criteria for transplant recipients. As a result, in 2001, more than 1500 LT procedures were performed worldwide, as reported to the International Society of Heart and Lung Transplantation (ISHLT) (5). Pulmonologists must understand the surgical procedures available to their patients, the selection criteria for transplantation, the immunosuppressive regimens, and the management of complications that commonly occur in transplant recipients. The first part of this chapter reviews each of these topics. The second part of this chapter reviews the more recently utilized surgical option for patients with end-stage emphysema: lung volume reduction surgery.

INDICATIONS FOR SINGLE LUNG TRANSPLANTATION

In 1983, the Toronto Group reported the first long-term survival of single lung transplantation (SLT) in a patient with idiopathic pulmonary fibrosis (IPF) (6). Restrictive parenchymal lung disease is ideal for SLT. The transplanted lung possesses normal compliance and vascular resistance and allows preferential ventilation and perfusion to the transplanted organ. SLTs have been performed for idiopathic and familial pulmonary fibrosis, drug- or toxin-induced lung disease, occupational lung disease, sarcoidosis, limited scleroderma, and other disorders resulting in end-stage fibrotic lung disease.

Initially, there was concern that patients with obstructive lung disease might develop severe ventilation–perfusion mismatch after SLT. These disorders are characterized by increased lung compliance and by destruction of the vascular bed. Perfusion could be diverted to the transplanted lung while ventilation remained in the native emphysematous lung. Early attempts at SLTs in patients with emphysema resulted in hyperinflation of the native lung with compression of the transplanted lung (7). Fortunately, careful management of mechanical ventilation and control of postoperative infections and rejection have resulted in successful SLTs in patients with obstructive lung disease (8). Although the patients have continued airway obstruction on pulmonary function testing, there is no significant ventilation–perfusion mismatch. This has allowed SLTs to be performed in patients with chronic obstructive pulmonary disease (COPD) and in patients with α_1-antitrypsin deficiency. The first successful SLT for COPD in the United States was performed in 1989 by Dr J. Kent Trinkle in San Antonio, Texas (9). Currently, COPD comprises the most common indication for SLT reported to the registry of the ISHLT at 53% (5).

SLT has also been successfully performed in patients with pulmonary vascular disease, although, in general, bilateral lung transplantations (BLTs) are preferred for this indication. A single lung allograft with normal pulmonary vasculature can accommodate the entire right ventricular output without elevation of pulmonary artery pressure (10). The right ventricle has been shown to be extremely resilient, and SLTs have been done in patients with right ventricular ejection fractions below 20%. The right ventricle shows significant improvement in function postoperatively. Patients with Eisenmenger syndrome (a cardiac abnormality resulting in pulmonary hypertension) and a repairable cardiac anomaly can also on occasion be candidates for SLT.

In general, the advantages of SLT include reduced surgical morbidity, shortened hospitalization, and often, the avoidance of cardiopulmonary bypass. This procedure also optimizes the use of donor organs, which are in critical shortage.

INDICATIONS FOR BILATERAL LUNG TRANSPLANTATION

Patients with suppurative pulmonary lung disease, such as cystic fibrosis (CF), are not candidates for SLTs. Once immunosuppressed, the native lung could infect the transplanted lung or could lead to systemic infection. Initially, patients with CF or bronchiectasis underwent heart–lung transplantation (HLT). Double lung transplantation (DLT) avoids concurrent or asynchronous rejection of the heart and may avoid the accelerated coronary artery disease seen with heart transplantation. Initially, this procedure was performed with an anastomosis at the level of the trachea; however, the rate of ischemic airway complications was prohibitive. Now transplant surgeons perform BLT or sequential SLT, with anastomoses performed at each mainstem bronchus.

Some transplant centers perform BLT for severe obstructive lung disease. In young patients with emphysema and with a longer posttransplant life expectancy or in patients with extensive bilateral bullae, BLT may be preferable. Similarly, patients with pulmonary hypertension with reduced right ventricular function undergoing SLT are the most difficult to manage in the intraoperative and postoperative periods. In addition, during times of graft dysfunction these patients can develop significant ventilation–perfusion mismatch such as acute or chronic rejection. Most centers, therefore, prefer BLT for pulmonary hypertension in an attempt to distribute blood flow equally to both lungs.

INDICATIONS FOR HEART–LUNG TRANSPLANTATION

Few centers are currently performing HLT. However, HLT remains the primary procedure for patients with combined end-stage lung disease and heart disease (e.g., emphysema with cardiomyopathy or irreparable coronary artery disease). Patients with Eisenmenger syndrome and irreparable cardiac lesions also require HLT. Most transplant centers require that patients be less than 55 years of age for HLT. There is an approximately 25% risk of major morbidity in the postoperative period with HLT (11). Opportunistic infections and bronchiolitis

TABLE 10-1. Transplantation Procedures for Various Disease States

Transplant Procedure	Disease State
Single lung	Restrictive fibrotic lung disease, COPD (emphysema, α_1-antitrypsin deficiency), pulmonary hypertension
Bilateral lung	Suppurative lung disease (cystic fibrosis, bronchiectasis), some patients with COPD, pulmonary hypertension
Heart–lung	End-stage cardiac and pulmonary disease

COPD, chronic obstructive pulmonary disease.
From Official ATS Statement—June 1992. Lung transplantation: report of the ATS workshop on lung transplantation. *Am Rev Respir Dis* 1993;147:772–776, with permission.

TABLE 10-2. General Recipient Selection Guidelines

Untreatable end-stage pulmonary disease of any etiology
No other significant medical diseases
Substantial limitation of daily activity
Limited life expectancy
Ambulatory with rehabilitation potential
Acceptable nutritional status
Satisfactory psychosocial profile and emotional support system

From Official ATS Statement—June 1992. Lung transplantation: report of the ATS workshop on lung transplantation. *Am Rev Respir Dis* 1993;147:772–776, with permission.

obliterans are major causes of mortality after this procedure. Despite the increased incidence of complications, HLT remains the only appropriate option for some patients with combined end-stage cardiac and pulmonary disease. A summary of transplantation procedures for various disease states is outlined in Table 10-1.

LIVING DONOR TRANSPLANTATION

Several institutions worldwide are now performing living donor transplantation. The primary indication for living donor transplantation is CF. Generally, each of the two blood group–compatible living donors provides a lower lobe to the recipient. Ideally, the donor lobes should be larger than that of the recipient's so that the donor lobes fill the hemithorax. This has not yet been performed at the majority of lung transplant centers because of certain technical and ethical issues involved in the procedure. Early data suggest that outcomes in these patients are comparable to those reported with cadaveric donor lung transplants (12).

GUIDELINES FOR RECIPIENT SELECTION

Any patient with end-stage pulmonary or cardiopulmonary disease with the capacity for rehabilitation can be considered for transplantation. Obviously, many patients will not be suitable candidates, and the patients most likely to survive the early postoperative transplant period are those who, although terminally ill, maintain an active lifestyle and an acceptable nutritional status. The patient should have untreatable end-stage pulmonary disease, no other significant medical illness, and a limited life expectancy. The candidate should be ambulatory with rehabilitation potential. Patients must be psychologically stable, committed to the idea of transplantation, and willing to comply with the rigorous medical protocols required for successful LT. These general guidelines have been accepted by the American Thoracic Society (13) and are outlined in Table 10-2.

AGE

The 1998 international guidelines for selection of transplant candidates suggested age limits of 55 years for HLT, 65 years for SLT, and 60 years for BLT procedures (14). Although this is somewhat arbitrary, numerous patients with end-stage pulmonary

disease are young to middle-aged, and there is a relative lack of available donors. A recent large survey of 50 North American transplant centers conducted by the Transplant Network of the American College of Chest Physicians found that most centers were adhering to these general age guidelines (15).

CONTRAINDICATIONS

The general relative and absolute contraindications to LT, as identified by the 1998 international guidelines, are listed in Table 10-3 (14).

Systemic or Multisystem Disease

Transplantation is not contraindicated in patients with systemic diseases limited to the lungs, such as scleroderma, systemic lupus erythematosus, polymyositis, and rheumatoid arthritis. These cases should be considered on an individual basis (16).

Patients with diabetes mellitus, poorly controlled hypertension, or neurologic disease should be evaluated carefully before being considered as candidates for LT and should be accepted only if their disease is well controlled and if there is no end organ damage.

Patients with active sites of infection are not considered good transplant candidates. Treated tuberculosis and fungal disease pose a particular problem but are not contraindications to LT. Some centers will not consider transplanting a patient

TABLE 10-3. Contraindications to Lung Transplantation

Relative	Mechanical ventilation
	Symptomatic osteoporosis
	Ideal body weight below 70% or over 130%
	Substance addiction in prior 6 mo (including tobacco use)
	Psychosocial problems
	Severe musculoskeletal disease
	Colonization with fungus or atypical mycobacteria
Absolute	Extrapulmonic disease, i.e., renal (creatine clearance below 50 mg/mL/min)
	HIV infection
	Malignancy within prior 2 yr
	Hepatitis B antigen positivity
	Hepatitis C, biopsy-proven liver disease

From Guidelines for the selection of lung transplant candidates. Joint Statement of the American Society for International Transplant Physicians/American Thoracic Society/European Respiratory Society/International Society for Heart and Lung Transplantation. *Am J Respir Crit Care Med* 1998;158:335–339, with permission.

who is chronically colonized with a resistant organism (e.g., *Burkholderia cepacia*, methicillin-resistant *Staphylococcus*, atypical *Mycobacterium*, or *Aspergillus*). Centers should try to eradicate these organisms in the pretransplant period, and patients should be considered on an individual basis (17). These patients should not be considered for SLT procedures because the colonized remaining lung could pose a serious threat to the new graft.

Corticosteroids

Initial data implicated corticosteroids as a cause of tracheal or bronchial dehiscence (18,19). At most centers, patients are required to completely discontinue corticosteroids. This eliminates a large number of patients with COPD and pulmonary fibrosis. Low-dose pretransplant corticosteroid therapy has proved to be acceptable in patients who cannot completely discontinue corticosteroids (9,19,20). Currently, transplant programs will consider patients who can be chronically maintained on 20 mg or less per day of prednisone, and may consider patients on higher doses.

Psychosocial Criteria

The patient must be well motivated and emotionally stable to withstand the extreme stress of the pretransplant and perioperative period. A history of noncompliance or a significant psychiatric illness is a relative contraindication, although many patients will present with reactive depression or anxiety in the terminal phase of their pulmonary illness. Prior to transplantation, a thorough psychiatric evaluation is required to exclude an underlying psychiatric diagnosis. The importance of a support system cannot be overemphasized.

Skeletal Disease

Osteoporosis has become a significant problem in the post-transplant period, and preexisting symptomatic osteoporosis has been identified as a relative contraindication to transplantation (21). Bone densitometry should be part of the pretransplant evaluation, and treatment should be initiated in those with evidence of osteoporosis, symptomatic or asymptomatic. Aggressive treatment with bisphosphonates has allowed patients with osteoporosis to proceed to transplant. Nonosteoporotic skeletal disease, such as kyphoscoliosis, is also a relative contraindication to transplantation.

Mechanical Ventilation

Requirement of invasive mechanical ventilation is a strong relative contraindication to transplantation. Patients who are on noninvasive ventilatory support can be considered for transplantation.

Nutritional Status

In order to be considered for transplantation, patients should have an ideal body weight of more than 70% or less than 130% of predicted, although there can be exceptions. Cachectic patients may be too weak to withstand the surgical procedure, and patients who are obese make more difficult surgical candidates.

Substance Abuse

Drug abuse or alcoholism is considered to be a contraindication to transplantation because these patients are at high risk for noncompliance. Patients who continue to smoke despite end-stage pulmonary disease are not candidates for LT. Most transplant centers require a patient to abstain from cigarette smoking, alcohol abuse, or narcotics for 6 months to 2 years before being considered for LT.

Absolute Contraindications

The 1998 international guidelines identify absolute contraindications to LT as including major organ dysfunction, that is, renal (creatinine clearance of <50 mg/mL/minute), human immunodeficiency virus (HIV) infection, hepatitis B antigen positivity, and hepatitis C with biopsy-documented liver disease (14). Active malignancy within the prior 2 years is also a contraindication to transplantation. For patients with a history of breast cancer beyond stage 2, colon cancer beyond Dukes A, renal carcinoma, or melanoma at or beyond level III, the waiting period should be at least 5 years. Patients with a prior malignancy should be restaged before they become transplant candidates.

DISEASE-SPECIFIC GUIDELINES FOR TIMING OF TRANSPLANTATION

Patients who meet all criteria for LT are usually placed on the active waiting list when their life expectancy is less than 18 to 24 months. This period of time has been referred to as the "transplant window," when the patient is ill enough to require transplantation and is healthy enough to assure a reasonable chance for success (22). Data from the United Network for Organ Sharing (UNOS) show that the mean waiting period ranges from 12 to 24 months. Guidelines for the timing of transplantation are difficult to determine but must be based on the natural history of each disease process. The 1998 international guidelines outline disease-specific criteria for transplant referral (see Table 10-4) (14).

CHRONIC OBSTRUCTIVE PULMONARY DISEASE

The variability in the natural course of COPD makes it especially difficult to predict when patients should be referred for lung transplantation. The National Institutes of Health's Intermittent Positive-Pressure Breathing (IPPB) trial demonstrated that patients less than 65 years old with an forced expiratory volume in one second (FEV_1) below 30% of predicted had a 3-year survival rate of 80% (23). This study excluded patients with hypoxemia. Nevertheless, this study confirmed prior reports that the postbronchodilator FEV_1 was the best predictor of survival. Another study reviewed two community-based populations with COPD during a 7- to 15-year study period (24). Again, the best predictor of survival was the percentage of predicted FEV_1 after the administration of bronchodilators. The presence or absence of cor pulmonale further improved the prediction of subsequent mortality. Cor pulmonale was clinically determined by history and physical examination, radiographic findings, and electrocardiogram. Poor nutritional status (assessed by serum albumin) and carbon monoxide

TABLE 10-4. Disease Specific Criteria for Lung Transplantation

COPD	FEV_1 under 25% of predicted (nonreversible)
	$PaCO_2$ at or over 55 mm Hg
	Cor pulmonale
	O_2-dependent hypercapnic patients (refer early)
IPF	Symptomatic disease despite medical therapy
	Abnormal pulmonary function:
	VC 60% to 70% of predicted
	Diffusing capacity 50% to 60% of predicted
CF	FEV_1 at or under 30% of predicted
	Clinical deterioration with FEV_1 >30% of predicted
	$PaCO_2$ over 50 mm Hg
	PaO_2 in room air under 55 mm Hg
	Young, female patients (refer early)
PPH	NYHA III–IV despite vasodilator treatment
	Cardiac index under 2 L/min/m^2
	Right atrial pressure over 15 mm Hg
	Mean pulmonary artery pressure over 55 mm Hg

CF, cystic fibrosis; COPD, chronic obstructive pulmonary disease; FEV_1, forced expiratory volume in one second; IPF, idiopathic pulmonary fibrosis; NYHA, New York Heart Association; $PaCO_2$, arterial carbon dioxide tension; PaO_2, arterial oxygen tension; PPH, primary pulmonary hypertension.

From Guidelines for the selection of lung transplant candidates. Joint Statement of the American Society for International Transplant Physicians/American Thoracic Society/European Respiratory Society/International Society for Heart and Lung Transplantation. *Am J Respir Crit Care Med* 1998;158:335–339, with permission.

diffusing capacity ($DLCO$) also showed some statistical significance. This study showed an overall 1-year survival of 65% when the postbronchodilator FEV_1 fell below 30% of predicted. Patients with cor pulmonale and an FEV_1 below 30% of predicted had a 2-year survival of 50% and a 3-year survival of only 20%.

Both studies showed wide individual variability in survival with COPD, and the decision to transplant in these patients is frequently based on the progression of disease. Analyses of registry and UNOS data have shown that this group of patients may achieve significant improvement in quality of life (QOL) without clear survival benefit with transplantation (25).

On the basis of the above data, the international guidelines (14) suggest that patients with COPD are in the transplant window if FEV_1 is less than 25% of predicted (nonreversible) and/or if $PaCO_2$ is at or over 55 mm Hg and/or if there is cor pulmonale. Those patients with hypercapnia and hypoxemia requiring oxygen supplementation should be given preference.

IDIOPATHIC PULMONARY FIBROSIS

Prospective longitudinal studies show that the mean survival in patients with usual interstitial pneumonia [idiopathic pulmonary fibrosis(IPF)] is 5.6 years after diagnosis (26). Although 10% of patients respond to therapy and 15% remain stable, this pattern is seen with only mild or moderate disease (26). Most patients have a progressive downhill course despite therapy. In one prospective randomized trial comparing prednisolone alone with cyclophosphamide and prednisolone, only the initial total lung capacity (TLC) and forced vital capacity (FVC) were associated with time of "failure." Patients

with a TLC below 60% of predicted did poorly regardless of the initial regimen and had a 50% 1-year survival (27).

On the basis of these high mortality statistics and the fact that many patients with IPF die while awaiting transplantation, the international guidelines suggest that these patients should be referred for transplantation early. Criteria include patients with symptomatic disease who have failed immunosuppressive therapy and/or patients with abnormal pulmonary function even with minimal symptoms, that is, vital capacity at or under 60% to 70% predicted and/or diffusing capacity at or under 50% to 60% of predicted (14).

CYSTIC FIBROSIS

Despite the improvement in life expectancy with CF, most patients still die from respiratory failure and cor pulmonale. A recent study followed almost 700 patients with CF for more than 12 years to determine whether the risk from respiratory failure could be predicted 1 or 2 years in advance (28). The study concluded that patients with an FEV_1 less than 30% predicted, a PO_2 below 55 mm Hg, or a PCO_2 above 50 mm Hg had a 2-year mortality of 50%.

The international guidelines (14) suggest that the following criteria should be used to define the transplant window for CF patients: an FEV_1 at or under 30% or an FEV_1 over 30% with progressive deterioration (including increasing hospitalizations, rapid fall in FEV_1, cachexia, and massive hemoptysis), and a PaO_2 under 55 mm Hg on room air and/or $PaCO_2$ over 50 mm Hg. Female patients and patients under the age of 18 years have a more progressive course and should be considered for LT at an earlier stage. The use of the FEV_1 criteria and the use of a more complicated multivariate logistic model to define transplant referral for CF have recently been evaluated in a large group of CF patients (29). The study found that these referral criteria had high negative predictive values (98% and 97%) but only modest positive predictive values (33% and 28%) and can result in premature transplant referral.

Patients with CF are often colonized with multiple-resistant organisms (resistance to all agents in two of the following antibiotic classes: the β-lactams, aminoglycosides, and/or quinolones) or panresistant organisms (resistant *in vitro* to all groups of antibiotics), particularly *Pseudomonas aeruginosa* and *B. cepacia*. Patients with multiple-resistant organisms can be successfully transplanted because of available synergistic use of antibiotics. However, panresistant organism colonization may be considered by some to be a strong relative contraindication. A recent study examined the outcome of CF patients with and without panresistant *P. aeruginosa* ($n = 21$) and *B. cepacia* ($n = 6$) versus those with sensitive organisms ($n = 39$) (17). Postoperative ventilator days, length of hospital stay, and antibiotic days were similar between the groups. The incidences of bronchitis and pneumonia were also comparable between the groups. One-year survival was comparable at 81% and 83%, respectively. However, when a subanalysis was performed, patients with *B. cepacia* had a lower 1-year survival of 50% in comparison to resistant *P. aeruginosa* (90%). The authors concluded that CF patients with panresistant *Pseudomonas* should not be excluded from transplantation on the basis of that criterion alone. More recent studies have suggested that those patients colonized with *B. cepacia* with the specific genomovar III have poorer outcomes (30).

PRIMARY PULMONARY HYPERTENSION

The natural median survival of patients with untreated primary pulmonary hypertension (PPH) is 2.8 years after diagnosis. The National Heart, Blood, and Lung Patient Registry followed approximately 200 patients for 3 to 7 years to characterize variables associated with poor survival (31). Median survival decreased from 58.6 months [for patients in New York Heart Association (NYHA) class I or II] to 31.5 months (for patients in functional class III) to 6 months (for patients in functional class IV). An increase in mean pulmonary artery pressure from <55 mm Hg to more than 85 mm Hg was associated with a decrease in mean survival from 48 months to 12 months. A decrease in cardiac index of 4 L/ minute/m^2 to 2 L/minute/m^2 was associated with a decrease in median survival from 43 months to 17 months. The presence of Raynaud phenomenon also predicted a poor prognosis, with a median survival of less than 1 year. More than 80% of patients were discharged on some drug therapy, usually a combination of vasodilators, anticoagulants, and diuretics.

The selection guidelines for transplantation suggested that PPH patients with NYHA class III or IV, despite optimal therapy, including vasodilators, that is, prostacyclin, endothelin antagonists, phosphodiesterase type V inhibitors, or calcium channel blockers, and those with significantly elevated pulmonary artery pressures (mean pulmonary artery pressures above 55 mm Hg), depressed cardiac index (below 2 L/minute/m^2), or right atrial pressure of over 15 mm Hg should be considered for transplantation. Others should be followed closely and reassessed for transplantation at 6-month intervals. Referral to a transplant center is usually made when the patient reaches NYHA class III.

EVALUATION

Once a patient is found to be a potential candidate for transplantation, a battery of studies is performed for further assessment. Typically, these include pulmonary function tests (PFT) including lung volumes, spirometry and diffusing capacity, and a measure of exercise performance. Cardiac evaluation includes an electrocardiogram and an echocardiogram, in addition to some functional cardiac study such as dobutamine echocardiography and/or coronary angiography in patients over the age of 40. A high-resolution computed tomography (HRCT) scan is usually obtained to look for bronchiectasis, which could indicate the necessity for a bilateral procedure, or to look for focal nodules not apparent on plain radiograph. Renal and liver functions are assessed by 24-hour creatinine clearance and liver function tests, respectively. A complete blood count and viral serologies are also obtained.

DONOR SELECTION

The shortage of donor organs continues to be the rate-limiting factor for the number of LT procedures performed. Most potential donors are brain-dead as a result of head trauma or a primary noninfectious central nervous system event. Standard donor criteria are shown in Table 10-5. The ideal donor should be less than 65 years of age and should have no history of lung disease and a low cumulative smoking history (fewer than 30 pack years). Serial chest radiographs should be grossly clear

TABLE 10-5. Guidelines for Donor Selection

Age under 65 yr

No history of significant lung disease

Limited cumulative cigarette smoking history (under 30 pack yr)

Clear lung field on chest radiograph

Acceptable lung compliance (peak inspiratory pressure under 30 cm H$_2$O)

Adequate oxygenation (Pa_{O_2} above 300 mm Hg at F_{IO_2} = 1.0 or Pa_{O_2}/F_{IO_2} above 250–300 mm Hg)[a]

Satisfactory gross appearance and bronchoscopic inspection

Pa_{O_2}, arterial oxygen tension; F_{IO_2}, fraction of inspired oxygen.

[a]At PEEP = 5 cm H$_2$O.

From Trulock EP. State of the art: lung transplantation. *Am J Respir Crit Care Med* 1997;155:789–818, with permission.

prior to consideration for lung donation. When donation is being considered for HLT or BLT, both lungs must meet criteria for donation. However, for SLT, unilateral lung injury secondary to trauma does not automatically exclude the contralateral lung from consideration for donation (32). The physiologic capacity of the potential donor graft is further assessed by gas exchange capability. Typically, a Pa_{O_2} above 300 mm Hg on an F_{IO_2} of 1 and 5 cm H$_2$O of positive end–expiratory pressure (PEEP) is required. Oxygenation not meeting the above criterion could indicate potential ventilation–perfusion mismatch following surgery.

Most lung transplant centers require a Gram stain of a tracheal aspirate and/or bronchoscopy to be performed on all potential donor candidates to minimize the possibility of transmitting infectious agents from an infected donor organ. Fiber-optic bronchoscopy is often a routine part of the organ harvest to assess blood, purulent secretions, or foreign bodies in the tracheobronchial tree that are not apparent on chest radiograph. If bronchoscopic examination is abnormal, the organ should be excluded from consideration for donation.

The donor evaluation process is completed by obtaining serologic tests for HIV, hepatitis B, and cytomegalovirus (CMV). The patient is not a donor candidate if hepatitis B surface antigen or HIV antibody is present.

Certain donor–recipient compatibility tests should be met following availability of an acceptable donor organ. Unlike other solid-organ donations, SLT, HLT, and DLT are only ABO blood groups matched and not human leukocyte antigen (HLA) matched. Currently, lung graft preservation time is limited to approximately 4 to 6 hours, and this short time precludes HLA typing prior to transplantation. Furthermore, retrospective analysis of HLA compatibility of SLT donors and recipients does not appear to correlate with subsequent episodes of rejection or mortality (33). Two recent retrospective studies dispute this and suggest that HLA matching may result in a reduced incidence of posttransplant rejection (34,35).

Several recent studies have examined the outcomes of LT in those patients receiving a graft or grafts from "marginal" or "extended" donors (i.e., those donors not meeting all of the above criteria) with similar outcome results (36–38). Widespread implementation of this strategy based on these findings can result in increased donor lungs for transplantation.

Size matching of the donor and the recipient is not handled uniformly at all transplant centers. Some centers measure the chest circumference of the transplant recipient and match it to the corresponding donor chest wall circumference within 3 inches in either direction (9). Other groups estimate the size match by determining the lung capacities of the donor and recipient with a height and sex nomogram (39). Some institutions perform size matching by estimating chest wall size by plain radiograph or by using a combination of measurements of body weight and chest wall circumference plus horizontal thoracic length (40). Regardless of the method of size matching used, the donor lung size approximates that of the recipient soon after transplantation (39,41).

SURGICAL TECHNIQUE: SINGLE LUNG TRANSPLANTATION

The donor lung is usually removed at the time of cardiac harvest via a median sternotomy incision. The pulmonary veins with a residual 5-mm cuff of left atrium are detached from the heart. The pulmonary artery is transected from the main pulmonary trunk, and the mainstem bronchus is transected between two staple lines (9). The donor lung graft is preserved in Perfadex solution (a crystalloid solution with intracellular electrolyte composition) at 4°C during transportation to the recipient site and is usually stored in a partially inflated position.

The recipient surgery is performed through a posterolateral thoracotomy incision. Initially, the donor pulmonary vein is anastomosed end to end to the recipient's left atrium. The technical details of the bronchial anastomosis vary among institutions. The lungs are the only solid organs that are transplanted without a complete vascular anastomosis (i.e., the bronchial circulation of the recipient and donor lungs are not anastomosed). Because of this lack of revascularization of the bronchial circulation, anastomotic complications, including bronchial dehiscence, bronchial stenosis, and bronchial infection, are major complications in LT. Some transplant centers perform an end-to-end anastomosis and wrap a piece of omentum with an intact vascular pedicle around the anastomosis to help in bronchial revascularization. Other institutions use the telescoping technique when performing the bronchial anastomosis. In the telescoping technique, the recipient and donor bronchi are overlapped by approximately one cartilaginous ring. This allows the intact bronchial circulation of the recipient to supply the donor bronchus. The use of the telescoping technique has significantly reduced the incidence of anastomotic complications as reported in some series, but other centers have obtained fewer anastomotic complications with the end-to-end procedure (42). SLT surgery is completed by performing an end-to-end anastomosis of the donor and recipient pulmonary arteries.

An interesting issue to consider when performing SLT is which side to transplant. This choice is based on a number of factors. For example, if the recipient's pleural space has been previously invaded by open lung biopsy or pneumothorax requiring chemical or surgical pleurodesis, the contralateral hemithorax should be chosen. If preoperative quantitative ventilation and perfusion ($\dot{V}/\dot{Q}$) scanning shows one lung functioning significantly better than the other lung, the less-functional lung should be transplanted. Assuming that the lungs function equally and that the recipient has had no prior surgery, the left side has traditionally been chosen for transplantation. Technically, the surgery is easier to perform on the left side because it is easier to clamp the left atrium proximal to the left pulmonary vein and it is possible to leave a larger donor atrial cuff and longer recipient bronchus (9). When performing SLT for COPD, radiographically, the transplanted left lung is apparently compressed by the native hyperinflated right lung. This compression is less dramatic when the transplant is placed on the right side. Despite the radiographic differences, the results of pulmonary function testing, exercise oximetry, and $\dot{V}/\dot{Q}$ lung scanning do not support a functional difference between the right and left graft position for the treatment of obstructive lung diseases (43).

THE POSTOPERATIVE PERIOD

GENERAL POSTOPERATIVE MANAGEMENT

Bilateral lung-transplant procedures are usually performed through a transverse thoracosternotomy (clamshell incision) or median sternotomy followed by sequential single lung procedures. Cardiopulmonary bypass may be required for cases of pulmonary hypertension. Following lung transplant surgery, patients remain intubated and require mechanical ventilation. Most patients are ventilated on a volume control mode, although some transplant centers have changed to pressure control ventilation in recent years. Airway pressures should be maintained as low as possible to avoid barotrauma and anastomotic dehiscence. Most institutions use routine pharmacologic sedation. Patients are generally maintained with tidal volumes of 6 to 10 mL per kg following surgery. At some institutions, a low level of PEEP is applied immediately after lung expansion in the operating room and continued following transplantation (9). Uncomplicated lung transplant recipients are extubated within the first 24 hours following transplantation. Both postural drainage and chest physiotherapy can be routinely employed without concern about mechanical complications at the anastomosis.

Certain patient populations require special ventilator management. In patients undergoing SLT for pulmonary hypertension, reperfusion pulmonary edema is often severe because nearly all perfusion is going to the newly implanted lung. Often, prolonged sedation and pharmacologic paralysis for up to two to three days are required following surgery. This patient population should have aggressive diuresis, and they may require higher levels of PEEP for longer periods of time. Some transplant centers have recommended that for the first few days following surgery, patients with significant pulmonary hypertension be positioned with the transplant side up to increase blood flow to the native lung, which is not as severely affected by the pulmonary reimplantation response (PRR).

In patients with obstructive lung disease, problems can be encountered if the delivered tidal volume or the required levels of PEEP are high. Occasionally, significant hyperinflation of the native lung can result, which can compromise the newly transplanted lung. To reduce this problem, many transplant centers avoid PEEP when performing SLT for obstructive disease. Several reports have described the use of selective independent ventilation with a double-lumen tube to prevent this possible complication (44).

Because many patients are nutritionally depleted prior to transplantation because of their underlying disease, postoperative nutritional needs are important. Ideally, immediate nutritional alimentation should be begun.

Antibiotics are routinely administered for the first 48 to 72 hours following transplantation. Routine antibiotic regimens vary between centers but include a broad-spectrum Gram negative agent. Several centers routinely use antifungal agents such as amphotericin B or itraconazole postoperatively. Empiric anaerobic coverage has been advocated by some centers. Gram stains and cultures of donor and recipient sputa may be used to choose appropriate antibiotics when available. Ganciclovir and, more recently, valganciclovir are administered for CMV prophylaxis in most transplant programs if either the patient or the donor is CMV-positive prior to surgery.

Induction immunosuppression is begun with cyclosporine preoperatively. Corticosteroids are administered as intravenous methylprednisolone at 0.5 to 1 g in the operating room (usually given at the time of reperfusion), then at 1 to 3 mg/kg/day for the subsequent 3 days, followed by 1 mg/kg/day, and then converted to an equivalent oral dose. Lympholytic medications such as antilymphocyte globulin (ALG) at 10 to 15 mg/kg/day intravenously or muromonab-CD3 (Orthoclone OKT3) 5 mg per day for the first 5 to 10 days following transplantation were commonly used as induction therapy; however, more recently their use has been very limited. Some centers are currently using IL-2 receptor blockers (Daclizumab and Basiliximab) for induction.

After the transplant surgery, most patients are then started on a triple immunosuppression protocol with a combination of prednisone, tacrolimus, or cyclosporine and mycophenolate mofetil or azathioprine (15).

POSTOPERATIVE PROBLEMS

Perhaps the most significant problem following LT is the development of PRR or primary graft failure (PGF). It is estimated that up to 80% of patients will experience some degree of reimplantation injury (45,46). To varying degrees, the PRR can persist for hours to days following lung transplant surgery. Clinically, the PRR is characterized by new radiographic alveolar and/or interstitial infiltrates, a decrease in pulmonary compliance, and disrupted gas exchange. Radiographic findings in these patients include a perihilar haze, patchy alveolar consolidations, and dense perihilar and basilar alveolar consolidations, with air bronchograms (see Fig. 10-1). The PRR usually worsens or stabilizes over the subsequent 2 to 4 days and then begins to resolve.

Although the mechanism for the PRR has not been completely delineated, several contributing factors have been postulated, including the disruption of lymphatics, bronchial vasculature, and/or nerves, as well as lung injury occurring either during preservation of the graft or following reperfusion. The PRR is thought to be a form of membrane permeability edema that develops to various degrees in all lung transplant recipients in whom warm ischemia persists for more than 30 minutes or those in whom cold ischemia persists for more than 2 hours (46,47). Animal studies have suggested that the severity of the PRR is related to the ischemic time and may relate to the production of toxic oxygen-free radicals (46).

In general, the PRR develops in the immediate postoperative period, whereas rejection and infection are more common after the first 24 hours. However, because the timing of these disorders may vary, differentiation may be difficult. The PRR may be minimized by the avoidance of prolonged ischemic

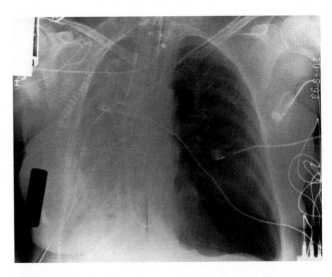

FIGURE 10-1. Anteroposterior portable chest radiograph of a 50-year-old woman with chronic obstructive lung disease taken 6 hours after a right single-lung transplant (SLT) procedure. Note the alveolar infiltrates caused by the pulmonary reimplantation response.

times, the optimization of organ preservation, the appropriate use of postoperative hemodynamic monitoring, and the timely use of diuretics, inotropic agents, and antibiotics or augmented immunosuppression if other diagnoses are suspected. There are several reports of the use of inhaled nitric oxide (48–50) and extracorporeal membrane oxygenation (ECMO) for severe early graft dysfunction (51).

A 1998 study documented a 15% incidence of PGF with associated prolonged hospital course, prolonged mechanical ventilation, poor 1-year survival (40% vs 69%), and compromised function among survivors (52). This study examined the findings in the 15 of 100 patients deemed by standard clinical criteria to have PGF. The authors found no clear risk factors for PGF, including age, sex, underlying disease, pulmonary artery pressure, type of transplant, ischemic times, or use of cardiopulmonary bypass. In those patients with PGF, induction immunosuppressive therapy was used less frequently than those patients who did not develop this complication. A more recent study found the incidence of severe PGF to be 11.8% among 255 transplant recipients. Risk factors associated with the development of PGF when subjected to multivariate analysis included a recipient diagnosis of PPH, donor female gender, donor African American race, and donor age less than 21 years and greater than 45 years (53). A French study concluded that the development of PGF, even in the mildest form, is associated with prolonged duration of mechanical ventilation and increased ICU morbidity and mortality (54).

MANAGEMENT AFTER THE POSTOPERATIVE PERIOD

After discharge, follow-up is performed in the outpatient clinic. A sample follow-up schedule would be weekly for the first two months, biweekly for the next month, and monthly thereafter. After three months of uncomplicated posttransplant observation, patients often return home and resume follow-up with their referring pulmonologists.

Weekly studies include a cyclosporine or tacrolimus level, a complete blood count to monitor the leukocyte count on azathioprine or mycophenolate mofetil, blood chemistries to follow creatinine while on cyclosporine or tacrolimus and to follow liver function tests, a chest radiograph, routine spirometry, and exercise oximetry. In addition, patients bring in their home spirometric measurements at each visit. Some institutions perform surveillance bronchoscopy on a routine schedule, whereas other institutions reserve this procedure for clinical deterioration.

Following transplantation, the most efficient and effective way to monitor the patient to detect early rejection, infection, or anastomotic complications remains controversial. Early in the transplant experience, quantitative ventilation and perfusion to the lung graft were examined as an indicator of graft rejection. Early acute rejection was often heralded by a decrease in perfusion to the lung graft (40). Subsequently, quantitative ventilation–perfusion lung scanning was found to be neither sensitive nor specific for graft complications.

Likewise, chest radiographs have been shown to be neither specific nor sensitive for early detection of infection or rejection (55–58). Seventy-four percent of cases of rejection or infection in HLT recipients were associated with abnormal chest radiographs in the first month following transplantation. However, after the first posttransplant month, only 23% of rejection episodes were associated with abnormal chest radiographs (57).

Close monitoring of pulmonary function has also been studied as a way of detecting graft complications (59,60). At most transplant centers, patients are given home spirometers and are instructed to document their $FEF_{25\%-75\%}$, FEV_1, and FVC twice a day. Patients are instructed to notify their local physician or the transplant center if these values decline by 10% to 15% on two subsequent measurements. If this decline is confirmed in the PFT laboratory, transbronchial biopsy is indicated because this degree of deterioration in pulmonary function has been associated with either rejection or infection (59,60). A study of HLT recipients comparing pulmonary function, chest radiographs, and transbronchial biopsies found pulmonary function testing to have 86% sensitivity in detecting rejection in the first 3 months following transplantation and 75% sensitivity subsequently. The sensitivity for detecting infection was 75%. Although pulmonary function testing was not able to distinguish between rejection and infection, pulmonary function testing did have 84% specificity for detecting complications in the lung graft. This study also reinforced prior data showing chest radiographs to be sensitive early following transplantation but having only 19% sensitivity for rejection subsequently (56). Desaturation of more than 4% or a drop below an absolute oxygen saturation of 90% on constant workload cycle exercise oximetry has also been suggested as an indicator of a complication in the lung graft (61).

Surveillance bronchoscopy has become a controversial issue in LT. Reports suggest that surveillance bronchoscopy may allow the early detection of asymptomatic complications such as acute rejection and could thus reduce future development of obliterative bronchiolitis (OB). A study using patients who had undergone surveillance bronchoscopy as historic controls did not support a difference in bronchiolitis obliterans syndrome (BOS) or in survival in comparison to a group of transplant recipients who did not undergo surveillance bronchoscopy (62). However, a recent large survey of 50 transplant centers reported that 69% continue to perform surveillance bronchoscopy on a regular basis (15).

OUTCOME

Lung function gradually improves and reaches a plateau by 3 months following surgery. SLT for obstructive lung disease results in residual mild-to-moderate obstructive pulmonary dysfunction secondary to the remaining native lung (63). SLT recipients with underlying restrictive lung disease have a residual mild restrictive defect (64–67). SLT recipients with pulmonary vascular disease maintain their normal pulmonary function and develop normal hemodynamics following transplantation (10). BLT or HLT performed for any indication results in improved spirometry following surgery (68,69).

Most of the ventilation and perfusion go to the transplanted lung following SLT for obstructive or restrictive lung disease (68). SLT for pulmonary hypertension results in a nearly equal division of ventilation between the transplanted and native lung, with nearly all perfusion going to the new lung graft (10). This ventilation–perfusion imbalance results in normal gas exchange under baseline conditions but can pose a problem during episodes of graft complications (70). Following BLT, or HLT, ventilation and perfusion are divided between the lungs.

All of the different lung-transplant procedures result in normal gas exchange following transplantation. Exercise testing uniformly results in reduced maximum exercise capacities with no evidence of ventilatory limitation or arterial oxygen desaturation. There is no significant difference in exercise capacities in patients undergoing SLT versus BLT, or HLT, despite the differences in spirometry for the SLT procedure (64–66,71). Proposed reasons for the reduced exercise capacity following transplantation include deconditioning, myopathy secondary to immunosuppressive medications, chronic anemia, and limited pulmonary vascular capacities in the case of SLT. Despite the reduced exercise capacities, all stable patients are able to carry out activities of daily living without compromise.

Although 1-, 2-, and 3-year survival rates of lung transplant recipients are 73%, 64%, and 57%, respectively (5)—lower than those achieved with heart or liver transplantation—some improvement in survival has been made over the last 10 years. Some lung transplant recipients are surviving 5 to 10 years or more and are maintaining a normal functional status. Mortality in the early postoperative period has been caused primarily by technical complications and by PGF. Mortality after the perioperative period (beyond 30 days) and up to 1 year is primarily due to infection. Mortality beyond the first year has been primarily related to bronchiolitis obliterans.

QOL issues are a relatively recent area of research in LT. Several small studies have shown improvement in overall and health-related QOL (72–75). The large majority of patients have expressed satisfaction with their transplant decision. Even if survival advantage is in question, the improvement in QOL is worth the sacrifice to many patients.

COMPLICATIONS FOLLOWING LUNG TRANSPLANTATION

AIRWAY COMPLICATIONS

Airway problems, a significant cause of morbidity and mortality following early attempts at LT, develop in 20% to 50% of transplant recipients (76–79). Airway complications can be divided into early and late time periods. Early complications typically develop in the first 1 to 2 months following transplantation and are characterized by anastomotic infection and/or partial or complete anastomotic dehiscence. Subsequently, anastomotic strictures and/or bronchomalacia can develop, which significantly compromise the function of the transplanted lung or lungs. Several theoretical causes of airway complications following LT have been postulated, including ischemia at the site of the anastomosis, infection of the anastomosis, poor organ preservation, pneumonia, graft rejection, early corticosteroid administration, and an excessively long donor bronchus. As stated previously, the lung is the only solid organ that is transplanted without complete revascularization of the systemic blood supply. Therefore, oxygenation of the new lung graft or grafts depends upon collateral blood flow from the pulmonary to the bronchial circulation.

Airway complications have been reduced with the development of the omental wrap and with the use of pericardial fat wrapped around the anastomosis. Experimental work in an animal model has been done on direct bronchial revascularization to decrease airway complications following transplantation (77,78). In contemporary series, airway complications have a prevalence of 10% to 20%, with a low mortality (42,80,81).

Clinically, bronchial stenosis can present with cough, shortness of breath, dyspnea on exertion, and worsening obstruction on pulmonary function testing. A characteristic flow–volume loop with an inspiratory and expiratory concave pattern has been noted (82). Radiographically, bronchial strictures may be seen on posteroanterior chest radiographs and can be clearly visualized by computed tomography (CT) and/or by the definitive test, bronchoscopy. Partial or complete bronchial dehiscence can present with mediastinal emphysema on chest radiograph or with air adjacent to the bronchial anastomosis on CT (58).

Many transplant centers advocate early routine surveillance bronchoscopy to evaluate the anastomosis and aid in early detection of complications. Anastomotic ischemia warrants close bronchoscopic observation. If an anastomotic infection is diagnosed, most commonly with *Staphylococcus aureus* or *P. aeruginosa*, appropriate antibiotics should be initiated. Several cases of *Aspergillus* tracheobronchitis involving the anastomosis have been described in HLT patients and more so in SLT patients (83). These have been successfully treated with amphotericin B followed by itraconazole.

Anastomotic strictures should be treated with balloon dilation, wire or silastic stent placement, laser, or surgery (81,84). Partial anastomotic dehiscence is managed conservatively. Complete dehiscence requires surgical revision of the anastomosis or retransplantation.

GRAFT REJECTION

Any solid organ transplanted into a genetically nonidentical recipient is an allograft and provokes an immunologic response called *rejection*. Rejection results from the activation, differentiation, and proliferation of effector T cells directed against the donor organ cells. The transplanted organ is rejected primarily because of differences between the donor and the recipient cell-surface molecules that are encoded by genes in the major histocompatibility complex (MHC). The MHC molecules allow the immune system to discriminate between "self" and "nonself." The human MHC was discovered in the mid-1950s, when leukoagglutination antibodies were found in the sera of multiparous women and were designated the HLA complex.

Traditionally, graft rejection has been classified according to the time of onset and has been defined by the histopathologic pattern as hyperacute, acute, or chronic rejection.

Acute Rejection

Hyperacute rejection in most other solid organ transplants occurs when preexisting alloantibodies bind to the vascular endothelium of the donor lung, activate complement, and cause widespread thrombosis of the vessels within the transplanted lung. Alloantibodies may be present in the donor's serum prior to transplantation through blood transfusions, pregnancy, or previous transplantation. Hyperacute rejection has been virtually eliminated by ABO blood group matching between the recipient and the donor and by pretransplantation screening of the recipients for panel-reactive antibodies (PRA). This panel uses a large group of antigens within the general donor population, and reactivity is measured between the panel and the serum of a prospective transplant recipient. Even though a recipient's serum shows no PRA, antibodies against donor alloantigens not represented in the screening panel could be present and could cause hyperacute rejection. Fortunately, hyperacute rejection is uncommon, and only a few pathologically proven cases have been documented following LT (79,85).

Acute rejection is a common immunologic response that affects the majority of LT recipients and usually occurs between 10 and 50 days after LT. Many patients experience two to three episodes within the first few months. Acute rejection is usually not seen as frequently after the first year posttransplantation (86). The risk factors for acute rejection remain poorly defined, but a recent study found that HLA-DR and HLA-B loci mismatches have a correlation with high-grade rejection episodes (34).

The clinical features of acute rejection include cough, dyspnea, malaise, fever, and adventitious lung sounds (rales, wheezes). The chest radiograph is usually abnormal during rejection in the first month posttransplantation but is abnormal in only one fourth of cases after the first month (57,87). The most common radiographic pattern has been a perihilar or lower lobe infiltrate, often associated with a small pleural effusion (88).

Hypoxemia and deterioration in pulmonary function studies frequently occur in the setting of acute rejection. Although pulmonary function abruptly improves in the early postoperative period, pulmonary function values continue to improve for 3 to 6 months. Once lung function has stabilized, the coefficient of variation for most PFT parameters remains below 5% (56). Thus, a decline of 10% or more in FVC or FEV_1 and a 10% to 15% decline in $FEF_{25\%-75\%}$ are significant changes and may signal either acute rejection or infection or an alternate graft complication (56).

Clinical criteria alone cannot differentiate acute rejection from infection. Transbronchial biopsy (TBB) with bronchoalveolar lavage (BAL) has emerged as the primary procedure in separating these entities. TBB has a positive predictive value of 69% to 83% in lung transplant patients with clinical deterioration (89,90). The sensitivity for diagnosing rejection has ranged from 70% to 95% and the specificity from 90% to 100% (90–92). A minimum of five transbronchial specimens containing pulmonary parenchyma should be obtained for histologic evaluation; however, 10 to 18 biopsies may be required to reach the 95% confidence level for the detection of rejection (92). Investigators have also examined exhaled nitric oxide as a possible marker of acute rejection (93).

Histologically, acute rejection is characterized by perivascular mononuclear infiltrates and may also have airway involvement, lymphocytic bronchitis, or bronchiolitis (94) (see Fig. 10-2). As rejection progresses, the perivascular lymphocytic infiltrate surrounding the venules and arterioles becomes dense and extends into the perivascular and peribronchiolar alveolar septa. With severe rejection, this process spills into the alveolar space and is usually associated with parenchymal necrosis, hyaline membranes, and a necrotizing vasculitis. A histologic grading system for acute pulmonary rejection, initially defined in 1990 and revised in 1996, is outlined in Table 10-6 (94). Although rejection and infection frequently coexist, a definitive diagnosis of acute rejection is difficult to make in the setting of an active infection. Perivascular and interstitial infiltrates may occur with infections, particularly CMV and *Pneumocystis* pneumonia, as well as with acute rejection. Because of the problem in differentiating these disorders, the clinician may have to initiate antimicrobials as well as increase immunosuppression in some cases.

Standard therapy for acute pulmonary rejection is high-dose corticosteroids. Methylprednisolone 7 to 15 mg/kg/day (not exceeding 1 g) for 3 days is a common regimen and usually leads to a dramatic improvement in the patient's condition within 24 hours if the diagnosis is correct. The maintenance immunosuppressive regimen should also be optimized, and frequently the dose of azathioprine is increased to 1.5 to 2 mg/kg/day and the prednisone escalated to 1 mg/kg/day

TABLE 10-6. Classification and Grading of Acute Pulmonary Rejection

Grade A0 — None
Grade A1 — Minimal: Infrequent perivascular infiltrates
Grade A2 — Mild: Frequent perivascular infiltrates
Grade A3 — Moderate: Dense perivascular infiltrates with alveolar involvement
Grade A4 — Severe: Diffuse perivascular and alveolar infiltrates with necrosis

From Yousem SA, Berry GJ, Cagle PT, et al. Revision of the 1990 working formulation for the classification of pulmonary allograft rejection: Lung Rejection Study Group. *J Heart Lung Transplant* 1996;15:1–15, with permission.

with a taper over several weeks. Some centers titrate azathioprine to maintain a total neutrophil count between 4,500 and 6,000 cells per mm³. Adjusting the immunosuppressive regimen is particularly important with severe episodes of rejection or when rejection occurs late in the posttransplant period (87). Conversion from a cyclosporine-based to a tacrolimus-based regimen may also result in improvement (decreased incidence and severity) of persistent or recurrent acute rejection (95). Lympholytic therapy, methotrexate, photophoresis, total lymphoid irradiation, and aerosolized cyclosporine have also been used for treatment of recurrent or persistent acute rejection (95–99).

Follow-up TBB following a diagnosis of acute rejection has been recommended by some investigators within 2 weeks to exclude persistent or recurrent acute rejection or infection resulting from augmented immunosuppression (100).

OBLITERATIVE BRONCHIOLITIS

OB following transplantation is defined clinically by an obstructive pulmonary function defect and histologically by the obliteration of terminal bronchioles (bronchiolitis obliterans syndrome, BOS). In the early HLT experience, 50% of recipients developed OB, a major cause of morbidity and mortality (101–103). With the use of increased immunosuppression, including corticosteroids and cyclosporine, and with the addition of azathioprine, the incidence of OB appeared to decrease (104). Furthermore, with augmented immunosuppression, the progression of disease has been slowed (101). Initially, it was thought that SLT and BLT procedures would result in a lower incidence of OB than would HLT procedures; however, when followed over time, it is apparent that the incidence of OB in SLT and BLT recipients is comparable to that currently seen in HLT patients (105). Many large transplant centers are reporting a 50% to 60% incidence of OB in LT recipients who survive 5 years posttransplant (5). OB remains a major problem in LT and is a leading cause of late mortality (106).

Although the etiology of OB remains unclear, several possible causes have been proposed, including uncontrolled acute rejection (102,107,108), CMV infection (109), HLA-A mismatches, total HLA mismatches, absence of donor antigen–specific hyporeactivity (108), bronchiolitis obliterans with organizing pneumonia (BOOP), and lymphocytic bronchiolitis (110,111). Acute rejection has been consistently identified as the most significant risk factor for BOS (112–116). Those patients with

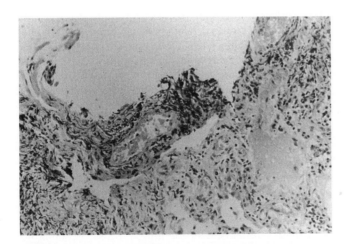

FIGURE 10-2. Transbronchial biopsy specimen revealing perivascular lymphocytic infiltration and necrosis around a small pulmonary artery, consistent with acute rejection.

recurrent, high-grade, acute rejection had a higher incidence of BOS in the Pittsburgh series.

Clinically, OB has been reported any time following the third month posttransplantation, but the typical onset is 16 to 20 months after surgery (114,117). The onset of OB may be heralded by an upper respiratory tract infection and can be mistakenly treated as such. Other patients present without clinical symptoms but with a gradual obstructive dysfunction on pulmonary function testing (118). FEV_1 has been the standard spirometric parameter used, but midexpiratory flow rates may be a more sensitive parameter for early detection (119).

Typically, chest radiographs are not helpful in the diagnosis of OB because most patients have radiographs that are unchanged from their baseline posttransplant film (118). Some investigators have described central bronchiectasis as a radiographic finding, suggesting a diagnosis of OB (120). HRCT in OB may reveal peripheral bronchiectasis, patchy consolidation, decreased peripheral vascular markings, air trapping, and bronchial dilatation, which investigators feel may aid in the early diagnosis of OB (121–124). Air trapping on expiratory HRCT has been shown to be a sensitive (91%) and accurate (86%) radiologic indicator of OB in LT patients but may not be able to provide an early diagnosis of this disorder. Specificity of this finding is reported to be 80% (125).

TBB is used in the evaluation of suspected OB (see Fig. 10-3). In addition to occasionally revealing histologic changes of OB, bronchoscopy is important in excluding other possible diagnoses such as acute rejection, infection, or airway complications as contributing causes of deteriorating pulmonary function. Unfortunately, it may be difficult to obtain diagnostic specimens of the terminal bronchioles by TBB. The sensitivity for detection of OB by TBB ranges from 15% to 87% (87,112,126–130). Because some patients are unable to tolerate open-lung biopsy, OB is sometimes a diagnosis of exclusion in a patient presenting with progressive obstruction on pulmonary function testing with an otherwise normal TBB.

Because of the variability in obtaining OB by TBB, the ISHLT has established a BOS staging system (131). This staging is based on the reduction in FEV_1 in comparison to a posttransplant baseline FEV_1, with or without the pathologic documentation of OB (see Table 10-7), and implies that other

TABLE 10-7. 2001 Clinical Staging System for Obliterative Bronchiolitis

Stage[a]		FEV_1
BOS 0	No OB	$FEV_1 > 90\%$ of baseline and $FEF_{25\%-75\%} > 75\%$ of baseline
BOS 0-p	Potential OB	FEV_1 81–90% of baseline and/or $FEF_{25\%-75\%} \leq 75\%$ of baseline
BOS 1	Mild OB	FEV_1 66% to 80% of baseline
BOS 2	Moderate OB	FEV_1 51% to 65% of baseline
BOS 3	Severe OB	$FEV_1 \leq 50\%$ of baseline

BOS, bronchiolitis obliterans syndrome; FEV_1, forced expiratory volume in one second; OB, obliterative bronchiolitis.

[a] Each stage is subdivided into *a* and *b*, where *a* is without histologic documentation of OB and *b* is with histologic documentation of OB.

From Estenne M, Maurer JR, Boehler A, et al. Bronchiolitis obliterans syndrome 2001: an update of the diagnostic criteria. *J Heart Lung Transplant* 2002;21:297–310, with permission.

causes of the physiologic changes have been excluded by bronchoscopy, such as acute rejection, airway complications, and infection. This staging system is currently under revision by the ISHLT, and the new system includes an earlier BOS category of potential BOS (BOS 0-p) using changes in FEV_1 and/or in midflows as compared to posttransplant baseline values (116). Several studies have examined the use of exhaled nitric oxide as a marker for BOS (132).

If OB has been diagnosed histologically or clinically by exclusion of alternate diagnoses, treatment is begun with high-dose methylprednisolone followed by a tapering course of oral corticosteroids. Lympholytic agents such as antilymphocyte globulin (ALG) or OKT3 can be considered if there is no clinical response to steroid treatment. Therapy may stabilize the pulmonary function but uncommonly results in significant improvement (133).

Mycophenolate mofetil and tacrolimus have also been associated with stabilization of pulmonary function when used as salvage treatment for BOS (134–136). Methotrexate, photophoresis, total lymphoid irradiation, inhaled cyclosporine, and newer immunosuppressive agents have been used in refractory cases of OB (137).

Unfortunately, infection frequently complicates intensive immunosuppression for OB and may result in death. Survival after diagnosis of OB was 74%, 50%, and 43% at 1 year, 3 years, and 5 years, respectively, in the Stanford series (138). Because most cases of OB can only be stabilized, strategies directed at prevention, early diagnosis, and treatments are necessary for preservation of lung function.

INFECTIOUS COMPLICATIONS

Infection is the leading cause of morbidity and mortality in recipients of LT or HLT (139,140). The act of surgically removing the donor lung, leaving it without blood supply for several hours, and then reimplanting it without reestablishing the lymphatic drainage or nerve supply dramatically diminishes the defense mechanisms of the lung. Mucosal ischemia impairs mucociliary clearance, and the anastomosis impairs the movement of mucus up the trachea. These factors, along with immunosuppression, explain why 30% to 80% of transplant

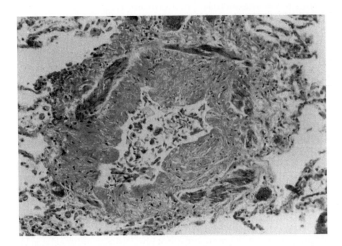

FIGURE 10-3. Transbronchial biopsy specimen revealing obliterative bronchiolitis.

recipients develop major infections within the first 4 months following transplantation (141). Pneumonia accounts for 50% to 80% of infections and is a leading cause of death in these patients (139,140).

Bacterial, candidal, and herpes simplex viral infections occur in the first month after transplantation. More than 90% of the infections occurring in this time period are the usual nosocomial infections of the surgical wound, vascular access, urinary tract, or lungs that occur in any postoperative patient.

Bacterial pneumonia is the most common life-threatening infection to occur in the early postoperative period. The risk of pneumonia in the first two postoperative weeks has been reported to be as high as 35% (142). *Pseudomonas aeruginosa* and *Staphylococcus* species have been the predominant pathogens. With the use of broad-spectrum antibiotic prophylaxis (usually an antipseudomonal cephalosporin and clindamycin) and routine culturing of the trachea of the donor and recipient at the time of surgery, the incidence of bacterial pneumonia has been significantly reduced to around 10%. If the cultures remain negative, prophylactic antibiotics are discontinued after 3 to 4 days.

The diagnosis of early bacterial pneumonia may be difficult because ischemic-reperfusion injury, pulmonary edema, rejection, and atelectasis may all present with similar clinical features. Gram-negative organisms are frequently found in the tracheal aspirate, and differentiating colonization from infection may require invasive procedures or semiquantitative bacterial cultures.

Atypical pneumonias, including *Pneumocystis carinii* pneumonia (PCP), *Legionella*, mycobacteria, and *Nocardia*, are uncommon in the first month and occur in 2% to 9% of lung and heart–lung transplant recipients (143,144). Other posttransplant infections include viral infections with herpes simplex virus and hepatitis B or C infections. Herpes simplex infections have almost been eliminated by the common use of acyclovir or ganciclovir, and the incidence of hepatitis B or C is minimal with better screening techniques of donors and blood products. Candidal infections are also seen in the early postoperative period, and the potential of this organism in causing invasive disease should always be considered when it is isolated from cultures.

In transplant centers in which trimethoprim–sulfamethoxazole prophylaxis is routinely used during the first year posttransplant and reinitiated when immunosuppression is augmented, the incidence of PCP is less than 1% (144–146). Nevertheless, lung transplant recipients have a fivefold higher prevalence of PCP than comparably immunosuppressed recipients of a cardiac allograft, and PCP must be considered in patients who are poorly compliant with their medications or are intolerant to trimethoprim–sulfamethoxazole (146).

Most opportunistic infections occur 1 to 6 months after transplantation. The combination of sustained immunosuppression and the immunomodulating viruses, particularly CMV, predisposes the patient to opportunistic organisms, including *Aspergillus*, *Mycobacterium*, *Nocardia*, *Listeria*, and geographically endemic fungi. During this time period, viral infections are a major cause of mortality and morbidity. CMV, a herpesvirus, accounts for the majority of the viral infections in these patients.

CMV is the most common cause of infections in the interval between 30 and 150 days postoperatively (142). The overall prevalence of CMV illness (infection or disease) in lung transplant recipients has been around 50% (106). The risk of developing CMV disease is dependent on the serologic status of the donor and the recipient, as well as on the use of high-intensity immunosuppressive therapy. CMV-positive recipients develop CMV disease approximately 25% to 35% of the time, whereas CMV-negative recipients have an 85% chance of developing disease when implanted with a CMV-positive lung (147). The case fatality rate for primary CMV disease (recipients that lack any intrinsic immunity) has been 20% to 25%.

CMV causes a wide spectrum of diseases ranging from asymptomatic infection (shedding of virus in urine or bronchoalveolar secretions) to widespread dissemination. CMV infection in transplant patients is characterized by active replication and shedding of virus that can be associated with unexplained fever or constitutional symptoms as well as laboratory abnormalities including mild atypical lymphocytosis, leukopenia, or thrombocytopenia. CMV disease is established by cytologic or histologic changes in cell preparations or tissue. Although CMV disease can be manifested by hepatitis, gastroenteritis, or colitis, CMV pneumonia is the most common presentation after LT.

CMV pneumonia typically presents insidiously with nonproductive cough, fever, malaise, hypoxemia, and a mild interstitial or alveolar infiltrate. Sputum smears and cultures are rarely diagnostic for CMV pneumonia. Fiber-optic bronchoscopy with TBB and BAL diagnoses 60% to 90% of patients with CMV pneumonia (141,144). A presumptive diagnosis is often made on the basis of a positive culture in a compatible clinical setting after other causes have been excluded.

The microscopic hallmark of CMV infection is the large (cytomegalic) 250-nm cell containing a large, central, basophilic intranuclear inclusion. The inclusion is referred to as an *owl's eye* because it is separated from the nuclear membrane by a halo. These inclusions are well seen on hematoxylin–eosin or on Papanicolaou stain (see Fig. 10-4). Cytologic identification of CMV inclusion cells is very specific (98%) but lacks sensitivity (21%) for the presence of infection (148). Biopsy specimens of the lung parenchyma contain CMV inclusion cells with a surrounding lymphocytic/mononuclear cell interstitial pneumonitis.

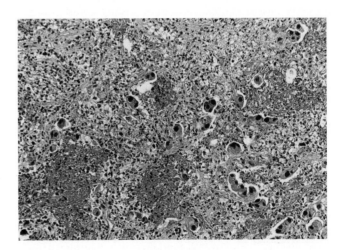

FIGURE 10-4. A photomicrograph revealing "owl's eye" intranuclear inclusions of cytomegalovirus (CMV) in the lung graft.

Ganciclovir, an acrylic guanine analog, is currently the mainstay of therapy for invasive CMV disease. Initial doses of 5 mg/kg twice daily for 2 to 4 weeks reduce mortality from 60%–80% to 15%–20% in symptomatic CMV pneumonitis (148). If CMV relapses, ganciclovir at 5 mg/kg/day may be required for 2 to 4 months. Some patients develop bone marrow toxicity on ganciclovir and require therapy with foscarnet. Major toxic reactions associated with foscarnet include renal failure and severe electrolyte disturbances. CMV-specific IgG or polyclonal IgG in combination with ganciclovir is associated with an improved survival among bone marrow transplant recipients with CMV pneumonitis (149). Because of the cost of immunoglobulin and the lack of data in solid-organ transplant recipients, IgG preparations are often reserved for life-threatening episodes of CMV infection. With any severe CMV infection, a reduction in the level of immunosuppression is recommended.

Although there is no consensus about the optimal regimen for prevention of CMV disease, prophylaxis against CMV infection has become a major strategy in most transplant centers. The easiest way to reduce CMV infections is to match CMV-negative recipients with CMV-negative donors whenever possible, but the severe limitation in grafts available for donation make this strategy impractical. Limited studies suggest that CMV hyperimmune globulin may prevent or ameliorate serious CMV infections in high-risk patients after renal, liver, or heart transplantation (150,151).

Ganciclovir is efficacious in preventing viral replication and delays the onset of CMV infection. This delay in onset of the infection reduces the severity of the illness because the patient's risk of morbidity and mortality is highest during the postoperative period and during the period of maximal immunosuppression.

A prospective study in liver transplant recipients demonstrated that a 3-month regimen of oral ganciclovir significantly reduced the incidence of CMV infection and disease (152). At least one small, open, comparative study also showed efficacy of intravenous followed by oral ganciclovir in the lung transplant population (153). Widespread use of prolonged antiviral therapy has the potential to lead to ganciclovir resistance (154). A preemptive strategy is attractive because it treats only those patients at higher risk for developing CMV disease. Surveillance cultures using sensitive assays, such as CMV antigenemia or polymerase chain reaction (PCR), offer significant advantages over previous methods. CMV antigen has been detected at a mean of 28 days prior to the development of CMV disease in heart and lung transplant recipients and should allow for sufficient time to initiate antiviral therapy and prevent disease (155–157). Standardization of quantitative antigenemia or PCR in blood or bronchoalveolar fluid may eliminate the need for universal prophylaxis for CMV in the near future.

Fungal infections are more common in lung and heart–lung transplant recipients than in those with other solid-organ transplants. The overall incidence of invasive fungal infections with LT or HLT ranges from 10% to 22% (158,159). Most fungal infections are caused by *Candida* or *Aspergillus* species, and more than 80% of fungal infections occur within the first 2 months (158). The overall mortality of fungal infections in heart–lung and lung transplant recipients is reported to be between 40% and 70% (158,159).

Aspergillus species (*A. fumigatus, A. flavus, A. terreus,* and *A. niger*) may present as an indolent progressive pneumonia or as an acute fulminant infection that rapidly disseminates. *Aspergillus* exhibits a propensity to invade blood vessels and may present as an infarct or with hemoptysis. The radiographic features of pulmonary aspergillosis include focal lobar infiltrates, patchy bronchopneumonic infiltrates, single or multiple nodules with or without cavitation, thin-walled cavities, and opacification of the entire lung graft. HRCT scan may reveal a halo sign felt to be pathognomonic for invasive aspergillosis (159). Prophylaxis with azoles or inhaled amphotericin has shown promise in decreasing the incidence of *Aspergillus* infections (160).

Definitive diagnosis of invasive aspergillosis requires identification of organisms within tissue. These organisms appear as septate hyphae that branch at acute angles and are visible on hematoxylin–eosin and methenamine–silver stains (see Fig. 10-5). Even with documented cases of invasive aspergillosis, cultures are positive in less than 50% of cases (141,161). Another form of *Aspergillus* infection is *Aspergillus* tracheobronchitis (83,162). These patients develop ulcerative tracheobronchitis that usually starts distal to the anastomosis and may result in progressive narrowing of the airway.

Improved survival has been achieved with the early initiation of high-dose amphotericin (1 mg/kg/day) and with the reduction of immunosuppressive therapy (163–165). Surgical resection as well as medical therapy may be required to maximize cure rates in patients with invasive aspergillosis, especially those with persistent signs of infections or necrotic tissue (161). Oral itraconazole (400 mg per day) compares favorably with amphotericin in uncontrolled studies (83,166). Newer azoles, such as voriconazole, are also of use in the lung transplant population. For life-threatening *Aspergillus* infections, amphotericin B remains the agent of choice. A lipid formulation of amphotericin B should be considered in the management of invasive fungal infections in patients who are intolerant of conventional amphotericin B and in patients with progressive fungal infection despite therapy with amphotericin deoxycholate (159).

Candida species cause a variety of syndromes, including mucocutaneous disease, line sepsis, wound infections, and

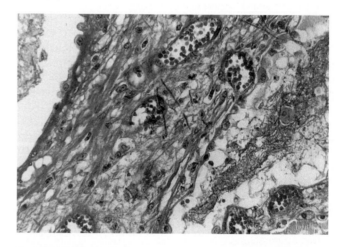

FIGURE 10-5. A photomicrograph revealing *Aspergillus* organisms in the lung graft.

pulmonary involvement associated with widespread dissemination. A heavy growth of *Candida* in the donor tracheal culture has been associated with the occurrence of dissemination in the recipient (167). This has led to some programs initiating low-dose amphotericin (0.3 mg/kg/day) for the first 14 postoperative days (142); other centers have tried another azole, fluconazole (168). Although amphotericin B remains the therapy of choice for life-threatening invasive candidiasis, fluconazole and caspofungin have emerged as effective alternatives for infections caused by *C. albicans*. Fluconazole is less active against *C. glabrata* and inactive against *C. krusei*; therefore, amphotericin should be used in severe candidal infections until the species is identified (159).

Less common causes of fungal infections in lung transplant recipients include *Cryptococcus neoformans* and the dimorphic fungi (*Coccidioides, Histoplasma, and Blastomyces*). Amphotericin B is the initial choice for therapy of serious infections with all these invasive mycoses. The dose, duration of therapy, and alternative therapy differ depending on the organism (165).

Mycobacterium tuberculosis (169), atypical mycobacteria (169–171), *Nocardia* (172–174), *Legionella* (143), and PCP (145,146) may all occur in lung transplant recipients, and the diagnosis and therapy of these organisms have been reviewed.

LYMPHOPROLIFERATIVE DISORDERS

Posttransplant lymphoproliferative disorders (PTLDs) are reported more frequently following LT than in other solid-organ transplant recipients (106). Lymphomas comprise the majority (22%) of posttransplant malignancies. The PTLDs comprise a heterogenous group of lymphoid proliferation of variable clonality. The B-cell non-Hodgkin lymphomas are the most frequent form of posttransplant lymphoma and have been associated with Epstein-Barr virus (EBV) activity, either serologically or by identification of viral DNA in tissue. No clear correlation has been made between episodes of rejection, specific immunosuppressive drugs, and development of PTLD. The incidence of PTLD following HLT and LT has been reported to be between 1.8% and 9.4% (175–183); however, patients who have negative EBV serology prior to transplantation may be at a significantly higher risk for developing PTLD (183). Clinical features of PTLD in LT recipients include development in the first posttransplant year, involvement of the allograft, and radiographic findings of solitary or multiple pulmonary nodules. Disseminated disease has also been reported. Treatment includes a reduction in immunosuppression as well as adjuvant treatment with radiation, chemotherapy, and/or surgery. Recently, the use of the CD20 monoclonal antibody, rituximab, for treatment of PTLD has been reported with some promising results (184).

Bronchogenic carcinoma either harbored or developing in the native lung following SLT has been described, with an incidence of 2.4% in one recent study (185).

IMMUNOSUPPRESSION

One of the most important factors in the successful evolution of LT has been advances in the area of immunosuppression. Currently, most transplant centers use triple immunosuppression regimens including cyclosporine or tacrolimus, azathioprine or mycophenolate mofetil, and prednisone (See Table 10-8). Cytolytic agents such as ALG or OKT3 may be used for induction and/or treatment of refractory rejection (186). More recently, human monoclonal antibodies to activated T cells have been developed because OKT3 may induce a capillary leak syndrome through cytokine release and ALG may induce serum sickness. Early studies have found that human monoclonal anti–T lymphocyte antibodies are effective as prophylaxis for rejection in solid-organ transplants, are well tolerated, and are easy to use because of prolonged half-life (187,188). A study from Duke University found a lower incidence of acute rejection with the use of antithymocyte globulin for induction therapy (189). However, there is no convincing evidence that induction therapy diminishes chronic rejection in LT (190) or results in improved survival, and prospective studies are needed to establish its role in this setting.

A typical maintenance immunosuppression regimen consists of cyclosporine (3 to 5 mg per kg twice daily) or tacrolimus (0.1 mg per kg twice daily) adjusted to serum levels, azathioprine (1 to 2 mg/kg/day adjusted to maintain a leukocyte count above 4500 per mm^3) or mycophenolate mofetil (1 to 1.5 g twice daily), and prednisone (approximately 0.5 mg/kg/day for the first 3 months, tapered over the next 3 months to 15 mg per day, then to 5 mg per day or 10 to 15 mg on alternate days by the 12th posttransplant month).

Cyclosporine and tacrolimus are the mainstays of immunosuppression. Each agent binds to intercellular proteins to create a complex that inhibits calcineurin (191). When calcineurin is inhibited, cytokine genes and other genes, such as the CD40 ligand, cannot be transcribed. Thus cyclosporine and tacrolimus functionally limit cytokine production and downstream lymphocyte proliferation (192,193). Tacrolimus is 50 to 100 times more potent than cyclosporine *in vitro* but its oral bioavailability is highly variable (194). The third-generation derivative of cyclosporine, cyclosporine microemulsion formulation, increases the absorption through the small bowel and reduces bile dependence and the effects of food on absorption. Assessment of blood levels is critical to the use of tacrolimus and cyclosporine because of the narrow therapeutic index.

Unfortunately, immunosuppressive medications have numerous toxicities. The toxicities of tacrolimus and cyclosporine are similar (195). Nephrotoxicity is the major clinical toxic manifestation and occurs in 25% to 75% of patients receiving the drugs (196); the acute renal toxicity is usually dose related and is typically reversible. The drugs can decrease renal blood flow by causing afferent arteriolar vasoconstriction, resulting in decreased glomerular filtration (197). Interstitial fibrosis, tubular changes, and vascular abnormalities can result with chronic use. Several other potentially nephrotoxic agents that can compound the nephrotoxicity include amphotericin B, aminoglycoside antibiotics, trimethoprim–sulfamethoxazole (even at low doses), and furosemide (198). The renal toxicity may resolve with a reduction in the dose or with the discontinuation of the drug, although this improvement is not universal. The concurrent administration of calcium channel blockers may diminish the vasoconstrictive effects of the agents (199).

A second serious complication of these agents is systemic hypertension, which develops in approximately 25% of lung

TABLE 10-8.   Common Immunosuppressive Drugs in Lung Transplantation

Drug	Dose[a]	Common Adverse Effects	Drug Interactions
Cyclosporine	For cyclosporine, the amount needed to achieve a whole-blood trough level of 250–350 ng/mL in the first 6 mo after transplantation and a trough level of 150–250 ng/mL thereafter[b] For tacrolimus, the amount needed to achieve a whole-blood trough level of 8–20 ng/mL	Nephrotoxicity, hypertension neurotoxicity (tremor, seizures, white-matter disease, headache), hyperlipidemia, hyperkalemia, hypomagnesemia, GI disturbance Hirsutism and gingival hyperplasia (with cyclosporine), hyperglycemia (with tacrolimus)	Blood levels are increased by azole antifungal agents, calcium channel blockers, cisapride, and macrolide antibiotics Blood levels are decreased by anticonvulsant drugs, rifampin, or rifabutin
Azathioprine	1–2 mg/kg of body wt/d	Leukopenia, macrocytic anemia, thrombocytopenia, hepatotoxicity, pancreatitis, nausea	Enhanced bone marrow toxicity when given with allopurinol
Mycophenolate mofetil	1000–1500 mg twice daily	Diarrhea, abdominal pain, emesis, leukopenia, anemia	No clinically significant interactions
Prednisone	0.5 mg/kg/d for 3 mo, followed by slow taper to 5 mg/d or 10–15 mg	Hyperglycemia, hypertension, hyperlipidemia, osteoporosis, myopathy, insomnia, cataracts, weight gain	No clinically significant interactions
Sirolimus	2–5 mg/d	Anemia, thrombocytopenia, leukopenia, anastomotic dehiscence (early postoperative period), hyperlipidemia, arthralgias, interstitial pneumonitis, lower extremity edema	Blood levels are increased by azole antifungal agents, calcium channel blockers, and macrolide antibiotics

[a]Doses are based on the protocol used at the University of Texas Health Science Center at San Antonio; the regimens may differ at other transplantation centers.

[b]Cyclosporine levels are measured by immunoassay.

transplant recipients. The most likely etiology of hypertension is a defect in renal sodium excretion (198). Many patients respond to sodium restriction and/or reduction in cyclosporine dose; approximately one third of patients require antihypertensive medications to achieve adequate blood pressure control. Hypercholesterolemia is also commonly reported and can develop in up to 75% of transplant recipients. The incidence of posttransplant hypertension and hypercholesterolemia is lower with tacrolimus (195).

Numerous less common side effects of cyclosporine and tacrolimus can develop. The spectrum of neurologic toxicity includes tremors, paresthesias, headaches, confusion, depression, somnolence, and seizures. Neurotoxicity is more common with tacrolimus than with cyclosporine. Posttransplant diabetes mellitus has been reported with both agents, but the incidence appears to be higher with tacrolimus. In some series, new-onset diabetes mellitus has been seen in up to 19% of patients on tacrolimus (200). Cosmetic changes that occur with cyclosporine, such as hirsutism and gingival hyperplasia, are uncommon with tacrolimus. Several electrolyte deficiencies have been reported with cyclosporine use, including hypomagnesemia in up to 50% of lung transplant patients (198) and hyperkalemia in 10% to 15% of transplant recipients. Cholestatic hepatotoxicity has also been reported (201).

Corticosteroids are the original drugs used in solid-organ transplantation (202). Corticosteroids bind to a cytoplasmic glucocorticoid receptor and undergo translocation into the nucleus, where they block the transcription of several genes. Corticosteroids exert inhibition of cytokine transcription (including IL-2), antigen presentation, eicosanoid production, and the expression of adherence molecules (203). The side effects of chronic corticosteroids seen in other patient populations occur in lung transplant recipients as well, including hyperglycemia, hypercholesterolemia, osteoporosis, cataracts, myopathy, exacerbation of peptic ulcer disease, Cushing syndrome, and mood changes. Many of these side effects are improved with a reduction in corticosteroid dosage.

Azathioprine is metabolized to 6-mercaptopurine, which inhibits nucleic acid synthesis and suppresses mitosis and proliferation of lymphocytes (202). Bone marrow toxicity and suppression are the most common toxic effects of azathioprine, and it is important to adjust the dose to maintain a leukocyte count above 4,500 per mm^3. Miscellaneous side effects related to azathioprine include pancreatitis, hepatitis, cholestatic jaundice, and an increased risk of malignancy (204).

Mycophenolate mofetil, like azathioprine, is an inhibitor of purine synthesis. Mycophenolate acts on a lymphocyte-selective enzyme to inhibit *de novo* purine synthesis. Because lymphocytes have a unique requirement for *de novo* purine synthesis, this effect selectively suppresses lymphocyte clonal expansion (191). The results of pooled analysis indicate that mycophenolate reduces acute rejection and prolongs graft survival in solid-organ transplant recipients (205). Well-controlled studies with mycophenolate in LT are lacking. Mycophenolate lacks the marrow toxicity of azathioprine at a dose of 2 g per day. Gastrointestinal symptoms of diarrhea and abdominal pain are the most common side effects of mycophenolate. The expense of mycophenolate and the inability to monitor drug levels are presently drawbacks to widespread use of this drug.

Sirolimus is one of the newer available immunosuppressant agents and is being used for cases of acute and chronic lung transplant rejection and in small studies as *de novo* therapy following LT. Sirolimus is a macrocyclic triene antibiotic (structurally related to tacrolimus) with immunosuppressive, antitumor, and antifungal properties. Sirolimus has been demonstrated to block the proliferative response and activation of T cells, B cells, and other cell lines by cytokines and growth factors, thus preventing cell-cycle progression and proliferation (206). In contrast, tacrolimus (FK-506) and cyclosporine inhibit the production of cytokines. The use of sirolimus in the immediate posttransplant period is discouraged because of the association with bronchial anastomotic dehiscence in combination with tacrolimus and corticosteroids. The major side effects of sirolimus include cytopenias (particularly thrombocytopenia and leukopenia), hyperlipidemia, arthralgias, and interstitial pneumonitis with components of alveolar hemorrhage, which can become a serious problem in the lung transplant recipient (207,208). Other side effects include those similar to side effects described with cyclosporine and tacrolimus, although, in general, the nephrotoxicity of this agent appears to be less than that of the other two agents. The role of sirolimus in the lung transplant armamentarium remains to be established.

Ongoing research in the field of immunosuppressive therapy as well as improvements in the prevention and treatment of infections and better graft preservation have made LT a therapeutic option for the treatment of end-stage lung disease and have extended the life of these patients.

LUNG VOLUME REDUCTION SURGERY

LT has provided a surgical option for patients with COPD who are relatively young and are able to find a donor match once they are listed as a possible recipient. Unfortunately, many people with emphysema are unable to qualify for LT or deteriorate during the time they have been listed as a possible lung transplant candidate with no donor available in the near future. For these types of patients, a second surgical option may be available. This option is known as lung volume reduction surgery (LVRS) (209–211).

LVRS is actually a rediscovered surgical approach to emphysema that was first performed in the 1950s by Dr. Otto Brantigan (212). He removed areas of emphysematous lung in patients with severe emphysema in order to allow the remaining lung to hyperinflate, thereby increasing lung elastic recoil and increasing airflow conductance. Dr. Brantigan also hypothesized that by reducing the amount of lung in the hyperinflated emphysema patient, the diaphragm would be allowed to return to a more normal configuration, and this could result in increased airflow because of an increase in the efficiency of the muscle. LVRS was performed on a number of patients, but the complication rate of bronchopleural fistula was very high, and the overall mortality rate from the surgery was unacceptable. For these reasons, the procedure was eventually abandoned (213).

In 1995, Dr. Joel Cooper et al. described the use of LVRS in 20 patients with severe emphysema (214). No mortality was reported from the surgery, and the patients improved their FEV_1 by a mean of 82% over a 6-month period. There was a significant increase in PaO_2 and a significant increase in exercise tolerance. The patients also reported an enhanced QOL. During this same time period, several reports of laser LVRS were also published, and enthusiasm for this "reborn" procedure became heightened.

Initially, Medicare reimbursed for the surgery, but in late 1995 the Health Care Financing Administration (HCFA) released a national policy not to reimburse for LVRS until more data could be collected on the procedure's efficacy and safety (210). In order to obtain these data, the National Emphysema Treatment Trial (NETT) began in 1998. The primary goals of this study included answering the following questions:

1. What are the benefits and risks of LVRS compared with good medical therapy alone?
2. How long do any benefits last?
3. Does LVRS benefit some patients more than others?

MECHANISMS OF DECREASED OBSTRUCTION AND IMPROVED EXERCISE TOLERANCE FOLLOWING LUNG VOLUME REDUCTION SURGERY

Patients who undergo LVRS have decreased chest wall elastic recoil and increased lung elastic recoil following surgery, which increases airway conductance. Diaphragm function is also improved because the flattened diaphragm is able to assume a more normal configuration postoperatively as lung hyperinflation is decreased and as the diaphragm ascends into the thorax (209). This allows the diaphragm to assume a resting position that is more favorably situated on the length–tension curve and thus permits the diaphragm to function more effectively as a pressure generator (211).

Improvement in the FEV_1 after LVRS can be primarily attributed to an increase in the vital capacity rather than to an increase in the FEV_1/FVC ratio. This clinical observation indicates that LVRS improves function principally by reducing the residual volume and by increasing vital capacity rather than by altering expiratory flows. At baseline, the lungs are too large for the chest cavity and are thus unable to expand to a volume at which the elastic recoil is sufficient to generate adequate expiratory flows. After LVRS, the elastic recoil improves, allowing a more complete emptying of the lungs; thus, one of the more important parameters to measure in order to evaluate the success of LVRS is the reduction in the residual volume (215).

Improvement in exercise performance may occur because of improved lung mechanics. Patients are capable of longer 6-minute walk distances and increased maximal oxygen uptake values. Ventilation–perfusion matching may also improve following LVRS because of the expansion of the compressed atelectatic lung.

SELECTION OF PATIENTS

Patients who are candidates for LVRS should have end-stage emphysema with debilitation due to either severe dyspnea at rest or exercise intolerance. They should have evidence of hyperinflation with a total lung capacity of $\geq 100\%$ of predicted with a residual volume = 150% of predicted. The high-resolution chest CT and $\dot{V}/\dot{Q}$ scans should reveal predominantly bilateral upper lobe emphysema, which provides target areas for resection. Their FEV$_1$ should be ≤45% of predicted. Alveolar hypoventilation is allowed, but the PaCO$_2$ should not exceed 60 mm Hg. The resting room air PaO$_2$ should be ≥45 mm Hg. Patients with a systolic pulmonary artery pressure ≥45 mm Hg or a mean pulmonary artery pressure ≥35 mm Hg are excluded. All patients must undergo a 6- to 10-week rehabilitation program prior to surgery during which they should receive maximum bronchodilator therapy, oxygen as needed, and a program of exercise and optimum breathing methods. Patients with significant comorbidity from nonrespiratory illnesses, especially cardiac disease, are excluded from LVRS treatment (see Table 10-9).

SURGICAL AND ENDOSCOPIC TECHNIQUES

LVRS has been performed by both thoracoscopic and median sternotomy approaches. Laser ablation of pulmonary tissue is used much less than the above approaches because of an increase in postoperative complications, including delayed pneumothorax (213). The use of video-assisted thoracoscopy with stapling seems to have results similar to median sternotomy, both in terms of operative mortality and functional outcome. This surgery is usually performed as a bilateral procedure in the vast majority of patients, but it can actually also be performed unilaterally. Simultaneous LVRS and resection of a suspected bronchogenic carcinoma in an upper lobe in patients with marginal pulmonary function are feasible and have been reported (216).

The physiologic principles and the clinical applications of LVRS have been demonstrated in a large group of patients, especially in patients with upper lobe emphysema; however, in some cases, the surgical management of these patients has been associated with a very high mortality, which has contraindicated LVRS in many patients who in theory should benefit from the procedure. This has motivated researchers as well as manufacturing companies to develop less invasive techniques to achieve volume reduction surgery without performing a thoracotomy.

The bronchoscopic possibilities include the use of valves or tissue-engineering glue to block the small airways and to collapse the emphysematous lung. Another endoscopic alternative is the formation of small channels between the emphysematous areas and the segmental airway using laser and stents (217). There are currently two commercially available endobronchial valves that have been studied in animals and small noncontrolled clinical studies. The results in patients undergoing this procedure are conflicting. Fifty percent of the patients have evidence of collapse of the targeted area, and positive spirometric results were seen in some patients, but it was not possible to define the patients deriving the most significant benefit prior to the procedure. There was no significant difference in symptoms or QOL following the procedure. The procedure can be performed safely without general anesthesia and with low complication rates. Reported complications include ipsilateral pneumothoraces in a minority of patients and COPD exacerbations in the peri-procedure period (218,219). A theoretical advantage of these procedures is that the procedure can be reversed and attempted in multiple areas, including bilateral application of the valves.

Ingenito described an alternative endoscopic management in the use of endoscopic valves (220). He theorized that the collapse of a target emphysematous region of the lung can be achieved using a washout solution to disrupt surfactant function followed by the use of a biocompatible "tissue sealant" to maintain the collapse and prevent reexpansion. This was tested in a sheep model with severe emphysema in which trypsin was instilled initially to remove epithelial cells followed by fibrin and thrombin to promote fibrosis of the affected area. The pulmonary function, radiographic findings, and pathology confirmed the collapse of the intended areas in most of the cases with no formation of lung abscesses (221). A different concept was recently described by Lausberg et al. in which fenestrations were produced in the segmental bronchi to enhance expiratory airflow in the emphysematous lung. These fenestrations were maintained with the use of small uncovered stents. The studies were done in explanted lungs from patients who underwent LT with some improvement in lung function (222).

At this time, bronchoscopic LVRS is in an early experimental phase and the clinical utility is unclear. In the next few years, there will be more studies with minimally invasive procedures that will help us establish the best techniques, select the ideal patients, and determine the risk/benefit ratio of these procedures.

CHANGES IN PULMONARY FUNCTION AND OTHER EFFECTS ON PATIENT OUTCOMES FOLLOWING LUNG VOLUME REDUCTION SURGERY

The reports of changes in FEV$_1$ by Cooper and associates (223) in 200 patients reveal an increase of 51%, 23%, and 9% in their FEV$_1$ at 6, 36, and 60 months, respectively, following surgery. There was a similar improvement in the residual volume. Most patients experienced subjective improvements in their exercise tolerance, dyspnea score, and patient satisfaction that correlated with the changes in pulmonary function. Other observational studies have also described changes in pulmonary function testing and QOL.

Gelb et al. (224) reported on a group of patients who received lung volume reduction by a video-assisted thoracoscopy with stapling in 10 patients with 1 year of follow-up. The group's FEV$_1$ improved 68% at 6 months, but this declined

TABLE 10-9.   Inclusion Criteria for Lung Volume Reduction Surgery

History, physical exam, and CT scan consistent with bilateral emphysema (heterogeneous)
Prerehabilitation FEV$_1$ ≤45% predicted, TLC ≥100% predicted, and RV ≥150% predicted
Prerehabilitation PaO$_2$ ≥45 mm Hg and PaCO$_2$ ≤60 mm Hg
Maximum medical therapy
Ambulatory with rehabilitation capabilities
No present cigarette use
No severe comorbid illness
No severe cardiac disease
No severe pulmonary hypertension (mean PA pressure ≤35 mm Hg or peak systolic PA pressure ≤45 mm Hg)
No severe obesity or cachexia
No history of recurrent infections or significant bronchiectasis

CT, computed tomography; FEV$_1$, forced expiratory volume in 1 second; TLC, total lung capacity; RV, residual volume; PaO$_2$, arterial oxygen tension; PaCO$_2$, arterial carbon dioxide tension.

to 34% by 1 year. Ingenito et al. (225) reported a 2-year follow-up in nine patients receiving LVRS. Their FEV$_1$ had declined by 19% at 2 years from their peak improvement, which occurred at 6 months following their surgery. All of these data suggest that maximum FEV$_1$ improvement occurs 6 months following the surgical procedure, but there is increasing obstruction recurring over the following 6- to 18-month period that even exceeds the rates reported in patients with severe COPD who continued to smoke. Brenner et al. (226) reported an average loss in FEV$_1$ of 163 mL per year in 180 patients who had undergone a variety of LVRS procedures. The most rapid loss was 255 mL per year, which occurred in a group of patients who had undergone bilateral thoracoscopic LVRS.

In the report by Cooper and associates (223), 39% of patients (101 patients) had been using oxygen preoperatively at rest and 16% were using it postoperatively. In that same group, 93% were using oxygen during exercise preoperatively and 49% were continuing to do the same postoperatively. Unfortunately, the improvements in terms of pulmonary function testing and oxygen requirements were not sustained for prolonged periods of time. At 3 years, there was worsening of both parameters, and by 5 years, 46% of the patients were on supplemental oxygen at rest and 71% required oxygen with exertion.

Cooper's report (223) has an annual Kaplan–Meier survival through 5 years after surgery of 93%, 88%, 83%, 74%, and 63%, respectively. Persistent bronchopleural fistula (over 7 days) is the most common postoperative complication and occurs in 30% to 50% of patients. Tracheostomy has been required in approximately 10% of patients during their postoperative course. At an average of 3.6 years after LVRS, 7.5% of patients underwent subsequent LT. Other significant complications include pneumonia and respiratory failure.

NATIONAL EMPHYSEMA TREATMENT TRIAL RESULTS

This selection of patients with severe emphysema and the results of LVRS in these patients has been an area of great debate and controversy. The initial results from the NETT brought very useful data in defining patients who clearly will not benefit from surgery (227). The group of patients who have an FEV$_1$ that was no more than 20% of their predicted volume and either a homogeneous distribution of emphysema on CT or a carbon monoxide diffusion capacity $\leq 20\%$ of their predicted value had a 30-day mortality rate after surgery of 16% as compared to a rate of 0% among medically treated patients. Even in the patients who survived the surgery, the results did not improve their QOL compared to the control group. On the basis of these results, these high-risk patients should be excluded from LVRS.

After the exclusion of the high-risk patients, a subgroup analysis of the large population of the NETT identified four additional groups of patients on the basis of the pattern of emphysema on CT scanning (homogeneous vs. upper lobe predominance) and the exercise capacity after rehabilitation (low vs. high maximal workload after rehabilitation) (228).

Group 1: This group with predominantly upper lobe emphysema and low maximal workload after rehabilitation had lower mortality and greater improvement in exercise capacity, symptoms, and QOL as compared to medical therapy.

Group 2: This group with predominantly upper lobe emphysema and high maximal workload after rehabilitation had

a greater chance of improvement in symptoms and exercise capacity than with medical therapy; however, the improvement was small and there was no difference in mortality as compared to medical therapy.

Group 3: This group with predominantly non–upper lobe emphysema and high maximal workload after rehabilitation had a higher mortality if they underwent LVRS than if they received medical therapy alone, and there was little functional improvement regardless of the treatment they received.

Group 4: This group with predominantly non–upper lobe emphysema and low maximal workload after rehabilitation had only a small chance of improvement in exercise capacity but a greater chance of symptomatic improvement after LVRS. There was no difference in mortality.

In general, the group that had surgery had some benefits in exercise capacity, lung function, QOL, and dyspnea, but the changes after surgery were variable in the different groups. The improvements in function also returned to the preoperative baseline by 2 years following surgery, although in the group receiving medical therapy, the functional parameters were considerably worse than the baseline values at the time of randomization.

The cost-effectiveness ratio for surgery as compared with medical therapy was very high—$190,000 per quality-adjusted life year gained. Excluding high-risk patients, the mean total financial cost per person at 3 years was $98,952 in the LVRS group versus $62,560 in the medically treated group. This is clearly a very expensive procedure, especially if the benefits are only sustained for a period of 2 or 3 years. However, if, in the long term, the benefits in the surgical group are sustained for a more prolonged period of time, then the cost-effectiveness ratio will be more favorable for the surgically treated group (229).

LVRS can drastically increase airflow in some patients with severe emphysema. The important questions concerning this new approach to emphysema include which patients are most likely to benefit from the surgery and how long the benefits will last. The cost-effectiveness of the procedure is also under intense scrutiny because of questions of long-term benefits and the large number of emphysema patients who could be potential candidates for this surgery. Overall, LVRS as a therapeutic modality for the general population with severe emphysema does not offer a survival benefit; however, the NETT results provide some guidance in the selection of patients who may benefit from such a procedure and help us to select the patients who have an increased risk of a poor outcome and who should be continued on medical therapy or referred for LT. In the future, clinical trials will be continued for nonsurgical techniques for volume reduction surgery and many more options will be offered to patients with advanced emphysema.

REFERENCES

1. Hardy JD, Webb WR, Dalton ML, et al. Lung homotransplantation in man: report of the initial case. *JAMA* 1963;186:1065–1074.
2. Derom F, Barbier F, Ringoir S, et al. Ten-month survival after lung homotransplantation in man. *J Thorac Cardiovasc Surg* 1971;61:835–846.
3. Nelems JM, Rebuck AS, Cooper JD, et al. Human lung transplantation. *Chest* 1980;78:569–573.
4. Borel JF, Feurer C, Gubler HB, et al. Biological effect of cyclosporine A: a new antilymphocyte agent. *Agents Actions* 1976;6:465–475.

5. Trulock EP, Edwards LB, Taylor DO, et al. The registry of the International Society for Heart and Lung Transplantation: twentieth official adult lung and heart-lung annual report—2003. *J Heart Lung Transplant* 2003;22:610–672.
6. Toronto Lung Transplant Group. Unilateral lung transplantation for pulmonary fibrosis. *N Engl J Med* 1986;314:1140–1145.
7. Stevens PM, Johnson PC, Bell RL, et al. Regional ventilation and perfusion after lung transplantation in patients with emphysema. *N Engl J Med* 1970;282(5):245–249.
8. Mal H, Andreassian B, Fabrice P, et al. Unilateral lung transplantation in end-stage pulmonary emphysema. *Am Rev Respir Dis* 1989;140:797–802.
9. Calhoon JH, Grover FL, Gibbons WJ, et al. Single lung transplantation—alternative indications and technique. *J Thorac Cardiovasc Surg* 1991;101(5):816–825.
10. Levine SM, Gibbons WJ, Bryan CL, et al. Single lung transplantation for primary pulmonary hypertension. *Chest* 1990;98:1107–1115.
11. Tuna I, Jamieson SW. Human heart and lung transplantation. *Adv Surg* 1989;22:251–276.
12. Barr ML, Baker CJ, Schenkel FA, et al. Living donor lung transplantation: selection, technique, and outcome. *Transplant Proc* 2001;33:3527–3532.
13. Official ATS Statement—June 1992. Lung transplantation. Report of the ATS workshop on lung transplantation. *Am Rev Respir Dis* 1993;147:772–776.
14. Joint Statement of the American Society for International Transplant Physicians/American Thoracic Society/European Respiratory Society/International Society for Heart and Lung Transplantation. Guidelines for the selection of lung transplant candidates. *Am J Respir Crit Care Med* 1998;158:335–339.
15. Levine SM, The Transplant/Immunology Network of the American College of Chest Physicians. A survey of clinical practice of lung transplantation in North America. *Chest* 2004;125:1224–1238.
16. Levine SM, Anzueto A, Peters JI, et al. Single lung transplantation in patients with systemic disease. *Chest* 1994;105:837–841.
17. Aris RM, Gilligan PH, Neuringer IP, et al. The effects of panresistant bacteria in cystic fibrosis patients on lung transplant outcome. *Am J Respir Crit Care Med* 1997;155:1699–1704.
18. Lima O, Cooper JD, Peters WJ, et al. Effects of methylprednisolone and azathioprine on bronchial healing following lung autotransplantation. *J Thorac Cardiovasc Surg* 1981;82:211–215.
19. Bryan CL, Anzueto A, Levine SM, et al. Corticosteroid therapy does not potentiate bronchial anastomotic complications in single lung transplantation (SLT) [Abstract]. *Am Rev Respir Dis* 1991;143(4):A461.
20. Shafers H-J, Wagner TOF, Dermertzis S, et al. Preoperative corticosteroids: a contraindication to lung transplantation? *Chest* 1992;102:1522–1525.
21. Aris RM, Neuringer IP, Weiner MA, et al. Severe osteoporosis before and after lung transplantation. *Chest* 1996;109:1176–1183.
22. Marshall SE, Kramer MR, Lewiston NJ, et al. Selection and evaluation of recipients for heart-lung transplantation. *Chest* 1990;98:1488–1494.
23. Anthonisen NR. Prognosis in chronic obstructive pulmonary disease: results from multicenter clinical trails. *Am Rev Respir Dis* 1989;140:S95–S99.
24. Traver GA, Cline MG, Burrows B. Predictors of mortality in chronic obstructive pulmonary disease. *Am Rev Respir Dis* 1979;119:895–902.
25. Hosenpud JD, Bennett LE, Keck BM, et al. Effect of diagnosis on survival benefit of lung transplantation for end-stage lung disease. *Lancet* 1998;351:24–27.
26. Carrington CB, Gaensler EA, Coutu RE, et al. Natural history and treated course of usual and desquamative interstitial pneumonia. *N Engl J Med* 1978;298:801–809.
27. Johnson MA, Kwan S, Snell NJC, et al. Randomised controlled trial comparing prednisolone alone with cyclophosphamide and low dose prednisolone in combination in cryptogenic fibrosing alveolitis. *Thorax* 1989;44:280–288.
28. Kerem E, Reisman J, Corey M, et al. Prediction of mortality in patients with cystic fibrosis. *N Engl J Med* 1992;326:1187–1191.
29. Mayer-Hamblett N, Rosenfeld M, Emerson J, et al. Developing cystic fibrosis lung transplant referral criteria using predictors of 2-year mortality. *Am J Respir Crit Care Med* 2002;166:1550–1555.
30. DeSoyza A, McDowell A, Archer L, et al. Burkholderia cepacia complex genomovars and pulmonary transplantation outcomes in patients with cystic fibrosis. *Lancet* 2001;358:1780–1781.
31. D'Alonzo GE, Barst RJ, Ayres SM, et al. Survival in patients with primary pulmonary hypertension. *Ann Intern Med* 1991;115:343–349.
32. Puskas JD, Winton TL, Miller JD, et al. Unilateral donor lung dysfunction does not preclude successful contralateral single lung transplantation. *J Thorac Cardiovasc Surg* 1992;103(5):1015–1017. Discussion;1017–1018.
33. Mohar DE, Bryan CL, Jenkinson SG, et al. HLA matching as a predictor of OB or death in SLT [Abstract]. *Chest* 1993;104(2):157S.
34. Schulman LL, Weinberg AD, McGregor C, et al. Mismatches at the HLA-DR and HLA-B loci are risk factors for acute rejection after lung transplantation. *Am J Respir Crit Care Med* 1998;157:1833–1837.
35. Sundaresan S, Mohanakumar T, Smith MA, et al. HLA-A locus mismatches and development of antibodies to HLA after lung transplantation correlate with the development of bronchiolitis obliterans syndrome. *Transplantation* 1998;65:648–653.
36. Bhorade SM, Vigneswaran W, McCabe MA, et al. Liberalization of donor criteria may expand the donor pool without adverse consequence in lung transplantation. *J Heart Lung Transplant* 2000;19:1199–1204.
37. Gabbay E, Williams TJ, Griffiths AP, et al. Maximizing the utilization of donor organs offered for lung transplantation. *Am J Respir Crit Care Med* 1999;160:265–271.
38. Orens JB, Boehler A, de Perrot M, et al. A review of lung transplant donor acceptability criteria. *J Heart Lung Transplant* 2003;22:1183–1200.
39. Otulana BA, Mist BA, Scott JP, et al. The effect of recipient lung size on lung physiology after heart-lung transplantation. *Transplantation* 1989;48(4):625.
40. The Toronto Lung Transplant Group. Experience with single-lung transplantation for pulmonary fibrosis. *JAMA* 1988;259(15):2258.
41. Lloyd KS, Holland VA, Noon GP, et al. Pulmonary function after heart-lung transplantation using larger donor organs. *Am Rev Respir Dis* 1990;142:1026.
42. Date H, Trulock EP, Arcidi JM, et al. Improved airway healing after lung transplantation: an analysis of 348 bronchial anastomoses. *J Thorac Cardiovasc Surg* 1995;110:1424–1433.
43. Levine SM, Anzueto A, Gibbons WJ, et al. Graft position and pulmonary function after single lung transplantation for obstructive lung disease. *Chest* 1993;103(2):444–448.
44. Bierman MI, Stein KL, Stuart RS, et al. Critical care management of lung transplant recipients. *Intensive Care Med* 1991;6:135.
45. Siegelman SS, Sinha SBP, Veith FT. Pulmonary reimplantation response. *Ann Surg* 1973;177:30.
46. Bryan CL, Cohen DJ, Gibbons WJ, et al. Lung transplantation: the reimplantation response. *Crit Care Rep* 1991;2:217.
47. Bryan CL, Cohen DJ, Dew JA, et al. Glutathione decreases the pulmonary reimplantation response in canine lung autotransplants. *Chest* 1991;100:1694–1702.
48. Ardehali A, Laks H, Levine M, et al. A prospective trial of inhaled nitric oxide in clinical lung transplantation. *Transplantation* 2001;72:112–115.
49. Meyer KC, Love RB, Zimmerman JJ. The therapeutic potential of nitric oxide in lung transplantation. *Chest* 1998;113:1360–1371.
50. Date H, Triantafillou AN, Trulock EP, et al. Inhaled nitric oxide reduces human lung allograft dysfunction. *J Thorac Cardiovasc Surg* 1996;111:913–919.
51. Glassman LR, Keenan RJ, Fabrizio MC, et al. Extracorporeal membrane oxygenation as an adjunct treatment for primary graft failure in adult lung transplant recipients. *J Thorac Cardiovasc Surg* 1995;110:723–727.
52. Christie JD, Bavaria JE, Palevsky HI, et al. Primary graft failure following lung transplantation. *Chest* 1998;114:51–60.
53. Christie JD, Kotloff RM, Pochettino A, et al. Clinical risk factors for primary graft failure following lung transplantation. *Chest* 2003;124:1232–1241.
54. Thabut G, Vinatier I, Stern JB, et al. Primary graft failure following lung transplantation: predictive factors of mortality. *Chest* 2002;121:1876–1882.

55. Herman SJ, Rappaport DC, Weisbrod GL, et al. Single-lung transplantation: imaging features. *Radiology* 1989;170:89–93.

56. Otulana BA, Higenbottam T, Scott J, et al. Lung function associated with histologically diagnosed acute lung rejection and pulmonary infection in heart-lung transplant patients. *Am Rev Respir Dis* 1990;14:329.

57. Millet B, Higenbottam TW, Flower CDR, et al. The radiographic appearances of infection and acute rejection of the lung after heart-lung transplantation. *Am Rev Respir Dis* 1989;140:62–67.

58. Herman SJ. Radiologic assessment after lung transplantation. *Clin Chest Med* 1990;11(2):333–347.

59. Otulana BA, Higenbottam TW, Scott JP, et al. Pulmonary function monitoring allows diagnosis of rejection in heart-lung transplant recipients. *Transplant Proc* 1989;21(1):2583.

60. Otulana BA, Higenbottam T, Ferrari L, et al. The use of home spirometry in detecting acute lung rejection and infection following heart-lung transplantation. *Chest* 1990;97(2):353.

61. Bryan CL, Levine SM, Anzueto A, et al. Exercise oximetry surveillance in single lung transplant recipients [Abstract]. *Am Rev Respir Dis* 1992;145(4):A702.

62. Tamm M, Sharples LD, Higenbottam TW, et al. Bronchiolitis obliterans syndrome in heart-lung transplantation. *Am J Respir Crit Care Med* 1997;155:1705–1710.

63. Levine SM, Anzueto A, Peters JI, et al. Medium term functional results of single lung transplantation for end-stage obstructive lung disease. *Am J Respir Crit Care Med* 1994;150:398–402.

64. Williams TJ, Patterson GA, McClean PA, et al. Maximal exercise testing in single and double lung transplant recipients. *Am Rev Respir Dis* 1992;145:101–105.

65. Miyoshi S, Trulock EP, Schaefers H-J, et al. Cardiopulmonary exercise testing after single and double lung transplantation. *Chest* 1990;97:1130–1136.

66. Gibbons SJ, Levine SM, Bryan CL, et al. Cardiopulmonary exercise responses after single lung transplantation for severe obstructive lung disease. *Chest* 1991;100:106–111.

67. Grossman RF, Frost A, Zamel N, et al. Results of single-lung transplantation for bilateral pulmonary fibrosis. *N Engl J Med* 1990;322:727–733.

68. Patterson GA, Maurer JR, Williams TJ, et al. Comparison of outcomes of double and single lung transplantation for obstructive lung disease. *J Thorac Cardiovasc Surg* 1991;101:623–632.

69. Theodore J, Jamieson SW, Burke CM, et al. Physiologic aspects of human heart-lung transplantation. Pulmonary function status of the post-transplanted lung. *Chest* 1984;86(3):349–357.

70. Levine SM, Jenkinson SG, Bryan CL, et al. Ventilation-perfusion inequalities during graft rejection in patients undergoing single lung transplantation for primary pulmonary hypertension. *Chest* 1992;101:401–405.

71. Levy RD, Ernst P, Levine SM, et al. Exercise performance after lung transplantation. *J Heart Lung Transplant* 1993;12(1):27–33.

72. Caine N, Sharples LD, Dennis C, et al. Measurement of health-related quality of life before and after heart-lung transplantation. *J Heart Lung Transplant* 1996;15:1047–1058.

73. Dennis C, Caine N, Sharples L, et al. Heart-lung transplantation for end-stage respiratory disease in patients with cystic fibrosis at Papworth Hospital. *J Heart Lung Transplant* 1993;12:893–902.

74. Gross CR, Savik K, Bolman RM III, et al. Long-term health status and quality of life outcomes of lung transplant recipients. *Chest* 1995;108:1587–1593.

75. Paris WP, Diercks M, Bright J, et al. Return to work after lung transplantation. *J Heart Lung Transplant* 1998;17:430–436.

76. de Hoyos AL, Patterson GA, Maurer JR, et al. Pulmonary transplantation: early and late results. *J Thorac Cardiovasc Surg* 1992;103:295–306.

77. Laks H, Louie HW, Haas GS, et al. New technique of vascularization of the trachea and bronchus for lung transplantation. *J Heart Lung Transplant* 1991;10(2):280–287.

78. Nazari S, Prati U, Berti A, et al. Successful bronchial revascularization in experimental single lung transplantation. *Eur J Cardiothorac Surg* 1990;4:561–567.

79. de Hoyos A, Maurer JR. Complications following lung transplantation. *Semin Thorac Cardovasc Surg* 1992;4(2):132–146.

80. Kshettry VR, Kroshus TJ, Hertz MI, et al. Early and late airway complications after lung transplantation: incidence and management. *Ann Thorac Surg* 1997;63:1576–1583.

81. Susanto I, Peters JI, Levine SM, et al. Use of balloon-expandable metallic stents in the management of bronchial stenosis and bronchomalacia after lung transplantation. *Chest* 1998;114:1330–1335.

82. Anzueto A, Levine SM, Tillis WP, et al. The use of the flow-volume loop in the diagnosis of bronchial stenosis after single lung transplantation. *Chest* 1994;105:934–936.

83. Kramer MR, Denning DW, Marshall SE, et al. Ulcerative tracheobronchitis after lung transplantation. *Am Rev Respir Dis* 1991;144:552–556.

84. Keller C, Frost A. Fiberoptic bronchoplasty. Description of a simple adjunct technique for the management of bronchial stenosis following lung transplantation. *Chest* 1992;102(4):995–998.

85. Frost AE, Jammal CT, Cagle PT. Hyperacute rejection following lung transplantation. *Chest* 1996;110:559–562.

86. Lawrence EC. Diagnosis and management of lung allograft rejection. *Clin Chest Med* 1990;11:269–277.

87. Trulock EP. Management of lung transplant rejection. *Chest* 1993;103:1566–1576.

88. Bergin CJ, Castellino RA, Blank N, et al. Acute lung rejection after heart-lung transplantation: correlation of findings on chest radiographs with lung biopsy results. *Am J Roentgenol* 1990;155:23–27.

89. Starnes VA, Theodore J, Oyer PE, et al. Pulmonary infiltrates after heart-lung transplantation: evaluation by serial transbronchial lung biopsies. *J Thorac Cardiovasc Surg* 1989;98:945–950.

90. Trulock EP, Ettinger NA, Brunt EM, et al. The role of transbronchial lung biopsy in the treatment of lung transplant recipients: an analysis of 200 consecutive procedures. *Chest* 1992;10:1049–1054.

91. Higenbottam T, Stewart S, Penketh A, et al. Transbronchial lung biopsy for the diagnosis of rejection in heart-lung transplant patients. *Transplantation* 1988;46:532–539.

92. Scott JP, Fradet G, Smyth RL, et al. Prospective study of transbronchial biopsies in the management of heart-lung and single lung transplant patients. *J Heart Lung Transplant* 1991;10:626–637.

93. Silkoff PE, Caramori M, Tremblay L, et al. Exhaled nitric oxide in human lung transplantation. *Am J Respir Crit Care Med* 1998;157:1822–1828.

94. Yousem SA, Berry GJ, Cagle PT et al., Lung Rejection Study Group. Revision of the 1990 working formulation for the classification of pulmonary allograft rejection. *J Heart Lung Transplant* 1996;15:1–15.

95. Horning NR, Lynch JP, Sundaresan SR, et al. Tacrolimus therapy for persistent or recurrent acute rejection after lung transplantation. *J Heart Lung Transplant* 1998;17:761–767.

96. O'Riordan TG, Iacono A, Keenan RJ, et al. Delivery and distribution of aerosolized cyclosporine in lung allograft recipients. *Am J Respir Crit Care Med* 1995;151:516–521.

97. Iacono A, Zeevi A, Keenan R, et al. Treatment of refractory acute lung allograft rejection with aerosolized cyclosporine A: evidence for a dose response relationship [Abstract]. *J Heart Lung Transplant* 1996;15(1;Part 2):S102.

98. Valentine VG, Robbins RC, Wehner JH, et al. Total lymphoid irradiation for refractory acute rejection in heart-lung and lung allografts. *Chest* 1996;109:1184–1189.

99. Andreu G, Achkar A, Couetil JP, et al. Extracorporeal photochemotherapy treatment for acute lung rejection episode. *J Heart Lung Transplant* 1995;14:793–796.

100. Aboyoun CL, Tamm M, Chhajed PN, et al. Diagnostic value of follow-up transbronchial lung biopsy after lung rejection. *Am J Respir Crit Care Med* 2001;164:460–463.

101. Glanville AR, Baldwin JC, Burke CM, et al. Obliterative bronchiolitis after heart-lung transplantation: apparent arrest by augmented immunosuppression. *Ann Intern Med* 1987;107:300–304.

102. Burke CM, Glanville AR, Theodore J, et al. Lung immunogenicity, rejection, and obliterative bronchiolitis. *Chest* 1987;92(3):547–549.

103. McCarthy PM, Starnes VA, Theodore J, et al. Improved survival after heart-lung transplantation. *J Thorac Cardiovasc Surg* 1990;99:54–60.

104. Scott JP, Sharples L, Mullins, P, et al. Further studies on the natural history of obliterative bronchiolitis following heart-lung transplantation. *Transplant Proc* 1991;23(1):1201–1202.

105. LoCicero J III, Robinson PG, Fisher M. Chronic rejection in single-lung transplantation manifested by obliterative bronchiolitis. *J Thorac Cardiovasc Surg* 1990;99:1059–1062.

106. Trulock EP. State of the art: lung transplantation. *Am J Respir Crit Care Med* 1997;155:789–818.
107. Griffith BP, Paradis IL, Zeevi A, et al. Immunologically mediated disease of the airways after pulmonary transplantation. *Ann Surg* 1988;208(3):371–378.
108. Kroshus TJ, Kshettry VR, Savik K, et al. Risk factors for the development of bronchiolitis obliterans syndrome after lung transplantation. *J Thorac Cardiovasc Surg* 1997;114:195–202.
109. Kennan RJ, Lega ME, Drummer JS, et al. Cytomegalovirus: serologic status and postoperative infection correlated with risk of developing chronic rejection after pulmonary transplantation. *Transplantation* 1991;51(2):433–438.
110. Girgis RE, Tu I, Berry GJ, et al. Risk factors for the development of obliterative bronchiolitis after lung transplantation. *J Heart Lung Transplant* 1996;15:1200–1208.
111. Ross DJ, Marchevsky A, Kramer M, et al. "Refractoriness" of airflow obstruction associated with isolated lymphocytic bronchiolitis/bronchitis in pulmonary allografts. *J Heart Lung Transplant* 1997;16:832–838.
112. Bando K, Paradis IL, Similo S, et al. Obliterative bronchiolitis after lung and heart-lung transplantation: an analysis of risk factors and management. *J Thorac Cardiovasac Surg* 1995;110:4–14.
113. Scott JP, Higenbottam TW, Sharples L, et al. Risk factors for obliterative bronchiolitis in heart-lung transplant recipients. *Transplantation* 1991;51:813–817.
114. Keller CA, Cagle PT, Brown RW, et al. Bronchiolitis obliterans in recipients of single, double, and heart-lung transplantation. *Chest* 1995;107:973–980.
115. Sharples LD, Tamm M, McNeil K, et al. Development of bronchiolitis obliterans syndrome in recipients of heart-lung transplantation—early risk factors. *Transplantation* 1996;61:560–566.
116. Estenne M, Maurer JR, Boehler A, et al. Bronchiolitis obliterans syndrome 2001: an update of the diagnostic criteria. *J Heart Lung Transplant* 2002;21:297–310.
117. Sundaresan RS, Trulock EP, Mohanakumar T, et al. Prevalence and outcome of bronchiolitis obliterans syndrome after lung transplantation. *Ann Thorac Surg* 1995;60:1341–1347.
118. Burke CM, Theodore J, Dawkins KD, et al. Post-transplant obliterative bronchiolitis and other late lung sequelae in human heart-lung transplantation. *Chest* 1984;86(6):824–829.
119. Patterson GM, Wilson S, Whang JL, et al. Physiologic definitions of obliterative bronchiolitis in heart-lung and double lung transplantation: a comparison of the forced expiratory flow between 25% and 75% of the forced vital capacity and forced expiratory volume in one second. *J Heart Lung Transplant* 1996;15:175–181.
120. Skeens JL, Fuhrman CR, Yousem SA. Bronchiolitis obliterans in heart-lung transplantation patients: radiologic findings in 11 patients. *Am J Roentgenol* 1989;153:253–256.
121. Halvorsen RA Jr, DuCret RP, Kuni CC, et al. Obliterative bronchiolitis following lung transplantation: diagnostic utility of aerosol ventilation lung scanning and high resolution CT. *Clin Nucl Med* 1991;16(4):256–258.
122. Morrish WF, Herman SJ, Weisbrod GL, et al. Bronchiolitis obliterans after lung transplantation: findings at chest radiography and high-resolution CT. *Radiology* 1991;179:487–490.
123. Worthy SA, Park CS, Kim JS, et al. Bronchiolitis obliterans after lung transplantation: high-resolution CT findings in 15 patients. *Am J Roentgenol* 1997;169:673–677.
124. Ikonen T, Kivisaari L, Tashinen E, et al. High-resolution CT in long-term follow-up after lung transplantation. *Chest* 1997;11:370–376.
125. Leung AN, Fisher K, Valentine V, et al. Bronchiolitis obliterans after lung transplantation. *Chest* 1998;113:365–370.
126. Yousem SA, Paradis IL, Dauber JH, et al. Efficacy of transbronchial lung biopsy in the diagnosis of bronchiolitis obliterans in heart-lung transplant recipients. *Transplantation* 1989;47:893–895.
127. Yousem SA, Ohori NP. Pathological classification of acute and chronic rejection of the lung. In: Shennib H, ed. *Immunology of the lung allograft*. Austin, TX: RG Landes Bioscience, 1989;29–44.
128. Kramer MR, Stoehr C, Whang JL, et al. The diagnosis of obliterative bronchiolitis after heart-lung and lung transplantation: low yield of transbronchial lung biopsy. *J Heart Lung Transplant* 1993;12:675–681.
129. Chamberlain D, Maurer J, Chaparro C, et al. Evaluation of transbronchial lung biopsy specimens in the diagnosis of bronchiolitis obliterans after lung transplantation. *J Heart Lung Transplant* 1994;13:963–971.
130. Yousem SA, Paradis I, Griffith BP. Can transbronchial biopsy aid in the diagnosis of bronchiolitis obliterans in lung transplant recipients? *Transplantation* 1994;57:151–153.
131. Cooper JD, Billingham M, Egan T, et al. A working formulation for the standardization of nomenclature and for clinical staging of chronic dysfunction in lung allografts. *J Heart Lung Transplant* 1993;12:713–716.
132. Gabbay E, Walters EH, Orsida B, et al. Post-lung transplant bronchiolitis obliterans syndrome (BOS) is characterized by increased exhaled nitric oxide levels and epithelial inducible nitric oxide synthase. *Am J Respir Crit Care Med* 2000;162:2182–2187.
133. Date H, Lynch JP, Sundaresan S, et al. The impact of cytolytic therapy on bronchiolitis obliterans syndrome. *J Heart Lung Transplant* 1998;17:869–875.
134. Ross DJ, Lewis MI, Kramer M, et al. FK 506 "rescue" immunosuppression for obliterative bronchiolitis after lung transplantation. *Chest* 1997;112:1175–1179.
135. Kesten S, Chaparro C, Scavuzza M, et al. Tacrolimus as rescue therapy for bronchiolitis obliterans syndrome. *J Heart Lung Transplant* 1997;16:905–912.
136. Whyte RI, Rossi SJ, Mulligan MS, et al. Mycophenolate mofetil for obliterative bronchiolitis syndrome after lung transplantation. *Ann Thorac Surg* 1997;64:945–948.
137. Iacono AT, Keenan RJ, Duncan SR, et al. Aerosolized cyclosporine in lung recipients with refractory chronic rejection. *Am J Respir Crit Care Med* 1996;153:1451–1455.
138. Valentine VG, Robbins RC, Berry GJ, et al. Actuarial survival of heart-lung and bilateral sequential lung transplant recipients with obliterative bronchiolitis. *J Heart Lung Transplant* 1996;15:371–383.
139. Brooks RG, Hofflin JM, Jamieson SW, et al. Infectious complications in heart-lung transplant recipients. *Am J Med* 1985;79:412.
140. Egan TM, Kaiser LR, Cooper JD. Lung transplantation. *Curr Probl Surg* 1989;26:675–751.
141. Lynch JP III, Chauncey JB III, Gyetko M. Pulmonary and infectious complications in organ transplant recipients. In: Tenholder MF, ed. *Approach to pulmonary infections in the immunocompromised host*. Mount Kisco: Futura Publishing, 1991:229–276.
142. Dauber JH, Paradis IL, Dummer JS. Infectious complications in pulmonary allograft recipients. *Clin Chest Med* 1990;11:291–308.
143. Ampel NM, Wing EJ. *Legionella* infection in transplant patients. *Semin Respir Infect* 1990;5:30–37.
144. Ettinger NA, Trulock EP. Pulmonary considerations of organ transplantation. *Am Rev Respir Dis* 1991;143:1386–1405; 144:213–223,433–454.
145. Davey RT, Masur H. Recent advances in the diagnosis, treatment, and prevention of *Pneumocystis carinii* pneumonia. *Antimicrob Agents Chemother* 1990;34:499–504.
146. Dummer JS. *Pneumocystis carinii* infections in transplant recipients. *Semin Respir Infect* 1990;5:50–57.
147. Paradis IL, William P. Infection after lung transplantation. *Semin Respir Infect* 1993;8:207–215.
148. Paradis H, Grgurick WF, Drummer JS, et al. Rapid detection of cytomegalovirus pneumonia by evaluation of bronchoalveolar cells. *Am Rev Respir Dis* 1988;138:697–702.
149. Snydman DR. Cytomegalovirus infection in solid organ transplantation. Prospects for prevention. *Transplant Rev* 1990;4:59–67.
150. Saliba F, Arulnaden JL, Gugenheim J, et al. CMV hyperimmune prophylaxis after liver transplantation: a prospective randomized controlled study. *Transplant Proc* 1989;21:2260–2262.
151. Havel M, Teufelsbauer H, Lackovics A, et al. Cytomegalovirus hyperimmunoglobulin prophylaxis in the prevention of cytomegalovirus infection in immunosuppressed heart transplant patients. *Transplant Proc* 1990;22:1805–1806.
152. Gane E, Saliba F, Valdecasas GJC, et al. Randomised trial of efficacy and safety of oral ganciclovir in the prevention of cytomegalovirus disease in liver transplant recipients. *Lancet* 1997;350:1729–1733.

153. Speich R, Thurnheer R, Gaspert A, et al. Efficacy and cost effectiveness of oral ganciclovir in the prevention of cytomegalovirus disease after lung transplantation. *Transplantation* 1999;67: 315–320.

154. Singh N, Yu VL. Oral ganciclovir usage for cytomegalovirus prophylaxis in organ transplant recipients. *Dig Dis Sci* 1998;43(6): 1190–1192.

155. Singh N, Yu VL, Gayowski T, et al. Cytomegalovirus antigenemia guided preemptive therapy with oral versus intravenous ganciclovir for the prevention of cytomegalovirus disease in liver transplant recipients [Abstract H5]. *37th international conference on antimicrobial agents and chemotherapy*, Toronto, 1997.

156. Schmidt CA, Oettle H, Peng R, et al. Comparison of polymerase chain reaction from plasma and buffy coat with antigen detection and occurrence of immunoglobulin M for the demonstration of cytomegalovirus infection after liver transplantation. *Transplantation* 1995;59:1133–1138.

157. Egan JJ, Barber L, Lomax J, et al. Detection of human cytomegalovirus antigenemia: a rapid diagnostic technique for predicting cytomegalovirus infection pneumonitis in lung and heart transplant recipients. *Thorax* 1995;50:9–13.

158. Paya CV. Fungal infections in solid-organ transplantation. *Clin Infect Dis* 1993;16:677–688.

159. Levine SM, Peters JI. Fungal infection in the lung transplant recipient. *Pulm Crit Care Update* 1998;13(12):17.

160. Minari A, Husni R, Avery RK, et al. The incidence of invasive aspergillosis among solid organ transplant recipients and implications for prophylaxis in lung transplants. *Transplant Infect Dis* 2002;4:195–200.

161. Denning DW, Stevens DA. Antifungal and surgical treatment of invasive aspergillosis: review of 2,121 published cases. *Rev Infect Dis* 1990;12:1147–1201.

162. Levine SM, Peters JI, Anzueto A, et al. *Aspergillus* infection in single lung transplant recipients [Abstract]. *Am Rev Respir Dis* 1993;147(4):A599.

163. Saral R. *Candida* and *Aspergillus* infection in immunocompromised patients: an overview. *Rev Infect Dis* 1991;13:487–492.

164. Wajszczuk CP, Dummer JS, Ho M, et al. Fungal infections in liver transplant recipients. *Transplantation* 1985;40:347–353.

165. Zeluff BJ. Fungal pneumonia in transplant recipients. *Semin Respir Med* 1992;13:216–233.

166. Denning D, Tucker RM, Hanson LH, et al. Treatment of invasive aspergillosis with itraconazole. *Am J Med* 1989;86:791–800.

167. Zenati M, Dowling RD, Dummer S, et al. Influence of the donor lung on development of early infections in lung transplant recipients. *J Heart Transplant* 1990;9:502–509.

168. Conti DJ, Tolkoff-Rubin NE, Baker GP, et al. Successful treatment of invasive fungal infection with fluconazole in organ transplant recipients. *Transplantation* 1989;48:692–695.

169. Sinnott JV IV, Emmanual PJ. Mycobacterial infections in the transplant patient. *Semin Respir Infect* 1990;5:65–73.

170. Novick RJ, Moreno-Cabral CE, Stinson EB, et al. Nontuberculous mycobacterial infections in heart transplant recipients: a seventeen-year experience. *J Heart Transplant* 1990;9:357–363.

171. Shelhamer JH, Toews GB, Masur H, et al. Respiratory disease in the immunosuppressed patient. *Ann Intern Med* 1992;117: 415–431.

172. Rolfe M, Strieter RM, Lynch JP III. Nocardiosis. *Semin Respir Med* 1992;13:216–233.

173. Wilson JP, Turner HR, Kirchner KA, et al. Nocardial infections in renal transplant recipients. *Medicine (Baltimore)* 1989;68:38–57.

174. Lynch JP III, Rolfe MW. Today's approach to managing and preventing nocardiosis. *J Respir Dis* 1993;14:112–121.

175. Nalesnik MA, Makowka L, Starzl TE. The diagnosis and treatment of lymphoproliferative disorders. *Curr Probl Surg* 1988;25: 371–472.

176. Randhawa PS, Yousem SA, Paradis IL, et al. The clinical spectrum, pathology, and clonal analysis of Epstein-Barr virus-associated lymphoproliferative disorders in heart-lung transplant recipients. *Am J Clin Pathol* 1989;92:177–185.

177. Yousem SA, Randhawa P, Locker J, et al. Posttransplant lymphoproliferative disorders in heart-lung transplant recipients: primary presentation in the allograft. *Hum Pathol* 1989;20:361–369.

178. Armitage JM, Kormos RL, Stuart RS, et al. Posttransplant lymphoproliferative disease in thoracic organ transplant patients: ten years of cyclosporine-based immunosuppression. *J Heart Lung Transplant* 1991;10:877–887.

179. Walker RC, Paya CV, Marshall WF, et al. Pretransplantation seronegative Epstein-Barr virus status is the primary risk factor for posttransplantation lymphoproliferative disorder in adult heart, lung, and other solid organ transplantations. *J Heart Lung Transplant* 1995;14:214–221.

180. Marshall WF, Strickler JG, Wiesner RH, et al. Pretransplantation assessment of the risk of lymphoproliferative disorder. *Clin Infect Dis* 1995;20:1346–1353.

181. Leblond V, Sutton L, Dorent R, et al. Lymphoproliferative disorders after transplantation: a report of 24 cases observed in a single center. *J Clin Oncol* 1995;13:961–968.

182. Levine SM, Angel L, Anzueto A, et al. A low incidence of posttransplant lymphoproliferative disorder in 109 lung transplant recipients. *Chest* 1999;116:1273–7.

183. Aris RM, Maia DM, Neuringer IP, et al. Post-transplantation lymphoproliferative disorder in the Epstein-Barr virus-naïve lung transplant recipient. *Am J Respir Crit Care Med* 1996;154: 1712–1717.

184. Verschuuren EA, Stevens SJ, van Imhoff GW, et al. Treatment of posttransplant lymphoproliferative disease with rituximab: the remission, the relapse, and the complication. *Transplantation* 2002;73:100–104.

185. Aracasoy SM, Hersh C, Christie JD, et al. Bronchogenic carcinoma complicating lung transplantation. *J Heart Lung Transplant* 2001;20:1044–1053.

186. Goldstein G. An overview of Orthoclone OKT3. *Transplant Proc* 1986;18(4):927–930.

187. Knight RJ, Kurrle R, McClain J, et al. Clinical evaluation of induction of immunosuppression with a murine IgG$_{2b}$ monoclonal antibody (BMA 031) directed toward the human α/β-T cell receptor. *Transplantation* 1994;57:1581–1588.

188. Vicente F, Lantz M, Birnbaum J, et al. A phase I trial of humanized anti-interleukin 2 receptor antibody in renal transplantation. *Transplantation* 1997;63:33–38.

189. Palmer SM, Miralles AP, Lawrence CM, et al. Rabbit antithymocyte globulin decreases acute rejection after lung transplantation: results of a randomized, prospective study. *Chest* 1999; 116:127–133.

190. Kriett JM, Smith CM, Hayden AM, et al. Lung transplantation without the use of antilymphocyte antibody preparations. *J Heart Lung Transplant* 1993;12:915–922.

191. Halloran PF. Immunosuppressive agents in clinical trials in transplantation. *Am J Med Sci* 1997;313(5):283–288.

192. US Renal Data System. *USRDS 1995 annual data report*. Bethesda: National Institutes of Health, National Institute of Diabetes and Digestive and Kidney Diseases, 1995.

193. Hunsicker LG, Bennett LE. Design of trials of methods to reduce late renal allograft loss: the price of success. *Kidney Int.* 1995; 48(Suppl.):S120–S123.

194. Briffa N, Morris RE. New immunosuppressive regimens in lung transplantation. *Eur Respir J* 1997;10:2630–2637.

195. Vasquez MA. New advances in immunosuppression therapy for renal transplantation. Southwestern Internal Medicine Conference. *Am J Med Sci* 1997;314:415–435.

196. Vine W, Bowers LD. Cyclosporine: structure, pharmacokinetics, and therapeutic drug monitoring. *Crit Rev Clin Lab Sci* 1988;25: 275–311.

197. Kaskel FJ, Devarajan P, Arbeit LA, et al. Effects of cyclosporine on renal hemodynamics and autoregulation in rats. *Transplant Proc* 1988;20(3):603–609.

198. Maurer JR. Therapeutic challenges following lung transplantation. *Clin Chest Med* 1990;11(2):279–291.

199. Mihatsch M, Thiel G, Ryffel B. Cyclosporin nephrotoxicity. *Adv Nephrol Necker Hosp* 1988;17:303.

200. 1996 Annual report of the U.S. scientific registry for transplant recipients and the organ procurement and transplantation network—transplant data. *1988–1995*. Rockville, MD: UNOS, Richmond, and the Division of Transplantation, Bureau of Health Resources Development, Health Resources and

Services Administration, U.S. Department of Health and Human Services, 1996.

201. Kahan BD. Cyclosporine. *Med Intell* 1989;321(25):1725–1737.

202. Bach JF, Strom TB. *The mode of action of immunosuppressive drugs,* 8th ed. New York: Elsevier, 1985.

203. Lu CY, Sicher SC, Vasquez MA. Prevention and treatment of renal allograft rejection: new therapeutic approaches and new insights into established therapies. *J Am Soc Nephrol* 1993;4:1239–1256.

204. Cameron DE, Traill TA. Complications of immunosuppressive therapy. In: Baumgartner WA, Reitz BA, Achuff SC, eds. *Heart and heart-lung transplantation.* Philadelphia: WB Saunders, 1990: 237–247.

205. The International MMF Renal Transplant Study Group. A pooled analysis of three randomized double-blind clinical studies in prevention of rejection with mycophenolate mofetil in renal allograft recipients. *Transplantation* 1997;63(1):39–47.

206. Knoop C, Haverich A, Fischer S. Immunosuppressive therapy after human lung transplantation *Eur Respir J* 2004;23:159–171.

207. Singer SJ, Tiernan R, Sullivan EJ. Interstitial pneumonitis associated with sirolimus therapy in renal-transplant recipients. *N Engl J Med* 2000;343:225–226.

208. McWilliams TJ, Levvey BJ, Russell PA, et al. Interstitial pneumonitis associated with sirolimus: a dilemma for lung transplantation. *J Heart Lung Transplant* 2003;22:210–213.

209. Fessler HE, Wise RA. Lung volume reduction surgery. Is less really more? *Am J Respir Crit Care Med* 1990;159:1031–1035.

210. Fein AM. Lung volume reduction surgery. Answering the crucial questions. *Chest* 1998;113:277S–282S.

211. Utz JP, Hubmayr RD, Deschamps C. Lung volume reduction surgery for emphysema: out on a limb without a NETT. *Mayo Clin Proc* 1998;73:552–566.

212. Brantigan OC, Mueller E. Surgical treatment of pulmonary emphysema. *Am Surg* 1957;23:789–804.

213. Payne DK, Markewitz BA, Owens MW. Surgical treatment of chronic obstructive pulmonary disease. *Am J Med Sci* 1993; 318(2):89–95.

214. Cooper JD, Trulock EP, Triantafillou AN, et al. Bilateral pneumectomy (volume reduction) for chronic obstructive pulmonary disease. *J Thorac Cardiovasc Surg* 1995;109:106–119.

215. Ingenito EP, Loring SH, Moy ML, et al. Physiological characterization of variability in response to lung volume reduction surgery. *J Appl Physiol.* 2003;94(1):20–30.

216. Ojo TC, Martinez F, Paine R III, et al. Lung volume reduction surgery alters management of pulmonary nodules in patients with severe COPD. *Chest* 1997;112:1494–1500.

217. Maxfield, R. New and emerging minimally invasive techniques for lung volume reduction. *Chest* 2004;125:777–783.

218. Snell GI, Holsworth LC, Borrill ZL, et al. The potential for bronchoscopic lung volume reduction using bronchial prostheses: a pilot study. *Chest* 2003;124(3):1073–1080.

219. Toma TP, Hopkinson NS, Hillier J, et al. Bronchoscopic lung volume reduction with implants in patients with severe emphysema. *Lancet* 2003;361:931–933.

220. Ingenito EP, Reilly JJ, Mentzer SJ, et al. Bronchoscopic lung volume reduction: a safe and effective alternative to surgical therapy for emphysema. *Am J Respir Crit Care Med* 2001;164:295–301.

221. Ingenito EP, Berger RL, Henderson AC, et al. Bronchoscopic lung volume reduction using tissue engineering principles. *Am J Respir Crit Care Med* 2003;167:771–778.

222. Lausberg HF, Chino K, Patterson GA, et al. Bronchial fenestration improves expiratory flow in emphysematous human lungs. *Ann Thorac Surg* 2003;75:393–397.

223. Yusen DY, Lefrak S, Gierada DS, et al. A prospective evaluation of lung volume reduction surgery in 200 consecutive patients. *Chest* 2003;123:1026–1037.

224. Gelb AF, Brenner M, McKenna RJ, et al. Lung function 12 months following emphysema resection. *Chest* 1996;10:1407–1415.

225. Ingenito EP, Evans RB, Loring SH, et al. Relation between preoperative inspiratory lung resistance and the outcome of lung volume reduction surgery for emphysema. *N Engl J Med* 1998;338: 1181–1185.

226. Brenner M, Kayaleh RA, Milne WN, et al. Thorascopic laser ablation of pulmonary bullae: radiographic selection and treatment response. *J Thorac Cardiovasc Surg* 1994;107:883–890.

227. National Emphysema Treatment Trial Research Group. Patients at high risk of death after lung-volume-reduction surgery. *N Engl J Med* 2001;345(15):1075–1083.

228. National Emphysema Treatment Trial Research Group. A randomized trial comparing lung volume reduction surgery with medial therapy for severe emphysema. *N Engl J Med* 2003; 348(21):2059–2073.

229. National Emphysema Treatment Trial Research Group. Cost effectiveness of lung volume reduction surgery for patients with severe emphysema. *N Engl J Med* 2003;348(21):2092–2102.

CHAPTER 11

Pulmonary Thromboembolism and Other Pulmonary Vascular Diseases

Alejandro C. Arroliga

Michael A. Matthay

Richard A. Matthay

The pulmonary blood vessels are frequently involved in diseases ranging from chronic obstructive pulmonary disease to interstitial fibrosis (1). If the disease is extensive, pulmonary hypertension may ensue (1). Pulmonary hypertension is also a feature of many congenital and acquired heart diseases and such systemic disorders as scleroderma and systemic lupus erythematosus (1). This chapter reviews the disorders associated with pulmonary vascular disease, focusing on pulmonary thromboembolism and infarction, primary pulmonary hypertension, and pulmonary heart disease (cor pulmonale). Congenital and acquired pulmonary arteriovenous malformations and neoplasia of the pulmonary vascular bed are also discussed briefly.

PULMONARY THROMBOEMBOLISM AND INFARCTION

Pulmonary thromboembolism is a common clinical entity frequently associated with significant morbidity and mortality (2). Because of its anatomy and location, the pulmonary circulation is frequently affected by emboli that lodge in the lungs. The most common type of embolus affecting the pulmonary circulation is a bland thromboembolus transported from its origin by the venous circulation (3).

INCIDENCE

Pulmonary thromboembolism is the most common acute pulmonary disorder among hospitalized patients in the United States, occurring in approximately 200,000 to 300,000 hospitalizations per year (2,4–7). The average annual incidence rate for pulmonary embolism (PE) is 69 per 100,000 (6).

It ranks third as a cause of death in this country, accounting for at least 50,000 to 100,000 deaths annually (4–6). However, the annual mortality decreased 30% from 1979 to 1998 (2).

Approximately one-third of the deaths from PE occur within 1 hour of the onset of symptoms, and the diagnosis is not even suspected in nearly 60% of the patients who die (6–8). Most of the deaths occur rapidly, before the appropriate diagnosis is made and the appropriate therapy is implemented; therefore, prevention is important (6). Patients in whom the diagnosis is made and therapy is instituted account for only about 7% of the deaths caused by thromboembolism; a simple, inexpensive screening test to detect asymptomatic deep venous thrombosis (DVT), the precursor of PE, would be invaluable.

In autopsy studies, major PE was seen in 13% to 25% of autopsies. Venous thromboembolism (PE and deep vein thrombosis) was significantly more common in patients who died in the hospital compared with nonhospital deaths (9). The prevalence of confirmed venous thromboembolism increases with age. The cumulative probability of suffering a first episode of venous thromboembolism is 10.7% by the age of 80 years (10). Multiple injuries, multiple surgical procedures, chronic immobilization, congestive heart failure, and bed rest put patients, especially the elderly, at high risk for DVT (see Tables 11-1 and 11-2) (9–12).

PATHOGENESIS

Most pulmonary emboli arise from detached portions of venous thrombi that form in the deep veins of the lower extremities or of the pelvis and in the right side of the heart (4,13,14). Thrombus formation is fostered by blood stasis, hypercoagulable states, and vessel wall abnormalities. Stasis may be caused by local pressure, venous obstruction, or immobilization after a fracture or surgery, and commonly occurs in patients with congestive heart failure, shock, hypovolemia, dehydration, and varicose veins.

Several conditions enhance the intravascular coagulability of blood (15–17). In some hypercoagulable states, abnormalities of the platelets and dysfunction of the endothelium mediated by cytokine activation may be important (15). Alteration of the endothelium may lead to loss of its normal anticoagulant surface functions, resulting in a proinflammatory thrombogenic phenotype (15). Certain abnormalities of the coagulation or fibrinolytic system are associated with recurrent venous thromboembolism, including increased platelet adhesiveness and survival time; abnormalities of the coagulation cascade, such as high levels of factor V or factor VII; or deficiency of antithrombin III, protein C, or protein S (15,16). The two most common thrombophilias

TABLE 11-1.   Independent Risk Factors for Deep Vein Thrombosis or Pulmonary Embolism

Baseline Characteristic	Odds Ratio	(95% Confidence Interval)
Institutionalization with or without recent surgery		
No institutionalization or recent surgery	1.00	—
Institutionalization without recent surgery	7.98	(4.49–14.18)
Institutionalization with recent surgery	21.72	(9.44–49.93)
Trauma	12.69	(4.06–39.66)
No malignancy	1.00	—
Malignancy without chemotherapy	4.05	(1.93–8.52)
Malignancy with chemotherapy	6.53	(2.11–20.23)
Prior central venous catheter or transvenous pacemaker	5.35	(1.57–19.58)
Prior superficial vein thrombosis	4.32	(1.76–10.61)
Neurologic disease with extremity paresis	3.04	(1.25–7.38)
Serous liver disease	0.10	(0.01–0.71)

From Heit SA, Silverstein MD, Mohr DN, et al. Risk factors for deep vein thrombosis and pulmonary embolism: a population-based case–control study. *Arch Intern Med* 2000;160:809–815, with permission.

TABLE 11-2. Conditions Predisposing to Venous Thrombosis and Pulmonary Thromboembolism

Advanced age
Postoperative status
Previous venous thrombosis
Trauma
Congestive heart failure
Central venous catheters
Cerebrovascular accidents
Thrombocytosis
Transvenous pacemakers
Erythrocytosis
Homocystinuria
Sickle cell anemia
Oral contraceptive use
Pregnancy
Prolonged bed rest
Long periods of travel (air or car)
Carcinoma
Obesity
Antiphospholipid syndrome

From Raskob GE, Hull RD. Diagnosis and management of pulmonary thromboembolism. *Q J Med* 1990;76:787–797, with permission.

(defined as a predisposition toward thrombotic events) are resistance to activated protein C (an anticoagulant protein) that is associated with an abnormal factor V gene (factor V Leiden) and a prothrombin gene variant (prothrombin G20210A). Activated protein C resistance accounts for almost 20% of cases of venous thrombosis, and prothrombin G20210A polymorphism is present in almost 7% of patients with venous thrombosis (17). The mutation in the factor V gene makes it resistant to inactivation by activated protein C, and the mutation in the prothrombin gene increases the levels of plasma prothrombin (16). Other groups at risk for venous hypercoagulability are patients with primary or secondary antiphospholipid syndrome (15,17). Patients with the antiphospholipid syndrome have antiphospholipid antibodies, including anticardiolipin antibodies and lupus anticoagulant. These antibodies are a heterogeneous group of immunoglobulins directed against protein-phospholipid complexes, mainly prothrombin and β_2-glycoprotein 1. The pathophysiologic mechanism in these patients is not fully understood; proposed mechanisms include inhibition of natural anticoagulant pathways, inhibition of fibrinolysis, and endothelial-cell activation (17). Severe hyperhomocysteinemia is known to be a risk factor for venous thromboembolism; even modest hyperhomocysteinemia is associated with a higher risk of developing venous thromboembolism (16).

Malignancy-associated phlebitis (Trousseau syndrome) should be considered in patients 50 years of age or older without risk factors who develop DVT and/or PE, or in whom thrombosis or embolism recurs during warfarin therapy (18). The pathophysiology in Trousseau syndrome is not understood, but tumor cells interacting with thrombin and plasmin-generating systems can influence thrombus formation (15). Patients who present with deep venous thromboses and with no known risk factors should have a minimal workup for malignancy, including measurement of serum carcinoembryonic antigen as well as a test for fecal occult blood, a chest radiograph or computerized

tomography (CT) of the chest, and measurement of prostate-specific antigen in men and mammography in women.

Local trauma or inflammation may damage a vessel wall. In instances of marked local phlebitis with tenderness, redness, warmth, and swelling, the thrombus may be more securely attached to the wall. When the thrombus fragment is released, it is carried into one of the pulmonary arteries (4). Large thrombi may become lodged in a large artery or may break up and block several smaller vessels. Distribution is probably related to the normal regional blood flow in the upright position; the lower lobes are predominantly involved because of their higher blood flow (5).

PATHOLOGY

Autopsies reveal that less than 10% of pulmonary emboli cause a pulmonary infarction. Infection and left heart failure increase the likelihood of pulmonary infarction, as do poor premortem functional status, emboli in multiple lobes, and lung cancer (14,19). In a pulmonary infarct, the necrotic tissue is hemorrhagic and the alveolar walls, bronchi, and vessels are necrotic. With time, the color of an infarct changes from dark red to brown when the hemosiderin pigment is ingested by alveolar macrophages. Finally, fibrosis occurs and a scar is formed (14).

PATHOPHYSIOLOGY

Whatever the source of the embolic material, the acute pathophysiologic results of a sudden pulmonary arterial branch obstruction are similar and have been well defined (20). A total cessation of blood flow to the distal lung zone is the initial effect of embolic obstruction, and this leads to respiratory and hemodynamic consequences.

Respiratory Consequences

Embolic obstruction of a pulmonary artery is followed by three primary respiratory events: an increase in alveolar dead space, bronchoconstriction, and loss of alveolar surfactant (20). Alveolar dead space is ventilated but receives no blood flow. Because gas exchange cannot occur in a nonperfused zone, any ventilation to it is wasted. Adequate alveolar ventilation requires an increase in total ventilation, which contributes to the patient's dyspnea. However, bronchoconstriction reduces the functional size of the ventilated, nonperfused lung zone.

Among the factors contributing to the development of bronchoconstriction is reduced carbon dioxide tension (P_{CO_2}) in the embolic zone. P_{CO_2} decreases in a lung zone that is ventilated with essentially CO_2-free inspired air and that receives no pulmonary blood flow. It has been demonstrated that severely hypocapnic areas constrict; inhalation of air containing carbon dioxide reverses this process, and inflation of the lungs overcomes the constriction temporarily (21). Additional studies have indicated that regional hypoxia is involved, because inhalation of oxygen can also reverse the constriction (22). It is also possible that agents released from the lung or embolus itself (serotonin, histamine) promote constriction (23). The activity of alveolar surfactant begins to decline shortly after pulmonary artery occlusion, resulting in alveolar collapse and regional atelectasis within 24 hours (24).

A secondary respiratory consequence of embolic obstruction is arterial hypoxemia (20). Not all patients with PE have arterial hypoxemia, but a wide alveolar–arterial oxygen tension gradient and a reduced arterial oxygen tension are common, particularly in massive embolism. Ventilation–perfusion mismatch, intrapulmonary shunting of mixed venous blood (perfusion of nonventilated lung units caused by atelectasis), alveolar hypoventilation, and preexistent cardiopulmonary disease may contribute to arterial hypoxemia. In massive embolic obstruction, hypoxemia may be aggravated by a reduction of cardiac output, with a subsequent drop in mixed venous oxygen tension (20). Right ventricular failure accompanied by a patent foramen ovale may contribute to severe hypoxemia in some patients.

Hemodynamic Consequences

The main hemodynamic consequence of PE is a decrease in the functional cross-sectional area of the pulmonary arterial bed, causing increased resistance to blood flow. To maintain the same flow at a higher pressure, the right ventricle must work harder. Therefore, in patients with substantial occlusion of the pulmonary vascular bed caused by PE, there is an increase in pulmonary arterial resistance, pulmonary artery pressure, and right ventricular work (20).

Pulmonary vascular resistance and right ventricular work correlate directly with the extent of pulmonary vascular bed obstruction (25). The presence of right ventricular afterload stress is associated with a higher in-hospital and within 1-year mortality (25). The substantial reserve capacity of the pulmonary vascular bed provides some protection to the right ventricle. However, when more than 50% of the pulmonary vascular bed is occluded, pulmonary arterial pressure rises, requiring additional right ventricular work to be done to maintain cardiac output. In patients with acute PE, pulmonary arterial pressures rarely exceed a mean of 40 mm Hg (20,26,27). The thin-walled right ventricle is not designed to accept acute heavy pressure loads, which may result in right ventricular failure and cardiovascular collapse (20). The role of reflex vasoconstriction in the pathogenesis of pulmonary hypertension associated with acute PE is uncertain. However, vasoconstrictors such as serotonin and thromboxane A_2 may play a role in the development of pulmonary hypertension after acute PE. Experimental evidence suggests that endothelin-1, the most potent vasoconstrictor described, mediates part of the hemodynamic alterations present in acute PE (27).

Infarction

A rare consequence of embolism is ischemic death of the pulmonary parenchyma (i.e., pulmonary infarction) (19). Less than 10% of all pulmonary emboli result in an infarct. Infarction is infrequent because the lung obtains oxygen from the bronchial arterial system and from the airways, in addition to the pulmonary arterial system. At least two of the three oxygen sources must be compromised to promote infarction. Infarction is most common in patients with preexisting left ventricular failure or pulmonary disease because bronchial arterial flow, pulmonary venous outflow, and ventilation are most likely to be compromised in these patients (14,19). Pulmonary infarction occurs more commonly in patients with occluded small pulmonary arteries.

Resolution of Pulmonary Thromboembolism

Like venous thrombi, pulmonary emboli tend to resolve rapidly. Beyond the acute stage, the most frequent course of thromboembolic obstruction is restoration of vascular patency (14,28–30). As with DVT, the removal of embolic material from the pulmonary vascular bed depends on thrombolysis, organization, and recanalization of the thrombus.

Emboli are lysed by the action of circulating fibrinolytic factors in the blood and of fibrinolytic factors released by the intima of pulmonary arteries. Several factors influence the speed of fibrinolytic dissolution, and a thrombus that has aged or has become organized before being released is less sensitive (or even completely resistant) to fibrinolytic attack (31).

Vascular patency is also restored by the organization of thrombus, a slower process than fibrinolysis, requiring days to weeks for completion. Organization is a reparative response, with invasion of fibroblasts and with neocapillarization of the embolus. After the embolus is converted to connective tissue, it shrinks and restores the original lumen (14).

The less thrombus that is removed through fibrinolysis, the more that remains for recanalization and organization and the more likely the residual pulmonary artery obstruction becomes. Regardless of the mechanisms involved in the removal of embolic material, vascular patency is generally restored to normal (7,14). Studies in dogs have demonstrated substantial resolution of emboli within hours and have established that administration of heparin can accelerate this rate (30,31). Perfusion lung scans and angiographic studies in humans have confirmed substantial resolution of emboli within a few days, with a progressive reduction in residual emboli within 4 to 6 weeks (28,29). Permanent residual emboli do occur, although the exact incidence is unknown (32,33). Less than 10% of patients appear to retain perfusion defects after 6 weeks (8). The rate and degree of resolution observed in humans are probably related to age, the composition and volume of the thrombus, and individual differences in fibrinolytic activity. Even massive emboli are likely to resolve within days or weeks, particularly in young persons who do not have coexisting cardiopulmonary disease.

Unresolved thromboembolic obstruction of the major pulmonary arteries occurs in 0.1% to 0.5% of the pulmonary thromboembolic patients who survive (34). Two groups of patients may develop late pulmonary hypertension: those with major "central" obstruction of main or lobar arteries and those with obstruction of multiple distal vessels. The embolic events in the latter group are not always recognized clinically, and incorrect diagnoses ranging from chronic lung disease to primary pulmonary hypertension are often made (3,33).

CLINICAL MANIFESTATIONS

It is important to maintain a high index of suspicion for DVT and pulmonary thromboembolism, particularly in patients at risk (Tables 11-1 and 11-2) (4,35). The diagnosis of DVT can be difficult, but nearly all patients with DVT have discomfort or swelling in the affected leg (36,37). Physical findings include erythema and warmth in one-third of patients and swelling and tenderness in three-fourths. The presence of a Homan sign or a palpable cord is variable. Moreover, proximal DVT is observed on venograms in only 42% of patients with two or more of the following clinical findings: swelling above and below the knee, fever, and a history of immobility and cancer (37).

Dyspnea is the most common symptom of PE (see Table 11-3) (8,38,39). Dyspnea was present in 73% of 117 patients with angiographically proven PE (38). The severity of dyspnea is related to the extent of embolic obstruction of the pulmonary vasculature, resulting primarily from the sudden appearance of alveolar dead space in the lung and likely being a response to changes in lung mechanics caused by the emboli. Massive embolism can produce syncope and hemodynamic instability besides causing dyspnea (6). Pleuritic chest pain and hemoptysis occur secondary to infarction or congestive atelectasis. Massive embolism can cause severe chest pain, mimicking coronary insufficiency. Although these clinical findings are nonspecific and can occur in various cardiopulmonary disorders, the context in which they occur (e.g., in the postoperative period, after lower-extremity trauma, or in the postpartum period) may increase the likelihood that they are caused by PE (3).

There are few characteristic physical findings associated with embolism (see Table 11-4) (8,37). Tachypnea and tachycardia may, like dyspnea, be transient. Sustained marked tachycardia and tachypnea occur in patients with extensive embolism (7,38). On lung examination, fine crackles arise from atelectasis, but the lungs are usually clear to auscultation and percussion (3,38). Additional physical findings may be present in up to 10% of patients in whom atelectasis or infarction occurs. These include pleural friction rub, pleural effusion, and fever (40).

Patients with massive embolism may have cardiac findings suggestive of acute cor pulmonale (right heart disease), including large A waves in the jugular venous pulse, a "lift" palpable over the right ventricle, a right ventricular diastolic gallop (S_3), a systolic murmur in the pulmonary valve area, and an accentuated pulmonary valve closure sound (loud P_2). However, the intensity of the closure sound may not reflect the extent of embolism. In massive obstruction, the right ventricle may fail, pulmonary blood flow may decrease, pulmonary arterial pressure may fall to or below normal values, and the pulmonic closure sound may be barely audible (7). Fixed splitting of the second heart sound is an ominous finding because it is present

TABLE 11-3. Symptoms in 117 Patients with Pulmonary Embolism and No Preexisting Cardiac or Pulmonary Disease

Symptom	Frequency (%)
Dyspnea	73
Pleuritic pain	66
Cough	37
Leg swelling	28
Leg pain	26
Hemoptysis	13
Palpitations	10
Wheezing	9
Angina-like pain	4

From Stein PD, Terrin MC, Hales CA, et al. Clinical, laboratory, roentgenographic and electrocardiographic findings in patients with acute pulmonary embolism and preexisting cardiac or pulmonary disease. *Chest* 1991;100:598–608, with permission.

TABLE 11-4. Signs in 117 Patients with Pulmonary Embolism and no Preexisting Cardiac or Pulmonary Disease

Sign	Frequency (%)
Tachypnea (respiration rate >20/min)	70
Rales (crackles)	51
Tachycardia (pulse >100/min)	30
Fourth heart sound	24
Increased pulmonary component of second sound	23
Deep venous thrombosis	11
Diaphoresis	11
Fever (temperature >38.5°C)	7
Wheezes	5
Homan sign	4
Right ventricular lift	4
Pleural friction rub	3
Third heart sound	3
Cyanosis	1

From Stein PD, Terrin MC, Hales CA, et al. Clinical, laboratory, roentgenographic and electrocardiographic findings in patients with acute pulmonary embolism and preexisting cardiac or pulmonary disease. *Chest* 1991;100:598–608, with permission.

only in patients with marked right ventricular compromise (41). Its development is controlled by two factors: premature closure of the aortic valve as the reduced volume of blood from the lungs rapidly flows out of the left ventricle, and delayed pulmonary valve closure as high resistance in the pulmonary vasculature delays the right ventricular ejection time (41).

Arterial Blood Gases and Electrocardiogram

Most patients with acute PE have hypoxemia and hypocapnia (39). Carbon dioxide retention is rare unless PE occurs in a comatose or paralyzed patient on assisted ventilation. The arterial oxygen tension (Pa_{O_2}) in patients with PE is frequently 80 mm Hg or less; however, in 15% to 25% of patients, the Pa_{O_2} values may exceed 80 mm Hg. A normal Pa_{O_2} does not help to exclude the diagnosis of PE. The main utility of determination of Pa_{O_2} is to document the severity of hypoxemia and direct oxygen therapy (42).

The electrocardiogram (ECG) can rule out other serious diagnoses, such as acute myocardial infarction or pericarditis, in patients with PE. The classic $S_1Q_3T_3$ occurs in only 15% of patients (43).

Chest Radiograph

The plain chest radiograph cannot be used by itself to diagnose or exclude PE, but it may rule out other potentially life-threatening conditions such as tension pneumothorax (44). In a dyspneic patient, however, a normal chest radiograph may be a clue to the presence of PE (44). A parenchymal density and an evidence of pleural reaction or effusion are often present in patients with PE who have infarction or atelectasis (38).

Subtle chest radiographic signs are common. Comparable vessels may be of unequal size (e.g., one main pulmonary artery may be enlarged, whereas the other may be smaller or normal). A major pulmonary artery with a "rat tail" appearance is indicative of an organizing thrombus within it. Oligemia of the lung zone also suggests embolic obstruction, particularly in association with increased flow to other lung areas. The presence of a prominent central pulmonary artery or cardiomegaly (in the absence of previous cardiopulmonary disease) is suggestive of pulmonary hypertension (44).

Thoracentesis

Pleural effusions are rarely massive. PE exhibits no diagnostic pleural fluid findings (45). Sixty-five percent of pleural effusions in patients with PE are sanguinous, and these are usually associated with infiltrates on the chest radiograph. Approximately 50% of the effusions are exudates, even in the absence of an infiltrate. Thoracentesis is used primarily to exclude empyema and to look for a grossly bloody pleural effusion, which occurs in up to 27% of patients with PE. Presence of a bloody pleural effusion is not a contraindication to anticoagulation (45).

By-products of Thrombin and Plasmin

Until anticoagulation therapy is initiated for PE, clot formation associated with thrombin generation occurs simultaneously with lysis secondary to plasmin action. Measurement of D-dimer, a specific degradation product of cross-linked fibrin, has been used to diagnose PE and DVT. The presence of D-dimer suggests that blood clotting has been initiated (46). After venous thromboembolism, D-dimer levels are elevated eightfold compared with controls, and the levels fall to one fourth between weeks 1 and 2, normalizing within 15 to 20 days (47). There are three methods of D-dimer detection: the enzyme linked immunosorbent assay (ELISA), the latex-agglutination assay, and the whole-blood agglutination (46). The sensitivity is high for the three methods, except for the first-generation latex-agglutination assay, which is intermediate. The specificity for all the three methods is low or intermediate for the whole-blood agglutination and for the first- and second-generation latex agglutination (47).

D-dimer assays have significant practical value; they are safe and cost effective when used with defined diagnostic strategies, in many cases reducing the number of imaging studies and minimizing the need for repeated investigation and for invasive studies. However, different assays are commercially available and cannot be used interchangeably. Clinicians should be familiar with the diagnostic performance of the assay used in their own institution (47).

LUNG SCANNING, COMPUTERIZED TOMOGRAPHY, AND PULMONARY ANGIOGRAPHY

The mortality of patients with untreated PE is as high as 30%; patients appropriately diagnosed and treated have a mortality of 2.5% to 8%, substantiating the need for prompt and accurate diagnosis (48). Because of the current emphasis on PE as the respiratory manifestation of venous thromboembolism, the diagnostic approach includes clinical evaluation, a combination of diagnostic modalities for PE ($\dot{V}/\dot{Q}$ scan, spiral CT,

and pulmonary angiogram), as well as noninvasive modalities for detecting DVT (impedance plethysmography [IPG] and B-mode imaging ultrasound) (48–54).

The perfusion lung scan is performed after intravenous injection of 10- to 50-μm particles radiolabeled with a γ-emitting isotope, usually Technetium 99m macroaggregate of albumin (48). The particles are trapped in the pulmonary arteriolar capillary bed, their distribution representing pulmonary blood flow. Embolic obstruction is manifested as zones of reduced or absent blood flow or of perfusion defects (see Fig. 5-25). However, any process that destroys or constricts pulmonary arterial vessels (e.g., old or recent necrotizing infection or regional hypoventilation) can also cause perfusion defects (48). Therefore, although the scan is a sensitive detector of changes in regional blood flow, it lacks specificity; however, a normal scan essentially eliminates clinically significant thromboembolic obstruction (48,49). The specificity of an abnormal perfusion scan may be improved when it is combined with a ventilation scan. Most ventilation scans are done with Xenon 133, but Xenon 127, Krypton 181m, and Technetium 99m aerosols have also been used (48). Embolism often causes regions of high or infinite $\dot{V}/\dot{Q}$ ratio—areas with reduced to absent blood flow but normal ventilation (see Fig. 5-25) (48). In contrast, parenchymal disorders that cause perfusion defects are generally associated with decreased or absent ventilation in the same lung zones (48). Thus, embolism tends to cause a ventilation–perfusion "mismatch," whereas parenchymal diseases result in "matched" ventilation–perfusion abnormalities (48). Furthermore, if the $\dot{V}/\dot{Q}$ scan is abnormal, the result can be classified as high probability, intermediate or indeterminate probability, and low probability for PE on the basis of the size of the defect and the degree of "mismatch" between the $\dot{V}/\dot{Q}$ scan and chest radiography abnormalities (see Table 11-5) (48–54). Concomitant cardiopulmonary disease does not diminish the diagnostic utility of a $\dot{V}/\dot{Q}$ scan in acute PE (55).

In the Prospective Investigation of PE Diagnosis (PIOPED) study, the usefulness of the $\dot{V}/\dot{Q}$ lung scan in the diagnosis of acute PE was assessed (56). The study protocol asked the clinicians to estimate the probability of PE before the $\dot{V}/\dot{Q}$ lung scan was performed, and the clinical estimate was combined with the findings of the lung scan to determine the probability of PE, with the pulmonary angiogram as the gold standard. The $\dot{V}/\dot{Q}$ lung scan interpretive criteria are shown in Table 11-5. The likelihood of PE diagnosed by angiography in the PIOPED study, as determined by the result of the scan and the clinical probability, is shown in Table 11-6. Patients with a high-probability $\dot{V}/\dot{Q}$ scan and a high clinical probability of PE had a 96% chance of having the PE confirmed by pulmonary angiogram; on the other hand, patients with a normal or near normal lung scan, independent of the clinical probability, had a very low likelihood of having a PE. Patients with an intermediate- or low-probability lung scan still had a substantial probability of having pulmonary embolic disease, independent of the clinical probability, and pulmonary angiography was critical in establishing the diagnosis.

The PIOPED study did not systematically evaluate the lower extremities for DVT (56). In 83% to 94% of cases in the diagnosis of proximal DVT (femoral and popliteal), IPG and B-mode ultrasound have been shown to correlate positively with the leg venogram (53,57–59). The correlation for distal (calf) venous

TABLE 11-5. Revised Prospective Investigation of Pulmonary Embolism Diagnosis (PIOPED) $\dot{V}/\dot{Q}$ Scan Interpretation Criteria

High probability: Two or more large (>75% of a segment) segmental perfusion defects without corresponding ventilation or abnormalities on chest radiograph

One large segmental perfusion defect and two or more moderate (25%–75% of a segment) segmental perfusion defects without corresponding ventilation or abnormalities on chest radiograph

Four or more moderate segmental perfusion defects without corresponding ventilation or abnormalities on chest radiograph

Intermediate probability: One moderate or up to two large segmental perfusion defects without corresponding ventilation defect or abnormalities on chest radiograph

Corresponding $\dot{V}/\dot{Q}$ defects and parenchymal opacity in lower lung zone on chest radiograph

Corresponding $\dot{V}/\dot{Q}$ defects and small pleural effusion

Single moderate matched $\dot{V}/\dot{Q}$ defects with normal findings on chest radiograph

Difficult to categorize as normal, low, or high probability

Low probability: Multiple matched $\dot{V}/\dot{Q}$ defects, regardless of size, with normal findings on chest radiograph

Corresponding $\dot{V}/\dot{Q}$ defects and parenchymal opacity in upper or middle lung zone on chest radiograph

Corresponding $\dot{V}/\dot{Q}$ defects and large pleural effusion

Any perfusion defects with substantially larger abnormality on chest radiograph

Defects surrounded by normally perfused lung (stripe sign)

Single or multiple small (<25% of a segment) segmental perfusion defects with a normal chest radiograph

Nonsegmental perfusion defects (cardiomegaly, aortic impression, enlarged hila)

Normal: No perfusion defects, and perfusion outlines the shape of the lung seen on chest radiograph

From Worsley DF, Alavi A, Palevsky JH. Role of radionuclide imaging in patients with suspected pulmonary embolism. *Radiol Clin N Am* 1993;31:849–858, with permission.

TABLE 11-6. Likelihood of Identifying Pulmonary Embolism on Pulmonary Angiogram on the Basis of $\dot{V}/\dot{Q}$ Lung Scan Reading and Clinical Probability Assessment

Scan Interpretation	Probability of Pulmonary Embolism (%)		
	High Clinical Probability	Intermediate Clinical Probability	Low Clinical Probability
High probability	96	88	56
Intermediate probability	66	28	16
Low probability	40	16	4
Near normal/ normal	0	6	2

From The PIOPED investigators. Value of the ventilation/perfusion scan in acute pulmonary embolism. Results of the prospective investigation of pulmonary embolism diagnosis (PIOPED). *JAMA* 1990;263:2753–2759, with permission.

thrombosis is less reliable (57). B-mode imaging has been used for the diagnosis of upper-extremity venous thrombosis, an increasing cause of PE (57); the sensitivity and specificity of duplex ultrasonography is 82% and 82%, respectively, when compared with contrast venography as the gold standard (60).

Recent studies suggest that spiral CT of the chest (CT angiography) may be a useful modality to diagnose PE (see Fig. 5-21) (50,52). A prospective study of the role of CT angiography in the diagnosis of PE (PIOPED II) was reported recently at a national meeting. The sensitivity of CT angiography was 83%. There was a significant rate of false negatives in patients with a high clinical probability for pulmonary thromboembolism and a significant rate of false positives in patients with a low clinical probability of pulmonary thromboembolism.

The pulmonary angiogram is the definitive test for diagnosing PE (53,61). The false-negative rate is only 1% to 2% (53), the death rate from the procedure is 0.5%, and 1% of patients develop major complications (61). On the pulmonary angiogram, the specific finding for PE is an abrupt cutoff of a major vessel, caused by full embolic obstruction. However, the most common angiographic abnormality is filling defects resulting from the flow of contrast medium around a partial obstruction (Fig. 5-25) (61). Additional angiographic signs that are less specific for PE include absent, decreased, or delayed filling of a lung zone; delayed venous emptying; "pruning" (absence of small branches); and abnormal vessel tapering; as well as dilation of the right ventricle and great vessels (61).

Pulmonary angiography also provides the opportunity to assess the hemodynamic status of the patient. Measurement of right heart pressures and of pulmonary artery wedge pressure and the assessment of cardiac output may provide information vital to therapeutic decisions (61). In those patients whose condition is unstable, segmental injection can be made into the abnormal area seen on the perfusion scan (6,62).

The diagnostic approach to pregnant patients is generally similar; however, the perfusion lung scan is done with a low dose of radioisotope (1 to 2 mCi), and if IPG or B-mode ultrasound of the lower extremities is positive, a venogram is obtained to rule out a false-positive result of the impedance study caused by the compression of the iliac vein by the gravid uterus, especially during the third trimester (63). During venography, the patient's abdomen is covered with a lead-lined apron. In a recent study of 121 suspected episodes of PE in 120 pregnant women, only 1.8% with suspected PE and no previous DVT had high-probability $\dot{V}/\dot{Q}$ scans, 25% had a nondiagnostic scan, and 74% had a normal scan. None of the group of pregnant women with normal or nondiagnostic scans was treated and none developed venous thromboembolism over the 20-month follow-up (64).

AN INTEGRATED APPROACH TO THE DIAGNOSIS OF SUSPECTED VENOUS THROMBOEMBOLISM

The evaluation of a patient with suspected venous thromboembolism is complex. Although the symptoms, signs, results of chest radiograph, electrocardiograms, and blood gases do not make the diagnosis or rule out the possibility of venous thromboembolism, the constellation of some symptoms (dyspnea, pleuritic chest pain, tachypnea, and tachycardia), in the presence of significant risk factors, indicate the need for further evaluation (65). There are several prediction rules for risk assessment of clinical probability of PE; a simple set of rules is shown in Table 11-7 (65,66).

In a recent systematic review (67) that included 25 studies involving more than 7,000 patients, the following diagnostic strategies were useful for excluding PE in all referred patients: (a) normal pulmonary angiography or normal perfusion lung scan, with or without normal compression ultrasonography or IPG, excluded PE with a failure rate of <3%; (b) using a standardized clinical model for clinical probability, the combination of low clinical probability and normal D-dimer safely excluded PE with a failure rate of 0.2%; (c) in patients with low to moderate clinical probability, a normal spiral CT and compression ultrasonography excluded PE (failure rate of 1.8%) (67).

When the first diagnostic test or tests did not exclude or confirm the diagnosis of PE, other strategies were evaluated in this systematic review (67). A normal pulmonary angiogram done after an abnormal or nondiagnostic perfusion lung scan was associated with a low failure rate (<1.3%). Serial compression ultrasonography done in 665 in- and outpatients with low to moderate clinical probability after a nondiagnostic perfusion scan had a failure rate of 0.5%. If the D-dimer level was elevated and if the patient had either a normal or nondiagnostic lung scan and low or moderate to high clinical probability and if the lung scan was normal, the failure rate was <1.4%.

Recently, the combination of a low clinical probability and a negative D-dimer has been proven to be useful in ruling out deep vein thrombosis (68–71). Wells et al. (71) evaluated patients with symptoms consistent with DVT using clinical probability and then randomly assigned them to have an ultrasound of the lower extremities or D-dimer testing (whole-blood and second-generation latex-agglutination assay) be performed on them. Those patients with a negative D-dimer testing and a low clinical probability could safely forgo serial

ultrasound testing; the failure rate in these patients was only 0.4%. However, in those patients with a moderate or high clinical probability of DVT, serial ultrasounds were needed when the D-dimer test was positive.

Finally, several reports (72–74) of management strategies to rule out PE suggest that a negative CT angiogram (in- and outpatient) has a false-negative rate of only 0.4% (72). Recently, Perrier et al. (74) studied a cohort of 965 outpatients using a noninvasive strategy: clinical assessment, D-dimer measurement (a rapid ELISA assay), ultrasonography of the extremities, and CT angiography. This noninvasive strategy had a diagnostic yield of 99%. A suggested diagnostic approach is shown in Figures 11-1–11-4.

DIFFERENTIAL DIAGNOSIS

The onset of an atrial arrhythmia in a patient with preexisting cardiac disease may be caused by PE, although the mechanisms involved are not clear. Sudden or progressive worsening of congestive heart failure also suggests embolic disease. Similarly, PE may occur in a patient with chronic obstructive pulmonary disease (COPD) whose condition suddenly deteriorates, or in a patient with worsening hypoxemia and dyspnea in the absence of infection or other obvious causes (8). Patients with other acute cardiopulmonary disorders (e.g., myocardial infarction, dissecting aortic aneurysm, and pneumothorax) can present with substernal discomfort, dyspnea, tachycardia, and electrocardiographic abnormalities (8). Episodes of syncope and dizziness in an apparently healthy person may indicate embolic phenomena, particularly in association with dyspnea (8), and recurrent attacks of hyperventilation should arouse suspicion.

Bacterial or viral pneumonitis may mimic embolism in a clinical context that predisposes to PE. For example, in the postoperative period, a low-grade fever, dyspnea, and tachycardia may develop and the chest radiograph may show a nonspecific infiltrate, possibly representing atelectasis, pneumonia, or PE (8). Infarction secondary to PE may be confused with any disorder capable of producing acute pleuritis, including collagen vascular diseases and infectious diseases (8).

PREVENTION AND TREATMENT

Prophylaxis of Deep Venous Thrombosis

Prophylaxis for venous thromboembolism is important for several reasons: the prevalence of venous thromboembolism is high in hospitalized patients, the clinical picture is frequently nonspecific, and it is associated with a high degree of morbidity and mortality (75). The patients at greater risk are those undergoing major lower extremity orthopedic surgery, patients who have had an ischemic stroke, and patients with major trauma or spinal cord injury. Patients admitted to the intensive care unit frequently have multiple risk factors and high incidences of DVT that vary between 25% and 31%.

Despite evidence of the efficacy of prophylaxis, it is used in less than 40% of hospitalized patients despite the presence of multiple risk factors (75,76). There are two basic kinds of prophylaxis of DVT: mechanical and pharmacologic. The mechanical approaches, which reduce venous stasis, include early ambulation (desirable in all patients at risk for venous thrombosis), the use of elastic stockings, pneumatic calf compression,

TABLE 11-7. Rules for Predicting the Probability of Embolism

Variable	No. of Points
RISK FACTORS	
Clinical signs and symptoms of deep venous thrombosis	3.0
An alternative diagnosis deemed less likely than pulmonary embolism	3.0
Heart rate >100 beats/min	1.5
Immobilization or surgery in the previous 4 wk	1.5
Previous deep venous thrombosis or pulmonary embolism	1.5
Hemoptysis	1.0
Cancer (receiving treatment, treated in the past 6 mo, or palliative care)	1.0
CLINICAL PROBABILITY	
Low	<2.0
Intermediate	2.0–6.0
High	>6.0

From Wells PS, Anderson DR, Rodger M, et al. Deviation of a simple clinical model to categorize patients probability of pulmonary embolism: increasing the model's utility with the SimpliRed D-dimer. *Thromb Haemost* 2000;83:416–420, with permission.

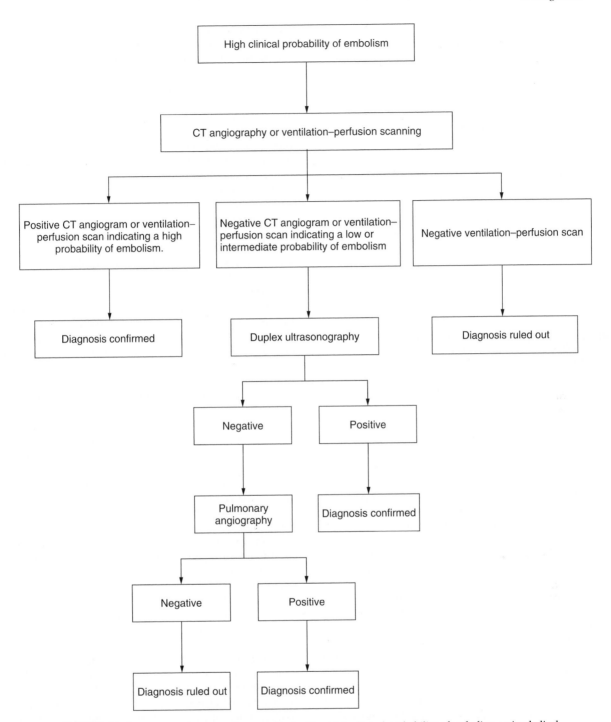

FIGURE 11-1. Diagnostic approach to a patient with a high clinical probability of embolism, using helical CT scanning or ventilation–perfusion scanning as the initial diagnostic study. (From Fedullo PF, Tapson VF. The evalution of suspected pulmonary embolism. *N Engl J Med* 2003;349:1247–1256, with permission.)

and electrical stimulation of calf muscles. The pharmacologic agents include warfarin, dextran, low-molecular weight heparin (LMWH), heparinoids, and unfractionated heparin (75). LMWHs have a restricted molecular weight distribution of around 5,000 daltons (77); heparinoids are a mixture of glycosaminoglycans, including heparin sulfate and dermatan sulfate (78). Table 11-8 summarizes the current recommendations for prophylaxis of DVT as set forth by the Seventh Consensus Conference of the American College of Chest Physicians (75).

Treatment of Acute Deep Venous Thrombosis

Subcutaneous LMWH, antifactor Xa inhibitors, intravenous unfractionated heparin, and adjusted dose subcutaneous heparin are effective drugs for the treatment of venous thromboembolism (79). Heparin catalyzes the effect of antithrombin III, a coagulation inhibitor that inactivates thrombin and factors Xa and IXa. Moreover, heparin inhibits the activation of factors V and VIII by thrombin (79). Heparin does not lyse

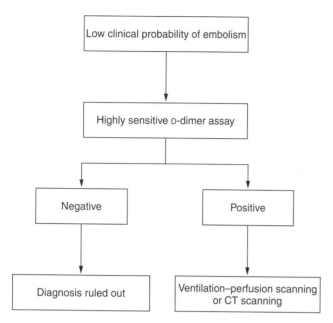

FIGURE 11-2. Diagnostic approach to an outpatient with a low clinical probability of pulmonary embolism, using a D-dimer assay as the initial diagnostic assay. (From Fedullo PF, Tapson VF. The evalution of suspected pulmonary embolism. *N Engl J Med* 2003;349:1247–1256, with permission.)

existing clots but prevents formation and propagation of further clots.

In patients with venous thromboembolic disease, intravenous heparin is effective but frequently underdosed (79). Nomograms have been used to facilitate dosing; a commonly used nomogram is shown in Table 11-9 (80). A frequently sought parameter to ensure adequate anticoagulation is the activated partial thromboplastin time (aPTT); however, the aPTT does not always correlate with plasma heparin levels or with antithrombotic activity (79). More importantly, the aPTT depends on the anticoagulation time and on the reagents used to perform the test. Because many hospitals cannot monitor plasma heparin levels and following the aPTT can result in under- or overdosing, each laboratory should correlate the therapeutic range of the aPTT in seconds that corresponds to plasma heparin levels of 0.2 to 0.4 IU per mL by protamine sulfate titration or of 0.3 to 0.7 IU per mL by an amidolytic assay (79). An alternative to aPTT is the thrombin clotting time (TCT). The TCT correlates well with plasma heparin levels, is reproducible (better than aPTT), and is not significantly affected by administration of warfarin. The TCT should also be correlated with plasma heparin levels.

Major bleeding occurs in 3% to 4% of patients receiving unfractionated heparin (81). Factors associated with an increased risk for bleeding complications are advanced age, uncontrolled hypertension, underlying coagulation abnormality, recent gastrointestinal hemorrhage, active vasculitis, chronic liver disease, uremia, and recent surgery or major arterial cannulation. Another potential side effect is heparin-induced thrombocytopenia (HIT). HIT occurs in <1% of cases with the administration of unfractionated heparin or LMWH, if either of these agents is administered for no more than 7 days

and the syndrome is unusual after 14 days of heparin administration. If the platelets count drops precipitously and is sustained, or if the platelet count falls to less than 100,000 μL, heparin therapy should be stopped (79). Alternative medications that can be used include heparinoids such as danaparoid and direct thrombin inhibitors such as argatroban, lepirudin, and ximelagatran.

LMWHs have been found to be safe and equivalent in efficacy to unfractionated heparin in the treatment of deep vein thrombosis and nonmassive PE. A large body of data suggests that treatment of venous thromboembolic disease with LMWHs may be associated with a lower incidence of major bleeding and an equal rate of recurrent major thromboembolic events compared to unfractionated heparin. LMWHs can be given as initial treatment and can be administered subcutaneously and without laboratory monitoring, making management simple and, in some patients, allowing management in the outpatient setting (79,81,82). The doses of some of the most commonly used LMWHs are shown in Table 11-10.

The coumarin derivatives are orally administered drugs that inhibit vitamin K–dependent clotting proteins in the liver (factors II, VII, IX, and X); the most commonly used coumarin derivative is racemic warfarin sodium (83). Because the antithrombotic effect of warfarin (a coumarin derivative) is related to its ability to reduce prothrombin levels, warfarin must be overlapped with heparin until the [International Normalized Ratio (INR)] is prolonged for 4 consecutive days for a full antithrombotic effect (83). Early introduction of warfarin at a dose of 5 mg will keep the total duration of heparin to less than a week (79,84). Coumarin derivatives are suitable for outpatient therapy and can provide long-term anticoagulation for patients with thrombotic problems. Coumarin therapy can be given to nursing mothers because the metabolite excreted in the milk is not an anticoagulant, but coumarin is contraindicated in pregnant patients. In those cases, LMWH or unfractionated adjusted-dose heparin that prolongs the aPTT to a level equal to a heparin level of 0.2 to 0.4 IU per mL is indicated (79).

The appropriate length of time for anticoagulation in patients with DVT is variable and depends on clinical circumstances. For example, patients developing DVT following transient immobilization or following a fracture in the lower extremity should be treated for 3 months. Other patients who have risk factors that cannot be modified (e.g., malignancy or patients with a hypercoagulable state and patients with recurrent venous thromboembolism) probably should be treated for at least a year and some patients should be treated indefinitely (79). Those patients with idiopathic venous thromboembolism present a special problem. These patients are vulnerable to recurrent episodes, some of them fatal (85). In patients with idiopathic venous thromboembolism, anticoagulant therapy should be given after a first episode for 6 to 12 months. However, the optimal duration is unknown (86,87).

Another important issue is the intensity of the anticoagulation (88,89). Two recent major studies evaluated the effectiveness of a low-intensity warfarin therapy (INR of 1.5 to 1.9) versus conventional intensity (INR of 2 to 3) and gave conflicting results. Until the issue is settled, patients with idiopathic venous thromboembolism should receive warfarin for 6 to 12 months, keeping the INR between 2 and 3.

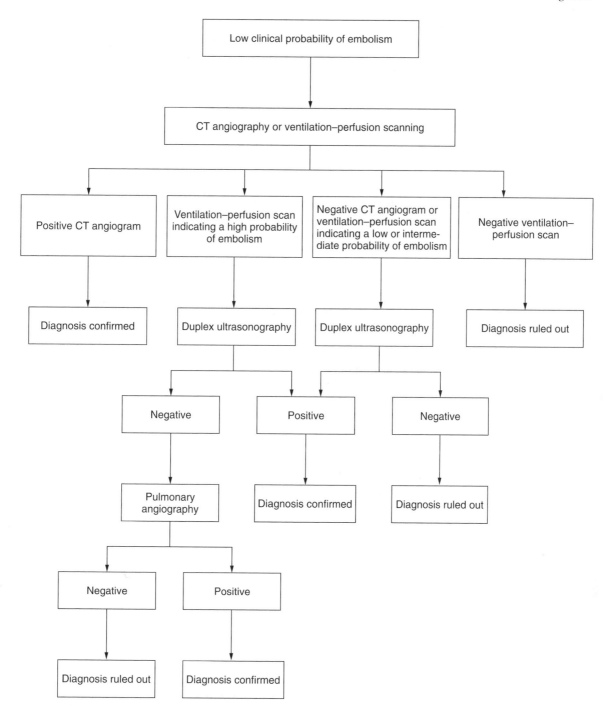

FIGURE 11-3. Diagnostic approach to a patient with a low clinical probability of embolism, using helical CT scanning or ventilation–perfusion scanning as the initial diagnostic study. (From Fedullo PF, Tapson VF. The evaluation of suspected pulmonary embolism. *N Engl J Med* 2003;349:1247–1256, with permission.)

Thrombolytic Therapy in Venous Thromboembolism

The role of thrombolytic therapy in DVT and PE is highly individualized. Because of the lack of proven mortality effect, thrombolysis is indicated in patients with PE and shock (79,90). Streptokinase, urokinase, and tissue plasminogen activator have been used (79). Proximal, massive thrombi (iliofemoral veins) respond better than distal thrombi. Streptokinase is given in a dose of 250,000 units in 30 minutes, followed by 100,000 units per hour for 24 hours in patients with PE and up to 72 hours through an intravenous line in patients with DVT. For PE, tissue plasminogen activator is given in a 100 mg infusion over 2 hours. Heparin should not be given concurrently with streptokinase or urokinase but can be given concurrently with tissue plasminogen activator. No laboratory test is recommended when tissue plasminogen activator or reteplase therapy is used. The thrombin time should be checked at 2 to 4 hours when streptokinase or urokinase is used. Prolongation of

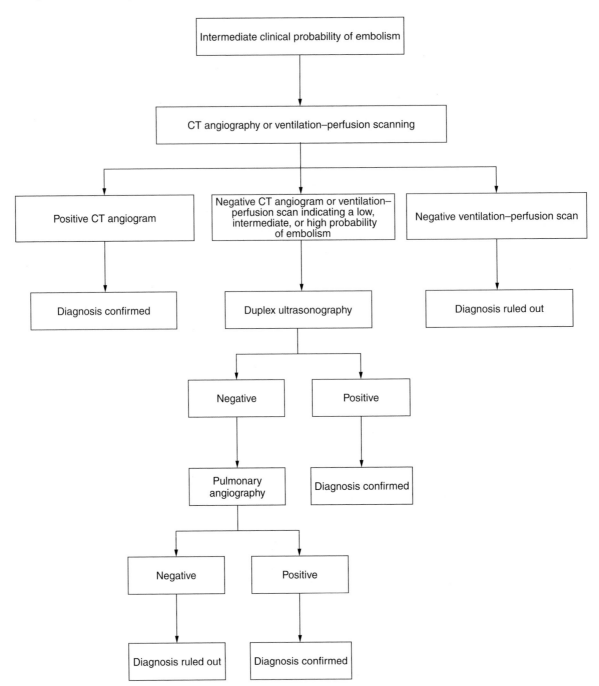

FIGURE 11-4.   Diagnostic approach to a patient with an intermediate clinical probability of embolism, using helical CT scanning or ventilation–perfusion scanning as the initial diagnostic study. (From Fedullo PF, Tapson VF. The evalution of suspected pulmonary embolism. *N Engl J Med* 2003;349:1247–1256, with permission.)

the thrombin time or the aPTT by 10 seconds indicate activation of fibrinolysis. In patients receiving streptokinase, the incidence of minor bleeding is increased; however, major bleeding episodes (requiring 2 or more units of blood) are apparently no more common than in patients receiving only heparin. Concomitant therapy with acetaminophen and intravenous corticosteroids is suggested to minimize allergic reactions (less than 5%) in patients receiving streptokinase therapy. After streptokinase therapy, heparin infusion (without a bolus) is needed.

Additional supportive measures may be necessary. If arterial hypoxemia is present, supplemental oxygen should be administered. Analgesia may be required to alleviate pain. In patients with hypotension and shock, fluid therapy to increase right ventricular preload is the first line of treatment. Second, vasopressor support is usually needed, and in patients in shock, norepinephrine is the vasopressor of choice to maintain systemic blood pressure, increase cardiac output, and maintain coronary perfusion of the right ventricle. Dobutamine can be

TABLE 11-8. Prophylaxis of Deep Venous Thrombosis and Pulmonary Embolism

Type of Operation	Usual-Risk Patient	High-Risk Patient (e.g., prior DVT or PE)
General abdominothoracic surgery	<40 y/o, no risk factors, no prophylaxis, early persistent ambulation All other patients: LDH, SCq 12h starting 2 h preoperatively *or* IPC or LMWH or ES	High-risk: LDH SCq 8 h, LMWH or IPC Very high risk with multiple risk factors and extensive gynecological surgery for malignancy: LMW[b], IPC/ES+LDH/LMWH
Major vascular surgery		LDH or LMWH
Orthopedic surgery[a]		
Hip replacement and elective knee arthroplasty	Warfarin (INR 2–3) preoperatively or immediately after surgery *or* LMWH (started 12 h before or 12–24 h after surgery) fondaparinux (2.5 mg 6–8 h after surgery)	IVCF in selected patients with contraindications to anticoagulants.
Hip fractures	Recommend LMW, adjusted dose of coumadin, fondaparinux	
Knee arthroscopy		
Neurosurgery intracranial	IPC, alternatives are: LDH, postoperative LMWH	
Elective spinal surgery		LDH or postoperative LMWH alone or perioperative IPC alone
Acute spinal cord injury with paralysis	LMWH after hemostasis *or* IPC or ES, contraindications to acute coagulants	
Multiple trauma	LMWH or IPC or ES in selected patients with contraindications to anticoagulants; continue prophylaxis after discharge in patients with impaired mobilization	
General medical patient		
Ischemic stroke and lower-extremity paralysis	LDH or LMWH IPC or ES if anticoagulant is contraindicated	
Other medical condition (heart failure, pneumonia, etc.)	LDH or LMWH	
Cancer patients who are bedridden	LDH or LMWH	
Critical care	LDH or LMWH; if patient is at risk of bleeding, IPC and/or ES	

LDH, low-dose heparin 5,000 units per dose; LMWH, low-molecular weight heparin; ES, graduated compression elastic stockings; INR, international normalized ratio; IVCF, inferior vena cava filter; IPC, intermittent pneumatic compression; DVT, deep venous thrombosis; PE, pulmonary embolism; y/o, years old.

[a]Consider maintaining prophylaxis for 24- to 35-day duration.

[b]LMWH should be used with caution if spinal tap is done or if epidural catheter is used.

From Geerts WH, Pineo GF, Heit JS, et al. Prevention of venous thromboembolism. *Chest* 2004; 126:338S–400S, with permission.

TABLE 11-9. Body Weight–Based Dosing of IV Heparin[a]

aPTT, s[b]	Dose Change IU/kg/h	Additional Action[c]	Next aPTT, h[d]
<35 (<1.2 × mean normal)	+4	Rebolus with 80 IU/kg	6
35–45 (1.2–1.5 × mean normal)	+2	Rebolus with 40 IU/kg	6
46–70 (1.5–2.3 × mean normal)	0	0	6
71–90 (2.3–3.0 × mean normal)	0	0	6
>90 (> × mean normal)	−3	Stop infusion 1 h	6

[a]Initial dosing: loading, 80 IU/kg; maintenance infusion: 18 IU/kg/h (aPTT in 6 h).

[b]The therapeutic range in seconds should correspond to a plasma heparin level of 0.2 to 0.4 IU/mL by protamine sulfate or of 0.3 to 0.6 IU/mL by amidolytic assay. When aPTT is checked at 6 hours or longer, steady state kinetics can be assumed.

[c]Heparin, 25,000 IU in 250 μL D5W. Infuse at the rate dictated by body weight through an infusion apparatus calibrated for low flow rates.

[d]During the first 24 hours, repeat aPTT every 6 hours. Thereafter, monitor aPTT once every morning unless it is outside the therapeutic range.

TABLE 11-10. Doses of Low-Molecular Weight Heparins and Indirect Factor Xa Inhibitors for Treatment of Venous Thromboembolism[a]

Agents	Doses
Nadroparin calcium	86 anti-Xa IU/kg twice a day or 171 anti-Xa IU/kg once a day subcutaneously for 10 days. Single dose should not exceed 17,100 IU
Enoxaparin sodium	1 mg/kg every 12 h or 1.5 mg/kg daily subcutaneously. Single dose should not exceed 180 mg
Dalteparin sodium	200 anti-Xa IU/kg daily or 100 anti-Xa IU/kg every 12 h subcutaneously. Single dose should not exceed 18,000 IU
Tinzaparin sodium	175 anti-Xa IU/kg daily subcutaneously
Fondaparinux	7.5 mg subcutaneously once a day. Dose should not exceed 10 mg in patients weighing >100 kg

[a] Warfarin should be started on day 1 and the LMWH or fondaparinux stopped when the INR is >2 for 4 days.

used in those patients with moderate hypotension and low cardiac output (91). Mechanical ventilation is often needed to support the patient because of the high work of breathing, increased dead-space fraction, and the metabolic acidosis that may be associated with a decline in cardiac output.

Thrombolytic therapy has been shown by angiography to result in early clot lysis, but it has not been shown to reduce the mortality from PE (90). A recent randomized study of 256 patients with submassive PE (right ventricular dysfunction without shock) compared heparin alone versus thrombolytic therapy with alteplase (92). The primary endpoint of the study was in-hospital death or clinical deterioration requiring an escalation of treatment. Escalation of treatment was more common in patients receiving heparin (24%) compared to 10% of patients receiving alteplase. There was no difference in mortality or in the rate of recurrence of PE.

Emergency surgical embolectomy is rarely done and can be considered only when other interventions have failed (e.g., patients with massive PE with a contraindication to or with a failure of therapy with thrombolytics). A report from a tertiary center suggests that there is an improvement in the survival (up to 89%) (93). Transvenous catheter extraction of emboli has a mortality rate of 27% to 33%. Catheter thrombectomy for high-risk PE patients may be useful in a small group of patients in whom heparin therapy is insufficient and thrombolysis is contraindicated (79).

In patients with proximal leg DVT in whom anticoagulation is contraindicated, has failed, or has caused complications, inferior vena cava (IVC) interruption is indicated. It is also indicated for chronic PE, in patients undergoing pulmonary embolectomy or pulmonary endarterectomy, and in patients developing recurrent PE in spite of adequate anticoagulation (79). In patients with an IVC filter, the reported rate of PE is less than 2%, and insertion of a filter causes fatal complications in approximately 0.1% (94). In the only prospective trial of patients considered to be at high risk for PE, patients were randomized to receive an IVC versus no filter. The patients who received a filter had less PE at day 12 compared with patients

who received only anticoagulation (95). However, no difference in survival was detected, and at 2 years, an increase in recurrent DVT was noted in patients with an IVC filter. Although patients with an IVC filter do not require anticoagulation, continuous warfarin therapy (if it is not contraindicated) is recommended to prevent the development and propagation of thrombi below the filter. Temporary filters and superior vena cava filters have been inserted and are undergoing testing (79).

CHRONIC THROMBOEMBOLIC PULMONARY HYPERTENSION

Chronic thromboembolic pulmonary hypertension, a chronic disease of the pulmonary arteries, is the result of extensive obstruction of the pulmonary vasculature (34). The cumulative incidence of symptomatic chronic thromboembolic pulmonary hypertension is 1% at 6 months and almost 4% at 2 years. Patients with idiopathic PE, those who are young, and those with a large perfusion defect in the lung scan are at high risk of developing pulmonary hypertension (96). When the pulmonary vessels become occluded, with extensive loss of cross-sectional area of the vascular bed, pulmonary hypertension develops at rest or with minimal exertion. Dyspnea on exertion and exercise intolerance are common; chest pain on exertion and syncope are late symptoms (34). Other physical findings late in the disease are suggestive of elevated right heart pressure (e.g., hepatomegaly, leg edema, loud P_2, or murmur of tricuspid insufficiency) (34). In 30% of patients, the physical examination reveals only a systolic or continuous murmur heard over the lung fields (34). The murmur, which is caused by partial obstruction of major pulmonary arteries, is rare in other pulmonary vascular diseases and absent in primary pulmonary hypertension (34).

Laboratory tests are unremarkable in general. Less than 1% of affected patients have deficiencies of antithrombin III and proteins C and S, and lupus anticoagulant is present in 10% of the patients (34). The chest radiograph may be normal, although such subtle findings as unequal central pulmonary vascular shadows and zones of avascularity are occasionally found. The electrocardiogram is normal early in the disease; later, right axis deviation, right ventricular hypertrophy, and T-wave inversion in the precordium may be present (34). Echocardiography shows an elevated pulmonary arterial systolic pressure and an increase in size of the right heart chambers (34). Pulmonary function tests are normal or show a restrictive ventilatory defect. The diffusing capacity for carbon monoxide (D_{LCO}) is normal or reduced. The arterial oxygen tension is normal at rest and declines during exercise. The most important noninvasive test in chronic thromboembolic pulmonary hypertension is the $\dot{V}/\dot{Q}$ lung scan (34). Affected patients have a segmental or larger perfusion–ventilation mismatch. In patients with primary pulmonary hypertension, the perfusion lung scan is normal or shows only patchy subsegmental defects. The pulmonary angiogram confirms the diagnosis; confirmatory findings include intraluminal bands, webs, intimal irregularities, vascular narrowing and obstruction, and "pouching defects" (occlusive thrombi that organize in a concave configuration) (34). The pulmonary arterial pressures are elevated with a normal wedge pressure. The role of CT in the evaluation of chronic thromboembolic disease is not defined (34). Other diagnostic techniques used in some centers include pulmonary angioscopy (34) and pulmonary intravascular ultrasound.

The prognosis of chronic thromboembolic disease is related to the degree of pulmonary hypertension. The only successful therapy is thromboendarterectomy of the pulmonary arteries. Thromboendarterectomy is indicated in symptomatic patients who have hemodynamic or ventilatory impairment at rest or with exercise. The presence of comorbid conditions, such as coronary disease, increases the risk but is not a contraindication of the surgical procedure (34). The overall perioperative mortality is 6.4% in leading centers (34). Lifelong anticoagulation is required after the surgery.

Thromboses are occasionally generated in the pulmonary arterial circulation itself. Decreased flow and increased blood viscosity typical of polycythemia and other myeloproliferative disorders probably contribute to their development. Pulmonary vascular changes caused by increased vasomotor tone, inflammation of the vessel wall, and sickling due to hemoglobin SC and hemoglobin SS disease are also contributing factors (97).

SEPTIC THROMBOEMBOLISM

Septic thromboembolisms are rare. They are usually important complications of bacterial endocarditis involving the tricuspid and, rarely, pulmonary valves, infected venous catheters, odontogenic infections, gynecologic–obstetric procedures, and intravenous drug use (98). Other sources of infected emboli are related to medical technology (e.g., infection may develop from catheters placed in peripheral and central veins, ventriculoatrial shunt catheters, transvenous pacemakers, and catheters for hemodialysis). Patients with the acquired immunodeficiency syndrome (AIDS) and organ transplant recipients are at risk for pulmonary septic emboli.

In septic thromboembolism, microorganisms invade a traumatized vein. In drug users, the vein is used for intravenous drug administration; in gynecologic–obstetric patients, the pelvic veins are involved; and in patients with catheters, the cannulated vein is affected. Mixtures of blood clot and bacteria occlude the involved veins, and small emboli are dislodged from such foci. The process may gradually resolve, with or without specific therapy, but if embolism develops, the already septic patient becomes more dyspneic; cough, sputum production, hemoptysis, and pleuritic chest pain often develop.

The chest radiograph characteristically shows multiple small, nodular densities, usually with fuzzy outlines (3). The number of these lesions may increase rapidly, and radiographs taken at 24-hour intervals often show striking changes that reflect the occurrence of repetitive, small, infected emboli. Pleural effusions and empyema may occur in up to 75% of patients with right-side infective endocarditis because of intravenous drug abuse (99). CT scans may show multiple peripheral nodules of various sizes, wedge-shaped peripheral lesions, and infiltrates (98). The nodules may be cavitated, may have air bronchograms, and can affect upper and lower lobes (98).

Both the infection and the thromboembolism must be treated with vigorous antibiotic therapy (99–101). Because blood cultures may be negative, antibiotic selection must be made empirically; antibiotic coverage should include gram-negative and gram-positive organisms, including penicillinase-producing staphylococci. Any indwelling venous catheter should be removed immediately and cultured.

The use of heparin in patients with right-sided endocarditis is controversial because of the risk of hemorrhage. The response to antibiotic is usually very good when the responsible organism is *Staphylococcus aureus*. If medical therapy fails to reverse the embolic process, surgical procedures should be considered. Patients with right-sided endocarditis required heart surgery in 6% of the cases (100).

PULMONARY EMBOLI OTHER THAN THROMBOEMBOLI

Fat Emboli

Of the many types of tissue that obstruct the lungs, fat has received the most attention (3,102). Fat cells and neutral fat are often found in the lungs of patients who have died after long-bone fractures and other types of severe trauma, pancreatitis, sickle cell disease and orthopedic surgery (102). Fat embolism with orthopedic surgery is common. Fat globules are detected in blood in 25% to 30% of patients that have undergone hip arthroplasty independently if the procedure was unilateral or bilateral or if the prosthesis was inserted with or without cement (103). The pathogenesis of fat embolism remains controversial and it is believed that the organ dysfunction seen in this syndrome is the result of the depot of fat globules from tissue into the bloodstream or is due to the production of inflammatory mediators—intermediaries of plasma-derived fat such as chylomicrons or infused lipids.

The typical case history is of a patient with long-bone fractures who, on admission, is alert, oriented, and in good condition with the exception of the traumatized areas. Within 12 to 36 hours, however, mental-status changes occur and progress to delirium and coma; high fever and marked dyspnea, tachypnea, and tachycardia occur and a petechial rash develops particularly over the thorax and upper extremities. Inspiratory rales fill the lungs, and the chest radiograph shows a diffuse alveolar filling-type pattern throughout both lung fields in 30% to 60% of patients. Arterial hypoxemia and hypocapnia develop; thrombocytopenia is common. Fat is recovered from sputum and urine, a nonspecific finding that may occur in other conditions as well. Bronchoalveolar lavage (BAL) specimens, when stained with oil red O, show fat droplets in 30% of the cells recovered from affected patients compared with less than 2% in patients who do not have fat embolism (104). In patients with sickle cell disease and acute chest syndrome, sputum samples stained with oil red O showed a high percentage of alveolar macrophages full of fat droplets that correlate well with a positive BAL, suggesting that sputum samples may be useful in diagnosing fat embolism in patients with sickle cell disease (105).

Treatment of suspected fat embolism is supportive, as with any form of adult respiratory distress syndrome. Infusion of heparin, ethanol, and low-molecular weight dextran seems to be ineffective, whereas corticosteroid therapy has been associated with ambiguous results (3,102).

Amniotic Fluid Embolism

Amniotic fluid embolism usually occurs during or shortly after delivery. The exact incidence is unknown; it ranges between 1 in 8,000 to 1 in 80,000 and the mortality is high (80% to 90%) (106). Among the survivors, only 15% recover neurologically intact. The clinical presentation consists of the sudden onset of dyspnea, restlessness, chills, and vomiting. Most patients are cyanotic, hypoxic, tachycardic, and hypotensive. Noncardiogenic pulmonary edema develops quickly, and grand mal seizures (30%) and disseminated intravascular coagulation occur frequently (10%).

There is no diagnostic test to confirm amniotic embolism (106). In patients with suspected amniotic fluid embolism, cytologic examination of a specimen obtained from a pulmonary artery catheter in the wedge position may reveal large numbers of fetal squamous cells coated with neutrophils and, less frequently, mucin and hair. The management of these patients is supportive and most require mechanical ventilation and hemodynamic support with inotropes to treat the frequently present cardiac dysfunction (106).

Foreign Body Emboli

Various irritant agents used to "cut" heroin may enter the circulation and pulmonary arteries of narcotic addicts. Talcum powder is one of these agents; it has a marked effect on the pulmonary vessels, causing a granulomatous reaction in the lumina of small pulmonary arteries or causing an interstitial granulomatous reaction with few granulomas in the pulmonary arteries. These insults may be extensive enough to cause pulmonary hypertension. Perfusion lung scans and pulmonary function tests are often abnormal, and thrombiobliterative changes are frequently seen at autopsy (3).

Air Emboli

Air can enter the pulmonary circuit after entering via the systemic veins or arteries. Small quantities of air are removed rapidly from the blood and lungs without causing symptoms, although repeated small air injections have induced pulmonary vascular lesions and even acute noncardiogenic pulmonary edema experimentally (107). Rapid entry of a large bolus of air into the heart can obstruct pulmonary blood flow. Neurosurgical procedures and neck and thorax wounds are particularly hazardous due to the strong suction exerted during inspiration on veins in these areas. Air embolism may complicate cardiopulmonary bypass procedures and is always a possibility when intravenous catheters or needles are in place, if the infusions are allowed to run out, or if leaks occur in the tubing (3). Patients treated with mechanical ventilation for the adult respiratory distress syndrome may be at high risk of developing arterial air embolism as a form of barotrauma. In these patients, a high index of suspicion is necessary, particularly in the presence of livedo reticularis, angioedema of the face or neck, and cerebral and cardiac dysfunction (108). Venous air embolism must be treated promptly to prevent air entering into the heart. The patient must be placed immediately in the left lateral decubitus position to allow collection of air in the superiorly placed right atrium. Maintaining intravascular volume and β-adrenergic agents may be beneficial. If this is unsuccessful, compression in a hyperbaric chamber may be useful (3). However, prevention of air embolism is of paramount importance.

PULMONARY HYPERTENSION

Pulmonary hypertension is present when the mean pulmonary artery pressure exceeds 20 mm Hg at rest and 30 mm Hg during exercise. Pulmonary hypertension could result from either increased pulmonary vascular resistance or increased pulmonary blood flow alone; however, even a large increase in pulmonary blood flow seldom leads to more than a mild elevation of the pressure as long as there are no pathologic vascular changes. Because of the elasticity of the pulmonary vasculature, the pulmonary vessels dilate in response to a large flow, causing the resistance to fall. The other factor explaining the low resistance of the pulmonary vessels is the capacity for recruitment of additional vessels (109). If flow increases, additional vessels open (usually in the upper lobes), decreasing pulmonary vascular resistance. Another important mediator of pulmonary vascular reactivity is nitric oxide (110). Nitric oxide is a potent vasodilator produced locally in the lung and has profound effects on smooth muscle relaxation. In patients with local hypoxemia (e.g., patients with atelectasis), the level of nitric oxide is reduced, causing a compensatory vasoconstriction that will shunt away the blood flow to areas of adequate ventilation, improving the overall ventilation–perfusion matching within the lung (110,111).

PATHOLOGIC CHARACTERISTICS

Pulmonary vessels undergo various pathologic changes in pulmonary hypertension; these changes depend on the cause of the hypertension and partially on the duration of exposure to high pressure (112). Both elastic and muscular pulmonary arteries are affected. In the elastic arteries, the muscular tunica media hypertrophies and the intimal connective tissues thicken. Medial hypertrophy may be followed by a form of mucoid degeneration, which, in conjunction with atrophy of the medial elastic tissue, may lead to aneurysmal dilation or even rupture. These conditions have been described in patent ductus arteriosus, mitral stenosis, and chronic pulmonary hypertension developing after corrective surgery for relief of tetralogy of Fallot. In addition to the medial changes, marked intimal atheromas usually develop, particularly at bifurcations. The atheroma may promote local thrombus formation from which distal embolism may develop. Focal media hyperplasia is an additional feature resulting either from the organization of mural thrombi or from the healing of mural necrosis secondary to hypertensive pulmonary polyarteritis (112).

Although morphologic characteristics of the vessels may vary depending on the cause of hypertension, some changes develop regardless of the cause. These changes are most striking in arterioles and in arteries <500 μm in diameter. In the arterioles, changes consist of muscular thickening and intimal proliferation. Whereas arterioles normally have no tunica media, in mild to moderate pulmonary hypertension, a distinct muscular tunica media develops, constituting up to 25% of the external diameter of the vessel and separated by internal and external elastic laminae. Later, intimal proliferation occurs, which is initially cellular but subsequently becomes fibrous. Finally, elastic tissue may develop and intimal proliferation may completely block the lumen. The tunica intima of the pulmonary trunk and the large elastic vessels become atherosclerotic, and muscular hyperplasia may thicken the tunica media.

PATHOGENESIS

The underlying process of pulmonary hypertension varies, and multiple factors are often responsible. The rise in pulmonary arterial pressure may be owing to vasoconstriction and, thus, should be reversible. In other cases, obstruction of the pulmonary vascular tree is largely or totally organic and thus irreversible. In Table 11-11, the causes of pulmonary hypertension are divided into five groups, each with somewhat different clinical, physiologic, and radiologic characteristics. In this chapter, selected entities of pulmonary hypertension are discussed.

TABLE 11-11. The 1998 WHO Evian Classification of Pulmonary Hypertension

1. Pulmonary arterial hypertension
   1.1 Primary pulmonary hypertension
      a. Sporadic
      b. Familial
   1.2 Related to:
      a. Collagen vascular disease
      b. Congenital systemic to pulmonary shunts
      c. Portal hypertension
      d. HIV infection
      e. Drugs/toxins (anorexigens or others)
      f. Persistent pulmonary hypertension of the newborn
      g. Other
2. Pulmonary venous hypertension
   2.1 Left-sided atrial or ventricular heart disease
   2.2 Left-sided valvular heart disease
   2.3 Extrinsic compression of central pulmonary veins
      a. Fibrosing mediastinitis
      b. Adenopathy/tumors
   2.4 Pulmonary veno-occlusive disease
   2.5 Other
3. Pulmonary hypertension associated with disorders of the respiratory system or hypoxemia
   3.1 Chronic obstructive pulmonary disease
   3.2 Interstitial lung disease
   3.3 Sleep-disordered breathing
   3.4 Alveolar hypoventilation disorders
   3.5 Chronic exposure to high altitude
   3.6 Neonatal lung disease
   3.7 Alveolar-capillary dysplasia
   3.8 Other
4. Pulmonary hypertension due to chronic thrombotic and/or embolic disease
   4.1 Thromboembolic obstruction of proximal pulmonary arteries
   4.2 Obstruction of distal pulmonary arteries
      a. Pulmonary embolism (thrombus, tumor, ova, parasites, foreign matter)
      b. *In situ* thrombosis
      c. Sickle cell disease
5. Pulmonary hypertension due to disorders directly affecting the pulmonary vasculature
   5.1 Inflammatory
      a. Schistosomiasis
      b. Sarcoidosis
      c. Other
   5.2 Pulmonary capillary hemangiomatosis

From Rich S. Primary pulmonary hypertension: executive summary from the world symposium on primary pulmonary hypertension. Geneva: World Health Organization, 1998; with permission.

PULMONARY ARTERIAL HYPERTENSION

Primary Pulmonary Hypertension

Primary pulmonary hypertension is a disease or group of diseases clinically characterized by a mean pulmonary artery pressure >25 mm Hg at rest and >30 mm Hg during exercise, with a normal pulmonary artery wedge pressure and absence of secondary causes (109,113). The mechanism is largely unknown but probably results from multiple noxious stimuli targeting a predisposed pulmonary vasculature (114). The best-known predisposing factors are the mutations in the BMPR2 gene (114) found in chromosome 2 in patients with familial pulmonary hypertension and in 26% of patients with sporadic disease.

Several factors contribute to the narrowing of the lumen of the pulmonary artery and increase the pressure and the vascular resistance: endothelial dysfunction/vasoconstriction, vascular wall remodeling (medial hypertrophy), and *in situ* thrombosis (114). Damage to the endothelium probably alters the balance between vasoconstrictive mediators, such as thromboxane and endothelin-1, and vasodilators, such as nitric oxide and prostacyclin, the end result being vasoconstriction (110,113–115). Vasoconstriction may not be the primary event, but it is an important component in the pathophysiology of primary pulmonary hypertension. Remodeling plays a major role in the increased vascular resistance. Abnormal proliferation of monoclonal endothelial cells occurs in plexogenic lesions, together with proliferation and hypertrophy of smooth muscle cells (114). Besides the abnormal proliferation of endothelial cells, an increase in extracellular matrix deposition contributes to the medial hypertrophy in patients with primary pulmonary hypertension. An additional factor that contributes to the narrowing of the lumen is the presence of thrombi in the small muscular arteries. It seems that this propensity for thrombosis is related to dysfunctional endothelium that has lost the normal anticoagulation properties (114).

Congenital Systemic to Pulmonary Shunts

The number of adults with surgically corrected and uncorrected congenital heart diseases is estimated to be 1 million in the United States (116). Disorders in this group include congenital heart defects with left-to-right shunt such as atrial septal defect, ventricular septal defect, patent ductus arteriosus, aortopulmonary window, and partial anomalous pulmonary venous return. In many of these conditions, there is initially shunting of blood from the left side of the heart to the right side (more complaint), causing an increase in pulmonary blood flow (116). A substantial increase in pulmonary artery flow may be undetected for an extended period before increased resistance results in pulmonary artery hypertension. The major chest radiographic sign is enlarged pulmonary arteries throughout the lungs; the corresponding hemodynamic change is increased flow, and the main and hilar pulmonary arteries usually are distended. The cardiac murmur may be distinctive, and specific signs may strongly suggest a particular anomaly, but accurate assessment often requires echocardiographic evaluation and cardiac catheterization, with or without angiocardiography.

Connective Tissue Disease and Other Causes of Pulmonary Arterial Hypertension

Pulmonary arterial hypertension occurs in 39% of patients with scleroderma (117). With the onset of scleroderma in a patient, the risk of pulmonary arterial hypertension increases with each decade of his or her life. In a subgroup of patients with limited scleroderma, isolated pulmonary hypertension occurs independent of the degree of fibrosis (118). Similar to patients with primary pulmonary hypertension, patients with isolated pulmonary hypertension and scleroderma have low levels of exhaled nitric oxide when compared with normal subjects and patients with scleroderma without pulmonary hypertension (119). Less frequently, rheumatoid arthritis, systemic lupus erythematosus, and mixed connective tissue disease can cause pulmonary hypertension.

Pulmonary artery involvement in Takayasu arteritis results in an uncommon and often unrecognized form of moderate pulmonary hypertension (120). Compression of the main pulmonary artery or its branches, sometimes as a result of an acquired mediastinal disorder, causes diffuse pulmonary oligemia of "central" origin. For example, a mediastinal mass exerting pressure on a pulmonary artery may compromise pulmonary artery flow. Dissecting aneurysms of the pulmonary artery or of the aorta, primary chondrosarcoma of the sternum, and fibrosing mediastinitis may have the same effect.

Pulmonary Hypertension Associated with Disorders of the Respiratory System or Hypoxemia

Numerous primary diseases of the lungs, pleura, chest wall, and respiratory control center may increase pulmonary arterial pressure and yet have no significant effect on pulmonary venous pressure (Table 11-11). Pulmonary artery pressures seldom reach the levels attained in cases of primary vascular disease.

Hypoxemia, with or without respiratory acidosis, may be the most important cause of pulmonary artery hypertension in this group of conditions. Ventilation–perfusion inequality or generalized alveolar hypoventilation may be the source of reduced oxygen saturation. Other contributory factors include hypervolemia and polycythemia, especially in cases of pulmonary emphysema and chronic bronchitis (121).

Pulmonary capillary destruction also may be associated with increased pulmonary artery pressure. The most common entities are emphysema and chronic bronchitis and diffuse interstitial or air-space disease of the lungs (112). Severe degrees of kyphoscoliosis or thoracoplasty may lead to pulmonary artery hypertension and cor pulmonale caused by a poorly ventilated but relatively well-perfused lung. Finally, there is a group of hypoventilation syndromes usually associated with sleep-disordered breathing or neuromuscular disorders that cause arterial hypoxemia and hypercapnia. Patients with these disorders may present clinically in right-sided heart failure (122,123).

Pulmonary hypertension has been described in humans and animals living at high altitude and is known as *chronic mountain sickness* or *Monge disease*. Pulmonary hypertension is present as well in subjects who live in low altitude areas and who develop high-attitude pulmonary edema. High-altitude pulmonary edema is probably a form of hydrostatic pulmonary edema (124) that occurs in genetically susceptible individuals with impairment of transepithelial sodium and water clearance

in the lungs and impaired synthesis of nitric oxide in the pulmonary circulation (125,126).

Pulmonary Venous Hypertension

The most common causes of cardiac-induced pulmonary hypertension are failure of the left ventricle, mitral valve disease, and myxoma (or thrombus) of the left atrium. The pulmonary venous causes of postcapillary hypertension include congenital stenosis at the origin of the pulmonary veins, mediastinal granulomas and neoplasms, idiopathic veno-occlusive disease (127), and anomalous pulmonary venous return. Any condition that raises pulmonary venous pressure above a critical level can result in postcapillary hypertension.

Symptoms related to postcapillary hypertension usually are distinguished from those of precapillary origin. In left ventricular failure, perhaps the most common cause of pulmonary venous hypertension, symptoms and signs predominantly arise from acute or subacute pulmonary edema. Postcapillary hypertension causes orthopnea, dyspnea, and, occasionally, paroxysmal nocturnal dyspnea, reflecting interstitial and air-space edema. In mitral stenosis, the pink frothy expectoration characteristic of acute cardiogenic pulmonary edema may be accompanied by bright red blood from hemorrhaging varicosities of the bronchial veins. Pulmonary vascular pressure remains steady until the mitral valve orifice shrinks to less than half its normal size (128). The symptoms and signs of pulmonary edema, the characteristic long opening snap of the first heart sound, and the soft, low-pitched, rumbling diastolic murmur permit differentiation between this form of hypertension and primary pulmonary hypertension (129).

Pulmonary venous hypertension may occur from blockage of the left atrium by a myxoma or a thrombus. Episodes of pulmonary edema or syncope that can be relieved by a change in position are frequent. Left atrial myxoma may be the source of systemic embolization or may be associated with fever, weight loss, increased sedimentation rate, anemia, or elevated γ-globulin levels.

DIAGNOSIS OF PULMONARY HYPERTENSION

Clinical Manifestations

Primary pulmonary hypertension is characterized by a slow, insidious onset of vague symptoms. On average, the diagnosis is delayed for almost 2 years, and, frequently, patients have been misdiagnosed as having hyperventilation and depression. Primary pulmonary hypertension is rare and can occur at any age, although it is more common in the third and fourth decades (109). The female-to-male ratio is 1.7:1, and familial disease represents 6% of all cases (114). The most common symptom is dyspnea, present in 60% of patients on initial presentation (109,113). Angina, probably as a result of underperfusion of the right ventricle or stretching of the large pulmonary arteries, is present in 47% of patients. Syncope is an early symptom in 8% of patients. Other symptoms include cough, hemoptysis, hoarseness (from compression of the recurrent laryngeal nerve by the pulmonary vessels), and Raynaud phenomenon in 10% of patients (130). Physical findings are similar in all patients with pulmonary hypertension. A loud second heart sound and right-sided fourth heart sounds are common. Other common signs are right ventricular heave, palpable systolic impulse of the pulmonary artery, pulmonary ejection murmur, and pulmonary tricuspid regurgitation murmur (109,130). Signs of right ventricular failure such as distended jugular veins, enlarged and pulsatile liver, ascites, and peripheral edema may be present. Cyanosis is present, owing to low cardiac output and right-to-left shunting across a patent foramen ovale. Clubbing does not occur in primary pulmonary hypertension (109).

Chest radiographic findings often include significant enlargement of the main and hilar pulmonary arteries, pruning of the peripheral arteries, and variable expansion of the right ventricle and atrium (113). Chest radiograph is normal in 6% of affected patients (109). Pleural effusions do not occur with right-sided heart failure alone (131).

In pulmonary veno-occlusive disease, a form of postcapillary hypertension, the signs and symptoms are similar (127). This form of primary pulmonary hypertension carries a poor prognosis (127). Radiographically, the main pulmonary artery and primary pulmonary branches are prominent, and there is evidence of increased bronchovascular markings and Kerley B lines (127). A CT scan shows smooth septal thickening, ground glass opacities, small nodules, pleural effusions, and areas of alveolar consolidation (127). The electrocardiographic findings in patients with pulmonary hypertension are right axis deviation and right ventricular hypertrophy with strain.

The physician must be aware of secondary forms of pulmonary hypertension because mitral valve disease or other treatable lesions may be present (129). Patients with rheumatic mitral stenosis may present with severe pulmonary hypertension; subtle findings may indicate the presence of mitral valve obstruction. The auscultatory findings of mitral disease may not be evident because of low cardiac output and the rotation of the heart caused by right ventricular hypertrophy. The chest radiograph may show only a prominent main pulmonary artery and right-sided enlargement, with little evidence of left atrial enlargement. Cardiac catheterization may reveal only increased pulmonary artery pressure, low cardiac output, and limited increase in pulmonary artery wedge pressure, which on rare occasions may be within normal limits.

Radiographic studies, including fluoroscopy, may help detect underlying lesions. Even minor enlargement of the left atrium suggests mitral stenosis; Kerley B lines, if present, are helpful, and the mitral valve area should be assessed for calcification, which generally confirms the presence of mitral valve disease. P waves compatible with left atrial enlargement are an electrocardiographic abnormality suggestive of mitral valve disease. Echocardiography has largely replaced catheterization of the left side of the heart for detecting mitral stenosis.

Differential Diagnosis

Frequently, severe pulmonary hypertension secondary to increased vascular resistance is the obvious diagnosis. However, the specific cause may be difficult to define clinically. Symptoms developing after pregnancy, DVT, or a surgical operation likely represent thromboembolic obstructive hypertension. In patients with cirrhosis and portal hypertension, significant pulmonary hypertension, so-called porto-pulmonary hypertension, may be present in 6% of patients evaluated for liver transplantation. Patients with porto-pulmonary hypertension

that have undergone liver transplantation have an elevated hospital mortality of 36% (132,133). Systemic lupus erythematosus, scleroderma, and schistosomiasis should be considered, and appropriate laboratory tests should be performed (134).

Excluding diseases of the pulmonary parenchyma requires careful assessment of the clinical picture and radiographic findings. Pulmonary function tests, particularly in the case of obstructive airways disease, may be helpful. High-resolution computed tomography (HRCT) may be useful in the group of patients with chronic interstitial lung disease and normal chest radiograph (135). A rise in pulmonary artery pressure, like that seen in patients with primary pulmonary hypertension, is rare in pulmonary parenchymal disease.

HEMODYNAMIC STUDIES IN PATIENTS WITH PULMONARY HYPERTENSION

Right and left cardiac catheterizations are necessary to diagnose cardiac causes of pulmonary hypertension and, in the absence of secondary causes, to make the diagnosis of primary pulmonary hypertension. Right heart catheterization is also useful to determine the degree of pulmonary hypertension and prognosis and the response to vasodilators (136,137). Patients with primary pulmonary hypertension, a high mean pulmonary arterial pressure and right atrial pressure, and a low cardiac index (less than 2 L/minute/m^2) have a very poor prognosis with a short survival (136).

TREATMENT OF PULMONARY HYPERTENSION

Primary pulmonary hypertension is progressive and often fatal (137). The goals of treatment are: vasodilatation of the pulmonary arteries to reduce the pulmonary pressures, treatment of right ventricular failure, improvement in the functional capacity and quality of life, and improvement in the survival (138). The mainstay of treatment consists of supplemental oxygen, anticoagulation, and vasodilators. Supplemental oxygen must be given to patients who are hypoxemic at rest or during exercise. The arterial oxygen saturation needs to be maintained above 90% to attenuate hypoxic pulmonary vasoconstriction. Chronic warfarin therapy has been shown to improve survival in patients with primary pulmonary hypertension (138). The prothrombin time must be monitored to maintain the INR in the range of 2. Diuretics may be used in low doses to control hepatic congestion and leg edema.

Vasodilators have been advocated as a treatment of primary pulmonary hypertension for decades; several of them have been tested with mixed results (138). The basis for vasodilator therapy in pulmonary hypertension is the assumption that reversible pulmonary vasoconstriction is present. The goal with vasodilator therapy is to reduce mean pulmonary artery pressure and pulmonary vascular resistance with a rise in cardiac output, while not inducing systemic hypotension (137,138). Unfortunately, only 26% of patients have a therapeutic response to oral vasodilators (137). Titration of nifedipine or diltiazem is done with hourly doses under close hemodynamic monitoring (pulmonary arterial catheter) until maximal effects or adverse effects are present. Patients who respond to calcium channel blocker therapy have a 5-year survival rate of 94% compared with 55% for nonresponders (137). The average daily dose of sustained-release nifedipine is 120 to 240 mg per day;

diltiazem in doses up to 900 mg per day is an alternative in tachycardiac patients. Intravenous prostacyclin (epoprostenol), initially used as a screening agent for vasoreactivity, has been used in a continuous infusion with significant success (138–140). Long-term therapy with epoprostenol improves survival, functional class, and duration of exercise (138–140). Epoprostenol reduces pulmonary vascular resistance and pressures and increases the cardiac output. Tachyphylaxis occurs with chronic use of epoprostenol. Treprostinil, a prostacyclin analog is available for subcutaneous infusion. Treprostinil improves the 6-minute walk distance, the mean right atrial pressure and mean pulmonary arterial pressure, cardiac index, and the quality of life (QOL) (138). The endothelin antagonist bosentan is currently the only oral therapy that has been proven effective in the treatment of primary pulmonary arterial hypertension, pulmonary hypertension related to collagen vascular disease, and some congenital heart disease (138).

Single or bilateral lung transplantation offers new hope for patients with primary pulmonary hypertension. Patients who need to be evaluated for transplantation include those with progressive disease despite optimal medical therapy (141).

COR PULMONALE (PULMONARY HEART DISEASE)

The terms "cor pulmonale" and "pulmonary heart disease" refer to enlargement of the right ventricle (hypertrophy or dilation) secondary to disorders affecting lung structure or function (111). In general, the manifestations of cor pulmonale vary from initial adaptations of the right ventricle in response to the demands of increased pulmonary artery pressures to frank right ventricular failure. In cor pulmonale, the cause may be either intrinsic pulmonary disease (e.g., interstitial lung disease or COPD), inadequate function of the chest bellows (e.g., kyphoscoliosis), or insufficient ventilatory drive from the respiratory centers. Anatomic adaptation (dilation or hypertrophy) is confined predominantly to the right ventricle. The degree and duration of pulmonary arterial hypertension determine the relative effects of dilation or hypertrophy on right ventricular enlargement (111).

INCIDENCE

Cor pulmonale is common; autopsy studies estimate that 40% of patients with chronic lung disease have cor pulmonale (111). Cor pulmonale is present in almost 40% of patients with an FEV_1 of <1 L (111). Furthermore, the presence of right ventricular dilatation in patients with COPD is a poor prognostic indicator (142). (Chronic bronchitis and pulmonary emphysema are discussed in detail in Chapter 9, Chronic Obstructive Lung Disease.)

SYMPTOMS AND SIGNS

Symptoms of cor pulmonale are nonspecific, although increases in pulmonary artery pressures frequently result in increasing dyspnea and easy fatigability. As the right ventricle loses its ability to meet mechanical work demands, symptoms related to fluid retention and weight gain may emerge. On physical examination, the patient is commonly cyanotic and dyspneic, often with audible wheezing and tachypnea (111,142). If considerable carbon dioxide is retained, the patient may be confused, somnolent, or even comatose. Hand flapping and tremors (asterixis) similar to those observed in hepatic decompensation are common. Examination of the ocular fundi occasionally reveals papilledema, a finding that is more likely if carbon dioxide retention has produced increased cerebral blood flow and increased intracranial pressure. Except in patients with overt right ventricular failure—who have cyanosis, peripheral edema, and hepatomegaly—important physical findings may be limited to the cardiovascular system. There may be a prominent left parasternal or epigastric lift owing to an enlarged right ventricle. The pulmonary second sound (P_2) may be palpable. Low frequency diastolic gallops arising from the right heart may be heard to the left of the sternum; a presystolic or right atrial gallop sound (S_4) indicates increased right ventricular filling pressures and may coincide with prominent A waves in the jugular venous pulse. A protodiastolic gallop (S_3) is evidence of right ventricular failure and is usually accompanied by other signs of right heart failure. Less frequently, a diastolic decrescendo murmur of pulmonary insufficiency indicates dilation of the pulmonary valve ring caused by excessive pulmonary artery pressure.

In patients with severe right ventricular failure, the functional insufficiency of the valve due to ventricular dilation gives rise to the holosystolic murmur of tricuspid regurgitation, a murmur that may increase with inspiration. Palpable pulsations in an enlarged, tender liver and prominent V waves in the jugular venous pulse are seen as well (111).

ELECTROCARDIOGRAPHIC ABNORMALITIES

The diagnostic value of the electrocardiogram in cor pulmonale depends on the underlying disorder. Electrocardiographic findings are reliable if pulmonary artery hypertension is caused by primary pulmonary vascular or interstitial disease. Characteristic patterns of right ventricular enlargement are less common when cor pulmonale complicates chronic bronchitis and emphysema because pulmonary hyperinflation rotates and displaces the heart and expands distances between electrodes. The presence of electrocardiographic signs of cor pulmonale and hypoxemia in patients with COPD is associated with a poor prognosis (143).

IMAGING STUDIES

In patients with pulmonary heart disease, manifestations of the underlying disease may dominate the chest radiograph. The chest radiograph is accurate (98%) in identifying pulmonary hypertension, although it cannot determine the severity of pulmonary hypertension. The most convincing evidence of the disorder is the combination of a large main pulmonary artery, a large right descending pulmonary artery (>16 mm) on the posteroanterior chest radiograph, and a large left descending pulmonary artery (>18 mm) on the lateral chest radiograph (Figs. 11-5 and 11-6) (111,144). An additional clue is an enlarged right ventricular silhouette. Generally, cardiomegaly is more readily detected through serial chest films than by a single examination. CT and magnetic resonance imaging (MRI) are accurate in the diagnosis of pulmonary hypertension. In CT, the pulmonary artery cross-sectional area

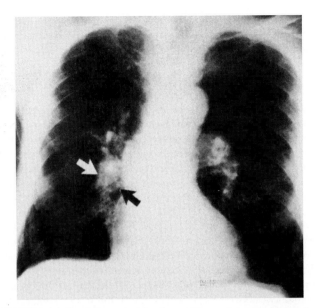

FIGURE 11-5. Enlarged right descending pulmonary artery (*arrows*) on posteroanterior chest radiograph in a patient with chronic obstructive pulmonary disease (COPD). Note also the large left main pulmonary artery. The mean pulmonary artery pressure is 57 mm Hg (normal is 18 to 20 mm Hg). (From Matthay RA, Schwarz MI, Ellis JH Jr, et al. Pulmonary hypertension in chronic obstructive pulmonary disease: determination by chest radiography. *Invest Radiol* 1981;16:95–100, with permission.)

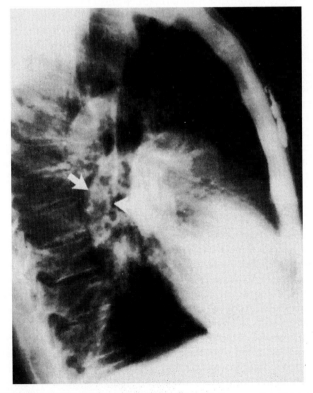

FIGURE 11-6. Enlarged left descending pulmonary artery (*arrows*) on left lateral chest radiograph in a patient with chronic obstructive pulmonary disease (COPD) and pulmonary artery hypertension. (From Matthay RA, Schwarz MI, Ellis JH Jr, et al. Pulmonary hypertension in chronic obstructive pulmonary disease: determination by chest radiography. *Invest Radiol* 1981;16:95–100, with permission.)

correlates well with mean pulmonary artery pressure. Pleural effusions do not occur in the setting of cor pulmonale alone (131). The presence of pleural effusions should suggest left heart failure or a primary pleural process such as infection, malignancy, or PE.

Echocardiography is more sensitive than a physical exam to detect cor pulmonale. Echocardiography shows structural changes, usually a decrease in the volume of the right ventricle relative to its mass. Echocardiography is sensitive in detecting severe elevation in pulmonary artery pressure but has limited value in detecting mild elevations (111). It is also important in the evaluation of left ventricular dysfunction, a common comorbid condition frequently present in patients with severe pulmonary diseases (145).

OTHER TESTS FOR EVALUATING PATIENTS WITH COR PULMONALE

Patients with cor pulmonale have arterial hypoxemia with a resting P_{O_2} usually ranging from below 60 mm Hg. In some patients, the P_{O_2} falls further during sleep; therefore, the patient has periods of marked oxygen desaturation. The hypoxemia aggravates the pulmonary hypertension, which then worsens the cor pulmonale. The arterial P_{CO_2} is usually in the range of 40 to 70 mm Hg. The degree of alveolar hypoventilation does not correlate well with the severity of airway obstruction. However, if the P_{CO_2} rises at night, then the acidemia (associated with the increase in P_{CO_2}) can potentiate the pulmonary hypertension and cor pulmonale (2).

Radionuclide ventriculography has been used to study the right and left ventricles in COPD. This method has provided reproducible values for right ventricular ejection fraction. The technique provides a noninvasive method for detection of right ventricular performance abnormalities secondary to pulmonary hypertension (142). In patients with severe lung disease, the right ventricular ejection fraction is frequently reduced because of the increase of the right ventricle afterload.

THERAPY FOR ACUTELY DECOMPENSATED COR PULMONALE

Oxygen

The initial treatment for acutely decompensated cor pulmonale is supplemental oxygen therapy to restore arterial oxygen to acceptable levels (146). An endpoint of 90% arterial oxygen saturation (or an arterial P_{O_2} of 60 mm Hg that corresponds to an arterial oxygen content of 18 vol%) is adequate in most settings (147). The coexistence of hypercapnia imposes constraint on administering oxygen; a practical approach consists of a trial of a modestly enriched oxygen mixture (e.g., 25% to 30% oxygen), monitored by a sampling of arterial blood to detect an unacceptable rise in arterial P_{CO_2} (147,148). Mechanical ventilation may be necessary to improve oxygenation and to avoid progressive respiratory acidosis.

Diuretics and Digitalis

Oxygen is the best diuretic. As arterial P_{O_2} rises, pulmonary hypertension decreases and cardiac output rises owing to a reduced right ventricular afterload. Diuretics must be administered cautiously to avoid volume depletion and possible reduction in cardiac output (2). Another potential complication of diuretic therapy is hypochloremic metabolic alkalosis, which can diminish the effect of the CO_2 stimulus on the respiratory centers and depress ventilatory drive. Therefore, serum electrolytes must be measured after diuretic administration or during periods of intensive salt and water retention. In some clinical circumstances, bed rest, modest salt restriction, and improved oxygenation alone may relieve significant water accumulation (2).

There is little proof that digitalis therapy is useful in patients with cor pulmonale. Digitalis therapy is considered appropriate only in the presence of coincident left heart failure or supraventricular arrhythmia (2,142,147). In patients with severe primary pulmonary hypertension, digoxin causes a modest increase in cardiac output (149).

Bronchodilators

Inhaled, short-acting β_2-agonists in combination with inhaled anticholinergics are the preferred bronchodilator treatment during acute exacerbations of COPD (148). Administration of aminophylline during an acute exacerbation is controversial. If used, close monitoring of serum theophylline is recommended (148).

Antibiotics

Antibiotic therapy must be considered early in patients with acutely decompensated cor pulmonale and chronic bronchitis who have a cough and increased production of purulent sputum (148). Sputum should be stained and cultured to identify the infecting organism and to determine appropriate drug therapy. Therapy directed at *Moraxella catarrhalis*, *Haemophilus influenzae*, and *Streptococcus pneumoniae* should be considered in the previously nonhospitalized patient with purulent sputum, with or without pulmonary infiltrates, until culture results or a clinical course indicates another pathogen or process.

Corticosteroids

Administration of systemic glucocorticosteroids (orally or intravenous) are recommended for patients with acute exacerbation of COPD because they are associated with reduction in treatment failure rates, duration of hospitalization, and improvement in airway function (148,150). Although the exact dose is not known, 30 to 40 mg of prednisolone or its equivalent for 10 to 14 days seems to be efficacious and safe (148).

Phlebotomy

Polycythemia impairs the vasodilatory response of the pulmonary artery in patients with severe chronic hypoxemic lung disease (121). The benefit of phlebotomy may be due to a reduction in total blood volume, a change in viscosity, and a restoration of the normal vasodilatory response in the pulmonary arteries (121). In chronic cor pulmonale, the reduction in hematocrit is accompanied by reduction in mean pulmonary artery pressure and pulmonary vascular resistance. However, in the setting of acute decompensation, the effect of phlebotomy is unknown. Accordingly, the procedure is best limited to patients with marked or refractory erythrocytosis (hematocrit greater

than 65%) in whom supplemental oxygen has failed to reduce the hematocrit or to patients in whom there is concern regarding thrombotic or central nervous system manifestations.

LONG-TERM MANAGEMENT OF COR PULMONALE

Persistent alveolar hypoxia contributes significantly to the chronic elevation of pulmonary artery pressure; in these cases, continuous low-flow oxygen therapy is a useful tool. Long-term continuous administration of supplemental oxygen to carefully selected patients to relieve hypoxia can significantly decrease hematocrit, stabilize resting pulmonary artery pressure in spite of progression of airflow abnormalities, and improve right ventricular performance, QOL, and mortality (148). Candidates for long-term oxygen therapy are patients with an arterial oxygen tension (Po_2) below 55 mm Hg or 88% arterial oxygen saturation with or without hypercapnia. Patients with a Po_2 above 55 mm Hg but below 59 mm Hg or oxygen saturation below 89% in the presence of cor pulmonale, heart failure, or erythrocytosis (hematocrit above 55%), are candidates for supplemental oxygen therapy as well. The Po_2 must be reevaluated at 1, 3, and 6 months to document the need for supplemental oxygen (148). The goal of long-term therapy is to increase the baseline Po_2 to at least 60 mm Hg or oxygen saturation to at least 90%.

CONGENITAL PULMONARY VASCULAR DISORDERS AND ACQUIRED ANEURYSMS

A variety of congenital abnormalities affect the pulmonary arteries and pulmonary veins (151). Atresia of the pulmonary veins refers to obliteration of the luminal continuity of the venous pathway but not to its absence. Atresias of the pulmonary veins are rare malformations that carry a high mortality of 40% if they are untreated. MRI is of great value in the definition of the anatomy in these complex patients (152). The treatment of unilateral pulmonary vein atresia is surgical—pneumonectomy. The functional results after pneumonectomy in these patients is good. Stenosis and atresia of the pulmonary arteries are common components of complex congenital heart diseases (152). Corrective or palliative surgery is frequently required in order to improve the pulmonary blood flow.

PULMONARY ARTERIOVENOUS MALFORMATIONS

Shunts between large blood vessels and between chambers of the heart normally exist during fetal life. Trauma, chest surgery, infection, metastatic carcinomas, and hepatic cirrhosis are the chief causes of abnormal vascular shunts after birth (153). Multiple arteriovenous and other intervascular connections may also develop in the lungs as a result of chronic infection, such as bronchiectasis.

In certain pathologic disorders, a large volume of blood may be shunted from the pulmonary artery to the pulmonary vein, resulting in considerable hypoxemia. Pulmonary arteriovenous malformation, a rare congenital lesion, is typical of true venous admixture. The shunt occurs from a pulmonary artery to a pulmonary vein. Such malformations may be single or multiple (153).

Pulmonary arteriovenous malformation may be isolated or, in 70% of cases, associated with hereditary hemorrhagic

telangiectasia (HHT) (Osler-Weber-Rendu disease) (153). Approximately 15% to 35% of patients with HHT have pulmonary arteriovenous malformation. In severe cases, up to 40% of the cardiac output may be shunted through the malformation. Genetic mapping has found that HHT is linked to loci on chromosomes 3, 9, and 12. It has been suggested that changes in endoglin, a binding protein for transforming growth factors β 1 and 3, may result in an abnormal response of endothelial cells during vascular remodeling, resulting in formation of arteriovenous malformation (HHT 1) (153). Endoglin also binds activin A, BMP 2, and BMP 7. Another mutation associated with HHT involves ALK1. ALK1 is a type 1 serine–threonine kinase receptor, which is expressed predominantly in endothelial cells (154). ALK1 mutations (HHT 2) are associated with fewer complications in patients that have endoglin mutations. The exact pathogenesis of pulmonary arteriovenous malformation is unknown.

Women are more affected than men, in a ratio of 2:1; symptoms usually start between the fourth and sixth decades and are more frequent in patients with multiple lesions or when the lesion is >2 cm (153). Epistaxis, dyspnea, and superficial telangiectasies are the most common findings in HHT. Dyspnea, platypnea, and hemoptysis are the most common symptoms in patients with pulmonary arteriovenous malformations. A bruit heard over the lung fields that increases with inspiration is present in almost 50% of the patients with pulmonary arteriovenous malformations. Clubbing and cyanosis are present in one-third of patients (153).

Neurologic effects of pulmonary arteriovenous shunts are headaches, confusion, dizziness, seizure, syncope, paresthesia, diplopia, thick speech, and paresis, as well as cerebrovascular accidents. Such complications have been attributed to cerebral hypoxia, polycythemia, and telangiectasia in the brain, with or without associated cerebral thrombosis. Brain abscess due to paradoxical emboli needs to be considered as well (153).

The pulmonary arteriovenous malformation may be so small as to be barely discernible on a chest radiograph, but a large pulmonary arteriovenous malformation can be seen on a routine posteroanterior chest radiograph. Typically, it is a lobulated or spherical opacity with smooth, discrete margins. It may be connected to the hilus by bandlike linear or sinuous opacities, although the afferent and efferent vessels may not be visible. The aneurysm may involve any segment of either lung, although there appears to be a predilection for the lower and middle lobes. Fluoroscopic examination may demonstrate pulsations in the lobulated density as well as in the hilus. Ultrafast contrast-enhanced chest CT, three-dimensional helical CT, contrast echocardiography, radionuclide perfusion lung scanning, and pulmonary angiography are important in the evaluation of patients with pulmonary arteriovenous malformations (153).

Physiologically, the presence of a true right-to-left shunt can be confirmed by the failure of the arterial P_{O_2} to rise above 500 mm Hg when a patient inhales 100% oxygen. Cardiac output is usually normal, although it may rise if the oxygen tension is very low. Pulmonary hypertension is present in 1% of affected patients (153). The suggested work-up for a patient suspected to have a pulmonary arteriovenous malformation is shown in Figure 11-7.

Therapy can range from conservative management to surgical resection (153,154). Embolization of the malformation has been achieved with low morbidity and no mortality (153,155). Coil embolization reduces the shunting, alleviates dyspnea, and improves exercise capacity and gas exchange (155). Therapeutic embolization is now the modality of choice in patients with a single pulmonary arteriovenous malformation that is symptomatic, when the malformation is >2 cm in diameter, in patients with multiple or bilateral malformations, or in patients who are at a poor surgical risk (153). It has also been recommended to treat patients with small pulmonary arteriovenous malformations (<2 cm) when a feeding artery is ≥3 mm in diameter, to reduce the risk of paradoxical embolization (153).

FIGURE 11-7. Algorithm for the evaluation of patients with pulmonary arteriovenous malformation. (From Gossage JR, Kanj G. Pulmonary arteriovenous malformations. *Am J Respir Crit Care Med* 1998; 158:643–661, with permission.)

PULMONARY ARTERY ANEURYSMS

Pulmonary artery aneurysms are rare saccular dilatations of the walls of the pulmonary artery that are usually detectable on a chest radiograph (156). Risk factors for acquired aneurysms are infection (bacterial, fungal, tuberculosis, and syphilis); congenital and acquired cardiac abnormalities; abnormalities of the vessel walls, such as cystic medionecrosis and atherosclerosis; vasculitis; trauma; and other conditions, such as Hughes–Stovin syndrome (DVT involving the vena cava and pulmonary arterial aneurysm, usually multiple), Behçet syndrome (157), Takayasu arteritis, and primary pulmonary hypertension (156). The clinical

presentation is nonspecific, but dyspnea, chest pain, cough, and hemoptysis may be present. Spiral CT and MRI are helpful in the noninvasive diagnosis of these patients (158,159). Surgical resection of the aneurysm is the treatment of choice in most cases (156).

NEOPLASIA OF THE PULMONARY VASCULAR BED

True neoplasms of the pulmonary arteries, veins, and lymphatic vessels are rare. Primary malignant tumors of the pulmonary arteries are usually sarcomatous (160). Sarcoma of the pulmonary arteries affects both sexes equally and the mean age of presentation is 52 years. The most common symptoms are dyspnea, chest pain, cough, and hemoptysis (161). On chest radiography, the most common abnormalities are hilar and pulmonary artery enlargement, pulmonary nodules, enlargement of the heart shadow, and decreased pulmonary vascularity. A CT scan shows large filling defects in the pulmonary blood vessels (161). Pulmonary angiography usually shows intraluminal masses and perfusion abnormalities. Surgical resection is the treatment of choice and the survival is 31% at 1 year. Adjuvant radiation and chemotherapy may be helpful (161).

REFERENCES

1. Gregoratos G, Karliner JS, Moser KM. Mechanisms of disease and methods of assessment. In: Moser KM, ed. *Pulmonary vascular diseases*. New York: Marcel Dekker Inc, 1979:279–339.
2. Horlander KT, Mannino DM, Leeper KV. Pulmonary embolism mortality in the United States, 1997–1998. An analysis using multiple-cause mortality data. *Arch Intern Med* 2003;163:1711–1717.
3. Moser KM. Pulmonary vascular obstruction due to embolism and thrombosis. In: Moser KM, ed. *Pulmonary vascular disease.* New York: Marcel Dekker Inc, 1979:341–386.
4. Raskob GE, Hull RD. Diagnosis and management of pulmonary thromboembolism. *Q J Med* 1990;76:787–797.
5. Silverstein MD, Heit JA, Mohr DN, et al. Trends in the incidence of deep vein thrombosis and pulmonary embolism. *Arch Intern Med* 1998;158:585–593.
6. Hyers TM. Venous thromboembolism. *Am J Respir Crit Care Med* 1999;159:1–14.
7. Moser K. State of the art: venous thromboembolism. *Am Rev Respir Dis* 1990;141:235–249.
8. Wolfe WB, Sabiston DC Jr. Pulmonary embolism. *Major Probl Clin Surg* 1980;25:1–180.
9. Nordstrom M, Linbland B. Autopsy-verified venous thromboembolism within a defined urban population. The city of Malmo, Sweden. *APMIS* 1998;106:378–384.
10. Hansson PO, Welin L, Tibblin G, et al. Deep vein thrombosis and pulmonary embolism in the general population. *Arch Intern Med* 1997;157:1665–1670.
11. Heit SA, Silverstein MD, Mohr DN, et al. Risk factors for deep vein thrombosis and pulmonary embolism: a population based case-control study. *Arch Intern Med* 2000;160:809–815.
12. Bosson JL, Labarere J, Sevestre MA, et al. Deep vein thrombosis in elderly patients hospitalized in subacute care facilities. *Arch Intern Med* 2003;163:2613–2618.
13. Morpurgo M, Schmid C. The spectrum of pulmonary embolism. Clinicopathologic correlation. *Chest* 1995;107:18S–20S.
14. Wagenvoort CA. Pathology of pulmonary thromboembolism. *Chest* 1995;107:10S–17S.
15. Nachman RL, Silverstein R. Hypercoagulable states. *Ann Intern Med* 1993;119:819–827.
16. Murin S, Marelich GP, Arroliga AC, et al. Hereditary thrombophilia and venous thromboembolism. *Am J Respir Crit Care Med* 1998;158:1369–1373.
17. Perry SL, Ortel TL. Clinical and laboratory evaluations of thrombophilia. *Clin Chest Med* 2003;24:153–170.
18. Sorensen HT, Mellemkjaer L, Steffensen FH, et al. The risk of diagnosis of cancer after primary deep venous thrombosis or pulmonary embolism. *N Engl J Med* 1998;338:1169–1173.
19. Schraufnagel DE, Tsao MS, Yao YT, et al. Factors associated with pulmonary infarction. A discriminant analysis. *Am J Clin Pathol* 1985;84:15–18.
20. Goldhaber SZ, Elliott GC. Acute pulmonary embolism: Part I. Epidemiology, pathophysiology and diagnosis. *Circulation* 2003; 108:2726–2729.
21. Severinghaus JW, Swenson EW, Finley TN, et al. Unilateral hypoventilation produced in dogs by occluding one pulmonary artery. *J Appl Physiol* 1961;15:53–60.
22. Tisi GM, Wolfe WG, Fallat RJ, et al. Effects of O₂ on airway smooth muscle following pulmonary vascular occlusion. *J Appl Physiol* 1970;28:570–573.
23. Thomas D, Stein M, Tanabe G, et al. Mechanisms of bronchoconstriction produced by thromboemboli in dogs. *Am J Physiol* 1964;206:1207–1212.
24. Finley TN, Swenson EW, Clements JA, et al. Changes in mechanical properties, appearance, and surface activity of extracts of one lung following occlusion of its pulmonary artery in the dog. *Physiologist* 1960;3:56.
25. Kasper W, Konstantinides S, Geibel A, et al. Prognostic significance of right ventricular after load stress detected by echocardiography in patients with clinically suspected pulmonary embolism. *Heart* 1997;77:346–349.
26. Dexter L, Smith GT. Quantitative studies of pulmonary embolism. *Am J Med Sci* 1964;247:641–648.
27. Lee JH, Chun YG, Lee IC, et al. Pathogenic role of endothelin 1 in hemodynamic dysfunction in experimental acute pulmonary embolism. *Am J Respir Crit Care Med* 2001;164:1282–1287.
28. Wessler S, Freeman DG, Ballon JS, et al. Experimental pulmonary embolism with serum-induced thrombi. *Am J Pathol* 1961;38:89–101.
29. Fred HL, Axelrod MA, Lewis JM, et al. Rapid resolution of pulmonary thromboemboli in man. *JAMA* 1966;196:1137–1139.
30. Moser KM, Guisan M, Bartimmo EE, et al. In vivo and postmortem dissolution rates of pulmonary emboli and venous thrombi in the dog. *Circulation* 1973;48:170–178.
31. Freiman DG, Wessler S, Lertzman M. Experimental pulmonary embolism with serum-induced thrombi aged in vivo. *Am J Pathol* 1961;39:95–102.
32. Moser KM, Daily PO, Peterson K, et al. Thromboendarterectomy for chronic, major-vessel thromboembolic pulmonary hypertension. Immediate and long-term results in 42 patients. *Ann Intern Med* 1987;107:560–565.
33. Rich S, Levitsky S, Brundage BH. Pulmonary hypertension from chronic pulmonary thromboembolism. *Ann Intern Med* 1988; 108:425–434.
34. Fedullo PF, Auger WR, Kerr KM, et al. Chronic thromboembolic pulmonary hypertension. *N Engl J Med* 2001;345:1465–1472.
35. Heit JA. Risk factors for venous thromboembolism. *Clin Chest Med* 2003;24:1–12.
36. Goldhaber SZ, Tapson VF, for the DVT FREE Steering Committee. A prospective registry of 5451 patients with ultrasound-confirmed deep vein thrombosis. *Am J Cardiol* 2004;93:259–262.
37. Landefeld CS, McGuire E, Cohen AM. Clinical findings associated with acute proximal deep vein thrombosis: a basis of quantifying clinical judgment. *Am J Med* 1990;88:382–388.
38. Stein PD, Terrin MC, Hales CA, et al. Clinical, laboratory, roentgenographic, and electrocardiographic findings in patients with acute pulmonary embolism and preexisting cardiac or pulmonary disease. *Chest* 1991;100:598–608.
39. Chunilal SD, Eikelboom JW, Attia J, et al. Does this patient have pulmonary embolism? *JAMA* 2003;290:2849–2858.
40. Hull RD, Raskob GE, Carter CJ, et al. Pulmonary embolism in outpatients with pleuritic chest pain. *Arch Intern Med* 1988;148:838–844.
41. Cobbs BW Jr, Logue RB, Dorney EG. The second heart sound in pulmonary embolism and pulmonary hypertension. *Am Heart J* 1966;71:843–844.
42. Stein PD, Goldhaber SZ, Henry JW. Alveolar-arterial oxygen gradient in the assessment of acute pulmonary embolism. *Chest* 1995;107:139–143.

43. Petruzzeli S, Palla A, Peeraccini F, et al. Routine electrocardiography in screening for pulmonary embolism. *Respiration* 1986;50:233–243.

44. Stein PD, Athanasoulis C, Greenspan RH, et al. Relation of plain chest radiographic findings to pulmonary arterial pressure and arterial blood oxygen levels in patients with acute pulmonary embolism. *Am J Cardiol* 1992;69:394–396.

45. Bynum LJ, Wilson JE III. Characteristics of pleural effusions associated with pulmonary embolism. *Arch Intern Med* 1976;136:159–162.

46. Bockenstedt P. D-dimer in venous thromboembolism (Editorial). *N Engl J Med* 2003;349:1203–1204.

47. Kelly J, Rudd A, Lewis RR, et al. Plasma D-dimers in the diagnosis of venous thromboembolism. *Arch Inter Med* 2002;162:747–756.

48. Worsley DF, Alavi A, Palevsky JH. Role of radionuclide imaging in patients with suspected pulmonary embolism. *Radiol Clin North Am* 1993;31:849–858.

49. Miniati M, Pistolesi M, Marini C, et al. Value of perfusion lung scan in the diagnosis of pulmonary embolism: Results of the prospective investigative study of acute pulmonary embolism diagnosis (PISA-PED). *Am J Respir Crit Care Med* 1996;154:1387–1391.

50. Mayo JR, Remy-Jardin M, Mueller NL, et al. Pulmonary embolism: prospective comparison of spiral CT with ventilation-perfusion scintigraphy. *Radiology* 1997;205:447–452.

51. Perrier A, Buswell L, Bounameaux H, et al. Cost-effectiveness of noninvasive diagnostic aids in suspected pulmonary embolism. *Arch Intern Med* 1997;157:2309–2316.

52. Ferretti GR, Bosson JL, Buffaz PD, et al. Acute pulmonary embolism: role of helical CT in 164 patients with intermediate probability at ventilation-perfusion scintigraphy and normal results at Duplex US of the leg. *Radiology* 1997;205:453–458.

53. Stein PD, Hull RS, Saltzman HA, et al. Strategy for diagnosis of patients with suspected acute pulmonary embolism. *Chest* 1993;103:1553–1559.

54. Wells PS, Ginsberg JS, Anderson DR, et al. Use of a clinical model for safe management of patients with suspected pulmonary embolism. *Ann Intern Med* 1998;129:997–1005.

55. Stein PD, Coleman RE, Gottschalk A, et al. Diagnostic utility of ventilation/perfusion lung scans in acute pulmonary embolism is not diminished by preexisting cardiac or pulmonary disease. *Chest* 1991;100:604–606.

56. The PIOPED Investigators. Value of the ventilation/perfusion scan in acute pulmonary embolism. Results of the prospective investigation of pulmonary embolism diagnosis (PIOPED). *JAMA* 1990;263:2753–2759.

57. Cronan JJ. Venous thromboembolic disease: the role of U.S. *Radiology* 1993;186:619–630.

58. Heijboer H, Buller HR, Lensing AWA, et al. A comparison of real-time compression ultrasonography with impedance plethysmography for the diagnosis of deep-vein thrombosis in symptomatic outpatients. *N Engl J Med* 1993;329:1365–1369.

59. Turkstra M, Pistolesi M, Marini C, et al. Diagnostic utility of ultrasonography of leg veins in patients suspected of having pulmonary embolism. *Ann Intern Med* 1997;126:775–780.

60. Baarslag HJ, van Beek EJR, Koopman MMW, et al. Prospective study of color duplex ultrasonography compared with contrast venography in patients suspected of having deep venous thrombosis of the upper extremities. *Ann Intern Med* 2002;136:865–872.

61. Stein PD, Athanasoulis C, Alavi A, et al. Complications and validity of pulmonary angiography in acute pulmonary embolism. *Circulation* 1992;85:462–468.

62. Quinn MF, Lundell CJ, Klotz TA, et al. Reliability of selective pulmonary arteriography in the diagnosis of pulmonary embolism. *Am J Roentgenol* 1987;149:469–471.

63. Lockshin MD. Venous thromboembolism during pregnancy. *N Engl J Med* 1996;335:108–114.

64. Chan WS, Ray JG, Murray S, et al. Suspected pulmonary embolism in pregnancy. Clinical presentation, results of lung scanning, and subsequent maternal and pediatric outcomes. *Arch Intern Med* 2002;162:1170–1175.

65. Fedullo PF, Tapson VF. The evaluation of suspected pulmonary embolism. *N Engl J Med* 2003;349:1247–1256.

66. Wells PS, Anderson DR, Rodger M, et al. Deviation of a simple clinical model to categorize patients probability of pulmonary embolism: increasing the model's utility with the SimpliRED D-dimer. *Thromb Haemost* 2000;83:416–420.

67. Kruip MJHA, Leclercq MGL, vander Heul C, et al. Diagnostic strategies for excluding pulmonary embolism in clinical outcome studies. A systematic review. *Ann Intern Med* 2003;138:941–951.

68. Bates SM, Kearon C, Crowther M, et al. A diagnostic strategy involving a quantitative latex D-dimer assay reliably excludes deep venous thrombosis. *Ann Intern Med* 2003;138:787–794.

69. Kearon C, Ginsberg JS, Douketis J, et al. Management of suspected deep venous thrombosis in outpatients by using clinical assessment and D-dimer testing. *Ann Intern Med* 2001;135:108–111.

70. Kraaijenhagen RA, Piovella F, Bernardi E, et al. Simplification of the diagnostic management of suspected deep venous thrombosis. *Arch Intern Med* 2002;162:907–911.

71. Wells PS, Anderson DR, Rodger M, et al. Evaluation of D-dimer in the diagnosis of suspected deep-vein thrombosis. *N Engl J Med* 2003;349:1227–1235.

72. Van Strijen MJL, deMonye W, Schiereck J, et al. Single-detector helical compute tomography as the primary diagnostic test in suspected pulmonary embolism: a multicenter clinical management study of 510 patients. *Ann Intern Med* 2003;138:307–314.

73. Musset D, Parent F, Meyer G, et al. Diagnostic strategy for patients with suspected pulmonary embolism: A prospective multicenter outcome study. *Lancet* 2002;360:1914–1920.

74. Perrier A, Roy PM, Aujesky D, et al. Diagnosing pulmonary embolism in outpatients with clinical assessment. D-dimer measurement, venous ultrasound, and helical computed tomography. A multicenter management study. *Am J Med* 2004;116:291–299.

75. Geerts WH, Pineo GF, Heit JA, et al. Prevention of venous thromboembolism. *Chest* 2004;126:338S–400S.

76. Gillies TE, Ruckley CV, Nixon SJ. Still missing the boat with fatal pulmonary embolism. *Br J Surg* 1996;83:1394–1395.

77. Weitz JI. Low-molecular-weight heparins. *N Engl J Med* 1997;337:688–698.

78. Salzman EW. Low-molecular-weight heparin and other new antithrombotic drugs (Editorial). *N Engl J Med* 1992;326:1017–1019.

79. Buller HR, Agnelli G, Hull RD, et al. Antithrombotic therapy for venous thromboembolic disease. *Chest* 2004;126:401S–428S.

80. Raschke RA, Reilly BM, Guidry JR, et al. The weight-based heparin-dosing nomogram compared with a "standard care" nomogram. A randomized controlled trial. *Ann Intern Med* 1993;119:874–881.

81. Hirsh J, Warkentin TE, Shaughnessy SG, et al. Heparin and low-molecular-weight heparin. Mechanism of action, dosing, monitoring, efficacy, and safety. *Chest* 2001;119:64S–94S.

82. Quinlan DJ, McQuillan A, Eikelboom JW. Low-molecular-weight heparin compared with intravenous unfractionated heparin for treatment of pulmonary embolism. *Ann Intern Med* 2004;140:175–183.

83. Hirsch J, Dalen JE, Anderson DR, et al. Oral anticoagulants: Mechanism of action, clinical effectiveness, and optimal therapeutic range. *Chest* 2001;119:8S–21S.

84. Crowther MA, Ginsberg JB, Kearon C, et al. A randomized trial comparing 5 mg and 10 mg warfarin loading doses. *Arch Intern Med* 1999;159:46–48.

85. Agnelli G, Prandoni P, Becattini C, et al. Extended oral anticoagulant therapy after a first episode of pulmonary embolism. *Ann Intern Med* 2003;139:19–25.

86. Hyers TM. Duration of anticoagulation in venous thromboembolism (Editorial). *Arch Intern Med* 2003;163:1265–1266.

87. Buller HR, Prins MH. Secondary prophylaxis with warfarin for venous thromboembolism (Editorial). *N Engl J Med* 2003;349:702–703.

88. Ridker PM, Goldhaber SZ, Danielson E, et al. Long-term, low-intensity warfarin therapy for the prevention of recurrent venous thromboembolism. *N Engl J Med* 2003;348:425–434.

89. Kearon C, Ginsberg JS, Kovacs MJ, et al. Comparison of low-intensity warfarin therapy with conventional-intensity warfarin therapy for long-term prevention of recurrent venous thromboembolism. *N Engl J Med* 2003;349:631–639.

90. Dalen JE. The uncertain role of thrombolytic therapy in the treatment of pulmonary embolism. *Arch Intern Med* 2002;162:2521–2523.

91. Layish DT, Tapson VF. Pharmacologic hemodynamic support in massive pulmonary embolism. *Chest* 1997;111:218–224.

92. Konstantinides S, Geibel A, Heusel G, et al. Heparin plus alteplase compared with heparin alone in patients with submassive pulmonary embolism. *N Engl J Med* 2002;347:1143–1150.

93. Aklog L, Williams CS, Byrne JG, et al. Acute pulmonary embolectomy. A contemporary approach. *Circulation* 2002;105:1416–1419.
94. Becker DM, Philbrick JT, Selby JB. Inferior vena cava filters. Indications, safety and effectiveness. *Arch Intern Med* 1992;52:1985–1994.
95. Decousus H, Leizorovicz A, Parent F, et al. A clinical trial of vena caval filters in the prevention of pulmonary embolism in patients with proximal deep-vein thrombosis. *N Engl J Med* 1998;338:409–415.
96. Pengo V, Lensing AWA, Prins MH, et al. Incidence of chronic thromboembolic pulmonary hypertension after pulmonary embolism. *N Engl J Med* 2004;350:2257–2264.
97. Sutton LL, Castro O, Cross DJ, et al. Pulmonary hypertension in sickle cell disease. *Am J Cardiol* 1994;74:626–628.
98. Iwasiki Y, Nagata K, Nakanishi M, et al. Spiral CT findings in septic emboli. *Eur J Radiol* 2001;37:190–194.
99. Miro JM, del Rio A, Mestres CA. Infective endocarditis in intravenous drug abusers and HIV-1 infected patients. *Infect Dis Clin North Am* 2002;16:273–295.
100. Olaison L, Pettersson G. Current best practices and guidelines. Indications for surgical intervention in infective endocarditis. *Infect Dis Clin North Am* 2002;16:453–475.
101. Le T, Bayer AS. Combination antibiotic therapy for infective endocarditis. *Clin Infect Dis* 2003;36:615–621.
102. Georgopoulos D, Bouros D. Fat embolism syndrome. Clinical examinations is still the preferable diagnostic method (Editorial). *Chest* 2003;123:982–983.
103. Kim YH, Oh SW, Kim JS. Prevalence of fat embolism following bilateral simultaneous and unilateral total hip arthroplasty performed with or without cement. *J Bone Joint Surg Am* 2002;84:1372–1379.
104. Mimoz O, Edourard A, Beydon L, et al. Contribution of bronehoalveolar lavage to the diagnosis of posttraumatic pulmonary fat embolism. *Int Care Med* 1995;21:973–980.
105. Lechapt E, Habibi A, Bachir D, et al. Induced sputum vs. bronchoalveoler lavage during acute chest syndrome in sickle cell disease. *Am J Respir Crit Care Med* 2003;168:1373–1377.
106. Davies S. Amniotic fluid embolus: A review of the literature. *Can J Anaesth* 2001;48:88–98.
107. Ohkuda K, Nakahara K, Binder A, et al. Venous air emboli in sheep: reversible increase in lung microvascular permeability. *J Appl Physiol* 1981;51:887–894.
108. Marini JJ, Culver BH. Systemic gas embolism complicating mechanical ventilation in the adult respiratory distress syndrome. *Ann Intern Med* 1989;110:699–703.
109. Olivari MT. Primary pulmonary hypertension. *Am J Med Sci* 1991;302:185–198.
110. Dweik RA, Laskowski D, Abou-soud HM, et al. Nitric oxide synthesis in the lung. Regulation by oxygen through a kinetic mechanism. *J Clin Invest* 1998;101:660–666.
111. Budev MM, Arroliga AC, Wiedemann HP, et al. Cor pulmonale: An Overview. *Semin Respir Crit Care Med* 2003;24:233–243.
112. Edwards WD. Pathology of pulmonary hypertension. *Cardiovasc Clin* 1988;18:321–359.
113. Rubin LJ. Primary pulmonary hypertension. *N Engl J Med* 1998;336:111–117.
114. Ghamra ZW, Dweik RA. Primary pulmonary hypertension: An overview of epidemiology and pathogenesis. *Cleve Clin J Med* 2003;70:2S–8S.
115. Kaneko FT, Arroliga AC, Dweik RA, et al. Biochemical reaction products of nitric oxide as quantitative markers of primary pulmonary hypertension. *Am J Respir Crit Care Med* 1998;158:917–923.
116. Brickner ME, Hills DL, Lange RA. Medical progress: Congenital heart disease in adults: First of two parts. *N Engl J Med* 2000;342:256–263.
117. Schachna L, Wigley FM, Chang B, et al. Age and risk of pulmonary arterial hypertension in scleroderma. *Chest* 2003;124:2098–2104.
118. Minai OA, Dweik RA, Arroliga AC. Manifestations of scleroderma pulmonary disease. *Clin Chest Med* 1998;19:713–731.
119. Kharitonov SA, Cailes JB, Black CM, et al. Decreased nitric oxide in the exhaled air of patients with systemic sclerosis with pulmonary hypertension. *Thorax* 1997;52:1051–1055.
120. Sullivan EJ, Hoffman GS. Pulmonary vasculitis. *Clin Chest Med* 1998;19:759–776.
121. Defouilloy C, Teiger E, Sediame S, et al. Polycythemia impairs vasodilator response to acetylcholine in patients with chronic hypoxemic lung disease. *Am J Respir Crit Care Med* 1998;157:1452–1460.
122. Krachman SL, Criner GJ, Chatila W. Cor pulmonale and sleep-disordered breathing in patients with restrictive lung disease and neuromuscular disorder. *Semin Respir Crit Care Med* 2003;24:297–305.
123. Laks L, Lehrhaft B, Grunstein RR, et al. Pulmonary artery pressure response to hypoxia in sleep apnea. *Am J Respir Crit Care Med* 1997;155:193–198.
124. Swenson ER, Maggiorani M, Mongovin S, et al. Pathogenesis of high-altitude pulmonary edema. Inflammation is not an etiologic factor. *JAMA* 2002;287:2228–2235.
125. Sartori C, Allemann Y, Duplain H, et al. Salmeterol for the prevention of high-altitude pulmonary edema. *N Engl J Med* 2002;346:1631–1636.
126. Droma Y, Hanaoka M, Ota M, et al. Positive association of the endothelial nitric oxide synthase gene polymorphisms with high-altitude pulmonary edema. *Circulation* 2002;106:826–830.
127. Mandel J, Mark EJ, Hales CA. Pulmonary veno-occlusive disease. *Am J Respir Crit Care Med* 2000;162:1964–1973.
128. Gorlin R, Gorlin SG. Hydraulic formula for circulation of the area of the stenotic mitral valve, other cardiac valves, and central circulatory shunts. *Am Heart J* 1951;41:1–29.
129. Carabello BA. Recognition and management of patients with valvular heart disease. In: Goldman L, Braunwald E, eds. *Primary cardiology*. Philadelphia, PA: WB Saunders, 1998.
130. Budev MM, Arroliga AC, Jennings CA. Diagnosis and evaluation of pulmonary hypertension. *Cleve Clin J Med* 2003;70:9s–17S.
131. Wiener-Kronish JP, Goldstein R, Matthay RA, et al. Lack of association of pleural effusion with chronic pulmonary arterial and right atrial hypertension. *Chest* 1987;92:967–970.
132. Colle IO, Moreau R, Godinho E, et al. Diagnosis of porto pulmonary hypertension in candidates for liver transplantation: a prospective study. *Hepatology* 2003;37:401–409.
133. Krowka MJ, Mandell MS, Ramsay MAE, et al. Hepatopulmonary syndrome and portopulmonary hypertension: a report of the multicenter liver transplant database. *Liver Transpl* 2004;10:174–182.
134. Barbosa MM, Lamounier JA, Oliveira EC, et al. Pulmonary hypertension in schisgtosomiasis mansonii. *Trans R Soc Trop Med Hyg* 1996;90:663–665.
135. Hansell DM. High-resolution computed tomography in the evaluation of fibrosing alveolitis. *Clin Chest Med* 1999;20:739–760.
136. D'Alonzo GE, Barst RJ, Ayres SM, et al. Survival in patients with primary pulmonary hypertension. Results from a national prospective registry. *Ann Intern Med* 1991;115:343–349.
137. Rich S, Kaufmann E, Levy PS. The effect of high doses of calcium-channel blockers on survival in primary pulmonary hypertension. *N Engl J Med* 1992;327:76–81.
138. Gildea TR, Arroliga AC, Minai OA. Treatments and strategies to optimize the comprehensive management of patients with pulmonary arterial hypertension. *Cleve Clin J Med* 2003;70:18S–27S.
139. Barst RJ, Rubin LJ, Long WA, et al. A comparison of continuous intravenous epoprostenol (prostacyclin) with conventional therapy for primary pulmonary hypertension. *N Engl J Med* 1996;334:296–301.
140. McLaughlin VV, Genthner DE, Parella MM, et al. Reduction in pulmonary vascular resistance with long-term epoprostenol (prostacyclin) therapy in primary pulmonary hypertension. *N Engl J Med* 1998;338:273–277.
141. Maurer JR, Frost AE, Glanville AR, et al. International guidelines for the selection of lung transplant candidates. *Am J Respir Crit Care Med* 1998;158:335–339.
142. Salvaterra CA, Rubin LJ. Investigation and management of pulmonary hypertension in chronic obstructive pulmonary disease. *Am Rev Respir Dis* 1993;148:1414–1417.
143. Incalzi RAA, Fuso L, De Rosa M, et al. Electrocardiographic signs of chronic cor pulmonaale. A negative prognostic finding in chronic obstructive pulmonary disease. *Circulation* 1999;99:1600–1605.
144. Matthay RA, Schwarz MI, Ellis JH Jr, et al. Pulmonary hypertension in chronic obstructive pulmonary disease: determination by chest radiography. *Invest Radiol* 1981;16:95–100.

145. Vizza CD, Lynch JP, Ochoa LL, et al. Right and left ventricular dysfunction in patients with severe pulmonary disease. *Chest* 1998;113:576–583.

146. Lee-Chiong TL, Matthay RA. Pulmonary hypertension and cor pulmonale in COPD. *Semin Respir Crit Care Med* 2003;24:263–272.

147. Celli BR, Snider GL, Heffner J, et al. Standards for the diagnosis and care of patients with chronic obstructive pulmonary disease. *Am J Respir Crit Care Med* 1995;152:S77–S120.

148. Pauwells RA, Buist AS, Calverley PMA, et al. Global strategy for the diagnosis, management, and prevention of chronic obstructive pulmonary disease. *Am J Respir Crit Care Med* 2001;163:1256–1276.

149. Rich S, Seidlitz M, Dodin E, et al. The short-term effects of digoxin in patients with right ventricular dysfunction from pulmonary hypertension. *Chest* 1998;114:787–792.

150. Singh JM, Palda VA, Stanbrook MB. Corticosteroid therapy for patients with acute exacerbations of chronic obstructive pulmonary disease. A systematic review. *Arch Intern Med* 2002;162:2527–2536.

151. Pourmoghadam KK, Moore JW, Khan M, et al. Congenital unilateral pulmonary venous atresia: definitive diagnosis and treatment. *Pediatr Cardiol* 2003;24:73–79.

152. Powell AJ, Chung T, Landzberg MJ, et al. Accuracy of MRI evaluation of pulmonary blood supply in patients with complex pulmonary stenosis and atresia. *Int J Card Imaging* 2000;16:169–174.

153. Gossage JR, Kanj G. Pulmonary arteriovenous malformations. *Am J Respir Crit Care Med* 1998;158:643–661.

154. Berg J, Porteous M, Reinhardt D, et al. Hereditary hemorrhagic telangiectasia: a questionnaire-based study to delineate the different phenotypes caused by endoglin and ALK 1 mutations. *J Med Genet* 2003;40:585–590.

155. Gupta P, Mordin C, Curtis J, et al. Pulmonary arteriovenous malformations: effect of embolization on right-to-left shunt, hypoxemia, and exercise tolerance in 66 patients. *Am J Roentgenol* 2002;179:347–355.

156. Bartter T, Irwin RS, Nash G. Aneurysms of the pulmonary arteries. *Chest* 1988;94:1065–1075.

157. Erkan F, Gul A, Tasali E. Pulmonary manifestations of Behcet's disease. *Thorax* 2001;56:572–5878.

158. Rankin SC. Spiral CT: vascular applications. *Eur J Radiol* 1998;28:18–29.

159. Berkmen T. MR angiography of aneurysm in Behcet disease: a report of four cases. *J Comput Assist Tomogr* 1998;22:202–206.

160. Kim JH, Gutierrez FR, Lee Ex, et al. Primary leiomyosarcoma of the pulmonary artery. A diagnostic dilemma. *J Clin Imaging* 2003;27:206–211.

161. Cox JE, Chiles C, Aquino SL, et al. Pulmonary artery sarcomas: a review of clinical and radiological features. *J Comput Assist Tomogr* 1997;21:750–755.

CHAPTER 12

Diffuse Parenchymal and Alveolar Lung Diseases

David G. Morris
Michael B. Gotway
Robert J. Homer
Paul W. Noble
Herbert Y. Reynolds
Richard A. Matthay

The interstitial lung diseases (ILD) are a diverse group of disorders characterized by fibrosis or inflammation or both. They involve the lung parenchyma or small airways (e.g., bronchioles). The interstitium of the lung includes the alveolar walls, pulmonary microvasculature, interstitial macrophages, fibroblasts, myofibroblasts, and extracellular matrix components such as collagen, elastin, and proteoglycans. The interstitium extends from the alveolar space proximal to the terminal and respiratory bronchioles. ILDs, therefore, can be located primarily in the conducting airways (e.g., constrictive bronchiolitis) or in the lung parenchyma [e.g., idiopathic pulmonary fibrosis (IPF)]. Some disorders that primarily affect the alveolar space [e.g., pulmonary alveolar proteinosis or cryptogenic organizing pneumonia (COP)] also typically fall under the heading of ILDs because of the nature of their clinical presentation and radiographic abnormalities. The clinical presentations of ILDs have many common features including similarities of patient symptoms, the development of diffuse radiographic abnormalities, and similar derangements in pulmonary physiology. Typically, ILDs also require histopathologic examination of lung tissue for diagnosis. For most, etiologies remain elusive.

This chapter reviews the essential points of the most frequently encountered diffuse ILDs. These include the idiopathic interstitial pneumonias, connective tissue (collagen vascular) diseases, systemic granulomatous and nongranulomatous vasculitis, sarcoidosis, hypersensitivity pneumonitis, drug-associated ILD, anti–basement membrane antibody disease (Goodpasture syndrome), pulmonary alveolar proteinosis, eosinophilic pulmonary syndromes, and lymphangioleiomyomatosis (LAM). Understandably, the information provided in this overview is far from encyclopedic, and interested readers are referred to several outstanding recent monographs, compendia, and reviews for more detailed information (1–6).

CLINICAL APPROACH TO PATIENTS WITH DIFFUSE PARENCHYMAL AND ALVEOLAR LUNG DISEASES

Clinical, Radiographic, and Physiologic Manifestations

The majority of patients with ILD complain of difficulty breathing. Depending on the nature of the underlying disease, this difficulty breathing may be acute (e.g., pulmonary hemorrhage syndromes), subacute over days to weeks (e.g., acute interstitial pneumonia), or so gradual as to have escaped notice until some precipitating event such as an incidental chest radiograph or a marked dyspnea following travel to an unaccustomed altitude prompts further medical evaluation (e.g., IPF). A substantial percentage of patients will also complain of cough. With most ILDs, constitutional complaints such as fevers, chills, and weight loss are notably absent. Their presence often suggests either an underlying collagen vascular disease or more acute diseases such as COP or acute interstitial pneumonia. Some specific clinical syndromes are nearly pathognomonic of particular diseases. Examples of this include the syndromes of uveitis, parotitis, erythema nodosum, and bilateral hilar adenopathy as initial presentation of typically self-limited sarcoidosis (1); or the characteristic

fevers, chills, and shortness of breath following exposure to moldy hay as characteristic of farmer's lung—a subtype of hypersensitivity pneumonitis (7,8). Such syndromes, while diagnostically helpful, are relatively rare.

With extremely rare exceptions, patients with clinically significant ILD have abnormalities detectable by radiologic imaging of the chest (9). Unfortunately, plain chest radiographs can be misleadingly negative in up to 10% of all patients with clinically significant ILD and in up to 90% of patients with hypersensitivity pneumonitis (10–15). Conventional computed tomography (CT) of the chest is a better but still relatively insensitive supplement (16). As a result, high-resolution computed tomographic (HRCT) imaging of the chest has been developed. In HRCT, selected images are acquired—generally without contrast—at 1- to 3-mm collimation ("slice thickness"), as opposed to the 5- to 10-mm collimation of a standard chest CT. HRCT images are also reconstructed using a high–spatial-resolution algorithm to minimize volume averaging of signal. Although this level of collimation and computerized image reconstruction is ideal for ILDs, it has previously been both time and cost prohibitive to image entire lung fields at this resolution. Additionally, because many more images were required, radiation exposure levels were substantially increased. As a result, many older HRCT scans of the chest have anatomic gaps between imaged levels, making them unacceptably insensitive for nodule detection. This situation has led to the practice of combining conventional CT imaging, which is superior for the detection of larger lung nodules by virtue of its contiguous 10-mm collimation images, with HRCT acquisition and of reconstructing selected regions. Increasingly, however, with the advent of faster helical multichannel CT scanners, improved computer technology, and increased detector sensitivity, the time and radiation dose required for high-resolution image acquisition and for data analysis have made contiguous high-resolution imaging possible in the majority of clinical centers. This, coupled with the fact that the diagnostic certainty associated with particular patterns of abnormality on HRCT scans of the chest can obviate lung biopsy in selected diseases such as IPF (17,18), sarcoidosis (19), and some forms of hypersensitivity pneumonitis (20), has made HRCT imaging of the chest the *de facto* standard of care in patients with known or suspected ILD. The diagnostic utility of HRCT is often substantially augmented by combining both inspiratory and expiratory imaging to increase the detection of coexisting airways disease as manifested by regional air trapping during exhalation (20). Nevertheless, the value of careful retrospective review of prior plain chest radiographs in patients with ILD cannot be overstated. These studies, even when obtained for other reasons, offer invaluable insight into the time of onset, clinical course, and current trajectory of a given patient's pulmonary disease.

Interstitial diseases alter mechanical and gas exchanging properties of the lungs. Restrictive pulmonary physiologic changes [reduced total lung capacity (TLC), reduced residual volume (RV), increased ratio of forced expiratory volume in 1 second to forced vital capacity (FEV_1/FVC), and decreased static compliance] and a reduced diffusing capacity for carbon monoxide (D_{LCO}) are hallmarks of ILDs in general. A select few also manifest substantial components of airflow obstruction. These include sarcoidosis, LAM, Langerhans cell histiocytosis (eosinophic granuloma), constrictive bronchiolitis, respiratory bronchiolitis (RB)–ILD, and hypersensitivity pneumonia. In some cases, the coincidence of both restrictive and obstructive components can lead to normalization of lung volumes. In these cases, careful examination of the flow–volume loop and chest imaging may be required to make the correct diagnosis. In diseases such as IPF, the DLCO is often depressed out of proportion to the restrictive defect. This reduced diffusing capacity is the result of compromised pulmonary capillary blood volume and abnormal membrane conductance of oxygen (21). In addition, substantial ventilation–perfusion mismatch occurs in ILDs, which is typically heterogeneously distributed throughout the lung parenchyma. Quantitative studies suggest that virtually all of the hypoxemia at rest in patients with ILD is due to this ventilation–perfusion inequality (21). In patients with apparently normal gas exchange at rest, exercise testing may be helpful in unmasking these defects and, therefore, useful in understanding patients' exertional dyspnea (21).

Diagnostic Approach

Beyond radiologic imaging and physiologic testing, most patients with suspected ILD require invasive studies to establish a final diagnosis. These studies range from bronchoscopy with bronchoalveolar lavage (BAL) to surgical lung biopsy. In bronchoscopy, a small flexible fiber-optic tube is passed through anesthetized vocal cords into the trachea and further on into the more distal airways. In general, fifth and sixth order airways can be examined with this technique (see also Chapter 7). Although some ILDs are occasionally associated with bronchoscopically obvious airway abnormalities [e.g., sarcoidosis, lung cancer with lymphangitic spread, and Kaposi sarcoma in the human immunovirus–infected (HIV–infected)], most of them are not so. BAL, endobronchial biopsy, and transbronchial biopsy augment the simple visual inspection of bronchoscopy.

In BAL, sterile saline is instilled through the bronchoscope that has been gently wedged into a distal subsegmental bronchus. Typically, three 50-mL volumes of saline are sequentially infused and immediately aspirated back through a port in the bronchoscope. The initial fluid recovered is often referred to as the *bronchial fraction* and reflects processes occurring in airways just distal to the bronchoscope. Fluid recovered after the third instillation and aspiration is most representative of the alveolar compartment. This distinction becomes important in certain infections and in diseases such as diffuse alveolar hemorrhage, where progressively bloody return on sequential lavage indicates an alveolar capillary rather than the more common bronchial vascular source of bleeding (22). Alveolar macrophage recovery, detected cytologically, is a useful indicator of adequate sampling of the alveolar compartment. Adequate alveolar sampling is necessary to confidently exclude certain infections from consideration—particularly, *Pneumocystis carinii* (23). In general, bronchoalveolar fluid analysis in patients with ILD should include cell counts and differentials (with particular attention to eosinophilia); cytologic examination both for neoplasia and for microorganisms such as *P. carinii*; culture for bacterial, fungal, and mycobacterial pathogens; and assays for viral and other "atypical" pathogens such as *Mycoplasma pneumoniae*. Specific clinical concerns will warrant more specialized testing such as cytologic analysis for hemosiderin-containing alveolar macrophages in cases of suspected acute or chronic

alveolar hemorrhage; periodic acid–Schiff (PAS) staining of the proteinaceous debris and vacuolated alveolar macrophages from the opalescent, milky lavage fluid of pulmonary alveolar proteinosis; cultures for unusual viral pathogens; and, very rarely, flow-cytometric analysis of lymphocyte subsets in cases of suspected hypersensitivity pneumonitis, sarcoidosis, or lymphoid malignancy. Generally speaking, in cases of ILDs, BAL is substantially more useful in ruling out particular conditions like infection than in determining a specific noninfectious cause (7,24–30).

Bronchoscopic biopsies of either bronchial tissue (endobronchial biopsy) or more distal lung (transbronchial biopsy) are of limited utility in the evaluation of ILDs in general. The notable exception to this is sarcoidosis. In sarcoidosis, endobronchial biopsy has a sensitivity of up to 90% in cases when bronchial abnormalities are seen, and "blind" transbronchial biopsies have a sensitivity of 80% or greater in cases where no bronchial abnormalities are seen (31). Instead, surgical biopsies are preferable in most cases of ILD because the amount of tissue obtained is substantially larger, allowing a vastly improved visualization of the pattern and the nature of the pathologic abnormalities. Multiple well-designed studies from surgical centers throughout the world have shown conclusively that video-assisted thoracoscopic (VATS) biopsies are equivalent to open lung biopsies in diagnostic yield, with improved morbidity and mortality rates (32–36). As a result of these improvements, lung biopsies have become outpatient surgical procedures in some centers (37,38). Recent studies have shown that sampling multiple lobes increases both the diagnostic yield and prognostic utility of surgical lung biopsies (39,40).

Clinicopathologic Correlation in the Diagnosis of Interstitial Lung Diseases

A multidisciplinary collaboration is generally required prior to beginning therapy on any patient with ILD because of the complexity and the interrelatedness of both the clinical, radiographic, and pathologic manifestations of illness and the lack of a truly diagnostic "gold standard" for the final diagnosis in many cases (41,42). This approach has been incorporated into the recommendations of the American Thoracic Society/European Respiratory Society (ATS/ERS) in their consensus statement on idiopathic interstitial pneumonias (3). Such collaboration typically necessitates person-to-person real-time interaction between a radiologist with an interest in diseases of the chest, a consulting pulmonologist, and a pathologist with expertise in the interpretation of nonneoplastic lung pathology. Substantial motivation is required to develop, coordinate, and nurture such high-intensity multispecialty collaboration. However, ongoing studies suggest a significant incremental impact of the interaction of radiologists and pathologists with clinicians in establishing the working clinical diagnosis in these diseases. As noted in the ATS/ERS consensus statement, further revision and refinement of the "final" clinical diagnosis is expected as further history or laboratory studies are obtained from patients (3). As tempting as the pathologic or radiologic diagnosis is, the responsibility for determining the final diagnosis and the management falls squarely on the shoulders of the clinician, who must be familiar with the myriad radiographic and histopathologic patterns associated with each of these diseases.

IDIOPATHIC INTERSTITIAL PNEUMONIAS

ACUTE INTERSTITIAL PNEUMONIA

Pathogenesis and Epidemiology

The original description of acute interstitial pneumonia is attributed to Hamman and Rich, who described the disease as a fulminant, fatal form of interstitial pneumonia in which proliferating fibrotic tissue virtually occludes the peripheral airways (43). Although acute interstitial pneumonia is pathologically similar in many respects to organizing pneumonia (OP), its defining features are the presence of hyaline membranes and a rather briskly deteriorating clinical course. In Hamman and Rich's initial description of four patients, the diagnosis was made at autopsy. For many years, acute interstitial pneumonia was considered to be a form of IPF, but in the most recent classification scheme it has been clearly separated and is considered to be a distinct pathologic entity (3,44,45). This syndrome can most easily be summarized as adult respiratory distress syndrome (ARDS) presenting in the absence of known precipitants such as trauma, sepsis, massive burns, or bone marrow transplantation (3). Acute interstitial pneumonitis is relatively uncommon; however, precise prevalence figures are lacking because all reported case series are retrospective (43,44,46–50). Though there is a clinical impression that patients who have survived a prior episode of acute interstitial pneumonitis are prone to developing it again, published literature on this is also lacking. Suspicion remains high for an inciting viral etiology based on the prodrome reported by many patients. However, this prodrome may also reflect a systemic inflammatory response related to the underlying cryptogenic lung injury itself. The high prevalence of respiratory failure among those infected with the severe acute respiratory syndrome–coronavirus (SARS–CoV) and the pathologic findings from the lungs of these patients show some interesting parallels to acute interstitial pneumonia. Nevertheless, efforts to identify specific viral pathogens or clear patterns of infectious outbreaks in idiopathic acute interstitial pneumonia have so far been unsuccessful (51,52). Unlike SARS–CoV–infected patients, giant cells are not typical of late-stage acute interstitial pneumonitis (52). Acute interstitial pneumonia occurs over a large age range. The mean age of onset is approximately 50 years and it is rare under the age of 40 (43,44,46–50). The precise molecular mechanisms remain elusive. Notably, the pathologic features of lung injury and fibrosis following bleomycin administration in animal models of pulmonary fibrosis most closely resemble acute interstitial pneumonia, suggesting that widespread alveolar epithelial injury followed by exuberant repair is critical in the pathogenesis of acute interstitial pneumonia.

Clinical Presentation and Evaluation

Patients with acute interstitial pneumonia frequently report a viral prodrome of malaise, fever, and cough that precede the development of hypoxemic respiratory failure by a few days to a few weeks (43,44,46–50). Patients typically present with bilateral interstitial pulmonary infiltrates suggestive of pulmonary edema in the absence of evidence of congestive heart failure. Examination of the chest may reveal crackles. The remainder of the physical examination is generally unrevealing. Most patients eventually require mechanical ventilatory support (43,44,46–50). Cultures and other studies for active bacterial, viral, and opportunistic infections at the time of clinical presentation are negative by definition. Hypotension and other signs of shock are rare. Surgical lung biopsies are required to definitively confirm the diagnosis, although bronchoscopy with BAL is often performed initially to confirm the absence of underlying infection.

Radiographic Features

The principal findings on chest radiographs are bilateral diffuse infiltrates, generally without dense consolidation or air bronchograms. Chest HRCT shows extensive areas of ground-glass attenuation (see Fig. 12-1). Traction bronchiectasis, airspace consolidation, and architectural distortion are also common (53). The CT findings of significant architectural distortion with bronchiectasis in association with ground-glass opacities and consolidation appear to be more common in groups of patients with acute interstitial pneumonia as compared with those with ARDS. An abundance of structural distortion presages a poor clinical outcome (54,55), though there is substantial overlap and the predictive utility of this finding in individual patients is unclear (56). Adenopathy and pleural effusion are not typical in acute interstitial pneumonia.

Pathologic Features

The characteristic pathologic findings of acute interstitial pneumonia are best appreciated on a surgical lung biopsy. These findings include intraalveolar buds of loosely organized collections of fibroblasts, loose matrix, and capillaries that are similar to Masson bodies seen in OP. Both intraalveolar and

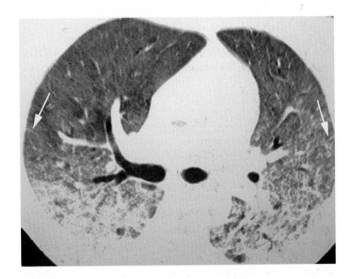

FIGURE 12-1. Acute interstitial pneumonia (Hamman–Rich syndrome). Axial high-resolution chest tomography (HRCT) image shows posterior predominant consolidation with multifocal ground-glass opacity anteriorly consistent with acute interstitial pneumonia. Minimal interlobular septal thickening (*arrows*) is present. The image quality is degraded by substantial motion artifact resulting from the patient's respiratory distress and rapid breathing.

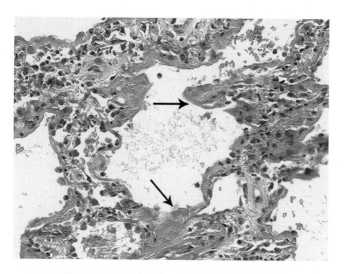

FIGURE 12-2. Acute interstitial pneumonia (Hamman–Rich syndrome). Surgical lung biopsy shows diffuse alveolar damage with sloughing of the epithelium lining and the alveolar space, exudation of proteinaceous fluid, and the formation of hyaline membranes (*arrows*) composed largely of fibrin. In later stages, these hyaline membranes are resorbed and are replaced with granulation tissue composed of proliferating fibroblasts, blood vessels, and provisional matrix that pathologically resemble the Masson body of cryptogenic organizing pneumonia (COP) (see Figure 12-10).

interstitial organizing connective tissue can be seen. Depending on the chronicity of the disease, intraalveolar eosinophilic fibrin deposition (hyaline membranes) will be more or less prominent (see Fig. 12-2). Type II alveolar epithelial cell hyperplasia is common later in the course of the disease. The proliferating connective tissue buds are generally of uniform age throughout the sample. Cytologic atypia of the Type II cells and mitogenic activity are also common. Microthrombi are also frequently seen (45). Dense collagen scar is generally not present. The specimen must be inspected carefully for viral inclusions, granulomas, necrosis, and polymorphonuclear leukocytic infiltrates that would each suggest underlying infection.

Treatment and Prognosis

The conventional therapy for acute interstitial pneumonia is high-dose corticosteroids. Generally, this means 2 mg per kg of methylprednisolone intravenously (or its equivalent) in 4 divided doses per day for 14 days followed by 7 days of 1 mg/kg/day in 2 divided doses followed by a 4-day taper. This regimen is based on the protocol developed as part of the National Institutes of Health–sponsored late steroid rescue study in ARDS (LaSRS trial), which has been reported to be successful in ARDS of greater than 1-week's duration (57,58). Also, by analogy to ARDS, a low tidal volume mechanical ventilation strategy of 6 mL per kg seems prudent in patients requiring support. Early reports of acute interstitial pneumonia emphasize a mortality rate exceeding 80%. More recent reviews suggest that the mortality may in fact be better than that of ARDS of known cause, with a retrospective mortality of 12.5% in acute interstitial pneumonia (50).

IDIOPATHIC PULMONARY FIBROSIS/USUAL INTERSTITIAL PNEUMONIA

Pathogenesis and Epidemiology

IPF is an uncommon chronic fibrotic ILD of unknown etiology. Despite several decades of intensive investigation, the pathogenesis of this disease remains unknown. Dysregulated apoptosis; abnormal fibroblast proliferation, differentiation, or synthetic function; fundamental alterations in extracellular matrix homeostasis; and a multitude of pro- and antiinflammatory mediators have all been variously invoked (59,60). No therapy has yet been devised that convincingly alters the clinical outcome of this disease.

Virtually all of the current data regarding the molecular pathogenesis of pulmonary fibrosis relies in one form or another on animal models that use bleomycin or other lung irritants to produce lung injury that is followed by fibrosis. This model was developed on the basis of observations of pulmonary fibrosis occurring in humans treated with bleomycin for malignancies. Pulmonary fibrosis was subsequently confirmed to occur in primates and in rodents exposed to bleomycin (61–77). Unfortunately, bleomycin-induced pulmonary fibrosis in most animal models relies first on the development of a sublethal acute lung injury followed by inflammation and subsequent repair. The comparability of these acute lung injury and repair models to human IPF remains an open question (78–80). Similarly, although many fundamental insights into the mechanisms underlying the initiation, maintenance, and resolution of pulmonary inflammation and repair have been gained using the bleomycin model, the precise connection of these inflammatory and noninflammatory pathways with the human disease remains speculative (59,81–104). Underlying genetic factors are also the subject of intense investigation, given the association of a usual interstitial pneumonia (UIP) histologic pattern with Hermansky–Pudlak albinism syndrome—for which many genes have been identified—and the recent association of mutations in the surfactant protein C gene and familial ILD of which some forms resemble UIP (105–107).

The incidence of IPF increases substantially with age. The prevalence among adults between the ages of 35 and 44 is 3 cases per 100,000 and increases to more than 175 cases per 100,000 in patients older than 75 (108,109). Factors associated with increased risk are male gender, smoking history, mining, residence in agricultural and polluted urban areas, and exposure to inhaled dust, solvents, livestock, and chemicals (109).

Clinical Presentation and Evaluation

The clinical presentation of IPF is characterized by cough and an insidious onset of progressive exertional breathlessness. Table 12-1 summarizes the clinical diagnostic criteria outlined in the recent American and European Consensus Statement (2,58,110). On average, 12 to 18 months elapse between the onset of dyspnea and its progression to the point of symptomatic breathlessness that is sufficient to bring the patient to medical attention (110,111). When noticeable dyspnea imposes physical limitation, other mild constitutional symptoms such as fatigue, poor appetite, and weight loss may be present. Fever is infrequent. Other respiratory symptoms such as pleurisy, chest pain, wheezing, or hemoptysis do not

TABLE 12-1. Clinical Diagnostic Criteria for Idiopathic Pulmonary Fibrosis

Major Criteria (All Four Required)

1. Exclusion of other known causes of interstitial lung disease (ILD) (associated drugs, environmental exposure, collagen vascular, or autoimmune diseases)
2. Abnormal pulmonary function studies (restrictive physiology) and impaired gas exchange (increased alveolar to arterial PO_2 difference at rest or with exercise; and decreased D_{LCO})
3. Bibasilar, reticular abnormalities with minimal ground-glass opacities on HRCT scans of the lungs
4. Transbronchial biopsy or bronchoalveolar lavage (BAL) showing no features to support an alternative diagnosis

Minor Criteria (Three of Four Required)

1. Age >50 yr
2. Insidious onset of otherwise unexplained dyspnea on exertion
3. Duration of illness >3 mo
4. Bibasilar, inspiratory crackles (dry or Velcro-type in quality)

From American Thoracic Society. Idiopathic pulmonary fibrosis: diagnosis and treatment. International Consensus Statement. *Am J Resp Crit Care Med* 2000;161:646–664, King TE Jr. Idiopathic interstitial pneumonia. In: Schwarz MI, King TE Jr., eds. *Interstitial lung diseases,* 4 ed. Hamilton, Ontario: B. C. Decker, 2003:701–786, and King TE Jr. Clinical features and differential diagnosis of IPF. In: Lynch JP III, ed. *Idiopathic pulmonary fibrosis.* New York: Marcel Dekker Inc, 2004:55–80, with permission.

usually occur. Patients may have an occupational history that includes exposure to one or a variety of toxic inhalation products, and this may add uncertainty to the precise time of disease onset and may suggest the contribution of other etiologic factors. A detailed work history, including each job dating back even to summer employment during school, is essential. Casual exposure to asbestos decades ago may provide a crucial link. Some will describe the onset of their breathlessness as coinciding with a viral syndrome. However, no clear viral etiologies have yet been established despite ongoing, active investigation (92).

Physical examination of a patient with IPF reveals crackles or rales on auscultation of chest in most. Vivid adjectives have been used to describe these lung sounds—"Velcro," crackling or cellophane paper, or "close to the ear." Other findings may include tachypnea at rest (50% of patients), finger clubbing (70%), and an ability to speak only a few words before being interrupted with breathlessness or cough (110,112). Pulmonary artery hypertension and right heart failure are noted as late complications in many patients (60% to 70%). They manifest as an augmented pulmonic second heart sound, a parasternal lift, and an S_3 gallop and peripheral signs of heart failure. Right ventricular ejection fraction is often depressed, although left ventricular function is typically preserved. Except for clubbing and evidence of heart failure, physical signs are limited to the chest, and other organ systems are not prominently involved.

Although the history and physical examination findings in IPF may be subtle, the physiologic derangements typically are not so. Resting arterial hypoxemia is relatively common but correlates poorly with stage—particularly early in the course

of disease. Hypoxemia is uniformly worsened by exertion (21). The alveolar–arterial oxygen difference [$P(A–a)O_2$] at rest and with exercise is elevated in virtually all patients. Resting arterial carbon dioxide tension (PCO_2) is characteristically normal or low, reflecting normal or slightly increased minute ventilation. Lung function tests reflect a pattern of restriction with a reduced TLC and reduced RV. FEV_1 and FVC are also typically reduced with an increased ratio of FEV_1 to FVC. In patients with a heavy smoking history, the restriction may be less pronounced because of coexistent emphysema. This "double whammy" is usually associated with an extremely reduced diffusing capacity. The rate and direction of change in patients' pulmonary function studies and performance on a standard 6-minute walk test during 6- and 12-month follow-up add substantial prognostic power to baseline physiologic measurements (111,113–118).

No blood test is diagnostic of IPF; however, serologic studies should be done in suspected patients primarily to rule out other coexisting diseases. Although serum rheumatoid factor, antinuclear antibodies, and autoimmune parameters can be detected in a minority of patients with IPF (10% to 20%), the titers are low. High levels suggest an occult collagen vascular disease. Pulmonary manifestations of autoimmune disease may precede the other defining clinical features of collagen vascular disease. However, patients with underlying connective tissue disease will typically note some suggestive premonitory syndromes such as symmetric inflammatory arthritis (rheumatoid arthritis), rashes (dermatomyositis), or muscle weakness (polymyositis), thus limiting ongoing clinical confusion to a few select cases (119).

Radiographic Features

Chest radiographs are abnormal in 90% of patients with IPF (see Fig. 12-3). A pattern of alveolar filling may evolve into reticular (linear) densities involving the peripheral (subpleural) and

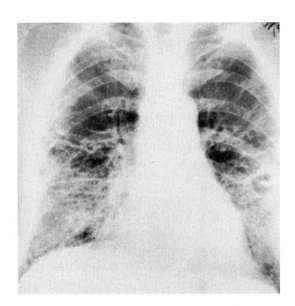

FIGURE 12-3. Idiopathic pulmonary fibrosis (IPF). Posteroanterior (PA) chest radiograph of a 71-year-old man with end-stage pulmonary fibrosis. There are diffuse, bilateral interstitial infiltrates with small cystic spaces within the infiltrates suggesting honeycombing.

basilar regions of the lung, producing distinctive but nondiagnostic chest radiographs. Lung volumes typically become obviously smaller on serial examinations. Pleural effusions and intrathoracic lymphadenopathy suggest alternative diagnoses such as malignancy, infection, or congestive heart failure. HRCT is superior to the conventional chest radiograph or CT in evaluating IPF (see Fig. 12-4) (13). Subpleural, basilar predominant, pallisading, 3 to 15 mm, thin-walled, air-filled cystic spaces referred to as *honeycombing* are strongly correlated with a pathologic diagnosis of UIP—the pathologic correlate of IPF (see Fig. 12-5). Reticular changes correlating with fibrosis and cystic changes of traction bronchiectasis can be seen in other regions as well. The HRCT findings can be highly distinctive for IPF and under certain circumstances can obviate the need for lung biopsy (17,120,121). Extensive honeycombing is associated with a poor prognosis (111,120,122,123).

Pathologic Features

The pathologic correlate of IPF is UIP (see Fig. 12-6). The characteristic histopathologic findings are subpleural areas of dense collagen scar abutting histologically normal lung with abundant interstitial fibroblastic foci and a relatively minor inflammatory component (2,45,124–126). Ultrastructural studies show substantial underlying epithelial injury (127). Perhaps the most characteristic aspect of UIP is its patchy nature. Considerable distortion of lung architecture occurs with thickening of alveolar septa and with formation of cystic spaces in the parenchyma. Additional features of advanced disease include type II pneumocyte proliferation and hyperplasia, traction bronchiolectasis, smooth muscle hypertrophy, and "muscularization" of pulmonary arteries. Pathologically, the distinction

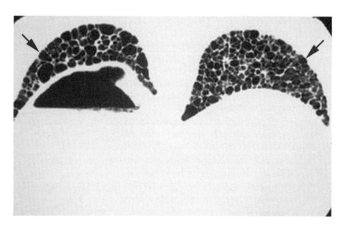

FIGURE 12-5. Idiopathic pulmonary fibrosis (IPF). Axial prone high-resolution computed tomography (HRCT) image shows extensive basilar subpleural honeycomb cysts (*arrows*) consistent with the histopathologic diagnosis of usual interstitial pneumonia.

between UIP and other forms of fibrosing interstitial diseases like nonspecific interstitial pneumonia (NSIP), COP, and ILD secondary to autoimmune collagen vascular disease is both important and challenging (39,104,111,115–117,126,128–134). Recent data suggest that substantial heterogeneity may exist within the lungs of a single patient with inflammatory changes consistent with NSIP (see section on nonspecific interstitial pneumonia) in one region and with histologic features diagnostic of UIP in others. Mortality in this group parallels that of patients with UIP in both lobes, thus the patient's prognosis is best predicted by the presence of UIP in any biopsied region (39,40).

Treatment and Prognosis

In virtually all cases, treatment should not be considered until a final diagnosis can be rendered with reasonable confidence

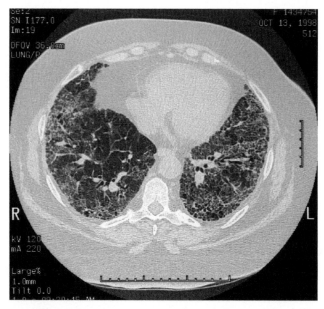

FIGURE 12-4. Idiopathic pulmonary fibrosis (IPF). High-resolution chest computed tomography (chest HRCT) of a 58-year-old woman with end-stage disease. The subpleural honeycomb changes, traction bronchiolectasis, and thickened interlobular septae are characteristic features.

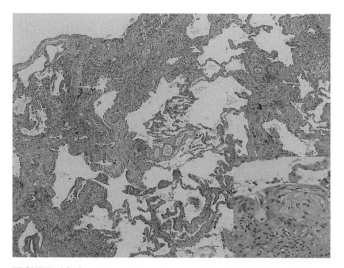

FIGURE 12-6. Idiopathic pulmonary fibrosis (IPF). Surgical lung biopsy shows usual interstitial pneumonia pathologically. Note the pleural-based fibrosis, alternating normal lung with dense scar, and relatively little inflammation. Interstitial fibroblast foci (*inset*) are interposed between these regions.

on the basis of the patient's history, physical examination, laboratory and radiologic studies, and, in most cases, a surgical lung biopsy. A decision not to pursue an adequate lung tissue biopsy to avoid the unpleasantness of chest surgery or thoracoscopic biopsy and instead to give the patient an empiric trial of corticosteroid therapy is generally ill-advised for several reasons. First, the toxicities of high-dose corticosteroid therapy alone, or in combination with another immunosuppressive agent, are not trivial. Secondly, a substantial number of patients with "steroid-responsive" ILDs such as sarcoidosis, cellular NSIP, COP, and some connective tissue disease–associated ILDs will require intensification of therapy with high-dose corticosteroids or cytotoxic therapy before a complete clinical response is seen. Such intensification of therapy is quite discomforting without having first undertaken a meticulous pretreatment evaluation, including a lung biopsy. Thirdly, IPF carries a 3-year mortality of approximately 50% from the time of diagnosis, similar, as should be noted, to Stage II non–small cell lung cancer, New York Heart Association (NYHA) Class II and III heart failure, and untreated acquired immunodeficiency syndrome (AIDS) from the time the peripheral blood CD4$^+$ lymphocyte count reaches 200 cells per mm^3 (135–137). These survival data stand in stark contrast to the 3- and 10-year survival rates in most other forms of chronic ILD with treatment. Therefore, in most circumstances, it is helpful for the patient and for the physician to be certain of the diagnosis for a more rapid consideration of lung transplantation in those who are otherwise eligible (e.g., age <65 years with no other serious or uncontrolled comorbid diseases), enrollment in a growing number of clinical trials, and for the purposes of appropriate prognostication.

Corticosteroids have been the mainstay of therapy for IPF for many years and still figure prominently in consensus treatment recommendations despite the lack of appropriate randomized, double-blind, placebo-controlled clinical trials (2,138). These consensus recommendations are based on data from studies prior to development of the current classification scheme, which showed that 10% to 30% of patients with IPF improved when treated with corticosteroids (2,139–142). However, retrospective analysis using the current classification scheme and separating patients with idiopathic interstitial pneumonias into IPF, NSIP, and others provides a strong suggestion that the "steroid-responders" in earlier trials would, by current standards, be classified as having NSIP or other histopathologic processes and not as having UIP characteristic of IPF (122,126,143–145). Nevertheless, because the natural course of IPF is an inexorable deterioration, many patients are "given the benefit of the doubt" and are offered a time-limited trial of immunosuppressive therapy in the hopes of realizing a measurable clinical improvement or a stabilization of pulmonary function.

The response to existing therapies is poor, and toxicities can be considerable; therefore, therapy must be individualized. Extremely high doses of corticosteroids have been advocated in the past, but more recent studies have suggested no advantage of high doses versus more moderate doses (146,147). The currently recommended approach to treatment—if treatment outside of a clinical trial is elected at all—is to institute prednisone at 40 to 60 mg daily (0.5 mg per kg) for 2 to 3 months along with a second steroid-sparing agent such as azathioprine

or cyclophosphamide (see below). Because of the substantially more favorable side-effect profile, azathioprine is generally preferred as the first adjunctive agent. The best methods for assessing response to therapy have not been definitively established, but recent data suggests that serial pulmonary function testing including D$_{LCO}$, serial 6-minute walk tests with attention to distance achieved and exercise-induced arterial oxygen desaturation, and room air blood gas analysis with monitoring of the alveolar–arterial oxygen difference at rest are most informative (111,113–118). Repeated imaging studies do not add significantly to the prognostication based on physiologic parameters (115).

Following a 2- to 3-month trial of therapy, prednisone should be tapered by 2.5 to 5 mg every 2 weeks until a dose of 15 to 30 mg is reached. These doses should be continued for an additional 6 months if the patient has shown some improvement. Some flexibility can be exercised in tailoring the maintenance therapy, and an alternate-day dose may be used if corticosteroid side effects are a significant management problem (2). In the absence of a response, steroids should be tapered more quickly to avoid side effects. Patients should receive preventative therapy against osteoporosis and dietary discretion should be encouraged to prevent excessive weight gain.

The use of adjunctive immunosuppressive agents in addition to prednisone for "steroid-sparing effect" is controversial. Although the use of these agents is advocated by many and is ensconced in current practice guidelines, clinical trials examining their efficacy are of generally poor quality and the effects that are reported are minor (2,148,149). Azathioprine is the least toxic of the cytotoxic immunosuppressive agents and there is some data to support modest efficacy (150–152). No direct studies have compared azathioprine to cyclophosphamide—the other cytotoxic agent often considered for treatment of IPF. Penicillamine and colchicine have been used as antifibrotic agents but results have been generally disappointing (153,154).

Several other agents are under active investigation. A recent study suggested a possible role for the antifibrotic agent perfenidone in patients with advanced IPF, but larger prospective studies are required to assess the efficacy of this new approach (155,156). Interest is also increasing for the therapeutic use of the antioxidant *N*-acetyl cysteine (NAC) on the basis of its tolerability and evidence of its efficacy in both animal models of pulmonary fibrosis and in small, nonrandomized clinical studies (88,157–160).

Cyclophosphamide, an alkylating drug, is a potent immunosuppressant that has been advocated by some as being effective in patients who are not controlled with corticosteroids (2,161,162). However, based on our current understanding of IPF, it is probably inappropriate for the vast majority of patients because there is considerable short-term and long-term toxicity without convincing evidence of a sustained improvement in outcome (149). Perhaps the most convincing data for the failure of immunosuppressive therapy, in general, for patients with IPF is from single lung transplant recipients, which shows progression of disease in the nontransplanted lung despite fairly intense immunosuppression (163). Single lung transplantation is the most definitive treatment option for patients failing medical therapy. Two-year survival following single lung transplantation approaches 70% and 5-year survival approaches 50%.

Survival following transplantation is substantially improved in younger patients and, in general, transplantation is not an option for patients older than 65 years (164–170).

Although patients can have relatively normal oxygen saturation at rest, with exercise there is frequently a marked drop in arterial oxygen tension (PaO_2). Therefore, exercise tolerance may be significantly improved with supplemental oxygen therapy. When oxygen requirements are high (more than 4 L per minute flow), direct administration of oxygen in the trachea may be preferred. Several modes of transtracheal catheter oxygen delivery are available (171). In addition to attaining a high local concentration of oxygen in the lungs, the cosmetic effect of not wearing obvious nasal prongs can be important.

As the pulmonary vascular bed is impaired by progressive fibrosis, pulmonary hypertension and cor pulmonale can develop. A recent study showed modest short-term (2.5 hour) improvement in pulmonary vascular resistance and in systemic oxygenation in patients with pulmonary hypertension due to pulmonary fibrosis who were given a single dose of 50 mg of sildenafil (172). No long-term data has been published. Currently, prospective, randomized, double-blind, placebo-controlled trials are under way to assess the therapeutic role of the oral endothelin-1 antagonist bosentan in this disease (173).

Some patients may also develop obstruction to airflow and may be troubled with wheezing and coughing that may respond to bronchodilators. As infection may occur during immunosuppressive therapy, it is important to maintain a high index of suspicion and to treat infection aggressively. Prophylactic use of pneumococcal and influenza vaccines is encouraged. Prophylaxis against *P. carinii* pneumonia is also advisable in patients on high-dose corticosteroids or on combination therapy with prednisone and another immunosuppressive agent.

Patients diagnosed with IPF currently face a rather grim reality and are extremely dependent upon their physicians to help them make the best of an extremely difficult situation. Pulmonary rehabilitation is certainly appropriate to minimize muscle and bone loss due to deconditioning and corticosteroid therapy. It improves subjective dyspnea, provides patients with an improved sense of control, and should be considered at an early stage—even at the time of initial diagnosis (174). Patients should also be counseled to stop smoking cigarettes, if necessary. Cough and dyspnea often become extremely refractory to therapy later in the course of the disease and narcotics should not be withheld. Clinicians should be candid about the prognosis of UIP and about the life-limiting nature of the diagnosis—even with therapy. Ongoing support to both the patient and the family, with open and frequent discussions concerning end-of-life care is appropriate. The vast majority of patients succumb to respiratory failure. Other causes of death include pulmonary emboli, cardiovascular disease, and infection. Lung cancer complicates IPF in up to 10% of patients (109,175,176). Intubation and mechanical ventilation for patients with advanced pulmonary fibrosis and superimposed acute respiratory failure is generally not indicated (177,178).

On a more hopeful note, both patients and clinicians should be somewhat encouraged by two facts. First, worldwide research interest in this disease at both a clinical and a molecular level has never been more intense. Secondly, pulmonary fibrosis has finally captured the attention of the pharmaceutical industry, meaning that new drugs and approaches to therapy are coming along rapidly. Although initial reports of a general beneficial effect of interferon-γ in pulmonary fibrosis were not borne out in a recently published prospective, randomized, double-blind, placebo-controlled trial (179,180), another trial is now under way assessing its efficacy in patients with less advanced disease. Clinicians caring for patients with IPF are strongly advised stay abreast of other ongoing clinical trials (*www.clinicaltrials.gov*) because many additional compounds are currently in various stages of clinical development and are aimed at interrupting the fibrotic process itself. These include a tyrosine kinase inhibitor directed at platelet-derived growth factor (PDGF) signaling, an inhibitor of tumor necrosis factor-α (TNF-α), and an inhibitor of connective tissue growth factor (CTGF). The Coalition for Pulmonary Fibrosis, a nonprofit patient support organization, maintains an updated list of ongoing clinical trials and educational materials for patients and clinicians.

NONSPECIFIC INTERSTITIAL PNEUMONIA

Pathogenesis and Epidemiology

In 1994, Katzenstein and Fiorelli described 64 cases of then unclassifiable interstitial pneumonia (181). They noted that the pathologic specimens revealed temporally homogeneous interstitial inflammation and fibrosis and that clinical outcomes appeared substantially better than those with UIP. They proposed that the term NSIP be applied to this entity, and this terminology was subsequently adopted by the ATS/ERS consensus classification (3). In the 10 years following this initial description, a deluge of manuscripts and chapters (more than 300 to date) have been published incorporating this term into the discussion of idiopathic interstitial pneumonia—excluding those using this term in the HIV–infected patient. This impressive prolificity is testament to the importance and utility of distinguishing this subtype of idiopathic interstitial pneumonia from the "bad actor," UIP.

In the 10 years since its clear delineation from the other forms of interstitial pneumonia, several points have been clearly made. First and foremost, like all pathologic diagnoses, NSIP is a pattern of lung response to a multitude of injuries—some currently known and probably many unknown. Diseases associated with NSIP include connective tissue diseases such as scleroderma (182,183), rheumatoid arthritis (133), and polymyositis-dermatomyositis (PM-DM) (182,184,185); pulmonary hypersensitivity responses to exogenous environmental agents (181,186); and drug-induced lung disease (4,187). Both the precise incidence and the prevalence of NSIP are unknown, though recent reviews and clinical experience suggest that it is a common cause of idiopathic interstitial pneumonia (188,189).

Clinical Presentation and Evaluation

In general, the clinical presentation and clinical evaluation of patients ultimately diagnosed as having NSIP is identical to that of patients with UIP or with suspected ILD. Given recent data showing that chest HRCT patterns have a high specificity and positive predictive value in predicting pathologic UIP, an increasing percentage of surgical lung biopsies can be expected to show other forms of idiopathic interstitial pneumonia such as NSIP (17,121). As of yet, no clinical characteristics—other than, perhaps, symptoms suggestive of an underlying connective tissue disease—are discriminatory.

Radiographic Features

The plain chest radiographic findings of NSIP are no different from any other interstitial pneumonias. Diffuse, symmetric interstitial peripheral reticular opacities predominate with low lung volumes, no adenopathy, and no pleural effusions or thickening. Volume loss is diffuse rather than focal and cystic changes are inconspicuous or entirely absent. The HRCT findings are characteristically those of ground-glass opacity, with a varying degree of structural distortion and reticulation suggestive of underlying fibrosis (see Fig. 12-7). Although patchy consolidation can mimic pneumonia, air bronchograms are typically absent in simple NSIP.

Pathologic Features

NSIP is characterized by varying degrees of inflammation and fibrosis that appear to be temporally related. That is, the strikingly patchy nature of UIP, with areas of extensive fibrosis abutting areas of normal lung, is not as pronounced. Foci of bronchiolitis obliterans with OP, denoting a tissue response to injury, are observed more frequently in NSIP than in UIP. NSIP is separated into three histologic subtypes: cellular (also called Type I), fibrosing (Type III), and mixed (Type II). Cellular NSIP shows diffuse mononuclear inflammatory cell infiltration—principally lymphocytes—that results in diffuse interstitial thickening without conspicuous collagen deposition (see Fig. 12-8). Fibrotic NSIP shows a similar, homogeneous alveolar septal thickening with a less striking inflammatory cell component and a more prominent fibroblastic proliferation and collagen deposition. Dense collagen scar is absent as is marked temporal heterogeneity. Fibroblastic foci are generally absent in cellular NSIP and less marked in fibrotic NSIP than in typical UIP (45,181).

Treatment and Prognosis

Because NSIP has only recently been separated clinically and pathologically from other forms of idiopathic interstitial pneumonia, no prospective studies are available to assess the efficacy of various therapies. Nevertheless, multiple studies using retrospective reclassifications of banked lung biopsies have shown that patients whose biopsies would be classified as NSIP by current classification standards have a substantially better survival than patients whose biopsies would be classified as UIP (126, 128,143–145,190–192). Further subdivision of cellular and fibrotic NSIP suggests that patients with cellular NSIP have a substantially improved survival compared to those with fibrotic NSIP and those with UIP (126,128,143–145,190–192). In these studies, which have followed patients with idiopathic interstitial pneumonia prospectively, large proportions of patients have been treated with corticosteroids and adjunctive immunosuppressive therapy, thus raising the possibility that these agents may have been important in the improved survival observed in these patients. Further, retrospective review of pathologic specimens of "responders" from prior trials of immunosuppressives in idiopathic interstitial pneumonias suggests that these patients would now be classified as having NSIP rather than UIP. In general, the recognition of NSIP as the underlying pathologic process in a patient with idiopathic interstitial pneumonia is a beginning rather than an end because NSIP can be a pathologic manifestation of a range of underlying diseases including hypersensitivity pneumonitis, collagen vascular disease, drug-induced lung disease, or it may be idiopathic—as emphasized in Kazenstein and Fiorelli's original description (181). Therefore, recognition of the underlying precipitant—particularly if NSIP is a response to an ongoing irritant, as in drug-induced lung

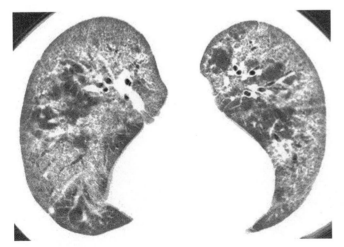

FIGURE 12-7. Nonspecific interstitial pneumonia (NSIP). Axial high-resolution computed tomography (HRCT) image taken with the patient in the prone position shows bilateral diffuse ground-glass opacities with relative subpleural sparing. There is no subpleural honeycomb-cyst formation.

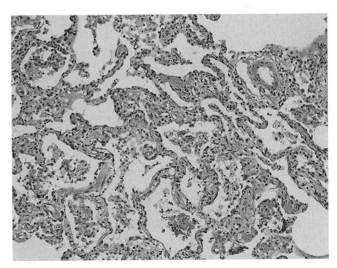

FIGURE 12-8. Nonspecific interstitial pneumonia (NSIP) cellular pattern (Type I). This surgical lung biopsy shows mild to moderate mononuclear cell infiltrate diffusely along septae without significant fibrosis.

disease or in hypersensitivity pneumonitis—is the single most important therapeutic intervention. On the basis of retrospective analysis, an underlying etiology is found in approximately 50% of patients with NSIP (190,193).

CRYPTOGENIC ORGANIZING PNEUMONIA

Pathogenesis and Epidemiology

OP is a pathologic process that follows a variety of pulmonary insults including bacterial pneumonia and acute lung injury. When the inciting event that caused the OP is unknown, or is cryptogenic, the syndrome is referred to as COP, a disease entity recognized only relatively recently (194,195). Though this disease was previously referred to as a bronchiolitis obliterans organizing pneumonia (BOOP), the most recent consensus conference has adopted the term COP to describe this entity (3,195). The disease is defined histologically by finding polypoid masses of granulation tissue in lumens of small airways, alveolar ducts, and some alveoli. These structures are referred to by some as *Masson bodies*. The pathogenesis of this syndrome is unknown but is thought to reflect the normal healing process of the lung following an injury that fails to resolve normally in some patients. The precise incidence of the disease is unknown (3). The mean age of onset is 55 years and there is an equal sex distribution, though the ratio of nonsmokers to smokers is 2:1 (196,197).

Clinical Presentation and Evaluation

The classic presentation of COP is similar to that of an infectious pneumonia that fails to respond to antibiotics. The course is usually subacute, developing over 2 weeks to 6 months. Half of patients with COP have detectable crackles on auscultation. Laboratory testing is nonspecific. Both the white blood cell count and erythrocyte sedimentation rate are elevated in most patients. Pulmonary function testing shows a restrictive ventilatory defect with reduced DLCO. This, along with the presence of alveolar filling opacities on imaging studies, differentiates COP from constrictive bronchiolitis and bronchiolitis obliterans, a complication of transplantation. Both constrictive bronchiolitis and bronchiolitis obliterans show obstructive ventilatory defects unresponsive to bronchodilators. A tissue diagnosis should be obtained and transbronchial biopsies may occasionally provide adequate tissue to secure the diagnosis (see below). However, if transbronchial biopsies are insufficient, as is typical, a surgical lung biopsy is the indicated procedure.

Radiographic Features

The chest radiograph can have a variety of manifestations, but the most frequent findings are patchy, hazy, peripheral infiltrates. Involvement may be unilateral or bilateral. Infiltrates may be fleeting and may resolve spontaneously. Therefore, the response of infiltrates to antibiotic therapy or to corticosteroid therapy may be difficult to assess except as they recur over time. COP can occasionally be confused with IPF because 20% to 30% of patients can present with bilateral lower lung zone reticular infiltrates. Pleural effusions are not characteristic of COP. The HRCT can be helpful in the evaluation of the infiltrates when a peripheral pattern of persistent multifocal infiltrates is observed (see Fig. 12-9) (198,199). Though COP may be confused with IPF, IPF has a poorer prognosis and does not respond in most cases to corticosteroids (195,200–203). Bronchioloalveolar carcinoma with lepedic spread should also be considered in the radiologic differential diagnosis. The honeycomb cysts that are characteristic of UIP and some forms of NSIP are not generally seen in COP (190). Importantly, OP is a pathologic diagnosis that can be seen in a number of clinical settings such as in connective tissue disease, in bone marrow and solid organ transplantation, following toxic fume exposure, and in the setting of chemotherapy or in infections such as *Legionella*. The pathologic identification of OP must be placed in the appropriate clinical setting. When no apparent cause is identified, the diagnosis is COP (3,203).

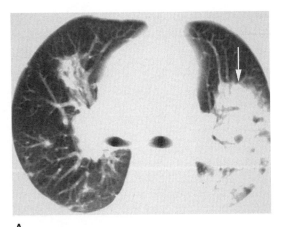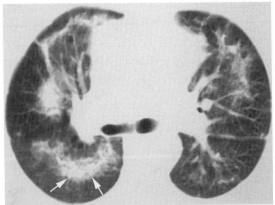

FIGURE 12-9. Migratory cryptogenic organizing pneumonia (COP). **A:** Axial computed tomography (CT) image at presentation shows bilateral consolidation, especially within the left lung (*arrow*). **B:** Axial high-resolution computed tomographic (HRCT) image 9 months after presentation shows that the left lower lobe consolidation has largely resolved and that peripheral right lower lobe consolidation (*small arrows*) has developed.

Pathologic Features

The pathologic findings of OP are an exuberant inflammatory response involving the terminal and respiratory bronchioles with extension of the tissue reaction into adjacent alveolar ducts. This is also referred to by some as proliferative bronchiolitis (204,205). The intraalveolar polypoid tufts are composed of loose, highly vascularized, myxoid connective tissue and proliferating fibroblasts resembling the granulation tissue found following severe epithelial injury elsewhere. These "Masson bodies" are conspicuous but not specific for COP (see Fig. 12-10). They are also commonly seen in ILD associated with an underlying connective tissue disease, in acute interstitial pneumonia, and in hypersensitivity pneumonia (45,206).

Treatment and Prognosis

Corticosteroid treatment is generally efficacious and approximately two-thirds of patients respond successfully to treatment with complete clinical and radiographic resolution (195,203). Spontaneous improvements have also been reported (195). Therapy should be initiated with prednisone at 1 mg/kg/day for at least 2 weeks. Treatment can be quite prolonged lasting 6 weeks to 30 months (203). Though patients may note improvement within the first week, slower response rates are also encountered frequently. The rate of tapering of prednisone is dictated by the radiographic response in accord with toxicities. Relapse is relatively frequent, occurring in nearly 50% of patients (207,208). Patients in whom OP is secondary to another underlying disease and in whom treatment is delayed appear to be particularly prone to relapse (207,208). A minority of patients (3% to 10%) may progress despite corticosteroids. Cytotoxic therapy should be considered early if there is a failure to resolve with corticosteroids.

RESPIRATORY BRONCHIOLITIS/DESQUAMATIVE INTERSTITIAL PNEUMONIA

Pathogenesis and Epidemiology

RB and desquamative interstitial pneumonia (DIP) are currently conceived as opposite extremes of smoking-related ILD (exclusive of emphysema and chronic bronchitis). RB is a relatively recently recognized clinical and pathologic entity

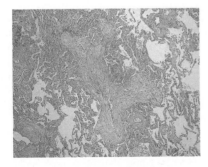

FIGURE 12-10. Cryptogenic organizing pneumonia (COP). Surgical lung biopsy shows extensive mononuclear cell interstitial inflammatory infiltration with a prominent intraalveolar bud of granulation tissue extending into the respiratory bronchioles. This loose assembly of connective tissue can resolve entirely with treatment in contrast to the dense collagenous scar observed in idiopathic pulmonary fibrosis.

(209,210). Initially described as an incidental finding at autopsy in the lungs of smokers, it is increasingly implicated as a cause of symptomatic breathlessness, particularly when it evolves into the more flagrant RB–ILD and its compatriot, DIP (211,212). Like most ILDs, the pathogenesis of this disorder is unknown. The typical age of onset is in the fourth or fifth decade in patients with an average cigarette exposure of 30 pack years or greater (212). The relationship between RB, RB–ILD, and DIP and the classic smoking-related lung diseases such as pulmonary emphysema, chronic bronchitis, and bronchogenic carcinoma remains unclear.

Clinical Presentation and Evaluation

Constitutional symptoms are not typically seen with RB, RB–ILD, or DIP. Patients usually have a near-normal physical examination even with a rather advanced disease state; faint inspiratory crackles occur in only about 50% of patients and clubbing is seen almost exclusively with DIP (210–212). Though patients with pure RB are typically not hypoxemic, patients with RB–ILD or DIP are more commonly so (211,212). Pulmonary function tests reveal a restrictive pattern with reduced D$_{LCO}$ in DIP, whereas in RB and RB–ILD, a mixed obstructive and restrictive defect is more common.

Radiographic Features

The chest radiograph demonstrates bibasilar reticulonodular infiltrates, although it may be normal. HRCT is critical to the diagnosis. The findings are fine peribronchiolar nodules (2 to 3 mm) and patchy ground-glass infiltrates. The subpleural honeycombing and traction bronchiectasis of IPF are not seen. Centrilobular emphysema is common, principally in the upper lobes (212). In RB, the fine—even subtle—nodular densities predominate, whereas in DIP, patchy or diffuse ground-glass opacities are the predominant finding.

Pathologic Features

Lung biopsy is required for a definite diagnosis and shows lightly pigmented macrophages filling the terminal and respiratory bronchioles. Although intraalveolar accumulations of macrophages are common in other ILD (so-called DIP-like reaction), in true DIP, on initial inspection, the alveolar architecture is nearly obscured by the exuberant macrophage infiltration (see Fig. 12-11). Although the interstitium may be modestly and diffusely thickened, this is due primarily to inflammatory cell accumulation rather than fibrosis (45). Fibroblastic foci are inconspicuous or absent altogether (45).

Treatment and Prognosis

The prognosis is generally good in patients who avoid exposure to tobacco smoke (211,213,214). Corticosteroids are generally employed with good results in patients with persistent symptoms despite cessation of smoking (142,215). Approximately 70% of patients survive ten years or longer (3). Of note, another pathologic entity also referred to as DIP occurs in children as a heritable form of ILD. This has recently been associated with mutations in the surfactant protein C gene (105–107). Family members of affected children appear to have a higher

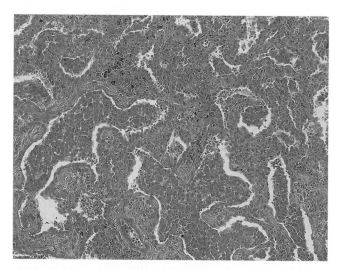

FIGURE 12-11. Desquamative interstitial pneumonia. Surgical lung biopsy shows complete filling of alveolar spaces with lightly pigmented alveolar macrophages. The interstitium is diffusely mildly thickened with a mononuclear cell inflammatory infiltrate. No fibroblastic foci are evident and the biopsy is temporally homogeneous.

incidence of other ILDs including pulmonary fibrosis and NSIP (105–107). The pediatric form of the disease is clinically distinct and relatively refractory to therapy (106).

LYMPHOCYTIC INTERSTITIAL PNEUMONIA

Pathogenesis and Epidemiology

Lymphocytic interstitial pneumonia (LIP) is rare and is unlike the other forms of idiopathic interstitial pneumonias in that in apparently all cases it is a primary disorder of lymphoid tissue proliferation and is part of a spectrum of disease that includes follicular bronchitis/bronchiolitis, nodular lymphoid hyperplasia, and low-grade malignant lymphoma (216,217). It has remained part of the classification scheme of idiopathic interstitial pneumonias both for historic reasons—because it was included in the original classification scheme introduced by Liebow and Carrington in 1969 (218)—and because its clinical presentation is that of an ILD (3). LIP occurs most commonly as a consequence of an underlying autoimmune disease—typically Sjögren syndrome, systemic lupus erythematosus (SLE), or rheumatoid arthritis—or in the setting of an underlying immunodeficiency disorder such as HIV infection or common variable immunodeficiency (217). It is rarely idiopathic, and in those situations, concern for underlying malignant lymphoma should remain high and clonality analysis using immunohistochemical, flow-cytometric, and molecular studies should be appropriate (3,217). Lymphoma can also occur in the setting of an underlying disease. This is particularly well documented in long-standing Sjögren syndrome, though its incidence appears to be below 1% (219–221).

Clinical Presentation and Evaluation

Patients with LIP typically present with the subacute onset of exertional breathlessness and dry cough in the absence of constitutional symptoms. Most patients are women between 40 and 70 years (217). Physical examination is generally normal except for the stigmata of underlying disease or subtle bibasilar inspiratory crackles. Generally speaking, patients with secondary LIP have had a long-standing primary disease, though it can be the initial presentation of common variable immunodeficiency syndrome. Therefore, checking immunoglobulin levels and subtypes is appropriate in all patients. Also, LIP can present as part of a dysproteinemia syndrome. Similarly, HIV testing in all patients is essential, though the HIV-associated variant is typically seen in children in whom it is part of the case definition of AIDS (217). Not surprisingly, pulmonary function findings are those of restrictive physiology with reduced DLCO (217).

Radiographic Features

Chest radiographs in LIP demonstrate bilateral reticulonodular infiltrates in most cases, but mixed alveolar filling patterns can also be seen. CT scan shows diffuse ground-glass attenuation, sometimes with a vaguely nodular appearance. The classic honeycomb changes of IPF are not seen; however, cystic airspace dilation can develop as a late complication (222). In addition, bronchovascular, interstitial, and interlobular septal thickening occur, as does lymphadenopathy (222).

Pathologic Features

Diffuse interstitial lymphoid infiltration is the hallmark of LIP. This infiltrate is manifested both as isolated lymphocytes percolating through the septae and, more strikingly, with the prolific formation of lymphoid aggregates often with germinal centers reminiscent of lymph node or spleen. This should be distinguished clearly from cellular NSIP in which interstitial mononuclear cells predominate but in which lymphoid aggregates are relatively sparse. The distinction between connective-tissue disease–associated ILD and LIP can be more difficult. In fact, in many cases this probably represents a distinction without a difference. Similarly, noncaseating granulomas may be seen, raising the possibility of hypersensitivity pneumonitis. As such, clinical diligence and ongoing healthy diagnostic skepticism should be maintained in both the initial workup and clinical follow-up of patients with these pathologic findings (217).

Treatment and Prognosis

The natural history of LIP is variable but generally less progressive than IPF. Lymphomas, when they develop, are low-grade marginal B-cell lymphomas (so-called MALT-omas or lymphomas of mucosa-associated lymphoid tissue). Mortality exceeds 30% in 5 years in LIP. Death occurs more commonly as a result of infectious complications, although respiratory failure can occur. Corticosteroids are considered the first line of therapy even in HIV-related cases, although dramatic improvement following institution of highly active antiretroviral therapy (HAART) has also been reported (217,223,224). Intravenous immunoglobulin therapy is indicated in patients with common variable immunodeficiency. The role of anti–B-cell therapy has not yet been evaluated in refractory forms of this disease.

NONINFECTIOUS GRANULOMATOUS INTERSTITIAL LUNG DISEASES

SARCOIDOSIS

Pathogenesis and Epidemiology

Sarcoidosis is enigmatic. It occurs frequently, is variable in its severity, can affect multiple organs but has a particular propensity for the respiratory tract, and remains of unknown cause (1,225,226). The diagnosis of pulmonary sarcoidosis is often made from a distinctive clinical presentation and a compatible chest radiographic pattern; laboratory studies and tissue histology are obtained to confirm and support the diagnosis (227). Its diagnosis requires exclusion of lymphoma, bronchogenic carcinoma, beryllium exposure, tuberculosis, histoplasmosis, coccidioidomycosis, and *P. carinii* in the immunocompromised patients because each may mimic the clinical picture and the tissue histology of sarcoidosis. The hallmark of the host's immune response in sarcoidosis is the activation of T cells and formation of typical nonnecrotizing (noncaseating) tissue granulomas in affected organs. Sarcoidosis features other abnormalities in lymphocyte function; in particular, anergy and peripheral lymphopenia associated with the accumulation of $CD4^+$ lymphocytes at sites of active disease (228–234). $CD4^+$-predominant lymphocytic inflammation is seen in the BAL fluid of patients with active disease (231). In the setting of HIV infection, a circulating $CD4^+$ lymphocyte count of approximately 200 cells per mm^3 or greater appears to be required to develop overt clinical disease (235). Studies of the cytokine profiles in lymphocytes from the lungs and in BAL fluid from patients with sarcoidosis show polarization toward a Th1 subtype (increased IFN-γ and IL-2 production) in both $CD4^+$ and $CD8^+$ cells (232,236–239). Alveolar macrophages from patients with sarcoidosis make large amounts of another key inflammatory cytokine, TNF-α, which is critical in granuloma formation (240–242).

Both environmental and infectious agents have been explored in sarcoidosis but none has proven etiologic. Studies focusing on mycobacteria have yielded mixed results. Recent data on propionibacteria are intriguing but await further confirmation (225,226). Genetic factors clearly play an important role and recent data suggest that familial clustering is more common in African Americans than in whites afflicted with sarcoidosis (243). Genetic association studies have linked polymorphisms in the chemokine receptor, CCR2, to Löfgren syndrome of erythema nodosum, hilar adenopathy, polyarthralgia, and fever (244). Multiple studies have shown various human leukocyte antigen (HLA) associations with particular clinical syndromes and clinical courses (1). Associations with mutations in the TNF-α promoter region have also been described (245). Although these findings are certainly suggestive that host factors play a critical role in the development of disease, the molecular mechanisms underlying these associations in disease have yet to be determined.

Sarcoidosis was once stereotyped as a disease that affected young African American people—often women—who lived in rural parts of the southern United States. This is now recognized as a faulty categorization because white Americans frequently have the disease and geography is not specific. In the United States, sarcoidosis has a prevalence of 35.5 per 100,000 for African Americans and 10.9 per 100,000 for whites (246). Temporal, spatial, and seasonal clustering of sarcoidosis has been noted worldwide (225,247).

Clinical Presentation and Evaluation

Sarcoidosis is protean in its clinical expression and at times can affect a variety of organs or can begin with recurrent fever and vague constitutional symptoms. However, respiratory tract findings are by far the most common (see Table 12-2) (1,248). In fact, the chest radiograph may provide the first clue, often in an asymptomatic person. Findings other than respiratory signs or symptoms are decidedly less frequent. Critical organ involvement may be striking and can confuse the diagnosis; when one is involved, this usually dictates prompt immunosuppressive therapy. Uveitis, cardiac arrhythmias, and neurologic signs—occasionally manifested as palsy of a single cranial nerve (the seventh nerve with Bell palsy)—and hypercalcemia are the major concerns and are more common in African American individuals (248–251). Although sarcoidosis as a cause of liver failure is exceedingly rare, asymptomatic liver enzyme elevations are quite common and this organ can be a source of diagnostic tissue in many patients (248,252). Respiratory symptoms are not distinctive for sarcoidosis and are similar to those noted with other interstitial pulmonary diseases—breathlessness, often with minimal exertion, and nonproductive cough. Signs of pleural involvement or wheezing are unusual.

Patients with adenopathy and ostensibly clear lung fields may have normal lung function. For patients with overt lung tissue involvement and radiographic changes of the parenchyma, tests of pulmonary function usually reveal a restrictive pattern, small lung volumes, and diminished DLCO, as found with other forms of diffuse interstitial pulmonary fibrosis. Obstructive patterns

TABLE 12-2. Presenting Clinical Manifestations of Sarcoidosis

Organ System	Percent
Lungs	95
Skin	16
Lymph node	15
Eye	12
Liver	12
Erythema nodosum	8
Spleen	7
Neurologic	5
Parotid/salivary	4
Bone marrow	4
Hypercalcemia	4
Ear, nose, or throat	3
Cardiac	2
Renal	<1
Bone and joint	<1
Muscle	<1

From Baughman RP, Teirstein AS, Judson MA, et al. Clinical characteristics of patients in a case control study of sarcoidosis. *Am J Respir Crit Care Med* 2001;164(10 Pt 1):1885–1889, with permission.

may also be seen, reflecting endobronchial disease or airways hyperresponsiveness (253–257). The diminished DLCO is more likely to correct for alveolar volume in sarcoidosis than in IPF (258). Other organs that require laboratory screening include the heart for possible arrhythmias, the liver with a liver enzyme profile, and the kidneys. Serum calcium should also be monitored. At one time, Kveim antigen skin testing and subsequent biopsy of the skin papule for typical sarcoid histology was useful for confirming the diagnosis. Now, both the general scarcity of a well-characterized and reliable antigen and the risks of transmitting disease by injection of human tissue extracts have resulted in the Kveim test not generally being performed, outside of very few centers. Skin test anergy to common fungal and tuberculin antigens is a usual feature of active sarcoidosis. This faulty delayed hypersensitivity probably reflects the paucity of circulating T lymphocytes among the blood mononuclear cells. Leukopenia (total white cell count <4000 per mm³) occurs in about 30% of patients (259).

Two enzymes, lysozyme and angiotensin-converting enzyme (ACE), have been found to be elevated in patients with sarcoidosis and are sometimes useful as diagnostic aids (260–266). ACE, which acts to convert serum angiotensin I to angiotensin II and to metabolize bradykinin, is primarily produced by capillary endothelial cells; however, other cells such as fibroblasts and alveolar macrophages can also produce it (264,267). Whereas serum ACE is more helpful in the diagnosis of sarcoidosis because it is elevated in 60% or more of patients with active disease, it is not specific. Other diseases that may have elevated levels are Gaucher disease; leprosy; coccidioidomycosis; some cases of silicosis, asbestosis, berylliosis, and *Mycobacterium intracellulare* infection; osteoarthritis; diabetes mellitus with retinopathy; miliary tuberculosis; primary biliary cirrhosis; or inflammatory bowel disease. Unfortunately, the list of diseases associated with elevated ACE levels is large, yet sarcoidosis continues to be the most common disease with high serum values. Several reports have indicated the usefulness of serial ACE values in monitoring sarcoid disease activity, although, typically, clinicians will not institute or intensify therapy on the basis of alterations in the ACE level alone (261,268). The ACE level in cerebrospinal fluid is helpful in the diagnosis of sarcoidosis affecting the central nervous system in the appropriate clinical setting (269). More recently, soluble interleukin-2 (IL-2) receptor and neopterin levels in the serum have been reported to correlate more accurately with progressive sarcoidosis (270).

Bronchoscopy is indicated to inspect the airways for possible endobronchial sarcoid and is quite useful in obtaining diagnostic tissue specimens. Endobronchial sarcoid can be recognized by a cobblestone appearance of whitish plaques on the airway mucosa. Endobronchial biopsies have a high yield when endobronchial abnormalities are visible bronchoscopically. In the absence of obvious endobronchial disease, "blind" transbronchial biopsies also have a high yield of granulomatous tissue in this disease—up to 70% to 80% (271). Even though the chest radiograph may not show parenchymal evidence of disease, it is usually present, and parenchymal biopsies contain distinctive tissue changes (272,273). In general at least four, and preferably five to six, transbronchial biopsy tissue fragments should be obtained to maximize diagnostic utility (274,275). Studies assessing the sensitivity of

transbronchial biopsies in the absence of parenchymal disease by chest HRCT have not been reported. In these situations, lymph node biopsy is typically also undertaken. In situations where lymph node sampling is required and cannot be achieved bronchoscopically, computed tomographically guided fine needle aspiration and core needle biopsies are gaining an ever-increasing role in diagnosis before proceeding to conventional mediastinoscopy (276).

Radiographic Features

Sarcoidosis in the chest is suggested by a pattern of symmetrically enlarged bilateral hilar lymph nodes with ostensibly clear lung parenchyma on the chest radiograph (see Fig. 12-12) (227,277). In such cases, about 50% of the chest radiographs also reveal enlarged paratracheal nodes (usually right-sided and unilateral). In fact, sarcoidosis is one of the few chest diseases that commonly involves nodes in the lung (hilar) and mediastinum simultaneously. In up to 60% of cases of sarcoidosis, bilateral hilar adenopathy found on a routine chest radiograph may be the only manifestation (226,259,278). Approximately 5% to 9% of patients present with only unilateral hilar adenopathy (279). In later stages of pulmonary sarcoidosis, the lymph node response diminishes and progressive involvement of the lung parenchyma ensues; end stages of lung sarcoidosis may leave upper-zone cystic spaces and extensive linear streaking and infiltrates throughout but may reveal little residual adenopathy. Such disease progression has led to a still-applicable radiographic classification of sarcoidosis (see Table 12-3).

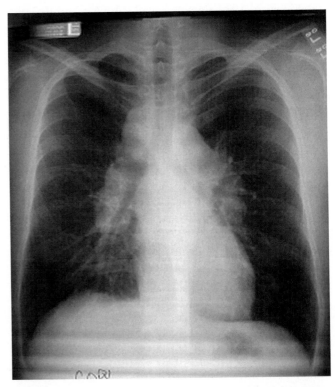

FIGURE 12-12. Sarcoidosis. Posteroanterior plain chest radiograph shows bilateral hilar, right paratracheal, and aortopulmonary window lymphadenopathy without radiographic evidence of parenchymal lung disease. This is chest radiographic stage I disease.

TABLE 12-3.   Radiographic Staging and Rates of Spontaneous Resolution of Sarcoidosis

Radiographic Stage	Lymphadenopathy	Parenchymal Disease	Spontaneous Resolution
O	—	—	>90%
I	+ +	0	60%–90%
II	+ − + +	+	40%–70%
III	+/−	+ +	10%–20%
IV	+/−	+ + +[a]	0%

[a]Honeycomb cyst formation

From American Thoracic Society. Statement on sarcoidosis. *Am J Respir Crit Care Med* 1999;160(2):736–755, Baughman RP, Teirstein AS, Judson MA, et al. Clinical characteristics of patients in a case control study of sarcoidosis. *Am J Respir Crit Care Med* 2001;164(10 Pt 1):1885–1889, Scadding JG. Prognosis of intrathoracic sarcoidosis in England. A review of 136 cases after five years' observation. *Br Med J* 1961;5261:1165–1172, Siltzbach LE, James DG, Neville E, et al. Course and prognosis of sarcoidosis around the world. *Am J Med* 1974;57(6):847–852, and Chappell AG, Cheung WY, Hutchings HA. Sarcoidosis: a long-term follow up study. *Sarcoidosis Vasc Diffuse Lung Dis* 2000;17(2):167–173, with permission.

Stage 0 is sarcoidosis in the absence of adenopathy or parenchymal disease. Stage I disease features symmetric, bilateral hilar adenopathy; stage II has hilar adenopathy and diffuse parenchymal changes; and stage III has diffuse pulmonary infiltrates without adenopathy (see Figs. 12-12 and 12-13). Stage IV is end-stage fibrotic lung disease with cysts or large cavities with marked structural distortion. This latter stage can be complicated by chronic airway infection and by the formation of intracavitary aspergillomas (280). The rate of spontaneous resolution of sarcoidosis roughly correlates with the radiographic stage (Table 12-3) (281,282).

The classic chest radiographic sequence is not observed in every patient. Dyspnea is roughly equated with higher radiographic stages of the disease that feature greater involvement of conducting airways and air-exchange tissue; however, some patients may not have respiratory symptoms despite obvious changes in the radiograph (282). The nonuniform, patchy distribution of sarcoid lesions in lung tissue can leave areas of parenchyma virtually normal, and this probably accounts for the preservation of good lung function and lack of symptoms in some patients. Unusual radiographic patterns can be present, and one must be alert to this possibility. Conglomerate infiltrates that give the appearance of pulmonary nodules or an alveolar filling pattern can occur, and pleural effusions may develop, though they are rare. In one series of 89 patients with an established tissue diagnosis of sarcoidosis, 15% had an atypical-appearing chest radiograph (279).

Chest HRCT is superior to plain chest radiographs in assessing the extent of parenchymal disease (Fig. 12-13) (19,283–289). It is also useful in defining the pattern of infiltration and the presence or absence of honeycombing, thereby providing some prognostic information. In addition, it can be quite useful in either adding or removing other interstitial disease from diagnostic consideration, hence influencing decisions of bronchoscopic versus surgical lung biopsy (19,283–289). The characteristic features of sarcoidosis by chest HRCT are peribronchovascular nodules, nodular opacities along septae (septal beading or "string of pearls"), and nodules abutting the pleural surface (19,283–289). These changes correlate with the tendency of granulomas to develop along lymphatic channels. Although physiologic evidence of obstruction is relatively common in sarcoidosis, it correlates better with the extent of parenchymal disease rather than with the airway-specific findings such as air trapping and mosaic attenuation, which are commonly seen in hypersensitivity pneumonia (290). The extent of ground-glass opacities does not seem to correlate as well with disease activity as the presence of nodules and consolidation, which often respond to therapy, or the degree of structural distortion, which is not as responsive (285,287–289).

Pathologic Features

Granulomatous inflammation without central necrosis (noncaseating) is a characteristic feature of sarcoidosis. The sarcoid granuloma is typically located in the interstitium along bronchovascular bundles, the pleural surface, and interlobular septae following the lymphatic channels of the lung (see Fig. 12-14). The sarcoid granuloma is made up of pallisading epithelioid histiocytes, which are derived from macrophages, with conspicuous multinucleated giant cells (see Fig. 12-15). Lymphocytes are typically arrayed around the outside of the

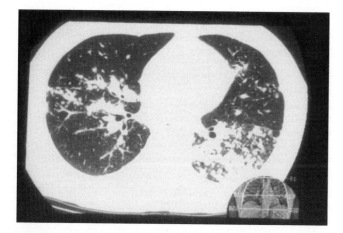

FIGURE 12-13.   Sarcoidosis. High-resolution computed tomography (HRCT) of the chest shows peribronchovascular infiltration with fissural beading and nodules abutting the pleural surface. No honeycomb-cyst formation is seen. Other images showed minimal adenopathy. This is stage III sarcoidosis.

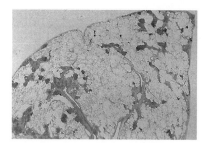

FIGURE 12-14. Sarcoidosis. A low magnification (4 × objective) view of lung tissue from a patient with sarcoidosis shows the peribronchovascular predominance of granulomatous inflammation and highlights the nodular nature of the inflammatory infiltrate.

granuloma and layering concentric fibrosis is often present in the periphery of the granuloma. Vasculitis, while often seen, is not the predominant finding in most patients (45). Special stains for mycobacteria and fungi should be routinely performed on biopsied tissue. Furthermore, tissue should routinely be cultured for bacteria, fungi, and mycobacteria. In immunocompromised hosts, particular diligence must be paid to a prior history of infections associated with granulomatous inflammation (235). Interstitial inflammation between granulomas is usually scant, and brisk interstitial inflammation should raise concern for hypersensitivity pneumonia (45). However, in hypersensitivity pneumonia, granulomas are typically less well formed, are scattered throughout the parenchyma, and are centered on airways rather than around lymphatic channels. Central necrosis can occasionally be seen in sarcoid granulomas but should certainly raise suspicion for an underlying infectious etiology—particularly in the immunocompromised patient. In this clinical situation, empiric therapy for tuberculosis while awaiting culture data and prior to consideration of immunosuppressive therapy is appropriate.

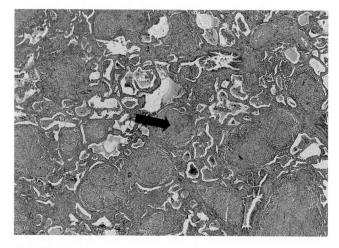

FIGURE 12-15. Sarcoidosis. This photomicrograph shows exuberant granulomatous inflammation in sarcoidosis. The granulomas are obvious and are well formed with abundant and conspicuous multinucleated giant cells (*arrow*). The surrounding lung parenchyma shows type II alveolar epithelial cell hyperplasia and mucous impaction. The typical concentric fibrosis of granulomas is also present.

Treatment and Prognosis

Once the diagnosis of sarcoidosis has been made, baseline radiographic, physiologic, and laboratory measurements should be obtained in all patients. The consensus recommendations are outlined in Table 12-4 (1). The clinical course of sarcoidosis is highly variable. In one study of 44 untreated, asymptomatic patients with symmetric hilar adenopathy and no parenchymal infiltrates, spontaneous resolution of the radiographic disease occurred in most of them; 73% remitted and most did so in 6 to 17 months after diagnosis (277). Rates of spontaneous resolution appear to vary among ethnic groups (291,292). Rates of progression between various radiographic stages also vary considerably (293). Thus, advocacy of a particular form of therapy for patients in the earliest stages of disease must be tempered by the fact that spontaneous regression of the pulmonary process is frequent (1,226,247,281,282,291,292,294,295). This does not remove the lingering question about persistence of an inciting agent in a dormant stage. Prevention or environmental control is not possible because the cause of the disease is unknown.

For extrapulmonary sarcoidosis involving such critical organs as eyes, heart, or nervous system, corticosteroid therapy is indicated (250,251,296,297). Eye disease can often be managed with topical rather than systemic corticosteroids. Cutaneous disease is often responsive to the antimalarial agent hydroxychloroquine (298). For disease confined to the lungs, the decision to treat is more difficult. Many studies have been done to assess the efficacy of corticosteroid therapy on pulmonary dysfunction in sarcoidosis. A recent meta-analysis showed that corticosteroids resulted in a small but statistically significant improvement in FVC and in the radiographic appearance of the disease. Notably, there was no obvious effect on the long-term outcome of the disease; the results were similar to a prospective British Thoracic Society study (299–301). These findings, along with some concern that patients treated with steroids may show an increased tendency for relapse and may have worse clinical outcomes overall, have tempered enthusiasm for corticosteroids in recent years (302–306).

As a general rule of thumb, a decrement of at least 20% below a patient's predicted values for lung volumes and spirometric parameters must be present along with a persistence of disease

TABLE 12-4. ATS/ERS Recommended Initial Evaluation of Patients with Sarcoidosis

History (occupational, environmental, and systemic symptoms)
Physical examination
Posteroanterior chest radiography
Pulmonary function testing: spirometry and D$_{LCO}$
Peripheral blood count: white blood cells, red blood cells, and platelets
Serum chemistries: calcium, liver enzymes, creatinine, and BUN
Urinalysis
ECG
Routine ophthalmologic examination
Tuberculin skin test

D$_{LCO}$, diffusing capacity of the lung for carbon monoxide; BUN, blood urea nitrogen; ECG, electrocardiogram.

From American Thoracic Society. Statement on sarcoidosis. *Am J Respir Crit Care Med* 1999;160(2):736–755, with permission.

for at least several months before any immunosuppressive therapy can be considered to control or arrest a decline in lung function barring other critical organ involvement (1,304). Nonsteroidal antiinflammatory agents are often helpful in controlling arthralgia and constitutional symptoms. However, if patients with pulmonary sarcoidosis have troublesome respiratory symptoms and a 20% to 30% reduction in pulmonary function parameters (lung volumes, DLCO, etc.), most clinicians institute a trial of corticosteroid therapy. This therapy consists of 3 months of prednisone at 20 to 40 mg per day with a formal assessment of clinical response at 3 months using clinical, physiologic, and radiographic assessments (1,307). Such therapy will generally improve symptoms, variably improve pulmonary function tests, and often improve the appearance of the chest radiograph. Long-term use of small doses of corticosteroid seems to be beneficial for many patients, and relapse and exacerbation of symptoms occurs in some if the drug is tapered or withdrawn. Inhaled corticosteroids are occasionally used—particularly for endobronchial disease—though controlled clinical trials of these agents in sarcoidosis are limited (300,308). Chloroquine has also shown efficacy in advanced pulmonary disease in one small randomized trial (309).

Other cytotoxic and immunosuppressive drugs have been used to treat sarcoidosis but rarely in a controlled trial; therefore, none can be recommended as proven therapy for the disease (301). One interesting trial suggests that weekly doses of 10 mg of methotrexate reduce the corticosteroid dose required to control disease at 6 months (310). A related, but apparently less toxic agent, leflunomide, may also prove useful as a steroid-sparing agent (311). Unfortunately, patients with sarcoidosis may be more prone to hepatic injury from chronic methotrexate than patients with rheumatoid arthritis may be—presumably related to underlying hepatic involvement of sarcoidosis—which complicates monitoring and management in these patients (312). Azathioprine and cyclophosphamide have both been used in patients with life-threatening progressive disease with some reported success (297,313). Cyclosporin A has been studied and has been shown to be without benefit in pulmonary disease. There is some evidence for benefit in refractory neurosarcoidosis (314,315).

By analogy to rheumatoid arthritis—another chronic inflammatory disease of unknown etiology associated with increased levels of the cytokine TNF-α, and in which anti-TNF-α therapy has been successful in refractory cases—recent interest has been focused on blockade of TNF-α in sarcoidosis (316,317). TNF-α has also been shown to be critical to granuloma formation in a range of diseases including tuberculosis and Crohn disease (318,319). Anti-TNF-α therapy with either thalidomide or infliximab has also been used for refractory sarcoidosis—particularly cutaneous disease—in several small studies (316,320–322). Another TNF-α antagonist, etanercept was tested and found to be ineffective alone in halting progressive sarcoidosis in a small prospective trial (323). An industry-sponsored phase-II trial evaluating the TNF-α antagonist, infliximab, which must be given intravenously, is currently under way in patients with well-preserved lung function, parenchymal infiltrates, and at least 3 months of therapy with corticosteroids or another immunosuppressant (*www.clinicaltrials.gov*).

For patients with established disease, the process eventually stabilizes and sarcoidosis is often said to have "burned out." In this advanced stage, there is usually widespread cystic and fibrotic destruction of lung tissue. Pulmonary function is invariably impaired. Aspergillomas can develop in cystic spaces left by advanced sarcoidosis (280). Significant or recurrent hemoptysis in this setting requires aggressive diagnostic and therapeutic intervention typically beginning with angiography and embolization of feeding bronchial arteries as well as with the initiation of antifungal therapy (324). Surgical resection may be required if the patient has sufficient pulmonary reserve, though postoperative recovery may be complicated (325). Management of these cases can become quite challenging and highly individualized.

Pulmonary hypertension is a substantial problem in patients with refractory or progressive sarcoidosis, and in some patients vasodilator therapy is helpful (326). In most cases, the pulmonary hypertension is thought to result from extensive parenchymal destruction. Nevertheless, granulomas obstructing the vasculature primarily have also been described (327). In rare instances, successful lung transplantation has been performed in sarcoidosis patients with respiratory insufficiency. Although recurrence of noncaseating granulomas has been described in the transplanted lung, progressive disease has not (326,328,329).

HYPERSENSITIVITY PNEUMONITIS (EXTRINSIC ALLERGIC ALVEOLITIS)

Pathogenesis and Epidemiology

Inhalation of a variety of organic dusts causes hypersensitivity pneumonitis, a disease that is likely underdiagnosed for several reasons (330). First, identifying the disease requires a high index of suspicion. Secondly, the manifestations of the disease mimic other common respiratory diseases such as asthma and community-acquired pneumonia. Thirdly, laboratory studies are relatively insensitive and nonspecific (41). Finally, the development of disease depends critically on unidentified host factors. This makes correlating exposures to the development of disease challenging. Although many people are exposed to these organic dusts and many become sensitized and develop precipitating serum antibodies to the causative antigens, only a few develop overt lung disease. Attack rates vary from 0.5% to up to 70% depending on the antigen and on the intensity of exposure (331). Initiating dusts can be derived from animal dander and proteins; from saprophytic fungi that contaminate vegetables, wood bark, or water-reservoir vaporizers; from environmental mycobacteria; and from dairy and grain products (see Table 12-5).

Colorful, descriptive names for the diseases underscore the frequent occupational nature of exposures underlying hypersensitivity pneumonitis (Table 12-5). Either the inhaled dust itself or a microbial contaminant passively carried with it may cause respiratory disease. Usually, a species of thermophilic actinomycetes is found. These ubiquitous sporulating bacteria thrive at the high ambient temperatures (45°C to 60°C range) reached during the decomposition of vegetable matter. About 10^9 mold spores per cubic millimeter of air must be inhaled on a daily basis for allergic alveolitis to develop, as was found for a group of Swedish farmers (332). For unknown reasons, tobacco smoke exposure appears to be protective against the development of hypersensitivity pneumonitis (330).

The lymphocyte accumulation in the alveoli in hypersensitivity pneumonitis is impressive. T cells predominate, especially

TABLE 12-5. Some Etiologic Agents in Hypersensitivity Pneumonitis

Disease	Source of Exposure	Major Antigens or Microbe
Farmer's lung	Moldy hay	*Micropolyspora faeni* (also *Faenia rectivirgula*)
Grain handler's lung	Moldy grain	*M. faeni, Thermoactinomyces vulgaris*
Bagassosis	Moldy sugar cane fiber	*T. sacchari*
Summer-type hypersensitivity	House dust or bird droppings	*Trichosporon cutaneum*
Humidifier or air conditioner lung	Contaminated forced-air system, heated water reservoirs	*M. faeni, T. vulgaris,* and occasionally amoebae are implicated
Maple bark stripper's lung	Moldy bark	*Cryptostroma corticale*
Malt worker's lung	Moldy malt	*Aspergillus clavatus*
Sequoiosis	Moldy redwood dust	*Aureobasidium pullulans* and *Graphium* spp.
Wheat weevil disease	Wheat weevil disease	*Sitophilus granarius*
Cheese worker's lung	Cheese mold	*Penicillium caseii*
Suberosis	Moldy cork dust	*P. frequentans*
Bird breeder's lung	Pigeons, parakeets, fowl, and rodents	Avian or animal proteins (in excreta)
Chemical worker's lung	Manufacture of plastics, polyurethane foam, or rubber	Trimellitic anhydride, diisocyanate, methylene diisocyanate

T suppressor (CD8$^+$) cells. Tissue granulomas develop in chronic forms of the disease. In striking contrast to sarcoidosis, there is the lack of marked hilar and mediastinal lymph node enlargement and an absence of splenomegaly. Recent studies on lymphocytes recovered from BAL in patients with hypersensitivity pneumonia and stimulated *in vitro* show Th1 differentiation with increased production of interferon-γ and with reduced levels of interleukin-10 (IL-10) (333).

Clinical Presentation and Evaluation

Some forms of occupational disease are easily recognized. When the clinical symptoms are temporally related to workplace exposure, suspicion for an environmental or inhalation source is high. However, subtle forms of exposure may occur among office personnel or among individuals in the home (called *sick building syndrome*). Putting clinical symptoms together with unsuspected and episodic exposure or with a lower dose but constant exposure can be difficult. A considerable amount of medical detective work may be required to find that a water-cooled air conditioning unit, a new down comforter, a hot tub, or an infant's cold-mist vaporizer is the culprit or that an orchid grower is inhaling fungal spores from the bark chips he or she uses to mulch his or her flowers. The source may be obscure (334). The list of potential antigens that can be inhaled and can cause airway sensitization is increasing, and recognition of these diseases is becoming more prevalent. Oftentimes, clinical consideration of hypersensitivity pneumonitis occurs after a lung biopsy is obtained as part of the evaluation of diffuse parenchymal lung disease, and characteristic histologic features are noted (see below).

Sensitization to an organic dust is usually insidious, and the patient is unaware of the detrimental effects it is causing. In certain avocations such as bird handling, almost all people intimately involved in care of the birds develop serum-precipitating antibodies to some avian antigens, but this immune response is not associated with disease in most of them (335).

Likewise, farm workers may have serum antibodies to certain thermophilic bacteria (336–338). The onset of respiratory symptoms may appear only after an exposure pattern is well established. In the acute form of hypersensitivity pneumonitis, respiratory and systemic symptoms develop explosively within 4 to 6 hours after dust is inhaled and consist of dyspnea, cough, chills, fever, and malaise. The symptoms may persist for 12 hours or so and abate spontaneously; with each reexposure, the acute episode occurs again. When observed, the patient is acutely ill and dyspneic, inspiratory crackles can be heard prominently in the lower lung zones. Temperature may be alarmingly elevated and the peripheral blood leukocyte count can be in excess of 25,000 per mm^3 with a shift toward immature white blood cell forms. The chest radiograph may appear normal but usually shows a fine, diffuse alveolar filling pattern and variable interstitial streaks.

Pulmonary function abnormalities in acute hypersensitivity pneumonitis can be measured in patients challenged with antigens in a pulmonary laboratory and can be followed with serial observations. Symptoms appear 4 to 6 hours following exposure. A decrease in FVC and FEV$_1$ occurs; air trapping and hyperinflation may be documented; and the D$_{LCO}$ is reduced. Also, pulmonary compliance decreases. These changes gradually normalize as the clinical picture improves. Another pattern of pulmonary dysfunction may occur, involving a two-phase reaction. Initially, just after aerosol exposure to antigen, an immediate asthmatic-type reaction develops that is characterized by air trapping and obstruction. This abates, to be followed in 4 to 6 hours by more restrictive and noncompliant lung function, as described above.

Acute phases of the disease are seen infrequently because a knowledgeable person will deduce the cause or make the connection between an airway exposure and subsequent respiratory symptoms. If the correlation is recognized, voluntary avoidance may solve the problem. On the other hand, if the exposure is continuous and protracted, a subacute or chronic form of disease may develop that does not include the acute exacerbations of respiratory symptoms (330,334,339). Instead, patients develop persistent symptoms of breathlessness, dyspnea with exertion, and cough that are indistinguishable from symptoms noted in other interstitial pulmonary diseases. Fatigue, poor appetite, and weight loss can be significant in this disease. Symptoms and evidence of constitutional effects of disease may be evident for months and occasionally for years before the patient presents for evaluation. Many patients with subacute and chronic hypersensitivity pneumonitis are not diagnosed until the more advanced stage of disease is present. At this stage, pulmonary function is characterized by a restrictive ventilatory pattern and by a deficit in DLCO. Patients with this chronic form of inhalational hypersensitivity disease are difficult to separate from those with IPF and a host of similar diseases unless an exposure history is elicited. Even at this stage, however, patients may note a significant symptomatic improvement when they are away from the source of the exposure if they are carefully questioned. A serum screen for hypersensitivity antigen precipitins will not establish a diagnosis but, if positive, it might orient the clinician toward a possible environmental exposure. Physical examination does not provide any signs not found in other ILD. Digital clubbing, initially considered an unusual occurrence, has been noted to develop in about 50% of the patients in one series of patients with bird-fancier's disease (340). It portends a poor prognosis.

Except for the consequences of weight loss and poor appetite, hypersensitivity pneumonitis is limited to the respiratory tract, and most laboratory abnormalities relate to that organ system. Blood parameters reflect the effects of chronic disease in patients with advanced illness but do not necessarily mirror immunologic events occurring in the airways. With the exception of acute episodes of pneumonitis, the white blood cell count is not elevated and eosinophilia is unusual. The erythrocyte sedimentation rate may be elevated and serum immunoglobulins are often increased. The presence of precipitating antibodies (in IgM, IgA, and IgG classes) in serum to antigens causing hypersensitivity disease can give a helpful clue. However, because many people develop such antibodies, this finding is not diagnostic but only indicates that prior exposure and sensitization have occurred. Skin testing with hypersensitivity antigens is not well standardized and can provide confusing conclusions. *Aspergillus* antigens may be useful in patients with bronchopulmonary aspergillosis but other fungal preparations are not. Peripheral blood lymphocytes can be stimulated with appropriate antigens to give mitogenic responses, but generally the lymphocytes, especially ones recovered from the alveoli by lavage, have not been studied in the same detail as those from patients with sarcoidosis. Environmental testing including air quality assessment with quantitative or qualitative microbiologic assessment may be useful in refractory cases. Routine site visits by both professional industrial hygienists and other members of the medical team to the home, workplace, and other locales frequented by affected individuals can be quite informative.

Most of the details about immune responses in the lungs have come from patients with farmer's lung with chronic hypersensitivity pneumonitis and from those with pigeon breeder's (bird-fancier's) lung (7,341). These patients are typically evaluated with bronchoscopy like others with diffuse ILD are, and bronchoalvelolar lavage and transbronchial biopsy help considerably to substantiate the diagnosis. Histologically, lung biopsy shows an infiltration with lymphocytes and inflammatory cells; granuloma formation and fibrosis are often evident as well. In patients with a chronic form of farmer's lung, the total recovery of cells from lung lavage is generally increased due primarily to an increased number of lymphocytes. A slight excess of T suppressor lymphocytes (CD8$^+$) is usually found (342–344). This is an interesting contrast to the striking increase in T helper (CD4$^+$) lymphocytes that is characteristic of active sarcoidosis. There is a possibility that an elevated CD4$^+$ T-cell response is found with a more insidious onset of hypersensitivity pneumonitis, but this needs further study (345). Moreover, lavage fluid from these patients contains high concentrations of immunoglobulin, especially IgG and IgM (346). The presence of IgM is unusual because this immunoglobulin class is rarely found in measurable amounts in normal lung fluid and is infrequently present in lavage fluid obtained in other lung diseases. Specific precipitating antibody to inciting antigens is found in sera and in the BAL fluid from a number of these patients. Although the marked difference in the ratios of CD4$^+$/CD8$^+$ lymphocytes has been touted as a feature that distinguishes hypersensitivity pneumonitis from sarcoidosis, other clinical factors such as exposure history, adenopathy, chest HRCT findings, pathologic findings, and the presence or absence of extrapulmonary disease are generally more helpful than BAL fluid lymphocyte subsets in differentiating these two diseases (347,348).

Patients with acute forms of hypersensitivity disease have not been studied extensively by lung lavage and biopsy because the illness is usually transient. Neutrophilic alveolitis, inflammation, and, occasionally, hyaline membranes are present in the early phase (129). Mononuclear cells are also seen with virtually no eosinophils (349). In more chronic stages of organic dust inhalation, the lung response in susceptible individuals is reminiscent of sarcoidosis, which is the prototype of a granulomatous cellular response, albeit with a different lymphocyte profile. An "asymptomatic" form in which the subject has no special symptoms of respiratory illness but has a subclinical form of alveolitis has been described, raising the question of unidentified host factors that confer resistance to progressive lung disease (350–352). An increased percentage of lung lymphocytes as well as specific precipitating antibody can be found in these patients. In such subjects, this form of benign alveolitis or lung inflammation is well tolerated for periods of at least 2 years without the development of overt disease (352). It appears that a lymphocytic alveolitis as sampled in BAL fluid from an asymptomatic farmer does not have any long-term clinical significance (353,354).

In a recent multinational study, six significant clinical predictors of hypersensitivity pneumonitis were identified in patients presenting with diffuse parenchymal lung disease of unknown etiology: exposure to a known offending antigen, positive precipitating antibodies to the offending antigen, recurrent episodes of symptoms, inspiratory crackles on physical examination, symptoms occurring 48 hours after exposure, and weight loss (7). Exposure to a known offending antigen was the strongest single predictor with an odds ratio of 38.8 (7). Of note, 84% of patients in this study had either bird-fancier's disease or farmer's lung, making the generalizability of these findings to all forms of hypersensitivity pneumonitis unclear (41).

Radiographic Features

Chest radiographs are abnormal in hypersensitivity pneumonitis. The radiographic pattern varies somewhat depending on the chronicity of the disease (20). In acute disease, the characteristic finding is upper-lobe–predominant hazy opacities without Kerley lines or cardiomegaly. Although the HRCT scan is substantially more sensitive and helpful in making the diagnosis of hypersensitivity pneumonitis in subacute and chronic hypersensitivity pneumonitis, in acute disease the pattern is indistinguishable from noncardiogenic pulmonary edema (355). Modest lymphadenopathy is also common in acute disease (355). In subacute disease, the most common chest HRCT findings are multiple fine nodules 2 to 4 mm in diameter with hazy, ground-glass opacities (see Fig. 12-16A) (12). Often, regional air trapping is appreciated on dynamic expiratory imaging—particularly in more chronic long-standing disease (Fig. 12-16B). In advanced chronic hypersensitivity pneumonitis, differentiation from IPF can be quite difficult (356). Reticulation is common in both. However, in IPF, reticulation is typically most pronounced at the bases of both lungs, whereas in hypersensitivity pneumonitis it tends to involve upper- and mid-lung zones at least as much as the bases (20,356). Micronodules, which are characteristic of hypersensitivity pneumonitis, are not a feature of IPF (121,356). Lymphadenopathy is not striking in either chronic hypersensitivity pneumonitis or in IPF and suggests an alternative diagnosis such as LIP or sarcoidosis.

Pathologic Features

The pathologic findings of hypersensitivity pneumonitis can be quite diverse. The most characteristic pattern is a lymphocytic infiltrate primarily focused around small airways with ill-formed, inconspicuous granulomas with occasional interstitial giant cells (see Fig. 12-17). Foci of OP are common but generally are not a dominant feature (45). Hyaline membranes also should be absent or rare in chronic disease, although they are a feature of acute hypersensitivity pneumonitis (45). A number

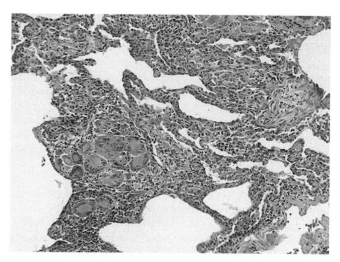

FIGURE 12-17. Hypersensitivity pneumonitis. Chronic extrinsic hypersensitivity pneumonitis is characterized pathologically by a mononuclear infiltrate with lymphocytes, plasma cells, foamy macrophages, and ill-defined collections of giant cells. Classically this infiltrate is centered on airways but this is commonly hard to appreciate. This example shows more conspicuous giant cells than is typical. Neutrophils and eosinophils are not major parts of this process.

of cases of hypersensitivity pneumonitis confidently diagnosed by clinical criteria show only features of cellular NSIP pathologically, making hypersensitivity pneumonitis an important consideration in cases of "idiopathic" NSIP (41,186).

Treatment and Prognosis

If the environmental source of an inhaled antigen is identified, simple avoidance is sufficient treatment. The acute form of disease generally abates without specific therapy. Preventing disease by avoiding the causative antigen is not always easy, especially if an occupational or pervasive household exposure is identified. A change of job or relocation within a factory to decrease exposure is often not a simple matter. Leaving one's

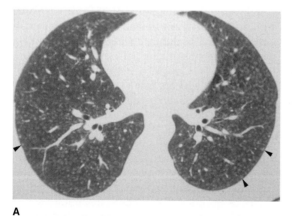
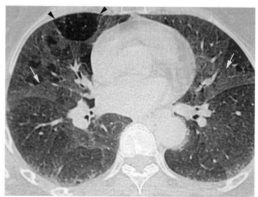

A   B

FIGURE 12-16. Hypersensitivity pneumonitis. **A:** Axial high-resolution computed tomographic (HRCT) image shows diffuse, bilateral ground-glass attenuation centrilobular nodules (*arrowheads*) characteristic of subacute hypersensitivity pneumonitis. The centrilobular distribution is easily identified by noting that the nodules closely approach, but do not touch, costal and fissural pleural surfaces. **B:** Axial HRCT image shows multifocal ground-glass opacity (*arrows*)—a characteristic appearance of chronic hypersensitivity pneumonitis. This is further associated with regions of decreased pulmonary parenchymal attenuation, representing mosaic perfusion (*arrowheads*).

home—either temporarily during extensive remodeling or permanently—is a decision never made lightly. Even the idea of eliminating exposure to a pet bird (or birds) is often unacceptable to many patients, even with biopsy-proven life-threatening hypersensitivity pneumonitis. With chronic forms of disease accompanied by respiratory symptoms and abnormal pulmonary function, a trial of corticosteroids can be given with a modest expectation that it will be effective. In general, however, if exposure continues, immunosuppressive therapy will be ineffective in preventing progression of disease. This can be a particular problem when avian antigens are the precipitant because they can linger in home ventilation systems long after the birds have been removed (330). In advanced chronic hypersensitivity pneumonitis, patients often become refractory even to aggressive immunomodulatory medications, and their clinical course parallels that of UIP (330). In patients who are otherwise eligible and show progressive disease, lung transplantation should be considered.

INTERSTITIAL LUNG DISEASE ASSOCIATED WITH COLLAGEN VASCULAR (CONNECTIVE TISSUE) DISEASES

The extracellular matrix is composed of a physiologically active ground substance containing fibrils of elastin, collagen, and reticulin. This, along with the cells that synthesize and support the extracellular matrix, comprises connective tissue. A host immune response against connective tissue leads to alterations in the chemical composition and physical constitution of the extracellular matrix and its supporting cells, causing edema, fibrinoid degeneration, and vascular lesions. The lungs may be the first organs involved. In this section, the pulmonary manifestations of four connective tissue diseases are reviewed in some detail. These are SLE, rheumatoid arthritis, diffuse progressive systemic sclerosis (scleroderma), and polymyositis-dermatomyositis (PM-DM). Sjögren syndrome and mixed connective tissue disease also have pleuropulmonary manifestations that are well reviewed elsewhere (119).

Our understanding of the biology, course, and response to therapy of connective tissue disease–associated ILD is rudimentary (119). Only recently, as a result of more rigorous classification of idiopathic interstitial pneumonias, are these diseases being pathologically separated from the UIP pattern referred to in older literature as the predominant pathologic finding in these diseases. In general, very little is known about the pulmonary response to therapies directed at controlling systemic connective tissue or autoimmune disease. Clinical experience suggests that the lung disease—particularly fibrosis—advances independently of systemic disease in many of these disorders and is often refractory to even aggressive immunosuppressive therapy. Rigorous prospective studies are sorely needed in these common disorders. These studies may also provide important insights into the links and differences between the regulation of inflammation and the regulation of fibrosis.

On a more practical note, the management of patients with connective tissue disease–associated interstitial disease is complicated as is the process of their rheumatologic classification. In many cases, rheumatologic syndromes evolve over time and treatment often involves toxic medications that require careful monitoring. Therefore, both the diagnosis and management of these patients typically requires patience and a close, ongoing collaboration between pulmonologists, rheumatologists, and patients' primary care physicians.

SYSTEMIC LUPUS ERYTHEMATOSUS

Pathogenesis and Epidemiology

SLE is a disease of unknown etiology that most often affects young women (357). Connective tissues of any organ in the body can be involved, but the vascular system, the epidermis, and the serous and synovial membranes are the most common (358,359). Pulmonary illness, however, may be the presenting manifestation of SLE (360). The most characteristic immunologic derangement in SLE is autoantibodies directed against components of the nucleosome, including nuclear and extractable nuclear antigens such as double- and single-stranded deoxyribonucleic acid (DNA), nuclear ribonucleoprotein, Smith antigen, Ro/SS-A, and La/SS-B. However, whether these autoantibodies are truly pathogenic or are markers of a more generalized derangement in immune regulation remains open to debate (361).

SLE is a relatively common autoimmune disease affecting 1 to 2 in 2,000 people with significant ethnic, racial, and socioeconomic variation (362). Up to 60% of these patients will have some pleuropulmonary complication of their underlying disease (360). Like the disease itself, the pathogenesis of the pulmonary manifestations remains incompletely understood but appears to relate to both the generalized immune hyperreactivity of both B and T cells and the deposition of immune complexes in the lung. Thrombophilic complications such as pulmonary embolism are common (360).

Clinical Presentation and Evaluation

Pleuropulmonary manifestations of SLE develop frequently and are summarized in Table 12-6 (119,360,363,364). Respiratory muscle dysfunction, including diaphragmatic muscle weakness, has also been described in patients with SLE (365,366). This may in part explain the well-described basilar atelectasis and the so-called vanishing lung syndrome noted in patients with this disease.

Winslow et al. emphasized the importance of pleuritis as an early manifestation of SLE (367). Pleural effusion occurred in 42 (81%) of their 57 patients; in 3 it was an isolated first sign, and in 16 others it was associated with only minor antecedent symptoms. Such pleural effusions are inflammatory exudates containing both mononuclear and polymorphonuclear cells. The glucose concentration and pH of the pleural fluid are within normal range. The finding of lupus erythematosus (LE)

TABLE 12-6. Pleuropulmonary Manifestations of Systemic Lupus Erythematosus

Pleurisy with or without effusion
Diaphragmatic dysfunction with reduced lung volume
Acute lupus pneumonitis
Diffuse alveolar hemorrhage
Diffuse interstitial disease
Pulmonary hypertension
Pulmonary thromboembolism

cells in the fluid is diagnostic (368). Moreover, a high pleural fluid antinuclear antibody (ANA) titer (1:160 or greater) and a pleural fluid to serum ANA titer ratio of greater than 1 strongly support the diagnosis (369). Low total and individual complement components are also characteristic (369,370). Fibrothorax and lung entrapment due to chronic pleural scarring are generally not seen.

Although many patients develop pulmonary infiltrates unrelated to infection, it still appears to be the most frequent cause of pulmonary infiltrates in SLE (119,360,363). Some patients with noninfectious pulmonary infiltrates have an acute onset; others have a more chronic onset. Acute lupus pneumonitis is characterized by severe dyspnea, a cough productive of scant sputum, fever (100°F to 104°F), negative sputum and blood cultures, hypoxemia, and a bilateral alveolar filling process on the chest radiograph (see Figs. 12-18 and 12-19) (119,360,363). Associated findings include cardiomegaly and pleuritis, with or without effusion. Acute lupus pneumonitis can develop during the course of the illness or can be the initial manifestation of SLE in 50% of cases with this complication (119,363). In 50% of the patients surviving the acute illness, the chest radiograph clears completely. In some reports, up to 50% of the surviving patients develop chronic interstitial pneumonitis with restrictive pulmonary function and decreased D$_{LCO}$, although this is not universally accepted (119,371).

Diffuse alveolar hemorrhage due to capillaritis, which can be confused with acute lupus pneumonitis, is characterized by the acute onset of fever, cough, dyspnea, and hemoptysis (372). The concomitant occurrence of a fall in hematocrit and a diffuse alveolar filling pattern on the chest radiograph supports the diagnosis. Unlike acute lupus pneumonitis, diffuse alveolar hemorrhage is not associated with pleural or pericardial disease and is not a presenting manifestation of SLE. The incidence of this complication is low (<5% of patients with SLE). In spite of treatment with corticosteroids, immunosuppressives, and plasmapheresis, the mortality rate can be high, varying from 25% to 68% in different series (119).

In 1973, Eisenberg et al. reported 18 patients, and in 1990, Weinrib, Sharma, and Quismorio reported 14 patients with SLE and chronic diffuse ILD (373). Pulmonary symptoms in these patients included dyspnea, a nonproductive cough, and pleuritic chest pain. Physical findings were poor diaphragmatic movement and basilar crackles, but clubbing was not a feature in these patients. Hypoxemia, a restrictive ventilatory defect, and reduced diffusing capacity were evident on pulmonary function tests. Huang et al. and Andonopoulos et al. noted that patients with SLE may demonstrate these abnormalities in the absence of clinical symptoms or abnormal chest radiographs (374,375). In fact, Andonopoulos et al. found normal function in only one-third of 70 nonsmoking patients with SLE, and an isolated reduction in D$_{LCO}$ was the most commonly detected functional abnormality (31% of patients) (375).

Pulmonary hypertension in SLE can be secondary to progressive interstitial pneumonitis with resultant lung destruction and hypoxemia, or it can be caused by a primary fibroproliferative pulmonary vasculopathy. It can occur either with or without the antiphospholipid antibody syndrome (119). In fact, even in the setting of detectable antiphospholipid antibodies, most patients with lupus and pulmonary hypertension (80%) do not have chronic thromboembolic disease (376). Raynaud phenomenon is present in 75% of the cases, and women are affected in more than 90% of the cases (360). There

is an associated glomerulonephritis in 63% of patients and cutaneous vasculitis in 33% (360).

Radiographic Features

Chest radiographic changes in patients with SLE include cardiac enlargement, pericardial effusion, pleuritis with or without effusion, and pulmonary infiltrates (Figs. 12-18 and 12-19) (119,360,363,364). The lung bases are most frequently involved with patchy areas of increased density, focal atelectasis with diaphragmatic elevation, and acute acinar or chronic interstitial infiltrates. The pulmonary infiltration tends to be recurrent and migratory in nature. Pleural effusions, usually small but sometimes massive, are frequently bilateral (Fig. 12-18) (119,364,367,369). Acute lupus pneumonitis is radiographically indistinguishable from other acute lung processes such as pneumonia, acute lung injury, or hemorrhage (363). In many cases, the plain chest radiograph is too insensitive to detect or to define the nature of the interstitial changes in lupus-related lung disease.

Chest HRCT is substantially more useful than plain chest radiographs. In fact, recent studies show a high prevalence of subclinical pulmonary abnormalities detected only by chest HRCT, with up to 32% having ILD even in the absence of pulmonary function abnormalities (377–379). Findings in these studies include interlobular septal thickening with honeycomb-cyst formation, airway wall thickening and bronchiectasis, ground-glass opacities, consolidation, and pleural thickening (377–379). Whether patients with these radiographic abnormalities are fated to develop progressive disease is currently unknown.

Pathologic Features

Although most patients who die of SLE have severe pathologic changes in their lungs, there are no features that are

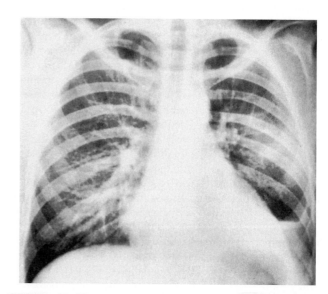

FIGURE 12-18.   Systemic lupus erythematosus. Posteroanterior (PA) chest radiograph of a 19-year-old man with an established diagnosis of systemic lupus erythematosus who developed fever and shortness of breath acutely. Note the left pleural effusion and enlarged cardiac silhouette. An echocardiogram revealed pericardial fluid. Corticosteroid therapy was instituted and the chest radiograph returned to normal within 5 days.

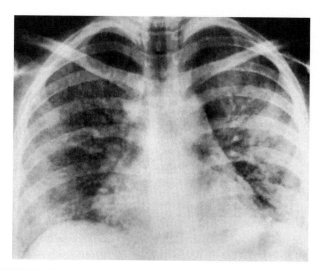

FIGURE 12-19. Systemic lupus erythematosus. Posteroanterior (PA) chest radiograph of an 18-year-old woman with acute lupus pneumonitis. Note the bilateral alveolar filling process. Two weeks after corticosteroid and azathioprine therapy was instituted, the chest radiograph had cleared markedly.

considered unique (373,380–384). Gross et al. found a high frequency of interstitial pneumonitis (98%), interstitial fibrosis (70%), and chronic pleuritis (95%) in 44 autopsy specimens (385). Acute inflammation of small pulmonary arteries and arterioles was found in 19% of specimens (385). In many patients, lung biopsies show histopathologic patterns consistent with what is now termed NSIP, although, notably, patients with underlying connective tissue disease were excluded from the development of the current classification scheme of idiopathic interstitial pneumonias (3,181). Foci of OP are also common (386,387). Other common but nonspecific changes in those who die of SLE include alveolar hyaline membranes, hemorrhage, and capillary thrombi (363,380–384). The pleural lesions often seen in this disease are usually manifested pathologically by a fibrinous pleuritis (385).

Treatment and Prognosis

Treatment of SLE is usually directed at control of the systemic disease and at preservation of renal function if the kidneys are seriously involved. In acute lupus pneumonitis, clearing of the pulmonary infiltrates in response to corticosteroids is frequently rapid. Azathioprine has been administered successfully to a small group of patients who had not responded to corticosteroids alone (363). Cyclophosphamide, methotrexate, and plasmapheresis have all also been reported to be successful in selected cases (388–390). The efficacy of therapy in chronic interstitial disease associated with SLE is unknown.

RHEUMATOID ARTHRITIS

Pathogenesis and Epidemiology

Rheumatoid arthritis is a symmetric inflammatory autoimmune polyarthritis that often results in severe progressive erosive arthropathy. In addition to being a disease of joints, it also involves other organs and tissues. Rheumatoid arthritis was first recognized clinically in the early 19th century, and nearly

150 years passed before the pleuropulmonary complications of the disease were described (391–400). The inciting pathophysiologic event in rheumatoid arthritis is unknown. Infectious etiologies have been aggressively pursued to no avail. Inflammation and vascular injury of the synovial lining of joints is the first articular manifestation of rheumatoid arthritis. This results in a reactive hypertrophy of synovial tissue and in infiltration by T lymphocytes, which form lymphoid aggregates along with a diffuse synovial inflammatory infiltrate. Immunophenotyping shows that $CD4^+$ lymphocytes predominate in the nodular lymphoid aggregates, whereas $CD8^+$ cells predominate in the intervening regions. As the disease progresses, lymphoid follicles with germinal centers may appear along with plasma cells—presumably responsible for the formation of the rheumatoid factor and other autoantibodies—and multinucleated giant cells. This chronic inflammation culminates in the development of an invasive synovial pannus composed of highly vascularized granulation tissue that erodes the articular surface and that undermines the structural integrity of the joint (401). These pathologic manifestations—particularly the lymphocytic infiltration and formation of lymphoid aggregates—are similar to those seen in the lungs of affected patients, raising the possibility of a shared antigenic stimulus. However, as with rheumatoid arthritis itself, the pathogenesis of "rheumatoid lung" remains unknown. Though the expression of many cytokines is dysregulated in rheumatoid arthritis, one in particular has emerged in recent years to play a critical role, the proinflammatory cytokine TNF-α (402). Selective inhibition of TNF-α using engineered neutralizing antibodies has proven remarkably effective at controlling articular disease (402). The role of this therapy in controlling the pulmonary manifestations remains unknown.

Rheumatoid arthritis is common. It affects 0.3% to 1.5% of the North American population, and approximately 20% of patients with rheumatoid arthritis develop extraarticular disease (401). Those who develop pulmonary disease have a shortened life expectancy (402), though the survival appears better than in patients affected by primary fibrotic lung diseases such as IPF (403). Pulmonary function abnormalities occur in about 10% of patients with rheumatoid arthritis, but the long-term clinical significance in most of them is unclear, and the prevalence does not appear to be changing over time (404,405).

Clinical Presentation and Evaluation

Though reports abound that pleuropulmonary disease is more common in patients with rheumatoid arthritis who have severe chronic articular disease; high titers of rheumatoid factor; subcutaneous nodules; and other systemic manifestations such as Felty syndrome, cutaneous vasculitis, myopericarditis, and ocular inflammation, it is increasingly being recognized in patients with more recent onset and with less severe disease (406). There are several pleuropulmonary abnormalities associated with the rheumatoid process (see Table 12-7) (364,391,392,394–396,398,407,408). Pleural involvement by the rheumatoid process is the most common thoracic complication of rheumatoid arthritis and accounts for attacks of pleurisy, with or without effusion. Such pleurisy has a remarkable predilection for men despite the fact that rheumatoid arthritis occurs predominantly in women in a ratio of 2:1.

TABLE 12-7. Pleuropulmonary Manifestations of
Rheumatoid Arthritis

Pleurisy with or without effusion
Interstitial lung disease
Pulmonary nodules
Bronchiolitis obliterans organizing pneumonia
Bronchiolitis obliterans
Pulmonary hypertension

Pleural disease rarely causes significant complications. Pulmonary restriction from pleuritis requiring decortication has been reported but is exceptionally rare (409,410). All patients with rheumatoid arthritis who present with pleurisy and effusion should have appropriate studies to exclude empyema, tuberculosis, and malignancy. An exceptionally low glucose concentration in pleural fluid recovered from patients with rheumatoid effusions is characteristic (411).

Restrictive ventilatory impairment and a reduction of the diffusing capacity have been found in as many as 41% of a group of patients with rheumatoid arthritis (396). More recent longitudinal data suggests a prevalence of about 9% to 13% (404,405,412). A higher prevalence of ILD occurs in men with rheumatoid arthritis than in women. Risk factors include smoking, high titers of rheumatoid factor, α-1-antitrypsin variants, subcutaneous nodules, or prominent extraarticular manifestations.

Asymptomatic fibrotic and inflammatory ILD is being increasingly recognized with more extensive use of HRCT scanning (396,405,406,408,413,414). No specific pattern of arthritis is associated with the development of ILD. Also, the prevalence of detectable rheumatoid factor is equivalent among patients who do and who do not develop parenchymal lung disease (119). Cough and dyspnea are often present, and clubbing is found in up to 75% of cases (393). In up to 20% of patients, the lung disease precedes the development of arthritis, although, characteristically, they both develop within 5 years of one another (119). The degree to which treatment of the underlying interstitial disease may prevent the complete unmasking of an underlying connective tissue disease is unknown.

Constrictive and follicular bronchiolitis, diseases of the terminal airways characterized by progressive airflow limitation with preservation or increase of lung volumes, have been described in patients with rheumatoid arthritis (397,412,415–417). These syndromes have previously been referred to as bronchiolitis obliterans but this term is now generally reserved for progressive, poorly reversible airflow limitation, which follows transplantation (3). Patients may complain of cough and dyspnea, and in most cases the chest radiograph is clear or shows hyperinflation. In many cases, these patients would have been diagnosed as having asthma but would fail to respond appropriately to bronchodilators and corticosteroids. Recent studies using HRCT suggest that airways disease associated with air trapping may occur in up to 20% of patients (412). Chest examination may reveal rhonchi with an inspiratory squeak, diminished breath sounds, or be entirely normal (205).

The intrapulmonary rheumatoid or necrobiotic nodule, which is pathologically identical to the subcutaneous nodule

in rheumatoid arthritis, is more common in men than in women (418,419). On the chest radiograph, necrobiotic nodules appear as single lesions or as bilateral, multiple, varying-sized coin lesions, with a predilection for the upper lung zones. Cavitation is common. Because the nodular form of rheumatoid lung disease may precede the arthritic manifestations, it must be differentiated from other granulomatous diseases. In the case of a single nodule, it may correlate with the activity and treatment status of the disease, but it must be differentiated from malignancy, which is generally more likely—particularly in the setting of tobacco smoke exposure (420). Therefore, histologic confirmation of benignity is generally advisable. Nodules may coexist with rheumatoid pleural effusions; spontaneous pneumothorax may also occur.

Caplan described a syndrome in coal miners with rheumatoid arthritis (392). This rheumatoid pneumoconiosis (Caplan syndrome) is characterized by the appearance of rounded densities on chest radiograph that evolve rapidly and can undergo cavitation—in contrast to the massive fibrosis of coal workers' pneumoconiosis. A similar syndrome has been reported in rheumatoid arthritis patients who are sandblasters, asbestos workers, potters, boiler scalers, and brass and iron workers (394,421). The pneumoconiotic nodule consists of layers of partially necrotic collagen and dust. Occasionally, there are foci of tuberculosis. The pulmonary disease may precede or coincide with the onset of the arthritis. Given improvements in industrial hygiene, this syndrome is now rarely seen, making the assessment for malignancy generally a more pressing concern.

In rare cases, pulmonary vasculitis may cause pulmonary hypertension in rheumatoid arthritis; more commonly, pulmonary hypertension is the result of advancing fibrosing alveolitis. Raynaud phenomenon has been present in a few reported cases of rheumatoid arthritis and pulmonary vasculitis (394,421). OP has also been reported in a few patients with rheumatoid arthritis, and its frequency in this disease remains unknown (133).

Radiographic Features

The prevalence of chronic ILD as detected by chest radiographic screening of rheumatoid patients is small. In one series of 516 cases, only 8 patients (2%) had radiographic evidence of ILD by chest radiograph (396). A much higher prevalence is detected by pulmonary function tests and chest HRCT (396,405,406,408,413,414). Recent data suggest that chest HRCT shows interstitial abnormalities in up to 20% to 30% of asymptomatic patients and in up to almost 70% of patients with respiratory symptoms (406,408,418).

The chest radiograph shows diffuse interstitial infiltrates, most marked in the lung bases; in the far-advanced disease, small cysts (honeycomb lung) appear accompanied by loss of lung volumes. Histopathologic examination of tissue may be helpful, especially when rheumatoid nodules are present in the lung interstitium in addition to the interstitial pneumonitis (363). HRCT shows a range of lesions. One large, well-controlled study of patients with and without respiratory symptoms found bronchiectasis or bronchiolectasis in 30% of patients, pulmonary nodules in 22%, pleural disease in 17%, ground-glass opacities in 14%, and honeycombing in 10%

(418). Not surprisingly, CT findings were significantly more common in symptomatic patients (418).

Pathologic Features

The most common interstitial pathologic pattern in rheumatoid arthritis is diffuse fibrosis with inflammation (422). Although many have referred to the pathologic findings of fibrosis in rheumatoid arthritis as UIP, by the current classification scheme, this pattern is only rarely seen. Rather, lympocytic infiltration, often with the formation of striking lymphoid aggregates, is common in ILD secondary to rheumatoid arthritis. When these well-developed lymphoid follicles with germinal centers are found adjacent to bronchioles, as is often the case, it is termed *follicular bronchiolitis*. This can be associated with significant airflow obstruction. Pulmonary vasculitis causing pulmonary hypertension has also been reported (423–427).

Treatment and Prognosis

In patients with rheumatoid arthritis and interstitial pneumonitis in whom a cellular lung biopsy is obtained, there is a positive objective response to corticosteroids or other immunosuppressive medications (395). Methotrexate is being used increasingly in the management of rheumatoid arthritis, and although interstitial pneumonitis has been reported as a complication of methotrexate, its incidence appears low on the basis of current practice (428–430). Hypoalbuminemia appears to be the major risk factor for developing methotrexate-associated lung injury, though other factors such as exposure to other disease-modifying agents and underlying lung disease also contribute to it (428).

The role of TNF-α antagonists is unknown. Similarly, other antifibrotic agents currently being studied in IPF have not been studied in interstitial disease related to rheumatoid arthritis. The bronchiolitis associated with rheumatoid arthritis is refractory to therapy and initial reports suggested less than a 2-year survival from the onset of symptoms (397). Recent studies have shown some benefit of macrolide antibiotics for other forms of constrictive and obliterative bronchiolitis (119,431). This has prompted its use in this disorder on a patient-by-patient basis. The median survival for all patients with rheumatoid arthritis and interstitial pneumonitis has been reported to be approximately 5 years (395,403,413,432). The effect of therapy on this survival has not been assessed nor has the course of asymptomatic patients with parenchymal disease, defined only by HRCT, been fully charted.

PROGRESSIVE SYSTEMIC SCLEROSIS (SCLERODERMA)

Pathogenesis and Epidemiology

Systemic sclerosis, or scleroderma, is a relatively rare inflammatory disorder of connective tissue that results in fibrosis and vascular abnormalities (433,434). The skin, gastrointestinal tract, musculoskeletal system, kidneys, heart, and lungs are frequently involved (433–435). The majority of patients are affected in their fourth through sixth decades; the disease is three times more common in women than in men. Prognosis is generally unfavorable once visceral disease develops. Significant advances in

the management of hypertensive renal crisis using ACE inhibitors early in the course of disease have resulted in elevating interstitial and pulmonary vascular diseases to being the major causes of morbidity and mortality in these patients (436–438).

Scleroderma is classified along three parameters: extent of skin involvement as manifested by thickening and atrophy; the presence and time course of significant visceral disease; and the presence of features suggestive of other connective tissue diseases such as SLE or rheumatoid arthritis (see Table 12-8) (433,439). The clinical course and prognosis associated with each of these variants is strikingly different. Most patients destined to develop pulmonary, gastrointestinal, or cardiac disease (45%–55%) and 70% of patients destined to develop renal or severe cutaneous disease do so within the first 3 years of disease (436). The extent of cutaneous disease does not separate those who will develop pulmonary disease from those who will not (440). Similarly, pulmonary involvement is not highly predictive of other visceral involvement except for cor pulmonale due to pulmonary hypertension (441). Cutaneous findings of scleroderma can also manifest themselves in other

TABLE 12-8. Classification of Systemic Sclerosis

DIFFUSE CUTANEOUS SCLERODERMA
- Skin thickening of face, neck, and trunk with symmetric involvement of fingers, hands, arms, and legs
- Raynaud phenomenon with rapid development and progression of disease
- Early development of visceral disease: pulmonary, renal, cardiac, or gastrointestinal
- Antinucleolar antibodies without anticentromere antibodies
- Poor but variable prognosis (40%–60% survival at 10 yr)

LIMITED CUTANEOUS SCLERODERMA
- Skin thickening limited to distal fingers (beyond proximal interphalangeal joint), distal arms, legs, face, and neck
- Raynaud syndrome precedes development or significant progression of disease
- Late visceral disease: hypertension and digit autoamputation
- Calcinosis, Raynaud syndrome, esophageal dysmotility, sclerodactyly, and telangectasia (CREST syndrome)
- Anticentromere antibodies
- Generally good prognosis (>70% at 10 yr)

OVERLAP SYNDROMES
- Diffuse or limited scleroderma with typical features of one or more other connective tissue diseases
- Mixed connective tissue disease with features of systemic lupus erythematosus, scleroderma, polymyositis, rheumatoid arthritis, and anti-U$_1$ RNP

LOCALIZED SCLERODERMA
- Morphea: plaques of fibrotic skin and fibrosis of subcutaneous tissue
- Linear scleroderma: longitudinal fibrotic bands on the extremities involving skin and deep soft tissue

From Subcommittee for scleroderma criteria of the American Rheumatism Association Diagnostic and Therapeutic Criteria Committee. Preliminary criteria for the classification of systemic sclerosis (scleroderma). *Arthritis Rheum* 1980;23(5):581–590 and Wigley FM. Systemic sclerosis and related syndromes: B. Clinical features. In: Klippel JH, ed. *Primer on the rheumatic diseases,* 11 ed. Atlanta: Arthritis Foundation, 1997:267–272, with permission.

connective tissue diseases such as SLE, complicating the classification of any given patient.

Scleroderma is a relatively rare disease. It has a prevalence of 26 cases per 100,000 in the United States (442,443). For comparison, this is 30 to 600 times less common than rheumatoid arthritis and one-quarter the frequency of SLE. Nevertheless, the high prevalence of lung involvement and the substantial morbidity and mortality associated with it make scleroderma lung disease fairly common in a referral setting.

Clinical Presentation and Evaluation

The most prominent respiratory symptoms are dyspnea and, less commonly, a cough, which may be slightly productive (119). The most frequent signs are fine basilar crackles and limited expansion of the chest. Signs of cor pulmonale may appear as a result of pulmonary vascular and interstitial disease (444).

Among the visceral organs involved in scleroderma, the lungs are second only to the esophagus (364,434,444,445). Clinical or autopsy evidence of pulmonary involvement is found in at least 70% of cases (446). Chest radiographic abnormalities have been reported in up to 25% of cases. Pulmonary symptoms have been found at some stage during the course of the illness in 20% to 50% of patients (436). One series using pulmonary function tests reported abnormalities in 21 of 22 patients (436). Postmortem studies on 196 cases revealed that only 18% were free of pleuropulmonary involvement (446). Pulmonary fibrosis was found in 77%, pulmonary vascular disease in 30%, and pleural disease in 32%. Three recent studies suggest an increased risk of malignancy, particularly lung cancer, in patients with scleroderma (447–449).

Pulmonary function abnormalities include a restrictive ventilatory pattern with reduction of vital capacity (VC) and normal flow rates (450,451). The compliance of the lung is reduced. A reduced D_{LCO} is frequently the earliest abnormality noted and may be present prior to recognized chest radiographic abnormalities (446). Owens et al. and Silver et al. found a significant correlation between BAL cellular recovery and the single-breath D_{LCO} (452,453). Sackner et al. showed that scleroderma involvement of the chest wall does not interfere with pulmonary function (450).

Patients with scleroderma can develop a range of autoantibodies including antinuclear, antinucleolar, anticentromere, and anti–tRNA synthase antibodies among others (454,455). Of these, the anticentromere antibody is associated with the best prognosis (455). Antitopoisomerase and antiribonucleic acid polymerase are associated with pulmonary hypertension and cor pulmonale (456,457). An increased prevalence of antitopoisomerase antibodies (also called Scl-70) is found in patients with ILD and systemic sclerosis (458,459).

Unlike IPF, the progressive ILD in scleroderma is currently thought to be preceded by significant, measurable lung inflammation or alveolitis. The concept of alveolitis, however, is somewhat vague and is defined by some as ground-glass opacities on chest HRCT and by others as an increase in total cell recovery or more often as a change in the percentage of various inflammatory cell components recovered by BAL (453,460–470). In a recent study by Witt et al., 11% of patients with scleroderma who met criteria for alveolitis by BAL fluid analysis

(defined as BAL differential cell counts of >15% lymphocytes, >3% neutrophils, and/or >0.5% eosinophils in nonsmokers; and of >7% lymphocytes, >3% neutrophils, and/or >0.5% eosinophils in smokers) had normal HRCT of the chest and 53% with an abnormal HRCT had a normal BAL fluid cell differential percentage. When the cohort of patients was followed for 2 years, only those with an excessive percentage of neutrophils showed progressively declining lung function (468). Nevertheless, when all published studies are considered together, they suggest that although the percentage of neutrophils is increased in BAL fluid in patients with scleroderma when compared to normal patients (5%–6% in scleroderma vs 2% in normal), the percentages do not differ significantly between patients with and without lung disease (119). Therefore, the role of screening bronchoscopy in this population remains controversial.

Pulmonary hypertension develops in 12% to 33% of patients with scleroderma, and there is increasing evidence that both acute and chronic vasodilator therapy are beneficial (471–482).

Radiographic Features

The most common abnormality on chest radiograph is an interstitial reticular pattern, particularly affecting the lung bases, reminiscent of IPF. As the disease progresses, the pulmonary infiltration becomes denser, with subsequent honeycombing and cyst formation (434). The cysts are most often subpleural in the basal and paravertebral areas and are usually bilateral. Although they tend to be small (5 mm or less in diameter), large cysts may form and rupture, resulting in a pneumothorax. Other findings include micronodulation, increased vascular markings, and pulmonary edema. Disseminated pulmonary calcification or calcification of the soft tissue of the thorax may be seen on the chest radiograph (363). The latter may also demonstrate the presence of pleural thickening, pleural effusion, and signs of pulmonary hypertension secondary to scleroderma lung disease. Disturbance of esophageal motility may result in retention of food and recurrent aspiration pneumonia. HRCT of the chest has been utilized to detect early ILD and to distinguish patients with predominantly fibrotic lung disease from those with significant inflammation (120,465,466,483). Moreover, HRCT has been successful in detecting mediastinal adenopathy and asymptomatic esophageal involvement in patients with scleroderma (484,485).

Pathologic Features

Pathologic changes in the lung occur frequently, with or without clinical or chest radiographic abnormalities (446,486). In an autopsy study, Weaver et al. found pulmonary abnormalities in all of their 28 cases of scleroderma (446). A progressive, nonspecific, bilateral lower-lobe interstitial fibrosis with bronchiectasis and cyst formation was the most prominent finding. Marked intimal thickening by loose myxomatous connective tissue occurred in small pulmonary arteries and arterioles.

In reviews of vascular disease in scleroderma, Norton and Nardo, and Shuck et al. point out that involvement of the arterioles and capillary bed in many tissues, particularly the lungs, is the basis of scleroderma (444,472). They conclude that scleroderma must be regarded as a vascular disease. It is clear that the pulmonary vascular lesions are not merely an extension of interstitial fibrosis because many scleroderma lungs have areas of severe interstitial fibrosis without arterial lesions as well as areas of vascular changes without interstitial disease (487). Thus, there are two predominant lung lesions in scleroderma: interstitial and pulmonary vascular (434). Other pathologic findings in patients with scleroderma include pleural thickening or effusion, cardiomegaly, vascular congestion, pulmonary edema, and pneumonitis. On the basis of the current classification scheme, the large majority of patients with ILD secondary to scleroderma show findings of NSIP, with approximately 75% of those showing the fibrotic (type III) pattern. Fifteen percent showed a UIP pattern or end-stage lung disease (488).

Treatment and Prognosis

The course of chronic interstitial lung disease in scleroderma is more indolent than IPF, and recent studies have suggested the 5-year mortality to be in the range of 15% (488,489). In general, corticosteroids are not thought to be beneficial in treating pulmonary disease in scleroderma (434). Two studies have demonstrated improvement in DLco following penicillamine therapy, whereas one study suggested this drug may arrest worsening of pulmonary dysfunction (460,490,491). In a 12-month trial of recombinant γ-interferon therapy in 14 patients, 9 of whom completed the trial, significant improvement was observed in skin involvement and in arterial oxygen tension (492). More recently, patients with evidence of alveolitis by BAL treated with low-dose prednisone and cyclophosphamide demonstrated clinical improvement (467,469,470,493–495). Although the 5-year survival rate for patients with scleroderma following the detection of lung disease has been previously reported to be less than 50%, the 5-year survival in all patients with scleroderma-associated ILD was substantially better in a more recent study from the Royal Brompton Hospital (82%–91%) (488). Of note, all patients in this series received therapy with corticosteroids and some received other unspecified immunosuppressive medications (488).

As noted above, pulmonary hypertension is both common and treatable in scleroderma (471–482). Prostacyclin, bosenten, nifedipine, and sildenafil have all been used successfully. In a recent study, the survival of patients with pulmonary hypertension and systemic sclerosis had a 1-, 2-, and 3-year survival of 81%, 63%, and 56%, respectively. The presence or absence of ILD did not alter survival probabilities in the setting of pulmonary hypertension (478).

POLYMYOSITIS-DERMATOMYOSITIS

Pathogenesis and Epidemiology

PM-DM are two manifestations of a diffuse inflammatory and degenerative disorder of striated muscle that causes symmetric weakness and atrophy of proximal muscle groups (496–501). This disease is twice as common in women as in men. It shows two peak age incidences: the first decade and the fifth and sixth decades (502). Patients commonly present with weakness and pain of proximal muscle groups (polymyositis) or muscle disease and erythematous skin lesions in a characteristic distribution (dermatomyositis).

The pulmonary complications of PM-DM may precede, follow, or occur simultaneously with the muscle and skin parenchymal disease (119). There are three mechanisms for the development of pulmonary parenchymal disease in polymyositis: primary interstitial pneumonitis; aspiration pneumonia due to a hypotonic esophagus; and hypostatic pneumonia secondary to chest wall involvement, with resultant hypoventilation (182,184,185,503–509). Interstitial disease is common in PM-DM and is present in 30% to 60% of patients at the time of their initial diagnosis of their connective tissue disease (184,506–509).

Respiratory muscle dysfunction caused by the inflammatory myopathy of PM-DM can lead to respiratory failure (alveolar hypoventilation) in up to 10% of patients. Subclinical respiratory muscle dysfunction is more frequent. These latter patients have tachypnea and dyspnea with exercise and may develop the aforementioned hypostatic pneumonia owing to failure to generate an adequate cough (119,496,498,499,503,510).

Clinical Presentation and Evaluation

The characteristic clinical features of PM-DM are marked muscular weakness, typically in proximal muscle groups, with marked elevation in the muscle enzymes creatine phosphokinase (CPK) and aldolase. The presence of eyelid erythema and edema (heliotrope rash), erythema and edema of the knuckles (Gottren papules), and digital ulceration or erosions (mechanic's hands) in association with muscular weakness are features of dermatomyositis. The clinical presentation of lung disease in PM-DM is quite variable. It may present as an acute pneumonitis with a mixed alveolar–interstitial pneumonitis in association with skin and muscle manifestations or as an asymptomatic finding on the chest radiograph. The most common presentation is one of gradual onset of dyspnea and cough, with development of diffuse pulmonary infiltrates most prominent at the lung bases. Diffuse soft tissue calcification may be present, a finding more often seen in children with PM-DM than in adults.

In approximately 40% of patients, the pulmonary disease precedes the skin and muscle manifestations by 1 to 24 months (511). Clubbing is not often present. In most cases, the lung disease is progressive, causing severe restrictive lung disease and cor pulmonale. Corticosteroids have caused remission, with either stabilization or improvement in the symptoms, chest films, and physiologic abnormalities in 50% of patients (511).

A subset of patients with PM present with ILD as the predominant manifestation with minimal muscle weakness. Raynaud phenomenon is often seen as well as arthralgias. Circulating autoantibodies to the amino-acyl tRNA synthetases are present. Most patients also have a positive ANA. The most common of the antisynthetase autoantibodies is against the histidyl-tRNA-synthetase (anti-Jo-1), but others have been described as well (497,512).

Radiographic Features

As in all other interstitial diseases, the HRCT of the chest offers significant advantages over plain chest radiographs in identifying the ILD associated with PM-DM. As noted above, pulmonary abnormalities can be visualized in 40% to 60% of patients at the time of presentation with their connective tissue disease. The CT pattern is nonspecific and consists of patchy areas of consolidation with other areas that show reticular changes. Air trapping and mosaic attenuation are not common, although ground-glass opacities are frequently seen scattered throughout the lung fields. Moderate structural distortion manifested by bronchiolectasis is common (184,185,507–509).

Pathologic Features

Lung tissue obtained from patients with PM-DM shows changes characteristic of connective tissue disease, that is, many different patterns within a single biopsy. These include foci of OP, vascular changes, a patchy lymphocytic infiltration with some lymphoid aggregates—generally with few or no giant cells—and, occasionally, foci of resolving acute lung injury. Often these biopsies are interpreted as NSIP because of the temporally homogeneous mononuclear cell infiltrate. In more acute cases, the changes may be exclusively those of diffuse alveolar damage (45,511). Fibrinous pleuritis may also be seen (45).

Treatment and Prognosis

Corticosteroids alone are generally insufficient and cyclophosphamide should be added in patients with ILD secondary to PM-DM once infection is satisfactorily excluded from consideration. Refractory cases should be considered for therapy with immunoglobulin, which has been shown to benefit some patients with classic PM (513–518). Patients who present with rapidly progressive respiratory failure and diffuse alveolar damage on biopsy have a poor prognosis (513–518). An unusual syndrome of spontaneous pneumomediastinum has also been reported in patients with PM-DM (519). It is associated with a rapid clinical decline and requires intensive immunosuppressive therapy to arrest it. Both pulse intravenous cyclophosphamide and cyclosporine A have been used successfully in progressive disease refractory to corticosteroids alone (513,516,518,520–522).

SYSTEMIC GRANULOMATOUS VASCULITIDES

WEGENER'S GRANULOMATOSIS

Pathogenesis and Epidemiology

Wegener's granulomatosis (WG) has a distinctive clinicopathologic triad of necrotizing granulomatous vasculitis of the upper and lower respiratory tracts; glomerulonephritis; and variable degrees of disseminated small-vessel vasculitis affecting arterioles, venules, and capillaries (523). A localized form of WG limited primarily to the respiratory tract has been reported, but it probably represents an early stage that, if not treated, eventually would involve the kidney and become a generalized WG (524). However, some patients may have a *forme fruste* of the disease that never disseminates. The etiology of WG remains unknown, although antineutrophilic cytoplasmic antibodies (ANCAs) are thought to play a role in the pathogenesis of this disease (525,526).

Fauci et al. have described the clinical features of WG (527,528). The mean age at diagnosis was 41, ranging 14 to 75 years. The disease occurs in men almost twice as frequently as in women (527). Initially, clinical presentations vary widely among patients but, generally, are related to the upper respiratory tract. Typical findings include sinusitis (67%), otitis media (29%), rhinitis or nasal symptoms (22%), epistaxis (11%), ulcers (6%), and hearing impairment (6%). Although chest radiographic abnormalities are present in 71%, less than 50% of Fauci's patients had noticed respiratory symptoms (cough in 33%, hemoptysis in 18%, chest pain in 8%, dyspnea in 7%, and pleurisy in 5%) (527). In one series, 8% of 77 patients with WG presented with diffuse hemorrhage (529). Pulmonary function studies show loss of lung volume with a restrictive ventilatory defect in association with significant parenchymal lesions. More than 50% of patients with WG also have an obstructive ventilatory abnormality that cannot be related to cigarette smoking (364). In patients with obstructive changes, granulomatous lesions that have blocked a major airway may be found during fiber-optic bronchoscopy, and the severity of airflow obstruction has been shown to correlate with the extent of endobronchial disease (530).

Renal disease is the *sine qua non* of generalized WG. Prior to the use of cytotoxic agents as therapy in this disorder, most patients had succumbed to renal disease, with a mean survival of 5 months from the onset of clinically evident renal involvement (531). The urinary findings in generalized WG are acute glomerulonephritis with hematuria, red blood cell casts, and proteinuria. Among systemic signs and symptoms at presentation are fever (34%), weight loss (16%), and anorexia or malaise (8%). Extrathoracic organ involvement at presentation includes arthritis (44%), skin rash (13%), ocular inflammation (6%), and proptosis (7%) (527,528).

Clinical Presentation and Evaluation

WG presents a characteristic complex of laboratory findings (527,528). The mild anemia of subacute or chronic diseases is seen frequently, as is mild leukocytosis. Thrombocytosis (up to 1 million platelets per cubic millimeter) can be present and probably represents an acute reaction. The results of ANA and LE cell preparation tests are uniformly negative. The total complement level is normal or mildly elevated. Mild hyperglobulinemia, particularly involving the serum IgA fraction, occurs commonly. Almost all patients have strikingly elevated erythrocyte sedimentation rates, usually 100 mm per hour or more (Westergren method). The C-reactive protein is almost always elevated. In 1982, a serum IgG against cytoplasmic components of polymorphonuclear leukocytes was described in eight patients with necrotizing granulonephritis (532). Subsequent studies have established the specificity of this antineutrophilic cytoplasmic antibody (c-ANCA or ANCA-PR3) for WG (533,534). Among 277 patients with WG and 1657 control patients, the specificity of ANCA was 99%. However, sensitivity is dependent on disease activity; thus, when only limited disease is present, the sensitivity drops to 67%, and in patients in remission, the sensitivity is between 32% and 40% (534). There is a good correlation between disease activity and c-ANCA titer (535). However, c-ANCA titers may persist in up to 40% of patients even after complete clinical remissions have been achieved. The antigen for the WG-specific c-ANCA is a 29-kilodalton (kd) molecule found in the azurophilic granules of human neutrophils (proteinase-3) (536). A second antibody, reacting to the myeloperoxidase, forms a perinuclear pattern (p-ANCA) by immunofluorescence. p-ANCA occurs in a wide range of necrotizing vasculitides such as Churg–Strauss syndrome, polyarteritis nodosa with visceral involvement, and microscopic polyangiitis (537–539).

An important aspect of WG is its pathologic and clinical similarity to a variety of other disorders characterized by granulomatous inflammation, vasculitis, or both (523). The diagnosis of WG is established when typical pathologic features accompany a characteristic clinical syndrome. The American College of Rheumatology criteria for WG include the presence of vasculitis (tissue or angiographically demonstrated) and any two of the following four findings: (a) painful or painless oral ulcers, or purulent or bloody nasal discharge; (b) chest radiograph showing the presence of nodules, fixed infiltrates, or cavities; (c) microhematuria (more than five red blood cells per high-power field) or red cell casts in urine sediment; (d) histologic changes showing granulomatous inflammation within the wall of an artery or in the perivascular or extravascular area (540). These criteria have an 88% sensitivity and a 92% specificity in recognizing WG (540). Although c-ANCA was not used in developing these criteria, the presence of this highly specific, moderately sensitive marker of WG may obviate the need for histologic confirmation (528).

Radiographic Features

The pulmonary infiltrates of WG are heterogeneous and may be of any size, shape, or lobar location (529). The most characteristic patterns (although not the most common) are solitary or multiple nodular densities or infiltrates, either poorly defined or sharply circumscribed (see Figs. 12-20 and 12-21) (527,528). These opacities vary in size from <1 cm to >9 cm, and, occasionally, air-fluid levels are found. The infiltrates may be transient, with one disappearing in one lung field and another appearing in a different location (541,542). Chest CT often discloses cavitation missed on a plain chest roentgenogram (529).

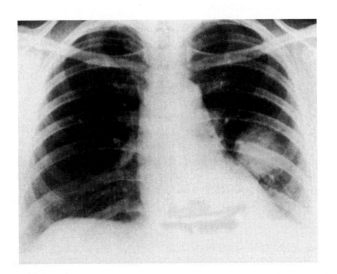

FIGURE 12-20. Wegener's granulomatosis. Posteroanterior (PA) chest radiograph shows bibasilar lung nodules.

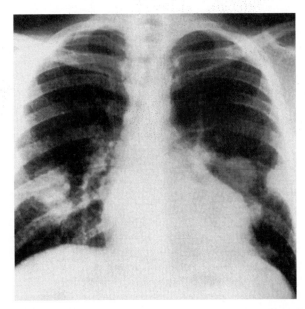

FIGURE 12-21. Wegener's granulomatosis. Posteroanterior (PA) chest radiograph shows multiple large bilateral lung nodules. No cavitation, adenopathy, or pleural effusion is present.

Pathologic Features

Lung biopsy (open or thoracoscopic) is the procedure of choice for histologic confirmation of WG. This method has the added advantage of making specimens available to rule out infectious diseases. Transbronchial biopsies establish a diagnosis in less than 10% of cases owing to small sample size. The outstanding pathologic feature in all cases is the presence of inflammatory masses (0.5 to 5 cm) within the parenchyma of one or both lungs (543). Generally, the masses are few and are sharply circumscribed on gross examination. Microscopically, they consist of necrotic areas surrounded by zones of granulation tissue. The earliest lesion in the kidney is a focal and segmental glomerulitis (543). If not treated properly, the lesions progress to a fulminant, necrotizing, and proliferative glomerulonephritis and eventually can lead to renal failure. At very early stages, glomerulitis may go undetected because the urinary sediment and renal function may be normal. Therefore, percutaneous renal biopsies are recommended when there is a high index of suspicion of WG, even when the urinary sediment is normal. Renal biopsies not only aid in establishing a diagnosis but also serve to monitor response to therapy, as measured by subsequent biopsies.

Treatment and Prognosis

Untreated, WG follows a rapidly fatal course, with a mean survival time of 5 months in most cases (527). Although prospective, randomized trials have not been performed in treating WG, oral cyclophosphamide plus corticosteroids is the mainstay of treatment (527,528,544–550). Fauci et al. reported a complete remission in 79 of 85 patients (93%) using cyclophosphamide (527). More recent data suggests a complete induction of remission in 75% of patients treated with combined cyclophosphamide and corticosteroids (528). The drug is administered orally or as a monthly intravenous infusion. A clinical response is usually seen after 1 to 3 weeks of therapy. The dose of cyclophosphamide must be monitored continually and must be adjusted to keep the white blood cell count above 3000 cells per mm³. In patients who cannot tolerate cyclophosphamide because of severe leukopenia or hemorrhagic cystitis or in young women who are not willing to accept the risk of ovarian damage associated with cyclophosphamide, azathioprine and methotrexate are alternative agents. Recent evidence has suggested that milder cases or those limited to the lung involvement may be treated effectively with methotrexate (550). A study from the National Institutes of Health cited favorable responses in 35 of 42 patients with non–life-threatening WG treated with oral methotrexate (mean dose 20 mg per week) plus prednisone (1 mg/kg/day, with gradual taper) (551). Also, a recent randomized controlled trial showed that azathioprine is as effective as cyclophosphamide in maintaining remission (552).

In 1985, De Remee et al. described improvement in 11 of 12 patients with WG treated with trimethoprim–sulfamethoxazole (T/S) (553). A recent study randomized patients with WG that had achieved complete remission with prednisone and cyclophosphamide to receive either T/S one double strength twice daily or placebo for 24 months in addition to their conventional therapy. There was an 18% relapse in the T/S group compared to 40% in the placebo (554). Other studies have found similar results (555).

ALLERGIC ANGIITIS AND GRANULOMATOSIS (CHURG–STRAUSS SYNDROME)

Pathogenesis and Epidemiology

Churg and Strauss in 1951 and Rose and Spencer in 1957 described an uncommon granulomatous inflammation and vascular necrosis primarily involving the heart, lungs, skin, nervous system, and kidneys (556,557). This entity, commonly referred to as allergic angiitis and granulomatosis, occurs primarily in patients with an allergic background, often with asthma. Characteristically, high degrees of blood eosinophilia are found (558). The cause is unknown. The syndrome is rare in the general population, with estimates ranging from 2 to 7 cases per million patients per year, though its prevalence is 10-fold higher among asthmatics (558).

Clinical Presentation and Evaluation

In the 30 cases of the Churg–Strauss syndrome reported by Chumbley et al., 21 were men and 9 were women (559). Ages ranged from 16 to 69 years; the average was 47 years. The mean duration of asthma was 8 years. In six cases, it began at the same time as the manifestations of systemic vasculitis but in all others, it preceded the manifestations. Allergic rhinitis occurred in 21 of the 30 cases (70%). Most patients with Churg–Strauss syndrome have a fever at some point in their clinical course. Anemia and weight loss are common, as is leukocytosis. Both p-ANCA and c-ANCA may be positive. The elevation of the erythrocyte sedimentation rate and the degree of peripheral blood eosinophilia are good indicators of disease activity.

Allergic granulomatosis (Churg–Strauss syndrome) strongly resembles classic polyarteritis nodosa, with some obviously distinguishing features (560–562). Churg–Strauss syndrome almost invariably is associated with an allergic diathesis, particularly severe asthma. Reports of the incidence of asthma with polyarteritis nodosa have ranged from 4% to as high as 54% (563). In general, unlike classic polyarteritis nodosa, in which pulmonary abnormalities are rare, lung involvement is invariable in Churg–Strauss syndrome. Also, this syndrome is characterized by high levels of peripheral eosinophilia (usually higher than 1500 per mm³), eosinophilic tissue infiltration, and granulomatous inflammation (558). In contrast, the predominant cellular infiltrate in polyarteritis nodosa is the polymorphonuclear leukocyte. In addition to the fibrinoid necrosis of small- and medium-sized muscular arteries that is the hallmark of classic polyarteritis nodosa, a substantial degree of involvement of small vessels such as capillaries and venules is present in Churg–Strauss syndrome. Apart from these differences, the presentation, clinicopathologic manifestations, organ system involvement, and clinical course of these two syndromes are similar.

Recently, a Churg–Strauss–like disease process has been described in patients receiving leukotriene antagonists for the treatment of steroid-dependent asthma (564). It remains controversial as to whether the disease process occurs because the steroid taper is allowing an underlying Churg–Strauss–like process to become exacerbated or as a consequence of the medication (558,564).

Radiographic Features

Chest radiographic abnormalities range from transient patchy densities to massive bilateral nodular infiltrates throughout the lung fields (543). New lesions may appear while older ones are disappearing; some remain stable after an initial period of improvement. Complete regression of a widespread active pulmonary process is sometimes seen with corticosteroids. The chest HRCT findings are of parenchymal consolidation and ground-glass opacities that vary over time in the setting of marked peripheral or BAL fluid eosinophilia (565).

Pathologic Features

Histologically, the lung typically shows fibrinoid, necrotizing, and eosinophilic granulomatous lesions, which frequently involve the pulmonary arteries and capillaries (543,563). In about 50% of their cases, Churg and Strauss found parenchymal lesions in the form of an extensive pneumonic process involving septa and alveoli (563). In the acute stage, the exudate in the lungs had a predominance of eosinophilic leukocytes mixed with giant cells. Frequently, healing terminated in focal fibrosis. Histologic evidence of bronchial asthma (hyalinization of basement membrane, increased mucous secretion, and eosinophilic infiltration of the bronchial walls) was present in most cases but generally was not very marked (563).

Treatment and Prognosis

Well-controlled experience with therapy for the Churg–Strauss syndrome is lacking. Chumbley et al. treated 27 of their 30 patients with prednisone; most received 40 to 60 mg daily, others received 100 to 120 mg daily (559). Fifteen of these 30 patients died, 3 within a year after symptoms of vasculitis appeared.

The interval from onset of signs and symptoms of vasculitis to death ranged from 6 months to 15 years; the average was 4.6 years. A recent prospective, randomized study failed to establish that plasma exchange adds to corticosteroids in preventing disease relapses (566). Cyclophosphamide and azathioprine therapy have theoretic rationale because they are effective in treating another necrotizing vasculitis, WG. Although experience with these agents is minimal, one prospective, randomized study showed that cyclophosphamide added to prednisone-plasma exchange therapy enhanced the relapse-free interval during long-term follow-up (562).

ALVEOLAR HEMORRHAGE SYNDROMES

Diffuse alveolar hemorrhage is a rare but potentially catastrophic event. It manifests radiographically by the rapid development of diffuse bilateral infiltrates, which, although they resemble pulmonary edema, occur in the absence of left atrial hypertension. The one exception to this is hemorrhage in mitral stenosis. Broadly speaking, alveolar hemorrhage syndromes can be divided into four groups: hemorrhage in the setting of pulmonary capillaritis; bland pulmonary hemorrhage; hemorrhage in the setting of diffuse alveolar damage; and hemorrhage due to vascular obstruction and other miscellaneous causes (567). Alveolar hemorrhage due to pulmonary capillaritis typically occurs in patients with an underlying connective tissue disease, although diffuse alveolar hemorrhage with capillaritis in the absence of autoantibodies has been reported (568). Of those syndromes associated with capillaritis, hemorrhage due to WG, microscopic polyangiitis, SLE, or anti–basement membrane antibody disease are discussed here. Many other associations have been made but the common factor among them is pathologic evidence of inflammation of the capillary bed with neutrophilic infiltration (567). In contrast, bland pulmonary hemorrhage occurs in the absence of vasculitis and is most often due to a drug or an exposure, although it can occur in patients with connective tissues diseases, particularly, antibasemement membrane antibody syndrome and SLE (567). Hemorrhage in the setting of diffuse alveolar damage is typically less severe than that which occurs in the other subtypes. It is most often detected only as slightly blood-tinged alveolar lavage fluid without the development of anemia or marked hemoptysis. Finally, hemorrhage in the setting of vascular obstruction is diagnostically the most challenging. In these cases, both pulmonary infiltrates and hemorrhage occur in the setting of apparent right ventricular volume overload and low left heart output, suggesting pulmonary hypertension. Pulmonary veno-occlusive disease is the exemplar but a number of other entities have been reported (567). Although lung biopsies are not required to make the diagnosis of alveolar hemorrhage—a diagnosis that is generally made when serial BALs reveal progressively bloodier aspirated fluid—biopsies are helpful in determining the etiology of the hemorrhage and in directing management. Although most alveolar hemorrhage syndromes are acute, interstitial fibrosis and hypoxemia develop in idiopathic pulmonary hemosiderosis, a rare disorder in which the etiology of recurrent and typically subclinical alveolar hemorrhage is unknown. In this syndrome, patients accumulate large numbers of hemosiderin-laden macrophages and develop diffuse interstitial thickening and chronic anemia. Lung biopsy is diagnostic (567).

ANTI–BASEMENT MEMBRANE ANTIBODY DISEASE (GOODPASTURE SYNDROME)

Pathogenesis and Epidemiology

Anti–basement membrane antibody syndrome (Goodpasture syndrome) is characterized by pulmonary hemorrhage with hemoptysis, diffuse alveolar filling on the chest radiograph, anemia, and glomerulonephritis (often rapidly progressive) (569). Although the catalyst is unknown, production of these antibodies is usually self-limited, and the syndrome apparently is inactive when the antibody is not detected. The presence of antibodies is clearly involved in the glomerulonephritis and probably in the pulmonary hemorrhage of Goodpasture syndrome (531). The mechanism responsible for the generation of these antibodies, however, is not known, although environmental factors are thought to be instrumental in triggering their production. For example, the influenza A2 virus might cause the production of antibodies that cross-react with the basement membrane structures. Many patients have a history of preceding viral syndromes, either of the upper respiratory tract or of the gastrointestinal tract. Infectious agents or chemical substances such as hydrocarbon solvents might uncover or alter some self-antigens so that they become immunogenic. Interestingly, Goodpasture described the syndrome at the height of the 1918 to 1919 influenza pandemic as part of an effort to define the lung pathology associated with the infection (569,570). There is a strong association with HLA-DR15 or -DR4 and an apparent protective effect of HLA-DR7 and -DR1 (571,572). The antigen has recently been identified as the α3 chain of Type IV collagen (572).

Clinical Presentation and Evaluation

Early reports on Goodpasture syndrome indicated a marked male predominance of 9:1, but more recent studies describe lower male-to-female ratios of 3.5:1 and 2:1 (569). Seventy-five percent of patients are between the ages of 17 and 27 years at the onset of the illness, whereas the remainder range in age up to 75 years (569).

In most cases, the initial symptom is hemoptysis, which occurs at some point during the course of the disease in 99% of cases (531,573–575). Bouts of hemoptysis range in severity from slightly blood-streaked sputum to massive hemorrhage (574). In about one-fifth of the patients, upper respiratory tract infections of a nonspecific (viral) nature precede the appearance of the syndrome (574). Chills and fever occur acutely with pulmonary hemorrhage but are not otherwise prominent. Substernal chest pain occurs without relation to activity, although coughing can aggravate it.

Renal abnormalities may occur before pulmonary symptoms. Urinary findings, present on admission in more than 80% of patients include proteinuria, microscopic hematuria, and, less commonly, pyuria. In 26 (81%) of Wilson and Dixon's patients, renal failure requiring dialysis occurred within 1 to 14 months of onset (mean 3.5 months) (576).

Anemia is universally present early in the disease. The anemia is apparently not hemolytic, although a decreased erythrocyte life span has been demonstrated (574). Neither hemolysis nor jaundice is present.

The D$_{LCO}$ may be useful in following the course of this disease (577). Because intraalveolar blood binds carbon monoxide, the D$_{LCO}$ may be raised above baseline levels during lung hemorrhage. Thus, serial measurements of D$_{LCO}$ may help distinguish fresh pulmonary hemorrhage from other causes of radiographic opacities (e.g., infection).

Radiographic Features

The radiographic appearance of Goodpasture syndrome is closely related to the distribution, volume, and temporal sequence of pulmonary hemorrhage. Both interstitial and alveolar involvement occurs. Confluent densities are seen shortly after hemorrhage and may be indistinguishable from hypervolemia associated with azotemia or from noncardiogenic pulmonary edema of another origin (see Fig. 12-22). All these conditions produce rapid alterations in the chest radiograph. Localized air space changes may progress to diffuse opacification within hours, whereas complete clearing may occur during remission. However, accentuated interstitial markings tend to persist in Goodpasture syndrome after repeated episodes of bleeding owing to the presence of siderophages in the interstitium. If the bleeding is of sufficient duration, permanent reticulonodular infiltrates develop, resembling those seen in idiopathic pulmonary hemosiderosis. Generally these changes are diffuse, but they may also be localized. The superimposition of fluffy alveolar filling densities on a reticulonodular background suggests recurrent pulmonary hemorrhage.

Goodpasture syndrome demonstrates a predilection for perihilar involvement, whereas, in contrast to the pulmonary venous congestion and edema of left ventricular failure, Kerley B lines and pleural effusions are not characteristic.

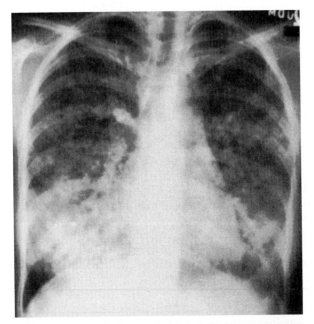

FIGURE 12-22.   Anti–glomerular basement membrane (anti–GBM) syndrome. Posteroanterior (PA) chest radiograph shows a characteristic alveolar filling pattern in a patient with hemoptysis and renal failure. The heart, pulmonary vascularity, and pleura are normal.

Pathologic Features

Diagnosis of Goodpasture syndrome depends on the demonstration of circulating anti–glomerular basement membrane antibodies (anti–GBM) and/or on the finding of linear deposits of immunoglobulin along glomerular or alveolar basement membranes (569,578). These findings are coupled with evidence of lung hemorrhage in a patient who typically presents with recurrent hemoptysis, dyspnea, and anemia. The erythrocyte sedimentation rate, although often slightly elevated, is usually not strikingly elevated as in most cases of systemic vasculitis (e.g., WG). The degree of renal injury is mirrored by elevations in serum creatinine and blood urea nitrogen (BUN), and active glomerulonephritis is almost always accompanied by proteinuria, hematuria (gross or microscopic), and red blood cell casts. Histologically, the renal abnormality in patients with Goodpasture syndrome is an actively proliferating, often necrotizing, crescent-forming type of glomerulonephritis. This is accompanied by variable, probably secondary tubular alterations and interstitial infiltrative processes (45).

Treatment and Prognosis

Historically, the prognosis for Goodpasture syndrome has been generally poor (579). Patients died of either renal failure or lung hemorrhage. In Wilson and Dixon's study, in which the diagnosis was based on the presence of circulating anti–GBM antibodies, 28 of 32 patients developed renal failure and more than 50% died within 1 year of diagnosis (576). Recently, with therapy and earlier intervention, the outlook has changed substantially.

The most successful therapy includes plasmapheresis, treatment of the inflammatory response in tissues, and suppression of further antibody production through the use of corticosteroids and cyclophosphamide or azathioprine (579). Because production of anti–GBM antibodies may be short-lived, plasma exchange appears to reduce damage to the glomerulus by lowering the levels of circulating anti–GBM antibody. Lockwood et al. reported on seven patients treated with plasma exchange, cytotoxic drugs, and corticosteroids (580). Recently, Levy et al. reported on a retrospective cohort of 71 patients treated identically and showed that patients who presented with a creatinine concentration <5.7 mg per dL had 100% patient survival and 95% renal survival at 1 year. In patients who presented with a creatinine concentration of >5.7 mg per dL but did not require immediate dialysis, patient and renal survival were 83% and 82%, respectively, at 1 year. In patients who presented with dialysis-dependent renal failure, patient and renal survival were 65% and 8%, respectively, at 1 year. All patients who required immediate dialysis and had 100% crescents on renal biopsy remained dialysis dependent (579). In general, plasma exchange is carried out every 1 to 3 days for 2 to 3 weeks. It is continued until anti–GBM antibodies are undetectable (579).

MICROSCOPIC POLYANGIITIS

Pathogenesis and Epidemiology

Microscopic polyangiitis causes pulmonary hemorrhage in the absence of anti–basement membrane antibodies. Renal disease with focal segmental glomerulonephritis is universal and antinuclear cytoplasmic antibodies are detectable in 75% of patients, usually (85%) in the perinuclear distribution (anti–myeloperoxidase antibodies and p-ANCA) (581). Other organ systems commonly involved include musculoskeletal system (arthritis and myositis), gastrointestinal tract (vasculitis and hemorrhage), and peripheral nervous system (neuropathy) (567). Antibodies to hepatitis B and C are seen in one-third of patients (561,582). The preponderance of evidence suggests a direct role of ANCA in activating neutrophils and monocytes, leading to vascular damage, vasculitis, and end-organ damage (526).

Microscopic polyangiitis is relatively rare, with an incidence between 8 to 25 cases per million (583,584). Alveolar hemorrhage occurs in approximately 11% of patients with microscopic polyangiitis (581).

Clinical Presentation and Evaluation

The presentation of microscopic polyangiitis is identical to anti–GBM syndrome; that is, rapidly progressive glomerulonephritis; hematuria with red blood cell casts; and, in the case of pulmonary hemorrhage, hemoptysis, anemia, and rapidly progressive hypoxemia. The severity of hemoptysis, as with all alveolar hemorrhage syndromes, is variable but is evident upon bronchoscopy with BAL. The clinical evaluation is identical to that outlined previously for pulmonary hemorrhage syndromes.

Radiographic Features

The chest radiograph shows bilateral fluffy or hazy opacities or even more dense consolidation with a characteristic rapid evolution and, if the bleeding is transient, a rapid clearing is seen within 1 to 2 days unless acute lung injury or pneumonia supervenes. Chest HRCT shows diffuse bilateral ground-glass opacities indistinguishable from pulmonary edema of a cardiogenic or noncardiogenic source. Scarring may develop with chronic hemorrhage. Honeycombing is not generally seen (567).

Pathologic Features

The pulmonary pathologic features are those of diffuse alveolar hemorrhage, with red blood cells densely filling the alveolar spaces. Evidence of a host response is critical for differentiating alveolar hemorrhage from surgical hemorrhage. Evidence of a host response includes evidence of acute vasculitis with polymorphonuclear leukocytes infiltrating the capillaries, alveolar macrophage influx into the alveolar space with ingestion of red blood cells (erythrophagocytosis), or a high percentage of hemosiderin-laden macrophages. In hemorrhage, the hemosiderin pigment is abundant, dark, and obvious. This should be distinguished from the lightly pigmented alveolar macrophages seen in DIP and RB–ILD. In these latter two conditions, red blood cells generally do not pack the alveolar spaces of a well-inflated lung and vasculitis is entirely absent (543).

Treatment and Prognosis

The treatment for microscopic polyangiitis is immunosuppression with high-dose corticosteroids (up to 7 mg per kg of intravenous methylprednisolone or its equivalent) for 3 days followed by a tapering dose, along with cyclophosphamide at a dose of 2 mg/kg/day by mouth or 0.5 mg per m^2 intravenously as a once-a-month dose, titrated upward to 1 mg per m^2 as tolerated on the basis of peripheral white blood cell count (585). As in WG, early treatment is critical to maintaining renal function. Mechanical ventilatory support may be needed if hemorrhage is severe.

EOSINOPHILIC SYNDROMES

Pathogenesis and Epidemiology

The presence of eosinophils in lung tissue is a common occurrence and indicates that these inflammatory cells are part of the host's normal cellular response to a variety of inciting agents and systemic immunologic diseases (586). Chemotactic factors released from degranulating mast cells attract eosinophils and localize them in sites of IgE-mediated reactions, whereupon eosinophils inactivate mediators actually seem to control the extent of the reaction. Eosinophils are found in the airways and in the lung tissue of patients with IPF. In other interstitial diseases that seem to have an allergic component (such as hypersensitivity pneumonitis, drug-induced lung syndromes, and sarcoidosis), eosinophils are a minor component of the tissue reaction but can usually be identified in tissue sections. In contrast, eosinophils can be the most conspicuous inflammatory cell in certain primary lung or systemic diseases that have frequent lung involvement, and these are grouped together as eosinophilic syndromes. There is considerable overlap among these syndromes, and precise separation is impossible because the etiology and pathogenesis are poorly understood. The current classification scheme is acute eosinophilic pneumonias, tropical pulmonary eosinophilia, chronic eosinophilic pneumonia, allergic bronchopulmonary aspergillosis, Churg–Strauss syndrome (discussed previously), and idiopathic hypereosinophilic syndrome (IHS).

Clinical Presentation and Evaluation

ACUTE EOSINOPHILIC PULMONARY SYNDROMES

Loeffler syndrome (simple pulmonary eosinophilia). Loeffler syndrome is usually a self-limited disease that features migratory, fleeting areas of infiltration in a peripheral pattern on the chest radiograph and is accompanied by minimal respiratory symptoms and blood eosinophilia (587,588). The disease seems to be an allergic response that can result from parasitic infection; the human parasite *Ascaris lumbricoides* and the nonhuman ones such as dog and cat ascarids that produce visceral larva migrans are known to be causative. Several other parasitic infections and exposure to numerous drugs such as sulfonamides have been implicated in a Loeffler-like syndrome (587,588). The clinical presentation is that of a dry cough, fever, and breathlessness. Peripheral eosinophilia can be striking and sputum frequently contains eosinophils. *Ascaris* larvae can be identified in sputum or in gastric lavage during the period when pulmonary infiltrates are present. Tissue diagnosis is not usually required, but BAL can show a marked increase in eosinophils (588). When *A. lumbricoides* is identified, mebendazole (100 mg twice daily for 3 days) is indicated to prevent the postpneumonic gastrointestinal manifestations. Numerous other parasitic infections can be associated with pulmonary infiltrates and peripheral eosinophilia (453). The more common offenders in the United States are *Strongyloides stercoralis*, *Toxocara canis* (visceral larva migrans), and *Ancylostoma brasiliensis*. *Strongyloides* infection has been associated with the "hyperinfection syndrome" (453). This typically occurs in individuals with a previous exposure who develop defects in host defense, either in association with an illness such as HIV infection or malignancy or when receiving systemic corticosteroids.

Drug-induced pulmonary eosinophilic syndromes. A variety of medications have been associated with pulmonary infiltrates and blood or pulmonary eosinophilia. Patients typically present with acute or subacute symptoms of cough and dyspnea. Careful questioning is required because nonprescription medications may be the culprit. Symptoms usually abate with cessation of the drug, but corticosteroids are occasionally required. Resolution of the pulmonary infiltrates is typically rapid (within 24 or 48 hours).

Idiopathic acute eosinophilic pneumonia. Eosinophilic pneumonia can present as rapidly progressive respiratory failure with a clinical presentation compatible with the ARDS. This has been termed *acute eosinophilic pneumonia* (589). Patients present with fever, myalgias, dyspnea, and significant hypoxemia that may require mechanical ventilation. Importantly, peripheral blood eosinophilia is not usually present. BAL is critical in delineating the diagnosis. Demonstration of abundant eosinophils in BAL fluid is diagnostic. There is typically a dramatic response to treatment with corticosteroids, with complete resolution of the pulmonary infiltrates.

Tropical pulmonary eosinophilia. Respiratory symptoms of cough, dyspnea, and, in some patients, attacks of asthma may be present in those with filarial infection. Systemic symptoms of malaise, fatigue, weight loss, and fever also occur; peripheral blood eosinophilia and high levels of antibody to filarial antigens are characteristic of laboratory abnormalities. The chest radiograph may reveal areas of patchy consolidation or bilateral streaking and increased parenchymal linearities in the hilar and lower lung zones. Histologically, microfilaria can be identified in areas of tissue nodules showing necrotic debris and eosinophils (590). A striking recovery of eosinophils in BAL fluid is typical. After therapy with diethylcarbamazine, these cells decrease and lung function tests improve (591).

CHRONIC EOSINOPHILIC PULMONARY SYNDROMES

Chronic eosinophilic pneumonia. As suggested by its name, chronic eosinophilic pneumonia disease differs from the acute form in that it is often chronic and accompanying pulmonary and systemic symptoms can be severe. If this disease persists, it can lead to a form of interstitial pulmonary fibrosis that radiographically shows honeycombed lung changes and lung function abnormalities characteristic of other diseases in this group.

Chronic eosinophilic pneumonia most commonly affects women and can present as a severe respiratory illness in which fever, night sweats, weight loss, and dyspnea are prominent symptoms (592–594). Presentation can be subacute or chronic. Blood eosinophilia is variable and often is not present. Extrapulmonary involvement does not occur. The disease is sometimes initially misdiagnosed as tuberculosis. A distinguishing feature described in the first cases of eosinophilic pneumonia was deterioration in the patient's condition despite a trial of

antituberculosis therapy (592). However, one helpful clue is often evident in the chest radiograph. Dense alveolar filling infiltrates develop that have a peculiar location in the peripheral portions of the lung, with a pronounced predilection for apical and axillary segments of the upper lobes. These peripheral infiltrates are not limited to a defined lobar or anatomic distribution but can extend across the usual anatomic barriers. Wheezing can be present or can develop *de novo* in some patients. The clinical, laboratory, and radiographic features are distinctive and an open or thoracoscopic biopsy is not usually required to establish the diagnosis. Fiber-optic bronchoscopy with transbronchial biopsy and BAL should be the first diagnostic test. Striking increases in BAL eosinophils (greater than 50%) are characteristic of chronic eosinophilic pneumonia (29). Infectious etiologies such as helminths need to be excluded. Once the diagnosis is established, treatment with corticosteroids causes a striking regression in the radiographic findings and in clinical symptoms; a chest radiograph taken a few weeks later may appear normal. Although the response to corticosteroid therapy is usually impressive, the disease may exacerbate after therapy is discontinued, and relapse can occur in about 50% of the patients during a 10-year follow-up period (593). The infiltrates tend to recur in the same locations on the chest radiograph.

Pulmonary eosinophilia with asthma. Asthma is a frequent complaint in many forms of lung disease, including the eosinophilic syndromes. Thus, it is difficult to separate a single disease entity on this basis alone. Two diseases, allergic bronchopulmonary aspergillosis and allergic angiitis with granulomatosis, as described by Churg and Strauss, can fit this description (556,595). Because the eosinophilic component to the diseases seems incidental, it can be argued that these diseases are best discussed with respective asthma syndromes and systemic vasculitides affecting the lung, such as Churg–Strauss syndrome (see prior discussion in this chapter).

Idiopathic hypereosinophilic syndrome. IHS is a rare disorder characterized by severe peripheral eosinophilia with diffuse organ infiltration with eosinophils in which no underlying cause for the eosinophilia can be identified (587). A variety of organs can be affected including the heart, central nervous system, bone marrow, visceral organs, gastrointestinal tract, skin, and eyes. The cardiac manifestations can be life-threatening, with congestive heart failure, intracardiac thrombi, mitral regurgitation, and cardiomyopathy all being described (587). Lung involvement occurs in about 50% of the cases, with pulmonary infiltrates with cough as the presenting manifestations. The disease was uniformly fatal prior to the advent of effective therapy with corticosteroids and hydroxyurea.

PULMONARY ALVEOLAR PROTEINOSIS

Pathogenesis and Epidemiology

Pulmonary alveolar proteinosis (PAP) is a disease of unknown etiology characterized by accumulation of PAS-positive, lipid-rich, proteinaceous material in the distal air spaces of the lungs (596,597). Rosen, Castleman, and Liebow first described this entity in 1958 on the basis of human lung biopsies (596). The age of onset is generally between 20 and 50 years, but the disorder also occurs in infants and in the elderly (597). There is a male preponderance of >3:1. Some patients are exposed to a variety of dusts and fumes, such as wood dust and silica, whereas in others the disease is idiopathic (597). Recent data from both animal and human studies have identified that deficiency of the cytokine granulocyte–monocyte–colony stimulating factor (GM–CSF), through either mutation or acquired inactivating antibodies, plays a critical role in the pathogenesis of this disease (597). GM–CSF appears to be a pivotal regulator of alveolar macrophage surfactant metabolism (597).

Pulmonary alveolar proteinosis is rare with an estimated prevalence of approximately 4 per million (597).

Clinical Presentation and Evaluation

The onset is usually gradual and insidious, but, occasionally, the disorder follows an acute febrile illness. Dyspnea during exertion is characteristically the first manifestation, gradually evolving into a dyspnea at rest. Cough is common and is often associated with the production of a thick, white to yellow sputum. In those with extensive lung involvement, fatigability and weight loss are common. Chest pain and hemoptysis are unusual.

Abnormal physical findings are few. The resonance of the percussion note over the thorax is diminished and breath sounds have a coarse bronchovesicular quality; coarse crackles are audible over affected areas. Fingers and toes become clubbed in some patients (598).

There are no distinctive hematologic abnormalities associated with pulmonary alveolar proteinosis. Anemia does not occur; in fact, polycythemia may result if hypoxemia is severe. Leukocyte counts vary from normal to a brisk leukocytosis (i.e., to as high as 15,000 to 20,000 cells per mm^3); this usually signifies the coexistence of an acute pulmonary infection. Hyperlipidemia, hyperglobulinemia, and elevated serum lactic dehydrogenase (LDH) levels occur in some patients with pulmonary alveolar proteinosis (598).

Pulmonary function tests characteristically show a restrictive ventilatory pattern (598). The accumulation of the proteinaceous material in the air spaces reduces the number of functioning lung units, thereby altering the overall pressure–volume relationships of the lung and causing pulmonary compliance to decrease. The VC, RV, and functional residual capacity (FRC) are all proportionally reduced. Flow rates are usually normal during a forced expiratory maneuver (599,600).

Marked ventilation–perfusion ratio abnormalities occur in pulmonary alveolar proteinosis. Many areas of lung are perfused with mixed venous blood but receive little or no ventilation. As a result, the alveolar–arterial difference for oxygen widens, and arterial hypoxemia is prominent. Moreover, because abnormal material in the alveolar spaces effectively amputates some gas-exchange surface and interferes with gas transfer across the alveolar axillary membrane, the D_{LCO} is reduced, and a fall in arterial oxygen saturation can be demonstrated regularly during exercise. Moreover, in most cases a shunt fraction greater than 17% is demonstrated while the patient is breathing 100% oxygen (601).

Serum laboratory values are usually within normal limits except for an elevation in the serum LDH level (602). In fact, the combination of an elevated shunt fraction and an elevated serum LDH level suggests the diagnosis of pulmonary alveolar proteinosis (306). Of note, elevated serum

LDH levels are also found in *P. carinii* pneumonia, as are foci of intraalveolar proteinaceous debris resembling pulmonary alveolar proteinosis.

On the basis of clinical, functional, and chest radiographic findings (i.e., dyspnea, diffuse alveolar filling on chest radiograph, elevated serum LDH level, and arterial hypoxemia with an increased shunt fraction), a presumptive diagnosis can often be made. BAL fluid demonstrates a thick opaque, milky effluent that sediments into multiple layers. However, definitive diagnosis is generally established by histologic examination of a lung biopsy obtained by bronchoscopy or thoracotomy (597–599). The diagnosis has also been made by the demonstration of PAS-positive material on light microscopic examination of sputum or lung washings. Electron microscopy of sputum or lung washings shows granular material and lamellar bodies (603). Findings on light microscopy and the clinical presentation can be confused with those of *P. carinii* infection; a methenamine–silver stain is needed to exclude this possibility. Secondary PAP (pseudo-PAP) may complicate hematologic malignancies and chronic infections.

Radiographic Features

The chest radiograph shows a diffuse alveolar filling process characterized by scattered patchy, confluent, nodular infiltrates (see Fig. 12-23) (596,598,599). The pattern and distribution are similar to those of cardiogenic pulmonary edema except that the cardiac silhouette is usually normal in alveolar proteinosis and that the alveolar filling pattern resembles a bat wing. The involvement is usually bilateral and symmetric, but asymmetric or unilateral patterns are seen occasionally. Hilar adenopathy, Kerley B lines, and pleural effusions do not occur. The chest HRCT scan shows the highly characteristic findings of diffuse ground-glass opacities with marked, symmetric septal thickening without adenopathy or effusion. This pattern is referred to as "crazy paving" because it resembles tiles with intervening grout (see Fig. 12-24) (598). A similar pattern can be seen with pulmonary edema and with *P. carinii* pneumonia (604).

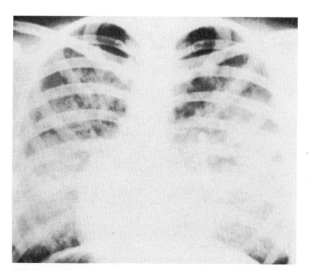

FIGURE 12-23. Pulmonary alveolar proteinosis. Posteroanterior (PA) chest radiograph of a 21-year-old woman with a diffuse, bilateral alveolar filling process and a normal cardiac silhouette.

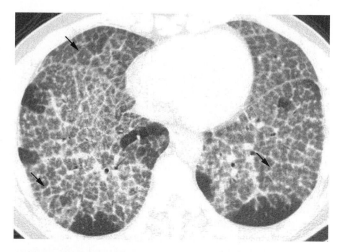

FIGURE 12-24. Pulmonary alveolar proteinosis. Axial high-resolution computed tomographic (HRCT) image shows multifocal bilateral ground-glass opacity associated with extensive interlobular septal thickening (*arrows*). The regions of abnormal lung have a sharp demarcation with normal lung regions. This pattern is called "crazy paving."

Pathologic Features

Grossly, the lungs contain multiple, firm, yellow nodules ranging in size from several millimeters to 2 or 3 centimeters in diameter. Microscopically, large groups of alveoli and small distal bronchioles are filled with a granular, floccular PAS-positive material (see Fig. 12-25). Generally, the alveolar walls are normal, but cellular infiltration and areas of fibrosis occur in the interstitial spaces of the lungs, particularly with long-standing disease. Electron microscopic examination of the proteinaceous material reveals alveolar macrophages that contain numerous lamellar osmiophilic inclusions within the cytoplasm. This lamellar material, rich in phospholipid, is found not only with macrophages but is also lying free in amorphous debris in the alveolar spaces. The marked PAS positivity of this material is probably due to the presence of

large amounts of surfactant protein A, a heavily glycosylated surfactant constituent (45).

Treatment and Prognosis

Spontaneous recovery with complete resolution of clinical findings and chest radiographic changes occurs in about 25% of patients with pulmonary alveolar proteinosis (598). In others, the disorder is progressive, although the rate of progression is variable. In about 15% to 20% of patients, this disease runs a rapid, fulminant course with marked arterial hypoxemia, cor pulmonale, and respiratory failure. In others, progression is over months to years, and in some patients with long-standing disease, interstitial fibrosis develops.

Pulmonary infections with mycotic organisms are common in alveolar proteinosis, which suggests impaired lung defenses. In fact, the alveolar macrophage, the principal cellular defense against intracellular organisms, has been found to be defective in this disease. The most frequently encountered infections are nocardiosis, cryptococcosis, aspergillosis, and mucormycosis (597,598). This dysfunction improves with lung lavage (605).

Assessment of therapeutic efficacy in pulmonary alveolar proteinosis is made difficult by the fact that many patients improve spontaneously (606). Corticosteroids seem to be of no benefit. A few patients appear to improve following administration of agents that presumably thin or liquefy bronchial secretions (e.g., potassium iodide; aerosolized streptokinase–streptodornase; trypsin; and a combination of saline, heparin, and acetylcysteine delivered by intermittent positive-pressure breathing). Recently, subcutaneous GM–CSF has shown some benefit in nonrandomized, open-label trials (607,608).

In patients with advanced disease and severe ventilatory compromise, lavage of an entire lung with large volumes of a saline solution remains the standard of care (597,605). The procedure is performed under general anesthesia using a double-lumen endotracheal tube for single lung ventilation during lavage of the contralateral lung. Usually, amelioration of symptoms, with improvement in pulmonary function, begins within hours after lavage, and by 24 to 48 hours pulmonary function and arterial P_{O_2} exceed prelavage levels.

LYMPHANGIOLEIOMYOMATOSIS

Pathogenesis and Epidemiology

LAM is a rare cystic lung disease causing progressive airflow obstruction in women of childbearing age. The histopathologic abnormality is a hamartomatous proliferation of atypical smooth muscle along lymphatics in a variety of organs but the most clinically evident are the lung and kidney (609,610). LAM occurs in two forms: arising in the setting of the tuberous sclerosis complex (TSC) or occurring sporadically. Tuberous sclerosis is an autosomal dominant neurocutaneous syndrome that results from mutations in one of two genes, TSC1 or TSC2. Tuberous sclerosis occurs in 1 in 6,000 to 1 in 10,000 births. Afflicted individuals have seizures, widespread hamartomatous lesions, and mental retardation. Approximately one-third of women with tuberous sclerosis develop the cystic lung lesions characteristic of LAM (611). The prevalence of known cases in North America is 400. These figures are kept by the LAM registry (612).

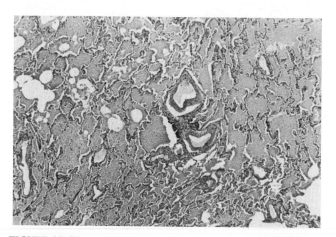

FIGURE 12-25. Pulmonary alveolar proteinosis. Surgical lung biopsy reveals diffuse alveolar filling with a granularlike material that stained periodic acid–Schiff (PAS) positive. Note the alveolar wall thickness is normal.

Clinical Presentation and Evaluation

Patients typically present in the third or fourth decade of life with breathlessness. LAM is most frequently misdiagnosed as asthma or chronic bronchitis owing to the marked airflow limitation observed on pulmonary function testing. Pneumothoraces are common. Chylous effusions occur in 7% to 39% (610). Hemoptysis occurs approximately 25% of the time. In addition to severe airflow limitation without responsiveness to bronchodilators, the diffusing capacity is severely reduced. Lung volumes are typically normal or are increased.

Radiographic Features

Chest radiographs show cystic or reticulonodular infiltrates with hyperinflation. Abnormalities on HRCT are highly distinctive and, given the clinical setting, virtually establish the diagnosis (see Fig. 12-26). Numerous thin-walled cysts are distributed throughout the lung fields. There is no predilection for the upper lobes. Unlike eosinophilic granuloma (EG), the nodular component is minimal. The cysts also are distinct from emphysematous changes. Angiomyolipomas occur in over one-third of patients and may cause severe hematuria.

Pathologic Features

Positive staining for melanoma-related marker (HMB-45) in smooth muscle is highly specific for LAM. The natural history is variable, but most patients die of respiratory failure within 10 years of the onset of symptoms (610).

Treatment and Prognosis

Major therapeutic approaches include oophorectomy or administration of antiestrogen regimens, but results have been disappointing. Medroxyprogesterone and/or oophorectomy are considered the major options for treatment. Lung transplantation has been performed in a few patients with a 2-year survival of approximately 60% (610).

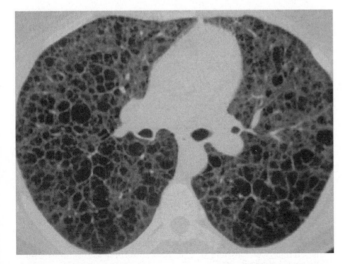

FIGURE 12-26. Lymphangioleiomyomatosis. Axial high-resolution computed tomographic (HRCT) image shows numerous, uniform, thin-walled cysts bilaterally, consistent with lymphangioleiomyomatosis.

PULMONARY LANGERHANS CELL HISTIOCYTOSIS (EOSINOPHILIC GRANULOMA)

Pathogenesis and Epidemiology

The histiocytoses are a group of diseases that feature proliferation and activation of mononuclear phagocytic cells, especially macrophages. The term *histiocyte* is synonymous with *macrophage* and emphasizes the fact that tissue macrophages can exist in many forms as alveolar or peritoneal cells, dermal Langerhans cells, hepatic Kupffer cells, osteoclasts, and microglial brain cells. Thus, the range of diseases and the principal organs affected are broad. Often, a form of cell-mediated immunity is evident and a granulomatous tissue reaction is found. Both findings suggest an intimate macrophage–lymphocyte interaction, as discussed already for sarcoidosis. Eosinophils may be contained in the granulomatous reaction. Immune complexes in blood can contribute to the lung reaction and can perhaps stimulate macrophages or histiocytes, but this too remains uncertain. The proliferation and accumulation of histiocytes in affected tissue, often producing a granulomatous lesion, are part of the disease process in the histiocytic disorders.

A comprehensive classification of the histiocytic diseases based on macrophage involvement presents obvious overlapping with other syndromes readily explained by etiology or easily recognized clinically. The spectrum includes (a) reactive histiocytic proliferation with a known microorganism (tuberculosis, fungal, or parasitic agents) or with inert particles; (b) reactive proliferation in which the inciting agent is unknown, which includes such diverse entities as eosinophilic granuloma, Wegener's and lymphomatoid granulomatosis of the lung, and sarcoidosis; (c) lipid storage diseases, which include Gaucher disease, Niemann–Pick disease, sea blue histiocytosis, and Fabry disease; and (d) neoplastic disorders such as acute monocytic leukemia, chronic myelomonocytic leukemia, and histiocytic lymphoma. EG is the only one that frequently affects the lungs except for other granulomatous vasculitides and sarcoidosis.

Langerhans cell histiocytosis (EG and histiocytosis X) can be a multifocal disease involving bones of the skull, extremities, ribs, pelvis, vertebrae, and mandible with lytic lesions. The triad of lytic skull lesions, exophthalmos, and pituitary involvement producing diabetes insipidus is known as *Hand–Schüller–Christian* disease. A diffuse form of histocytosis of the Letterer–Siwe type is a fulminant disease generally unresponsive to therapy. A unifocal or local extraosseous form of Langerhans cell histiocytosis involves the lungs. Only this entity is discussed here in detail (613).

Langerhans cell histiocytosis is rare with estimated prevalence of two to five cases per million. It can affect all ages, but young adults, especially men, develop the disease most frequently.

Clinical Presentation and Evaluation

Symptoms may have an insidious onset, with cough and breathlessness with exertion as initial complaints. A spontaneous pneumothorax can be the presenting manifestation, although this is more likely to occur in advanced fibrotic stages of the disease when localized areas of airway obstruction lead to cyst formation and overdistention. Few constitutional symptoms may be present. Greater than 90% of cases occur in smokers. Blood eosinophilia is unusual, but circulating immune complexes can be measured in serum in many patients with active disease, and the titer reflects the degree of cellular reactivity in a lung biopsy (614).

Radiographic Features

The chest radiograph usually reveals a diffuse micronodular and interstitial-appearing infiltrate, initially involving the middle and lower lung zones; later, small cystic air spaces develop in the infiltrate, producing a honeycomb pattern (see Fig. 12-27) (615). Adenopathy or pleural disease is unusual. The radiographic appearance differs from the one described for eosinophilic pneumonia, in which migratory infiltrates in the periphery of the lung are characteristic. Pneumothoraces occur in 10% to 30% of patients. The HRCT scan is highly distinctive, showing peribronchial cystic and nodular lesions predominantly in the mid- and upper-lung zones. Numerous thin-walled cysts are observed, with micronodules coexistent in most cases (see Fig. 12-28) (616).

Pathologic Features

Lung biopsies reveal a mixture of inflammatory, cystic, nodular, and fibrotic abnormalities. Light microscopy shows a stellate pattern of fibrosis that is distinctive. The characteristic feature of Langerhans cell histiocytosis is, not surprisingly, aggregates of Langerhans cells, which are large histiocytes derived from

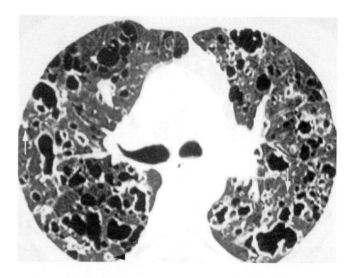

FIGURE 12-28. Pulmonary Langerhans cell histiocytosis. Axial high-resolution computed tomographic (HRCT) image shows numerous bilateral irregular cysts characteristic of Langerhans cell histiocytosis. Centrilobular nodules (*arrows*), one of which is cavitating (*arrowhead*), are also present.

dendritic cells (see Fig. 12-29) (617–619). They stain positively for S-100 protein or OKT6 antigen (45). Electron microscopy demonstrates the Birbeck granule (pentolaminar body) but is of marginal clinical utility because of expense. Diagnosis usually requires a thoracoscopic biopsy but the presence of more than 5% Langerhans cells in BAL fluid by S-100 or OKT6 strongly supports the diagnosis.

Treatment and Prognosis

The course of pulmonary Langerhans cell histiocytosis is quite variable in adults, and the prognosis is generally better for focal disease limited to the lungs than for multifocal disease

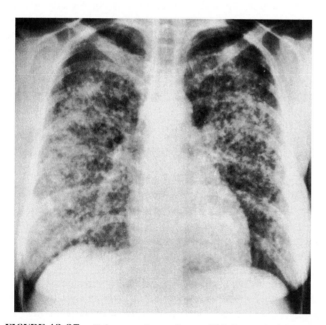

FIGURE 12-27. Pulmonary Langerhans cell histiocytosis. A 31-year-old woman had a viral upper respiratory infection 3 months previously (a chest radiograph was not obtained), and a dry, nonproductive cough persisted. Dyspnea developed in the interim and shortness of breath limited her daily activities. Her chest radiograph shows extensive alveolar filling and interstitial infiltrates in all lung zones; also, small cystic spaces are evident. Tissue from an open lung biopsy revealed eosinophilic granuloma and evidence of cystic changes, suggesting that the disease process was chronic. Corticosteroid therapy improved the appearance of the chest radiograph and her symptoms. She also discontinued cigarette smoking, which is an essential part of the therapy.

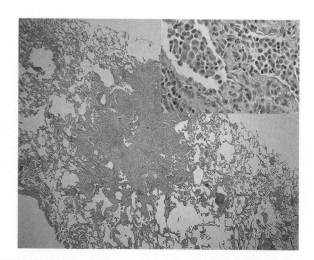

FIGURE 12-29. Pulmonary Langerhans cell histiocytosis. Langerhans cell histiocytosis (histiocytosis X, eosinophilic granuloma) is most easily recognized at low power in the surgical lung biopsy by forming a stellate lesion centered on an airway. At high power (*inset*), numerous macrophages are seen accumulated within alveoli. Eosinophils and Langerhans cells are seen in the pulmonary interstitium.

and bone involvement. A bone scan is advisable as part of the initial evaluation of a patient with focal Langerhans cell histiocytosis and should certainly be made if bone symptoms occur later because approximately 20% of patients eventually develop a lytic bone lesion. Rarely, diabetes insipidus occurs. The lung disease does have a significant rate of spontaneous remission. Regression of pulmonary symptoms and chest radiographic infiltrates may occur in 10% to 25% of patients within several months of diagnosis, although the disease does not disappear entirely without some residual symptoms. As most patients are cigarette smokers, cessation of smoking greatly helps. Corticosteroid treatment is not especially effective in suppressing the disease, except for the initial boost in subjective well-being associated with the "steroid effect." In many cases, the lung disease stabilizes and in effect burns out, leaving the patient with moderate pulmonary symptoms (dyspnea on exertion), residual lung fibrosis, cystic spaces in the parenchyma, and a restrictive pattern of lung function (620). Therapy at this stage of disease is symptomatic. Pulmonary hypertension is also common (621). Some patients are troubled with persisting bronchitis, which is superimposed on the quiescent interstitial fibrosis. If wheezing or obstructive airway changes on pulmonary testing are noted, judicious use of antibiotics and bronchodilators can be effective. In refractory disease, lung transplantation may be required. Unfortunately, recurrence after transplantation has been well documented (622–624).

DRUG-INDUCED PULMONARY DISEASE

The development of antibiotics, cytotoxic antineoplastic agents, and various immunosuppressive drugs has had a remarkable impact on medical therapeutics and has made the control of infection, cancer, collagen vascular diseases, and organ transplant rejection everyday realities in medicine. One undesirable by-product of drug therapy, albeit a rather minor one in the overall scheme, is related to iatrogenic and adverse complications of their use. Development of an allergy to drugs is common, and specific drug-induced pulmonary reactions occur frequently. In fact, almost every therapeutic agent used has (or may have) been noted to cause pulmonary disease; the lists compiled are impressive (187,625–637). A list of some of these drugs is provided in Table 12-9; the antineoplastic chemotherapy drugs and immunosuppressants are the most prominent offenders. Occasionally, lung toxicity results from a very commonly used drug such as hydrochlorothiazide or from an antibiotic such as nitrofurantoin, penicillin, or a sulfonamide drug.

The host reaction often seems to be hypersensitivity, for contact with the drug may eventually cause sensitization to occur. Subsequently, an immune response develops in the form of antibody or an exaggerated lymphocytic mitogenic response when the host is challenged with the offending drug antigen. However, the precise mechanisms are poorly understood, and for this reason experimental models have been difficult to develop except for bleomycin.

Most drugs are organic compounds of low molecular weight (less than 1,000). To become "antigenic" they must couple to larger carrier substances, which are usually serum proteins; in the process of drug–protein binding, the structure of the protein is denatured in that its tertiary molecular configuration is altered. The immune response that is elicited, however, is usually directed to the drug determinant, although a metabolite of the drug might be the actual antigen. Because the antigenic form is usually not known, this complicates selection of the correct metabolite to be used in assaying the reaction *in vitro* or in an experimental model. Most of the drug reactions that affect the lung do not elicit IgE-antibody or cause a type I immediate hypersensitivity reaction as they do in other reactions, for example, to penicillin, in which immediate or accelerated allergic reactions occur. Although asthmatic symptoms can be severe, it is the insidious onset of cough and dyspnea that characterizes most of the reactions caused by the drugs listed in Table 12-9.

Principal emphasis will be given to pulmonary disease caused by cytotoxic, immunosuppressive drugs because the clinical setting of patients receiving them is complicated and the specific effect of drug toxicity is often difficult to factor out (626,636). Pulmonary infection (often with nosocomial or opportunistic microorganisms), radiation therapy to the thorax and lung, or progression of the disease under treatment can confuse and compound the issue of drug toxicity. For example, gold or penicillamine, both of which can cause interstitial lung injury, may be used to treat patients with rheumatoid arthritis, a disease with a 0% to 15% incidence of associated interstitial pulmonary fibrosis; whether disease progression or concomitant pulmonary drug toxicity is responsible may be difficult to decide (625). Moreover, a latent period may occur between the cessation of drug therapy and the onset of pulmonary symptoms that are in retrospect attributed to a toxic drug effect. A period of months to perhaps years, as noted with busulfan use, may elapse before the untoward drug reaction is evident.

Gradual development of shortness of breath and a nagging, dry, nonproductive cough are characteristic complaints of most patients with drug-related pulmonary disease (625–629, 632,636,637). Tachypnea and lung crackles may be found on physical examination. The connection between the drug and the symptoms may be overlooked if the patient has progressive signs of the primary lung disease process or a systemic disease. Subtle development of congestive heart failure may occur from use of potentially myotoxic drugs such as adriamycin, now used frequently in multiple-agent chemotherapy protocols. Chest radiographic abnormalities are not usually noted until the patient experiences respiratory symptoms; then, diffuse linear densities and streaks occur, predominantly in the lower lung zones. However, certain drug-induced pulmonary reactions have individual features that can heighten one's suspicion that they are causative or are contributing to lung symptoms.

CYTOTOXIC AGENTS

Bleomycin, a mixture of glycopeptides isolated from *Streptomyces verticillus*, is a versatile and effective drug used against squamous cell carcinoma, malignant lymphomas, and testicular tumors and is a popular drug to be included in multiple-agent regimens (626). It is a rather predictable cause of interstitial pulmonary fibrosis, and for this reason it has provided one of the best experimental models of this disease. Toxicity correlates with the total dose of bleomycin given, for significant drug-related pulmonary illness is infrequent

TABLE 12-9.   Drugs or Drug Groups that Cause Pulmonary Reactions

Drug	Syndrome(s)	Frequency
CYTOTOXIC DRUGS		
Azathioprine	HP	<1%
Bleomycin	PF, NPE, HP, AP	3% to 25% (PF)
Busulfan	PF	<1%
Carmustine	PF, AP	10% to 30%
Cyclophosphamide	PF, NPE, HP	<1%
Cytosine arabinoside	NPE	<1%
Methotrexate	HP, NPE, PF, pleuritis	7% (HP)
Mitomycin	PF, AP	3% to 12%
Procarbazine	HP	<1%
Vinca alkaloids[a]	AP	20% to 40%
NONCYTOTOXIC DRUGS		
Amiodarone	PF, NPE, AP	6% to 15%
Aspirin	NPE,[a] bronchospasm	22%[b] (NPE)
β-Adrenergic blockers	Bronchospasm	Variable
Bromocriptine	PF, pleuritis	<1%
Captopril	Cough	10%
Carbachol	Bronchospasm	<1%
Carbamazepine	HP	<1%
Chlorambucil	PF	<1%
Chlordiazepoxide	NPE[b]	<1%
Dantrolene	Pleuritis	<1%
Diphenylhydantoin	HP	<1%
Enalapril	Cough	10% to 20%
Ethchlorvynol	NPE[b]	<1%
Gold salts	HP, PF, BO	<1%
Hydrochlorothiazide	NPE	<1%
Lidocaine	NPE	<1%
Methysergide	Pleuritis	<1%
Naloxone	NPE	<1%
Neuromuscular blocking agents	Bronchospasm	<1%
Nitrofurantoin	HP, PF	<1%
Nonsteroidal antiinflammatory agents	Bronchospasm, HP	4% to 20%
Opiates	NPE	<1%
Penicillamine	BO, PRS, PF, HP	<1%
Protamine	NPE	<1%
Pyrimethamine–chloroquine	HP	<1%
Pyrimethamine–dapsone	HP	<1%
Sulfasalazine	PF, HP, BO	<1%
Tocolytic agents	NPE	<1%
Tocainide	PF, NPE	<1%

HP, hypersensitivity pneumonitis; PF, pulmonary fibrosis; NPE, noncardiogenic pulmonary edema; AP, acute pneumonitis; BO, bronchiolitis obliterans; PRS, pulmonary renal syndrome.

[a]Not as a single agent but in conjunction with mitomycin only.

[b]Overdose only.

From Cooper JA Jr. Drug-related pulmonary diseases. In: Bone RC, Dantzker DR, George RB, et al., eds. *Pulmonary and critical care medicine*, vol 2. Chicago: Mosby-Year Book, 1993:1–9, with permission.

(less than 10%) if the cumulative dose is <150 to 200 mg; for doses of >300 to 500 mg, toxicity may approach 50% with approximately 10% mortality (61). Several factors seem to enhance pulmonary toxicity from bleomycin, and these should alert the physician to expect complications. Older people have more toxicity. Simultaneous administration of bleomycin and thoracic radiation increases the likelihood of toxicity, which also occurs at a lower cumulative dose of the drug. Prior use of radiation also increases the risk. Administration of high oxygen concentrations produces synergistic toxicity with bleomycin, and a fulminant form of interstitial pneumonitis and fibrosis can develop. Oxygen given during surgical procedures seems sufficient to trigger the response. Patients with esophageal carcinoma who have received radiation and bleomycin therapy and who undergo subsequent surgery are at high risk to develop lung toxicity (638).

Whereas interstitial fibrosis is the usual manifestation of pulmonary toxicity, an apparent hypersensitivity form of toxicity can develop that is more amenable to improvement with corticosteroid therapy than the fibrotic form (639). Finally, the route of bleomycin administration accounts for a striking difference in lung susceptibility to injury. In experimental animals, a single intratracheal dose may cause a progressive form of pulmonary fibrosis to develop (62). In contrast, if the drug is given parenterally, much larger and repetitive doses can be tolerated; in fact, continuous intravenous administration of the drug in low doses may lower the incidence of toxicity to some extent. Pulmonary function abnormalities generally include arterial hypoxemia and a restrictive ventilatory pattern with decreased lung volumes and a diminished DLco (61).

The lung response to the three cytotoxic agents busulfan, cyclophosphamide, and methotrexate shows similarities and is different from other forms of pulmonary toxicity. A considerable latent period may occur before pulmonary symptoms suggesting toxicity develop; often the patient is under treatment for a hematologic malignancy, and several years of rather stable drug usage may have elapsed before toxicity appears for inapparent reasons. Cough, dyspnea, and fever set in and the chest radiograph may show a combined alveolar filling and interstitial pattern and, occasionally, a pleural effusion. The troublesome differential is that of a drug reaction versus a leukemic infiltration of the lung, and an opportunistic infection may be present as well. The onset of illness in patients taking methotrexate can be variable, occurring within a few days of beginning therapy or after a latent period; the dosage of drug per week may be an important determinant of this illness (626). Bleomycin may also cause nodular lesions and the pathology in these circumstances can disclose BOOP. In all these drug reactions, fever is an important part of the toxic syndrome. Sputum or bronchial washings may yield unusual-appearing type II pneumocytes that can be identified by cytology and are characteristic of these particular drug-induced toxic pulmonary reactions. Histopathologic features of cytotoxic lung disease include type II pneumocyte proliferation, macrophage infiltration of the interstitium, and fibrosis.

Mitomycin can cause chronic interstitial fibrosis in a pattern similar to bleomycin. Rarely, mitomycin C can cause a syndrome characterized by noncardiogenic pulmonary edema, vasculopathy, microangiopathic hemolytic anemia, and acute renal failure (626).

NONCYTOTOXIC AGENTS

Amiodarone, a powerful antiarrhythmic agent, causes lung disease in 4% to 27% of patients (627). Pulmonary fibrosis and hypersensitivity or acute pneumonitis can be induced by this drug. A major risk factor is maintenance dose(s) of more than 400 mg per day. Diffuse reticular infiltrates are most commonly seen on the chest radiograph, although diffuse acinar infiltrates have also been described. HRCT scans demonstrate localized or diffuse areas of very high attenuation that can be highly characteristic of amiodarone toxicity (640). A restrictive ventilatory defect with a diffusion impairment is the most common physiologic abnormality (627). The DLco is highly sensitive for amiodarone toxicity. Moreover, a DLco greater than 80% of pretreatment level virtually excludes amiodarone toxicity (627). The major histologic finding is abundant, intraalveolar "foamy" macrophages. Amiodarone inhibits phospholipases, leading to accumulation of lamellar inclusions that can be demonstrated by electron microscopy. However, foamy macrophages can be seen in patients without clinical evidence of lung disease; thus, their presence does not confirm toxicity. Discontinuation of the drug or reduction in drug dosage in conjunction with corticosteroid therapy can reduce the pulmonary disease. Recovery may be slow owing to the prolonged half-life (greater than 1 month) (627).

The antibiotic nitrofurantoin is one of the most widely recognized drugs causing pulmonary toxicity (629,630,635). The acute onset of fever, chills, cough, and dyspnea can occur after a few days of therapy or within a few hours of the first dose in patients who have received the drug on previous occasions. Blood eosinophilia is likely and the symptom complex points to an allergic or hypersensitivity-type lung reaction, although the response has not been well characterized histologically. The pulmonary response seems to be one of pulmonary edema, with diffuse crackles heard in the lungs. A chest radiograph supports the impression of noncardiogenic pulmonary edema. Pleural effusion may be noted. The reaction clears within 48 hours after discontinuing the drug; the disease is self-limited without mortality. Episodes of recurrent pneumonia can occur if the patient resumes use of the drug. To conclusively prove the drug–disease relationship, a challenge dose will elicit the reaction. A chronic form of nitrofurantoin disease can occur that does not include fever, pleural effusion, and eosinophilia but, rather, includes an insidious onset of cough and dyspnea months after the drug has been taken on a regular basis, usually for suppression of chronic bacteriuria. In this form, the lung disease is virtually indistinguishable from interstitial pneumonitis and fibrosis. Discontinuance of the drug plus corticosteroid therapy arrests the process.

Interstitial pulmonary fibrosis has been described following the treatment of prostate cancer with the antiestrogen medications leuprolide and nilutamide. Progressive disease can usually be avoided with cessation of therapy and with institution of corticosteroids (641).

A variety of drugs are known to induce SLE; among the more than 20 drugs incriminated, procainamide, hydralazine, diphenylhydantoin, and sulfonamides are among the ones most frequently encountered (635,642). Drug-induced SLE differs from the spontaneous disease in that there is less kidney and skin involvement and more pleuropulmonary reaction. Antihistone antibodies are frequently positive. The lung reaction and the entire syndrome remit if the causative drug is discontinued.

Acknowledgment

This work was supported by grant K08 HL04465 from the National Institutes of Health and by an unrestricted educational grant C-03-010 from the ATS and from the Respiratory Institute, a Division of GlaxoSmithKline.

REFERENCES

1. American Thoracic Society. Statement on sarcoidosis. *Am J Respir Crit Care Med* 1999;160(2):736–755.
2. American Thoracic Society. Idiopathic pulmonary fibrosis: diagnosis and treatment. International Consensus Statement. *Am J Resp Crit Care Med* 2000;161:646–664.
3. American Thoracic Society. American Thoracic Society/European Respiratory Society international multidisciplinary consensus classification of the idiopathic interstitial pneumonias. *Am J Respir Crit Care Med* 2002;165:277–304.
4. Travis WD, Colby TV, Koss MN, et al. *Non-neoplastic disorders of the lower respiratory tract*, 1st ed. Washington, DC: Armed Forces Institute of Pathology and the American Registry of Pathology, 2002.

5. Schwarz MI, King TE Jr. *Interstitial lung disease*, 4th ed. Hamilton, Ontario Canada: B. C. Decker, 2003.

6. Lynch JP III. *Idiopathic pulmonary fibrosis*, 1st ed. New York: Marcel Dekker Inc, 2004.

7. Lacasse Y, Selman M, Costabel U, et al. Clinical diagnosis of hypersensitivity pneumonitis. *Am J Respir Crit Care Med* 2003; 168(8):952–958.

8. Richerson HB, Bernstein IL, Fink JN, et al. Guidelines for the clinical evaluation of hypersensitivity pneumonitis. Report of the subcommittee on hypersensitivity pneumonitis. *J Allergy Clin Immunol* 1989;84(5 Pt 2):839–844.

9. Nasser-Sharif FJ, Balter MS. Hypersensitivity pneumonitis with normal high-resolution computed tomography scans. *Can Respir J* 2001;8(2):98–101.

10. Nishimura K, Izumi T, Kitaichi M, et al. The diagnostic accuracy of high-resolution computed tomography in diffuse infiltrative lung diseases. *Chest* 1993;104(4):1149–1155.

11. Sant SM, Doran M, Fenelon HM, et al. Pleuropulmonary abnormalities in patients with systemic lupus erythematosus: assessment with high-resolution computed tomography, chest radiography and pulmonary function tests. *Clin Exp Rheumatol* 1997;15(5):507–513.

12. Lynch DA, Rose CS, Way D, et al. Hypersensitivity pneumonitis: sensitivity of high-resolution CT in a population-based study. *Am J Roentgenol* 1992;159(3):469–472.

13. Lynch D. Chapter 4: Imaging of diffuse parenchymal lung diseases. In: Schwarz MI, King TE Jr., eds. *Interstitial lung disease*. Hamilton, Ontario, Canada: B. C. Decker, 2003:75–113.

14. Epler GR, McLoud TC, Gaensler EA, et al. Normal chest roentgenograms in chronic diffuse infiltrative lung disease. *N Engl J Med* 1978;298(17):934–939.

15. Hodgson MJ, Parkinson DK, Karpf M. Chest X-rays in hypersensitivity pneumonitis: a metaanalysis of secular trend. *Am J Ind Med* 1989;16(1):45–53.

16. Remy-Jardin M, Remy J, Deffontaines C, et al. Assessment of diffuse infiltrative lung disease: comparison of conventional CT and high-resolution CT. *Radiology* 1991;181(1):157–162.

17. Hunninghake GW, Zimmerman MB, Schwartz DA, et al. Utility of a lung biopsy for the diagnosis of idiopathic pulmonary fibrosis. *Am J Respir Crit Care Med* 2001;164(2):193–196.

18. Tung KT, Wells AU, Rubens MB, et al. Accuracy of the typical computed tomographic appearances of fibrosing alveolitis. *Thorax* 1993;48(4):334–338.

19. Wells A. High-resolution computed tomography in sarcoidosis: a clinical perspective. *Sarcoidosis Vasc Diffuse Lung Dis* 1998;15(2): 140–146.

20. Patel RA, Sellami D, Gotway MB, et al. Hypersensitivity pneumonitis: patterns on high-resolution CT. *J Comput Assist Tomogr* 2000;24(6):965–970.

21. O'Donnell DE, Fitzpatrick MF. Physiology of interstitial lung disease. In: Schwartz MI, King TE Jr., eds. *Interstitial lung disease*. Hamilton, Ontario, Canada: B. C. Decker, 2003:54–74.

22. Green RJ, Ruoss SJ, Kraft SA, et al. Pulmonary capillaritis and alveolar hemorrhage. Update on diagnosis and management. *Chest* 1996;110(5):1305–1316.

23. Broaddus C, Dake MD, Stulbarg MS, et al. Bronchoalveolar lavage and transbronchial biopsy for the diagnosis of pulmonary infections in the acquired immunodeficiency syndrome. *Ann Intern Med* 1985;102(6):747–752.

24. Costabel U, Donner CF, Haslam PL, et al. Clinical guidelines and indications for bronchoalveolar lavage (BAL): occupational lung diseases due to inhalation of inorganic dust. *Eur Respir J* 1990;3(8): 946–9–961–9.

25. Veeraraghavan S, Latsi PI, Wells AU, et al. BAL findings in idiopathic nonspecific interstitial pneumonia and usual interstitial pneumonia. *Eur Respir J* 2003;22(2):239–244.

26. Schnabel A, Holl-Ulrich K, Dalhoff K, et al. Efficacy of transbronchial biopsy in pulmonary vaculitides. *Eur Respir J* 1997; 10(12):2738–2743.

27. Latsi PI, Wells AU. Evaluation and management of alveolitis and interstitial lung disease in scleroderma. *Curr Opin Rheumatol* 2003;15(6):748–755.

28. Costabel U, Guzman J. Chapter 5: Bronchoalveolar lavage. In: Schwarz MI, King TE Jr., eds. *Interstitial lung disease*, 4th ed. Hamilton, Ontario, Canada: B. C. Decker, 2003:114–133.

29. Allen JN, Davis WB, Pacht ER. Diagnostic significance of increased bronchoalveolar lavage fluid eosinophils. *Am Rev Respir Dis* 1990;142(3):642–647.

30. Allen JN, Pacht ER, Gadek JE, et al. Acute eosinophilic pneumonia as a reversible cause of noninfectious respiratory failure. *N Engl J Med* 1989;321(9):569–574.

31. Lynch JP 3rd, Kazerooni EA, Gay SE. Pulmonary sarcoidosis. *Clin Chest Med* 1997;18(4):755–785.

32. Bensard DD, McIntyre RC Jr., Waring BJ, et al. Comparison of video thoracoscopic lung biopsy to open lung biopsy in the diagnosis of interstitial lung disease. *Chest* 1993;103(3):765–770.

33. Mouroux J, Clary-Meinesz C, Padovani B, et al. Efficacy and safety of videothoracoscopic lung biopsy in the diagnosis of interstitial lung disease. *Eur J Cardiothorac Surg* 1997;11(1):22–4–25–6.

34. Rena O, Casadio C, Leo F, et al. Videothoracoscopic lung biopsy in the diagnosis of interstitial lung disease. *Eur J Cardiothorac Surg* 1999;16(6):624–627.

35. Ayed AK, Raghunathan R. Thoracoscopy versus open lung biopsy in the diagnosis of interstitial lung disease: a randomised controlled trial. *J R Coll Surg Edinb* 2000;45(3):159–163.

36. Miller JD, Urschel JD, Cox G, et al. A randomized, controlled trial comparing thoracoscopy and limited thoracotomy for lung biopsy in interstitial lung disease. *Ann Thorac Surg* 2000;70(5): 1647–1650.

37. Blewett CJ, Bennett WF, Miller JD, et al. Open lung biopsy as an outpatient procedure. *Ann Thorac Surg* 2001;71(4):1113–1115.

38. Chang AC, Yee J, Orringer MB, et al. Diagnostic thoracoscopic lung biopsy: an outpatient experience. *Ann Thorac Surg* 2002;74(6): 1942–1946; discussion 1946–1947.

39. Flaherty KR, Travis WD, Colby TV, et al. Histopathologic variability in usual and nonspecific interstitial pneumonias. *Am J Respir Crit Care Med* 2001;164(9):1722–1727.

40. Monaghan H, Wells AU, Colby TV, et al. Prognostic implications of histologic patterns in multiple surgical lung biopsies from patients with idiopathic interstitial pneumonias. *Chest* 2004;125(2):522–526.

41. Morris DG. Gold, silver, and bronze: metals, medals, and standards in hypersensitivity pneumonitis. *Am J Respir Crit Care Med* 2003;168(8):909–910.

42. Nicholson AG. Classification of idiopathic interstitial pneumonias: making sense of the alphabet soup. *Histopathology* 2002;41(5): 381–391.

43. Hamman L, Rich AR. Fulminating diffuse interstitial fibrosis of the lungs. *Trans Am Clin Climatol Assoc* 1935;51:154–163.

44. Katzenstein AL, Myers JL, Mazur MT. Acute interstitial pneumonia. A clinicopathologic, ultrastructural, and cell kinetic study. *Am J Surg Pathol* 1986;10(4):256–267.

45. Travis WD, Colby TV, Koss MN, et al. Chapter 3: Idiopathic interstitial pneumonia and other diffuse parenchymal lung diseases. *Non-neoplastic disorders of the lower respiratory tract*, 1st ed. Washington, DC: American Registry of Pathology and the Armed Forces Institute of Pathology, 2002:49–232.

46. Olson J, Colby TV, Elliott CG. Hamman-Rich syndrome revisited. *Mayo Clin Proc* 1990;65(12):1538–1548.

47. Primack SL, Hartman TE, Ikezoe J, et al. Acute interstitial pneumonia: radiographic and CT findings in nine patients. *Radiology* 1993;188(3):817–820.

48. Ichikado K, Johkoh T, Ikezoe J, et al. Acute interstitial pneumonia: high-resolution CT findings correlated with pathology. *Am J Roentgenol* 1997;168(2):333–338.

49. Vourlekis JS, Brown KK, Cool CD, et al. Acute interstitial pneumonitis. Case series and review of the literature. *Medicine (Baltimore)* 2000;79(6):369–378.

50. Quefatieh A, Stone CH, DiGiovine B, et al. Low hospital mortality in patients with acute interstitial pneumonia. *Chest* 2003; 124(2):554–559.

51. Peiris JSM, Yuen KY, Osterhaus ADME, et al. The severe acute respiratory syndrome. *N Engl J Med* 2003;349(25):2431–2441.

52. Franks TJ, Chong PY, Chui P, et al. Lung pathology of severe acute respiratory syndrome (SARS): a study of 8 autopsy cases from Singapore. *Hum Pathol* 2003;34(8):743–748.

53. Johkoh T, Muller NL, Taniguchi H, et al. Acute interstitial pneumonia: thin-section CT findings in 36 patients. *Radiology* 1999; 211(3):859–863.

54. Ichikado K, Suga M, Muller NL, et al. Acute interstitial pneumonia: comparison of high-resolution computed tomography

findings between survivors and nonsurvivors. *Am J Respir Crit Care Med* 2002;165(11):1551–1556.

55. Tomiyama N, Muller NL, Johkoh T, et al. Acute respiratory distress syndrome and acute interstitial pneumonia: comparison of thin-section CT findings. *J Comput Assist Tomogr* 2001;25(1):28–33.

56. Hansell DM. Acute interstitial pneumonia: clues from the white stuff. *Am J Respir Crit Care Med* 2002;165(11):1465–1466.

57. Meduri GU, Chinn AJ, Leeper KV, et al. Corticosteroid rescue treatment of progressive fibroproliferation in late ARDS. Patterns of response and predictors of outcome. *Chest* 1994;105(5):1516–1527.

58. King TE Jr. Idiopathic interstitial pneumonia. In: Schwarz MI, King TE Jr., eds. *Interstitial lung diseases,* 4th ed. Hamilton, Ontario: B. C. Decker, 2003:701–786.

59. Crystal RG, Bitterman PB, Mossman B, et al. Future research directions in idiopathic pulmonary fibrosis: summary of a National Heart, Lung, and Blood Institute working group. *Am J Respir Crit Care Med* 2002;166(2):236–246.

60. Kaminski N, Belperio JA, Bitterman P, et al. Idiopathic pulmonary fibrosis. *Am J Respir Cell Mol Biol* 2003;29:S1–105.

61. Pascual RS, Mosher MB, Sikand RS, et al. Effects of bleomycin on pulmonary function in man. *Am Rev Respir Dis* 1973;108(2):211–217.

62. McCullough B, Collins JF, Johanson WG Jr., et al. Bleomycin-induced diffuse interstitial pulmonary fibrosis in baboons. *J Clin Invest* 1978;61(1):79–88.

63. Collins JF, McCullough B, Coalson JJ, et al. Bleomycin-induced diffuse interstitial pulmonary fibrosis in baboons. II. Further studies on connective tissue changes. *Am Rev Respir Dis* 1981;123(3):305–312.

64. Thrall RS, Barton RW, D'Amato DA, et al. Differential cellular analysis of bronchoalveolar lavage fluid obtained at various stages during the development of bleomycin-induced pulmonary fibrosis in the rat. *Am Rev Respir Dis* 1982;126(3):488–492.

65. Phan SH, Armstrong G, Sulavik MC, et al. A comparative study of pulmonary fibrosis induced by bleomycin and an O2 metabolite producing enzyme system. *Chest* 1983;83(5 Suppl):44S–45S.

66. Phan SH, Schrier D, McGarry B, et al. Effect of the beige mutation on bleomycin-induced pulmonary fibrosis in mice. *Am Rev Respir Dis* 1983;127(4):456–459.

67. Schrier DJ, Phan SH, McGarry BM. The effects of the nude (nu/nu) mutation on bleomycin-induced pulmonary fibrosis. A biochemical evaluation. *Am Rev Respir Dis* 1983;127(5):614–617.

68. Schrier DJ, Kunkel RG, Phan SH. The role of strain variation in murine bleomycin-induced pulmonary fibrosis. *Am Rev Respir Dis* 1983;127(1):63–66.

69. Thrall RS, Barton RW. A comparison of lymphocyte populations in lung tissue and in bronchoalveolar lavage fluid of rats at various times during the development of bleomycin-induced pulmonary fibrosis. *Am Rev Respir Dis* 1984;129(2):279–283.

70. Hay JG, Haslam PL, Dewar A, et al. Development of acute lung injury after the combination of intravenous bleomycin and exposure to hyperoxia in rats. *Thorax* 1987;42(5):374–382.

71. Hay JG, Haslam PL, Turner-Warwick M, et al. The effects of iron and desferrioxamine on the lung injury induced by intravenous bleomycin and hyperoxia. *Free Radical Res Commun* 1987;4(2):109–114.

72. Rossi GA, Szapiel S, Ferrans VJ, et al. Susceptibility to experimental interstitial lung disease is modified by immune- and non-immune-related genes. *Am Rev Respir Dis* 1987;135(2):448–455.

73. Filderman AE, Genovese LA, Lazo JS. Alterations in pulmonary protective enzymes following systemic bleomycin treatment in mice. *Biochem Pharmacol* 1988;37(6):1111–1116.

74. Harrison JH Jr., Lazo JS. Plasma and pulmonary pharmacokinetics of bleomycin in murine strains that are sensitive and resistant to bleomycin-induced pulmonary fibrosis. *J Pharmacol Exp Ther* 1988;247(3):1052–1058.

75. Filderman AE, Lazo JS. Murine strain differences in pulmonary bleomycin metabolism. *Biochem Pharmacol* 1991;42(1):195–198.

76. Haston CK, Amos CI, King TM, et al. Inheritance of susceptibility to bleomycin-induced pulmonary fibrosis in the mouse. *Cancer Res* 1996;56(11):2596–2601.

77. Haston CK, Travis EL. Murine susceptibility to radiation-induced pulmonary fibrosis is influenced by a genetic factor implicated in susceptibility to bleomycin-induced pulmonary fibrosis. *Cancer Res* 1997;57(23):5286–5291.

78. Harrison JJ, Lazo J. High-dose continuous infusion of bleomycin in mice: a new model for drug-induced pulmonary fibrosis. *J Pharmacol Exp Ther* 1987;243(3):1185–1194.

79. Borzone G, Moreno R, Urrea R, et al. Bleomycin-induced chronic lung damage does not resemble human idiopathic pulmonary fibrosis. *Am J Respir Crit Care Med* 2001;163(7):1648–1653.

80. Gabazza EC, Taguchi O, Adachi Y. Bleomycin-induced pulmonary fibrosis. *Am J Respir Crit Care Med* 2002;165(6):845b–8846.

81. Kuwano K, Hagimoto N, Kawasaki M, et al. Essential roles of the Fas-Fas ligand pathway in the development of pulmonary fibrosis. *J Clin Invest* 1999;104(1):13–19.

82. Munger JS, Huang X, Kawakatsu H, et al. The integrin alpha v beta 6 binds and activates latent TGF beta 1: a mechanism for regulating pulmonary inflammation and fibrosis. *Cell* 1999;96(3):319–328.

83. Kaminski N, Allard JD, Pittet JF, et al. Global analysis of gene expression in pulmonary fibrosis reveals distinct programs regulating lung inflammation and fibrosis. *Proc Natl Acad Sci U S A* 2000;97(4):1778–1783.

84. Pittet JF, Griffiths MJ, Geiser T, et al. TGF-beta is a critical mediator of acute lung injury. *J Clin Invest* 2001;107(12):1537–1544.

85. Haston CK, Zhou X, Gumbiner-Russo L, et al. Universal and radiation-specific loci influence murine susceptibility to radiation-induced pulmonary fibrosis. *Cancer Res* 2002;62(13):3782–3788.

86. Zuo F, Kaminski N, Eugui E, et al. Gene expression analysis reveals matrilysin as a key regulator of pulmonary fibrosis in mice and humans. *Proc Natl Acad Sci U S A* 2002;99(9):6292–6297.

87. Teder P, Vandivier RW, Jiang D, et al. Resolution of lung inflammation by CD44. *Science* 2002;296(5565):155–158.

88. Behr J. Oxidants and antioxidants in idiopathic pulmonary fibrosis. In: Lynch JP III, ed. *Idiopathic pulmonary fibrosis.* New York: Marcel Dekker Inc, 2004:379–396.

89. Chapman HA. Disorders of lung matrix remodeling. *J Clin Invest* 2004;113(2):148–157.

90. Chilosi M, Murer B, Doglioni C. Bronchiolar epithelium in idiopathic pulmonary fibrosis/usual interstitial fibrosis. In: Lynch JP III, ed. *Idiopathic pulmonary fibrosis.* New York: Marcel Dekker Inc, 2004:631–664.

91. Idell S. Fibrin turnover in pulmonary fibrosis. In: Lynch JP III, ed. *Idiopathic pulmonary fibrosis.* New York: Marcel Dekker Inc, 2004:397–417.

92. Geist LJ, Hunninghake GW. Role of viruses in the pathogenesis of pulmonary fibrosis. In: Lynch JP III, ed. *Idiopathic pulmonary fibrosis.* New York: Marcel Dekker Inc, 2004:665–673.

93. Gharaee-Kermani M, Phan SH. Role of fibroblasts and myofibroblasts in idiopathic pulmonary fibrosis. In: Lynch JP III, ed. *Idiopathic pulmonary fibrosis.* New York: Marcel Dekker Inc, 2004:507–561.

94. Kim HJ, Bitterman PB. Peptide and provisional matrix signals in idiopathic pulmonary fibrosis. In: Lynch JP III, ed. *Idiopathic pulmonary fibrosis.* New York: Marcel Dekker Inc, 2004:563–572.

95. Koth LL, Sheppard D. Integrins and pulmonary fibrosis. In: Lynch JP III, ed. *Idiopathic pulmonary fibrosis.* New York: Marcel Dekker Inc, 2004:359–378.

96. Kunkel SL, Lukacs NW, Chensue SW. Cytokine phenotypes and the progression of chronic pulmonary fibrosis. In: Lynch JP III, ed. *Idiopathic pulmonary fibrosis.* New York: Marcel Dekker Inc, 2004:303–320.

97. Peters-Golden M. Arachidonic acid metabolites: potential mediators and therapeutic targets in fibrotic lung disease. In: Lynch JP III, ed. *Idiopathic pulmonary fibrosis.* New York: Marcel Dekker Inc, 2004:419–449.

98. Portnoy J, Mason RJ. Role of alveolar type II epithelial cells in pulmonary fibrosis. In: Lynch JP III, ed. *Idiopathic pulmonary fibrosis.* New York: Marcel Dekker Inc, 2004:573–608.

99. Rishikof DC, Ricupero DA. Extracellular matrix. In: Lynch JP III, ed. *Idiopathic pulmonary fibrosis.* New York: Marcel Dekker Inc, 2004:481–506.

100. Selman M, Pardo A. Matrix metalloproteinases and tissue inhibitors of metalloproteinases in pulmonary fibrosis. In: Lynch JP III, ed. *Idiopathic pulmonary fibrosis.* New York: Marcel Dekker Inc, 2004:451–480.

101. Strieter RM, Belperio JA, Keane MP. CXC chemokines in angiogenesis related to pulmonary fibrosis. In: Lynch JP III, ed. *Idiopathic pulmonary fibrosis.* New York: Marcel Dekker Inc, 2004:321–339.

102. Takahashi H. Surfactant proteins in the pathophysiology of pulmonary fibrosis. In: Lynch JP III, ed. *Idiopathic pulmonary fibrosis.* New York: Marcel Dekker Inc, 2004:609–630.

103. White ES, Standiford TJ. Role of polymorphonuclear leukocytes in the pathogenesis of idiopathic pulmonary fibrosis. In: Lynch JP III, ed. *Idiopathic pulmonary fibrosis.* New York: Marcel Dekker Inc, 2004:341–357.

104. King TE Jr., Schwarz MI, Brown K, et al. Idiopathic pulmonary fibrosis: relationship between histopathologic features and mortality. *Am J Respir Crit Care Med* 2001;164(6):1025–1032.

105. Thomas AQ, Lane K, Phillips J III, et al. Heterozygosity for a surfactant protein c gene mutation associated with usual interstitial pneumonitis and cellular nonspecific interstitial pneumonitis in one kindred. *Am J Respir Crit Care Med* 2002;165(9):1322–1328.

106. Nogee LM, Dunbar AE, Wert SE, et al. A mutation in the surfactant protein c gene associated with familial interstitial lung disease. *N Engl J Med* 2001;344(8):573–579.

107. Wahidi MM, Schwartz DA, Raghu G. Genetics of familial pulmonary fibrosis and other variants. In: Lynch JPI, ed. *Idiopathic pulmonary fibrosis.* New York: Marcel Dekker Inc, 2004:31–54.

108. Coultas DB, Zumwalt RE, Black WC, et al. The epidemiology of interstitial lung diseases. *Am J Respir Crit Care Med* 1994;150(4):967–972.

109. Coultas DB, Hubbard R. Epidemiology of idiopathic pulmonary fibrosis. In: Lynch JP III, ed. *Idiopathic pulmonary fibrosis.* New York: Marcel Dekker Inc, 2004:1–30.

110. King TE Jr. Clinical features and differential diagnosis of IPF. In: Lynch JP III, ed. *Idiopathic pulmonary fibrosis.* New York: Marcel Dekker Inc, 2004:55–80.

111. King TE Jr., Tooze JA, Schwarz MI, et al. Predicting survival in idiopathic pulmonary fibrosis: scoring system and survival model. *Am J Respir Crit Care Med* 2001;164(7):1171–1181.

112. Schwarz MI, King TE Jr., Raghu G. Chapter 1: Approach to the evaluation and diagnosis of interstitial lung disease. In: Schwarz MI, King TE Jr., eds. *Interstitial lung disease.* 4th ed. Hamilton, Ontario, Canada: B. C. Decker, 2003:1–30.

113. Hanson D, Winterbauer RH, Kirtland SH, et al. Changes in pulmonary function test results after 1 year of therapy as predictors of survival in patients with idiopathic pulmonary fibrosis. *Chest* 1995;108(2):305–310.

114. Collard HR, King TE Jr., Bartelson BB, et al. Changes in clinical and physiologic variables predict survival in idiopathic pulmonary fibrosis. *Am J Respir Crit Care Med* 2003;168(5):538–542.

115. Flaherty KR, Mumford JA, Murray S, et al. Prognostic implications of physiologic and radiographic changes in idiopathic interstitial pneumonia. *Am J Respir Crit Care Med* 2003;168(5):543–548.

116. Lama VN, Flaherty KR, Toews GB, et al. Prognostic value of desaturation during a 6-minute walk test in idiopathic interstitial pneumonia. *Am J Respir Crit Care Med* 2003;168(9):1084–1090.

117. Latsi PI, du Bois RM, Nicholson AG, et al. Fibrotic idiopathic interstitial pneumonia: the prognostic value of longitudinal functional trends. *Am J Respir Crit Care Med* 2003;168(5):531–537.

118. Noble PW, Morris DG. Time will tell: predicting survival in idiopathic interstitial pneumonia. *Am J Respir Crit Care Med* 2003;168(5):510–511.

119. Freemer MM, King TE Jr. Chapter 21: Connective tissue diseases. In: Schwarz MI, King TE Jr., eds. *Interstitial lung disease.* 4th ed. Hamilton, Ontario, Canada: B. C. Decker, 2003:535–598.

120. Wells AU, Hansell DM, Rubens MB, et al. The predictive value of appearances on thin-section computed tomography in fibrosing alveolitis. *Am Rev Respir Dis* 1993;148(4 Pt 1):1076–1082.

121. Hunninghake GW, Lynch DA, Galvin JR, et al. Radiologic findings are strongly associated with a pathologic diagnosis of usual interstitial pneumonia. *Chest* 2003;124(4):1215–1223.

122. Gay SE, Kazerooni EA, Toews GB, et al. Idiopathic pulmonary fibrosis. Predicting response to therapy and survival. *Am J Respir Crit Care Med* 1998;157(4):1063–1072.

123. Wells AU, Desai SR, Rubens MB, et al. Idiopathic pulmonary fibrosis: a composite physiologic index derived from disease extent observed by computed tomography. *Am J Respir Crit Care Med* 2003;167(7):962–969.

124. Kuhn C 3rd, Boldt J, King TE Jr., et al. An immunohistochemical study of architectural remodeling and connective tissue synthesis in pulmonary fibrosis. *Am Rev Respir Dis* 1989;140(6):1693–1703.

125. Hyde DM, King TE Jr., McDermott T, et al. Idiopathic pulmonary fibrosis. Quantitative assessment of lung pathology. Comparison of a semiquantitative and a morphometric histopathologic scoring system. *Am Rev Respir Dis* 1992;146(4):1042–1047.

126. Katzenstein AL, Myers JL. Idiopathic pulmonary fibrosis: clinical relevance of pathologic classification. *Am J Respir Crit Care Med* 1998;157(4 Pt 1):1301–1315.

127. Myers JL, Katzenstein AL. Epithelial necrosis and alveolar collapse in the pathogenesis of usual interstitial pneumonia. *Chest* 1988;94(6):1309–1311.

128. Flaherty KR, Toews GB, Travis WD, et al. Clinical significance of histological classification of idiopathic interstitial pneumonia. *Eur Respir J* 2002;19(2):275–283.

129. Travis WD, Colby TV, Koss MN, et al. Idiopathic interstitial pneumonia and other diffuse parenchymal lung diseases. *Atlas of nontumor pathology: non-neoplastic disorders of the lower respiratory tract.* Washington, DC: American Registry of Pathology and the Armed Forces Institute of Pathology, 2002:49–233.

130. Flaherty KR, Thwaite EL, Kazerooni EA, et al. Radiological versus histological diagnosis in UIP and NSIP: survival implications. *Thorax* 2003;58(2):143–148.

131. Flaherty KR, Colby TV, Travis WD, et al. Fibroblastic foci in usual interstitial pneumonia: idiopathic versus collagen vascular disease. *Am J Respir Crit Care Med* 2003;167(10):1410–1415.

132. Cohen AJ, King TE Jr., Downey GP. Rapidly progressive bronchiolitis obliterans with organizing pneumonia. *Am J Respir Crit Care Med* 1994;149(6):1670–1675.

133. Yousem SA, Colby TV, Carrington CB. Lung biopsy in rheumatoid arthritis. *Am Rev Respir Dis* 1985;131(5):770–777.

134. Grau JM, Miro O, Pedrol E, et al. Interstitial lung disease related to dermatomyositis. Comparative study with patients without lung involvement. *J Rheumatol* 1996;23(11):1921–1926.

135. Mountain C. Revisions in the international system for staging lung cancer. *Chest* 1997;111(6):1710–1717.

136. The SOLVD Investigators. Effect of enalapril on survival in patients with reduced left ventricular ejection fractions and congestive heart failure. *N Engl J Med* 1991;325(5):293–302.

137. Osmond D, Charlebois E, Lang W, et al. Changes in AIDS survival time in two San Francisco cohorts of homosexual men, 1983 to 1993. *JAMA* 1994;271(14):1083–1087.

138. Richeldi L, Davies HR, Ferrara G, et al. Corticosteroids for idiopathic pulmonary fibrosis. *Cochrane Database Syst Rev* 2003(3):CD002880.

139. Turner-Warwick M, Burrows B, Johnson A. Cryptogenic fibrosing alveolitis: clinical features and their influence on survival. *Thorax* 1980;35(3):171–180.

140. Turner-Warwick M, Burrows B, Johnson A. Cryptogenic fibrosing alveolitis: response to corticosteroid treatment and its effect on survival. *Thorax* 1980;35(8):593–599.

141. Rudd RM, Haslam PL, Turner-Warwick M. Cryptogenic fibrosing alveolitis. Relationships of pulmonary physiology and bronchoalveolar lavage to response to treatment and prognosis. *Am Rev Respir Dis* 1981;124(1):1–8.

142. Carrington CB, Gaensler EA, Coutu RE, et al. Natural history and treated course of usual and desquamative interstitial pneumonia. *N Engl J Med* 1978;298(15):801–809.

143. Bjoraker JA, Ryu JH, Edwin MK, et al. Prognostic significance of histopathologic subsets in idiopathic pulmonary fibrosis. *Am J Respir Crit Care Med* 1998;157(1):199–203.

144. Daniil ZD, Gilchrist FC, Nicholson AG, et al. A histologic pattern of nonspecific interstitial pneumonia is associated with a better prognosis than usual interstitial pneumonia in patients with cryptogenic fibrosing alveolitis. *Am J Respir Crit Care Med* 1999;160(3):899–905.

145. Nicholson AG, Colby TV, du Bois RM, et al. The prognostic significance of the histologic pattern of interstitial pneumonia in patients presenting with the clinical entity of cryptogenic fibrosing alveolitis. *Am J Respir Crit Care Med* 2000;162(6):2213–2217.

146. Keogh BA, Bernardo J, Hunninghake GW, et al. Effect of intermittent high dose parenteral corticosteroids on the alveolitis of idiopathic pulmonary fibrosis. *Am Rev Respir Dis* 1983;127(1):18–22.

147. Gulsvik A, Kjelsberg F, Bergmann A, et al. High-dose intravenous methylprednisolone pulse therapy as initial treatment in cryptogenic fibrosing alveolitis. A pilot study. *Respiration* 1986;50(4):252–257.

148. Dayton CS, Schwartz DA, Helmers RA, et al. Outcome of subjects with idiopathic pulmonary fibrosis who fail corticosteroid therapy. Implications for further studies. *Chest* 1993;103(1):69–73.

149. Davies HR, Richeldi L, Walters EH. Immunomodulatory agents for idiopathic pulmonary fibrosis. *Cochrane Database Syst Rev* 2003(3):CD003134.

150. Cegla UH. [Treatment of idiopathic fibrosing alveolitis. Therapeutic experiences with azathioprine-prednisolone and D-penicillamine-prednisolone combination therapy]. *Schweiz Med Wochenschr* 1977;107(6):184–187.

151. Raghu G, Depaso WJ, Cain K, et al. Azathioprine combined with prednisone in the treatment of idiopathic pulmonary fibrosis: a prospective double-blind, randomized, placebo-controlled clinical trial. *Am Rev Respir Dis* 1991;144(2):291–296.

152. Winterbauer RH. The treatment of idiopathic pulmonary fibrosis. *Chest* 1991;100(1):233–235.

153. Selman M, Carrillo G, Salas J, et al. Colchicine, D-penicillamine, and prednisone in the treatment of idiopathic pulmonary fibrosis: a controlled clinical trial. *Chest* 1998;114(2):507–512.

154. Douglas WW, Ryu J, Schroeder D. Idiopathic pulmonary fibrosis. Impact of oxygen and colchicine, prednisone, or no therapy on survival. *Am J Respir Crit Care Med* 2000;161(4):1172–1178.

155. Raghu G, Johnson WC, Lockhart D, et al. Treatment of idiopathic pulmonary fibrosis with a new antifibrotic agent, pirfenidone: results of a prospective, open-label Phase II study. *Am J Respir Crit Care Med* 1999;159(4 Pt 1):1061–1069.

156. Nagai S, Hamada K, Shigematsu M, et al. Open-label compassionate use one year-treatment with pirfenidone to patients with chronic pulmonary fibrosis. *Intern Med* 2002;41(12):1118–1123.

157. Shahzeidi S, Sarnstrand B, Jeffery PK, et al. Oral N-acetylcysteine reduces bleomycin-induced collagen deposition in the lungs of mice. *Eur Respir J* 1991;4(7):845–852.

158. Meyer A, Buhl R, Magnussen H. The effect of oral N-acetylcysteine on lung glutathione levels in idiopathic pulmonary fibrosis. *Eur Respir J* 1994;7(3):431–436.

159. Meyer A, Buhl R, Kampf S, et al. Intravenous N-acetylcysteine and lung glutathione of patients with pulmonary fibrosis and normals. *Am J Respir Crit Care Med* 1995;152(3):1055–1060.

160. Behr J, Maier K, Degenkolb B, et al. Antioxidative and clinical effects of high-dose N-acetylcysteine in fibrosing alveolitis. Adjunctive therapy to maintenance immunosuppression. *Am J Respir Crit Care Med* 1997;156(6):1897–1901.

161. Turner-Warwick M, Haslam PL. The value of serial bronchoalveolar lavages in assessing the clinical progress of patients with cryptogenic fibrosing alveolitis. *Am Rev Respir Dis* 1987;135(1):26–34.

162. Baughman RP, Lower EE. Use of intermittent, intravenous cyclophosphamide for idiopathic pulmonary fibrosis. *Chest* 1992;102(4):1090–1094.

163. Wahidi MM, Ravenel J, Palmer SM, et al. Progression of idiopathic pulmonary fibrosis in native lungs after single lung transplantation. *Chest* 2002;121(6):2072–2076.

164. Grossman RF, Frost A, Zamel N, et al. Results of single-lung transplantation for bilateral pulmonary fibrosis. The Toronto Lung Transplant Group. *N Engl J Med* 1990;322(11):727–733.

165. Meyers BF, Lynch JP, Trulock EP, et al. Single versus bilateral lung transplantation for idiopathic pulmonary fibrosis: a ten-year institutional experience. *J Thorac Cardiovasc Surg* 2000;120(1):99–107.

166. Mogulkoc N, Brutsche MH, Bishop PW, et al. Pulmonary function in idiopathic pulmonary fibrosis and referral for lung transplantation. *Am J Respir Crit Care Med* 2001;164(1):103–108.

167. The Toronto Lung Transplant Group. Experience with single-lung transplantation for pulmonary fibrosis. *JAMA* 1988;259(15):2258–2262.

168. American Thoracic Society, Medical Section of the American Lung Association. Lung transplantation. Report of the ATS workshop on lung transplantation. *Am Rev Respir Dis* 1993;147(3):772–776.

169. Chacon RA, Corris PA, Dark JH, et al. Comparison of the functional results of single lung transplantation for pulmonary fibrosis and chronic airway obstruction. *Thorax* 1998;53(1):43–49.

170. Trulock EP, Cooper JD, Kaiser LR, Pasque MK, Ettinger NA, Dresler CM, Washington University Lung Transplantation Group. The Washington University-Barnes Hospital experience with lung transplantation. *JAMA* 1991;266(14):1943–1946.

171. Hoffman LA, Wesmiller SW, Sciurba FC, et al. Nasal cannula and transtracheal oxygen delivery. A comparison of patient response after 6 months of each technique. *Am Rev Respir Dis* 1992;145(4 Pt 1):827–831.

172. Ghofrani HA, Wiedemann R, Rose F, et al. Sildenafil for treatment of lung fibrosis and pulmonary hypertension: a randomised controlled trial. *Lancet* 2002;360(9337):895–900.

173. Park S, Saleh D, Giaid A, et al. Increased endothelin-1 in bleomycin-induced pulmonary fibrosis and the effect of an endothelin receptor antagonist. *Am J Respir Crit Care Med* 1997;156(2):600–608.

174. De Vries J, Kessels BL, Drent M. Quality of life of idiopathic pulmonary fibrosis patients. *Eur Respir J* 2001;17(5):954–961.

175. Turner-Warwick M, Lebowitz M, Burrows B, et al. Cryptogenic fibrosing alveolitis and lung cancer. *Thorax* 1980;35(7):496–499.

176. Hubbard R, Venn A, Lewis S, et al. Lung cancer and cryptogenic fibrosing alveolitis. A population-based cohort study. *Am J Respir Crit Care Med* 2000;161(1):5–8.

177. Blivet S, Philit F, Sab JM, et al. Outcome of patients with idiopathic pulmonary fibrosis admitted to the ICU for respiratory failure. *Chest* 2001;120(1):209–212.

178. Stern JB, Mal H, Groussard O, et al. Prognosis of patients with advanced idiopathic pulmonary fibrosis requiring mechanical ventilation for acute respiratory failure. *Chest* 2001;120(1):213–219.

179. Ziesche R, Hofbauer E, Wittmann K, et al. A preliminary study of long-term treatment with interferon gamma-1b and low-dose prednisolone in patients with idiopathic pulmonary fibrosis. *N Engl J Med* 1999;341(17):1264–1269.

180. Raghu G, Brown KK, Bradford WZ, et al. A placebo-controlled trial of interferon gamma-1b in patients with idiopathic pulmonary fibrosis. *N Engl J Med* 2004;350(2):125–133.

181. Katzenstein AL, Fiorelli RF. Nonspecific interstitial pneumonia/fibrosis. Histologic features and clinical significance. *Am J Surg Pathol* 1994;18(2):136–147.

182. Douglas WW, Tazelaar HD, Hartman TE, et al. Polymyositis-dermatomyositis-associated interstitial lung disease. *Am J Respir Crit Care Med* 2001;164(7):1182–1185.

183. Bouros D, Wells AU, Nicholson AG, et al. Histopathologic subsets of fibrosing alveolitis in patients with systemic sclerosis and their relationship to outcome. *Am J Respir Crit Care Med* 2002;165(12):1581–1586.

184. Cottin V, Thivolet-Bejui F, Reynaud-Gaubert M, et al. Interstitial lung disease in amyopathic dermatomyositis, dermatomyositis and polymyositis. *Eur Respir J* 2003;22(2):245–250.

185. Arakawa H, Yamada H, Kurihara Y, et al. Nonspecific interstitial pneumonia associated with polymyositis and dermatomyositis: serial high-resolution CT findings and functional correlation. *Chest* 2003;123(4):1096–1103.

186. Vourlekis JS, Schwarz MI, Cool CD, et al. Nonspecific interstitial pneumonitis as the sole histologic expression of hypersensitivity pneumonitis. *Am J Med* 2002;112(6):490–493.

187. Flieder DB, Travis WD. Pathologic characteristics of drug-induced lung disease. *Clin Chest Med* 2004;25:37–45.

188. Demedts M, Wells AU, Anto JM, et al. Interstitial lung diseases: an epidemiological overview. *Eur Respir J Suppl* 2001;32:2s–16s.

189. Martinez FJ, Flaherty KR, Travis WD. Chapter 5: Nonspecific interstitial pneumonia. In: Lynch JP, ed. *Idiopathic pulmonary fibrosis.* New York: Marcel Dekker Inc, 2004:101–136.

190. Nagai S, Kitaichi M, Itoh H, et al. Idiopathic nonspecific interstitial pneumonia/fibrosis: comparison with idiopathic pulmonary fibrosis and BOOP. *Eur Respir J* 1998;12(5):1010–1019.

191. Travis WD, Matsui K, Moss J, et al. Idiopathic nonspecific interstitial pneumonia: prognostic significance of cellular and fibrosing patterns: survival comparison with usual interstitial pneumonia and desquamative interstitial pneumonia. *Am J Surg Pathol* 2000;24(1):19–33.

192. Riha RL, Duhig EE, Clarke BE, et al. Survival of patients with biopsy-proven usual interstitial pneumonia and nonspecific interstitial pneumonia. *Eur Respir J* 2002;19(6):1114–1118.

193. Cottin V, Donsbeck A, Revel D, et al. Nonspecific interstitial pneumonia. Individualization of a clinicopathologic entity in a series of 12 patients. *Am J Respir Crit Care Med* 1998;158(4):1286–1293.

194. Davison AG, Heard BE, McAllister WA, et al. Cryptogenic organizing pneumonitis. *Q J Med* 1983;52(207):382–394.

195. Epler GR, Colby TV, McLoud TC, et al. Bronchiolitis obliterans organizing pneumonia. *N Engl J Med* 1985;312(3):152–158.

196. Izumi T, Kitaichi M, Nishimura K, et al. Bronchiolitis obliterans organizing pneumonia. Clinical features and differential diagnosis. *Chest* 1992;102(3):715–719.

197. King TE Jr., Mortenson RL. Cryptogenic organizing pneumonitis. The North American experience. *Chest* 1992;102(1 Suppl): 8S–13S.

198. Lee KS, Kullnig P, Hartman TE, et al. Cryptogenic organizing pneumonia: CT findings in 43 patients. *Am J Roentgenol* 1994; 62(3):543–546.

199. Akira M, Yamamoto S, Sakatani M. Bronchiolitis obliterans organizing pneumonia manifesting as multiple large nodules or masses. *Am J Roentgenol* 1998;170(2):291–295.

200. Katzenstein AL, Myers JL, Prophet WD, et al. Bronchiolitis obliterans and usual interstitial pneumonia. A comparative clinicopathologic study. *Am J Surg Pathol* 1986;10(6):373–381.

201. Guerry-Force ML, Muller NL, Wright JL, et al. A comparison of bronchiolitis obliterans with organizing pneumonia, usual interstitial pneumonia, and small airways disease. *Am Rev Respir Dis* 1987;135(3):705–712.

202. Muller NL, Guerry-Force ML, Staples CA, et al. Differential diagnosis of bronchiolitis obliterans with organizing pneumonia and usual interstitial pneumonia: clinical, functional, and radiologic findings. *Radiology* 1987;162(1 Pt 1):151–156.

203. Alasaly K, Muller N, Ostrow DN, et al. Cryptogenic organizing pneumonia. A report of 25 cases and a review of the literature. *Medicine (Baltimore)* 1995;74(4):201–211.

204. King TE Jr. Overview of bronchiolitis. *Clin Chest Med* 1993;14(4): 607–610.

205. King TE Jr. Chapter 26: Bronchiolitis. In: Schwarz MI, King TE Jr., eds. *Interstitial lung disease*, 4th ed. Hamilton, Canada: B. C. Dekker; 2003:787–824.

206. Colby TV. Pathologic aspects of bronchiolitis obliterans organizing pneumonia. *Chest* 1992;102(1 Suppl):38S–43S.

207. Watanabe K, Senju S, Wen FQ, et al. Factors related to the relapse of bronchiolitis obliterans organizing pneumonia. *Chest* 1998;114(6): 1599–1606.

208. Lazor R, Vandevenne A, Pelletier A. Cryptogenic organizing pneumonia. Characteristics of relapses in a series of 48 patients. The Groupe d'Etudes et de Recherche sur les Maladies "Orphelines" Pulmonaires (GERM"O"P). *Am J Respir Crit Care Med* 2000; 162(2 Pt 1):571–577.

209. Niewoehner DE, Kleinerman J, Rice DB. Pathologic changes in the peripheral airways of young cigarette smokers. *N Engl J Med* 1974;291(15):755–758.

210. Myers JL, Veal CF Jr., Shin MS, et al. Respiratory bronchiolitis causing interstitial lung disease. A clinicopathologic study of six cases. *Am Rev Respir Dis* 1987;135(4):880–884.

211. Yousem SA, Colby TV, Gaensler EA. Respiratory bronchiolitis-associated interstitial lung disease and its relationship to desquamative interstitial pneumonia. *Mayo Clin Proc* 1989;64(11):1373–1380.

212. Ryu JH, Myers JL, Swensen SJ. Bronchiolar disorders. *Am J Respir Crit Care Med* 2003;168(11):1277–1292.

213. Matsuo K, Tada S, Kataoka M, et al. Spontaneous remission of desquamative interstitial pneumonia. *Intern Med* 1997;36(10): 728–731.

214. Heyneman LE, Ward S, Lynch DA, et al. Respiratory bronchiolitis, respiratory bronchiolitis-associated interstitial lung disease, and desquamative interstitial pneumonia: different entities or part of the spectrum of the same disease process? *Am J Roentgenol* 1999;173(6):1617–1622.

215. Gaensler EA, Goff AM, Prowse CM. Desquamative interstitial pneumonia. *N Engl J Med* 1966;274(3):113–128.

216. Kennedy JL, Nathwani BN, Burke JS, et al. Pulmonary lymphomas and other pulmonary lymphoid lesions. A clinicopathologic and immunologic study of 64 patients. *Cancer* 1985;56(3):539–552.

217. Travis WD, Colby TV, Koss MN, et al. Chapter 5: Reactive lymphoid lesions. *Non-neoplastic disorders of the lower respiratory tract*, 1st ed. Washington, DC: American Registry of Pathology and the Armed Forces Institute of Pathology, 2002:265–289.

218. Liebow AA, Carrington CB. The interstitial pneumonias. In: Simon M, Potchen EJ, LeMay M ed. *Frontiers in pulmonary radiology*, 1st ed. New York: Grune & Stratton, 1969:102–141.

219. Cain HC, Noble PW, Matthay RA. Pulmonary manifestations of Sjogren's syndrome. *Clin Chest Med* 1998;19(4):687–699, viii.

220. Skopouli FN, Dafni U, Ioannidis JP, et al. Clinical evolution, and morbidity and mortality of primary Sjogren's syndrome. *Semin Arthritis Rheum* 2000;29(5):296–304.

221. Pertovaara M, Pukkala E, Laippala P, et al. A longitudinal cohort study of Finnish patients with primary Sjogren's syndrome: clinical, immunological, and epidemiological aspects. *Ann Rheum Dis* 2001;60(5):467–472.

222. Johkoh T, Muller NL, Pickford HA, et al. Lymphocytic interstitial pneumonia: thin-section CT findings in 22 patients. *Radiology* 1999;212(2):567–572.

223. Principi N, Marchisio P, Massironi E, et al. Effect of zidovudine in HIV-infected children with lymphocytic interstitial pneumonitis. *AIDS* 1991;5(4):468–469.

224. Scarborough M, Lishman S, Shaw P, et al. Lymphocytic interstitial pneumonitis in an HIV-infected adult: response to antiretroviral therapy. *Int J STD AIDS* 2000;11(2):119–122.

225. Baughman RP, Lower EE, du Bois RM. Sarcoidosis. *Lancet* 2003; 361(9363):1111–1118.

226. Thomas KW, Hunninghake GW. Sarcoidosis. *JAMA* 2003; 289(24):3300–3303.

227. Carr PL, Singer DE, Goldenheim P, et al. Noninvasive testing of asymptomatic bilateral hilar adenopathy. *J Gen Intern Med* 1990;5(2):138–146.

228. Hunninghake GW, Fulmer JD, Young RC Jr., et al. Localization of the immune response in sarcoidosis. *Am Rev Respir Dis* 1979; 120(1):49–57.

229. Daniele RP, Dauber JH, Rossman MD. Immunologic abnormalities in sarcoidosis. *Ann Intern Med* 1980;92(3):406–416.

230. Hunninghake GW, Gadek JE, Young RC Jr., et al. Maintenance of granuloma formation in pulmonary sarcoidosis by T lymphocytes within the lung. *N Engl J Med* 1980;302(11):594–598.

231. Hunninghake GW, Crystal RG. Pulmonary sarcoidosis: a disorder mediated by excess helper T-lymphocyte activity at sites of disease activity. *N Engl J Med* 1981;305(8):429–434.

232. Hunninghake GW, Bedell GN, Zavala DC, et al. Role of interleukin-2 release by lung T-cells in active pulmonary sarcoidosis. *Am Rev Respir Dis* 1983;128(4):634–638.

233. Hunninghake GW. Release of interleukin-1 by alveolar macrophages of patients with active pulmonary sarcoidosis. *Am Rev Respir Dis* 1984;129(4):569–572.

234. Hunninghake GW. Role of alveolar macrophage- and lung T cell-derived mediators in pulmonary sarcoidosis. *Ann N Y Acad Sci* 1986;465:82–90.

235. Morris DG, Jasmer RM, Huang L, et al. Sarcoidosis following HIV infection: evidence for CD4+ lymphocyte dependence. *Chest* 2003;124(3):929–935.

236. Baumer I, Zissel G, Schlaak M, et al. Th1/Th2 cell distribution in pulmonary sarcoidosis. *Am J Respir Cell Mol Biol* 1997;16(2):171–177.

237. Prasse A, Georges CG, Biller H, et al. Th1 cytokine pattern in sarcoidosis is expressed by bronchoalveolar CD4+ and CD8+ T cells. *Clin Exp Immunol* 2000;122(2):241–248.

238. Wahlstrom J, Katchar K, Wigzell H, et al. Analysis of intracellular cytokines in CD4+ and CD8+ lung and blood T cells in sarcoidosis. *Am J Respir Crit Care Med* 2001;163(1):115–121.

239. Moller DR. Treatment of sarcoidosis - from a basic science point of view. *J Intern Med* 2003;253(1):31–40.

240. Ziegenhagen MW, Benner UK, Zissel G, et al. Sarcoidosis: TNF-alpha release from alveolar macrophages and serum level of sIL-2R are prognostic markers. *Am J Respir Crit Care Med* 1997;156(5): 1586–1592.

241. Ziegenhagen MW, Rothe ME, Zissel G, et al. Exaggerated TNFalpha release of alveolar macrophages in corticosteroid resistant sarcoidosis. *Sarcoidosis Vasc Diffuse Lung Dis* 2002;19(3):185–190.

242. Fehrenbach H, Zissel G, Goldmann T, et al. Alveolar macrophages are the main source for tumour necrosis factor-alpha in patients with sarcoidosis. *Eur Respir J* 2003;21(3):421–428.

243. Rybicki BA, Iannuzzi MC, Frederick MM, et al. Familial aggregation of sarcoidosis. A case-control etiologic study of sarcoidosis (ACCESS). *Am J Respir Crit Care Med* 2001;164(11):2085–2091.

244. Spagnolo P, Renzoni EA, Wells AU, et al. C-C chemokine receptor 2 and sarcoidosis: association with Lofgren syndrome. *Am J Respir Crit Care Med* 2003;168(10):1162–1166.

245. Grutters JC, Sato H, Pantelidis P, et al. Increased frequency of the uncommon tumor necrosis factor -857T allele in British and

Dutch patients with sarcoidosis. *Am J Respir Crit Care Med* 2002; 165(8):1119–1124.

246. Rybicki BA, Major M, Popovich J Jr., et al. Racial differences in sarcoidosis incidence: a 5-year study in a health maintenance organization. *Am J Epidemiol* 1997;145(3):234–241.

247. James DG, Neville E, Siltzbach LE. A worldwide review of sarcoidosis. *Ann N Y Acad Sci* 1976;278:321–334.

248. Baughman RP, Teirstein AS, Judson MA, et al. Clinical characteristics of patients in a case control study of sarcoidosis. *Am J Respir Crit Care Med* 2001;164(10 Pt 1):1885–1889.

249. Roberts WC, McAllister HA Jr., Ferrans VJ. Sarcoidosis of the heart. A clinicopathologic study of 35 necropsy patients (group 1) and review of 78 previously described necropsy patients (group 11). *Am J Med* 1977;63(1):86–108.

250. Sharma OP, Sharma AM. Sarcoidosis of the nervous system. A clinical approach. *Arch Intern Med* 1991;151(7):1317–1321.

251. Sharma OP. Cardiac and neurologic dysfunction in sarcoidosis. *Clin Chest Med* 1997;18(4):813–825.

252. Devaney K, Goodman ZD, Epstein MS, et al. Hepatic sarcoidosis. Clinicopathologic features in 100 patients. *Am J Surg Pathol* 1993;17(12):1272–1280.

253. Bechtel JJ, Starr T 3rd, Dantzker DR, et al. Airway hyperreactivity in patients with sarcoidosis. *Am Rev Respir Dis* 1981;124(6): 759–761.

254. Benjamin RG, Sackner MA. Pulmonary function in sarcoidosis. *Sarcoidosis* 1984;1(1):50–52.

255. Sharma OP, Johnson R. Airway obstruction in sarcoidosis. A study of 123 nonsmoking black American patients with sarcoidosis. *Chest* 1988;94(2):343–346.

256. Loddenkemper R, Kloppenborg A, Schoenfeld N, et al. Clinical findings in 715 patients with newly detected pulmonary sarcoidosis—results of a cooperative study in former West Germany and Switzerland. WATL Study Group. Wissenschaftliche Arbeitsgemeinschaft fur die Therapie von Lungenkrankheitan. *Sarcoidosis Vasc Diffuse Lung Dis* 1998;15(2):178–182.

257. Lavergne F, Clerici C, Sadoun D, et al. Airway obstruction in bronchial sarcoidosis: outcome with treatment. *Chest* 1999;116(5): 1194–1199.

258. Dunn TL, Watters LC, Hendrix C, et al. Gas exchange at a given degree of volume restriction is different in sarcoidosis and idiopathic pulmonary fibrosis. *Am J Med* 1988;85(2):221–224.

259. Mayock RL, Bertrand P, Morrison CE, et al. Manifestations of Sarcoidosis. Analysis of 145 Patients, with a Review of Nine Series Selected from the Literature. *Am J Med* 1963;35:67–89.

260. Lieberman J. Elevation of serum angiotensin-converting-enzyme (ACE) level in sarcoidosis. *Am J Med* 1975;59(3):365–372.

261. Lieberman J, Schleissner LA, Nosal A, et al. Clinical correlations of serum angiotensin-converting enzyme (ACE) in sarcoidosis. A longitudinal study of serum ACE, 67gallium scans, chest roentgenograms, and pulmonary function. *Chest* 1983;84(5): 522–528.

262. Ainslie GM, Benatar SR. Serum angiotensin converting enzyme in sarcoidosis: sensitivity and specificity in diagnosis: correlations with disease activity, duration, extra-thoracic involvement, radiographic type and therapy. *Q J Med* 1985;55(218): 253–270.

263. Lieberman J. Enzymes in sarcoidosis. Angiotensin-converting-enzyme (ACE). *Clin Lab Med* 1989;9(4):745–755.

264. Allen RK. A review of angiotensin converting enzyme in health and disease. *Sarcoidosis* 1991;8(2):95–100.

265. Allen RK, Pierce RJ, Barter CE. Angiotensin-converting enzyme in bronchoalveolar lavage fluid in sarcoidosis. *Sarcoidosis* 1992; 9(1):54–59.

266. Tomita H, Sato S, Matsuda R, et al. Serum lysozyme levels and clinical features of sarcoidosis. *Lung* 1999;177(3):161–167.

267. Hinman LM, Stevens C, Matthay RA, et al. Angiotensin convertase activities in human alveolar macrophages: effects of cigarette smoking and sarcoidosis. *Science* 1979;205(4402):202–203.

268. Fanburg BL, Schoenberger MD, Bachus B, et al. Elevated serum angiotensin I converting enzyme in sarcoidosis. *Am Rev Respir Dis* 1976;114(3):525–528.

269. Tahmoush AJ, Amir MS, Connor WW, et al. CSF-ACE activity in probable CNS neurosarcoidosis. *Sarcoidosis Vasc Diffuse Lung Dis* 2002;19(3):191–197.

270. Ziegenhagen MW, Rothe ME, Schlaak M, et al. Bronchoalveolar and serological parameters reflecting the severity of sarcoidosis. *Eur Respir J* 2003;21(3):407–413.

271. Wall CP, Gaensler EA, Carrington CB, et al. Comparison of transbronchial and open biopsies in chronic infiltrative lung diseases. *Am Rev Respir Dis* 1981;123(3):280–285.

272. Morales CF, Patefield AJ, Strollo PJ Jr., et al. Flexible transbronchial needle aspiration in the diagnosis of sarcoidosis. *Chest* 1994;106(3):709–711.

273. Trisolini R, Agli LL, Cancellieri A, et al. The value of flexible transbronchial needle aspiration in the diagnosis of stage I sarcoidosis. *Chest* 2003;124(6):2126–2130.

274. Milman N, Faurschou P, Munch EP, et al. Transbronchial lung biopsy through the fibre optic bronchoscope. Results and complications in 452 examinations. *Respir Med* 1994;88(10):749–753.

275. Descombes E, Gardiol D, Leuenberger P. Transbronchial lung biopsy: an analysis of 530 cases with reference to the number of samples. *Monaldi Arch Chest Dis* 1997;52(4):324–329.

276. Zwischenberger JB, Savage C, Alpard SK, et al. Mediastinal transthoracic needle and core lymph node biopsy: should it replace mediastinoscopy? *Chest* 2002;121(4):1165–1170.

277. Winterbauer RH, Belic N, Moores KD. Clinical interpretation of bilateral hilar adenopathy. *Ann Intern Med* 1973;78(1):65–71.

278. Pietinalho A, Ohmichi M, Hiraga Y, et al. The mode of presentation of sarcoidosis in Finland and Hokkaido, Japan. A comparative analysis of 571 Finnish and 686 Japanese patients. *Sarcoidosis Vasc Diffuse Lung Dis* 1996;13(2):159–166.

279. Littner MR, Schachter EN, Putman CE, et al. The clinical assessment of roentgenographically atypical pulmonary sarcoidosis. *Am J Med* 1977;62(3):361–368.

280. Wollschlager C, Khan F. Aspergillomas complicating sarcoidosis. A prospective study in 100 patients. *Chest* 1984;86(4):585–588.

281. Scadding JG. Prognosis of intrathoracic sarcoidosis in England. A review of 136 cases after five years' observation. *Br Med J* 1961; 5261:1165–1172.

282. Siltzbach LE, James DG, Neville E, et al. Course and prognosis of sarcoidosis around the world. *Am J Med* 1974;57(6):847–852.

283. Brauner MW, Grenier P, Mompoint D, et al. Pulmonary sarcoidosis: evaluation with high-resolution CT. *Radiology* 1989; 172(2):467–471.

284. Lynch DA, Webb WR, Gamsu G, et al. Computed tomography in pulmonary sarcoidosis. *J Comput Assist Tomogr* 1989;13(3):405–410.

285. Brauner MW, Lenoir S, Grenier P, et al. Pulmonary sarcoidosis: CT assessment of lesion reversibility. *Radiology* 1992;182(2):349–354.

286. Lenique F, Brauner MW, Grenier P, et al. CT assessment of bronchi in sarcoidosis: endoscopic and pathologic correlations. *Radiology* 1995;194(2):419–423.

287. Oberstein A, von Zitzewitz H, Schweden F, et al. Non-invasive evaluation of the inflammatory activity in sarcoidosis with high-resolution computed tomography. *Sarcoidosis Vasc Diffuse Lung Dis* 1997;14(1):65–72.

288. Leung AN, Brauner MW, Caillat-Vigneron N, et al. Sarcoidosis activity: correlation of HRCT findings with those of 67Ga scanning, bronchoalveolar lavage, and serum angiotensin-converting enzyme assay. *J Comput Assist Tomogr* 1998;22(2):229–234.

289. Abehsera M, Valeyre D, Grenier P, et al. Sarcoidosis with pulmonary fibrosis: CT patterns and correlation with pulmonary function. *Am J Roentgenol* 2000;174(6):1751–1757.

290. Hansell DM, Milne DG, Wilsher ML, et al. Pulmonary sarcoidosis: morphologic associations of airflow obstruction at thin-section CT. *Radiology* 1998;209(3):697–704.

291. Pietinalho A, Ohmichi M, Lofroos AB, et al. The prognosis of pulmonary sarcoidosis in Finland and Hokkaido, Japan. A comparative five-year study of biopsy-proven cases. *Sarcoidosis Vasc Diffuse Lung Dis* 2000;17(2):158–166.

292. Judson MA, Baughman RP, Thompson BW, et al. Two year prognosis of sarcoidosis: the ACCESS experience. *Sarcoidosis Vasc Diffuse Lung Dis* 2003;20(3):204–211.

293. Hunninghake GW, Gilbert S, Pueringer R, et al. Outcome of the treatment for sarcoidosis. *Am J Respir Crit Care Med* 1994;149(4 Pt 1): 893–898.

294. Teirstein AS, Siltzbach LE, Berger H. Patterns of sarcoidosis in three population groups in New York City. *Ann N Y Acad Sci* 1976;278:371–376.

295. Chappell AG, Cheung WY, Hutchings HA. Sarcoidosis: a long-term follow-up study. *Sarcoidosis Vasc Diffuse Lung Dis* 2000; 17(2):167–173.

296. Gullapalli D, Phillips LH 2nd. Neurologic manifestations of sarcoidosis. *Neurol Clin* 2002;20(1):59–83, vi.

297. Doty JD, Mazur JE, Judson MA. Treatment of corticosteroid-resistant neurosarcoidosis with a short-course cyclophosphamide regimen. *Chest* 2003;124(5):2023–2026.

298. English I, Joseph C, Patel PJ, et al. Sarcoidosis. *J Am Acad Dermatol* 2001;44(5):725–743.

299. Gibson GJ, Prescott RJ, Muers MF, et al. British Thoracic Society Sarcoidosis study: effects of long-term corticosteroid treatment. *Thorax* 1996;51(3):238–247.

300. Paramothayan S, Jones PW. Corticosteroid therapy in pulmonary sarcoidosis: a systematic review. *JAMA* 2002;287(10):1301–1307.

301. Paramothayan S, Lasserson T, Walters EH. Immunosuppressive and cytotoxic therapy for pulmonary sarcoidosis. *Cochrane Database Syst Rev* 2003(3):CD003536.

302. Reich JM, Johnson RE. Course and prognosis of sarcoidosis in a nonreferral setting. Analysis of 86 patients observed for 10 years. *Am J Med* 1985;78(1):61–67.

303. Gottlieb JE, Israel HL, Steiner RM, et al. Outcome in sarcoidosis. The relationship of relapse to corticosteroid therapy. *Chest* 1997;111(3):623–631.

304. Hunninghake GW. Goal of the treatment for sarcoidosis. Minimize harm for the patient. *Am J Respir Crit Care Med* 1997; 156(5):1369–1370.

305. Reich JM. Corticosteroid therapy and relapse in sarcoidosis. *Chest* 1998;113(2):559–561.

306. Reich JM. Mortality of intrathoracic sarcoidosis in referral vs population-based settings: influence of stage, ethnicity, and corticosteroid therapy. *Chest* 2002;121(1):32–39.

307. Judson MA. An approach to the treatment of pulmonary sarcoidosis with corticosteroids: the six phases of treatment. *Chest* 1999;115(4):1158–1165.

308. Baughman RP, Iannuzzi MC, Lower EE, et al. Use of fluticasone in acute symptomatic pulmonary sarcoidosis. *Sarcoidosis Vasc Diffuse Lung Dis* 2002;19(3):198–204.

309. Baltzan M, Mehta S, Kirkham TH, et al. Randomized trial of prolonged chloroquine therapy in advanced pulmonary sarcoidosis. *Am J Respir Crit Care Med* 1999;160(1):192–197.

310. Baughman RP, Winget DB, Lower EE. Methotrexate is steroid sparing in acute sarcoidosis: results of a double blind, randomized trial. *Sarcoidosis Vasc Diffuse Lung Dis* 2000;17(1):60–66.

311. Baughman RP, Lower EE. Leflunomide for chronic sarcoidosis. *Sarcoidosis Vasc Diffuse Lung Dis* 2004;21(1):43–48.

312. Baughman RP, Koehler A, Bejarano PA, et al. Role of liver function tests in detecting methotrexate-induced liver damage in sarcoidosis. *Arch Intern Med* 2003;163(5):615–620.

313. Muller-Quernheim J, Kienast K, Held M, et al. Treatment of chronic sarcoidosis with an azathioprine/prednisolone regimen. *Eur Respir J* 1999;14(5):1117–1122.

314. Stern BJ, Schonfeld SA, Sewell C, et al. The treatment of neurosarcoidosis with cyclosporine. *Arch Neurol* 1992;49(10):1065–1072.

315. Wyser CP, van Schalkwyk EM, Alheit B, et al. Treatment of progressive pulmonary sarcoidosis with cyclosporin A. A randomized controlled trial. *Am J Respir Crit Care Med* 1997;156(5): 1371–1376.

316. Baughman RP, Lower EE. Infliximab for refractory sarcoidosis. *Sarcoidosis Vasc Diffuse Lung Dis* 2001;18(1):70–74.

317. O'Connor TM, Shanahan F, Bredin CP. Infliximab therapy for complicated sarcoidosis. *Ann Intern Med* 2002;137(4):296–297.

318. Keane J, Gershon S, Wise RP, et al. Tuberculosis Associated with Infliximab, a Tumor Necrosis Factor {alpha}-Neutralizing Agent. *N Engl J Med* 2001;345(15):1098–1104.

319. Podolsky DK. Inflammatory bowel disease. *N Engl J Med* 2002;347(6):417–429.

320. Baughman RP, Judson MA, Teirstein AS, et al. Thalidomide for chronic sarcoidosis. *Chest* 2002;122(1):227–232.

321. Haley H, Cantrell W, Smith K. Infliximab therapy for sarcoidosis (lupus pernio). *Br J Dermatol* 2004;150(1):146–149.

322. Pritchard C, Nadarajah K. Tumour necrosis factor {alpha} inhibitor treatment for sarcoidosis refractory to conventional treatments: a report of five patients. *Ann Rheum Dis* 2004;63(3):318–320.

323. Utz JP, Limper AH, Kalra S, et al. Etanercept for the treatment of stage II and III progressive pulmonary sarcoidosis. *Chest* 2003; 124(1):177–185.

324. Stevens DA, Kan VL, Judson MA, et al. Practice guidelines for diseases caused by Aspergillus. Infectious Diseases Society of America. *Clin Infect Dis* 2000;30(4):696–709.

325. Battaglini JW, Murray GF, Keagy BA, et al. Surgical management of symptomatic pulmonary aspergilloma. *Ann Thorac Surg* 1985; 39(6):512–516.

326. Shorr AF, Davies DB, Nathan SD. Predicting mortality in patients with sarcoidosis awaiting lung transplantation. *Chest* 2003; 124(3):922–928.

327. Smith LJ, Lawrence JB, Katzenstein AA. Vascular sarcoidosis: a rare cause of pulmonary hypertension. *Am J Med Sci* 1983; 285(1):38–44.

328. Judson MA. Lung transplantation for pulmonary sarcoidosis. *Eur Respir J* 1998;11(3):738–744.

329. Shorr AF, Davies DB, Nathan SD. Outcomes for patients with sarcoidosis awaiting lung transplantation. *Chest* 2002;122(1):233–238.

330. Selman M. Chapter 19: Hypersensitivity pneumonitis. In: Schawarz MI, King TE Jr., eds. *Interstitial lung disease*, 4th ed. Hamilton, Canada: B. C. Dekker, 2003:452–484.

331. Rose C. Chapter 14: Hypersensitivity pneumonitis. In: Harber P, Schenker MB, Balmes JR, eds. *Occupational and environmental respiratory disease*, 1st ed. New York: Mosby, 1996:201–215.

332. Malmberg P, Rask-Andersen A, Rosenhall L. Exposure to microorganisms associated with allergic alveolitis and febrile reactions to mold dust in farmers. *Chest* 1993;103(4):1202–1209.

333. Yamasaki H, Ando M, Brazer W, et al. Polarized type 1 cytokine profile in bronchoalveolar lavage T cells of patients with hypersensitivity pneumonitis. *J Immunol* 1999;163(6):3516–3523.

334. Reynolds HY, Fulmer JD, Kazmierowski JA, et al. Analysis of cellular and protein content of broncho-alveolar lavage fluid from patients with idiopathic pulmonary fibrosis and chronic hypersensitivity pneumonitis. *J Clin Invest* 1977;59(1):165–175.

335. Patterson R, Wang JL, Fink JN, et al. IgA and IgG antibody activities of serum and bronchoalveolar fluid from symptomatic and asymptomatic pigeon breeders. *Am Rev Respir Dis* 1979;120(5): 1113–1118.

336. Treuhaft MW, Roberts RC, Hackbarth C, et al. Characterization of precipitin response to Micropolyspora faeni in farmer's lung disease by quantitative immunoelectrophoresis. *Am Rev Respir Dis* 1979;119(4):571–578.

337. Cormier Y, Belanger J, Durand P. Factors influencing the development of serum precipitins to farmer's lung antigen in Quebec dairy farmers. *Thorax* 1985;40(2):138–142.

338. Cormier Y, Belanger J. The fluctuant nature of precipitating antibodies in dairy farmers. *Thorax* 1989;44(6):469–473.

339. Braun SR, doPico GA, Tsiatis A, et al. Farmer's lung disease: long-term clinical and physiologic outcome. *Am Rev Respir Dis* 1979;119(2):185–191.

340. Sansores R, Salas J, Chapela R, et al. Clubbing in hypersensitivity pneumonitis. Its prevalence and possible prognostic role. *Arch Intern Med* 1990;150(9):1849–1851.

341. Reynolds HY. Hypersensitivity pneumonitis: correlation of cellular and immunologic changes with clinical phases of disease. *Lung* 1988;166(4):189–208.

342. Leatherman JW, Michael AF, Schwartz BA, et al. Lung T cells in hypersensitivity pneumonitis. *Ann Intern Med* 1984;100(3):390–392.

343. Costabel U, Bross KJ, Ruhle KH, et al. Ia-like antigens on T-cells and their subpopulations in pulmonary sarcoidosis and in hypersensitivity pneumonitis. Analysis of bronchoalveolar and blood lymphocytes. *Am Rev Respir Dis* 1985;131(3):337–342.

344. Semenzato G, Chilosi M, Ossi E, et al. Bronchoalveolar lavage and lung histology. Comparative analysis of inflammatory and immunocompetent cells in patients with sarcoidosis and hypersensitivity pneumonitis. *Am Rev Respir Dis* 1985;132(2):400–404.

345. Murayama J, Yoshizawa Y, Ohtsuka M, et al. Lung fibrosis in hypersensitivity pneumonitis. Association with CD4+ but not CD8+ cell dominant alveolitis and insidious onset. *Chest* 1993; 104(1):38–43.

346. Calvanico NJ, Ambegaonkar SP, Schlueter DP, et al. Immunoglobulin levels in bronchoalveolar lavage fluid from pigeon breeders. *J Lab Clin Med* 1980;96(1):129–140.

347. Winterbauer RH, Lammert J, Selland M, et al. Bronchoalveolar lavage cell populations in the diagnosis of sarcoidosis. *Chest* 1993;104(2):352–361.

348. Drent M, Grutters JC, Mulder PG, et al. Is the different T helper cell activity in sarcoidosis and extrinsic allergic alveolitis also reflected by the cellular bronchoalveolar lavage fluid profile? *Sarcoidosis Vasc Diffuse Lung Dis* 1997;14(1):31–38.

349. Fournier E, Tonnel AB, Gosset P, et al. Early neutrophil alveolitis after antigen inhalation in hypersensitivity pneumonitis. *Chest* 1985;88(4):563–566.

350. Solal-Celigny P, Laviolette M, Hebert J, et al. Immune reactions in the lungs of asymptomatic dairy farmers. *Am Rev Respir Dis* 1982;126(6):964–967.

351. Cormier Y, Belanger J, Beaudoin J, et al. Abnormal bronchoalveolar lavage in asymptomatic dairy farmers. Study of lymphocytes. *Am Rev Respir Dis* 1984;130(6):1046–1049.

352. Cormier Y, Belanger J, Laviolette M. Persistent bronchoalveolar lymphocytosis in asymptomatic farmers. *Am Rev Respir Dis* 1986;133(5):843–847.

353. Gariepy L, Cormier Y, Laviolette M, et al. Predictive value of bronchoalveolar lavage cells and serum precipitins in asymptomatic dairy farmers. *Am Rev Respir Dis* 1989;140(5):1386–1389.

354. Lalancette M, Carrier G, Laviolette M, et al. Farmer's lung. Long-term outcome and lack of predictive value of bronchoalveolar lavage fibrosing factors. *Am Rev Respir Dis* 1993;148(1):216–221.

355. Cormier Y, Brown M, Worthy S, et al. High-resolution computed tomographic characteristics in acute farmer's lung and in its follow-up. *Eur Respir J* 2000;16(1):56–60.

356. Lynch DA, Newell JD, Logan PM, et al. Can CT distinguish hypersensitivity pneumonitis from idiopathic pulmonary fibrosis? *Am J Roentgenol* 1995;165(4):807–811.

357. Steinberg AD, Gourley MF, Klinman DM, et al. NIH conference. Systemic lupus erythematosus. *Ann Intern Med* 1991;115(7):548–559.

358. Boumpas DT, Austin HA 3rd, Fessler BJ, et al. Systemic lupus erythematosus: emerging concepts. Part 1: Renal, neuropsychiatric, cardiovascular, pulmonary, and hematologic disease. *Ann Intern Med* 1995;122(12):940–950.

359. Boumpas DT, Fessler BJ, Austin HA 3rd, et al. Systemic lupus erythematosus: emerging concepts. Part 2: Dermatologic and joint disease, the antiphospholipid antibody syndrome, pregnancy and hormonal therapy, morbidity and mortality, and pathogenesis. *Ann Intern Med* 1995;123(1):42–53.

360. Keane MP, Lynch JP 3rd. Pleuropulmonary manifestations of systemic lupus erythematosus. *Thorax* 2000;55(2):159–166.

361. Rekvig OP, Nossent JC. Anti-double-stranded DNA antibodies, nucleosomes, and systemic lupus erythematosus: a time for new paradigms? *Arthritis Rheum* 2003;48(2):300–312.

362. Ruiz-Irastorza G, Khamashta MA, Castellino G, et al. Systemic lupus erythematosus. *Lancet* 2001;357(9261):1027–1032.

363. Matthay RA, Schwarz MI, Petty TL, et al. Pulmonary manifestations of systemic lupus erythematosus: review of twelve cases of acute lupus pneumonitis. *Medicine (Baltimore)* 1975;54(5):397–409.

364. Hunninghake GW, Fauci AS. Pulmonary involvement in the collagen vascular diseases. *Am Rev Respir Dis* 1979;119(3):471–503.

365. Martens J, Demedts M, Vanmeenen MT, et al. Respiratory muscle dysfunction in systemic lupus erythematosus. *Chest* 1983;84(2):170–175.

366. Wilcox PG, Stein HB, Clarke SD, et al. Phrenic nerve function in patients with diaphragmatic weakness and systemic lupus erythematosus. *Chest* 1988;93(2):352–358.

367. Winslow WA, Ploss LN, Loitman B. Pleuritis in systemic lupus erythematosus: its importance as an early manifestation in diagnosis. *Ann Intern Med* 1958;49(1):70–88.

368. Naylor B. Cytological aspects of pleural, peritoneal and pericardial fluids from patients with systemic lupus erythematosus. *Cytopathology* 1992;3(1):1–8.

369. Good JT Jr., King TE, Antony VB, et al. Lupus pleuritis. Clinical features and pleural fluid characteristics with special reference to pleural fluid antinuclear antibodies. *Chest* 1983;84(6):714–718.

370. Halla JT, Schrohenloher RE, Volanakis JE. Immune complexes and other laboratory features of pleural effusions: a comparison of rheumatoid arthritis, systemic lupus erythematosus, and other diseases. *Ann Intern Med* 1980;92(6):748–752.

371. Brasington RD, Furst DE. Pulmonary disease in systemic lupus erythematosus. *Clin Exp Rheumatol* 1985;3(3):269–276.

372. Onomura K, Nakata H, Tanaka Y, et al. Pulmonary hemorrhage in patients with systemic lupus erythematosus. *J Thorac Imaging* 1991;6(2):57–61.

373. Eisenberg H, Dubois EL, Sherwin RP, et al. Diffuse interstitial lung disease in systemic lupus erythematosus. *Ann Intern Med* 1973;79(1):37–45.

374. Huang CT, Hennigar GR, Lyons HA. Pulmonary dysfunction in systemic lupus erythematosus. *N Engl J Med* 1965;272:288–293.

375. Andonopoulos AP, Constantopoulos SH, Galanopoulou V, et al. Pulmonary function of nonsmoking patients with systemic lupus erythematosus. *Chest* 1988;94(2):312–315.

376. Alarcon-Segovia D, Deleze M, Oria CV, et al. Antiphospholipid antibodies and the antiphospholipid syndrome in systemic lupus erythematosus. A prospective analysis of 500 consecutive patients. *Medicine (Baltimore)* 1989;68(6):353–365.

377. Bankier A, Kiener H, Wiesmayr M, et al. Discrete lung involvement in systemic lupus erythematosus: CT assessment. *Radiology* 1995;196(3):835–840.

378. Fenlon HM, Doran M, Sant SM, et al. High-resolution chest CT in systemic lupus erythematosus. *Am J Roentgenol* 1996;166(2):301–307.

379. Ooi GC, Ngan H, Peh WC, et al. Systemic lupus erythematosus patients with respiratory symptoms: the value of HRCT. *Clin Radiol* 1997;52(10):775–781.

380. Haupt HM, Moore GW, Hutchins GM. The lung in systemic lupus erythematosus. Analysis of the pathologic changes in 120 patients. *Am J Med* 1981;71(5):791–798.

381. Carette S, Macher AM, Nussbaum A, et al. Severe, acute pulmonary disease in patients with systemic lupus erythematosus: ten years of experience at the National Institutes of Health. *Semin Arthritis Rheum* 1984;14(1):52–59.

382. Desnoyers MR, Bernstein S, Cooper AG, et al. Pulmonary hemorrhage in lupus erythematosus without evidence of an immunologic cause. *Arch Intern Med* 1984;144(7):1398–1400.

383. Abud-Mendoza C, Diaz-Jouanen E, Alarcon-Segovia D. Fatal pulmonary hemorrhage in systemic lupus erythematosus. Occurrence without hemoptysis. *J Rheumatol* 1985;12(3):558–561.

384. Myers JL, Katzenstein AA. Microangiitis in lupus-induced pulmonary hemorrhage. *Am J Clin Pathol* 1986;85(5):552–556.

385. Gross M, Esterly JR, Earle RH. Pulmonary alterations in systemic lupus erythematosus. *Am Rev Respir Dis* 1972;105(4):572–577.

386. Gammon RB, Bridges TA, al-Nezir H, et al. Bronchiolitis obliterans organizing pneumonia associated with systemic lupus erythematosus. *Chest* 1992;102(4):1171–1174.

387. Mana F, Mets T, Vincken W, et al. The association of bronchiolitis obliterans organizing pneumonia, systemic lupus erythematosus, and Hunner's cystitis. *Chest* 1993;104(2):642–644.

388. Isbister JP, Ralston M, Hayes JM, et al. Fulminant lupus pneumonitis with acute renal failure and RBC aplasia. Successful management with plasmapheresis and immunosuppression. *Arch Intern Med* 1981;141(8):1081–1083.

389. Eiser AR, Shanies HM. Treatment of lupus interstitial lung disease with intravenous cyclophosphamide. *Arthritis Rheum* 1994;37(3):428–431.

390. Fink SD, Kremer JM. Successful treatment of interstitial lung disease in systemic lupus erythematosus with methotrexate. *J Rheumatol* 1995;22(5):967–969.

391. Ellman P, Ball RE. Rheumatoid disease with joint and pulmonary manifestations. *Br Med J* 1948;2:816–820.

392. Caplan A. Certain unusual radiological appearances in the chest of coal-miners suffering from rheumatoid arthritis. *Thorax* 1953;8(1):29–37.

393. Lee FI, Brain AT. Chronic diffuse interstitial pulmonary fibrosis and rheumatoid arthritis. *Lancet* 1962;2:693–695.

394. Walker WC, Wright V. Pulmonary lesions and rheumatoid arthritis. *Medicine (Baltimore)* 1968;47(6):501–520.

395. Walker WC, Wright V. Diffuse interstitial pulmonary fibrosis and rheumatoid arthritis. *Ann Rheum Dis* 1969;28(3):252–259.

396. Frank ST, Weg JG, Harkleroad LE, et al. Pulmonary dysfunction in rheumatoid disease. *Chest* 1973;63(1):27–34.

397. Geddes DM, Corrin B, Brewerton DA, et al. Progressive airway obliteration in adults and its association with rheumatoid disease. *Q J Med* 1977;46(184):427–444.

398. Hunder GG, McDuffie FC, Hepper NG. Pleural fluid complement in systemic lupus erythematosus and rheumatoid arthritis. *Ann Intern Med* 1972;76(3):357–363.

399. DeHoratius RJ, Abruzzo JL, Williams RC Jr. Immunofluorescent and immunologic studies of rheumatoid lung. *Arch Intern Med* 1972;129(3):441–446.

400. Short CL. The antiquity of rheumatoid arthritis. *Arthritis Rheum* 1974;17(3):193–205.

401. Goronzy JJ, Weyand CM. Rheumatoid arthritis: epidemiology, pathology, and pathogenesis. In: Klippel JH, ed. *Primer on the rheumatic diseases*, 11th ed. Atlanta: Arthritis Foundation, 1997:155–161.

402. Choy EHS, Panayi GS. Cytokine pathways and joint inflammation in rheumatoid arthritis. *N Engl J Med* 2001;344(12):907–916.

403. Saravanan V, Kelly CA. Survival in fibrosing alveolitis associated with rheumatoid arthritis is better than cryptogenic fibrosing alveolitis. *Rheumatology* 2003;42(4):603–604.

404. Fuld JP, Johnson MK, Cotton MM, et al. A longitudinal study of lung function in nonsmoking patients with rheumatoid arthritis. *Chest* 2003;124(4):1224–1231.

405. Biederer J, Schnabel A, Muhle C, et al. Correlation between HRCT findings, pulmonary function tests and bronchoalveolar lavage cytology in interstitial lung disease associated with rheumatoid arthritis. *Eur Radiol* 2004;14(2):272–280.

406. Gabbay E, Tarala R, Will R, et al. Interstitial lung disease in recent onset rheumatoid arthritis. *Am J Respir Crit Care Med* 1997;156(2 Pt 1):528–535.

407. Jones FL, Blodgett RC Jr. Empyema and rheumatoid pleuropulmonary disease. *Ann Intern Med* 1978;89(1):139–140.

408. Dawson JK, Fewins HE, Desmond J, et al. Fibrosing alveolitis in patients with rheumatoid arthritis as assessed by high-resolution computed tomography, chest radiography, and pulmonary function tests. *Thorax* 2001;56(8):622–627.

409. Yarbrough JW, Sealy WC, Miller JA. Thoracic surgical problems associated with rheumatoid arthritis. *J Thorac Cardiovasc Surg* 1975;69(3):347–354.

410. Brunk JR, Drash EC, Swineford O Jr. Rheumatoid pleuritis successfully treated with decortication. Report of a case and review of the literature. *Am J Med Sci* 1966;251(5):545–551.

411. Lillington GA, Carr DT, Mayne JG. Rheumatoid pleurisy with effusion. *Arch Intern Med* 1971;128(5):764–768.

412. Cortet B, Perez T, Roux N, et al. Pulmonary function tests and high-resolution computed tomography of the lungs in patients with rheumatoid arthritis. *Ann Rheum Dis* 1997;56(10):596–600.

413. Hakala M. Poor prognosis in patients with rheumatoid arthritis hospitalized for interstitial lung fibrosis. *Chest* 1988;93(1):114–118.

414. Rajasekaran BA, Shovlin D, Lord P, et al. Interstitial lung disease in patients with rheumatoid arthritis: a comparison with cryptogenic fibrosing alveolitis. *Rheumatology* 2001;40(9):1022–1025.

415. Corrin B, Turner-Warwick M, Geddes DM, et al. Bronchiolitis obliterans. A new form of rheumatoid lung? *Chest* 1978;73(2):244.

416. Herzog CA, Miller RR, Hoidal JR. Bronchiolitis and rheumatoid arthritis. *Am Rev Respir Dis* 1981;124(5):636–639.

417. Howling SJ, Hansell DM, Wells AU, et al. Follicular bronchiolitis: thin-section CT and histologic findings. *Radiology* 1999;212(3):637–642.

418. Cortet B, Flipo RM, Remy-Jardin M, et al. Use of high-resolution computed tomography of the lungs in patients with rheumatoid arthritis. *Ann Rheum Dis* 1995;54(10):815–819.

419. White DA, Mark EJ. Case 10-2001- A 53-year-old woman with arthritis and pulmonary nodules. *N Engl J Med* 2001;344(13):997–1004.

420. Jolles H, Moseley PL, Peterson MW. Nodular pulmonary opacities in patients with rheumatoid arthritis. A diagnostic dilemma. *Chest* 1989;96(5):1022–1025.

421. Scadding JG. The lungs in rheumatoid arthritis. *Proc R Soc Med* 1969;62(3):227–238.

422. Cervantes-Perez P, Toro-Perez AH, Rodriguez-Jurado P. Pulmonary involvement in rheumatoid arthritis. *JAMA* 1980;243(17):1715–1719.

423. Kay JM, Banik S. Unexplained pulmonary hypertension with pulmonary arteritis in rheumatoid disease. *Br J Dis Chest* 1977;71(1):53–59.

424. Baydur A, Mongan ES, Slager UT. Acute respiratory failure and pulmonary arteritis without parenchymal involvement: demonstration in a patient with rheumatoid arthritis. *Chest* 1979;75(4):518–520.

425. Morikawa J, Kitamura K, Habuchi Y, et al. Pulmonary hypertension in a patient with rheumatoid arthritis. *Chest* 1988;93(4):876–878.

426. Young ID, Ford SE, Ford PM. The association of pulmonary hypertension with rheumatoid arthritis. *J Rheumatol* 1989;16(9):1266–1269.

427. Balagopal VP, da Costa P, Greenstone MA. Fatal pulmonary hypertension and rheumatoid vasculitis. *Eur Respir J* 1995;8(2):331–333.

428. Alarcon GS, Kremer JM, Macaluso M, et al. Risk factors for methotrexate-induced lung injury in patients with rheumatoid arthritis. A multicenter, case-control study. Methotrexate-Lung Study Group. *Ann Intern Med* 1997;127(5):356–364.

429. Kremer JM, Alarcon GS, Weinblatt ME, et al. Clinical, laboratory, radiographic, and histopathologic features of methotrexate-associated lung injury in patients with rheumatoid arthritis: a multicenter study with literature review. *Arthritis Rheum* 1997;40(10):1829–1837.

430. Dawson JK, Graham DR, Desmond J, et al. Investigation of the chronic pulmonary effects of low-dose oral methotrexate in patients with rheumatoid arthritis: a prospective study incorporating HRCT scanning and pulmonary function tests. *Rheumatology* 2002;41(3):262–267.

431. Gerhardt SG, McDyer JF, Girgis RE, et al. Maintenance azithromycin therapy for bronchiolitis obliterans syndrome: results of a pilot study. *Am J Respir Crit Care Med* 2003;168(1):121–125.

432. Hubbard R, Venn A. The impact of coexisting connective tissue disease on survival in patients with fibrosing alveolitis. *Rheumatology* 2002;41(6):676–679.

433. Subcommittee for scleroderma criteria of the American Rheumatism Association Diagnostic and Therapeutic Criteria Committee. Preliminary criteria for the classification of systemic sclerosis (scleroderma). *Arthritis Rheum* 1980;23(5):581–590.

434. Arroliga AC, Podell DN, Matthay RA. Pulmonary manifestations of scleroderma. *J Thorac Imaging* 1992;7(2):30–45.

435. Jimenez SA, Derk CT. Following the molecular pathways toward an understanding of the pathogenesis of systemic sclerosis. *Ann Intern Med* 2004;140(1):37–50.

436. Steen VD, Medsger TA Jr. Severe organ involvement in systemic sclerosis with diffuse scleroderma. *Arthritis Rheum* 2000;43(11):2437–2444.

437. King TE Jr. Nonspecific interstitial pneumonia and systemic sclerosis. *Am J Respir Crit Care Med* 2002;165(12):1578–1579.

438. King TE Jr. Nonspecific interstitial pneumonia and systemic sclerosis. *Am. J. Respir. Crit. Care Med* 2002;165(12):1578–1579.

439. Wigley FM. Systemic sclerosis and related syndromes: Clinical features. In: Klippel JH, ed. *Primer on the rheumatic diseases*, 11th ed. Atlanta: Arthritis Foundation, 1997:267–272.

440. Morelli S, Barbieri C, Sgreccia A, et al. Relationship between cutaneous and pulmonary involvement in systemic sclerosis. *J Rheumatol* 1997;24(1):81–85.

441. Tashkin DP, Clements PJ, Wright RS, et al. Interrelationships between pulmonary and extrapulmonary involvement in systemic sclerosis. A longitudinal analysis. *Chest* 1994;105(2):489–495.

442. Kurland LT, Hauser WA, Ferguson RH, et al. Epidemiologic features of diffuse connective tissue disorders in Rochester, Minn., 1951 through 1967, with special reference to systemic lupus erythematosus. *Mayo Clin Proc* 1969;44(9):649–663.

443. Arnett FC, Cho M, Chatterjee S, et al. Familial occurrence frequencies and relative risks for systemic sclerosis (scleroderma) in three United States cohorts. *Arthritis Rheum* 2001;44(6):1359–1362.

444. Norton WL, Nardo JM. Vascular disease in progressive systemic sclerosis (scleroderma). *Ann Intern Med* 1970;73(2):317–324.

445. Owens GR, Follansbee WP. Cardiopulmonary manifestations of systemic sclerosis. *Chest* 1987;91(1):118–127.

446. Weaver AL, Divertie MB, Titus JL. Pulmonary scleroderma. *Dis Chest* 1968;54(6):490–498.

447. Rosenthal AK, McLaughlin JK, Linet MS, et al. Scleroderma and malignancy: an epidemiological study. *Ann Rheum Dis* 1993;52(7):531–533.

448. Abu-Shakra M, Guillemin F, Lee P. Cancer in systemic sclerosis. *Arthritis Rheum* 1993;36(4):460–464.

449. Rosenthal AK, McLaughlin JK, Gridley G, et al. Incidence of cancer among patients with systemic sclerosis. *Cancer* 1995;76(5):910–914.

450. Sackner MA, Akgun N, Kimbel P, et al. The Pathophysiology of Scleroderma Involving the Heart and Respiratory System. *Ann Intern Med* 1964;60:611–630.

451. Ritchie B. Pulmonary function in scleroderma. *Thorax* 1964;19:28–36.

452. Silver RM, Metcalf JF, Stanley JH, et al. Interstitial lung disease in scleroderma. Analysis by bronchoalveolar lavage. *Arthritis Rheum* 1984;27(11):1254–1262.

453. Owens GR, Paradis IL, Gryzan S, et al. Role of inflammation in the lung disease of systemic sclerosis: comparison with idiopathic pulmonary fibrosis. *J Lab Clin Med* 1986;107(3):253–260.

454. White B. Systemic sclerosis and related syndromes: epidemiology, pathology and pathogensis. In: Klippel JH, ed. *Primer on rheumatic diseases*, 11th ed. Atlanta: Arthritis Foundation, 1997:263–266.

455. Jacobsen S, Halberg P, Ullman S, et al. Clinical features and serum antinuclear antibodies in 230 Danish patients with systemic sclerosis. *Br J Rheumatol* 1998;37(1):39–45.

456. Kuwana M, Kaburaki J, Mimori T, et al. Longitudinal analysis of autoantibody response to topoisomerase I in systemic sclerosis. *Arthritis Rheum* 2000;43(5):1074–1084.

457. Jacobsen S, Ullman S, Shen GQ, et al. Influence of clinical features, serum antinuclear antibodies, and lung function on survival of patients with systemic sclerosis. *J Rheumatol* 2001;28(11):2454–2459.

458. Catoggio LJ, Bernstein RM, Black CM, et al. Serological markers in progressive systemic sclerosis: clinical correlations. *Ann Rheum Dis* 1983;42(1):23–27.

459. Briggs DC, Vaughan RW, Welsh KI, et al. Immunogenetic prediction of pulmonary fibrosis in systemic sclerosis. *Lancet* 1991;338(8768):661–662.

460. Edelson JD, Hyland RH, Ramsden M, et al. Lung inflammation in scleroderma: clinical, radiographic, physiologic and cytopathological features. *J Rheumatol* 1985;12(5):957–963.

461. Pesci A, Bertorelli G, Manganelli P, et al. Bronchoalveolar lavage analysis of interstitial lung disease in CREST syndrome. *Clin Exp Rheumatol* 1986;4(2):121–124.

462. Wallaert B, Hatron PY, Grosbois JM, et al. Subclinical pulmonary involvement in collagen-vascular diseases assessed by bronchoalveolar lavage. Relationship between alveolitis and subsequent changes in lung function. *Am Rev Respir Dis* 1986;133(4):574–580.

463. Harrison NK, Glanville AR, Strickland B, et al. Pulmonary involvement in systemic sclerosis: the detection of early changes by thin-section CT scan, bronchoalveolar lavage and 99mTc-DTPA clearance. *Respir Med* 1989;83(5):403–414.

464. Wallaert B, Rossi GA, Sibille Y. Clinical guidelines and indications for bronchoalveolar lavage (BAL): collagen-vascular diseases. *Eur Respir J* 1990;3(8):942–3–961–9.

465. Wells AU, Hansell DM, Corrin B, et al. High-resolution computed tomography as a predictor of lung histology in systemic sclerosis. *Thorax* 1992;47(9):738–742.

466. Wells AU, Hansell DM, Rubens MB, et al. Fibrosing alveolitis in systemic sclerosis. Bronchoalveolar lavage findings in relation to computed tomographic appearance. *Am J Respir Crit Care Med* 1994;150(2):462–468.

467. Behr J, Vogelmeier C, Beinert T, et al. Bronchoalveolar lavage for evaluation and management of scleroderma disease of the lung. *Am J Respir Crit Care Med* 1996;154(2 Pt 1):400–406.

468. Witt C, Borges AC, John M, et al. Pulmonary involvement in diffuse cutaneous systemic sclerosis: broncheoalveolar fluid granulocytosis predicts progression of fibrosing alveolitis. *Ann Rheum Dis* 1999;58(10):635–640.

469. White B, Moore WC, Wigley FM, et al. Cyclophosphamide is associated with pulmonary function and survival benefit in patients with scleroderma and alveolitis. *Ann Intern Med* 2000;132(12):947–954.

470. Giacomelli R, Valentini G, Salsano F, et al. Cyclophosphamide pulse regimen in the treatment of alveolitis in systemic sclerosis. *J Rheumatol* 2002;29(4):731–736.

471. Ungerer RG, Tashkin DP, Furst D, et al. Prevalence and clinical correlates of pulmonary arterial hypertension in progressive systemic sclerosis. *Am J Med* 1983;75(1):65–74.

472. Shuck JW, Oetgen WJ, Tesar JT. Pulmonary vascular response during Raynaud's phenomenon in progressive systemic sclerosis. *Am J Med* 1985;78(2):221–227.

473. Alpert MA, Pressly TA, Mukerji V, et al. Acute and long-term effects of nifedipine on pulmonary and systemic hemodynamics in patients with pulmonary hypertension associated with diffuse systemic sclerosis, the CREST syndrome and mixed connective tissue disease. *Am J Cardiol* 1991;68(17):1687–1691.

474. Bartosik I, Eskilsson J, Scheja A, et al. Intermittent iloprost infusion therapy of pulmonary hypertension in scleroderma—a pilot study. *Br J Rheumatol* 1996;35(11):1187–1188.

475. Hesselstrand R, Scheja A, Akesson A. Mortality and causes of death in a Swedish series of systemic sclerosis patients. *Ann Rheum Dis* 1998;57(11):682–686.

476. Channick RN, Simonneau G, Sitbon O, et al. Effects of the dual endothelin-receptor antagonist bosentan in patients with pulmonary hypertension: a randomised placebo-controlled study. *Lancet* 2001;358(9288):1119–1123.

477. Rubin LJ, Badesch DB, Barst RJ, et al. Bosentan therapy for pulmonary arterial hypertension. *N Engl J Med* 2002;346(12):896–903.

478. Mukerjee D, St George D, Coleiro B, et al. Prevalence and outcome in systemic sclerosis associated pulmonary arterial hypertension: application of a registry approach. *Ann Rheum Dis* 2003;62(11):1088–1093.

479. Paramothayan NS, Lasserson TJ, Wells AU, et al., Prostacyclin for pulmonary hypertension. *Cochrane Database Syst Rev* 2003(2):CD002994.

480. Rosenkranz S, Diet F, Karasch T, et al. Sildenafil improved pulmonary hypertension and peripheral blood flow in a patient with scleroderma-associated lung fibrosis and the raynaud phenomenon. *Ann Intern Med* 2003;139(10):871–873.

481. Sitbon O, Badesch DB, Channick RN, et al. Effects of the dual endothelin receptor antagonist bosentan in patients with pulmonary arterial hypertension: A 1-year follow-up study. *Chest* 2003;124(1):247–254.

482. Liefeldt L, van Giersbergen PL, Dingemanse J, et al. Treatment of secondary pulmonary hypertension with bosentan and its pharmacokinetic monitoring in ESRD. *Am J Kidney Dis* 2004;43(5):923–926.

483. Pignone A, Matucci-Cerinic M, Lombardi A, et al. High-resolution computed tomography in systemic sclerosis. Real diagnostic utilities in the assessment of pulmonary involvement and comparison with other modalities of lung investigation. *Clin Rheumatol* 1992;11(4):465–472.

484. Bhalla M, Silver RM, Shepard JA, et al. Chest CT in patients with scleroderma: prevalence of asymptomatic esophageal dilatation and mediastinal lymphadenopathy. *Am J Roentgenol* 1993;161(2):269–272.

485. Garber SJ, Wells AU, duBois RM, et al. Enlarged mediastinal lymph nodes in the fibrosing alveolitis of systemic sclerosis. *Br J Radiol* 1992;65(779):983–986.

486. Harrison NK, Myers AR, Corrin B, et al. Structural features of interstitial lung disease in systemic sclerosis. *Am Rev Respir Dis* 1991;144(3 Pt 1):706–713.

487. Naeye RL. Pulmonary vascular lesions in systemic scleroderma. *Dis Chest* 1963;44:374–379.

488. Bouros D, Wells AU, Nicholson AG, et al. Histopathologic subsets of fibrosing alveolitis in patients with systemic sclerosis and their relationship to outcome. *Am J Respir Crit Care Med* 2002;165(12):1581–1586.

489. Wells AU, Cullinan P, Hansell DM, et al. Fibrosing alveolitis associated with systemic sclerosis has a better prognosis than lone cryptogenic fibrosing alveolitis. *Am J Respir Crit Care Med* 1994;149(6):1583–1590.

490. Steen VD, Owens GR, Redmond C, et al. The effect of D-penicillamine on pulmonary findings in systemic sclerosis. *Arthritis Rheum* 1985;28(8):882–888.

491. Akesson A, Blom-Bulow B, Scheja A, et al. Long-term evaluation of penicillamine or cyclofenil in systemic sclerosis. Results from a two-year randomized study. *Scand J Rheumatol* 1992;21(5):238–244.

492. Hein R, Behr J, Hundgen M, et al. Treatment of systemic sclerosis with gamma-interferon. *Br J Dermatol* 1992;126(5):496–501.

493. Silver RM, Warrick JH, Kinsella MB, et al. Cyclophosphamide and low-dose prednisone therapy in patients with systemic sclerosis (scleroderma) with interstitial lung disease. *J Rheumatol* 1993;20(5):838–844.

494. Akesson A, Scheja A, Lundin A, et al. Improved pulmonary function in systemic sclerosis after treatment with cyclophosphamide. *Arthritis Rheum* 1994;37(5):729–735.

495. Pakas I, Ioannidis JP, Malagari K, et al. Cyclophosphamide with low- or high-dose prednisolone for systemic sclerosis lung disease. *J Rheumatol* 2002;29(2):298–304.

496. Dickey BF, Myers AR. Pulmonary disease in polymyositis/dermatomyositis. *Semin Arthritis Rheum* 1984;14(1):60–76.

497. Hochberg MC, Feldman D, Stevens MB, et al. Antibody to Jo-1 in polymyositis/dermatomyositis: association with interstitial pulmonary disease. *J Rheumatol* 1984;11(5):663–665.

498. Hochberg MC, Feldman D, Stevens MB. Adult onset polymyositis/dermatomyositis: an analysis of clinical and laboratory features and survival in 76 patients with a review of the literature. *Semin Arthritis Rheum* 1986;15(3):168–178.

499. Tuffanelli DL, Lavoie PE. Prognosis and therapy of polymyositis/dermatomyositis. *Clin Dermatol* 1988;6(2):93–104.

500. Kasper CS, White CL 3rd, Freeman RG. Pathology and immunopathology of polymyositis/dermatomyositis. *Clin Dermatol* 1988;6(2):64–75.

501. Sontheimer RD, Ziff M. Questions pertaining to the etiology and pathophysiology of polymyositis/dermatomyositis. *Clin Dermatol* 1988;6(2):105–119.

502. Olsen NJ, Wortmann RL. Chapter 21: Inflammatory and metabolic diseases of muscle. In: Kippel JH, ed. *Primer on the rheumatic diseases*, 11th ed. Atlanta: Arthritis Foundation, 1997:276–288.

503. Lakhanpal S, Lie JT, Conn DL, et al. Pulmonary disease in polymyositis/dermatomyositis: a clinicopathological analysis of 65 autopsy cases. *Ann Rheum Dis* 1987;46(1):23–29.

504. Takizawa H, Shiga J, Moroi Y, et al. Interstitial lung disease in dermatomyositis: clinicopathological study. *J Rheumatol* 1987;14(1):102–107.

505. Hirakata M, Nagai S. Interstitial lung disease in polymyositis and dermatomyositis. *Curr Opin Rheumatol* 2000;12(6):501–508.

506. Lee CS, Chen TL, Tzen CY, et al. Idiopathic inflammatory myopathy with diffuse alveolar damage. *Clin Rheumatol* 2002;21(5):391–396.

507. Marie I, Hachulla E, Cherin P, et al. Interstitial lung disease in polymyositis and dermatomyositis. *Arthritis Rheum* 2002;47(6):614–622.

508. Schnabel A, Reuter M, Biederer J, et al. Interstitial lung disease in polymyositis and dermatomyositis: clinical course and response to treatment. *Semin Arthritis Rheum* 2003;32(5):273–284.

509. Fathi M, Dastmalchi M, Rasmussen E, et al. Interstitial lung disease, a common manifestation of newly diagnosed polymyositis and dermatomyositis. *Ann Rheum Dis* 2004;63(3):297–301.

510. Marie I, Hachulla E, Hatron PY, et al. Polymyositis and dermatomyositis: short-term and long-term outcome, and predictive factors of prognosis. *J Rheumatol* 2001;28(10):2230–2237.

511. Schwarz MI, Matthay RA, Sahn SA, et al. Interstitial lung disease in polymyositis and dermatomyositis: analysis of six cases and review of the literature. *Medicine (Baltimore)* 1976;55(1):89–104.

512. Kiely JL, Donohoe P, Bresnihan B, et al. Pulmonary fibrosis in polymyositis with the Jo-1 syndrome: an unusual mode of presentation. *Respir Med* 1998;92(9):1167–1169.

513. Tanaka F, Origuchi T, Migita K, et al. Successful combined therapy of cyclophosphamide and cyclosporine for acute exacerbated interstitial pneumonia associated with dermatomyositis. *Intern Med* 2000;39(5):428–430.

514. Ito M, Kaise S, Suzuki S, et al. Clinico-laboratory characteristics of patients with dermatomyositis accompanied by rapidly progressive interstitial lung disease. *Clin Rheumatol* 1999;18(6):462–467.

515. Yoshida T, Koga H, Saitoh F, et al. Pulse intravenous cyclophosphamide treatment for steroid-resistant interstitial pneumonitis associated with polymyositis. *Intern Med* 1999;38(9):733–738.

516. Nawata Y, Kurasawa K, Takabayashi K, et al. Corticosteroid resistant interstitial pneumonitis in dermatomyositis/polymyositis: prediction and treatment with cyclosporine. *J Rheumatol* 1999;26(7):1527–1533.

517. Yamanishi Y, Maeda H, Konishi F, et al. Dermatomyositis associated with rapidly progressive fatal interstitial pneumonitis and pneumomediastinum. *Scand J Rheumatol* 1999;28(1):58–61.

518. Maeda K, Kimura R, Komuta K, et al. Cyclosporine treatment for polymyositis/dermatomyositis: is it possible to rescue the deteriorating cases with interstitial pneumonitis? *Scand J Rheumatol* 1997;26(1):24–29.

519. Barvaux VA, Van Mullem X, Pieters TH. et al. Persistent pneumomediastinum and dermatomyositis: a case report and review of the literature. *Clin Rheumatol* 2001;20(5):359–361.

520. Sauty A, Rochat T, Schoch OD, et al. Pulmonary fibrosis with predominant CD8 lymphocytic alveolitis and anti-Jo-1 antibodies. *Eur Respir J* 1997;10(12):2907–2912.

521. Schnabel A, Reuter M, Gross WL. Intravenous pulse cyclophosphamide in the treatment of interstitial lung disease due to collagen vascular diseases. *Arthritis Rheum* 1998;41(7):1215–1220.

522. Kurasawa K, Nawata Y, Takabayashi K, et al. Activation of pulmonary T cells in corticosteroid-resistant and -sensitive interstitial pneumonitis in dermatomyositis/polymyositis. *Clin Exp Immunol* 2002;129(3):541–548.

523. Savage CO, Harper L, Adu D. Primary systemic vasculitis. *Lancet* 1997;349(9051):553–558.

524. Carrington CB, Liebow A. Limited forms of angiitis and granulomatosis of Wegener's type. *Am J Med* 1966;41(4):497–527.

525. Jennette JC, Ewert BH, Falk RJ. Do antineutrophil cytoplasmic autoantibodies cause Wegener's granulomatosis and other forms of necrotizing vasculitis? *Rheum Dis Clin North Am* 1993;19(1):1–14.

526. Heeringa P, Tervaert JWC. Pathophysiology of ANCA-associated vasculitides: Are ANCA really pathogenic? *Kidney Int* 2004;65(5):1564–1567.

527. Fauci AS, Haynes BF, Katz P, et al. Wegener's granulomatosis: prospective clinical and therapeutic experience with 85 patients for 21 years. *Ann Intern Med* 1983;98(1):76–85.

528. Hoffman GS, Kerr GS, Leavitt RY, et al. Wegener's granulomatosis: an analysis of 158 patients. *Ann Intern Med* 1992;116(6):488–498.

529. Cordier JF, Valeyre D, Guillevin L, et al. Pulmonary Wegener's granulomatosis. A clinical and imaging study of 77 cases. *Chest* 1990;97(4):906–912.

530. Rosenberg DM, Weinberger SE, Fulmer JD, et al. Functional correlates of lung involvement in Wegener's granulomatosis. Use of pulmonary function tests in staging and follow-up. *Am J Med* 1980;69(3):387–394.

531. Salant DJ. Immunopathogenesis of crescentic glomerulonephritis and lung purpura. *Kidney Int* 1987;32(3):408–425.

532. Davies DJ, Moran JE, Niall JF, et al. Segmental necrotising glomerulonephritis with antineutrophil antibody: possible arbovirus aetiology? *Br Med J (Clin Res Ed)* 1982;285(6342):606.

533. van der Woude FJ, Rasmussen N, Lobatto S, et al. Autoantibodies against neutrophils and monocytes: tool for diagnosis and marker of disease activity in Wegener's granulomatosis. *Lancet* 1985;1(8426):425–429.

534. Nolle B, Specks U, Ludemann J, et al. Anticytoplasmic autoantibodies: their immunodiagnostic value in Wegener's granulomatosis. *Ann Intern Med* 1989;111(1):28–40.

535. Kallenberg CG, Mulder AH, Tervaert JW. Antineutrophil cytoplasmic antibodies: a still-growing class of autoantibodies in inflammatory disorders. *Am J Med* 1992;93(6):675–682.

536. Goldschmeding R, van der Schoot CE, ten Bokkel Huinink D, et al. Wegener's granulomatosis autoantibodies identify a novel diisopropylfluorophosphate-binding protein in the lysosomes of normal human neutrophils. *J Clin Invest* 1989;84(5):1577–1587.

537. Savige J, Dimech W, Fritzler M, et al. Addendum to the International Consensus Statement on testing and reporting of antineutrophil cytoplasmic antibodies. Quality control guidelines, comments, and recommendations for testing in other autoimmune diseases. *Am J Clin Pathol* 2003;120(3):312–318.

538. Savige J, Davies D, Falk RJ, et al. Antineutrophil cytoplasmic antibodies and associated diseases: a review of the clinical and laboratory features. *Kidney Int* 2000;57(3):846–862.

539. Savige J, Gillis D, Benson E, et al. International consensus statement on testing and reporting of antineutrophil cytoplasmic antibodies (ANCA). *Am J Clin Pathol* 1999;111(4):507–513.

540. Leavitt RY, Fauci AS, Bloch DA, et al. The American College of Rheumatology 1990 criteria for the classification of Wegener's granulomatosis. *Arthritis Rheum* 1990;33(8):1101–1107.

541. Kornblum D, Fienberg R. Roentgen manifestations of necrotizing granulomatosis and angiitis of the lungs. *Am J Roentgenol Radium Ther Nucl Med* 1955;74(4):587–592.

542. McGregor MB, Sandler G. Wegener's Granulomatosis. A Clinical and Radiological Survey. *Br J Radiol* 1964;37:430–439.

543. Travis WD, Colby TV, Koss MN. Chapter 4: Pulmonary vasculitis. In: King DW, ed. *Atlas of nontumor pathology*, 1st ed. Washington, DC: Armed Forces Institute of Pathology and the American Registry of Pathology, 2002:233–264.

544. Langford CA, Talar-Williams C, Barron KS, et al. A staged approach to the treatment of Wegener's granulomatosis: induction of remission with glucocorticoids and daily cyclophosphamide switching to methotrexate for remission maintenance. *Arthritis Rheum* 1999;42(12):2666–2673.

545. Langford CA, Talar-Williams C, Sneller MC. Use of methotrexate and glucocorticoids in the treatment of Wegener's granulomatosis. Long-term renal outcome in patients with glomerulonephritis. *Arthritis Rheum* 2000;43(8):1836–1840.

546. Langford CA, Talar-Williams C, Barron KS, et al. Use of a cyclophosphamide-induction methotrexate-maintenance regimen for the treatment of Wegener's granulomatosis: extended follow-up and rate of relapse. *Am J Med* 2003;114(6):463–469.

547. Langford CA, Talar-Williams C, Sneller MC. Mycophenolate mofetil for remission maintenance in the treatment of Wegener's granulomatosis. *Arthritis Rheum* 2004;51(2):278–283.

548. Fauci AS, Wolff SM, Johnson JS. Effect of cyclophosphamide upon the immune response in Wegener's granulomatosis. *N Engl J Med* 1971;285(27):1493–1496.

549. Fauci AS, Katz P, Haynes BF, et al. Cyclophosphamide therapy of severe systemic necrotizing vasculitis. *N Engl J Med* 1979; 301(5):235–238.

550. Hoffman GS, Leavitt RY, Kerr GS, et al. The treatment of Wegener's granulomatosis with glucocorticoids and methotrexate. *Arthritis Rheum* 1992;35(11):1322–1329.

551. Sneller MC, Hoffman GS, Talar-Williams C, et al. An analysis of forty-two Wegener's granulomatosis patients treated with methotrexate and prednisone. *Arthritis Rheum* 1995;38(5):608–613.

552. Jayne D, Rasmussen N, Andrassy K, et al. A randomized trial of maintenance therapy for vasculitis associated with antineutrophil cytoplasmic autoantibodies. *N Engl J Med* 2003;349(1):36–44.

553. DeRemee RA, McDonald TJ, Weiland LH. Wegener's granulomatosis: observations on treatment with antimicrobial agents. *Mayo Clin Proc* 1985;60(1):27–32.

554. de Groot K, Reinhold-Keller E, Tatsis E, et al. Therapy for the maintenance of remission in sixty-five patients with generalized Wegener's granulomatosis. Methotrexate versus trimethoprim/sulfamethoxazole. *Arthritis Rheum* 1996;39(12):2052–2061.

555. Stegeman CA, Tervaert JW, de Jong PE, et al., Dutch Co-Trimoxazole Wegener Study Group. Trimethoprim-sulfamethoxazole (co-trimoxazole) for the prevention of relapses of Wegener's granulomatosis. *N Engl J Med* 1996;335(1):16–20.

556. Churg J, Strauss L. Allergic granulomatosis, allergic angiitis and periarteritis nodosa. *Am J Pathol* 1951;27:277–301.

557. Rose GA, Spencer H. Polyarteritis nodosa. *Q J Med* 1957;26(101): 43–81.

558. Noth I, Strek ME, Leff AR. Churg-Strauss syndrome. *Lancet* 2003;361(9357):587–594.

559. Chumbley LC, Harrison EG Jr., DeRemee RA. Allergic granulomatosis and angiitis (Churg-Strauss syndrome). Report and analysis of 30 cases. *Mayo Clin Proc* 1977;52(8):477–484.

560. Guillevin L, Lhote F, Jarrousse B, et al. Treatment of polyarteritis nodosa and Churg-Strauss syndrome. A meta-analysis of 3 prospective controlled trials including 182 patients over 12 years. *Ann Med Interne (Paris)* 1992;143(6):405–416.

561. Guillevin L, Lhote F, Gayraud M, et al. Prognostic factors in polyarteritis nodosa and Churg-Strauss syndrome. A prospective study in 342 patients. *Medicine (Baltimore)* 1996;75(1):17–28.

562. Guillevin L, Cohen P, Gayraud M, et al. Churg-Strauss syndrome. Clinical study and long-term follow-up of 96 patients. *Medicine (Baltimore)* 1999;78(1):26–37.

563. Churg J. Allergic granulomatosis and granulomatous-vascular syndromes. *Ann Allergy* 1963;21:619–628.

564. Wechsler ME, Garpestad E, Flier SR, et al. Pulmonary infiltrates, eosinophilia, and cardiomyopathy following corticosteroid withdrawal in patients with asthma receiving zafirlukast. *JAMA* 1998;279(6):455–457.

565. Worthy SA, Muller NL, Hansell DM, et al. Churg-Strauss syndrome: the spectrum of pulmonary CT findings in 17 patients. *Am J Roentgenol* 1998;170(2):297–300.

566. Guillevin L, Fain O, Lhote F, et al. Lack of superiority of steroids plus plasma exchange to steroids alone in the treatment of polyarteritis nodosa and Churg-Strauss syndrome. A prospective, randomized trial in 78 patients. *Arthritis Rheum* 1992;35(2):208–215.

567. Fontenot AP, Schwarz MI. Chapter 23: Diffuse alveolar hemorrhage. In: Schwarz MI, King TE Jr., eds. *Interstitial lung disease*, 4th ed. Hamilton, Canada: B. C. Dekker; 2003.

568. Jennings CA, King TE Jr., Tuder R, et al. Diffuse alveolar hemorrhage with underlying isolated, pauciimmune pulmonary capillaritis. *Am J Respir Crit Care Med* 1997;155(3):1101–1109.

569. Salama AD, Levy JB, Lightstone L, et al. Goodpasture's disease. *Lancet* 2001;358(9285):917–920.

570. Goodpasture EW. The significance of certain pulmonary lesions in relation to the etiology of influenza. *Am J Med Sci* 1919; 158:863–870.

571. Fisher M, Pusey CD, Vaughan RW, et al. Susceptibility to anti-glomerular basement membrane disease is strongly associated with HLA-DRB1 genes. *Kidney Int* 1997;51(1):222–229.

572. Turner N, Mason PJ, Brown R, et al. Molecular cloning of the human Goodpasture antigen demonstrates it to be the alpha 3 chain of type IV collagen. *J Clin Invest* 1992;89(2):592–601.

573. Schwartz EE, Teplick JG, Onesti G, et al. Pulmonary hemorrhage in renal disease: Goodpasture's syndrome and other causes. *Radiology* 1977;122(1):39–46.

574. Teague CA, Doak PB, Simpson IJ, et al. Goodpasture syndrome: an analysis of 29 cases. *Kidney Int* 1978;13(6):492–504.

575. Leatherman JW, Davies SF, Hoidal JR. Alveolar hemorrhage syndromes: diffuse microvascular lung hemorrhage in immune and idiopathic disorders. *Medicine (Baltimore)* 1984;63(6):343–361.

576. Wilson CB, Dixon FJ. Anti-glomerular basement membrane antibody-induced glomerulonephritis. *Kidney Int* 1973;3(2):74–89.

577. Ewan PW, Jones HA, Rhodes CG, et al. Detection of intrapulmonary hemorrhage with carbon monoxide uptake. Application in goodpasture's syndrome. *N Engl J Med* 1976;295(25):1391–1396.

578. Hudson BG, Kalluri R, Gunwar S, et al. Molecular characteristics of the Goodpasture autoantigen. *Kidney Int* 1993;43(1):135–139.

579. Levy JB, Turner AN, Rees AJ, et al. Long-term outcome of anti-glomerular basement membrane antibody disease treated with plasma exchange and immunosuppression. *Ann Intern Med* 2001;134(11):1033–1042.

580. Lockwood CM, Boulton-Jones JM, Lowenthal RM, et al. Recovery from Goodpasture's syndrome after immunosuppressive treatment and plasmapheresis. *Br Med J* 1975;2(5965):252–254.

581. Guillevin L, Durand-Gasselin B, Cevallos R, et al. Microscopic polyangiitis: clinical and laboratory findings in eighty-five patients. *Arthritis Rheum* 1999;42(3):421–430.

582. Guillevin L, Lhote F, Cohen P, et al. Polyarteritis nodosa related to hepatitis B virus. A prospective study with long-term observation of 41 patients. *Medicine (Baltimore)* 1995;74(5):238–253.

583. Gonzalez-Gay MA, Garcia-Porrua C, Guerrero J, et al. The epidemiology of the primary systemic vasculitides in northwest Spain: implications of the Chapel Hill Consensus Conference definitions. *Arthritis Rheum* 2003;49(3):388–393.

584. Mahr A, Guillevin L, Poissonnet M, et al. Prevalences of polyarteritis nodosa, microscopic polyangiitis, Wegener's granulomatosis, and Churg-Strauss syndrome in a French urban multiethnic population in 2000: a capture-recapture estimate. *Arthritis Rheum* 2004;51(1):92–99.

585. Jennette JC, Falk RJ. Small-vessel vasculitis. *N Engl J Med* 1997; 337(21):1512–1523.

586. Rothenberg ME. Eosinophilia. *N Engl J Med* 1998;338(22): 1592–1600.

587. Allen JN, Davis WB. Eosinophilic lung diseases. *Am J Respir Crit Care Med* 1994;150(5 Pt 1):1423–1438.

588. Pope-Harman AL, Davis WB, Allen ED, et al. Acute eosinophilic pneumonia. A summary of 15 cases and review of the literature. *Medicine (Baltimore)* 1996;75(6):334–342.

589. Badesch DB, King TE Jr., Schwarz MI. Acute eosinophilic pneumonia: a hypersensitivity phenomenon? *Am Rev Respir Dis* 1989;139(1):249–252.

590. Travis WD, Colby TV, Koss MN, et al. Chapter 12: Lung infections. *Non-neoplastic disorders of the lower respiratory tract*, 1st ed. Washington, DC: American Registry of Pathology and the Armed Forces Institute of Pathology, 2002:691–692.

591. Pinkston P, Vijayan VK, Nutman TB, et al. Acute tropical pulmonary eosinophilia. Characterization of the lower respiratory

tract inflammation and its response to therapy. *J Clin Invest* 1987;80(1):216–225.

592. Carrington CB, Addington WW, Goff AM, et al. Chronic eosinophilic pneumonia. *N Engl J Med* 1969;280(15):787–798.

593. Jederlinic PJ, Sicilian L, Gaensler EA. Chronic eosinophilic pneumonia. A report of 19 cases and a review of the literature. *Medicine (Baltimore)* 1988;67(3):154–162.

594. Naughton M, Fahy J, FitzGerald MX. Chronic eosinophilic pneumonia. A long-term follow-up of 12 patients. *Chest* 1993; 103(1):162–165.

595. Soubani AO, Chandrasekar PH. The clinical spectrum of pulmonary aspergillosis. *Chest* 2002;121(6):1988–1999.

596. Rosen SH, Castleman B, Liebow AA. Pulmonary alveolar proteinosis. *N Engl J Med* 1958;258(23):1123–1142.

597. Trapnell BC, Whitsett JA, Nakata K. Pulmonary alveolar proteinosis. *N Engl J Med* 2003;349(26):2527–2539.

598. Vourlekis JS, Greene KE. Chapter 30: Pulmonary alveolar proteinosis. In: Schwarz MI, King TE Jr., eds. *Interstitial lung diseases*, 4th ed. Hamilton, Ontario: B. C. Dekker, 2003:865–876.

599. Du Bois RM, McAllister WA, Branthwaite MA. Alveolar proteinosis: diagnosis and treatment over a 10-year period. *Thorax* 1983;38(5):360–363.

600. Goldstein LS, Kavuru MS, Curtis-McCarthy P, et al. Pulmonary alveolar proteinosis: clinical features and outcomes. *Chest* 1998;114(5):1357–1362.

601. Martin RJ, Rogers RM, Myers NM. Pulmonary alveolar proteinosis: shunt fraction and lactic acid dehydrogenase concentration as aids to diagnosis. *Am Rev Respir Dis* 1978;117(6):1059–1062.

602. Hoffman RM, Rogers RM. Serum and lavage lactate dehydrogenase isoenzymes in pulmonary alveolar proteinosis. *Am Rev Respir Dis* 1991;143(1):42–46.

603. Costello JF, Moriarty DC, Branthwaite MA, et al. Diagnosis and management of alveolar proteinosis: the role of electron microscopy. *Thorax* 1975;30(2):121–132.

604. Webb WR, Muller N, Naidich DP. Chapter 6: Parenchymal opacification. *High-resolution CT of the chest*, 2nd ed. New York: Lippincott–Raven Publishers, 1996:202–206.

605. Hoffman RM, Dauber JH, Rogers RM. Improvement in alveolar macrophage migration after therapeutic whole lung lavage in pulmonary alveolar proteinosis. *Am Rev Respir Dis* 1989;139(4): 1030–1032.

606. Wilson DO, Rogers RM. Prolonged spontaneous remission in a patient with untreated pulmonary alveolar proteinosis. *Am J Med* 1987;82(5):1014–1016.

607. Kavuru MS, Sullivan EJ, Piccin R, et al. Exogenous granulocyte-macrophage colony-stimulating factor administration for pulmonary alveolar proteinosis. *Am J Respir Crit Care Med* 2000; 161(4):1143–1148.

608. Seymour JF, Presneill JJ, Schoch OD, et al. Therapeutic efficacy of granulocyte-macrophage colony-stimulating factor in patients with idiopathic acquired alveolar proteinosis. *Am J Respir Crit Care Med* 2001;163(2):524–531.

609. Taylor JR, Ryu J, Colby TV, et al. Lymphangioleiomyomatosis. Clinical course in 32 patients. *N Engl J Med* 1990;323(18):1254–1260.

610. Sullivan EJ. Lymphangioleiomyomatosis: a review. *Chest* 1998; 114(6):1689–1703.

611. Kristof AS, Moss J. Chapter 29: Lymphangioleiomyomatosis. In: Schwarz MI, King TE Jr., eds. *Interstitial lung disease*, 4th ed. Hamilton, Ontario: B. C. Decker, 2003:851–876.

612. Sullivan EJ, Beck GJ, Peavy HH, et al. Lymphangioleiomyomatosis Registry. *Chest* 1999;115(1):301.

613. Marcy TW, Reynolds HY. Pulmonary histiocytosis X. *Lung* 1985;163(3):129–150.

614. King TE Jr., Schwarz MI, Dreisin RE, et al. Circulating immune complexes in pulmonary eosinophilic granuloma. *Ann Intern Med* 1979;91(3):397–399.

615. Lacronique J, Roth C, Battesti JP, et al. Chest radiological features of pulmonary histiocytosis X: a report based on 50 adult cases. *Thorax* 1982;37(2):104–109.

616. Webb WR, Muller N, Naidich DP. Chapter 7: Diseases characterized primarily by decreased lung opacity, including cystic abnormalities, emphysema and bronchiectasis. *High-resolution CT of the chest*, 2nd ed. New York: Lippincott–Raven Publishers, 1996:227–269.

617. Chollet S, Dournovo P, Richard MS, et al. Reactivity of histiocytosis X cells with monoclonal anti-T6 antibody. *N Engl J Med* 1982;307(11):685.

618. Casolaro MA, Bernaudin JF, Saltini C, et al. Accumulation of Langerhans' cells on the epithelial surface of the lower respiratory tract in normal subjects in association with cigarette smoking. *Am Rev Respir Dis* 1988;137(2):406–411.

619. Tazi A, Bonay M, Grandsaigne M, et al. Surface phenotype of Langerhans' cells and lymphocytes in granulomatous lesions from patients with pulmonary histiocytosis X. *Am Rev Respir Dis* 1993;147(6 Pt 1):1531–1536.

620. Crausman RS, Jennings CA, Tuder RM, et al. Pulmonary histiocytosis X: pulmonary function and exercise pathophysiology. *Am J Respir Crit Care Med* 1996;153(1):426–435.

621. Fartoukh M, Humbert M, Capron F, et al. Severe pulmonary hypertension in histiocytosis X. *Am J Respir Crit Care Med* 2000;161(1): 216–223.

622. Gabbay E, Dark JH, Ashcroft T, et al. Recurrence of Langerhans' cell granulomatosis following lung transplantation. *Thorax* 1998; 53(4):326–327.

623. Habib SB, Congleton J, Carr D, et al. Recurrence of recipient Langerhans' cell histiocytosis following bilateral lung transplantation. *Thorax* 1998;53(4):323–325.

624. Etienne B, Bertocchi M, Gamondes J-P, et al. Relapsing pulmonary Langerhans' cell histiocytosis after lung transplantation. *Am J Respir Crit Care Med* 1998;157(1):288–291.

625. Lock BJ, Eggert M, Cooper JAD Jr. Infiltrative lung disease due to noncytotoxic agents. *Clin Chest Med* 2004;25(1):47–52.

626. Limper AH. Chemotherapy-induced lung disease. *Clin Chest Med* 2004;25(1):53–64.

627. Camus P, Martin WJ II, Rosenow EC III. Amiodarone pulmonary toxicity. *Clin Chest Med* 2004;25(1):65–75.

628. Allen JN. Drug-induced eosinophilic lung disease. *Clin Chest Med* 2004;25(1):77–88.

629. Epler GR. Drug-induced bronchiolitis obliterans organizing pneumonia. *Clin Chest Med* 2004;25(1):89–94.

630. Lee-Chiong T Jr., Matthay RA. Drug-induced pulmonary edema and acute respiratory distress syndrome. *Clin Chest Med* 2004; 25(1):95–104.

631. Kopko PM, Popovsky MA. Pulmonary injury from transfusion-related acute lung injury. *Clin Chest Med* 2004;25(1):105–111.

632. Babu KS, Marshall BG. Drug-induced airway diseases. *Clin Chest Med* 2004;25(1):113–122.

633. Higenbottam T, Laude L, Emery C, et al. Pulmonary hypertension as a result of drug therapy. *Clin Chest Med* 2004;25(1):123–131.

634. Schwarz MI, Fontenot AP. Drug-induced diffuse alveolar hemorrhage syndromes and vasculitis. *Clin Chest Med* 2004;25(1):133–140.

635. Huggins JT, Sahn SA. Drug-induced pleural disease. *Clin Chest Med* 2004;25(1):141–153.

636. White DA. Drug-induced pulmonary infection. *Clin Chest Med* 2004;25(1):179–187.

637. Wolff AJ, O'Donnell AE. Pulmonary effects of illicit drug use. *Clin Chest Med* 2004;25(1):203–216.

638. Goldiner PL, Carlon GC, Cvitkovic E, et al. Factors influencing postoperative morbidity and mortality in patients treated with bleomycin. *Br Med J* 1978;1(6128):1664–1667.

639. Holoye PY, Luna MA, MacKay B, et al. Bleomycin hypersensitivity pneumonitis. *Ann Intern Med* 1978;88(1):47–49.

640. Kuhlman JE. The role of chest computed tomography in the diagnosis of drug-related reactions. *J Thorac Imaging* 1991;6(1):52–61.

641. Wieder JA, Soloway MS. Interstitial pneumonitis associated with neoadjuvant leuprolide and nilutamide for prostate cancer. *J Urol* 1998;159(6):2099.

642. Cush JJ, Goldings EA. Drug-induced lupus: clinical spectrum and pathogenesis. *Am J Med Sci* 1985;290(1):36–45.

CHAPTER 13

Occupational and Environmental Lung Disease

Carrie A. Redlich

John R. Balmes

In the past decade, there has been a marked increase in concern about the adverse health effects of hazardous exposures in both workplaces and elsewhere in the environment. The lung with its extensive surface area, high blood flow, and thin alveolar epithelium is an important site of contact with substances in the environment. Such agents can cause direct toxicity, can be absorbed by or deposited in the respiratory tract, or can cause an immunologic reaction. Because of the seemingly endless array of substances or lack of toxicologic, epidemiologic, or industrial hygiene expertise, many clinicians feel ill-prepared to recognize, diagnose, and treat occupational lung diseases.

This chapter discusses major occupational respiratory tract disorders, emphasizing certain basic principles and recognition and diagnosis of such disorders. It also reviews the adverse health effects of environmental exposures such as passive smoking, air pollution, and domestic radon. Almost all respiratory diseases may be caused or exacerbated by factors in the workplace or environment. Thus, it is important to maintain a high level of suspicion when evaluating patients with any respiratory disorder. Several excellent recent occupational and environmental medicine textbooks provide an extensive review of this topic (1–5).

PRINCIPLES OF OCCUPATIONAL AND ENVIRONMENTAL LUNG DISEASE

Certain principles apply broadly to all respiratory disorders caused by inhalational exposure to agents in the workplace or environment.

1. Environmental and occupational lung diseases are difficult to distinguish from those of nonenvironmental origin. Almost any defined lung disease may have an environmental cause. Conversely, few environmental lung diseases will present with obvious or pathognomonic features.

2. A given substance in the workplace or environment can cause more than one clinical or pathologic entity. For example, cobalt can cause interstitial lung disease and airways disease.

3. The etiology of many lung diseases may be multifactorial, and occupational factors may interact with other factors. For example, asbestos-exposed workers who smoke have a greater risk of developing lung cancer than those exposed to either asbestos or cigarettes alone.

4. The respiratory effects of occupational and environmental lung exposures occur following exposure with a latent interval that depends on the given exposure. For acute diseases, there is a short and usually predictable time between exposure and resultant clinical manifestations, which should suggest an association. For chronic diseases such as cancer or most pneumoconioses, long latency between first exposure and subsequent clinical manifestations is common. Consequently, the patient's exposure to the offending agent(s) may have ceased long before the onset of the disease, making the diagnosis of such diseases much more challenging.

5. The dose of exposure is an important determinant of the proportion of individuals affected or the severity of disease. Higher doses usually result in more affected individuals or greater disease severity.

6. Individual differences in susceptibility to exposures exist. Adverse effects may occur in some individuals, whereas others are spared. Host factors that determine susceptibility to environmental agents are poorly understood but likely include both inherited genetic factors and acquired factors, such as diet, the presence of other lung disease, and other exposures.

There are several compelling reasons to pursue the search for an occupational or environmental cause in all cases of pulmonary disease. Knowledge of cause may affect patient management and prognosis, and may prevent further disease progression. New associations between exposure and disease may be identified, such as new agents that can cause occupational asthma. A larger population at risk that may benefit from preventive measures may be identified. Finally, establishing the cause may have significant legal and financial implications for the patient.

CLINICAL APPROACH TO THE PATIENT

There are two distinct phases in the workup of any patient with a potential occupational or environmental lung disease. First, as with any patient presenting with a potential disorder of the respiratory tract, its nature and extent must be defined and characterized, regardless of the suspected etiology.

Second, whether the disease or symptom complex was caused or exacerbated by any exposures at work or in the environment must be determined.

The initial approach to all such patients includes a detailed history, physical examination, appropriate laboratory testing, chest radiograph, and pulmonary function testing. Initial exposure information can be used to direct the sequence of the workup and to obviate unnecessary procedures when the diagnosis is straightforward. If the initial evaluation does not fully explain the patient's symptomatology, other tests are available to better characterize the nature and extent of the respiratory disorder, such as computed chest tomography, laryngoscopy, flow-volume loops, cardiopulmonary exercise studies, nonspecific inhalation challenge testing, bronchoscopy, open lung biopsy, and various immunologic studies. However, few are specific for any given occupational or environmental diagnosis.

Prior medical records can be helpful in the evaluation of a patient with a potential occupational or environmental lung disease. Such records can establish the patient's earlier complaints, provide objective data such as prior pulmonary function tests or chest radiographs for comparison, and clarify temporal relationships between exposure and effect, an important component of biologic plausibility.

DIAGNOSTIC CRITERIA

After the disease process is characterized, whether any occupational or environmental exposures are causative or contributory must be determined. The following criteria are used to determine whether a disease is caused or exacerbated by agents in the workplace or environment.

1. The clinical presentation and workup are consistent with the diagnosis.

2. A causal relationship (biologic plausibility) between the exposure and the diagnosed condition has been previously established or strongly suggested in the medical or toxicologic literature. Several different types of data can be used to establish a causal relationship. Epidemiologic studies (such as cohort or case control studies) can demonstrate associations between certain exposures or jobs and adverse effects. Clinical studies or case reports of similarly exposed patients can be used to determine the adverse effects of an exposure. Such studies may also provide useful information about the magnitude of the risk, the amount of exposure necessary for disease, and the latency between exposure and disease. Data from animal toxicologic studies can also be helpful, especially when human data are not available.

3. There is sufficient exposure to cause the disease, as assessed below.

4. The details of the particular case, such as the temporal relationship between exposure and disease, are consistent with known information about the exposure–disease association.

5. There is no other more likely diagnosis.

Exposure Assessment

The occupational and environmental history is the single most helpful tool to determine whether exposure to one or more environmental agents has occurred and the magnitude and extent of the exposure. A detailed occupational history consists of a chronologic list of all jobs and includes the job title, a description of the job activities, potential toxins at each job, and an assessment of the extent and duration of exposure. The length of time exposed to the agent, the use of personal protective equipment such as respirators, and a description of the ventilation and overall hygiene are helpful in attempting to quantify exposure from the patient's history.

Patients should be asked whether they think their problem is related to anything in the environment. Temporal associations between the patient's symptoms and exposures and the presence of similar symptoms among co-workers should be determined. Information about potential exposures outside the workplace, such as in the home or encountered with hobbies, should also be obtained.

There are a number of sources available for obtaining additional exposure information. These are Material Safety Data Sheets (MSDSs) (federal law requires employers to provide employees with information about the potential toxicity of the materials used in the workplace); exposure records from the employer or insurance companies; information from inspections by health and regulatory agencies such as the Occupational Safety and Health Administration (OSHA), unions and community groups, and direct site visits. For recent or current exposures, a site visit is usually helpful in providing information about the nature and extent of potential exposures and other exposed workers. Epidemiologic data on co-workers or previous workers with similar types of jobs can be used to assess the nature and extent of exposures for a given patient. Finally, further information about the patient's exposure can be obtained from certain diagnostic tests, such as a positive radioallergosorbent test (RAST) or skin test to a specific antigen or tissue mineralogic analysis. For acute diseases such as occupational asthma, reproducing the disease manifestations by reexposure to the suspected environmental agent is additional evidence that supports the diagnosis.

Once this additional information is obtained, the clinician has to determine whether any occupational or environmental exposures are causing or contributing to the patient's disease process. Although some diagnoses such as asbestosis are frequently straightforward, others may be diagnostically challenging and easily overlooked. There is always some degree of uncertainty in medical decision making. In most workers' compensation cases, the standard of certainty is usually whether the patient's problem is more probably than not (a >50% likelihood) related to an occupational or environmental exposure. This is a much lower standard of certainty than physicians generally use in making diagnostic decisions. Occupational or environmental diseases can be diagnosed even when there is significant uncertainty. After such a diagnosis, the physician should consider the public health issues involved (i.e., that other individuals in that same environment may also be similarly affected) and contemplate appropriate action.

CLASSIFICATION OF OCCUPATIONAL AND ENVIRONMENTAL LUNG DISEASE

Environmentally induced lung diseases can be classified by several schemes. Because these diseases so closely resemble other lung diseases, it may be helpful to classify them by the clinical presentation, as shown in Table 13-1. An overview of these acute and chronic disorders, and the adverse health effects of indoor and outdoor air pollutants, can be found in this chapter, except hypersensitivity pneumonitis (HP) and infectious diseases, which are discussed in Chapters 12, Diffuse Parenchymal and Alveolar Lung Diseases, and 15, Respiratory Tract Infections, respectively.

MAJOR ACUTE AND SUBACUTE DISEASES

UPPER RESPIRATORY TRACT IRRITATION AND OCCUPATIONAL RHINITIS

Symptoms of eye, nose, and throat irritation are frequently associated with environmental exposures and can present as upper respiratory tract irritation and/or rhinitis. Numerous workplace irritants can cause upper respiratory tract irritation, including dusts, such as coal or manmade vitreous fibers (MMVF); chemicals such as ammonia, chlorine, and solvents; and metal fumes. Presenting symptoms can mimic common disorders such as upper respiratory infection, rhinitis, acute bronchitis, sinusitis, or hay fever. Many of these exposures can also cause lower respiratory tract disease, such as occupational asthma, toxic pneumonitis, chronic bronchitis, or interstitial lung disease, depending on the particular agent and the dose and duration of exposure.

Occupational rhinitis is a common disorder that has received little attention and is closely related to occupational asthma (discussed in the following section). The term refers to rhinitis or inflammation of the nose caused by workplace allergen and irritant exposures (6–8). The primary symptoms are nasal congestion, rhinorrhea, sneezing, itching, and overlap with upper respiratory tract irritation, which is believed to be an irritant rather than an allergic response. Occupational rhinitis is much more common than occupational asthma; more than 50% of patients with immune-mediated occupational asthma can have rhinitis, which commonly predates the development of asthma (8).

The diagnosis of either upper respiratory tract irritation or occupational rhinitis is usually made on the basis of a temporal association between exposure to the irritant or allergen and symptoms. Improvement in symptoms away from work and similar symptoms in co-workers are helpful clues. Atopic individuals appear to be at increased risk. It is important to determine whether there is any lower respiratory tract involvement, which can usually be done by reading a patient's history and spirometry or methacholine challenge testing. RAST testing may be helpful if the history suggests IgE-mediated allergies. Successful treatment involves reducing or eliminating the offending exposures.

AIRWAY DISORDERS

Occupational Asthma

DEFINITION AND CAUSES. Occupational asthma has been defined as variable airflow obstruction or airway hyperresponsiveness caused by a specific agent or process encountered in the workplace (9–12). This definition presumes nothing about pathogenic mechanism and includes bronchospasm due to nonspecific irritant stimuli (irritant-induced asthma), in addition to asthma caused by agents to which specific "sensitization" has developed. A broader definition includes aggravation

TABLE 13-1.   Classification of Occupational Lung Disorders

Disease/Problem	Example of Causative Agent
Major acute or subacute diseases	
Upper respiratory tract irritation	Irritant gases, solvents
Airway disorders	
Occupational asthma	
Sensitization	Diisocyanates, animal dander
Irritant-induced, RADS	Irritant gases, World Trade Center dust
Work-aggravated asthma	Irritants, allergens
Byssinosis	Cotton dust
Grain dust effects	Grain
Inhalation injury	
Toxic pneumonitis	Irritant gases, metals
Metal fume fever	Metal oxides—zinc, copper
Polymer fume fever	Plastics
Smoke inhalation	
Hypersensitivity pneumonitis	Microbial agents
Infectious disorders	Tuberculosis
Acute pleural disease	Asbestos
Major chronic diseases	
Interstitial fibrotic diseases (pneumoconioses)	Asbestos, silica, coal
Beryllium/hard metal-related disease	Beryllium, cobalt
Chronic bronchitis/COPD	Mineral dusts, coal
Malignancies of the respiratory tract and pleura	
Sinonasal cancer	Wood dust
Laryngeal cancer	Asbestos
Lung cancer	Asbestos, radon
Mesothelioma	Asbestos
Air pollution	
Ambient air pollution	Sulfur oxides, particulates
Indoor air pollution	Environmental tobacco smoke

RADS, reactive airways dysfunction syndrome; COPD, chronic obstructive pulmonary disorder.

of preexisting asthma by exposures in the workplace or work-aggravated asthma. Work-related asthma is a broader term used to include asthma caused or aggravated by workplace exposures.

Immune-mediated or sensitizer-induced occupational asthma is caused by sensitizing agents, which include both high-molecular weight (more than 1,000 daltons) and low-molecular weight compounds (see Table 13-2). High-molecular weight compounds are animal, plant, and fungal proteins. Low-molecular weight compounds are usually chemicals; most common are the diisocyanates, anhydrides, and plicatic acid (the putative cause of western red cedar-induced asthma). This distinction by size is justified by the differing clinical characteristics and pathogenic features of asthma induced by agents in the respective categories. The number of agents or processes that have been shown to cause occupational asthma is large (over 300 agents) and constantly growing (13). The role of environmental exposures in atopic asthma is discussed in Chapter 8, Asthma. Irritant-induced asthma and work-aggravated asthma are discussed below.

PREVALENCE. It has been estimated that 5% to 20% of adult-onset asthma is attributable to workplace exposures (14,15). The

incidence of occupational asthma in different industrial settings varies. For example, 5% to 20% of isocyanate-exposed persons, 5% to 10% of those exposed to western red cedar, and up to 25% of workers exposed to grain dusts have been reported to develop occupational asthma (9,10,14,16).

The single most important factor determining the prevalence of occupational asthma is exposure to a sensitizing agent. Only a portion of workers exposed to a sensitizing agent ever develop asthma. However, host susceptibility factors for occupational asthma are not well understood. Atopy is often a predisposing factor for the development of asthma due to high-molecular weight compounds such as animal- or plant-derived material. However, atopy does not appear to be an important risk factor when low-molecular weight compounds such as diisocyanates or plicatic acid are the causative agents (16). Cigarette smoking and preexisting nonspecific airway hyperresponsiveness do not appear to be strong risk factors (16).

CLINICAL FEATURES. The most easily recognized presentation of occupational asthma consists of wheezing and dyspnea, which occur within minutes after contact with the offending agent at the workplace and typically disappear after work, the

TABLE 13-2. Occupational Asthma[a]

Asthma-inducing Agents	Common Occupations
High-molecular-weight compounds	
Animal-derived material (dander, excreta, secretions)	
Laboratory animals	Laboratory workers
Birds, bats	Breeders
Shellfish	Food processors
Insects	Laboratory workers
Plants and vegetable products	
Castor beans	Food processors
Coffee beans	Food processors
Grain dust	Grain handlers
Cotton dust	Textile workers
Flour	Bakers
Psyllium	Laxative manufacturers
Vegetable gums	Printers
Latex	Hospital and dental workers
Enzymes	
Alcalase	Detergent manufacturers, food processors
Papain	Pharmaceutical workers
Pancreatic extracts	Pharmaceutical workers
Low-molecular-weight compounds	
Wood dusts	Woodworkers, carpenters
Western red cedar	
California redwood	
Mahogany	
Oak	
Diisocyanates	Painters, printers, foam manufacturers
Toluene (TDI)	
Diphenylmethane (MDI)	
Hexamethylene (HDI)	
Acid anhydrides	Epoxy resin, paint, chemical workers
Trimellitic (TMA)	
Phthalic (PA)	
Maleic (MA)	
Amines	
Ethylenediamine	Plastic workers
Drugs	Pharmaceutical workers
Cimetidine	
Cephalosporins	
Psyllium	
Penicillins	
Sulfonamides	
Other chemicals	
Azo dyes	Dye workers
Formaldehyde	Nurses, laboratory workers
Glutaraldehyde	Nurses, hospital workers
Insecticides (organophosphates)	Manufacturers, farmers
Persulfates	Hairdressers
Polyvinyl chloride (decomposition)	Food wrappers
Metal fumes and salts platers,	Metal workers, metal welders
Chromium	
Cobalt	
Nickel	
Platinum salts	

[a]For a more comprehensive list, see Chan-Yeung M, Malo JL. Aetiological agents in occupational asthma. *Eur Respir J* 1994;7:346–371.

so-called immediate reaction. Cough or chest tightness rather than wheezing is also common. A delayed reaction, particularly common with low-molecular weight compounds, may begin up to 12 hours after exposure, so that wheeze, cough, or chest tightness at night may be the only presenting symptoms. Patients can have both immediate and delayed symptoms (i.e., a dual reaction). Symptoms frequently worsen over the course of a workweek and improve on weekends and vacation. Sensitizer-induced occupational asthma develops after a latent period that can vary from months to years following the onset of exposure, but typically occurs in the first 2 years of exposure.

The relationship between symptoms and exposure tends to be less clear after asthma has been present for several years. Continued exposure to the causative agent may result in persistent airway obstruction and/or hyperresponsiveness, such that symptoms may persist after cessation of exposure. Lack of improvement off work does not exclude the diagnosis of occupational asthma. However, lack of any improvement during a vacation of several weeks is unusual. Nonspecific triggers such as upper respiratory tract infections, exercise, cold, and emotional stimuli may precipitate asthmatic attacks in patients with occupational asthma, just as in those with asthma not related to the workplace.

DIAGNOSIS. The diagnosis of occupational asthma involves first establishing the diagnosis of asthma, and then determining whether it is associated with exposure to some substance or process in the workplace. There is no single simple diagnostic test for occupational asthma, and the diagnosis may be difficult to make. A high index of suspicion is key to the correct diagnosis.

A careful occupational history is the most effective, useful, and practical means of identifying workers with possible occupational asthma. The following should raise the suspicion for occupational asthma: new-onset asthma in an adult, worsening symptoms at or after work with deterioration over the course of the week, improvement away from work, and the presence of an agent in the workplace known to cause occupational asthma. The timing of asthma symptoms in relationship to work is frequently clearest when the symptoms first started. Additional helpful information is the use of any new agents or processes at the worksite, similar symptoms in co-workers, and the presence of preexisting asthma or atopy.

The diagnosis of asthma is confirmed, as with any asthmatic patient, by demonstrating reversible airflow obstruction. Tests for nonspecific airway hyperresponsiveness, such as methacholine challenge, can be used to document hyperreactive airways if spirometry is normal.

Several methods are available to document the association between airflow obstruction and exposure to the suspected agent (10,14,17,18).

1. Preshift and postshift measurement in the forced expiratory volume in 1 second (FEV_1). Demonstration of a decrement of more than 10% in the FEV_1 across the work shift is a relatively specific test, but it is insufficiently sensitive because of the relatively frequent occurrence of delayed responses, and it can be logistically difficult to perform.
2. Serial measurements of peak expiratory flow rates (PEFR). A worker can make serial measurements of peak expiratory flow throughout the work shift and later at home by means of a handheld instrument, a Mini-Wright peak flowmeter. A reduction in peak flows associated with exposure to the suspected agent supports a diagnosis of occupational asthma. Visual interpretation is as useful as quantitative analysis. An example of a PEFR record supporting a diagnosis of occupational asthma is shown in Figure 13-1. Good-quality PEFR recordings with adequate off-work and workdays may be difficult to obtain.

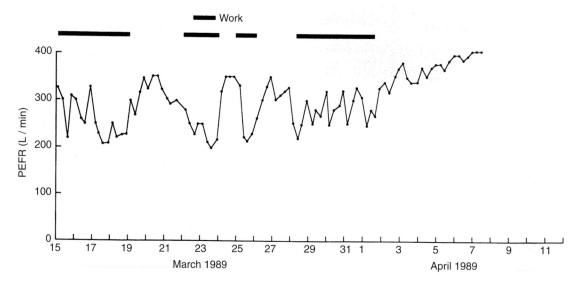

FIGURE 13-1.   Peak expiratory flow rates (PEFR) record of a hairdresser who developed symptoms of asthma from exposure to a bleaching reagent she used at work. PEFR showed improvement when she was away from work. (From Rosenstock L, Cullen MR, eds. *Textbook of clinical occupational and environmental medicine.* Philadelphia, PA: WB Saunders, 1994, with permission.)

3. Workplace or specific inhalation challenge. Workplace challenges can be performed under actual exposure conditions, but because multiple exposures are common, they may not identify the specific agent. Specific challenge testing with the suspected agent(s), with a fall in FEV_1 following exposure, is considered the "gold standard" for diagnosing occupational asthma. However, such testing requires a specialized chamber, is time consuming, expensive, and carries certain risks, and false negatives can occur. Specific inhalation challenge is helpful in documenting a previously unrecognized cause of occupational asthma and in establishing a specific etiologic diagnosis when multiple exposures are present. However, specific challenge is not necessary for the diagnosis of most cases of occupational asthma and is rarely available in the United States.

In practice, objective evidence of variable airflow obstruction in relation to workplace exposure can be difficult to obtain for multiple reasons, especially if the patient has changed jobs. It may also be difficult to identify a single specific causative agent. For the purposes of a worker's compensation in the United States (>50% likelihood), a temporal association between asthmatic symptoms and workplace exposure(s) may provide sufficient evidence of work-relatedness if the suspect exposure or process is a documented cause of asthma (Table 13-2).

IMMUNOLOGIC TESTS. Skin tests and detection of specific IgE antibodies to the suspected agent in the serum by immunoassays such as the RAST have varying degrees of usefulness. In the case of high-molecular weight allergens, such as flours or rodent proteins, the demonstration of a positive skin test or specific IgE antibodies is highly confirmatory of exposure but does not distinguish exposure from disease. For low-molecular weight compounds, such as diisocyanates or plicatic acid, negative tests are common, and the application of these techniques has limited clinical utility (19).

OUTCOME AND MANAGEMENT. Studies of workers with sensitizer-induced occupationally induced asthma have shown that many of these workers (up to 80%) have persistent symptoms and airway hyperresponsiveness, even after removal from further exposure (12,20). Persistent asthma following removal has been associated with longer duration of symptoms and exposure and greater severity of asthma (abnormal spirometry and more marked airway hyperresponsiveness). These patients can be clinically indistinguishable from intrinsic, nonoccupationally induced asthmatics with acute exacerbations following viral infections and nonspecific stimuli.

A better prognosis is associated with early diagnosis and removal from further exposure (9,12,21). However, the socioeconomic consequences of removal from work can be substantial and should be considered in patient management (21). Exposure to minute quantities of sensitizing agents, even below regulatory permissible limits, can induce bronchospasm in sensitized workers, and complete avoidance is preferable once occupational asthma has been diagnosed. However, sufficient reductions in exposure within the same workplace can sometimes be achieved, which can avoid the severe socioeconomic consequences of removal from work. A change in job within the same workplace, industrial hygiene modifications

to reduce exposure, and use of respiratory protective devices for selected tasks can be tried but require close monitoring of the worker's respiratory status. Medications used to treat occupational asthma are the same as those used with nonoccupational asthma but should not be used in lieu of reducing exposure.

REACTIVE AIRWAYS DYSFUNCTION SYNDROME OR IRRITANT-INDUCED ASTHMA AND WORK-AGGRAVATED ASTHMA. Brooks originally termed the persistence of symptoms consistent with asthma and nonspecific airway hyperresponsiveness in some individuals following exposure to a high dose of an irritating vapor, fume, gas, or smoke as *reactive airways dysfunction syndrome* (RADS), and it is more recently known as *irritant-induced asthma* (12,22,23). Although the literature on irritant-induced asthma is more limited and controversial than that on sensitizer asthma, recent data suggests that recurrent exposures to lower levels of irritant can cause new-onset asthma, in addition to exacerbating preexisting asthma, although these can be difficult to distinguish. Recent studies of firefighters following the World Trade Center collapse in 2001 have demonstrated the development and persistence of airway hyperreactivity and asthmatic symptoms in these workers that was associated with the extent of exposure (24). The effects of chronic irritant exposures on chronic airways disease are discussed further below. Work-aggravated asthma refers to work-related asthma symptoms in workers with preexisting or coincident asthma. Work-related symptoms can occur in response to relatively low levels of a number of exposures at work, such as respiratory irritants (dusts, fumes, vapors, mists, cigarette smoke), allergens, cold, and exercise.

The incidence, relative risk, and natural history of irritant-induced and work-aggravated asthma are not well defined and can be difficult to distinguish from irritant aggravation of preexisting asthma. Typically, less than 20% of reported cases of occupational asthma are attributed to acute irritant exposures, although this may reflect diagnostic and/or compensation practices (25). The risk of persistent airway hyperresponsiveness reported following acute inhalation accidents is variable, and likely depends on the extent and nature of the inhalation exposure, as well as a host of factors such as atopy, ranging from less than 10% to more than 50% of subjects with asthma-like symptoms. Work-aggravated asthma is likely quite common, although data is limited. A recent Canadian study found that 50% of all work-related asthma claims were for work-aggravated asthma (9).

The diagnosis of RADS or irritant-induced asthma is based on the following considerations:

1. Absence of preceding asthmalike respiratory disease or complaints.
2. Documentation of asthma (reversible airflow obstruction) using spirometry or methacholine challenge.
3. Onset of symptoms after a single or multiple high-level exposure(s) to a known irritant gas, vapor, fume, aerosol, or dust. Industrial hygiene data documenting such exposures typically are not available, as the episodes are frequently accidental or sporadic.
4. Onset of symptoms shortly after (typically within 24 hours) the high exposure and lasting for at least 3 months, usually longer.

5. With more chronic, ongoing irritant exposures at work, documentation of new-onset asthma symptoms associated with the irritant exposures. Worsening of asthma at work and improvement away from the irritant exposures should be documented by work-related changes in symptoms and/or medication use, and preferably changes in lung function, such as PEFRs, although the latter can be difficult to obtain.

6. Other asthmalike illnesses are ruled out.

Work-aggravated asthma is typically based on a history of asthma symptoms that are worse at work and improve to some extent away from work (11). Asthma should be objectively confirmed, as with other types of work-related asthma, and the association between asthma aggravation and work documented as thoroughly as possible, as noted above.

With irritant-induced asthma and work-aggravated asthma, the worker can return frequently to the workplace if the aggravating exposures are limited (9,26). However, this can be difficult to accomplish. Close follow-up is necessary to monitor for persistent or progressive symptoms and airflow obstruction.

PATHOGENESIS OF OCCUPATIONAL ASTHMA. Similar to non–work-related asthma, airway inflammation likely plays a crucial role in the pathogenesis of occupational asthma (13,27). Components of airway inflammation include alterations in airway epithelial and smooth muscle cells; airway infiltration by inflammatory cells such as T lymphocytes, mast cells, eosinophils, and neutrophils; and airway remodeling. How different exposures cause airway inflammation is not well understood but likely involves both immunologic and nonimmunologic mechanisms and numerous different mediators and cell types. Airways may be injured directly by intense exposure to irritant chemicals such as chlorine or sulfur dioxide, resulting in epithelial damage, airway inflammation, and hyperresponsiveness. Such a mechanism is likely involved in the pathogenesis of irritant-induced asthma. Airway injury, repair, and remodeling are also likely involved in immune-mediated asthma.

In most cases of sensitizer-induced occupational asthma, airway inflammation likely involves immune-mediated processes. High-molecular weight animal- and plant-derived compounds can induce specific IgE responses in a high proportion of exposed symptomatic individuals. With low-molecular weight chemicals such as diisocyanates, specific antibodies are detected in only a fraction of such patients, and both immunologic and nonimmunologic mechanisms are likely involved.

Byssinosis: Textile Dust-related Disease

DEFINITION, CLINICAL FEATURES, AND PATHOGENESIS. Excessive inhalation of certain vegetable fiber dusts causes byssinosis, an acute and chronic obstructive lung disease of textile workers. First described by Ramazzini, it was essentially rediscovered by Schilling in the 1950s yet remains poorly understood (28–30). The disease originally was recognized in cotton workers but has been reported among other textile workers. In its early more acute stages, byssinosis is characterized by symptoms of chest tightness, cough, wheezing, and dyspnea that are especially prominent on the first day back to work and are correlated with a reversible decline in FEV$_1$.

These symptoms initially tend to improve over the first few days of the workweek, but as the disease progresses, chronic chest tightness can develop, and respiratory symptoms and chronic airflow obstruction can persist, even away from exposure. The risk of developing byssinosis is related to the intensity of dust exposure, duration of exposure, job, and type of fiber. Exposure to the end product (e.g., cotton cloth) does not cause byssinosis. In addition to byssinosis, textile workers can also develop HP, chronic bronchitis, and febrile syndromes such as mill fever and mattress makers' fever.

The mechanisms by which cotton and other dusts cause byssinosis remain unclear, despite substantial investigation. Cotton dust contains a large number of potentially toxic components, such as bacteria, fungi, inorganic material, and organic chemicals. Endotoxin from bacteria has been suspected as the primary causative agent, but its role is uncertain (28,31).

DIAGNOSIS AND PREVENTION. The diagnosis of byssinosis depends primarily on the occupational history of the characteristic symptom pattern in association with exposure to cotton or other natural textile dusts (28). Spirometry documenting a cross-shift decline in FEV$_1$ supports the diagnosis. Patients with more advanced chronic disease may have evidence of irreversible airflow obstruction. In the United States, the implementation of the OSHA cotton dust standard and the closure of older mills have reduced dust levels. However, in less developed countries, dusty conditions still exist.

Agricultural Lung Diseases: Respiratory Effects of Organic Dusts

Agricultural work is associated with a high prevalence of respiratory symptoms. Organic dusts such as grain dust are respiratory exposures in agricultural work. Grain dust is a complex mixture consisting of various grains contaminated with fungi, bacteria, insects and mites, animal matter, endotoxins, various agricultural chemicals such as fungicides and pesticides, and inorganic matter, mainly soil. Acute and chronic respiratory disease in grain workers was first recognized by Ramazzini almost three centuries ago. Grain dust and other organic dusts can cause asthma, acute febrile syndromes [organic dust toxic syndrome (ODTS)], HP, asthma, chronic bronchitis, and accelerated decline in lung function (FEV$_1$) (31,32).

Most grain workers who complain of respiratory symptoms do not have a history of atopy, possibly because of the healthy worker effect. Grain workers who are atopic are at increased risk of developing grain dust asthma. The combined effects of cigarette smoking and grain on lung function are probably additive.

ODTS was recently coined to describe grain fever and other acute self-limited febrile illnesses associated with heavy exposure to organic dusts (32). Patients present with symptoms of fever, chills, dry cough, malaise, dyspnea, and headache 4 to 12 hours after exposure, similar to acute HP, but without the typical lung pathology or radiographic changes. Organic dusts contain a number of potential toxic substances, with endotoxin considered a likely causative agent. Exposure to grain dusts less commonly causes HP (farmer's lung), likely due to thermophilic actinomycetes. The diagnosis and management of HP are discussed in Chapter 12, Diffuse Parenchymal and Alveolar Lung Diseases.

Agricultural workers also develop asthma, likely caused by sensitization to any of a number of different allergens associated with grain dust and animal exposures. Irritant exposures that can aggravate asthma are also common, such as ammonia, nitrogen dioxide, organic dusts, and various chemicals. Inhalation challenge tests with grain dusts or their extracts have documented classic immediate or delayed reactions. The diagnosis and management of occupational asthma in agricultural workers is similar to occupational asthma in other settings (discussed above).

Chronic grain dust exposure is associated with chronic bronchitic symptoms and reduced lung function (31,32). Early, the initial decrements in lung function appear to be reversible, but with continued exposure, chronic irreversible changes in lung function can occur. Workers who experience acute respiratory symptoms and airway obstruction in response to grain dust, as well as those more heavily exposed, may be at increased risk of developing chronic airflow obstruction and an accelerated decline in lung function (31,33).

INHALATION INJURY

Toxic Lung Injury and Toxic Pneumonitis

Excessive inhalational exposure to a large number of different irritant gases, mists, and fumes may produce inflammation of any portion of the respiratory tract, depending on the dose and duration of exposure and the anatomic level at which the toxin is deposited or absorbed (34). The latter is determined largely by the size of the particles and the solubility of gases in water. Highly soluble gases (such as ammonia) and large particles affect the conjunctivae, pharynx, larynx, trachea, and major bronchi; small particles and insoluble gases (such as phosgene or nitrogen dioxide) affect smaller distal airways and alveoli predominantly. Common irritant gases are listed in Table 13-3.

Clinical Presentation and Long-term Effects

Clinical signs appear after variable delays from the time of exposure; latency is shortest for the mucous membranes of the face and becomes progressively longer as one moves distally. Thus, the eyes, nose, and throat are likely to become inflamed shortly after exposure, whereas evidence of pneumonitis may appear hours to days later. Because of variable latency, early results of blood gas analyses, chest radiographs, and lung function tests must be interpreted with caution.

Most patients who survive recover completely. Chronic sequellae of injury to the airways are chronic bronchitis and tracheitis, usually with gradual improvement over many months. RADS can develop and persist following acute irritant exposures, as discussed above. Chronic sequellae of lower respiratory tract injury are rare and include progressive interstitial fibrosis, bronchiolitis obliterans, and bronchiolitis obliterans organizing pneumonia (34,35).

Evaluation and Treatment

There is no specific treatment for acute inhalational injury (34). Evaluation should include a careful history of the exposure event and assessment of risk factors for excessive exposure. A careful physical exam, chest radiograph, and oximetry should be obtained. Specific exposures such as smoke inhalation or certain metals may warrant additional studies. Support and expectant management are the keys to treatment. The role of steroids is controversial, with few clinical trials. Unless cardiorespiratory failure is imminent, emergency attention should proceed from the upper tract downward. Inflamed mucosal surfaces, especially the eyes, should be rinsed first. If hoarseness, stridor, or other signs are present, the vocal cords should be visualized and endotracheal intubation considered. Reactive airways disease is treated with bronchodilators and commonly a course of steroids, despite limited data. Pneumonitis, with onset as late as 72 hours after exposure, should be anticipated, especially if bronchospasm is present. Noncardiogenic pulmonary edema due to chemical pneumonitis should be managed in the same manner as other causes of severe pneumonitis and respiratory failure.

Specific Agents

IRRITANT GASES. Common irritant gases are listed in Table 13-3. Ammonia is highly water soluble and thus extremely irritating to mucous membranes. Most cases of severe lower respiratory tract injury due to ammonia involve entrapment in confined spaces. Sulfur dioxide is generated during a wide range of industrial operations, such as the refining of petroleum products and paper manufacturing. It is relatively water soluble and causes sufficient upper respiratory tract irritation to warn anyone exposed to a high concentration. Chlorine, also widely used, is less soluble and is associated with a correspondingly increased risk of bronchiolitis or alveolitis. Nitrogen dioxide, reddish in color, is liberated whenever nitrogen-containing material is burned; it is also a by-product of welding, store silage, and mining, as well as numerous chemical operations. It is relatively insoluble; therefore, the risk of parenchymal lung injury is high. Recurrent episodes after exposure have been reported.

Ozone is a highly toxic gas normally found in the atmosphere at very low concentrations. It can be generated by welding, and increased amounts are found at high altitude (airplanes) and in urban smog. It can cause substernal burning and transient changes in lung function (decreased FEV_1 and increased nonspecific airway responsiveness), but rarely pneumonitis or

TABLE 13-3. Common Irritant Gases and Vapors

Gas	Water Solubility	Lethality
Ammonia	High	Low
Acetaldehyde	High	Low
Chlorine	Medium	Medium
Hydrogen fluoride	High	Low
Hydrogen sulfide	High	Low
Methylisocyanate	(Highly reactive)	High
Oxides of nitrogen (NO, NO_2, N_2O_4)	Low	High
Ozone	Low	Low
Phosgene	Very low	Very high
Sulfur dioxide	High	Low

pulmonary edema. Phosgene is a poorly soluble gas originally developed for chemical warfare. It penetrates to the distal lung, where it causes parenchymal injury.

TOXIC METAL AND POLYMER FUMES. Several irritant metals are encountered in industrial environments. Cadmium fumes from primary smelting, electroplating, or welding can cause severe lower respiratory tract inflammation (27). Bronchitis and emphysema have been associated with chronic cadmium exposure (28). Mercury vapor and beryllium compounds can cause acute pneumonitis, and persistent symptoms can occur. Fumes and dusts of manganese, inhaled by welders, have been associated with acute airway and parenchymal lung inflammation.

METAL FUME FEVER. Fumes of zinc and copper, generated from smelting, welding, or foundry work, contain fine particles of zinc and copper oxides (36). Several hours after an intense exposure, a flulike illness with fever, myalgia, headache, and leukocytosis, called *metal fume fever*, can occur. Thirst and a metallic taste may also occur. Chest infiltrates are not seen, and the illness generally runs a benign 24-hour course. "Tolerance" occurs with daily or continuous exposure; workers usually get the "fever" on Mondays after a few days away from exposure.

POLYMER FUME FEVER. Closely related to metal fume fever is *polymer fume fever* from inhaling pyrolysis products of Teflon (polytetrafluorethylene). Infiltrates do occur but clear spontaneously, along with the fever and constitutional symptoms. Symptoms may persist for weeks but typically resolve completely, although long-term studies have not been performed.

SMOKE INHALATION. Smoke inhalation injury is common among burn patients, including firefighters (34). The pulmonary effects of smoke inhalation depend on the magnitude of the exposure and the specific chemical fumes released during combustion. The major components of fire smoke are toxic irritants such as acrolein and hydrogen chloride and chemical asphyxiants such as hydrogen cyanide (see Table 13-4). Less commonly, thermal injury from high temperature can also occur, especially with aerosolized liquids (i.e., steam) or particles (i.e., metallic oxides), which have a greater heat capacity than dry air and can cause thermal injury to the lower airways.

TABLE 13-4. Toxic Inhalants Commonly Encountered in Fires

Chemical irritants
  Aldehydes (acrolein, formaldehyde)
  Ammonia
  Aromatic hydrocarbons (benzene)
  Hydrogen chloride
  Isocyanates
  Metals (lead, chromium, arsenic)
  Nitrogen dioxide
  Sulfur dioxide
Chemical asphyxiants
  Hydrogen cyanide
  Carbon monoxide
  Hydrogen sulfide

Persons affected by fire are typically exposed to a number of different toxic inhalants because of the many potentially combustible products present at the site of a fire, such as furniture, plastics, carpets, and polyurethane materials.

Treatment of smoke inhalation is similar to other inhalational injuries. Smoke-exposed individuals should receive oxygen and an arterial blood gas and carboxyhemoglobin level should be obtained. Physical examination should include a careful assessment for facial or oropharyngeal burns, wheezing, or any neurologic abnormalities. A chest radiograph, electrocardiogram (ECG), and spirometry or peak flow determination are recommended. Patients with clinically significant smoke exposures need close observation for delayed pulmonary effects, even if initially asymptomatic. Chronic sequellae similar to other acute inhalational injuries can occur, in particular, hyperreactive airways and bronchiolitis obliterans. The risk of developing chronic airflow obstruction is not resolved. Individual firefighters can show accelerated loss of lung function, and removal from further exposure may be indicated.

ACUTE PLEURAL DISEASE

Asbestos exposure can result in transient pleural effusions and, less commonly, recurrent attacks of pleurisy (37). Asbestos-induced pleural effusions are typically exudative and may be hemorrhagic and/or eosinophilic (38). The diagnosis depends on the history of asbestos exposure, the presence of an effusion, no other cause for the effusion, and no development of malignancy within 3 years of diagnosis. Benign asbestos effusions are frequently asymptomatic and occur with a latency of 10 years or more. They may result in the development of diffuse pleural thickening.

MAJOR CHRONIC DISEASES

INTERSTITIAL FIBROSING DISEASES: OVERVIEW

Occupational and environmental interstitial lung diseases are a group of heterogeneous lung diseases that diffusely involve the lung parenchyma with varying degrees of chronic alveolitis and fibrosis. The term *pneumoconioses* has traditionally been defined as the accumulation of dust in the lung and the resulting tissue reaction. Originally used to describe inorganic dust-induced diseases such as asbestosis or silicosis, the term is also used loosely to describe diseases resulting from the inhalation of other substances that may not accumulate in the lung, such as cobalt. There are a large number of occupational and environmental causes of pulmonary interstitial fibrosis. Major causes are listed in Table 13-5.

The fibrogenic potential of inorganic dusts varies considerably, with silica and asbestos having greater fibrogenic potential than coal dust or more benign agents such as iron. Most inorganic dusts, such as coal, asbestos, or silica, require prolonged exposure for at least 6 months, usually many years, at relatively high levels, for significant pulmonary disease to develop. However, disease can occur following shorter, more intense exposures. The response to agents such as beryllium or cobalt is much more idiosyncratic, and disease can occur after much lower exposure. The fibrogenic potential of a given

TABLE 13-5. Common Causes of Occupational Interstitial Lung Diseases

Free silica
Silicates
Fibrous–asbestos
Mixed dust
Coal
Metals
Beryllium
Hard metal (cobalt)

exposure depends on various factors such as the agent's ability to reach the lower respiratory tract; the dose, durability, and various physical and chemical properties of the agent; and individual host susceptibility factors.

Airway involvement in most pneumoconioses has traditionally been felt to be nonexistent or related to smoking. However, certain exposures such as asbestos can result in peribronchial fibrosis and mild airflow obstruction, and many can cause chronic bronchitis, which may be associated with chronic airways disease.

The overall prevalence of pneumoconioses in the United States is unknown but varies significantly among different exposed populations. Historically, the most common interstitial lung diseases were owing to inhalation of mineral dusts such as silica, asbestos, and coal dust (39). Worldwide, silicosis remains the most common pneumoconiosis (40). With improved industrial hygiene and reduced use in the United States, heavy exposure to these dusts has declined. However, several recent reports demonstrate that moderate and high levels of exposure can still exist, frequently in small uncontrolled workplaces, and can result in miniepidemics of disease (41,42). Even with overall improved control measures, the prevalence of these diseases remains high in many exposed populations because of the latency between exposure and disease (42,43).

Fibrotic lung diseases caused by agents that appear to involve immune-mediated mechanisms and which have less clear dose–response relationships, such as beryllium or hard metal, are more difficult to both diagnose and control, as disease may occur at lower exposure levels and in a more sporadic fashion.

Chest Radiography

The chest radiograph is the most important diagnostic test for occupational fibrotic disorders. It is critical that radiographs of high technical quality be obtained. The chest radiograph can be highly suggestive of a pneumoconiosis and is frequently sufficient, along with an appropriate exposure history, to establish a diagnosis. Chest radiography can be normal in approximately 10% to 20% or more of patients with interstitial lung disease.

An international uniform classification system, under the auspices of the International Labour Office (ILO) in Geneva, Switzerland, has evolved to evaluate chest radiographs for epidemiologic studies, clinical evaluation, and screening (44). The system classifies radiographic opacities according to shape, size, extent, and concentration. Pleural changes are also graded according to site, pleural thickening, and pleural calcification.

Computed Tomography

Much has been written about the role of computed tomography (CT) scanning in the evaluation of patients with occupational interstitial lung disease, primarily asbestosis (45,46). Conventional CT scanning (8- to 10-mm-thick slices) and high-resolution computed tomographic scanning (HRCT) (1- to 3-mm-thick slices) can be used to better evaluate pleural and parenchymal abnormalities, such as pleural plaques or focal pulmonary masses. In patients with suspected interstitial lung disease but a normal chest radiograph, HRCT can be helpful in identifying parenchymal abnormalities. When the diagnosis of an occupational interstitial lung disease is clear on the basis of the chest radiograph and history, CT and HRCT scanning may not be indicated.

Pulmonary Function and Cardiopulmonary Exercise Testing

Resting lung function testing is the most important tool to assess functional respiratory status (18). As with any interstitial fibrotic disease, physiologic testing in diffuse fibrotic occupational diseases typically shows a restrictive pattern with reduced lung volumes and decreased diffusing capacity (D_{LCO}). Airflow rates and FEV_1/FVC ratio are preserved unless there is coexisting airways disease. The findings on physiologic testing are not specific for a particular etiology, but they are important for evaluating dyspnea and assessing the degree of pulmonary impairment. In a given patient, chest radiographic findings, lung volumes, and D_{LCO} may or may not be correlated in assessing the extent of disease and functional impairment.

Cardiopulmonary exercise testing is helpful in evaluating a select group of patients with dyspnea and normal pulmonary function tests or dyspnea that appears out of proportion to the changes in lung function, and can help distinguish between cardiac, pulmonary, and deconditioning causes of dyspnea, as discussed in Chapter 6, Clinical Pulmonary Function Testing, Exercise Testing, and Disability Evaluation. However, in most patients with occupational interstitial lung disease, exercise testing is not necessary for diagnosis or management.

Bronchoscopy

Under certain circumstances when the diagnosis is not straightforward, bronchoscopy with transbronchial biopsy and bronchoalveolar lavage (BAL) may be helpful. Transbronchial biopsies yield small tissue samples that may be adequate to diagnose the presence of interstitial fibrosis but usually cannot determine specific etiology. They are most helpful in diagnosing granulomatous processes such as beryllium disease or HP. Although not routinely performed in many institutions, under certain circumstances BAL can be helpful, such as in the diagnosis of beryllium disease, for which a positive beryllium lymphocyte proliferation test (BeLPT) is diagnostic. Cells obtained from BAL contain dust particles such as asbestos, which may reflect current and possibly past exposures, and can confirm the exposure history.

Lung Biopsy

Open lung biopsy can be helpful when there is no clear cause of interstitial lung disease or an atypical presentation. To establish a diagnosis, histopathologic changes should be consistent with the known disease, and the suspected causative dusts or particles can, in most cases, be detectable in the lung. A number of methods to analyze dust content of tissue are available including light microscopic evaluation with polarization, bulk analytic techniques such as x-ray fluorescence, and microanalytic techniques such as scanning electron microscopy (47,48). If a patient with an interstitial lung disease of unclear etiology in whom an occupational or environmental cause is being considered undergoes open lung biopsy, more extensive particle analysis should be considered if light microscopic histologic examination is nondiagnostic. There are some limitations that should be remembered. Only particulates that are insoluble, retained in tissue, and at sufficient concentration will be detected. In addition, a positive finding indicates some degree of exposure, but not necessarily disease.

SILICOSIS

Silicosis is a chronic fibrosing disease of the lungs, produced by excessive inhalation of free crystalline silica dust. The ores of most minerals, from coal to gold, are generally found embedded in silica-containing rock in the earth's crust. Mining and quarrying have long been associated with a high incidence of silicosis. Hazardous exposure to silica dust also may occur in a wide variety of other industries such as foundry work, tunneling, sandblasting, pottery making, polishing, and the manufacture of glass, tiles, and bricks (39).

Silica, or silicon dioxide, can exist unbound to other minerals (free silica) and in either crystalline or amorphous states. Silicates are minerals containing silicon dioxide combined with other elements, such as talc, asbestos, mica, or kaolin. Inhalational exposure to most silica-containing minerals has been associated with some risk of pneumoconiosis. However, free crystalline silica dust is more likely to cause pulmonary fibrosis than either amorphous silica or nonasbestiform silicates.

Pathogenesis and Histologic Features

Respirable-sized silica particles deposited in the distal airways are readily ingested by scavenging alveolar macrophages or penetrating the interstitium. The alveolar macrophages become activated, then release a number of inflammatory mediators that initiate and perpetuate the processes of inflammation and fibrosis. Neutrophils, T lymphocytes, and other inflammatory cells contribute to the inflammatory and fibrotic processes, eventually resulting in the silicotic nodule (49).

Three types of silicosis have been described: (a) ordinary or simple chronic silicosis, in which exposure to relatively low concentrations of free silica dust has continued for 20 years or more; (b) accelerated silicosis, in which exposure to moderately high dust concentrations occurs, usually over a shorter time (4 to 8 years); and (c) acute silicosis, in which there is massive exposure to high concentrations of dust.

The formation of silicotic nodules in the pulmonary parenchyma and the hilar lymph nodes characterizes simple silicosis. The development of progressive massive fibrosis (PMF) may complicate simple silicosis. The lesions of PMF tend to be found in the upper lung zones and are composed of confluent nodules, often with obliterated blood vessels and bronchioles as well. With accelerated silicosis, the rate of progression is more rapid, and PMF occurs more frequently.

Acute silicosis is a relatively rare condition occurring only in workers exposed to very high concentrations of fine, particulate-free silica dust without adequate ventilation or personal protective equipment. Unlike the situation in chronic silicosis, the lungs show consolidation without silicotic nodules, and the alveolar spaces are filled with fluid similar to that found in pulmonary alveolar proteinosis (50).

Clinical Presentation

The most common form of silicosis is uncomplicated chronic simple silicosis, which is usually asymptomatic and is diagnosed on the basis of chest radiographic findings. Pulmonary function testing in patients with simple silicosis can be normal or demonstrate abnormalities consistent with mild restrictive or obstructive abnormalities (43). Significant dyspnea generally is seen only with patients who have complicated disease characterized by PMF. Complicated silicosis is associated with reduced lung volumes and diffusing capacity, nonreversible airflow obstruction, and arterial oxygen desaturation with exercise. Nodular lesions >1 cm in diameter are seen on chest radiography and can become confluent and retract the hila upward. Constitutional symptoms such as malaise, anorexia, and weight loss can occur with complicated disease. The major features of accelerated silicosis are similar to those of complicated chronic silicosis, but the course of the disease is abbreviated, and there is a greater chance that significant disability and respiratory failure will develop. Patients with acute silicosis present with marked dyspnea, fever, cough, and weight loss and usually progress rapidly to respiratory failure.

Diagnosis

The diagnosis of silicosis is based on (a) a history of sufficient silica exposure, (b) chest radiographic abnormalities consistent with silicosis, and (c) absence of other illnesses that mimic silicosis. Silica exposure occurs in a number of occupational settings, and the history of exposure may not always be obvious. The presence of diffuse nodular opacities on the chest radiograph of an individual known to have sustained prolonged exposure to silica is usually sufficient (see Fig. 13-2). Calcification of hilar lymph nodes and a classic "eggshell" pattern is not a consistent finding in silicosis, but when it is seen in patients with diffuse nodular lung disease, it generally excludes other diagnoses (see Fig. 13-3). Histologic evaluation is usually not necessary in these settings.

Associated Illnesses

Patients with silicosis have an increased risk of mycobacterial infection (involving atypical mycobacterial organisms as well as *Mycobacterium tuberculosis*) (51). The decreased resistance of the silicotic lung to mycobacterial infection appears related to impaired macrophage function. Tuberculosis should be suspected in any patient with silicosis whose symptoms or chest radiograph change more acutely. Various connective tissue disorders, particularly scleroderma, have been noted to occur with greater frequency in patients with silicosis (51). Caplan

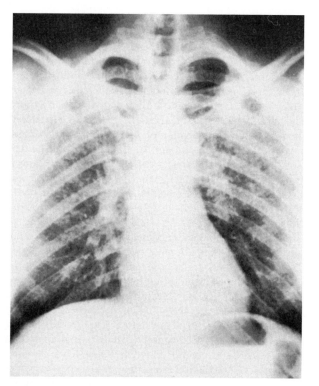

FIGURE 13-2. Typical simple silicosis with diffuse, bilateral nodular densities.

syndrome (rheumatoid arthritis and large lung nodules) occurs with silicosis as well as with coal workers' pneumoconiosis (CWP). There is an increased prevalence of circulating autoantibodies, such as antinuclear antibody and rheumatoid factor, among silicotic patients. Patients with silicosis are at increased risk of developing lung cancer (discussed in the following).

Treatment

There is no specific treatment for silicosis except removal from further exposure, which may not affect progression of the disease. Supportive therapy with the aim of preventing

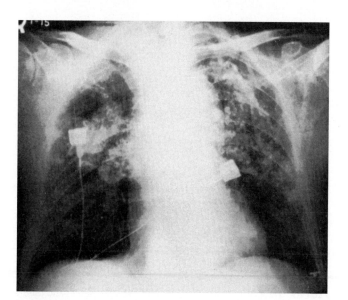

FIGURE 13-3. Eggshell calcification of hilar lymph nodes.

complications such as tuberculosis can be offered. Patients with silicosis should have annual screening for mycobacterial infection [i.e., purified protein derivative (PPD) skin testing] and prophylaxis is recommended for patients with positive PPD tests. Establishing the diagnosis of tuberculosis in a patient with silicosis can be challenging; a high index of suspicion remains important. Tuberculosis should be suspected if any rapid changes occur on the chest radiograph. When tuberculosis is superimposed on complicated silicosis, there may be no obvious radiographic changes. The use of induced sputum and fiber-optic bronchoscopy to obtain specimens for acid-fast staining and mycobacterial culture may increase the diagnostic yield. Because of the decreased responsiveness of silicotuberculosis to chemotherapy, multidrug regimens are recommended (51).

The treatment of silica-associated bronchitis and airflow obstruction is similar to that offered to any patient with chronic bronchitis (Chapter 9, Chronic Obstructive Lung Disease). Bronchodilator therapy can be effective for patients in whom a reversible obstructive component is present. The cessation of cigarette smoking is of obvious importance. Whole-lung lavage has been reported to be helpful in patients with acute silicosis presenting with a clinicopathologic picture consistent with pulmonary alveolar proteinosis.

NONMALIGNANT ASBESTOS-RELATED PULMONARY DISEASE

Asbestos is the generic name for a group of naturally occurring fibrous silicates. There are three main commercial types of asbestos: chrysotile, crocidolite, and amosite. Chrysotile fibers are somewhat curved or serpentine; crocidolite and amosite are needlelike or amphibole. Asbestos may cause several different types of disease involving the lungs and pleura and may also increase the risk of extrapulmonary neoplasms such as colon cancer. *Asbestosis* refers to the diffuse interstitial pulmonary fibrosis caused by asbestos exposure.

Epidemiology

Although asbestos has been valued since antiquity because of its resistance to fire, only during the last century has its mining and commercial use been extensive. Not until the 1930s did the magnitude of the asbestos hazard begin to be recognized. Use of asbestos in the United States has declined sharply since the mid-1970s, but worldwide use continues (39). Workers with potentially significant asbestos exposure include asbestos miners and millers; persons employed in the building trades and shipyards, such as insulation workers, pipe fitters, sheet metal workers, welders, asbestos removal workers; and workers involved in the manufacture or repair of automotive friction products. Although exposure to small amounts of asbestos fiber may contribute to the risk of malignancy, it is not generally associated with clinically significant, nonmalignant, asbestos-related pulmonary disease.

Asbestos-Related Pleural Disease

Asbestos exposure can cause discrete pleural thickening (pleural plaques), diffuse pleural thickening, rounded atelectasis, and benign exudative effusions (discussed in the preceding section) (38). All types of asbestos have the potential to induce asbestos-related pleural disease.

PLEURAL THICKENING. Circumscribed areas of pleural thickening or fibrosis, called *pleural plaques*, are the most common radiographic findings caused by chronic asbestos exposure and most commonly occur without asbestosis. Individuals with isolated pleural plaques are usually asymptomatic. Pathologically, plaques usually involve the parietal pleural surface, are composed mostly of collagen, and may become calcified. They have a latency of about 15 to 20 years following first exposure. Pleural plaques are most often visible on the PA chest radiograph along the lower lateral borders of the thoracic cavity and the central portions of the hemidiaphragms. Although there are other causes of unilateral pleural thickening and calcification (empyema, hemothorax, and thoracic trauma), the presence of bilateral pleural thickening is almost always due to asbestos exposure. Circumscribed plaques, in the absence of parenchymal asbestosis, are usually not associated with respiratory impairment. However, workers with radiographic evidence of plaques but no asbestosis can have mildly reduced lung volumes (37).

Diffuse pleural thickening, involving visceral as well as parietal pleura, is less common than circumscribed plaques but is more likely to be associated with mildly reduced lung volumes and interstitial changes on HRCT. Diffuse pleural thickening is believed to be a sequela of benign asbestos pleural effusions. Chest CT scanning provides the most sensitive and specific technique for identifying pleural plaques and diffuse pleural thickening.

Progression of pleural thickening to advanced asbestosis is not common. There is no evidence that pleural plaques undergo malignant transformation to mesothelioma.

ROUNDED ATELECTASIS. Localized fibrosis of the pleura involving the visceral as well as the parietal surfaces can entrap the adjacent lung parenchyma and mimic the radiographic appearance of a solitary pulmonary nodule. This phenomenon, known as *rounded atelectasis*, occurs with asbestos-related pleural disease. Rounded atelectasis may be recognized radiographically by an irregular shadow that tapers toward the hilum, the so-called comet tail sign, and can usually be differentiated from a more serious mass lesion by use of CT scanning.

Asbestosis

PATHOGENESIS, CLINICAL PRESENTATION, EVALUATION, AND DIAGNOSIS. Inhaled asbestos can generate reactive oxygen species, and also become phagocytosed by alveolar macrophages that become activated and can release various cytokines and inflammatory mediators that can recruit additional inflammatory and mesenchymal cells, resulting in an alveolitis and peribronchiolitis. In the early stages of asbestosis, a mixed leukocyte infiltration of the interstitial spaces, accompanied by varying degrees of organizing fibrosis, is typically present. The parenchymal interstitial fibrosis is similar to other interstitial lung diseases. All major types of asbestos are fibrogenic, although some studies have provided support for the concept that long, thin asbestos fibers have the greatest fibrogenic potential.

The clinical presentation of asbestosis is indistinguishable from that of other forms of interstitial pulmonary fibrosis. The most common symptom is progressive dyspnea, usually over a period of years. Cough, either nonproductive or productive, is common. The physical examination findings are nonspecific;

for example, bibasilar crackles and clubbing of the fingers can occur.

The diagnosis of asbestosis is usually based on a history of sufficient asbestos exposure with appropriate latency, duration, and intensity, and certain clinical, radiographic, and pulmonary function features. Moderate exposure with a latency of greater than 15 years and duration of greater than 6 months can result in asbestosis. The intensity of asbestos exposure can be determined by information on the job, industry, and use of personal protective equipment. Chest radiographic evidence of small, irregular opacities, a restrictive pattern of lung impairment; a reduced diffusing capacity; and bilateral crackles not cleared with cough are seen with the classic presentation. The certainty of the diagnosis of asbestosis increases as more of the criteria are met.

Chest radiographic evidence is the most important criteria in addition to the occupational history. The characteristic chest radiograph shows irregular or linear opacities with ILO profusion abnormalities (grade 1/0 or higher) distributed throughout the lung fields but more prominent in the lower zones (see Fig. 13-4). The most useful finding in the differential diagnosis is the presence of pleural thickening (Fig. 13-4). Diaphragmatic or pericardial calcification is almost a pathognomonic sign of asbestos exposure. However, asbestosis can occur without any visible pleural thickening. When chest x-ray findings are equivocal, HRCT is more sensitive and can provide evidence of interstitial fibrosis (45). However, when the diagnosis is clear on the basis of the chest radiograph and history, HRCT usually is not necessary for diagnosis.

Pulmonary function abnormalities usually indicate the presence of a restrictive defect with reduced lung volumes, diffusing capacity, and exercise tolerance. Asbestos, in the absence of cigarette smoking, can result in a mild degree of airflow

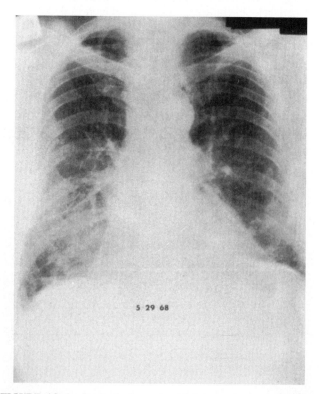

FIGURE 13-4. Typical asbestosis with "shaggy heart" and pleural plaques with diaphragm calcification.

obstruction (52). Although in population studies there is a correlation between pulmonary function and radiographic severity of asbestosis, in individual cases, such correlation may not be present.

OTHER TESTS. Bronchoscopy and lung biopsy are usually not necessary to make the diagnosis of asbestosis, but may be indicated in atypical presentations. BAL and transbronchial biopsy can rule out other causes of abnormality such as infection, sarcoidosis, or HP. Histopathologic material from lung biopsy can be used to identify and characterize the presence of fibrosis, inflammatory changes, and identify and quantify asbestos bodies or fibers. The presence of numerous asbestos bodies and asbestos fibers confirms the exposure history and suggests that the pulmonary fibrosis seen is related to asbestos exposure (see Fig. 13-5). However, asbestos can also be found in lung tissue from individuals without significant histories of occupational exposure (47).

PROGNOSIS AND TREATMENT. The natural history of patients with asbestosis is variable. Marked accelerated loss of pulmonary function can occur, but more stable disease with minimal or mild progression is more common (53). Progression of disease can occur following removal from exposure. A major concern is the increased risk of lung cancer, which is discussed below. Smoking cessation for active smokers is crucial.

Further asbestos exposure should be minimized. Steroids and immunosuppressive therapy probably have little beneficial effect on the course of the disease, although no controlled trials have been reported in the literature. Appropriate therapy of superimposed respiratory tract infections is important, and bronchodilator therapy is indicated if there is evidence of

a reversible obstructive component. Although there is no evidence that ongoing medical surveillance with annual chest radiography and spirometry is beneficial, such surveillance is commonly recommended.

COAL WORKERS' PNEUMOCONIOSIS

Chronic inhalation of coal dust can result in coal worker's pneumoconiosis (CWP) and chronic bronchitis without CWP, the latter discussed below (43). CWP occurs in either simple or, less commonly, complicated forms. Only a small percentage of miners with simple CWP ever develop complicated disease. The chest radiographic pattern of simple CWP is typically one of small nodular opacities. The opacities visible on chest radiographs of simple CWP are due to the presence of coal macules in the lungs. The diagnosis of complicated CWP is made when larger opacities (1 cm or larger in diameter) are seen on a chest radiograph (see Fig. 13-6). These large opacities represent masses of confluent fibrous tissue and may undergo cavitation secondary to either ischemic necrosis or superimposed tuberculous infection. It is unusual to see significant pneumoconiosis in miners who have spent less than 20 years underground. Chronic bronchitis from inhalation of coal dust is common among miners.

Pathology and Pathogenesis

The initial response to the inhalation of coal dust involves phagocytosis of the deposited dust by alveolar macrophages. Coal appears to be less fibrogenic than asbestos or silica but similar to these exposures, coal dust can result in increased reactive oxygen species and macrophage activation with production of various cytokines and growth factors (54). The

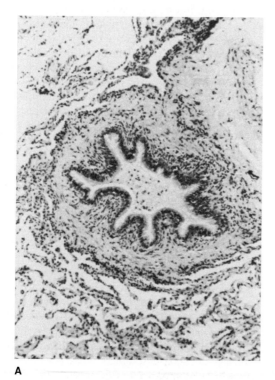

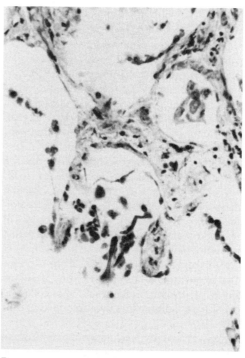

A **B**

FIGURE 13-5. A: Lung biopsy from a patient with asbestos showing peribronchiolar fibrosis. **B:** Intraalveolar asbestos bodies.

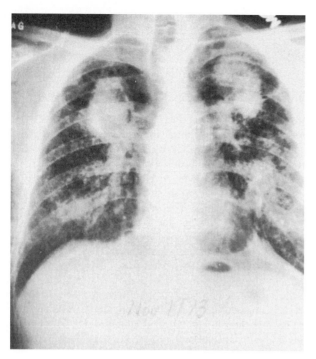

FIGURE 13-6. Coal workers' pneumoconiosis with progressive massive fibrosis.

factors that determine whether simple CWP progresses to complicated CWP are not well understood. The presence of silica in the retained dust and superimposed tuberculous infection can stimulate fibrosis. However, cases of complicated CWP can occur in the absence of either of these factors.

Clinical Evaluation and Diagnosis

Simple CWP is usually a relatively benign process. Symptoms of cough and dyspnea are common among coal miners and may be present in a given individual miner regardless of whether the chest radiograph shows pneumoconiosis. Complicated disease is now uncommon. Once the process of complicated disease begins, however, it generally results in PMF, even if there is no further exposure to coal dust. Miners with PMF are usually dyspneic to the point of being disabled. Pulmonary hypertension and cor pulmonale may be late sequelae.

The results of pulmonary function testing vary with the stage of CWP. With simple CWP, there are usually no gross abnormalities. However, significant reductions in lung function in coal miners have been documented in a number of epidemiologic studies (43,55). Decline in FEV_1 and the presence of irregular opacities have been correlated with cumulative dust exposure. Miners with complicated CWP can have obstructive, restrictive, or mixed ventilatory defects. There is an increased prevalence of autoantibodies in the serum of miners with CWP, usually without clinical manifestation of collagen-vascular disease. Caplan syndrome was first described in conjunction with CWP.

A diagnosis of CWP can usually be made on the basis of the exposure history and characteristic chest radiograph findings. A lung biopsy is rarely needed. Bronchitis and chronic obstructive pulmonary disease (COPD) can occur from exposure to coal mine dust in the absence of complicated pneumoconiosis

or smoking (43,55,56). Miners with CWP or bronchitis should try to minimize further mining exposures but do not necessarily have to leave mining, depending on the extent of their disease. Bronchospasm should be treated with standard bronchodilator therapy. For miners who smoke, smoking cessation should be strongly recommended.

BERYLLIUM- AND HARD METAL–RELATED DISEASE

Beryllium and cobalt are metals that can cause interstitial lung disease, probably through immunologically mediated mechanisms. Although more is known about the pathogenesis of chronic beryllium disease (CBD) than about hard metal (cobalt)-related lung disease, these diseases have several features in common: only a fraction of exposed workers appear to be susceptible; disease can occur at relatively low exposure levels, compared with those necessary to cause traditional pneumoconioses; and the exposure history is frequently less obvious than with exposures such as asbestos or coal dust. Thus, both the diagnosis and prevention of beryllium- and hard metal–related disease can be more challenging than with the traditional pneumoconioses.

Chronic Beryllium Disease

CBD is a chronic pulmonary and systemic granulomatous disease that is similar to sarcoidosis but is caused by chronic beryllium exposure. Acute high beryllium exposures can cause an acute pneumonitis, which is rarely seen.

EPIDEMIOLOGY. CBD was first recognized in the United States among employees frosting fluorescent light bulbs with beryllium oxide (BeO) during World War II. As beryllium use has increased in aerospace, electronics, and other high-technology industries, cases have become more widely dispersed. The reported prevalence of CBD in exposed workers is low, around 5% in most settings, but can be higher (57–59). As exposure is decreased, the incidence, but not necessarily the severity, appears to decrease. Cases of CBD from a metal refinery in which exposures may have been below OSHA standards have been reported (57–59). Beryllium is usually present as an alloy with other metals such as copper, aluminum, and nickel, and workers may not be aware of beryllium exposure.

PATHOGENESIS AND NATURAL HISTORY. Noncaseating granulomas identical to those seen in sarcoidosis are the pathologic hallmark of CBD (see Fig. 13-7). Although predominantly in the lung, these granulomas can be found in peripheral sites such as the liver and skin. CBD results from a beryllium-specific cell-mediated immune response, which can be demonstrated by the *in vitro* proliferative response of cultured T lymphocytes from BAL fluid or peripheral blood to beryllium (the BeLPT). Following exposure, beryllium is phagocytosed by macrophages and presented to lymphocytes, resulting in sensitization and proliferation of beryllium-specific CD4+ T cells and a T-helper 1-type cytokine response, which eventually leads to granuloma formation.

BeLPT is increasingly being used in workplace surveillance and can identify asymptomatic workers with beryllium sensitivity, which can progress to CBD, even in the absence of ongoing exposure (57). The natural history of beryllium sensitivity and CBD can be variable and difficult to predict (60). The latency

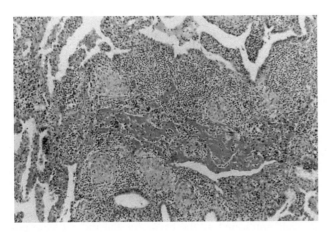

FIGURE 13-7. Lung biopsy from a patient with chronic beryllium disease showing lymphocytic alveolitis and noncaseating granulomas (H&E).

between exposure and manifestation of disease can range from months to more than 20 years. Susceptibility to beryllium sensitization appears to be related to polymorphisms in major histocompatibility complex (MHC) genes involved in beryllium presentation to T cells; a glutamic acid substitution at position 69 in the β chain of HLA DP1 has been associated with increased risk for CBD (61–63).

DIAGNOSIS AND TREATMENT. The most common symptoms of CBD are progressive exertional dyspnea and cough. Systemic complaints such as fatigue or weight loss can occur. Chest radiographs typically show diffuse interstitial infiltrates and bilateral hilar adenopathy in less than half the cases. Obstructive, restrictive, or mixed restrictive-obstructive patterns can be seen on pulmonary function testing. Diagnosis is based on a consistent clinical presentation, a history of beryllium exposure, beryllium-specific immune response (an abnormal BeLPT), and consistent lung histopathology. The history of beryllium exposure can be difficult to obtain because beryllium is frequently present as an alloy with other metals. Furthermore, because of the latency between exposure and clinical presentation, the relevant exposure history may have occurred many years in the past. The clinical presentation can include respiratory symptoms, compatible abnormalities on chest radiograph or chest CT scan, or altered pulmonary physiology (64).

Fiber-optic bronchoscopy with BAL and transbronchial biopsy are used to confirm sensitization and granulomatous inflammation. As noted, a positive BeLPT using peripheral blood or BAL lymphocytes is a specific test for beryllium sensitization. The test is more sensitive when performed on BAL lymphocytes (close to 100% sensitivity) than on peripheral blood lymphocytes (60% to 95%) (65,66).

Clinically, CBD can be difficult to distinguish from sarcoidosis. The presence of uveitis, erythema nodosum, and asymptomatic hilar adenopathy favor a diagnosis of sarcoidosis; a history of beryllium exposure and evidence of beryllium sensitization strongly support the diagnosis of CBD.

Patients with symptomatic CBD should be removed from further exposure. Spontaneous improvement after removal from further exposure can occur. Therapy follows the principles for sarcoidosis, including a trial of systemic steroids for symptomatic disease.

Hard Metal Disease

Exposure to hard metal, a cemented alloy of tungsten carbide with cobalt, can result in interstitial pulmonary fibrosis and asthma. Cobalt is probably the etiologic agent for both processes but may require the concomitant inhalation of other compounds such as metallic carbides or diamond dust (67). Cobalt dust has been shown experimentally to cause acute alveolitis, fibrosis, and bronchitis, whereas tungsten carbide without cobalt appears to be nontoxic (67,68). Diamond workers exposed to cobalt without any tungsten carbide have developed an interstitial disease histologically identical to hard metal disease, as well as specific airway sensitization to cobalt (67).

EPIDEMIOLOGY AND PATHOGENESIS. Exposure to cobalt is common and can occur during production or use of hard-metal tools and in industries such as diamond polishing. The reported prevalence of interstitial disease in exposed workers is relatively low, ranging from less than 1% (most studies) to more than 10% (67). Cobalt-induced asthma is probably more common, around 5% to 10%. Although usually occurring separately, cobalt-induced interstitial lung disease and asthma can occur in the same patient. An association of hard-metal disease with an HLA polymorphism has been reported (69).

The histologic finding is a fibrosing alveolitis, with characteristic multinucleated giant cells consisting of macrophages and alveolar epithelial cells. Multinucleated macrophages can be seen on BAL but can be a nonspecific finding.

CLINICAL PRESENTATION, DIAGNOSIS, AND MANAGEMENT. Cobalt-exposed workers can present with symptoms of occupational asthma, slowly progressive interstitial lung disease, or rapidly progressive interstitial pneumonitis. The latency from exposure to onset of hard-metal disease is variable, from a few to more than 20 years. Chest radiographs in patients with hard-metal disease typically demonstrate a diffuse reticulonodular pattern that tends to be more prominent in the mid- and lower-lung fields. Most commonly restrictive, but also obstructive or mixed, defects can be seen on pulmonary function testing.

A high level of suspicion and a careful occupational history are key to the diagnosis of hard metal disease. An open lung biopsy may be required. The characteristic lung pathology showing multinucleated giant cells is helpful. The detection of tungsten on lung biopsy confirms exposure. Cobalt, because it is more soluble than tungsten, is usually not detected. Cobalt in the blood and urine indicates current or recent exposure.

Hard-metal disease can progress after removal from exposure. Removal from further exposure, steroids, and bronchodilator therapy if airflow obstruction is present are the mainstay of therapy.

LESS COMMON PNEUMOCONIOSES

A number of other silicates, dusts, and metals can also cause pneumoconioses. Several of these are discussed below.

Talcosis

Talc is a hydrated magnesium silicate that is chemically related to asbestos. Because asbestos and silica are found in conjunction with talc, there is some uncertainty about the magnitude of the fibrogenic potential of pure talc. Significant talc exposure can occur during the mining of soapstone; the manufacture of ceramics, roofing materials, and rubber goods; and use of talcum powder. Pulmonary fibrosis can occur after many years of exposure to talc dust (70). Pulmonary fibrosis also may result from a microembolization process secondary to the intravenous injection of talc-containing pills by drug abusers. Pathologically, lesions similar to those of silicosis and asbestosis as well as foreign-body granulomas containing talc particles may be seen.

The clinical presentation is one of progressive dyspnea and productive cough. The initial chest radiographic appearance of talcosis is similar to that of asbestosis: The upper lung zones tend to be relatively spared, and mild pleural thickening and calcification may occur. However, talcosis may progress in a manner similar to that of silicosis with regard to the coalescence of lesions and the development of PMF. Studies of pulmonary function in patients with talcosis have demonstrated decreases in lung volumes and diffusing capacity.

Kaolin Pneumoconiosis

Kaolin, also called *China clay*, is a hydrated aluminum silicate used in the manufacture of ceramics, paint, paper, and cement. Epidemiologic studies are conflicting, but radiographic changes owing to excessive kaolin dust exposure (diffuse nodular opacities) are more prominent than clinical manifestations of disease. However, cases of kaolin-associated PMF have been reported.

Other Silicates

Fuller's earth (attapulgite) is an absorbent aluminum silicate clay now used primarily in oil refining and in the building of foundry molds. Although massive fibrosis can occur, the pneumoconiosis associated with fuller's earth is relatively benign.

Micas are a group of complex aluminum silicates that have been associated with the development of interstitial pulmonary fibrosis in heavily exposed workers. Mica also has been associated with pleural thickening. It is unclear whether these findings may be caused by contamination with silica or asbestos.

Mixed-dust pneumoconiosis refers to lung disease seen in workers exposed to crystalline silica and other dusts, such as coal or iron oxides. The disease is similar to silicosis, the amount of fibrosis depending on the amount of free silica exposure.

Manmade Vitreous Fibers

A variety of synthetic silicate mineral fibers (MMVFs) have increasingly been used as substitution for asbestos. There are several types of MMVFs: mineral (slag or rock) wools, glass fibers, and ceramic fibers. Most common are mineral wools and glass fiber, which can cause skin and respiratory tract irritation and bronchitis but have not been shown to cause pneumoconiosis (71). There is concern that the less common refractory ceramic fibers may be more fibrogenic and carcinogenic, based on animal data and fiber shape (72). A possible relationship between refractory ceramic fiber exposure and pleural plaques and a small reduction in forced vital capacity (FVC) has been reported (73). Epidemiologic studies in populations exposed to MMVF have not clearly demonstrated that

symptomatic pneumoconiosis is a consequence of such exposure, although there may not yet be adequate follow-up time to entirely exclude the possibility (74). The carcinogenic potential is discussed below.

Graphite Pneumoconiosis

Graphite is pure crystallized carbon that can be either natural or synthetic. Most natural deposits are contaminated with some free silica, whereas synthetic graphite is relatively pure. Graphite is used in the manufacture of steel, pencils, electric equipment, and in the printing industry. Excessive graphite dust exposure may lead to chest radiographic changes identical to those of simple CWP, and concomitant silica exposure has been implicated as the cause for the more severe pulmonary fibrosis occasionally seen in graphite-exposed workers. An uncommon pneumoconiosis has also been associated with inhalation of pure synthetic graphite dust.

Aluminum Pneumoconiosis

Aluminum is produced from bauxite, a naturally occurring hydrous aluminum oxide ore. Pulmonary fibrosis has been reported in workers exposed to aluminum oxide dust and fumes. This condition, known as *Shaver disease*, typically presents as progressive dyspnea, and has been attributed to free silica contamination. However, exposure to aluminum powder that does not contain silica can result in pulmonary fibrosis and is associated with an increased incidence of spontaneous pneumothorax. The pathologic features of this uncommon pneumoconiosis are interstitial fibrosis, initially in the upper lobes, and emphysematous bleb formation on pleural surfaces. The aluminum content in the lung is greatly increased. Pulmonary function testing reveals a restrictive disorder.

Work in aluminum potrooms has been associated with obstructive lung disease, termed *potroom asthma*, although the exact causative agent is not clear (75,76).

Flock Worker's Lung

A unique interstitial lung disease has been reported in workers in nylon flock plants (77,78). Nylon flock is finely cut nylon filaments used to make fabrics such as upholstery covering. Exposed workers have developed interstitial lung disease with typical symptoms, reduced lung volumes and D_{LCO}, and increased interstitial markings on chest radiographs. Histopathologic findings have revealed a characteristic lesion, a lymphocytic bronchiolitis, and peribronchiolitis with lymphoid hyperplasia (77,78). Most have improved away from work although recovery has not always been complete. Recent clinical, epidemiologic, and toxicologic studies suggest that the causative agent is respirable fragments of nylon.

Miscellaneous Dusts

Exposure to the dusts of metals such as iron, barium, tin, antimony, and titanium may lead to radiographically visible deposits in the lungs without corresponding parenchymal fibrosis and pulmonary function impairment. Pneumoconiosis can also occur as a result of chronic exposure to dusts of synthetic materials such as Bakelite and polyvinyl chloride, but there is some controversy about the degree of functional impairment that may result.

CHRONIC BRONCHITIS AND CHRONIC AIRWAYS DISEASE

Occupational or industrial bronchitis is defined as bronchitis that is caused or aggravated by exposures at work. The pathophysiology and interrelationships between chronic bronchitis, emphysema, and asthma, all of which are associated with airflow obstruction, are discussed in Chapter 8, Asthma, and Chapter 9, Chronic Obstructive Lung Disease. A wide range of different occupational exposures to gases, mineral dusts, metals, fumes, and organic substances (see Table 13-6) can cause bronchitic symptoms. Irritant exposures can cause airway inflammation and mucous hypersecretion, both of which can be associated with airflow obstruction.

A growing literature now supports the conclusion that occupational exposure to chronic irritant exposures can cause airflow obstruction and accelerated loss of ventilatory function, not just bronchitic symptoms, recently summarized in an American Thoracic Society (ATS) Statement (15). A number of both community- and workforce-based epidemiologic studies have shown an association between chronic irritant exposures and airflow obstruction, chronic obstructive lung disease, or accelerated loss of lung function in populations occupationally exposed to irritating dusts, gases, and fumes, such as miners or cotton workers (15,79–82). However, this occupational effect is usually of lesser magnitude than the detrimental effect of cigarette smoke on lung function. Epidemiologic studies suggest that the interaction between smoking and occupational exposures in causing bronchitic symptoms and reduced lung function may be additive or multiplicative (15,82). Certain host susceptibility factors such as preexisting nonspecific airway hyperresponsiveness may predispose certain workers to chronic airways obstruction.

Pathologic data support the notion that occupational exposure to certain dusts is capable of causing chronic airflow obstruction (83). Coal miners, for example, had more centrilobular

TABLE 13-6. Partial List of Agents That Can Cause Chronic Bronchitis

Minerals
  Coal
  Oil mist
  Silica
  Silicates
  MMVF
Metals
  Welding fumes
Organic substances
  Cotton
  Grain
  Wood
Irritant gases
  Sulfur dioxide
  Chlorine
  Nitrogen dioxide
Smoke
Diesel exhaust

MMVF, manmade vitreous fibers.

emphysema than controls in an autopsy study, and severity of emphysema was related to lung burden of coal dust (84). Autopsy studies in South African gold miners exposed to silica have also documented a risk of emphysema related to dust exposure, even in nonsmoking miners (82).

Common exposures that can cause chronic bronchitis and which have also been documented to cause accelerated loss of lung function are asbestos, silica, coal, grain, wood, and cotton dusts. Chronic exposures that can cause chronic bronchitic symptoms and that are suspected of causing respiratory impairment are MMVF, welding fumes, firefighting exposures, irritant gases, and diesel exhaust.

Clinical Evaluation

The clinical evaluation of a patient with suspected occupational bronchitis is similar to that of any patient with chronic bronchitic symptoms. It is important to assess whether bronchitic symptoms alone are present or whether asthma, emphysema, or some other pulmonary process is involved. Any environmental or occupational exposures that may be contributing to the patient's pulmonary condition should be identified. No specific diagnostic tests are available for occupational bronchitis, and a causal role for occupational exposures can be difficult to establish, especially in a smoker. The presence of eye and upper respiratory tract irritation and inflammation, a temporal association between symptoms and workplace exposures (especially early in the course), and co-workers with similar symptoms suggest work-relatedness. Chronic bronchitic symptoms can persist after removal from exposure.

Pulmonary function testing, such as D_{LCO}, is useful both diagnostically and to assess level of impairment. Methacholine challenge testing may be indicated if the history suggests asthma and spirometry is normal. Chest radiography should also be performed.

When a patient's bronchitis is suspected to be work-related, interventions to reduce or eliminate exposure to the putative agent(s) or process are justified. Engineering controls are preferable to the use of respirators. If the patient improves with such intervention, then the diagnosis of work-relatedness is supported. However, symptoms may persist after cessation of exposure. Commonly, bronchitis is of multifactorial etiology, with smoking playing a role. Smoking cessation is key. Medical surveillance to detect accelerated loss of ventilatory function or airway hyperresponsiveness is recommended. The medical management of work-related chronic bronchitis is similar to that caused by smoking alone.

Data available concerning prognosis in patients with irritant-induced chronic bronchitis are limited. However, as discussed, exposure to inhaled irritants may be associated with both symptoms of chronic bronchitis and small decrements in lung function.

MALIGNANCIES OF THE RESPIRATORY TRACT AND PLEURA

This section addresses the occupational and environmental causes of lung carcinoma and other cancers of the respiratory tract and pleura. (See Chapter 14, Lung Neoplasms, for an extensive discussion of the pathogenesis, evaluation, and treatment of lung cancer.)

SINONASAL CANCERS

Sinonasal cancers are rare in the general population but have been associated with several different occupational exposures, most strongly with nickel and wood dust (85,86). Increased risk has also been reported with exposure to chromium and formaldehyde (87,88). Cigarette smoking and alcohol use are not major causes of sinonasal cancers.

LARYNGEAL CANCER

Laryngeal cancer, nearly all squamous histology, usually is attributed to tobacco smoke and alcohol exposure. Epidemiologic studies suggest an increased risk of laryngeal cancer in workers exposed to asbestos, nickel, and metal working fluids (89,90).

LUNG CANCER

Lung cancer, once a rare tumor, is now the leading cause of cancer death in both men and women in the United States. Starting with the demonstration by Doll in the 1950s of a causal role for cigarette smoke, epidemiologic techniques have identified a number of respiratory tract carcinogens (91–3). Although cigarette smoking is the single greatest risk factor for lung cancer, occupational and environmental exposures are important preventable causes. Estimates of the percentage of lung cancers attributable to occupational and environmental factors have varied widely, ranging from 5% to more than 30% of all cases, with more recent estimates around 9% of lung cancer among men and 2% among women (91,92). A number of agents are considered known or suspected human lung carcinogens (see Table 13-7). Additionally, studies have shown an excess risk of lung cancer among members of several trades and industries, although identification of specific carcinogenic agents has not been possible.

There is considerable evidence that diet is also an important factor in the etiology and prevention of lung cancer. Most consistently, a diet high in fruit and vegetables has been shown to be associated with a reduced risk of lung cancer (94). What component(s) of such a diet produce(s) the protective effect remains unclear. Clinical chemoprevention trials of vitamin A and β-carotene in preventing lung cancer among high-risk smokers and asbestos-exposed workers found either no effect

TABLE 13-7. Known Occupational Lung Carcinogens

Substance	Examples of Exposure Settings
Asbestos	Insulation workers, shipyard workers
Arsenic	Smelting of copper, zinc, lead; pesticide production
Beryllium	Beryllium production, processing
Chloromethyl ether	Production workers
Chromium	Chromate production, pigment manufacture, electroplating
Mustard gas	Production workers, soldiers
Nickel	Nickel refining, plating
Polycyclic aromatic hydrocarbons	Coke oven workers, rubber workers, aluminum reduction workers, roofers
Radon	Uranium mining, hard rock mining
Silica	Mining, foundries

or increased risk of lung cancer in those taking the vitamin supplementation (95,96).

From a public health standpoint, recognition of risk factors can lead to prevention. For those already exposed, recognition of the degree of risk allows the intelligent application of screening strategies or interventions to reduce risk of lung cancer.

Clinical Evaluation and Management

The evaluation of any patient with lung cancer should include a careful occupational and environmental exposure history. To determine whether a given exposure caused the patient's cancer, the following guidelines are recommended. The clinician must determine what potential lung carcinogens the patient was exposed to and assess the dose of exposure and latency as best as possible. A thorough smoking history, including passive smoke exposure, is essential. When more than one carcinogen is present, dose, timing, and relative risk of each exposure should be considered. It can be difficult to quantify risk because of more than exposure, and it is common to conclude that both exposures contributed to the patient's cancer. The management of a patient with occupationally induced lung cancer is similar to that of any patient with lung cancer.

Known Lung Carcinogens

ARSENIC. Arsenic has been shown to increase lung cancer risk in workers engaged in smelting, pesticide manufacturing, and other industries with arsenic exposure, with a clear dose–response relationship and a latency of about 25 years (93). Arsenic is believed to be a late-stage promoter of lung cancer.

ASBESTOS. Numerous studies have established that asbestos causes lung cancer, which is a far more important cause of death than mesothelioma in asbestos-exposed workers (72,97–102). However, several areas of debate remain, such as the carcinogenic potential of different types of asbestos fibers, the magnitude of the synergistic effect between asbestos and cigarette smoke, whether asbestosis or asbestos exposure is the risk factor, and the risks of low-level exposures.

Asbestos-related lung cancer is indistinguishable from lung cancer owing to smoking alone or other causes. Latency between exposure and disease peaks at 20 to 30 years with a distribution of cell types comparable to that among the general population (103). Although the location of tumors is more frequently in the lower lobes, this feature is insufficiently specific to determine etiology in an individual patient. Although estimates have varied, the risk of lung cancer clearly increases with the extent of asbestos exposure and is more common in smokers. Smokers with asbestosis are clearly at highest risk, with up to 40% developing lung cancer (72,97). However, studies have shown that individuals with occupational asbestos exposure without parenchymal changes also have an increased risk of lung cancer (97). Cigarette smoke clearly potentiates the carcinogenic effects of asbestos, with studies showing both additive and synergistic effects. Among nonsmoker asbestos-exposed workers, the relative risk of lung cancer is increased by a factor of approximately 5; among smokers, the risk is increased by a factor of approximately 10; and among smoking asbestos-exposed workers, the relative risk is increased by a factor of at least 15 (additive) to greater than 50 (synergistic)

(97,100,104). Cessation of smoking is the most important step in cancer prevention for previously exposed individuals, although control of asbestos exposure is also imperative.

The dose–response relationship at low levels of asbestos exposure is less clear. In some cohort studies, the dose–response relationship does not include zero risk, suggesting that there is no threshold or "safe" level of exposure. Other data favors the existence of a safe threshold, such as cohort mortality studies showing no increased risk at low exposure, low-dose animal studies, negative studies among residents with low-level exposure, and studies suggesting that asbestos-related lung cancers occur only in those with asbestosis. If there is an increased risk of lung cancer at low doses, the risk is small.

The mechanism of asbestos-related carcinogenesis is probably linked to the processes of oxidant generation, lung inflammation, and fibrosis (105). Asbestos likely acts primarily as a promoting rather than an initiating agent. There is mounting evidence that both the physical dimensions and surface chemical characteristics of the fibers are important. All major forms of asbestos appear to be associated with an increased risk of lung cancer, although chrysotile may be less hazardous than the amphiboles (amosite, crocidolite, and tremolite).

BERYLLIUM. The epidemiologic data linking beryllium to lung cancer has been controversial, based primarily on a limited number of cohort and case control studies of beryllium production workers exposed to very high, historic levels, or patients with CBD (91,106,107). Questions concerning small relative risks, exposure misclassification, lack of adequate smoking data, other confounders, and relevance to current exposures have been raised (106,108,109). The association between beryllium and lung cancer has been supported by animal studies, and the International Agency for Research on Cancer (IARC) has classified beryllium as "definitely carcinogenic to humans."

CHLOROMETHYL ETHERS AND MUSTARD GAS. Alkylating agents used in the chemical and pharmaceutical industries, such as bischloromethyl ether (BCME) and mustard gas [bis(2-chloroethyl) sulfide], are highly carcinogenic. A number of studies have documented that BCME exposure is strongly associated with an increased risk of lung cancer, especially small-cell carcinomas at a young age. Smoking does not appear to further increase the risk of cancer among BCME-exposed workers (110).

CHROMIUM. Hexavalent chromium, used in chromate production, electroplating, pigment manufacture, and the ferrochromium industry, has been associated with an increased relative risk of lung cancer (106).

NICKEL. Nickel exposure (among nickel mining and refinery workers) has been associated with excess lung cancer rates, with a mean latency of about 20 years (86,91,106). Metallic nickel has not been associated with an increased risk of lung cancer. Nickel oxides and sulfides appear to be most carcinogenic.

POLYAROMATIC HYDROCARBONS. Polyaromatic hydrocarbons (PAHs) are a complex mix of a number of widespread substances generated during the incomplete combustion of carbonaceous products such as coal, oil, pitch, and tar. PAHs are also present in cigarette smoke and diesel exhaust. A number of studies have demonstrated that a variety of workers exposed to PAHs—such as coke oven workers, printers, roofers, aluminum production workers, railroad workers, and truck drivers—have an increased risk of lung cancer (111,112).

RADON. Radon is an inert gas that is a decay product of uranium-238. Radon decays with a particle emission to various short-lived radon daughters. Underground uranium miners exposed to radon and its decay products have a marked increased risk of developing lung cancer, with a preponderance of small cell carcinoma, although other cell types are also increased (91,93,113). Cigarette smoke and radon most likely interact more than additively in increasing the risk for lung cancer. Excess lung cancer rates have been found in other types of miners such as tin, iron, and lead miners (113). The potential risk of domestic radon is discussed in the following section.

CRYSTALLINE SILICA. In 1996, the IARC reclassified crystalline silica as a definite human carcinogen (43,72,114). Several recent studies have reported an increased risk of lung cancer among miners, foundry workers, and other silica-exposed workers (72). The risk of lung cancer is highest in those with chronic silicosis compared with those with only silica exposure, but it is unclear whether silicosis is required for silica-associated lung cancer (115).

Suspected Lung Carcinogens

Vinyl chloride monomer and acrylonitrile, both animal carcinogens, are suspected human respiratory tract carcinogens. Excess lung cancer mortality in human populations exposed to acrylonitrile has been shown, but the magnitude of the effect is relatively small and variable. There is also evidence that cadmium exposure as well as occupational exposure to diesel exhaust is associated with increased risk of lung cancer (91). MMVFs include rock and slag wool, glass fibers, and ceramic fibers. Some excess lung cancer risk has been reported in MMVF-exposed cohorts, but without a strong dose–response relationship (72). Ceramic fibers can cause malignant mesothelioma in rodents, but there are insufficient human data. A small increased risk of lung cancer in formaldehyde-exposed workers has also been reported.

Workers in several industries such as foundries, rubber industry, welding, and printing have been shown to be at increased risk of lung cancer in some studies. However, the etiologic agents are unclear, and confounding by smoking and other exposures can limit the findings.

Risk Factors for Lung Cancer in the Environment

There has been increasing interest in the role of environmental exposures such as environmental tobacco smoke (ETS), air pollution, and domestic radon in the causation of lung cancer. The nonmalignant respiratory effects of these and other exposures present in indoor and ambient air are discussed in the final section of this chapter.

DOMESTIC RADON. Exposure to radon in homes, derived primarily from rock, soil, and drinking water, is a potential risk factor for lung cancer (116–118). Average domestic radon exposures in the United States range from 0.8 to 1.5 pCi per L, well below the levels experienced by miners. However, cumulative lifetime exposures comparable to those of miners probably exist in a small percentage of American homes. Most estimates of the risk of domestic radon are based on extrapolations from studies of miners to lower indoor levels. These risk assessments estimate that about 5,000 to 20,000 deaths annually in the United States (approximately 3% to 15% of all lung cancer deaths) are attributable to radon (116–118). Case–control studies have found both an increased relative risk of lung cancer associated with increased domestic radon levels and no increased risk (116–118). In smokers, the best way to reduce the risk of lung cancer is to stop smoking, regardless of domestic radon levels. If very high domestic radon measurements are found (e.g., above 5 to 10 pCi per L in a living area), it is reasonable to consider home mitigation techniques such as improved ventilation.

ENVIRONMENTAL TOBACCO SMOKE. ETS contains sidestream smoke (SS) released from the burning cigarette and mainstream smoke (MS) exhaled by the smoker. Passive smokers are exposed to the same carcinogenic constituents of tobacco smoke as smokers, although generally at lower doses and in different relative concentrations. A large number of epidemiologic studies have shown a significantly increased risk of lung cancer (typically 20% to 25%) in nonsmokers from exposure to ETS, typically 20% to 25% (116,119–122). Workplace ETS has also been shown to be a risk factor for lung cancer (120). Because of the large number of people exposed to ETS and the relatively high incidence of lung cancer, a small increase in lung cancer risk owing to ETS exposure is of great public health importance.

AIR POLLUTION. Outdoor ambient air pollution is a complex and variable mixture of natural and manmade pollutants such as products of combustion such as oxides of nitrogen, sulfur oxides, fine particulate matter, and carbon monoxide, photochemically derived agents such as ozone, and so-called hazardous pollutants (primarily carcinogens such as asbestos, benzene, or PAH). Methodologic challenges such as quantification of air pollution exposures and controlling for confounders such as cigarette smoking and occupational exposures have hampered epidemiologic studies of lung cancer risk and other diseases associated with air pollution, discussed in the following section. Despite these challenges, there is growing evidence suggesting an increased risk of lung cancer associated with air pollution (123,124). With regard to specific agents, recent meta-analyses of occupational studies have suggested that ambient exposure to diesel exhaust may pose a potential problem (111,112).

Another concern is whether indoor air pollution such as household coal smoke or other heating or cooking smoke increases the risk of lung cancer. Studies from China suggest that household cooking smoke may increase this risk (116).

ASBESTOS IN BUILDINGS. Low-level asbestos exposure is ubiquitous. Exposures in buildings, especially schools and public buildings, which frequently contain friable and decaying asbestos, have created great anxiety. The primary concern about low-level exposure is the risk of mesothelioma and lung cancer. As discussed, the magnitude of this risk, if any, is controversial. Although the risk of cancer from such exposures is undoubtedly extremely low, it is unlikely to be zero. In considering public policy and personal decisions, the risks of low-level asbestos exposure should be considered in the context of other risks in life, and the costs of remediation likewise need to be weighed against other costs and financial decisions.

MALIGNANT MESOTHELIOMA

Malignant mesotheliomas are rare tumors of the pleura or peritoneum that in most cases are associated with a history of asbestos exposure (38,125,126). Additional risk factors may include radiation, viruses, and genetic factors (125). Although there is some dose–response relationship, mesotheliomas may occur with relatively short-term and low-level asbestos exposures. Mesotheliomas have been reported to occur in family members of asbestos workers and persons living near shipyards. Patients can be free of obvious radiographic evidence of asbestos exposure, unlike the situation with asbestos-related lung cancer. The latency period is in the range of 30 to 40 years. Pleural cases are more common than peritoneal (126).

The relative carcinogenicity of the different asbestos fiber types is an area of debate. Although all types probably can cause mesothelioma, chrysotile, the most common fiber type in the United States, is the least likely to cause mesothelioma, whereas the amphiboles crocidolite and amosite appear to have the highest potential for inducing mesotheliomas (38). In contrast to what has been observed with bronchogenic carcinoma, cigarette smoking does not increase the risk of mesothelioma.

The most common presenting symptom in patients with pleural mesothelioma is chest pain. Dyspnea, weight loss, and cough may also be present (38). A pleural effusion is frequently seen on the chest radiograph. CT scanning can confirm the presence of a pleural-based mass(es). The pleural fluid is exudative, and cytology examination frequently is insufficiently sensitive or specific to confirm the diagnosis. Histologic differentiation from poorly differentiated adenocarcinoma metastatic to the pleura or reactive mesothelial cells can be difficult. Open pleural biopsy with adequate tissue specimens and an experienced pathologist are often required to make the diagnosis. Mesotheliomas extend locally and can also metastasize. New therapeutic options are under investigation, but the prognosis remains poor (38).

AIR POLLUTION: NONMALIGNANT RESPIRATORY EFFECTS

There has been increasing concern about the adverse health effects of both outdoor ambient and indoor air pollution (127–129). Patients and the public frequently turn to physicians with questions and advice concerning the risks of radon, ETS, and other air pollutants. This section reviews the known nonmalignant pulmonary health effects of ambient (outdoor) and indoor air pollution and which populations may be more susceptible to these effects. The role of these exposures in contributing to lung cancer is addressed in the preceding section.

AMBIENT AIR POLLUTION

Numerous natural and manmade sources contribute to outdoor air pollution. There are three broad groups of exposures that may have adverse respiratory health effects: (a) combustion of fossil fuels that often contain sulfur [fine particulate matter ($PM_{2.5}$), oxides of nitrogen, sulfur oxides, acidic aerosols]; (b) photochemically generated pollution [e.g., ozone from oxides of nitrogen and volatile organic compounds (VOCs)]; and (c) hazardous air pollutants (primarily carcinogens as noted above, but some VOCs have been associated with increased asthma symptoms) (130). The Environmental Protection Agency (EPA) regulates the ambient levels of six so-called criteria pollutants under the Clean Air Act for which there is sufficient scientific knowledge of health effects at specific exposure levels (see Table 13-8). Three major types of research have contributed to such knowledge (epidemiologic studies, controlled human exposure studies, and inhalational toxicologic studies using animals). Exposures to air pollutants almost always occur as part of a complex mixture, not individually, and interactions between different exposures probably exist but are difficult to determine.

Epidemiologic studies have shown that air pollution can be associated with increased respiratory symptoms and exacerbations of asthma and bronchitis, although which particular component, such as fine particles or ozone, is responsible can be difficult to determine (128–130). Multiple studies have shown an association between air pollution (primarily fine particles) and daily mortality, largely from cardiopulmonary causes (124). The effects of specific pollutants at ambient levels of exposure are summarized (127–129).

Sulfur oxides and particulate matter are produced by sulfur-containing fuels such as coal and petroleum. Particulate matter is also produced by other types of combustion; motor vehicle emissions are an important source. Particulate matter can exacerbate asthma and COPD and increase respiratory symptoms in children. Asthmatics are especially sensitive to the bronchoconstrictor effects of sulfur dioxide. Children exposed to acid vapor (e.g., nitric acid) in Southern California may have decreased growth of lung function (131).

Acute exposure to ambient levels of ozone has been shown to result in lung inflammation and transient reductions in lung function. Although the chronic effects of such exposures remain unclear, there is evidence suggesting that childhood exposures may lead to airway remodeling (132,133). Persons with asthma appear to have enhanced airway inflammatory responses to ozone, and multiple epidemiologic studies have demonstrated that ozone exposure is associated with increased risk of asthma exacerbations and possibly developing asthma (127,134–136).

Carbon monoxide (CO) can bind to hemoglobin and carboxyhemoglobin, reducing oxygen delivery to tissues. In patients with coronary artery disease, CO may exacerbate myocardial ischemia and arrhythmias.

In summary, current data suggest that ambient levels of certain pollutants may increase respiratory symptoms and exacerbate underlying respiratory or cardiac diseases, primarily in children, asthmatics, and persons with COPD, ischemic heart disease, or congestive heart failure. Cigarette smoking may have additive or synergistic effects with air pollutants, and exercise may also increase the likelihood of adverse effects (by increasing the effective dose).

INDOOR AIR POLLUTION

Increasing concern is being raised about the adverse health effects of indoor air, and various symptoms have been attributed to exposures in the indoor environment. Illnesses that have been related to building exposures are allergic respiratory diseases such as sinusitis, rhinitis, asthma, and HP caused by exposures to molds, spores, chemicals, or other substances (137,138). Building-related infectious diseases such as Legionnaires' disease are well recognized. It is important to obtain a careful occupational and environmental exposure history in any patient presenting with such an illness. Nonindustrial environments should not be assumed to be clean and free of significant exposures.

Sick Building Syndrome

Since the 1970s, nonspecific symptoms among employees in indoor, nonindustrial environments have increasingly come to medical attention. The term *Sick Building Syndrome* (SBS) refers to nonspecific complaints that usually involve mucous membrane and upper respiratory irritative symptoms, headaches, fatigue, difficulty concentrating, and odor complaints, which are associated with a particular building(s) (137,138). Symptoms generally improve away from that indoor environment. Other causes for the patient's complaints should be evaluated and ruled out. The cause of these symptoms is typically multifactorial with inadequate ventilation systems an important contributing factor in most cases. Other factors such as indoor air pollutants (i.e., ETS, particulates, and cleaning agents), job satisfaction, and work stress may be involved. Physician recommendations concerning the workplace environment may facilitate ventilation improvements or other beneficial interventions in the work environment.

Environmental Tobacco Smoke

Children of parents who smoke are at increased risk of respiratory infections, respiratory symptoms, asthma exacerbations, and reduced lung function, compared with children of nonsmoking parents (139–141). More recently, ETS exposure has been associated with respiratory tract disease in adults, including exacerbation of asthma, sensory irritation symptoms, lower respiratory tract symptoms, lung function impairment and increased risk of lung cancer, as noted above (121,122,140).

TABLE 13-8. United States Ambient Air Quality Criteria Pollutants and Principal Health Effects

Pollutant	Health Effects
Ozone	Acute respiratory symptoms, decrements in lung function, respiratory tract inflammation, and asthma exacerbation
Particulate matter ($PM_{2.5}$, PM_{10})	Asthma, COPD exacerbation, increased cardiopulmonary mortality
Sulfur oxides	Asthma exacerbation
Nitrogen dioxide	Asthma/COPD exacerbation; increased susceptibility to respiratory tract infections
Carbon monoxide	Ischemic heart disease exacerbation
Lead	Decreased cognitive function in children

COPD, chronic obstructive pulmonary disease.

Biomass and Fossil Fuels

Indoor use of wood, coal, kerosene, or gas for heating and cooking releases various combustion products. Epidemiologic studies have shown an association between these exposures and childhood respiratory symptoms and also possibly an increased risk of childhood infections, asthma, and reduced lung function (142,143).

Carbon Dioxide

Carbon dioxide, which is produced primarily by human respiration, is frequently measured as an indicator of adequate indoor ventilation CO_2 results that are commonly presented to physicians caring for patients with complaints of SBS. Normal CO_2 levels are frequently measured despite inadequate ventilation, and such measurements are frequently not helpful in managing complaints of inadequate indoor air quality or SBS.

Molds

"Mold" is the common term for multicellular fungi that grow as a mat of intertwined microscopic filaments (hyphae). Molds are pervasive in the outdoor environment and may also be present indoors under certain conditions, primarily excessive moisture from leaks in roofs or walls, plant pots, or pet urine. The most common indoor molds are *Cladosporium*, *Penicillium*, *Aspergillus*, and *Alternaria*. Other molds that can grow indoors are *Fusarium*, *Trichoderma*, and *Stachybotrys*; the presence of these molds usually indicates a problem with water leakage or damage. Recently, there has been substantial public concern about the health effects of indoor molds, particularly when *Stachybotrys chartarum* has been identified (144–148).

Molds and other fungi may adversely affect human health through three processes: (a) allergy, (b) infection, and (c) toxicity from mycotoxins. Allergic responses to mold are common and include allergic asthma, rhinitis, and HP. Serious fungal infections are primarily a concern with immunocompromised subjects. Some species of fungi, such as some molds, can produce secondary metabolites, or mycotoxins. Mycotoxins can cause acute intoxication if ingested in moldy food or inhaled in high concentration in occupational settings (ODTS). Current evidence does not support the concern that residential or office-building exposures to toxigenic mold species can result in disease in humans.

The public furor over indoor molds began in 1994 when the Centers for Disease Control (CDC) reported that a cluster of cases of acute idiopathic pulmonary hemorrhage (AIPH) in infants was associated with home contamination by *S. chartarum*. After a subsequent detailed reevaluation of the original data, the CDC concluded that there was insufficient evidence to causally link the cluster of AIPH to *S. chartarum* exposure (149). Recent critical reviews of the literature have concluded that a causal relationship has not been established between building-related symptoms and indoor exposures to *S. chartarum* or other molds that can produce mycotoxins (144,145,147,150).

Homes and buildings that have excessive moisture or water damage can lead to enhanced growth of fungi. Allergic and hypersensitivity responses such as asthma, rhinitis, and less commonly HP can occur related to indoor mold exposures. For any patient with asthma, rhinitis, or HP, the health care provider should inquire about home, school, or work-building conditions associated with the patient's symptoms. If the conditions suggest indoor mold contamination, further evaluation by an individual trained in the evaluation of building environments (e.g., an industrial hygienist) is warranted, as well as measures to reduce moisture and mold contamination.

REFERENCES

1. Rosenstock L, Cullen MR, eds. *Textbook of clinical occupational and environmental medicine*. Philadelphia, WB Saunders, 1994.
2. Rom WN *Environmental and occupational medicine*, 3rd ed. Boston: Little, Brown and Company, 1998.
3. Harber P, Schenker MB, Balmes JR, eds. *Occupational and environmental respiratory disease*. St. Louis, Mosby–Year Book, 1996.
4. Hendrick DJ, Burge PS, Beckett WS, Churg A, eds. *Occupational disorders of the lung: recognition, management and prevention*. London: WB Saunders, 2002.
5. Bernstein IL. *Asthma in the workplace*, 2nd ed. New York: Marcel Dekker Inc, 1999.
6. Hellgren J, Karlsson G, Toren K. The dilemma of occupational rhinitis: management options. *Am J Respir Med* 2003;2:333–341.
7. Siracusa A, Desrosiers M, Marabini A. Epidemiology of occupational rhinitis: prevalence, aetiology and determinants. *Clin Exp Allergy* 2000;30:1519–1534.
8. Slavin RG. Occupational rhinitis. *Ann Allergy Asthma Immunol* 2003;90:2–6.
9. Tarlo SM, Liss GM. Occupational asthma: an approach to diagnosis and management. *CMAJ* 2003;168:867–871.
10. Malo JL, Chan-Yeung M. Occupational asthma. *J Allergy Clin Immunol* 2001;108:317–328.
11. Arnaiz NO, Kaufman JD. New developments in work-related asthma. *Clin Chest Med* 2002;23:737–747.
12. Vandenplas O, Malo JL. Definitions and types of work-related asthma: a nosological approach. *Eur Respir J* 2003;21:706–712.
13. van Kampen V, Merget R, Baur X. Occupational airway sensitizers: an overview on the respective literature. *Am J Ind Med* 2000; 38:164–218.
14. Lombardo LJ, Balmes JR. Occupational asthma: a review. *Environ Health Perspect* 2000;108(Suppl 4):697–704.
15. Balmes J, Becklake M, Blanc P, et al. American Thoracic Society Statement: Occupational contribution to the burden of airway disease. *Am J Respir Crit Care Med* 2003;167:787–797.
16. Venables KM, Chan-Yeung M. Occupational asthma. *Lancet* 1997;349:1465–1469.
17. Anees W. Use of pulmonary function tests in the diagnosis of occupational asthma. *Ann Allergy Asthma Immunol* 2003;90:47–51.
18. Sood A, Redlich CA. Pulmonary function tests at work. *Clin Chest Med* 2001;22:783–793.
19. Cullinan P. Occupational asthma, IgE and IgG [editorial; comment]. *Clin Exp Allergy* 1998;28:668–670.
20. Perfetti L, Cartier A, Ghezzo H, et al. Follow-up of occupational asthma after removal from or diminution of exposure to the responsible agent: relevance of the length of the interval from cessation of exposure. *Chest* 1998;114:398–403.
21. Vandenplas O, Toren K, Blanc PD. Health and socioeconomic impact of work-related asthma. *Eur Respir J* 2003;22:689–697.
22. Brooks SM, Hammad Y, Richards I, et al. The spectrum of irritant-induced asthma: sudden and not-so-sudden onset and the role of allergy. *Chest* 1998;113:42–49.
23. Tarlo SM. Workplace irritant exposures: do they produce true occupational asthma? *Ann Allergy Asthma Immunol* 2003;90:19–23.
24. Nemery B. Reactive fallout of World Trade Center dust. *Am J Respir Crit Care Med* 2003;168:2–3.
25. Alberts WM, do Pico GA. Reactive airways dysfunction syndrome. *Chest* 1996;109:1618–1626.
26. Tarlo SM. Workplace respiratory irritants and asthma. *Occup Med* 2000;15:471–484.
27. Redlich CA, Karol MH. Diisocyanate asthma: clinical aspects and immunopathogenesis. *Int Immunopharmacol* 2002;2:213–224.
28. Castellan RM. Cotton dust. In: Harper P, Schenker M, Balmes J, eds. *Occupational and environmental respiratory disease*. St. Louis: Mosby–Year Book, 1996:401–419.

29. Niven RM, Fletcher AM, Pickering CA, et al. Chronic bronchitis in textile workers. *Thorax* 1997;52:22–27.

30. Schachter EN Byssinosis and other textile dust-related lung diseases. In: Rosenstock L, Cullen MR, eds. *Textbook of clinical occupational and environmental medicine*. Philadelphia, WB Saunders, 1994.

31. Chan-Yeung M, Enarson DA, Kennedy SM. State of the art: the impact of grain dust on respiratory health. *Am Rev Respir Dis* 1992;145:476–487.

32. Spurzem JR, Romberger DJ, Von Essen SG. Agricultural lung disease. *Clin Chest Med* 2002;23:795–810.

33. Huy T, De Schipper K, Chan-Yeung M, et al. Grain dust and lung function. Dose-response relationships. *Am Rev Respir Dis* 1991; 144:1314–1321.

34. Rabinowitz PM, Siegel MD. Acute inhalation injury. *Clin Chest Med* 2002;23:707–715.

35. Schwartz DA. Acute inhalational injury. *Occup Med* 1987;2:297–318.

36. Sferlazza SJ, Beckett WS. The respiratory health of welders. *Am Rev Respir Dis* 1991;143:1134–1148.

37. Rudd RM. New developments in asbestos-related pleural disease. *Thorax* 1996;51:210–216.

38. Cugell DW, Kamp DW. Asbestos and the pleura: a review. *Chest* 2004;125:1103–1117.

39. Wagner GR. Asbestosis and silicosis. *Lancet* 1997;349:1311–1315.

40. van Sprundel MP. Pneumoconioses: the situation in developing countries. *Exp Lung Res* 1990;16:5–13.

41. Nugent K, Perrotta D, Dodson RF, et al. A cluster of silicosis in sandblasters. *Am Rev Respir Dis* 1990;142:1466.

42. Rosenman KD, Reilly MJ, Kalinowski DJ, et al. Silicosis in the 1990s. *Chest* 1997;111:779–786.

43. Cohen R, Velho V. Update on respiratory disease from coal mine and silica dust. *Clin Chest Med* 2002;23:811–826.

44. ILO. Guidelines for the use of ILO international classification or radiographs of pneumoconioses. *Occup. Safety Health* 1980;22:48.

45. Akira M. High-resolution CT in the evaluation of occupational and environmental disease. *Radiol Clin North Am* 2002;40: 43–59.

46. Begin R, Ostiguy G, Filion R, et al. Computed tomography in the early detection of asbestosis. *Br J Ind Med* 1993;50:689–698.

47. Churg A, Green FHY. *Pathology of occupational lung disease*, 2nd ed. New York: Igaku-Shoin Medical Publishers, 1998.

48. Abraham JL, Burnett BR, Hunt A. Development and use of a pneumoconiosis database of human pulmonary inorganic particulate burden in over 400 lungs. *Scanning Microsc* 1991;5:95–104; discussion 5–8.

49. Mossman BT, Churg A. Mechanisms in the pathogenesis of asbestosis and silicosis. *Am J Respir Crit Care Med* 1998;157: 1666–1680.

50. Xipell JM, Ham KN, Price CG, et al. Acute silicoproteinosis. *Thorax* 1977;32:104–111.

51. American Thoracic Society Committee of the Scientific Assembly on Environmental and Occupational Health. Adverse effects of crystalline silica exposure. *Am J Respir Crit Care Med* 1997; 155:761–768.

52. Griffith DE, Garcia JG, Dodson RF, et al. Airflow obstruction in nonsmoking, asbestos- and mixed dust-exposed workers. *Lung* 1993;171:213–224.

53. Beckett WS. Diagnosis of asbestosis. Primum non nocere. *Chest* 1997;111:1427–1428.

54. Schins RP, Borm PJ. Mechanisms and mediators in coal dust induced toxicity: a review. *Ann Occup Hyg* 1999;43:7–33.

55. Coggon D, Newman Taylor A. Coal mining and chronic obstructive pulmonary disease: a review of the evidence. *Thorax* 1998;53: 398–407.

56. Attfield MD, Hodous TK. Pulmonary function of U.S. coal miners related to dust exposure estimates. *Am Rev Respir Dis* 1992; 145:605–609.

57. Maier LA. Genetic and exposure risks for chronic beryllium disease. *Clin Chest Med* 2002;23:827–839.

58. Henneberger PK, Cumro D, Deubner DD, et al. Beryllium sensitization and disease among long-term and short-term workers in a beryllium ceramics plant. *Int Arch Occup Environ Health* 2001; 74:167–176.

59. Kreiss K, Mroz MM, Zhen B, et al. Risks of beryllium disease related to work processes at a metal, alloy, and oxide production plant. *Occup Environ Med* 1997;54:605–612.

60. Newman LS, Lloyd J, Daniloff E. The natural history of beryllium sensitization and chronic beryllium disease. *Environ Health Perspect* 1996;104(Suppl 5):937–943.

61. McCanlies EC, Kreiss K, Andrew M, et al. HLA-DPB1 and chronic beryllium disease: a HuGE review. *Am J Epidemiol* 2003; 157:388–398.

62. Richeldi L, Sorrentino R, Saltini C. HLA-DPB1 glutamate 69: a genetic marker of beryllium disease. *Science* 1993;262:242–244.

63. Wang Z, White PS, Petrovic M, et al. Differential susceptibilities to chronic beryllium disease contributed by different Glu69 HLA-DPB1 and -DPA1 alleles. *J Immunol* 1999;163:1647–1653.

64. Maier LA, Newman LS. Beryllium disease. In: Rom WN, ed. *Environmental and occupational medicine*, 3rd ed. Philadelphia: Lippincott-Raven Publishers, 1998:1021–1035.

65. Rossman MD, Kern JA, Elias JA, et al. Proliferative response of bronchoalveolar lymphocytes to beryllium. A test for chronic beryllium disease. *Ann Intern Med* 1988;108:687–693.

66. Kreiss K, Wasserman S, Mroz MM, et al. Beryllium disease screening in the ceramics industry. Blood lymphocyte test performance and exposure-disease relations. *J Occup Med* 1993;35:267–274.

67. Cugell DW. The hard metal diseases. *Clin Chest Med* 1992;13: 269–279.

68. Lison D, Lauwerys R, Demedts M, et al. Experimental research into the pathogenesis of cobalt/hard metal lung disease. *Eur Respir J* 1996;9:1024–1028.

69. Potolicchio I, Mosconi G, Forni A, et al. Susceptibility to hard metal lung disease is strongly associated with the presence of glutamate 69 in HLA-DP beta chain. *Eur J Immunol* 1997;27: 2741–2743.

70. Gibbs AE, Pooley FD, Griffiths DM, et al. Talc pneumoconiosis: a pathologic and mineralogic study. *Hum Pathol* 1992;23:1344–1354.

71. De Vuyst P, Dumortier P, Swaen GM, et al. Respiratory health effects of man-made vitreous (mineral) fibres. *Eur Respir J* 1995;8: 2149–2173.

72. Steenland K, Stayner L. Silica, asbestos, man-made mineral fibers, and cancer. *Cancer Causes Control* 1997;8:491–503.

73. Lockey J, Lemasters G, Rice C, et al. Refractory ceramic fiber exposure and pleural plaques. *Am J Respir Crit Care Med* 1996;154: 1405–1410.

74. Cowie HA, Wild P, Beck J, et al. An epidemiological study of the respiratory health of workers in the European refractory ceramic fibre industry. *Occup Environ Med* 2001;58:800–810.

75. Kongerud J, Boe J, Soyseth V, et al. Aluminium potroom asthma: the Norwegian experience. *Eur Respir J* 1994;7:165–172.

76. Soyseth V, Boe J, Kongerud J. Relation between decline in FEV_1 and exposure to dust and tobacco smoke in aluminium potroom workers. *Occup Environ Med* 1997;54:27–31.

77. Kern DG, Crausman RS, Durand KT, et al. Flock worker's lung: chronic interstitial lung disease in the nylon flocking industry. *Ann Intern Med* 1998;129:261–272.

78. Eschenbacher WL, Kreiss K, Lougheed MD, et al. Nylon flock-associated interstitial lung disease. *Am J Respir Crit Care Med* 1999;159:2003–2008.

79. Trupin L, Earnest G, San Pedro M, et al. The occupational burden of chronic obstructive pulmonary disease. *Eur Respir J* 2003; 22:462–469.

80. Balmes JR. Occupational airways diseases from chronic low-level exposures to irritants. *Clin Chest Med* 2002;23:727–35–vi.

81. Hnizdo E, Sullivan PA, Bang KM, et al. Association between chronic obstructive pulmonary disease and employment by industry and occupation in the US population: a study of data from the Third National Health and Nutrition Examination Survey. *Am J Epidemiol* 2002;156:738–746.

82. Hnizdo E, Vallyathan V. Chronic obstructive pulmonary disease due to occupational exposure to silica dust: a review of epidemiological and pathological evidence. *Occup Environ Med* 2003;60:237–243.

83. Churg A, Wright JL. Airway wall remodeling induced by occupational mineral dusts and air pollutant particles. *Chest* 2002; 122:306S–309S.

84. Cockcroft A, Seal RM, Wagner JC, et al. Post-mortem study of emphysema in coalworkers and non-coalworkers. *Lancet* 1982;2: 600–603.

85. Demers PA, Boffetta P, Kogevinas M, et al. Pooled reanalysis of cancer mortality among five cohorts of workers in wood-related industries. *Scand J Work Environ Health* 1995;21:179–190.

86. Doll R, Mathews JD, Morgan LG. Cancers of the lung and nasal sinuses in nickel workers: a reassessment of the period of risk. *Br J Ind Med* 1977;34:102–105.

87. Luce D, Gerin M, Leclerc A, et al. Sinonasal cancer and occupational exposure to formaldehyde and other substances. *Int J Cancer* 1993;53:224–231.

88. Satoh N, Fukuda S, Takizawa M, et al. Chromium-induced carcinoma in the nasal region. A report of four cases. *Rhinology* 1994;32:47–50.

89. Smith AH, Handley MA, Wood R. Epidemiological evidence indicates asbestos causes laryngeal cancer. *J Occup Med* 1990;32:499–507.

90. Calvert GM, Ward E, Schnorr TM, et al. Cancer risks among workers exposed to metalworking fluids: a systematic review. *Am J Ind Med* 1998;33:282–292.

91. Steenland K, Loomis D, Shy C, et al. Review of occupational lung carcinogens. *Am J Ind Med* 1996;29:474–490.

92. Doll R, Peto R. The causes of cancer: quantitative estimates of avoidable risks of cancer in the United States today. *J Natl Cancer Inst* 1981;66:1191–1308.

93. Samet JM, ed. *Epidemiology of lung cancer*. New York: Marcel Dekker Inc, 1994.

94. Ziegler RG, Mayne ST, Swanson CA. Nutrition and lung cancer. *Cancer Causes Control* 1996;7:157–177.

95. The Alpha-Tocopherol, Beta Carotene Cancer Prevention Study Group. The effect of vitamin E and beta carotene on the incidence of lung cancer and other cancers in male smokers. *N Engl J Med* 1994; 330:1029–1035.

96. Omenn GS, Goodman GE, Thornquist MD, et al. Effects of a combination of beta carotene and vitamin A on lung cancer and cardiovascular disease. *N Engl J Med* 1996;334:1150–1155.

97. Hillerdal G, Henderson DW. Asbestos, asbestosis, pleural plaques and lung cancer. *Scand J Work Environ Health* 1997;23:93–103.

98. Nurminen M, Tossavainen A. Is there an association between pleural plaques and lung cancer without asbestosis? *Scand J Work Environ Health* 1994;20:62–64.

99. Landrigan PJ, Nicholson WJ, Suzuki Y, et al. The hazards of chrysotile asbestos: a critical review. *Ind Health* 1999;37:271–280.

100. Lee PN. Relation between exposure to asbestos and smoking jointly and the risk of lung cancer. *Occup Environ Med* 2001;58:145–153.

101. Goodman M, Morgan RW, Ray R, et al. Cancer in asbestos-exposed occupational cohorts: a meta-analysis. *Cancer Causes Control* 1999;10:453–465.

102. Weiss W. Asbestosis: a marker for the increased risk of lung cancer among workers exposed to asbestos. *Chest* 1999;115:536–549.

103. Brodkin CA, McCullough J, Stover B, et al. Lobe of origin and histologic type of lung cancer associated with asbestos exposure in the Carotene and Retinol Efficacy Trial (CARET). *Am J Ind Med* 1997;32:582–591.

104. Hammond EC, Selikoff IJ, Seidman H. Asbestos exposure, cigarette smoking and death rates. *Ann N Y Acad Sci* 1979;330:473–490.

105. Manning CB, Vallyathan V, Mossman BT. Diseases caused by asbestos: mechanisms of injury and disease development. *Int Immunopharmacol* 2002;2:191–200.

106. Hayes RB. The carcinogenicity of metals in humans. *Cancer Causes Control* 1997;8:371–385.

107. Sanderson WT, Ward EM, Steenland K, et al. Lung cancer case-control study of beryllium workers. *Am J Ind Med* 2001;39:133–144.

108. Levy PS, Roth HD, Hwang PM, et al. Beryllium and lung cancer: a reanalysis of a niosh cohort mortality study. *Inhal Toxicol* 2002;14:1003–1015.

109. Gordon T, Bowser D. Beryllium: genotoxicity and carcinogenicity. *Mutat Res* 2003;533:99–105.

110. Blair A, Kazerouni N. Reactive chemicals and cancer. *Cancer Causes Control* 1997;8:473–490.

111. Lipsett M, Campleman S. Occupational exposure to diesel exhaust and lung cancer: a meta-analysis. *Am J Public Health* 1999;89:1009–1017.

112. Kagawa J. Health effects of diesel exhaust emissions—a mixture of air pollutants of worldwide concern. *Toxicology* 2002;181-182:349–353.

113. Reger RB, Morgan WK. Respiratory cancers in mining. *Occup Med* 1993;8:185–204.

114. Wilbourn JD, McGregor DB, Partensky C, et al. IARC reevaluates silica and related substances. *Environ Health Perspect* 1997;105:756–759.

115. Checkoway H, Franzblau A. Is silicosis required for silica-associated lung cancer? *Am J Ind Med* 2000;37:252–259.

116. Boffetta P, Nyberg F. Contribution of environmental factors to cancer risk. *Br Med Bull* 2003;68:71–94.

117. Lubin JH, Boice JD Jr. Lung cancer risk from residential radon: meta-analysis of eight epidemiologic studies. *J Natl Cancer Inst* 1997;89:49–57.

118. Neuberger JS, Gesell TF. Residential radon exposure and lung cancer: risk in nonsmokers. *Health Phys* 2002;83:1–18.

119. Leonard CT, Sachs DP. Environmental tobacco smoke and lung cancer incidence. *Curr Opin Pulm Med* 1999;5:189–193.

120. Adlkofer F. Lung cancer due to passive smoking—a review. *Int Arch Occup Environ Health* 2001;74:231–241.

121. Jaakkola MS. Environmental tobacco smoke and health in the elderly. *Eur Respir J* 2002;19:172–181.

122. Brownson RC, Figgs LW, Caisley LE. Epidemiology of environmental tobacco smoke exposure. *Oncogene* 2002;21:7341–7348.

123. Katsouyanni K, Pershagen G. Ambient air pollution exposure and cancer. *Cancer Causes Control* 1997;8:284–291.

124. Pope CA 3rd, Burnett RT, Thun MJ, et al. Lung cancer, cardiopulmonary mortality, and long-term exposure to fine particulate air pollution. *JAMA* 2002;287:1132–1141.

125. Carbone M, Kratzke RA, Testa JR. The pathogenesis of mesothelioma. *Semin Oncol* 2002;29:2–17.

126. Britton M. The epidemiology of mesothelioma. *Semin Oncol* 2002;29:18–25.

127. Vedal S. Update on the health effects of outdoor air pollution. *Clin Chest Med* 2002;23:763–75–vi.

128. Committee of the Environmental and Occupational Health Assembly of the American Thoracic Society. Health effects of outdoor air pollution. Part 2. *Am J Respir Crit Care Med* 1996;153:477–498.

129. Committee of the Environmental and Occupational Health Assembly of the American Thoracic Society. Health effects of outdoor air pollution. *Am J Respir Crit Care Med* 1996; 153:3–50.

130. Delfino RJ Epidemiologic evidence for asthma and exposure to air toxics: linkages between occupational, indoor, and community air pollution research. *Environ Health Perspect* 2002;110(Suppl 4):573–589.

131. Gauderman WJ, Gilliland GF, Vora H, et al. Association between air pollution and lung function growth in southern California children: results from a second cohort. *Am J Respir Crit Care Med* 2002;166:76–84.

132. Kunzli N, Lurmann F, Segal M, et al. Association between lifetime ambient ozone exposure and pulmonary function in college freshmen—results of a pilot study. *Environ Res* 1997;72:8–23.

133. Schelegle ES, Miller LA, Gershwin LJ, et al. Repeated episodes of ozone inhalation amplifies the effects of allergen sensitization and inhalation on airway immune and structural development in Rhesus monkeys. *Toxicol Appl Pharmacol* 2003;191:74–85.

134. Salvi S. Pollution and allergic airways disease. *Curr Opin Allergy Clin Immunol* 2001;1:35–41.

135. Delfino RJ, Gong H Jr, Linn WS, et al. Asthma symptoms in Hispanic children and daily ambient exposures to toxic and criteria air pollutants. *Environ Health Perspect* 2003;111:647–656.

136. McConnell R, Berhane K, Gilliland F, et al. Asthma in exercising children exposed to ozone: a cohort study. *Lancet* 2002;359:386–391.

137. Menzies D, Bourbeau J. Building-related illnesses. *N Engl J Med* 1997;337:1524–1531.

138. Redlich CA, Sparer J, Cullen MR. Sick-building syndrome. *Lancet* 1997;349:1013–1016.

139. Tutka P, Wielosz M, Zatonski W. Exposure to environmental tobacco smoke and children health. *Int J Occup Med Environ Health* 2002;15:325–335.

140. Eisner MD. Environmental tobacco smoke and adult asthma. *Clin Chest Med* 2002;23:749–761.

141. Chan-Yeung M, Dimich-Ward H. Respiratory health effects of exposure to environmental tobacco smoke. *Respirology* 2003;8:131–139.

142. Zhang J, Smith KR. Indoor air pollution: a global health concern. *Br Med Bull* 2003;68:209–225.

143. Boman BC, Forsberg AB, Jarvholm BG. Adverse health effects from ambient air pollution in relation to residential wood

combustion in modern society. *Scand J Work Environ Health* 2003; 29:251–260.

144. Chapman JA, Terr AI, Jacobs RL, et al. Toxic mold: phantom risk vs science. *Ann Allergy Asthma Immunol* 2003;91:222–232.

145. Hardin BD, Kelman BJ, Saxon A. Adverse human health effects associated with molds in the indoor environment. *J Occup Environ Med* 2003;45:470–478.

146. Kolstad HA, Brauer C, Iversen M, et al. Do indoor molds in nonindustrial environments threaten workers' health? A review of the epidemiologic evidence. *Epidemiol Rev* 2002;24:203–217.

147. Kuhn DM, Ghannoum MA. Indoor mold, toxigenic fungi, and Stachybotrys chartarum: infectious disease perspective. *Clin Microbiol Rev* 2003;16:144–172.

148. Rogers CA. Indoor fungal exposure. *Immunol Allergy Clin North Am* 2003;23:501–518.

149. Update: Pulmonary hemorrhage/hemosiderosis among infants—Cleveland, Ohio, 1993-1996. *MMWR* 2000; 49:180–184.

150. Nordness ME, Zacharisen MC, Fink JN. Toxic and other non-IgE-mediated effects of fungal exposures. *Curr Allergy Asthma Rep* 2003;3:438–446.

CHAPTER 14

Lung Neoplasms

Lynn T. Tanoue
Darryl C. Carter
Richard A. Matthay

EPIDEMIOLOGY
Tobacco Smoking
Environmental Tobacco Smoke
Gender
Environmental Air Pollution
Occupational Factors
Chemoprevention
Diet
Genetic Factors

PATHOLOGY
Bronchogenic Carcinoma
Other Pulmonary Neoplasms

CLINICAL MANIFESTATIONS
Symptoms and Signs
Metabolic Manifestations
Neurologic Manifestations
Skeletal Manifestations
Dermatologic Manifestations

DIAGNOSIS
Screening Techniques for Early Diagnosis of Lung Cancer
Chest Imaging

Sputum Cytology
Bronchoscopy
Needle Aspiration Biopsy
Pleural Biopsy

STAGING CLASSIFICATION

STAGING PROCEDURES
Noninvasive Staging
Invasive Staging
Evaluation for Extrapulmonary Metastasis

APPROPRIATE INVESTIGATION OF A SOLITARY PERIPHERAL PARENCHYMAL MASS

TREATMENT
Non–Small Cell Lung Cancer
Small Cell Lung Cancer
Palliative Care

Lung cancer is the leading cause of death from cancer in the United States and worldwide (1,2). It is estimated that in 2004, in the United States, cancer of the lung and bronchus will account for 13% of all new cancer diagnoses (1). Lung cancer is responsible for 28% of deaths attributable to cancer in this country. It is anticipated that in 2004 in the United States, 91,930 deaths in men and 68,510 deaths in women will be due to lung cancer (1) (see Figs. 14-1 and 14-2). The relative significance of lung cancer as a cause of mortality in the United States is evident when one appreciates that it is the cause of more deaths annually than the three next most common causes of cancer death (colon and rectum, breast, and prostate) combined.

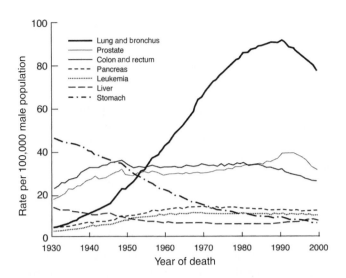

FIGURE 14-1. Annual age-adjusted cancer death rates at selected sites for men in the United States from 1930 to 1990. Age is adjusted to the 2000 US standard population. (From Jemal A, Tiwari RC, Murray T, et al. Cancer statistics. *CA Cancer J Clin* 2004;54:8–29, with permission.)

The World Health Organization (WHO) International Agency for Research on Cancer (IARC) estimated that approximately 900,000 deaths related to lung cancer occurred worldwide in the year 2000, with more than 50% of these deaths occurring in developed nations (2). A wide geographic range of lung cancer incidence rates is well documented and is demonstrated in Table 14-1. This global variation may be related to such factors as differences in occupational or environmental exposures or in local cancer reporting mechanisms, but it almost surely reflects differences in the degree of cigarette use by different populations (3). Although public health interventions, litigation, and education have contributed to a decline

TABLE 14-1. Lung Cancer: Worldwide Crude Incidence Rate, 2000 (Cases per 100,000 Population)

Region	Men	Women
World	29.57	11.22
More developed countries	91.49	28.74
Less developed countries	17.44	6.75
Africa		
Eastern	1.39	1.04
Middle	2.72	0.46
Northern	9.01	1.93
Southern	12.43	7.32
Western	1.05	0.35
Carribbean	25.29	9.56
Central America	13.89	5.94
South America	18.41	7.25
North America	78.39	54.75
Asia		
Eastern	38.60	55.48
Southeastern	18.34	7.07
South Central	7.76	1.75
Western	20.15	3.56
Europe		
Eastern	87.18	15.10
Northern	73.47	37.52
Southern	95.90	15.22
Western	83.90	19.44
Australia/New Zealand	58.56	28.18

From Ferlay J, et al. Cancer incidence, mortality, and prevalence worldwide. In: *Globocan 2000*. Lyon: IARC Press, 2001, with permission.

in smoking and in lung cancer rates in the United States, the potential for the lung cancer epidemic to be sustained in developing countries presents a daunting challenge to global public health efforts.

EPIDEMIOLOGY

The dramatic increases in lung cancer incidence through the 20th century strongly suggest the influences of new exposures to carcinogenic substances. Landmark epidemiologic studies conducted in the United States and Britain in the 1950s were the first in a now enormous body of evidence unequivocally linking lung cancer to cigarette smoking (4–6). Although the risk of lung cancer is related primarily to active cigarette smoking, other etiologic entities have been identified as well, including a number of occupational carcinogenic agents, passive inhalation of environmental tobacco smoke (ETS), domestic exposure to radon, and air pollution. In a recent review on the epidemiology of lung cancer, Alberg and Samet have summarized current epidemiologic evidence for lung cancer risk factors (3). On the basis of the available data, they have concluded that active smoking is responsible for 90% of lung cancer cases, occupational exposure to carcinogens for 9% to 15% of cases, radon for 10% of cases, and outdoor air pollution for 1% to 2% of cases, with the combined risk of these factors exceeding 100% because of interactions that can occur between the various exposures (3). However, it is increasingly clear that the etiology of lung cancer is multifactorial, involving more than a simple association with a single exposure. The influence

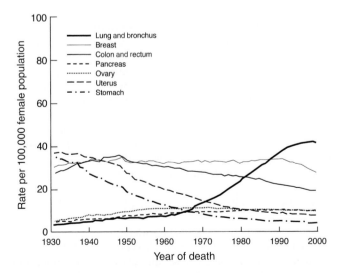

FIGURE 14-2. Annual age-adjusted cancer deaths at selected sites for women in the United States from 1930 to 2000. Age is adjusted to the 2000 US standard population. (From Jemal A, Tiwari RC, Murray T, et al. Cancer statistics. *CA Cancer J Clin* 2004;54:8–29, with permission.)

of environmental carcinogens may have additive or even synergistic effects, and other influences undoubtedly contribute to the risk for the development of lung cancer. Dietary factors, for example, may contribute both risk to and protection from lung cancer. Further, new molecular biologic techniques may allow us in the future to understand the role of genetic susceptibility in the development of lung cancer. Perhaps the most powerful message from the vast literature about lung cancer epidemiology is that many of the most important factors relating to lung cancer risk are modifiable and are therefore potentially preventable.

TOBACCO SMOKING

Tobacco smoking is the most important risk factor for the development of lung cancer. Evidence incriminating tobacco as a causative agent for cancer in humans began accumulating in the early 1920s and 1930s. The carcinogenic effect of burning tobacco has been known since 1930 (7). Since the landmark case-control studies reported by Wynder and Graham and Doll and Hill demonstrating an association between cigarette smoking and carcinoma of the lung, a vast amount of evidence has incriminated smoking of tobacco, especially cigarettes, as the main cause of the progressive rise in mortality from lung cancer (3,4,6,8). A steadily increasing body of retrospective and prospective data indicate the following: a dose-response relationship exists between cigarette smoking and lung cancer, the demographic distribution of lung cancer correlates with long-term smoking habits, reduced lung cancer rates are found among ex-smokers, and lung cancer has been induced by the administration of tar or inhaled cigarette smoke in experimental animals (3,8).

Overall, male smokers exhibit an average of a ten-fold increase in relative risk of death from lung cancer when compared with lifelong nonsmokers (8,9). The severity of risk varies with several factors, including total exposure to cigarette smoke as measured by the number of cigarettes smoked, the duration of smoking in years, the age of initiation of smoking, and the tar and nicotine levels in the cigarettes smoked (3,10). In a review of 3,070 new patients with lung cancer, the Edinburgh Lung Cancer Group found only 74 lifelong nonsmokers (2.4%), of whom 19 were men (0.6%) and 55 were women (1.8%) (11).

The Cancer Prevention Study II (CPSII) prospectively followed more than one million participants for over 6 years (9). Compared with lifelong nonsmokers, men who smoked one pack of cigarettes per day had 22 times the risk of dying from lung cancer, whereas men who smoked greater than two packs per day had 45 times the risk. A model proposed by Peto and colleagues based on the observations of a prospective cohort of British physicians for two decades, predicted that a tripling of the duration of smoking increased lung cancer risk 100-fold (12,13). Whether the age of initiation of smoking is a separate risk factor or is related to duration of smoking is not clear. In a case-control study of 282 patients with lung cancer reported by Hegmann et al., the odds ratio for the development of lung cancer among men who began smoking before the age of 20 was twice that of those who began smoking after the age of 20 (14). However, this increase in risk has not been consistently observed in other studies evaluating the age of

smoking initiation as a risk factor for the subsequent development of lung cancer. Nonetheless, it is clear that persons who begin smoking at younger ages are more likely to become habitual smokers, and, thus, are more likely to smoke for longer durations (9).

Over the past several decades, the composition of cigarettes has changed. Most cigarettes are now filtered with reduced tar content. However, cigarettes still contain more than 50 identifiable carcinogens. It is thus not surprising that changing the composition of cigarettes has not resulted in any measurable health benefit (15–17).

Smoking cessation is associated with health benefits in both cardiovascular disease and lung cancer. On the basis of two large case-control studies in 1950 and in 1990, Peto et al. reported that smoking cessation nearly halved the expected number of lung cancer cases (12). In men who stopped smoking at ages 60, 50, 40, and 30, the cumulative risk of death from lung cancer was 10%, 6%, 3%, and 2%, respectively, as compared to 16% in men who continued to smoke until the age of 75. Thus, despite frustrating statistics relating to the small number of smokers who become sustained nonsmokers, efforts must be continued in the arena of smoking cessation. Benefit as measured by a decrease in lung cancer risk can definitely be achieved. Despite intensive antismoking campaigns, limitation of tobacco advertising, tobacco awareness education in schools, and widespread public appreciation of the health risks associated with smoking, 20% to 25% of the American population continue to be committed smokers. Although this figure is unacceptably high, it does represent a substantial decrease in smoking percentage compared to several decades ago. Adult cigarette consumption in the United States from 1900 to 1999 is shown graphically in Figure 14-3. The steady rise in the number of cigarettes consumed per adult per year from the beginning of the century through the two World Wars continued until the landmark 1964 Surgeon General's report on the health consequences of smoking (18). This report definitively linked cigarette smoking with increases in age-specific death rates, lung cancer, and coronary artery disease and was the first major event that contributed to the declining use of cigarettes. Continued public health efforts, nonsmokers' rights movements, increases in cigarette taxes, and limiting the distribution of tobacco products to minors (Synar Amendment) have all likely contributed to the declining use of cigarettes. Brown and Kessler have projected reductions in lung cancer mortality in the 21st century that depend primarily on the effectiveness of the current efforts to reduce smoking prevalence (19). Figure 14-4 shows their projections of the age-adjusted lung cancer death rate in the United States with (*solid lines*) and without (*dashed lines*) additional successful interventions targeted at smoking prevention.

ENVIRONMENTAL TOBACCO SMOKE

Over the last several decades, considerable controversy relating to the risks of ETS has arisen. ETS consists of both exhaled mainstream smoke and sidestream smoke from smoldering tobacco. The Environmental Protection Agency (EPA) and the IARC both classify ETS as containing lung carcinogens, including benzene, benzo[a]pyrene, and 4-(methylnitrosamino)-1-(3-pyridyl)-1-butanone (20,21). In a study reported by Hecht

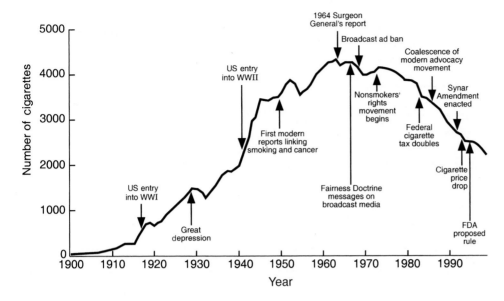

FIGURE 14-3. Adult per capita cigarette consumption and major smoking and health events per capita in the United States from 1900 to 1999. (From U.S. Department of Health and Human Services, *Reducing Tobacco Use: A Report of the Surgeon General.* Atlanta, Georgia: U.S. Department of Health and Human Services, Centers for Disease Control and Prevention, National Center for Chronic Disease Prevention and Health Promotion, Office on Smoking and Health, 2000:p. 33, with permission.)

et al., the urine collected from nonsmokers exposed to machine-generated sidestream smoke demonstrated excreted metabolites of the latter carcinogen, confirming that these compounds are absorbed by inhalation of ETS (22).

The 1986 US Department of Health and Human Services Report on the health consequences of involuntary smoking concluded that passive smoking is a cause of lung cancer and other diseases in nonsmokers (23). In an examination of data provided by the American Cancer Society CPSII, Cardanus

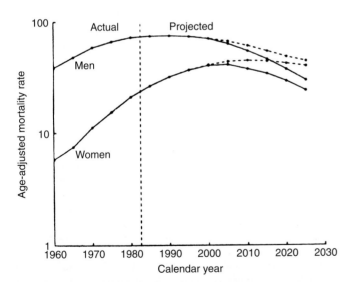

FIGURE 14-4. Actual (up to 1982) and projected age-adjusted lung cancer mortality rates for US white men and women for the years 1960 to 2025. *Dashed lines* indicates projections based on current trends in smoking prevalence, per capita consumption, initiation, age, and cigarette tar content. *Solid lines* represent projections assuming achievement of a reduction in overall smoking prevalence to 15% of US adults in 1990, according to the National Cancer Institute (NCI) Year 2000 Project. (This national goal in smoking cessation was not reached in 2000.) (From Brown CC, Kessler LG. Projections of lung cancer mortality in the United States: 1986–2025. *JNCI* 1988;80:43–51, with permission.)

et al. determined that the relative risk of lung cancer in women with smoking husbands was 1.2 times greater than that of women with nonsmoking husbands (24). Furthermore, the risk of lung cancer in these women was higher if their husbands smoked more than two packs of cigarettes a day. Similarly, in a report pooling data from eight studies published between 1981 and 1991, Pershagen determined a 1.25 times higher risk of lung cancer in nonsmokers living with smokers (25). These studies imply that living with a smoking spouse increases the risk of lung cancer by approximately 20%.

The burden of scientific information addressing the health effects of passive smoking indicates that there is no safe level of ETS. An estimated 3,000 cases of lung cancer related to ETS occur each year in the United States (3). Efforts to eliminate passive smoking from public places seem completely justifiable under these circumstances.

GENDER

Since 1950, a greater than 500% increase in lung cancer mortality has been noted in women (16,26). Although most of this increase has been attributed to the dramatic increase in the prevalence of cigarette smoking among women since the 1940s, several additional disturbing facts have emerged. The first is that dose for dose, women appear to have an increased susceptibility to carcinogens when compared with men. This in turn may translate into an increased risk for lung cancer. A number of studies suggest that women may be more vulnerable to tobacco carcinogens than men may be (27–31). In a case-control study by Risch et al., male-female differences in lung cancer covering the period from 1981 to 1985 in Ontario, Canada, were assessed (30). Among individuals with 40 years of cigarette smoking relative to lifelong nonsmokers, the odds ratio for developing lung cancer was 27.9 in women versus 9.6 in men. In another large case-control study on 1,889 lung cancer subjects and 2,070 controls, Zang and Wynder showed that the dose-response odds for development of lung cancer were 1.2- to 1.7-fold higher in women than in men (31). In both studies, the increase in lung cancer risk was present in all major histologic types. The causes of the apparent gender difference in susceptibility are unknown but may be related to a number of factors, including hormonal effects, sex-related differences in nicotine metabolism, or metabolic activation or detoxification of lung carcinogens (31).

Lung cancer also appears to occur more commonly in nonsmoking women than in nonsmoking men. In the above case-control study reported by Zang and Wynder, the proportion of never-smoking lung cancer patients was more than twice as high in women than in men (31). A case-control study reported by Taioli and Wynder demonstrated an increased risk of adenocarcinoma of the lung in women using estrogen replacement therapy, with a reported odds ratio of 1.7 (32). Although the reasons for such sex-related differences are not clear, women may have greater exposure to nontobacco environmental carcinogens, such as radon; increased exposure to ETS; or sex-related differences in the metabolism of nontobacco environmental carcinogens(3,30,33,34).

ENVIRONMENTAL AIR POLLUTION

The association between environmental air pollution and lung cancer has historically been difficult to examine because of the inherent challenges posed in measuring exposure to air pollutants over long periods of time, changes in air content related to changing transportation means and heavy industry, implementation of air quality regulation, and the confounding contributions of other risk factors for lung cancer. However, it is widely believed that an association between urbanization and lung cancer does exist.

An estimated 1% to 2% of lung cancer cases are related to air pollution (3,35). The atmosphere contains known human carcinogens including polycyclic aromatic hydrocarbons, such as benzene and benzo[a]pyrene; arsenic; nickel; and chromium (3,36). Recent studies have also demonstrated an association between fine particulate (particles <2.5 mm) air pollution and cardiopulmonary disease including lung cancer (37,38). These particles are by-products of the burning of fossil fuels and wood and can be small enough to be respirable (39). Carcinogens as well as other compounds including ozone, nitrogen dioxide, and oxides of sulfur and nitrogen can be adsorbed on these particles, which are found in higher concentrations in urban areas and in regions with close proximity to fossil fuel-burning plants. A recent report by Pope et al. evaluated the relationship between long-term exposure to fine particulate air pollution and mortality from lung cancer and other cardiopulmonary diseases (38). This study included data on 16 years of follow-up in approximately 500,000 adults entered in the American Cancer Society CPSII and linked the individual risk factor data to information on exposure to fine particulate and chemical air pollutants. After adjusting for other lung cancer risk factors, such as smoking, age, and socioeconomic status, fine particulate and sulfur oxide-related pollution were associated with increases in all-cause, lung cancer, and cardiopulmonary mortality. Each 10 mg per m^3 increment in fine particle concentration was associated with an 8% increase in lung cancer mortality.

Though it has been difficult to prove, it seems clear that long-term exposure to air pollution is an important independent risk factor for lung cancer. Standards for air pollutants, including fine particle concentration, were established in 1997 by the EPA under the Clean Air Act and have been upheld recently by the Supreme Court (39).

TABLE 14-2. Substances Encountered in Workplace Exposures Categorized as Causative for Bronchogenic Carcinoma

Arsenic
Asbestos
Bis(chloromethyl) ether and chloromethyl methyl ether
Chromium and certain chromium compounds (hexavalent chromium)
Ionizing radiation, γ -radiation x-rays
Synthetic mineral fibers (certain kinds only)
Mustard gas
Nickel in nickel refining
Radon progeny (decay products)
Soots, tars, mineral oils (polycyclic aromatic hydrocarbons)
Vinyl chloride

From Beckett WS. Epidemiology and etiology of lung cancer. *Clin Chest Med* 1993;14(1):1–15, with permission.

OCCUPATIONAL FACTORS

Specific agents found during industrial exposure have been related to the development of bronchial carcinoma and are listed in Table 14-2 (40). The most notorious ones are radioactive material, asbestos, chromates, nickel, mustard gas, isopropyl oil, hydrocarbons, arsenic, hematite, vinyl chloride, and bis(chloromethyl) ether (3,31,36,40–45).

Radioactive Materials

All types of radiations may be carcinogenic. The lung cancer risk increases from 3 to 30 times depending on the degree of exposure (42). The latent period (interval between beginning of exposure and onset of lung cancer) is more than 10 years, the mean value being 16 to 17 years. There is a strong association between exposure to uranium and development of bronchogenic carcinoma, particularly small cell carcinoma (43–46). It is well documented that the combination of smoking and uranium exposure markedly increases the risk of developing lung cancer (see Fig. 14-5) (43–47).

Radon 222 is a naturally occurring decay product of radium 226, which is a decay product of radium 238. The carcinogenic effect of uranium has been documented for over a century (8,46,48). Uranium mining has ceased in the United States. However, uranium and radium are commonly present in soil and in rock in highly variable concentrations, and, thus, radon is also ubiquitously present in the environment.

Radon is released as a radioactive gas. It has a half-life of 3.82 days and eventually decays into "radon daughters." These include polonium 218 and polonium 214, which emit α-particles. α-particles can cause tissue damage. At a cellular level, a single α-particle transversal can result in gene mutation and cell death (49). Inhalation of radon or its decay products can result in α-product emission in the lungs. As genetic mutations are thought to play an important role in the multiple-step pathways leading to neoplasia in the lung, radon may contribute to lung cancer pathogenesis by this mechanism.

The concentration of radon in an environment depends on the intensity of its source and on the ventilation around that source. A poorly ventilated environment that is rich in radium or uranium is likely to be associated with high radon levels, a

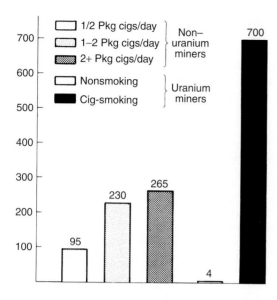

FIGURE 14-5. Lung cancer due to smoking and uranium exposure. (From Wright ES, Hammond EC. Radiation-induced carcinoma of the lung—the St. Lawrence tragedy. *J Thorac Cardiovasc Surg* 1977; 74:496, with permission.)

situation, for instance, that is likely to occur in underground mines. Miners in uranium and nonuranium mines have demonstrated higher lung cancer risk independent of cigarette smoking (28,43,50–52). Domestic radon exposure is related to ventilation and to the concentration of radium in the soil and in the rock over which a house is built. Low level α-radiation likely occurs in this setting, and this has raised concern about the carcinogenic effects of radon within the house. There has been a great deal of interest in the role of domestic radon exposure in lung cancer. Lubin and Boice reported a meta-analysis of eight studies of domestic radon exposure including over 4000 persons with lung cancer that concluded that higher residential radon exposure levels are associated with an increased risk of lung cancer (53). The effects of low-dose radiation related to radon exposure continue to be a controversial area. Nonetheless, at present, an estimated 15,000 to 20,000 lung cancer deaths per year in the United States are thought to be related to radon (54).

Asbestos

Asbestos is a class of fibrous minerals whose strength and fire-retardant qualities are useful in construction and insulation. Asbestos is now a universally recognized carcinogen and has historically been an important occupational cause of human lung cancer (36,40,55,56). Asbestos is causally linked to both bronchogenic lung cancer and mesothelioma. The latent period between the initiation of exposure and the development of malignancy is usually 20 years or more (36,40,55).

There are differences in the carcinogenic potential of various types of asbestos. People exposed to chrysotile asbestos have a respiratory tract cancer mortality 2 to 4 times higher than that in controls, whereas those exposed to a combination of chrysotile and crocidolite asbestos have a mortality rate 5.3 times higher than that in controls. For amosite asbestos, the death rate due to respiratory cancer is more than 10 times higher than that in

controls. In the United States, chrysotile asbestos is the most commonly used type. Tobacco is a critical cofactor (3,36,40,56,57). Lung cancer in asbestos-exposed nonsmokers is uncommon (57). Most cases of lung cancer in occupationally exposed workers occur in smokers with asbestos-related pulmonary interstitial disease, that is, smokers with asbestosis (58). There is controversy as to whether asbestos exposure alone is a risk factor for lung cancer or whether asbestosis is required for the risk to be present. From a public health perspective, this question is particularly relevant because of concern in the general population about asbestos present in buildings and homes. Asbestos fibers (ferruginous bodies) are ubiquitously found in the lungs of city dwellers. The atmosphere in New York City contains 10×10^{-9} grams of asbestos per cubic meter of air, which corresponds to millions of respirable submicroscopic fibrils (36). The significance of prolonged exposure to such low-level concentrations of asbestos remains uncertain, particularly as this low intensity exposure is extremely unlikely to lead to asbestosis.

The use of asbestos has precipitously declined since its adverse health consequences have been identified. The most important intervention for lung cancer prevention in individuals who have had asbestos exposure is smoking prevention or smoking cessation.

Other Occupational Factors

Workers engaged in handling chromates from chromium-containing iron ore have approximately a 4 to 15 times greater incidence of lung cancer than the general population do (36). There is usually a long latent period similar to the 20 years that commonly elapses between asbestos exposure and tumor occurrence. Nickel refinery workers were once noted to have a 3 to 5-fold increased lung cancer mortality and a 150-fold increased risk of nasal cancer. Nickel dust was the likely responsible carcinogen, although generally adopted changes in the refinery process made before World War II not only drastically reduced nickel dust levels but also reduced worker exposure to arsenic. Arsenic is a known carcinogen that has been implicated in the development of lung cancer in individuals who are given arsenic-containing drugs or who are engaged in the manufacture and use of pesticides.

The mining of hematite (an iron ore containing ferric oxide and silica) is associated with an increased risk of lung cancer. In addition, a number of other industrial operations in which exposure to iron and silica is common may be responsible for a poorly quantified but increased risk of lung cancer. These include metal grinding, sandblasting, and iron and steel foundry work.

CHEMOPREVENTION

There is enormous interest in the development of compounds that may be beneficial as chemopreventive agents against neoplasms. For example, potential chemopreventive benefit of nonsteroidal anti-inflammatory drugs in colorectal cancer is being evaluated (59–61). Finasteride, an inhibitor of 5-α-reductase, is being evaluated as a possible chemopreventive agent for prostate cancer (62). A wide number of classes of therapeutic agents are currently under investigation as potential lung cancer chemopreventive agents. These include carotenoids, selenium, COX-2 inhibitors, epidermal growth factor receptor (EGFR) inhibitors, lipoxygenase inhibitors, inhibitors of angiogenesis, cell cycle inhibitors, and demethylation agents (63). Thus far, none has proven to be beneficial, but chemoprevention is actively and intensively being pursued as an area of investigation.

DIET

Several epidemiologic studies have shown a relation between greater dietary intake of vegetables and modestly lower risk for lung and other cancers (40,64–66). β-carotene (a precursor to the class of retinoids, including retinol or vitamin A, which are found in many green, yellow, and orange fruits and vegetables) may be associated with lower lung cancer risk (40,63,64,66). The protective effect is particularly evident in current or past cigarette smokers (40). A variety of studies in several countries have shown that (a) low dietary intake of these fruits and vegetables is associated with an increased lung cancer risk and (b) a low serum level of β-carotene is associated with increased risk for development of lung cancer at a later stage (see Fig. 14-6) (40,64–67). Similarly, in epidemiologic studies, high intake of lycopene, found in tomatoes, has been shown to be associated with lower risk of lung cancer (66).

Three important prospective, randomized, controlled large-scale epidemiologic studies were performed recently to address whether supplemental β-carotene and vitamin A might be useful as cancer chemopreventive agents (65,68,69). Unfortunately, none of these trials established that administration of either β-carotene or vitamin A decreased mortality due to lung cancer. In fact, in the study reported by the Alpha-Tocopherol, Beta Carotene Cancer Prevention Study Group from Finland, there was an unsuspected higher than expected mortality primarily due to lung cancer and heart disease in a group receiving β-carotene (68). Similarly, in the study reported by Omenn et al., patients receiving both vitamin A and β-carotene experienced a 17% increase in mortality and a 28% increase in the number of lung cancers compared with the placebo group (69).

The study by Hennekens et al. evaluating the effects of β-carotene in subjects enrolled in the Physicians' Health Study revealed neither benefit nor harm in terms of malignancy or cardiovascular disease (65). On the basis of the findings of these three trials, the use of supplemental β-carotene and vitamin A should be discouraged. Instead, a balanced dietary intake of fruits and vegetables, including those containing β-carotene, should be encouraged.

GENETIC FACTORS

A minority of heavy cigarette smokers (approximately one in eight) develops lung cancer, suggesting that other factors are important in determining the risk (40). Family studies have repeatedly shown a slightly greater lung cancer risk, approximately two- to threefold, in nonsmokers who are relatives of lung cancer patients compared with nonsmokers who have no family history of lung cancer (70–73). Environmental factors are probably superimposed on genetic patterns that predispose to lung cancer (40). In fact, genetic factors may exert an influence on the development of lung cancer equal to that of cigarette smoking (15,31,74–76).

The genetically determined ability to metabolize carcinogens may have a direct role in lung cancer risk (15,40). Molecular epidemiology is a rapidly expanding field that may elucidate genetic determinants of lung cancer susceptibility both in patients with innate familial risk as well as in patients with acquired susceptibility related to exposures to tobacco-related or other carcinogens. Genotype analysis of enzymatic pathways involved in carcinogen detoxification is one example of this new avenue addressing the molecular basis of lung cancer. Enzymes of the cytochrome P-450, the glutathione *S*-transferase, and the arylhydrocarbon hydroxylase systems are all involved in metabolic detoxification or inactivation of carcinogenic substances in tobacco smoke, including polycyclic aromatic hydrocarbons. The cytochrome P-450 system is responsible for metabolism of debrisoquine, the glutathione *S*-transferase

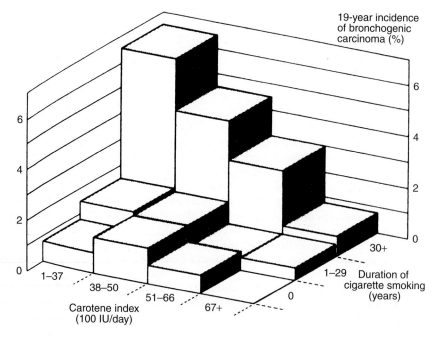

FIGURE 14-6. Association of an index of dietary β-carotene and the duration of cigarette smoking with the 19-year index of cigarette smoking in the Western Electric Study. Dietary index was based on questionnaires about food intake over a 28-day period given to 2100 men aged 40 to 55 years during two examinations separated by 1 year. Intake of preformed retinol (vitamin A) and other nutrients was not significantly associated with lung cancer risk. (From Shekelle RB, Liu S, Raynor WJ, et al. Dietary vitamin A and risk of cancer in the Western Electric Study. *Lancet* 1981;2:1185–1190, with permission.)

system detoxifies metabolites of polycyclic aromatic hydrocarbons, and the arylhydrocarbon hydroxylase system converts the polycyclic aromatic hydrocarbons of cigarette smoke into carcinogenic epoxides (77,78,79,3,74,80–82). Polymorphisms in these and likely other enzymes may alter the balance between detoxification and activation of carcinogens, with resultant alterations in lung cancer risk. The identification of these types of polymorphisms by molecular epidemiologic techniques are important in understanding mechanisms of carcinogenesis, but may also be useful in identifying patients for targeted treatment strategies (83).

Oncogenes, tumor suppressor genes, and genes involved in DNA repair are also likely involved in determining lung cancer susceptibility in individuals (84). Several genetic changes have already been associated with small cell and non-small cell carcinomas of the lung. These include loss of DNA sequences on the short arm of chromosome 3 (3p) or 11 (11p), amplification of a number of oncogenes (tumor-promoting genes) including the *myc* family (c-*myc*, N-*myc*, and L-*myc*) and the *ras* family (K-*ras*, H-*ras*, and N-*ras*), and the p53 tumor suppressor gene (15,57,75,76,84). Whereas the association of genetic markers with lung cancer strongly supports the concept that susceptibility is partially determined at the molecular level, it is not clear that such mutations are necessary for carcinogenesis to occur. However, if high-risk genotypes can be identified, this type of information may potentially be useful in the future in selecting populations of patients who could receive focused screening or even genotype-directed treatment.

PATHOLOGY

BRONCHOGENIC CARCINOMA

Classification

A committee of pathologists convened by the WHO established the standard classification system for lung cancer (85,86). As new data becomes available on the natural history of treated and untreated lung cancer, this comprehensive system continues to be updated (87). According to this classification, the four major cell types of lung cancer and their approximate relative incidences include adenocarcinoma (31% to 34%), squamous cell carcinoma (30%), small cell carcinoma (20% to 25%), and large cell carcinoma (10% to 16%). Bronchoalveolar carcinomas (so-called alveolar cell carcinomas) are considered adenocarcinomas; as a group, they comprise approximately 3% to 4% of all lung carcinomas (88,89).

Pathogenesis

Squamous cell bronchogenic carcinomas arise most commonly in segmental and subsegmental bronchi in response to repetitive carcinogenic stimuli, inflammation, or irritation (90). The mucosal lining is most susceptible to injury, particularly at the bifurcation of bronchial structures. Ciliary mechanisms and superficial columnar lining cells tend to shed or become denuded, a process abetted by the physiologically altered airflow and reduced mucous flow rates at these sites. Carcinogenic agents are more likely to be deposited, absorbed, and retained in these zones. Basal (reserve) cells are stimulated to proliferate.

In some cases, hyperplasia of mucin-secreting columnar epithelial cells is followed by replacement of the bronchial lining by an orderly arrangement of metaplastic, stratified squamous epithelium. Metaplasia is a response to injury by either carcinogenic or noncarcinogenic agents. In the course of carcinogenesis, the basal half of the metaplastic epithelium may become disorganized. Cells lose their usual polarity and individual cells develop atypical, irregular, hyperchromatic nuclei. Abnormal mitoses may be identified, whereas the superficial layers of the mucosa retain a stratified, flattened, but unified pattern. These changes are termed *atypical metaplasia* or *dysplasia* (91). Eventually, the entire thickness of the mucosa may be replaced by proliferating neoplastic cells (carcinoma *in situ*).

Infiltrating neoplasms may develop at some unpredictable future time when the integrity of the basal membrane has been lost. This mechanism pertains particularly to bronchial squamous cell malignancies in experimental animals as well as in humans. Factors associated with these changes include smoking and occupational exposure to arsenic, uranium, chromium, asbestos, or other minerals (40,41). The pathogenesis of small cell carcinoma is not as well understood, but this tumor may also originate in the basal cells of the bronchial epithelium.

Multiple exogenous and endogenous factors are associated with adenocarcinomas, which likely arise from the mucin-secreting cells in the more peripheral bronchi. Among the exogenous factors are tobacco smoke, asbestos, cadmium, chromium, beryllium, and pneumoconiotic dusts. Endogenous conditions include chronic interstitial pneumonitis and fibrosis and progressive systemic sclerosis (scleroderma).

Histology

SQUAMOUS CELL CARCINOMA. Squamous cell carcinoma is the second most common bronchogenic carcinoma (see Figs. 5-23, 14-7, and 14-8) (57,85,86,90,91). These tumors are predominantly composed of flattened or polygonal neoplastic epithelial cells that tend to stratify, form intercellular bridges, and elaborate keratin on an individual cell basis or in the complex of an epithelial pearl. On the basis of the degree of differentiation, these tumors are divided into three subtypes: well-differentiated, moderately differentiated, and poorly differentiated. They usually arise from the mucosa of large bronchi and are frequently associated with adjoining foci of intraepithelial malignancy or dysplasia. In about two-thirds of cases, they present as a proximal or hilar lesion, and it is uncommon for them to metastasize early (57). The tumors tend to be bulky, encroach on bronchial lumen with the production of obstructing intraluminal granular or polypoid masses, and invade cartilage and adjoining lymph nodes. Fifty percent of differentiated squamous cell lung carcinomas are confined to the thorax at autopsy (87). Gail et al. found squamous cell carcinomas to have the most favorable prognosis of all the non-small cell carcinomas (92).

ADENOCARCINOMA. Adenocarcinoma, the most prevalent carcinoma of the lung in both sexes, forms acinar or glandular structures (see Fig. 14-9) (57,86,90,91,93,94). Histologically, this tumor is divided broadly into well differentiated, moderately well differentiated, poorly differentiated, and bronchoalveolar types.

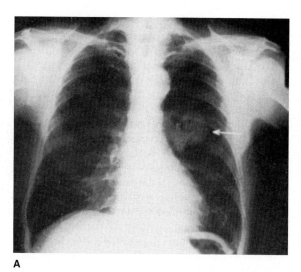
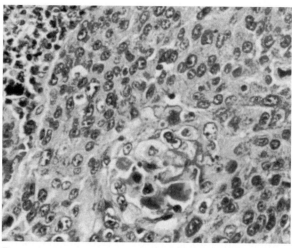

FIGURE 14-7. **A:** Squamous cell carcinoma. A posteroanterior (PA) chest radiograph shows a 3-cm mass adjacent to the left hilum *(arrow)*. **B:** Squamous cell carcinoma histology. Squamous cell carcinomas are characterized by the presence of keratin in the cytoplasm of the malignant cell. The malignant cells are frequently connected by an extensive series of intercellular bridges and may form small "pearls" in which the squamous cells are arranged in small groups. In this figure, the cells at the periphery do not show differentiation, but the central portion contains some cells with markedly hyperchromatic nuclei and keratinized cytoplasm characteristic of squamous cell carcinoma.

Fifty-five to 60 percent of adenocarcinomas are limited to the periphery of lung, not obviously related to any bronchus. Peripheral adenocarcinomas are frequently circumscribed and subpleural with central pigmented fibrotic cores. Classic bronchoalveolar carcinomas, whether single, multicentric, or lobar in type, tend to use existing alveolar septa as a framework for their growth and are not scar-associated.

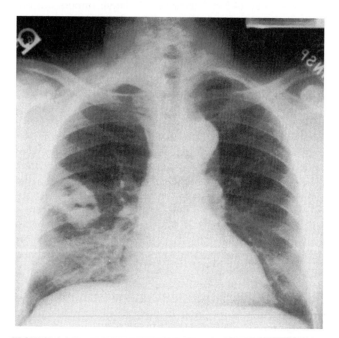

FIGURE 14-8. Squamous cell carcinoma. Posteroanterior (PA) chest radiograph shows a large cavitating peripheral squamous cell carcinoma in the right hemithorax.

The liver, adrenals, bone, and central nervous system (CNS) are frequent sites of metastases (57). In more than 50% of the cases studied at autopsy, the brain is involved, and in 12% the brain is the sole site of metastasis (95).

LARGE CELL CARCINOMA. Large cell carcinoma, also called *undifferentiated carcinoma*, includes all tumors that show no evidence of differentiation to small cell, squamous cell, or adenocarcinoma (see Fig. 14-10) (57,90,91). In general, these tumors are composed of pleomorphic cells with variably enlarged nuclei and prominent nucleoli with abundant cytoplasm. The tumors tend to form large, bulky, somewhat circumscribed, and necrotic masses; are frequently subpleural in origin; invade locally; and disseminate widely. About 60% of the tumors are limited to the periphery of the lung. The metastatic pattern of large cell carcinoma is similar to that of the adenocarcinomas, with cerebral metastases in more than 50% of the cases (57).

The giant cell variant of large cell carcinoma is composed of huge, multinucleated, bizarre cells that are frequently associated with an extensive inflammatory cell infiltrate (57). These tumors are usually large and peripheral, aggressive, and most often found at a late stage but are amenable to surgical cure when resected in stage I or II (96). They show an ability to metastasize widely, curiously with a predilection for the small intestine (57,97).

SMALL CELL CARCINOMA. Small cell carcinomas have been divided by the WHO into two groups: pure small cell and combined (see Fig. 14-11) (86,98). Histologic variants include oat cell (lymphocytelike) carcinoma, which is composed of cells with round-to-oval nuclei. The nucleoli are always indistinct, and the cytoplasm is scanty. The intermediate (polygonal) variant is the most common and is characterized by cells with somewhat larger, fusiform or spindled nuclei. Nuclear

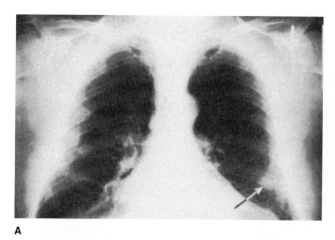

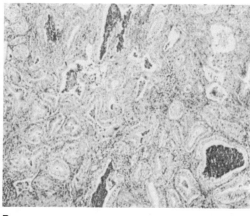

FIGURE 14-9. **A**: Adenocarcinoma. Posteroanterior (PA) chest radiograph shows a 1.5-cm solitary lesion in the lingula (*arrow*). Note also rib fractures in the right hemithorax, a finding attributable to previous trauma. **B:** Histology of adenocarcinoma. Adenocarcinomas of the lung are characterized by gland formation in a fibrous background. Numerous glands are formed in this well-differentiated adenocarcinoma.

chromatin has a dense but even distribution, and nucleoli are usually absent and always indistinct. Cytoplasm is minimal. In the combined type, small cell carcinoma is combined with a non-small cell type—large cell, squamous cell, or adenocarcinoma. The most important combined variant is the small cell plus large cell variant (99,100).

Although 75% to 80% of the small cell carcinomas present as proximal lesions, they may arise in any part of the tracheobronchial tree; they tend to lift the mucosa slightly to form a velvety, thickened lining; they rapidly invade vascular channels, mediastinal lymph nodes, and soft tissue; and they disseminate widely, often before pulmonary symptoms are

recognized or provoked. In contrast to squamous cell carcinoma, the lumen is usually not filled with tumor but is compressed externally through the submucosa and by the hilar lymph node spread.

Small cell carcinoma is extrathoracic when discovered in 70% of cases, with little chance of 5-year survival (57). When limited to the thoracic cavity, small cell carcinoma has a complete response to chemotherapy and radiation therapy in more than 50% of the cases, with approximately 30% of these remissions sustained beyond 2 years. The most common sites of metastatic involvement at initial presentation are listed in Table 14-3 (101).

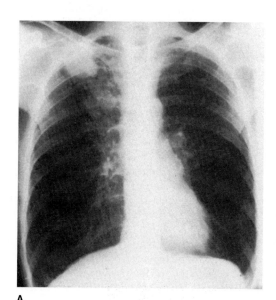

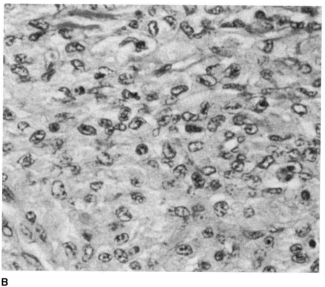

FIGURE 14-10. **A**: Large cell carcinoma. Posteroanterior (PA) chest radiograph shows a right apical density adjacent to the pleura and the chest wall and a proximal density adjacent to the right tracheal wall. **B:** Histology of large cell carcinoma. The cells of a large cell undifferentiated carcinoma are characterized by a moderate amount of cytoplasm, nuclei that are usually oval or round with some chromatin clearing, and the presence of one or several nucleoli, which may be markedly irregular in shape. These cells contain neither keratin nor mucin.

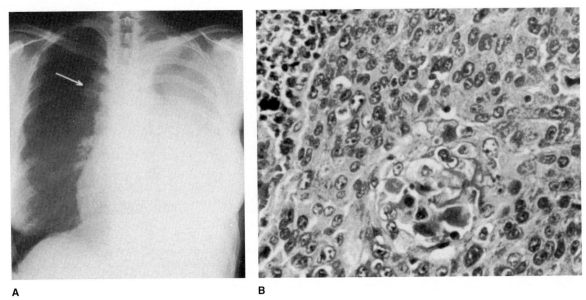

FIGURE 14-11. **A:** Small cell carcinoma. Posteroanterior (PA) chest radiograph showing a large left pleural effusion opacifying the left hemithorax. Note the mediastinal adenopathy manifested on the chest radiograph by a density in the right paratracheal area (*arrow*). Pleural fluid analysis revealed malignant cells, and bronchoscopy revealed a large endobronchial mass identified as small cell carcinoma on biopsy. **B:** Histology of small cell carcinoma. The nucleus of small cell carcinoma is different from that of other types of lung cancer. It is characterized by the relatively even distribution of chromatin throughout the nucleus. There is no clearing of the chromatin, and nucleoli are never prominent. The cytoplasm of the cell varies from the small rim of cytoplasm seen in the oat cell variant (shown in this photomicrograph) to a moderate amount of eosinophilic cytoplasm seen in the polygonal variant. The subtyping of various types of small cell carcinoma has been shown to have a profound effect on prognosis or response to therapy.

OTHER PULMONARY NEOPLASMS

Carcinoid Tumor (Bronchial Adenoma)

Bronchopulmonary carcinoid tumors constitute 1% to 4% of all primary lung neoplasms (102). These highly vascularized lesions arise in submucosal glands in the bronchial wall; grow slowly; invade locally; and occasionally metastasize to the lymph nodes, mediastinum, vertebra, and liver (57,103). The red or pink carcinoid appears as a polypoid or sessile mass protruding from the bronchial wall and is covered by intact bronchial mucosa. Of these lesions, 90% of typical carcinoids are located in a major or segmental bronchus and about 10% are present as peripheral lesions. Carcinoids are composed of small uniform cuboidal cells with fine granular homogeneous cytoplasm. The nuclei are round or oval and deeply staining

TABLE 14-3.   Sites of Metastases in Patients Presenting with Small Cell Lung Cancer

Site	Percentage
Bone	35
Liver	25
Bone marrow	20
Brain	10
Extrathoracic lymph nodes	5
Subcutaneous masses	5

From Johnson BE. Management of small cell lung cancer. *Clin Chest Med* 1993;14(1):173–187, with permission.

and are usually in the center of the cell. Little pleomorphism is seen, and mitoses and necrosis are absent. Neuroendocrine markers—chromogranin, syntoptophysin, or hormones—are demonstrable by immunohistochemistry, and dense core granules are evident ultrastructurally.

Carcinoids occur slightly more frequently in women (103). Most patients are in their thirties and have had symptoms for over 5 years prior to diagnosis. Signs and symptoms are secondary to bronchial obstruction or to the extreme vascularity of the tumor. Hemoptysis occurs in one-third of patients, but signs and symptoms of pulmonary infection behind the obstructed bronchus are more frequently noted (104). Occasionally, a patient is asymptomatic and the tumor is discovered after routine radiography of the chest.

Three types of chest radiographic abnormalities are seen in patients with carcinoid tumor (103). Most frequently there is pneumonia or the sequela of such an infection, with poor bronchial drainage. A smooth, rounded hilar mass may be present, or rarely, a peripheral nodule is seen.

The diagnosis is usually made on the basis of the history of frequent hemoptysis or repeated bouts of pneumonia and on the basis of observation of the characteristic tumor by bronchoscopy. Biopsy is usually inadvisable because of the possibility of severe hemorrhage. Also, it may be difficult to make a definite histologic diagnosis from the small pieces of tissue obtained by bronchial biopsy. Cytologic study of sputum or bronchial washings is usually not diagnostic because the mucous membrane over the tumor is usually intact. Operative removal is indicated because this is the only means of preventing the severe hemoptysis and infection that can accompany these tumors. Moreover, early removal may prevent the late metastatic spread that occurs in a few instances (103). The 5-year survival rate after resection is more than 90% (57).

Atypical Carcinoid Tumors

In 1972, Arrigoni et al. described an atypical carcinoid tumor that accounted for most but not all of the mortality of pulmonary carcinoids (105). Fifty percent of these lesions were large and peripherally located. Histologically, they are carcinoids with necrosis, numerous mitotic figures, and more anaplastic nuclei of the large cell type (58,105,106). A 41% survival rate has been reported (57). Travis et al. have divided the atypical carcinoids into low grade, which they call *atypical carcinoid*, and high grade, which they refer to as *large cell neuroendocrine carcinoma* (LCNEC) (107). The 5-year survival of LCNEC is poor.

Bronchial Tumors of the Salivary Gland Type

Neoplasms that are similar to those of the major and minor salivary glands infrequently arise in bronchial submucosal glands. These include mucoepidermoid carcinoma, adenoid cystic carcinoma, and pleomorphic adenomas (108–110). All are present as endobronchial or endotracheal masses. The mucoepidermoid carcinomas are divided into high and low grade, according to both size and histology. High-grade mucoepidermoid carcinomas are larger and more invasive, with both epidermoid glandular and intermediate cell elements that have more anaplastic nuclei, numerous mitotic figures, and foci of necrosis. The treatment is resection; survival is good for low-grade but not as good for high-grade lesions (111). Adenoid cystic carcinomas are composed of cells that form a characteristic cylindromatous pattern of regular glands (108). Resection is the preferred treatment, if possible, and survival is good at 5 years (85%), lower at 10 years (55%), and poor at 20 years (20%) (102,108,112).

Papillomas of the Bronchus

Papillomas are exceedingly rare lung tumors that are often associated with generalized papillomatosis of the upper respiratory tract (103). They are usually wart-like growths and have a well-developed connective tissue stroma (113). Bronchial papillomas in adults are often solitary growths but may be associated with papillomas elsewhere in the bronchial tree (114,115). Approximately 50% of the solitary adult tumors become malignant (115). They are associated with the human papilloma virus immunohistochemically demonstrated in these tumors (113,116).

Sclerosing Hemangioma

In 1956, Liebow and Hubbell described a lesion of the periphery of the lung, often found in women and at a younger age than is usual (117). Because of the strikingly vascular pattern associated with the lesion, it was named a *sclerosing hemangioma*. Grossly, the lesions are usually sharply circumscribed and present a hemorrhagic appearance.

Microscopically, there are three distinct patterns, which are a vascular pattern with numerous small and large spaces filled with red blood cells, a papillary pattern, and a solid pattern. The cells making up the lesion are large, with centrally placed nuclei that often contain small nucleoli. Although the lesion is quite cellular, mitotic figures are rarely, if ever, seen. The mingling of patterns, cellularity, and vascularity may suggest a diagnosis of malignancy, especially adenocarcinoma. The histogenesis of the lesion was debated primarily because of its original designation as a hemangioma. Electron microscopic studies showed the cells lining the blood-filled space to be type II pneumocytes (118). Subsequently, immunohistochemical studies have confirmed their epithelial nature (119,120). Although it is unusual, it is important to recognize this lesion because it has a benign course, distinctly different from the much more common adenocarcinoma that it mimics.

Alveolar Adenoma

In 1986, Yousem and Hochholzer described six cases of an alveolar adenoma (121). These presented as solitary nodules in basically asymptomatic patients, they were resected by wedge biopsy or lobectomy, and all of the patients did well. Grossly, the lesions were strikingly well circumscribed. Histologically, they were composed of proliferating alveolar pneumocytes, far less cellular than those seen in the sclerosing hemangioma, and were accompanied by an interstitial spindle cell component of benign-appearing stromal cells.

Intravascular Bronchioloalveolar Tumor

In 1983, Dail et al. described a lesion by the name *intravascular bronchioloalveolar tumor* (122). This lesion occurs predominantly in women with an age range of 12 to 60. Most patients present with cough, dyspnea, and chest pain. On chest radiograph, multiple peripheral, usually bilateral pulmonary nodules, measuring up to 3 cm in diameter are seen. Grossly, the lesions are circumscribed and are often multiple, even in a small wedge biopsy. Microscopically, the polygonal tumor cells are characterized by nuclei with an evenly dispersed chromatin pattern and rare mitotic figures. They are often found in a slightly basophilic matrix, apparently filling the alveolar spaces in a polypoid fashion. Despite the epithelial appearance of the cells, it has been shown both ultrastructurally and immunohistochemically that the lesion is endothelial in character. Corrin et al. described the presence of Weibel-Palade bodies characteristic of endothelial cells, and several studies have immunohistochemically demonstrated the presence of factor VIII-related antigen (123). Its appearance is similar to that of the histiocytoid hemangioma, or epithelioid hemangioendothelioma, another vascular lesion that may be mistaken for carcinoma. The clinical course is one of slow progression with an overall mortality rate of 40%.

Mesodermal Tumors of the Bronchi and Lung

Mesodermal tumors of the lung as a group are rare and account for a small percentage of all pulmonary neoplasms (103). The following is a classification of these neoplasms (124):

1. *Benign parenchyma tumors:* hamartomas
2. *Benign intrabronchial tumors:* chondroma, osteochondroma, lipoma, and leiomyoma

3. *Malignant intrabronchial tumors:* fibrosarcoma and leiomyosarcoma

4. *Malignant parenchyma tumors:* sarcomas and lymphomas

Hamartoma

Hamartomas are the most common benign tumors of the lung (102). They are composed of disorganized elements of tissue normally present in the lung (103,115,125). The term hamartoma is applied inappropriately to an interstitial mesenchymal tumor composed primarily of cartilage, with focal ossification in some cases. Septae of connective tissue extend from the periphery to the central portion of the nodule, near the edge of which bronchial or alveolar epithelium is entrapped. No capsule is present, and the tumor does not invade the surrounding tissue. The cartilage found within the tumor is not related to the cartilage found normally in bronchi, but 8% to 10% of the lesions arise within a major or segmental bronchus; the remainder are found in the periphery of the lung.

Most hamartomas are discovered on routine chest radiography (103). Characteristically, the lesion is round, has sharply defined margins, and varies in size from a few millimeters to 4 to 5 centimeters in diameter. As it grows, it may become lobulated. On chest radiograph, it is most likely to be confused with a tuberculoma or a metastatic lesion from elsewhere in the body. Calcification is evident on chest radiograph in 10% of cases and appears as small flecks throughout the lesion rather than in a ring form (102).

Definite diagnosis can be made only by histologic examination of the lesion (125–127). Adequate tissue can be obtained through the bronchoscope or by transthoracic needle biopsy; however, thoracotomy is often required.

Histologic confirmation is necessary to eliminate the possibility of a malignant lesion. Simple excision of the lesion is adequate, but follow-up has been undertaken in small, slowly growing, well-documented hamartomas.

Chondroma and Osteochondroma

Chondromas and osteochondromas are very rare neoplasms that arise in the trachea or a major bronchus in association with normal cartilaginous rings (103,128,129). They are usually slow growing but may reach great size and may cause obstruction and destruction of the pulmonary parenchyma. Histologically, they differ from hamartoma in containing only cartilage. If extensive lung destruction distal to the tumor occurs, pulmonary resection is indicated.

Lipoma

Lipomas originate from fatty tissue normally present in the fibrous tissue external to cartilaginous plates and to a lesser extent in the connective tissue and in the muscular layers of the bronchi (103,130,131). They occur more frequently in men than in women, usually in the fifth or sixth decade of life, and are more common in the left bronchial tree (130,131). They present as soft, smooth, often lobulated masses. Removal of the tumor can usually be accomplished by the straight-tube bronchoscope with satisfactory results, unless bronchial obstruction has produced destruction of lung tissue.

Leiomyoma

Nearly all of the smooth muscle tumors, leiomyomas, in the lung are well-differentiated metastases from leiomyosarcomas of the uterus. Primary leiomyoma is extremely rare (132–134). In one series of 14 cases, 12 were in women. This tumor likely arises from the smooth muscle of the interstitium and is composed of bands of amitotic smooth muscle cells. Surgical removal is the treatment of choice.

Sarcomas

Sarcomas in the lung show the spectrum of histologies seen in malignant tumors of soft tissue from which they are more often metastatic than primary in the lung. Two sarcomas, malignant fibrous histiocytoma and leiomyosarcoma, are mentioned briefly here. As in soft tissue, the most common sarcoma is malignant fibrous histiocytoma. On histologic examination, this tumor is composed of elongated spindle-shaped malignant cells, many of which are arranged in bands (135–137). A variable component of histiocytes is present. The tumor is relatively slow growing and metastasizes late. If complete removal of the primary tumor can be accomplished surgically, the prognosis is good (136–138).

In a study of 20 patients with pulmonary leiomyosarcoma, the age at presentation varied from 4 to 83 years, with 11 patients over 40 (139). Signs and symptoms of bronchial obstruction had been present from 1 month to 3.5 years. Most of the tumors were encapsulated and their cut surface was gray or white. Histologically, leiomyosarcomas are composed of spindle-shaped cells with elongated nuclei and abundant cytoplasm with myofibrils. Mitotic figures are frequent. Five of the patients had metastases when the cases were reported. Of the 11 patients in whom the tumor was resected, 9 were alive and were well 6 years after operation. In two patients, radiation therapy had no effect on their disease (134).

Lymphoma

Most lymphomas occur in several sites and secondary pulmonary involvement is a frequent finding (103). Lymphomas that are primary in the lung include the so-called lymphomatoid granulomatosis (LYG) and the low-grade lymphomas of bronchial mucosa-associated lymphoid tissue (baltomas) of B-cell type (140,141). LYG occurs over a broad age range; presents with cough, fever, and shortness of breath; and may also involve skin, CNS sinuses, and peripheral nerves. Lymph node involvement is unusual. Radiographically, it presents with multiple, often cavitary, nodules. Histologically, it is characterized by necrosis secondary to vascular invasion and destruction by abnormal lymphocytes. LYG has been separated into three grades according to increasing numbers of malignant lymphocytes that mark as both clonal B cells with evidence of Epstein-Barr virus and a larger number of nonclonal T lymphocytes, although some histologically and clinically similar cases mark as clonal T cells. The outcome is generally poor (142).

Baltomas are often found radiographically in asymptomatic patients, although symptomatic patients may present with cough, fever, and shortness of breath. Most cases (70%) present as solitary masses and are localized to the lung without nodal involvement, but multiple pulmonary nodules may be present. Histologically, there are sheets of small round lymphocytes that may be admixed with plasma cells and germinal centers with features of the previously diagnosed pseudolymphoma. The B cells are monoclonal and lack CD-5 and CD-10 staining, and do not show BCL-1 gene rearrangement. The 5-year survival is excellent, with or without chemotherapy, but progression to higher-grade lymphoma has been observed.

Large cell lymphomas also occur primarily in the lungs but are more often secondary to lymph node-based lymphomas. Lymphomas in the setting of transplant patients are often associated with Epstein-Barr virus residues.

CLINICAL MANIFESTATIONS

SYMPTOMS AND SIGNS

The overwhelming majority of patients with lung cancer present with advanced disease and are symptomatic at diagnosis (143). In a series of 678 patients with newly diagnosed lung cancer, only 6% were asymptomatic at initial presentation (144). Most patients have one or more symptoms and/or signs related to the presence of the tumor, although the symptomatology may not be specific to the primary tumor site. The presence of symptoms is a less favorable prognostic sign. Shimizu et al. reported a 5-year survival of only 25% among patients with lung cancer who presented with symptoms, in contrast with 56% for asymptomatic patients detected by screening (145). As symptoms and signs may be highly variable, it may be clinically useful to group them in the following categories: bronchopulmonary, intrathoracic extrapulmonary, metastatic, and paraneoplastic symptoms.

Bronchopulmonary Symptoms and Signs

Cough is the most common symptom in patients with lung cancer; it is present in 45% to 75% of patients (146). Irritation of the bronchus induces a cough, which may be productive or nonproductive and is frequently described by the patient as being a "cigarette cough." Ulceration of the tumor can result in hemoptysis, which most often presents as episodic blood streaking of the sputum. Hemoptysis occurs in approximately 60% of patients; massive hemoptysis is rare (146–148). Airway obstruction, complete or partial, may lead to wheezing, dyspnea, and occasionally, stridor. Such airway obstruction may lead to atelectasis with infection of the distal pulmonary parenchyma. The associated inflammatory process, obstructive pneumonitis, or abscess formation often leads to febrile respiratory symptoms, which may be present in as many as one third of patients (147). Unfortunately, the febrile episode may be misinterpreted by the physician because it may be ameliorated by antibiotic therapy and may thus lead to delay in diagnosis. Airway obstruction may also result in wheezing or, less commonly, stridor. The presence of a localized wheeze should always raise the suspicion of a localized obstructing lesion. Dyspnea may accompany atelectasis, particularly in patients with underlying lung disease with limited pulmonary reserve. This may particularly be the case in patients with obstructive airway disease related to cigarette use or in those who have interstitial lung disease. Dyspnea may also be an indication of lymphangitic spread of tumor or of the presence of pleural effusion.

Extrapulmonary Intrathoracic Symptoms and Signs

Approximately 15% of patients complain of symptoms caused by growth of the tumor outside the lung into the pleura, chest wall, mediastinal structures, and contiguous nerves (147). Vague chest pains, often described as a dull ache, occur in up to 50% of patients (146,147). This chest pain may be caused by inflammatory involvement of the parietal pleura and chest wall. Involvement of the chest wall intercostal nerves may result in severe radicular pain. Metastatic involvement of the vertebrae may also result in posterior chest pain. Hoarseness occurs in 1% to 18% of patients and raises concern about involvement of the left or, rarely, the right recurrent laryngeal nerve in tumor (149,150). The left recurrent laryngeal nerve is particularly susceptible to compression by lymph node metastases in the aortopulmonary window or in the subaortic space, though, occasionally, compression or invasion from a primary tumor site may be responsible. The superior vena cava (SVC) syndrome occurs in approximately 5% of patients with carcinoma of the lung (147). SVC syndrome is usually related to compression or invasion of the SVC by neoplastic tissue from related lymph nodes but, occasionally, may be due to direct invasion by a primary tumor in the right upper lobe. A sensation of fullness in the head, headaches, dizziness, and dyspnea are frequent presenting features. Cough, pain, and dysphagia occur less often (151). Physical signs include dilated neck veins, a prominent venous pattern on the anterior chest wall, upper-extremity and facial edema, and a plethoric appearance (146). Pleural effusion of varying amounts occurs in 7% to 10% of patients and most commonly indicates obstruction to pulmonary lymph flow or metastatic involvement of the pleura (146,147,152). Malignant pleural effusions may be serous, serosanguineous, or grossly bloody in appearance and are more common in patients with adenocarcinoma (146,153).

Partial obstruction of the esophagus by tumor in paraesophageal lymph nodes causes dysphagia in rare patients with lung cancer (147). Involvement of the branches of the brachial plexus from tumors located in the superior sulcus can cause pain and weakness of the arm and shoulder. Horner syndrome may also be present in the latter situation (147).

Symptoms and Signs of Metastatic Disease

Symptoms of metastatic disease may be nonspecific, including anorexia, weight loss, and fatigue. In the series of 678 patients reported by Carbone et al., 27% of patients presented with such "constitutional" symptoms (144). In the same series, 32% of patients presented with symptoms referable to specific sites of metastatic disease. The patterns of symptoms and signs of this disease thus reflect patterns of metastatic spread. By histologic type, small cell lung carcinoma has the highest propensity for involvement of the CNS and squamous cell carcinoma has the least propensity for the same (154). Neurologic abnormalities caused by intracranial metastases are present in 3% to 6% of cases. These include hemiplegia, epilepsy, personality changes, confusion, speech defects, and headache. In a study of causes of symptomatic brain metastases reported by Merchut, lung cancer was the most common primary site of disease (155). Bone pain and pathologic fracture from metastatic involvement are variably reported on presentation in as few as 1% or in as many as 22% of patients (147,149). Though the liver and adrenal glands are included with the brain and the bones as being the more frequent sites of metastatic disease, symptomatic liver or adrenal disease related to such metastases is relatively uncommon. Disease in these organs is typically identified by imaging studies rather than by symptoms. Rarely, jaundice, ascites, or an abdominal mass is a major complaint. Neck, muscle, or subcutaneous tissue masses are present infrequently.

Paraneoplastic Syndromes

Ten to 20 percent of patients with lung cancer have systemic symptoms and signs not related either to the primary tumor site or to identifiable metastatic spread of the tumor (see Table 14-4) (57,146,147,156–158). These "paraneoplastic syn-

TABLE 14-4. Classification of Extrapulmonary Manifestations of Carcinoma of the Lung

Endocrine and metabolic
  Carcinoid syndrome
  Cachexia
  Antidiuretic hormone secretion
  Hypercalcemia
  Ectopic adrenocorticotropic hormone secretion
  Ectopic gonadotropic stimulating hormone secretion
  Gynecomastia
  Insulinlike activity
Neuromuscular
  Hoarseness
  Horner syndrome
  Seizures
  Cranial nerve abnormalities
  Carcinomatous myopathy
  Peripheral neuropathies
  Eaton–Lambert syndrome
  Cortical–cerebellar degeneration
  Encephalomyelopathy
  Autonomic overactivity
  Dementia and psychosis
Skeletal
  Clubbing
  Pulmonary hypertrophic osteoarthropathy
  Monoarticular arthritis
Dermatologic
  Acanthosis nigricans
  Scleroderma
  Dermatomyositis and polymyositis
Cardiovascular
  Migratory thrombophlebitis
  Nonbacterial verrucous endocarditis
  Arterial thrombosis
Hematologic
  Anemia
  Thrombocytosis
  Red cell aplasia
  Fibrinolytic purpura
  Nonspecific leukocytosis
  Polycythemia
  Gastrointestinal
  Jaundice
  Abnormal liver function tests
Renal
  Proteinuria
  Nephrotic syndrome

dromes" more frequently occur with small cell lung cancer, (SCLC) but can also be seen with non-small cell lung cancer (NSCLC). In some cases, paraneoplastic syndromes are the result of secretion of identified biologically active molecules acting in an endocrinelike fashion on distant tissues. However, the pathophysiology of all of these syndromes is not known, and they may present with widely variable and clinically profound consequences.

METABOLIC MANIFESTATIONS

The majority of metabolic manifestations are the result of secretion of endocrine or endocrinelike substances by the tumor. At times, these syndromes may be produced by tumors that are still resectable, and treatment of the primary tumor may result in complete or partial remission of the paraneoplastic syndrome. Most of the syndromes are found in association with small cell carcinoma, but NSCLC may also cause endocrine-related metabolic derangements (101,146,147,159).

Cushing Syndrome

Approximately 50% of patients with paraneoplastic Cushing syndrome have bronchogenic carcinoma, with small cell lung cancer and bronchial carcinoid being the most commonly associated tumor types (160). In patients with lung carcinoma, this syndrome differs from the classic syndrome (147,159). In small cell carcinoma patients, for instance, it is characterized by an older age of incidence; the prominence of hypokalemic alkalosis and hyperglycemia; fewer physical stigmata of typical Cushing syndrome; and a more rapid, fulminating course. This syndrome is clinically apparent in approximately 2% to 10% of patients with small cell carcinoma (101,146,158). Adrenocorticotropic hormone (ACTH) has been demonstrated in the tumor tissue and in the blood of many of these patients. This ectopic ACTH is indistinguishable from the normal hormone. Tumors have physiologic autonomy because dexamethasone fails to suppress the levels of ACTH end products in the urine. Excessive quantities of hydroxycorticosteroids (17-OHCS) are demonstrable in the urine. Treating the carcinoma is the most important therapy for patients with ectopic ACTH production. The presence of clinically apparent Cushing syndrome in patients with small cell lung cancer is associated with poorer prognosis (161,162).

Syndrome of Inappropriate Antidiuretic Hormone

The syndrome of inappropriate antidiuretic hormone (SIADH) secretion due to excessive antidiuretic hormone secretion is associated with symptoms of water intoxication—anorexia, nausea, and vomiting accompanied by increasingly severe neurologic complications (158,159,160,163–165). SIADH is characterized by hyponatremia (serum sodium concentration <135 mmol per L), hyposmolality (plasma osmolality < 275 mOsm per kg), and impaired water excretion in the absence of other identifiable causes, including hypovolemia; hypotension; ineffective intravascular volume; or abnormalities of cardiac, renal, thyroid, and adrenal function (146,163). SCLC is estimated to account for more than 75% of all tumors associated with SIADH (164,165). Treating the carcinoma is the most important therapy for patients with paraneoplastic SIADH

(165). Water restriction is the primary form of treatment for patients who are asymptomatic or for those who have modest hyponatremia. Symptoms related to hyponatremia are generally neurologic in nature, ranging from nausea, lethargy, and headaches with moderate hyponatremia to seizures and obtundation in patients with more severe degrees of hyponatremia. Water restriction with salt administration may be necessary in patients with severe hyponatremia associated with symptoms. The effect of water restriction and of salt administration can be enhanced by the use of loop diuretics, demeclocycline, or urea (166–170). In the treatment of patients with hyponatremia, care should be taken that the rate of correction of hyponatremia is moderated to avoid the development of osmotic demyelination (171,172).

Carcinoid Syndrome

Carcinoid syndrome is a well-defined clinical entity characterized by cutaneous, cardiovascular, gastrointestinal, and respiratory manifestations (57,173). Classically, the syndrome includes episodic signs and symptoms related to the release of various vasoactive amines. Neurosecretory granules have been described in small cell tumors that are similar to those seen in carcinoid tumors and are thought to be the source of these mediators (174). Flushing and/or edema of the face and upper body, hyperperistalsis and diarrhea, tachycardia, wheezing, pruritus, paresthesia, and vasomotor collapse may occur in varying combinations. Vasoactive substances including serotonin (5-hydroxytryptamine), 5-hydroxytryptophan, bradykinin and its precursor enzyme kallikrein, and various catecholamines are produced by these tumors and are thought to contribute to the development of the clinical features (173).

Carcinoid syndrome is usually associated with small cell carcinoma. Treatment is palliative. In addition to treatment of the tumor itself, corticosteroids, phenothiazines, antihistamines, and kallikrein inhibitors have been used in the management of flushing with varying degrees of success (173).

Hypercalcemia

Hypercalcemia in lung cancer is most often associated with squamous cell tumors (57,147,158,175–178). Two mechanisms by which hypercalcemia can occur with lung cancer have been described: (a) direct osteolysis by bony metastases and (b) tumor hypercalcemia of malignancy mediated by parathyroid hormone-related protein (PTHrP) (158,175,179,180). Clinically, the hypercalcemic patient may have somnolence and mental status changes as well as anorexia, nausea, vomiting, abdominal discomfort, and weight loss. In resectable cases, removal of the tumor usually results in blood calcium levels returning to normal. Medical treatments used to control hypercalcemia include volume replacement and the use of loop diuretics to increase urinary calcium excretion and medications to inhibit bone resorption (calcitonin, bisphosphonates, and gallium nitrate) (158,175,176).

Ectopic Gonadotropin

Ectopic gonadotropin production has rarely been found in association with carcinoma of the lung. Most of these tumors have been large cell carcinomas. Usually, the patient is a man with tender gynecomastia, often with hypertrophic osteoarthropathy, in whom production of gonadotropin has been documented (147,159).

NEUROLOGIC MANIFESTATIONS

Paraneoplastic neurologic syndromes are uncommon but potentially morbid complications of lung cancer, particularly small cell carcinoma (181). The mechanisms of these syndromes are poorly understood, but at least two are antibody-mediated, suggesting that there may be common antigens shared by tumors and the nervous system (181,158).

Paraneoplastic Encephalomyelitis

Paraneoplastic encephalomyelitis is associated with neuronal loss in the absence of metastatic invasion of the nervous system. Sensory or motor neuropathy, cerebellar degeneration, brainstem encephalomyelitis, or limbic encephalomyelitis may ensue (158,182). Patients with sensory neuropathy or evidence of encephalomyelopathy should have serum and cerebrospinal fluid (CSF) examined for anti-Hu antibodies. Eighty percent of patients with anti-Hu antibody syndrome have small cell carcinoma (183). In 70% of cases, the syndrome predates the diagnosis of the underlying malignancy (182,184).

Lambert-Eaton Myasthenic Syndrome

Lambert-Eaton Myasthenic syndrome (LEMS) affects approximately 3% of patients with SCLC. It is associated with antibodies directed against P/Q-type presynaptic voltage-gated calcium channels (185). These antibodies interrupt the normal calcium flux required for uptake of acetylcholine at the neuromuscular junction (186). Patients typically present with lower extremity weakness as the initial symptom. Upper extremity weakness and oculobulbar symptoms tend to be less severe in this syndrome than in classical myasthenia. Autonomic dysfunction, especially dry mouth, is frequent. Like anti-Hu antibody syndrome, neurologic symptoms of LEMS often antedate identification of the underlying malignancy.

SKELETAL MANIFESTATIONS

The most frequent peripheral sign of bronchial carcinoma is clubbing of the fingers, which, at times, is associated with generalized hypertrophic pulmonary osteoarthropathy (146,147). This clinical syndrome consists of swelling of the soft tissues of the terminal phalanges with curvature of the nails, pain and swelling of the joints, and periostitis with elevation of the periosteum and new bone formation. The mechanism of development of the tissue changes is not well known, although an increase in blood flow in the affected portions of the limbs has been reported. A prompt fall in the blood flow to normal levels occurs following successful treatment of the underlying condition. The cause of increased flow is unknown.

Both humoral and neurogenic factors have been implicated as the cause of the osteoarthropathy. Elevated levels of estrogen have been described, but the significance of this finding has been questioned. An efferent and afferent neurologic reflex has been postulated, with the afferent fibers running in the vagus or the intercostal nerves. This theory is supported by the observation that the osteoarthropathy may be reversed by cutting either the vagi or intercostal nerves without removal of the underlying disease (187,188).

The incidence of hypertrophic pulmonary osteoarthropathy in patients with carcinoma of the lung has been reported to be from 2% to 12% (147,189). It occurs only rarely, if ever, in small cell tumors. Its occurrence is distributed equally among the other three major cell types (squamous, adenocarcinoma, and large cell). The removal of the pulmonary lesion may give dramatic remission of the arthralgia and peripheral edema; however, osseous radiographic changes regress much more slowly. Recurrence of the pulmonary neoplasm is not necessarily accompanied by return of the symptoms of osteoarthropathy.

DERMATOLOGIC MANIFESTATIONS

Dermatologic disease related to lung cancer is relatively uncommon. A number of skin conditions have been described in association with lung cancer, including acanthosis nigricans, dermatomyositis, pruritus, tylosis, urticaria, angioedema, scleroderma, erythema gyratum, acquired ichthyosis, and other nonspecific dermatoses (147).

DIAGNOSIS

SCREENING TECHNIQUES FOR EARLY DIAGNOSIS OF LUNG CANCER

It has been widely appreciated that the vast majority of patients with lung cancer have advanced disease at presentation. Most are symptomatic in some way. Only a minority of cases are identified at early stages when surgical resection offers a reasonable chance for cure. Screening programs for other solid tumors including breast, colon, and prostate cancer are widely accepted and practiced, though controversies persist about efficacy, accuracy, and overdiagnosis. Screening for lung cancer has understandably generated great interest as early detection would be expected to substantively improve survival outcomes. However, such survival benefit has not been demonstrated using chest radiography or sputum cytology, though there continue to be ongoing efforts in reexamining these tools as well as the more recent interest in screening with low-dose computed tomography (LDCT) scanning.

In the 1970s and early 1980s, the National Cancer Institute (NCI) Cooperative Early Lung Cancer Detection Program sponsored three large randomized studies in the United States examining lung cancer screening with chest radiograph and sputum cytology (190–194). The Mayo Clinic, Memorial Sloan-Kettering Cancer Center (MSKCC), and Johns Hopkins University conducted multiyear clinical trials assessing the impact of these techniques on mortality and numbers of cancers detected (195). The MSKCC and Johns Hopkins studies were designed to assess the impact of adding sputum cytology to annual chest radiograph screening. The Mayo Clinic Lung Project compared an intervention group screened with chest radiograph and sputum cytology with a control group who were advised to have these studies performed annually. These studies did indicate that (a) lung cancer was detected more frequently in the screened groups, (b) more cancers were detected at an early stage, and (c) early detection failed to demonstrate any improvement in mortality (191,192,195–198). The failure of these large randomized studies to demonstrate a

survival benefit related to screening with chest radiograph or sputum cytology has resulted in a lack of support for lung cancer screening with either of these techniques. However, as recently summarized by Bach et al., these studies have been criticized for two important reasons (199,200). First, the control subjects of the MSKCC and Johns Hopkins studies received annual chest radiographs. From these studies it was concluded that the addition of sputum cytology to annual chest radiograph was of no mortality benefit, but the issue of whether annual chest radiograph itself is of benefit is not clear. In the Mayo Clinic Lung Project, control subjects were advised to have "usual medical care," which included annual chest radiograph. In sum, none of these studies had a "no screening" arm. Thus, the conclusion that screening was of no benefit, which evolved into current recommendations that serial chest radiograph for the purposes of lung cancer screening should not be performed, continues to be questioned. Second, the Mayo Lung Project, which was the only one of the three studies to not actually include a chest radiograph in its control group, was powered to detect a 50% reduction in lung cancer mortality (192,193). Detection of a smaller reduction in mortality would have required substantially larger numbers of subjects. Because even a 10% to 20% reduction in lung cancer mortality is considered clinically significant in many currently active treatment protocols, the 50% mortality reduction endpoint could be considered unrealistically high (199,200). However, the economic realities of powering a screening study to detect a smaller reduction could understandably be prohibitive. Nonetheless, such studies are still necessary. The NCI-sponsored Prostate, Lung, Colorectal, and Ovarian Trial currently being completed will again address the issue of chest radiographic screening for lung cancer and is powered to detect a 10% reduction in lung cancer mortality in smokers (201). Hopefully, this study will shed new light on this important topic.

Recently, interest in radiographic screening for lung cancer has been refueled by reports on the use of LDCT scanning as a tool for early detection (202–206). Interpretation of the results of a number of studies evaluating the utility of LDCT has been controversial. It is clear that LDCT is much more sensitive than chest radiography in identifying early lung cancers. However, LDCT also identifies large numbers of lesions that are not malignant, with the potential to precipitate enormous costs related to the evaluation and follow-up necessary once such lesions are identified and with the potential harm related to evaluation for false-positive lesions. Further, the concept of "overdiagnosis" of indolent lung cancers that would not have resulted in mortality has been raised (200,207). For example, the first LDCT screening trial in the United States, the Early Lung Cancer Action Project (ELCAP), reported its initial data in 1999 (204). In 1,000 volunteers, aged 60 years or older, with at least 10 pack years of cigarette smoking, noncalcified nodules were detected in 233 (23%) participants by LDCT at baseline, compared with 68 (7%) by chest radiography. Malignant disease was detected in 27 (2.7%) by computed tomography (CT) and in 7 (0.7%) by chest radiography. Twenty-three of the 27 CT-detected cancers and four of the seven chest radiography-detected lesions were stage I. These data suggest LDCT can greatly improve the detection of lung cancer at an earlier and potentially curable stage. However, these data also demonstrate the large percentage of patients in whom lesions are identified, which, after further evaluation, are felt likely to be benign. The evaluation of such lesions inevitably generates cost, both economic and emotional, which is substantial. A mathematic model to predict the cost related to screening for persons with cigarette smoking-related lung cancer risk in the United States was reported by Mahadevia et al. (208). This computer-simulated model evaluated hypothetical cohorts or current, quitting, and former heavy smokers 60 years and older. Cost-effectiveness was measured as dollars spent per quality-adjusted life year (QALY) gained from screening. The projected cost for current smokers was $116,300 per QALY gained, whereas for former smokers the cost projected was $2,322,700 per QALY gained. The projected cost for annual screening in the United States for the estimated 50 million ever smokers was $115 billion. This type of projection raises grave concerns about the potential economic burden of lung cancer screening programs in this country and argues that the role of LDCT as a screening technique will need careful definition. The NCI is currently sponsoring a new study evaluating yearly screening of current and former smokers with chest radiograph versus CT scan. The study will evaluate the mortality, cost, and impact of screening on smoking behavior; is anticipated to enroll an estimated 50,000 persons; and is projected to be completed in 2009.

Whether mass screening programs will ultimately have a beneficial impact on augmenting survival for lung cancer is not clear. At this time, there are no official recommendations that advocate screening patients for lung cancer by chest radiograph, sputum cytology, or LDCT. However, the reasonable expectation that early detection should result in improved survival outcomes justifiably continues to drive research interest and efforts in this important area.

CHEST IMAGING

Most lung cancers are detected by the standard chest radiograph. Although a small percentage of patients have a stage 0 lesion (endobronchial tumor and negative chest film), most will have a detectable lesion on chest radiograph. It is possible to visualize lesions as small as 3 mm, but generally lesions <5 to 6 mm in diameter are unlikely to be detected (192,196). It is usually not possible to reliably differentiate between benign and malignant lesions on a chest radiograph, yet certain radiographic signs may suggest malignancy (209,210). Spiculation or poorly defined margins of lesions are more indicative of a malignancy; however, a sharply defined or smooth margin does not rule out malignancy (211–213). The presence of calcification within a lesion suggests a benign diagnosis when it is central, homogeneous, ring-like, or popcornlike in distribution (214). Eccentric calcification may occur in bronchogenic carcinoma.

Certain radiographic patterns characterize the different cell types (115,211,212). Squamous cell carcinoma is centrally located two-thirds of the time but may arise in the lung periphery, often as a cavitating lesion (Fig. 14-8). It is the lung cancer cell type that cavitates most frequently. Small cell carcinoma is also a central lesion in most cases, often with central adenopathy at presentation (Fig. 14-11). It is peripheral in less than 20% of cases and does not cavitate. As stated, in 55% to 60% of cases, adenocarcinoma is a peripheral lesion (Fig. 14-9). Frequently, there is associated pleural involvement, and in 50% of patients, hilar or mediastinal adenopathy is identified at initial presentation. Bronchoalveolar carcinoma, a subtype of adenocarcinoma, may have a variety of radiographic manifestations.

Most commonly, it appears as a solitary peripheral nodule on the chest radiograph, but it may present as numerous small nodules resembling metastatic disease or as an infiltrate or consolidation with air bronchograms. Large cell carcinomas are more likely to be peripheral than central and are sharply defined, lobulated masses that occasionally cavitate (Fig. 14-10).

SPUTUM CYTOLOGY

Sputum cytology may be particularly helpful in diagnosing central squamous cell and small cell carcinomas (215,216). However, there are several potential problems in accurately interpreting sputum cytology specimens. Among these are inadequate sample number (less than three or four), inadequate specimen sample (without alveolar macrophages), purulent sputum causing degeneration of malignant cells prior to examination, poor sample preparation, or an inexperienced cytopathologist. Accordingly, a negative sputum cytologic examination in a suspicious setting should never terminate further evaluation. Sputum immunostaining with monoclonal antibodies offers considerable promise in detecting early, localized cancers.

BRONCHOSCOPY

Flexible fiber-optic bronchoscopy is used widely for diagnosing both central airway and peripheral parenchymal lesions (217–224). For endobronchial lesions that are endoscopically visible, bronchial washings have a diagnostic yield of 79%, bronchial brushings 92%, and forceps biopsies 93% (219). Occasionally, in the setting of deeper submucosal lesions (e.g., small cell carcinoma), false-negative results occur because of an inability to grasp and bite tissue with biopsy forceps. Transbronchial needle aspiration in association with transbronchial biopsy may improve the diagnostic yield in these lesions (220,224). Bronchoscopy is less helpful in peripheral lesions, particularly in lesions <2 cm in diameter (218,221, 222). For lesions <2 cm, the diagnostic yield is in the range of 20% or less; however, lesions larger than 4 cm may be diagnosed by transbronchial biopsy in 50% to 80% of cases (218,221,222,223).

Complications of fiber-optic bronchoscopy have been minimal. In one report, among 24,521 bronchoscopies performed by 192 bronchoscopists, mortality was only 0.1% (225) and there were no deaths in a series of 600 procedures performed by Zavala (225,226). Other potential complications include laryngospasm (0.13%), pneumothorax (up to 10%), hypoxemia (0.3%), and significant hemorrhage (0.2%) (224–226).

NEEDLE ASPIRATION BIOPSY

Transbronchial needle aspiration for both central and peripheral lesions was introduced for use with the fiber-optic bronchoscope by Wang and Terry (227). When used in conjunction with transbronchial biopsy, the diagnostic yield may be as high as 95% for central lesions and somewhat lower for peripheral lesions. Complications of this procedure include minor bleeding or pneumothorax.

Percutaneous transthoracic thin-needle aspiration biopsy has proven to be a safe and reliable method for diagnosing nonendobronchial lung carcinomas (218,228,229). A 95% or greater accuracy for diagnosing malignant lesions has been reported (229,230). CT or fluoroscopy is used to guide most biopsies. A positive cytologic examination appears to be diagnostic for lung malignancy because there have been only a few reported cases of false-positive results. However, because false-negative results may occur, a negative cytologic examination of a fine-needle aspirate of a lung lesion cannot be used to diagnose a "benign lesion" unless the pathologist can provide a specific benign diagnosis such as hamartoma. Twenty-nine percent of lesions initially diagnosed as negative on percutaneous needle aspiration were subsequently found to be malignant in one recent study (231). In most of these cases, the initial needle aspiration biopsy reading was nonspecifically benign (i.e., no specific benign diagnosis, such as hamartoma or granuloma, could be made). Serial follow-up chest radiographs should still be obtained by transthoracic needle biopsy in patients with a specific benign diagnosis. When a high-risk patient has a nonspecific diagnosis by percutaneous needle biopsy, a further invasive diagnostic workup is necessary until either malignancy or a specific benign process has been diagnosed.

Pneumothorax, the major complication of transthoracic needle aspiration (TTNA), develops in 25% to 30% of patients and usually resolves spontaneously (218,229,232). The most important contributing factor for the development of a pneumothorax is the presence of chronic obstructive pulmonary disease (COPD) (229). In one study, there was a 46% incidence of pneumothorax in patients with COPD compared with a 7% incidence in patients without COPD (233). The placement of a chest tube or a small catheter connected to a Heimlich (one-way) valve may be required (229). Other infrequent complications include hemoptysis and transient parenchymal hemorrhage (229). Cardiac tamponade and fatal air embolism are rare complications. There have been only two reports of implantation of the needle tract with malignant cells (234,235).

PLEURAL BIOPSY

Combined thoracentesis and pleural biopsy will provide up to a 90% yield in patients with carcinoma of the lung and malignant pleural involvement (236). Thoracoscopy, which involves introduction of either a flexible or a rigid bronchoscope into the pleural space with biopsy taken under direct vision, may augment the diagnostic yield in patients with pleural effusions (237).

STAGING CLASSIFICATION

After the tissue diagnosis of lung carcinoma is made, staging is performed to assess extent of disease, to select correct therapy, and to determine prognosis (238–241). Accurate staging is critical for these clinical purposes as well as to identify groups of patients in whom new therapies can be evaluated rigorously. The accepted staging system for non-small cell carcinoma of the lung is the tumor-node-metastasis (TNM) classification, originally proposed in 1946 by Denoix (240). In 1986 and in 1997, the TNM classification was revised and updated (239,241). The details of each subset under the new system are given in Table 14-5 and stage groupings for TNM subsets and outcome by clinical and surgical-pathologic stage are given in Table 14-6 (241). The TNM system can be employed at any time from the initial clinical diagnosis to the time of autopsy (238,240,241). The critical distinction is between

the clinical TNM staging made prior to the institution of any therapy and the surgical-pathologic staging determined from histologic examination of resected specimens (238–241). The recent changes in TNM classification were designed to include within stage groupings and subgroupings patients with tumor characteristics with somewhat similar outcomes (241). It has long been recognized that patients with T1N0M0 (stage IA) lesions have significantly better survival than patients with T2N0M0 (stage IB) lesions. Clinical estimates of the extent of disease reveal that 61% of patients with clinical stage IA and 38% of patients with clinical stage IB tumors are expected to survive for 5 years or more after treatment (Table 14-6) (241). Similarly, within stage II, patients with T1N1M0 (stage IIA) lesions have a significantly better survival than patients with T2N1M0 or T3N0M0 (stage IIB) lesions. Thirty-four percent of patients with clinical T1N1M0 tumors (stage IIA) and 24% of those who have clinical T2N1M0 (stage IIB) disease are expected to survive for 5 or more years after treatment (Table 14-6) (241). The substantial difference in survival between clinical and surgical stage represents the underappreciation of extent of disease with our current clinical staging techniques. Surgical staging reveals occult disease that is not appreciated in clinical staging methods. With either clinical or surgical stage, patients with stage IA (T1N0M0) lesions have the best overall survival and stage IV patients with distant metastasis (M1) have the worst survival (Table 14-6) (241). Most pleural effusions associated with lung cancer are caused by tumor. There are, however, a few patients in whom multiple cytopathologic examinations (on more than one specimen) are negative for tumor; the fluid is nonbloody and is not an exudate. In such cases where these elements and clinical judgment dictate that the effusion is not related to the tumor, the effusion should be excluded as a staging element (241). Pericardial effusion is classified according to the same rules.

The TNM classification has been less useful in staging small cell carcinoma because of the rapid extrathoracic spread of tumor (101,242,243). At the time of diagnosis, more than 85% of patients are stage III or stage IV, and even for those considered to be stage I or stage II, the prognosis is poor because of the frequent presence of undetectable but present metastatic disease (242). The staging system most commonly used for small cell carcinoma is that of the Veterans Administration Lung Cancer Study Group, in which disease is simply classified as either limited or extensive (101,242,243). Limited disease refers to tumor confined to the ipsilateral hemithorax with or without SVC obstruction or involvement of supraclavicular nodes. Extensive disease is defined as a spread beyond the ipsilateral hemithorax and adjacent lymph nodes, recurrent disease after radiation to the primary tumor, or cytologically positive pleural effusion. With limited stage disease, complete response to therapy and prolonged survival are more likely, although less than one third of patients fall into this category at the time of diagnosis.

STAGING PROCEDURES

The staging process commences with a complete history and physical examination; attention is given to signs and symptoms suggesting CNS, bone, liver, chest wall, or mediastinal involvement (218,244). It is unusual for a patient with metastatic disease to be completely asymptomatic. A comprehensive

TABLE 14-5. Definitions in the Revised International Staging System for Lung Cancer

PRIMARY TUMOR (T)

TX	Primary tumor cannot be assessed or tumor proven by the presence of malignant cells in sputum or bronchial washings but not visualized by imaging or bronchoscopy
T0	No evidence of primary tumor
Tis	Carcinoma *in situ*
T1	Tumor ≤3 cm in greatest dimension, surrounded by lung or visceral pleura, without bronchoscopic evidence of invasion more proximal than the lobar bronchus[a] (i.e., not in the main bronchus)
T2	Tumor with any of the following features of size or extent: >3 cm in greatest dimension Involves main bronchus, ≥2 cm distal to the carina Invades the visceral pleura Associated with atelectasis or obstructive pneumonitis that extends to the hilar region but does not involve the entire lung
T3	Tumor of any size that directly invades any of the following: chest wall (including superior sulcus tumors), diaphragm, mediastinal pleura, parietal pericardium; or tumor in the main bronchus <2 cm distal to the carina, but without involvement of the carina; or associated atelectasis or obstructive pneumonitis of the entire lung
T4	Tumor of any size that invades any of the following: mediastinum, heart, great vessels, trachea, esophagus, vertebral body, carina; or tumor with a malignant pleural or pericardial effusion,[b] or with satellite tumor nodule(s) within the ipsilateral primary-tumor lobe of the lung

REGIONAL LYMPH NODES (N)

NX	Regional lymph nodes cannot be assessed
N0	No regional lymph node metastasis
N1	Metastasis to ipsilateral peribronchial and/or ipsilateral hilar lymph nodes, and intrapulmonary nodes involved by direct extension of the primary tumor
N2	Metastasis to ipsilateral mediastinal and/or subcarinal lymph node(s)
N3	Metastasis to contralateral mediastinal, contralateral hilar, ipsilateral or contralateral scalene, or supraclavicular lymph node(s)

DISTANT METASTASIS (M)

MX	Presence of distant metastasis cannot be assessed
M0	No distant metastasis
M1	Distant metastasis present[c]

[a] The uncommon superficial tumor of any size with its invasive component limited to the bronchial wall, which may extend proximal to the main bronchus, is also classified T1.

[b] Most pleural effusions associated with lung cancer are due to tumor. However, there are a few patients in whom multiple cytopathologic examinations of pleural fluid show no tumor. In these cases, the fluid is nonbloody and is not an exudate. When these elements and clinical judgment dictate that the effusion is not related to the tumor, the effusion should be excluded as a staging element and the patient's disease should be staged T1, T2, or T3. Pericardial effusion is classified according to the same rules.

[c] Separate metastatic tumor nodule(s) in the ipsilateral nonprimary tumor lobe(s) of the lung also are classified M1.

From Mountain CF. Revisions in the International system for staging lung cancer. *Chest* 1997;111:1710–1717, with permission.

history is thus critical to the initial evaluation as more than 90% of patients in some series have symptoms at presentation (143). A full laboratory examination should include a complete blood count, liver function tests, determination of calcium level, and other chemistry evaluation based on the presence of symptoms. Hematologic abnormalities such as anemia, thrombocytopenia, or leukoerythroblasts in the peripheral blood may result from direct bone marrow involvement by the tumor. Hypercalcemia may be present in relation to metastatic spread of tumor to bone or, more commonly, to parathyroidlike hormone released by the malignancy (175–178). Abnormal liver function may reflect intrahepatic spread or extrahepatic obstruction.

NONINVASIVE STAGING

Thoracic Imaging Techniques

The crucial element in staging is determining whether mediastinal lymph node involvement with tumor has occurred (218). Except in special cases, the presence or absence of mediastinal metastases will determine whether surgery is performed.

The conventional chest radiograph is only about 40% sensitive for detecting mediastinal lymph node involvement (245). Tomography may increase the yield, but the most sensitive, widely utilized technique is the chest CT scan, which is up to 60% to 75% sensitive for detecting malignant mediastinal disease (218,244,246-248). Chest CT scan is the most widely used noninvasive technique for imaging the mediastinum in patients with lung cancer. Most centers use a lymph node short axis of >1 cm as the cutoff for defining abnormal nodes. However, the reliability and accuracy of CT scanning for detecting malignant mediastinal lymph node involvement is imperfect. Toloza et al. rigorously evaluated the accuracy of CT scanning for identifying mediastinal lymph node metastases (248). In their review of the medical literature, 23 studies addressing this issue were identified that met the following criteria: (a) publication in a peer-reviewed journal, (b) size greater than 50 patients, (c) histologic or cytologic confirmation of the primary tumor as well as mediastinal node involvement, (d) patient data not reproduced in a subsequent update, and (e) raw data available. The 23 studies included nearly 5,000 evaluable patients. The overall sensitivity of CT scanning for identifying

TABLE 14-6. Stage Grouping of TNM Subsets and Outcome by Clinical and Pathologic Stage

Stage	TNM Subset	Clinical Stage[a]	Surgical Pathology Stage[b]
		5 Years After Treatment (Cumulative % Surviving)	
IA	T1N0M0	61	67
IB	T2N0M0	38	57
IIA	T1N1M0	34	55
IIB	T2N1M0	24	39
	T3N0M0	22	38
IIIA	T3N1M0	9	25
	T1N2M0 ⎫		
	T2N2M0 ⎬	13	23
	T3N2M0 ⎭		
IIIB	T4N0M0 ⎫		
	T4N1M0 ⎬	7	ND
	T4N2M0 ⎭		
	T1N3M0 ⎫		
	T2N3M0 ⎬	3	ND
	T3N3M0 ⎭		
IV	Any T any N M1	1	ND

ND, No Data.

[a] Percentage distribution of cell types: adenocarcinoma, 47.2% (2,466/5.230); squamous cell carcinoma, 33.9% (1,773/5.230); large cell carcinoma, 3.1% (163/5.230); small cell carcinoma, 11.9% (624/5.230); NOS (carcinoma not specified), 3.9% (204/5.230).

[b] Percentage distribution of cell types: adenocarcinoma, 53.0% (1,012/1,910); squamous cell carcinoma, 41.6% (794/1,910); large cell carcinoma, 3.6% (68/1,910); NOS (carcinoma not specified), 1.9% (36/1,910).

From Mountain CF. Revisions in the International system for staging lung cancer. *Chest* 1997;111:1710–1717, with permission.

mediastinal lymph node involvement was 60% and the overall specificity was 81%. Thus, an unacceptably large percent of patients with either present or absent mediastinal malignant disease are misdiagnosed by CT scanning. In the past, patients were typically sent directly to thoracotomy for tumor resection when the mediastinum appeared to be without disease on chest CT. However, 5% to 15% of patients with clinical T1N0M0 lesions as judged by CT criteria are found to have lymph node involvement by surgical sampling, highlighting the need for more accurate noninvasive lymph node staging (218). Conversely, enlarged lymph nodes may be the result of inflammatory, nonneoplastic processes (249). In these cases, accepting CT evidence of malignancy without histologic confirmation of disease might deny the patient potentially curative surgery. Thus, patients with "normal" lymph nodes by CT scan should not be assumed to be free of mediastinal disease and, further, patients with "abnormal" lymph nodes by CT scan should not be assumed to have mediastinal lymph node spread of tumor. Both of these findings require further evaluation and, preferably, histologic confirmation of the presence or absence of disease (247).

Magnetic resonance imaging (MRI) has also been evaluated for imaging the mediastinum (213,218,250). However, because the sensitivity of MRI appears to be similar to that of CT, the latter remains the initial procedure of choice for evaluating the mediastinum, and MRI is reserved for patients in whom CT results are equivocal. MRI is the procedure of choice for evaluating superior sulcus tumors and for assessing chest wall extension of lung cancer. Moreover, tumor invasion of the pericardium or heart (the latter indicating tumor unresectability) is best demonstrated with MRI (213). Multiplanar imaging capability provides accurate evaluation of involvement of the brachial plexus, spinal canal, chest wall, and subclavian artery in such tumors (218).

Positron emission tomography (PET) has emerged as a useful noninvasive method for diagnosing and staging lung cancer (251,252). PET scanning is becoming more widely available, though many areas of the United States are still gaining experience in its use. Images are based on measurements of uptake of positron emitting radiotracers such as ^{18}F–fluorodeoxy–glucose (FDG), a glucose analog that is utilized to track glucose uptake and phosphorylation. FDG is transported into the cells and phosphorylated by hexokinase but cannot undergo further significant metabolism or diffusion out of the cell. Concentration of the radiolabeled compound in cells can be imaged using a PET camera. Certain malignant tissues, including lymphoma, tumors of the brain, and lung cancer, demonstrate increased glucose metabolism that can be observed by using PET and FDG. PET imaging is thus primarily a metabolic rather than an anatomic study and has added greatly to the ability to identify abnormal tissues. Toloza et al. evaluated the medical literature for PET scanning in lung cancer in a parallel fashion to their examination of CT scanning (248). Using criteria similar to those described above for studies on CT scanning, they identified 19 appropriate studies evaluating the accuracy of PET scanning in patients with lung cancer. These 19 studies combined yielded 1,111 evaluable patients. The sensitivity of PET scanning in these patients was 85%, with specificity being 88%. Thus, PET scanning had both higher sensitivity and specificity for identifying mediastinal lymph node involvement in lung cancer than CT scanning did.

A further advantage of PET is that it is a whole body test. It provides information beyond the thorax that may be important in evaluating for extrathoracic spread of lung cancer. For example, PET can detect metastases in distant organs including bone, liver, extrathoracic nodes, and adrenal glands. PET scanning is usually not useful in detecting metastases in the brain as normal brain tissue is FDG avid. False-negative PET findings have been reported in patients with slow-growing or well-differentiated tumors, such as bronchoalveolar lung carcinoma (253,254). Furthermore, FDG uptake is not limited to malignant cells. Other metabolically active abnormal tissues, including infected or inflamed cells, as well as some normal tissues, such as the brain and heart, avidly take up glucose and will be positive on PET imaging. A patient with pneumonia or pulmonary tuberculosis, for example, will likely have a positive PET scan in the affected area of the lung (255). Most importantly, PET scanning should not replace histologic confirmation of disease. Positive PET findings in the mediastinum suggesting malignant disease should always be confirmed by biopsy. Moreover, the small but present false-negative rate indicates that a full surgical exploration of the mediastinum should be performed in patients undergoing lung cancer resection, even in the absence of identifiable disease in the mediastinum by PET or CT scanning. Two further important limitations of PET scanning include the current lack of wide availability of PET scanners and the high cost of the test.

The combination of the anatomic accuracy of CT scanning and the functional information provided by PET scanning will likely become the standard for noninvasive evaluation of patients with lung cancer. Studies evaluating PET combined with CT versus CT or PET alone for intrathoracic lymph node staging in NSCLC are still few in number (251,252). In one such report, Vansteenkiste et al. (252) showed that utilizing PET plus CT scanning for staging the mediastinum improved the sensitivity of CT scanning alone from 75% to 93%. Moreover, the specificity was improved from 63% for CT alone to 95% for PET plus CT. The recent American College of Chest Physicians (ACCP) Guidelines for the Diagnosis and Management of Lung Cancer recommend that CT scan of the chest be performed in all patients and, if available, PET scanning be performed to evaluate the mediastinum in all patients who are potential candidates for surgery (247).

INVASIVE STAGING

A number of invasive techniques are available that provide histologic confirmation of malignancy, either at the primary site or at sites of suspected spread. Establishing metastatic disease does not necessarily require that the presence of tumor at the presumed primary site in the lung has been proved. In some cases, both diagnosis and staging can be established by biopsying a site separate from the primary tumor. In most patients, evaluation of the mediastinum is the first priority. However, in patients in whom noninvasive evaluation suggests metastatic disease at an extrathoracic site, evaluation of that site may be the most efficient means of establishing a disease stage as well as a diagnosis.

Invasive Staging of the Mediastinum

The indication for mediastinoscopy in patients with carcinoma of the lung is to determine the presence or absence of metastatic tumor in the mediastinal nodes (see Fig. 14-12). Such information may be of considerable prognostic significance and may also be helpful in planning the appropriate therapeutic approach. The accuracies of invasive staging techniques of the mediastinum are highly variable. Confirmation of metastatic disease in mediastinal nodes is inherently only as accurate as the noninvasive techniques that identify those nodes as being suspicious. As noted above, both chest CT and PET scanning have imperfect sensitivity and specificity. Nodes that are not identified as abnormal by either of these imaging techniques will not be biopsied except by nondirected mediastinoscopy or at the time of surgical resection. The choice of which technique to utilize will depend on the location of the abnormal nodes as indicated by noninvasive imaging and by the local expertise in each of the invasive techniques (see Fig. 14-13).

BRONCHOSCOPY AND TRANSBRONCHIAL NEEDLE ASPIRATION. Bronchoscopy is typically utilized in obtaining tissue from a suspected primary site. Bronchoscopy for staging is useful in assessing the proximity of endobronchial tumor to the main carina. Tumors involving the carina or located within 1 to 2 cm of the carina are often considered to be inoperable because of the technical difficulty of the surgical resection and the poorer

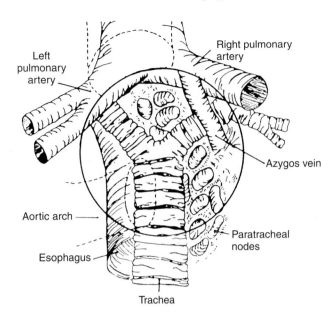

FIGURE 14-12. Representation of the view through a mediastinoscope at the level of the tracheal bifurcation with subcarinal lymph nodes and right pulmonary artery and azygous vein. (From Straus MJ. *Lung cancer: clinical diagnosis and treatment.* New York: Grune & Stratton, 1977:123, with permission.)

prognosis associated with lesions in this location. Transbronchoscopic needle aspiration biopsy has been used as a mediastinal staging technique (218,223,224,227). The sensitivity of this procedure is variable. Use of this technique may provide the ability to establish histologic confirmation both at the primary site as well as in the mediastinum during a single procedure.

TRANSTHORACIC NEEDLE ASPIRATION; ENDOSCOPIC ULTRASOUND-GUIDED NEEDLE ASPIRATION. TTNA and endoscopic ultrasound (EUS)-guided needle aspiration have been used to sample enlarged mediastinal lymph nodes. TTNA is also utilized to biopsy peripheral lung lesions (229). The sensitivity of these procedures for mediastin nodes is reported to be as high as 90% (256,257). However, TTNA and EUS-guided needle aspirations provide a sampling of only a limited number of nodes. Because these aspirations are typically directed by CT or PET scanning, these techniques are unlikely to be utilized in patients who have malignant disease in the mediastinum but whose lymph nodes are small. EUS-guided needle aspiration is particularly useful in sampling nodes that are difficult to reach by traditional mediastinoscopy, including the subcarinal area and the aortopulmonary window.

MEDIASTINOSCOPY AND MEDIASTINOTOMY. Mediastinoscopy has been considered the gold standard for evaluation of mediastinal lymph node involvement in lung cancer (218,244,257–260). However, this technique has a sensitivity of approximately 80% to 85%, with a false-negative rate of approximately 20% and, like needle aspirations, has limitations due to its reliance on imperfect noninvasive imaging techniques to identify suspicious nodes (256,257). There are also mechanical limitations to this technique. In general, only the superior aspects of the mediastinum can be fully evaluated by cervical mediastinoscopy. The presence of large vessels, airways, and nerves may limit access to the mediastinum. Lymph nodes

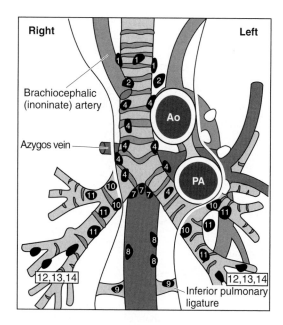

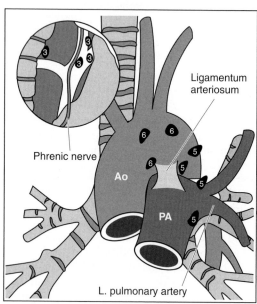

FIGURE 14-13. Regional lymph node stations for lung cancer staging. (From Mountain CF, Dresler CM. Regional lymph node classification for lung cancer staging. *Chest* 1997;111:1718–1723, with permission.)

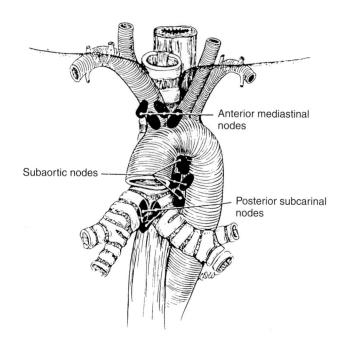

FIGURE 14-14. Diagrammatic representation of thoracic lymph nodes inaccessible to mediastinoscopy. The anterior mediastinal lymph nodes and subaortic lymph nodes may be reached by anterior mediastinotomy (Chamberlain procedure). (From Shields TW, Ritts RE. *Bronchial carcinoma.* Springfield, IL: Charles C Thomas, 1974, with permission.)

in the posterior subcarinal and inferior mediastinal stations and in the aortopulmonary window are generally not accessible by this technique (see Fig. 14-14). Aortopulmonary lymph nodes are amenable to biopsy by anterior mediastinotomy, also known as the *Chamberlain procedure*, or to extended cervical mediastinoscopy. Anterior mediastinotomy provides a more direct approach to the mediastinal lymph nodes than mediastinoscopy does. This approach is typically used for left lung tumors when the major lymph node groups to be evaluated are in the subaortic anterior mediastinal areas. Neoplasms of the left upper lobe, in particular, may spread directly to the anterior mediastinal group of lymph nodes without involving the inferior tracheal bronchial, superior tracheal bronchial, or paratracheal nodal chain (Fig. 14-14) (249,258,260,261).

Opinion is divided as to whether mediastinoscopy should be performed in all patients with apparent clinically resectable disease. Even with its limitations, mediastinoscopy is still the most comprehensive pathologic evaluation of the mediastinal nodes. Mediastinoscopy may not be recommended in patients who have received mediastinal irradiation, who have had a tracheotomy, or who have SVC syndrome. Detterbeck et al. writing for the ACCP Evidence-Based Lung Cancer Guidelines suggest that mediastinoscopy should be performed in all patients with NSCLC who appear to have resectable disease (257). In patients without evidence of mediastinal lymph node disease by noninvasive imaging and in those without evidence of distant metastases, lymph node sampling by directed biopsy (such as would be performed with TTNA or EUS-guided aspiration) will be of poor yield. In patients with evidence of mediastinal node enlargement but with no evidence of distant metastases, mediastinoscopy still provides the best overall node sampling, though in these cases lymph node sampling by directed needle aspiration biopsy may be less invasive but may still establish the presence of disease. It should be emphasized that pathologic confirmation of mediastinal lymph nodes deemed abnormal by CT or PET imaging must be pursued. No patient should be denied surgery solely on the basis of noninvasive imaging of the mediastinum.

VIDEO-ASSISTED THORACOSCOPIC SURGERY. Video-assisted thoracoscopic surgery (VATS) may sometimes be utilized to biopsy lymph nodes in the mediastinum that are not accessible by cervical mediastinoscopy. With the availability of EUS-guided needle aspiration, it may not be necessary to proceed to VATS to sample nodes in the subcarinal space or in the aortopulmonary window.

THORACOTOMY FOR DIAGNOSIS AND STAGING. Historically, 5% to 20% of patients with NSCLC had undergone surgery without a positive histologic or cytologic diagnosis. Today, because of widespread use of bronchoscopy and needle biopsy techniques, at least 95% of patients with lung cancer who undergo thoracotomy have a histologic or cytologic diagnosis established prior to surgery. Thoracotomy should not be used for establishing the diagnosis when there appears to be no hope that the lesion is resectable; this is especially true in the elderly or in patients with limited functional pulmonary reserve (147).

A formal thoracotomy for diagnosis alone is usually not justified in patients with a superior sulcus tumor or SVC syndrome. In the former situation, a tissue diagnosis may be obtained prior to institution of a therapeutic regimen by bronchoscopy with fluoroscopic guidance, by percutaneous needle aspiration biopsy, or by a more limited surgical approach. In patients with SVC obstruction, tissue diagnosis may usually be obtained by bronchoscopy or by mediastinotomy; however, mediastinoscopy could be hazardous due to increased pressure in large veins (147).

EVALUATION FOR EXTRAPULMONARY METASTASIS

Lung cancer staging requires a thorough search for metastatic disease. The presence of extrathoracic spread of disease to distant organs indicates that the patient is not a candidate for surgical resection. It should be emphasized that patients with clinical stage I or II disease who are found to be asymptomatic after comprehensive history and physical examination do not require further imaging. Such patients should proceed to lung resection if they can physiologically tolerate surgery. The Canadian Lung Oncology Group performed a prospective, randomized clinical trial in patients with early clinical stage NSCLC by assigning each to either CT scan of the chest and mediastinoscopy or CT scan of the chest; mediastinoscopy; bone scan; and CT scan of the liver, adrenal glands, and head (262). No differences in recurrence rates or survival was demonstrated between the two groups. Routinely performing extensive imaging in these patients is more likely to produce false-positive results, which may lead to further noninvasive or invasive studies, cost, and delay of appropriate treatment (247,218,263,264). Conversely, the presence of abnormal symptoms, signs, or laboratory findings is associated with a significant yield of identifying metastatic disease with further evaluation (265,266). Patients with such abnormalities should have selective imaging or invasive evaluation directed by the specific abnormality.

Certain groups of patients have been identified who are more likely to have metastatic disease. These include patients with stage IIIA and IIIB disease, and patients with N2 disease in the mediastinum (218,247,267,268). These patients are much less likely to be asymptomatic and should in general be evaluated for metastatic disease by routine imaging studies (247). Metastases can be detected by CT scan, PET scan, radionuclide scans of specific organs, or MRI. A CT scan or MRI of the head is useful for detecting CNS spread and may reveal asymptomatic metastasis. CT scanning of the liver and adrenal glands or whole body PET imaging may also detect metastatic lesions in these organs (247,249,251,269). Bone scans and radionuclide liver–spleen scans are also of utility in determining tumor spread.

In summary, the search for metastatic disease in patients with NSCLC should be symptom-directed whenever possible.

Asymptomatic patients with early stage NSCLC, with no evidence of mediastinal spread by chest CT scanning, and who have negative PET scanning outside the primary tumor site should proceed to surgical resection if they have adequate pulmonary reserve. Patients with Stage III disease, or who have symptoms, should have a directed metastatic evaluation performed.

As with NSCLC, the radiographic staging of small cell tumors focuses on the presence or absence of extrathoracic disease. The approach remains the same as that for non–small cell tumors, but some clinicians recommend routine multiorgan (i.e., head, bone, liver, and adrenal) scanning because of the frequent spread of disease. In addition, many investigators recommend routine bone marrow investigation with bone marrow aspiration and biopsy because bone marrow involvement occurs in up to 50% of cases even in the absence of peripheral blood abnormalities or a bone scan with positive findings. Certainly, patients who are considered for locoregional therapy (chest radiotherapy and/or surgical resection) or for participation in clinical trials should undergo these additional staging studies to identify asymptomatic metastatic sites (101).

APPROPRIATE INVESTIGATION OF A SOLITARY PERIPHERAL PARENCHYMAL MASS

A circumscribed, solitary, peripheral lung mass (the pulmonary coin lesion) in the asymptomatic patient frequently represents a relatively early primary carcinoma of the lung. However, it may be an inflammatory mass, a vascular lesion, a benign tumor, or even a solitary metastasis to the lung. On chest radiograph, the actual margins of the lesion may vary from being ill defined to being sharply demarcated, and the size may vary, although, in general, no lesion >3 cm in diameter should be included in this category (218,270,271). Table 14-7 shows some of the benign causes of the solitary pulmonary nodule.

The percentage of benign and malignant lesions in any given series of coin lesions varies with patient selection and

TABLE 14-7. Common Nonmalignant Lesions Presenting as Solitary Pulmonary Nodules

Very common
  Granulomas
    Histoplasmoma, tuberculoma, and coccidioidoma
    Cryptococcosis, blastomycosis, and actinomycosis
    Unidentified granulomas
Common
  Lung abscess before evacuation into a bronchus
  Slowly resolving circumscribed pneumonia
  Lipoid pneumonia
  Hamartoma
Less common
  Bronchogenic cyst
  Pulmonary infarct
  Bronchial adenoma
  Arteriovenous fistula
  Enlarged pulmonary artery
  Infected, fluid-filled bulla
  Rheumatoid nodule

with the definition of such a lesion. In the general population, 5% of such masses discovered by a routine radiographic survey are carcinomas. However, in the series in which resections have been performed, 50% of such masses in patients over 50 years of age are carcinomas (147). Furthermore, this percentage increases with advancing age of the patient group.

Of the malignant lesions, approximately 8% to 10% are metastatic (147). Less than 0.5% of all patients with coin lesions have metastatic disease in the lungs from an unknown, asymptomatic tumor elsewhere in the body (272). Consequently, in a patient with a coin lesion, any extensive radiographic examination for a possible primary tumor hidden in another organ system has little potential reward. As stated, investigation of a specific organ system is indicated only when the patient has a history of a previous malignant tumor or has symptoms related to that system or when the routine laboratory studies reveal an abnormality that suggests the presence of a silent tumor (147,249). Because the sensitivity of PET scans ranges from 95% to 100%, the failure to demonstrate increased FDG uptake in a solitary lung lesion (≥ 1 cm in widest diameter), in most cases, warrants watchful waiting. However, exceptions to this exist as well-differentiated tumors may not take up FDG avidly. For example, if the solitary lesion contains an air bronchogram, suggesting a bronchoalveolar cell carcinoma, the PET scan may be false negative, and further investigation may be warranted (253,254). It should also be noted that nonneoplastic inflammatory or infectious processes, including sarcoidosis or tuberculosis, may be FDG avid and may generate positive PET scans.

In the evaluation of a coin lesion following a standard history, physical examination, and routine laboratory and radiographic studies of the chest, skin tests should be performed for *Mycobacterium tuberculosis*. Sputum smears for detection of acid-fast organisms and cytologic studies should be carried out. Any available previous radiographs of the chest should be reviewed. Chest CT should be performed to confirm that the lesion is solitary and to assess for presence of calcification. When the lesion is found to have been present and unchanged for a period of 24 months or more or when any one of four specific types of calcification (central, ring-like, homogeneous, or popcorn-like) is seen, the lesion may be judged to be benign and be observed radiographically at periodic intervals (210,218,249). When acid-fast organisms are demonstrated in the sputum, the patient should receive appropriate antituberculous chemotherapy, and the lesion as well as sputum cultures should be reevaluated within 2 to 3 months. When none of these features is present, particularly when the patient is over 40 years of age, is a cigarette smoker, or has any other features suggesting an increased risk of lung cancer, further invasive evaluation is warranted. In some cases, if the risk for lung cancer is felt to be high, the lesion should be surgically removed to establish a diagnosis and to decide on treatment (147,271).

TREATMENT

NON–SMALL CELL LUNG CANCER

Therapy for NSCLC depends primarily on the stage of the cancer at diagnosis. Multiple host factors including age, general condition, and the presence of concomitant diseases, particularly COPD and atherosclerotic cardiac disease, influence decisions about treatment choices. Therapeutic interventions including surgical resection, radiation therapy, chemotherapy, and palliative modalities will be dictated by tumor stage and by the global health of the individual patient. In general, resection is the treatment of choice for early stage or localized NSCLC, whereas combined modality regimens are typically offered to patients with Stage III disease. Past and recent clinical trials continue to contribute to an evolving approach to patients with all stages of lung cancer. It is only through the efforts of such clinical trials that the current abysmal 5-year survival of 14% of patients with NSCLC will improve.

Early Stage Non–small Cell Lung Cancer

A small number of patients are found to have radiographically occult lung cancers, usually detected by cytologic examination of sputum or by bronchoscopy. These tumors are typically treated with surgical resection of the lobe or the lung containing the bronchus with tumor. Photodynamic therapy (PDT) may also be a treatment option, particularly in patients who have marginal pulmonary reserve and in those who may not be able to tolerate lobectomy or pneumonectomy. PDT involves administration of a tumor-selective photosensitizer to the patient. The agent is taken up by the malignant tissue and subsequently activated by intrabronchial exposure to light of a specific wavelength. A number of series have demonstrated complete response rates with PDT of 64% to 86% (273–278). PDT, thus, should be considered a therapeutic alternative to surgery for patients who are felt to be poor surgical candidates for resection (273).

Stage I Non–small Cell Lung Cancer

Approximately 15% of all persons with lung cancer present with Stage I disease (241,279). For these patients, surgical resection is the treatment of choice. The best long-term survival results have been obtained in patients who have true Stage I disease (i.e., by pathologic staging) and small primary tumors (i.e., T1N0M0, Stage IA) (241,249,280–284). Mountain (Table 14-6) and Naruke et al. have reported 5-year survivals of 67.5% and 75.5%, respectively, in this subgroup (241,281). Patients with tumors larger than 3 cm (Stage 1B, T2N0M0), have a lower survival rate than patients with tumors ≤ 3 cm (Stage 1A, T1N0M0) (Table 14-6) (241). Following complete resection of Stage I NSCLC in 598 patients, Martini and Battie reported overall 5- and 10-year survival rates of 75% and 67%, respectively (285). Survival rates in patients with T1 tumors were 82% at 5 years and 74% at 10 years, in contrast with 68% at 5 years and 60% at 10 years, respectively, for patients with T2 lesions. Hence, the smaller the tumor, the better the outcome.

If possible, patients with confirmed Stage I NSCLC should be offered surgical resection. Full anatomic resection requires lobectomy or pneumonectomy. However, many of these patients have significant comorbidities, including severe COPD with imperfect pulmonary reserve, which may preclude full anatomic resection. Approaches to the assessment of "operability" of such patients have been proposed by several groups on the basis of algorithms of physiologic assessment (286-288). In patients with severe COPD who cannot tolerate full anatomic resection, sublobar (wedge) resection should be considered. A number of studies including a prospective randomized control trial from the Lung Cancer Study Group have demonstrated that lung cancer recurrence rates are higher in patients who undergo limited resection compared to patients who have complete anatomic resections (289–292). However, lobectomy and, particularly, pneumonectomy may not be possible in patients with limited pulmonary reserve, and therefore, sublobar resection may be appropriate treatment in some cases.

The selection of radiation therapy as the primary modality for curative therapy is indicated in an occasional patient with Stage I NSCLC. Typically, these are patients who cannot physiologically tolerate surgical resection, who are felt to be poor surgical candidates for other medical reasons, or who refuse surgery (293–296). Radical radiation therapy (local dosage of 50 to 65 Gy) is capable of sterilizing carcinoma of the lung (293,297,298). Thus, local control of a bronchial carcinoma may be accomplished. Patients who seem to benefit most from this approach are those with small peripheral lesions (i.e., T1N0M0); this is the same group with the best survival outcome from surgical resection (296). Approximately 15% of these patients will be long-term survivors, 25% will die of complications related to other medical disease, 30% will die of distant metastatic disease, and 30% will die after local failure only (296).

In general, treatment modalities (chemotherapy or radiation therapy) given in addition to surgery have not been felt to be of additional benefit to surgical resection in patients with stage I disease. However, ongoing clinical trials as well as two recently published studies suggest there may be a role for chemotherapy in patients with completely resected stage IB disease (299–301). This represents a change in approach to these patients. For these patients, the use of adjuvant chemotherapy following surgical resection is still probably best done in the context of a clinical trial. This area represents one that will continue to be a focus of intense scrutiny in the near future.

Stage II Non–small Cell Lung Cancer

Stage II NSCLC is a relatively uncommon presentation of disease. In surgical series, less than 5% of patients undergoing lung cancer resection for NSCLC present with Stage IIA disease, whereas Stage IIB tumors account for another 15% to 25% (241,302). As outlined in Table 14-6, Stage II is divided into Stage IIA (T1N1M0) and Stage IIB (T2N1M0 or T3N1M0) disease. In Mountain's original revisions to the International Staging System for lung cancer in 1997, 5-year survival for clinical pathologic stage IIA disease was 55%, whereas that for Stage IIB was 38% to 39% (Table 14-6) (241). These outcomes were based on a database of more than 5,000 patients from the MD Anderson Cancer Center and the Lung Cancer Study Group. Other large series evaluating survival in patients with Stage II NSCLC indicate 5-year survival between 52% and 57% for patients with pathologic Stage IIA disease and from 33% to 48% for Stage IIB patients (303–305).

Patients with T1N1M0 or T2N1M0 disease require complete anatomic resection, including the intrapulmonary (N1) nodes. These patients should also undergo evaluation of the mediastinal lymph nodes. Complete anatomic resection will therefore require lobectomy or pneumonectomy. When feasible, sleeve lobectomy allows preservation of lung tissue and should spare patients the greater physiologic impairment related to a pneumonectomy. Patients with chest wall involvement (T3) must undergo *en bloc* resection of the chest wall unless it is clear that the tumor does not extend beyond the

parietal pleura. In the latter case, extrapleural resection may be possible (302). At present, there is no evidence that adjuvant radiation therapy for patients with T3 tumors (where the primary lesion extends either into the chest wall or into the mediastinum, or is within 2 cm of the carina) is of any benefit (306–308). However, in patients who undergo incomplete resection of T3 lesions, postoperative radiation therapy may be of some benefit (302,309–311).

Patients with Stage II NSCLC and N1 nodal disease have been studied with regard to efficacy of adjuvant treatment. Routine administration of postoperative radiation has not been demonstrated to have any influence on survival. However, postoperative radiation does decrease local recurrence rates. At present, adjuvant radiation therapy is not generally recommended, but there continues to be interest in adjuvant chemotherapy after surgical resection for stage II disease. A meta-analysis of eight studies evaluating cisplatin-based regimens suggested a survival benefit of approximately 5% at 5 years in patients receiving adjuvant chemotherapy for N1 disease (312). These results have been supported recently by the International Adjuvant Lung Cancer Trial collaborative group (299,301). This multicenter study demonstrated an approximately 4% higher disease-free survival rate in patients given cisplatin-based chemotherapy after complete resection of NSCLC. The results of these studies cannot yet be extrapolated to recommend that adjuvant chemotherapy can be given to all patients with resected NSCLC. Issues relating to toxicity of adjuvant chemotherapy, the role of adjuvant radiation therapy, and questions about the appropriate timing of the various modalities are yet to be answered (301). Ongoing clinical trials addressing these issues should define the role of adjuvant therapy for patients with resectable Stage II disease.

Stage IIIA Non–small Cell Lung Cancer

The revised international lung cancer–staging system classified Stage IIIA disease into two major groups (Table 14-6). Approximately 10% of patients with NSCLC present with stage IIIA disease (241). The first group includes patients with primary tumors with chest wall involvement and N1 nodal disease (i.e., T3, N1). These patients are treated in similar fashion to patients with T3N0M0 (i.e., Stage IIB) disease and will not be discussed in further detail here. The second and larger group includes patients with ipsilateral mediastinal lymph node metastases (i.e., T1–3, N2). The remainder of this section will address this group of patients.

PATIENTS WITH OCCULT N2 DISEASE. Careful evaluation of patients with a diagnosis of NSCLC should focus on the exclusion of metastatic disease to the mediastinal lymph nodes and to distant sites. The identification of mediastinal lymph node disease can be challenging and should take advantage of the various diagnostic procedures outlined previously. Despite careful preoperative evaluation, up to one-fourth of patients undergoing thoracotomy for lung cancer resection will be found to have occult N2 disease (313–315). This emphasizes the critical importance of thorough mediastinal lymph node dissection in all patients undergoing thoracotomy for resection. The best of preoperative evaluations will still miss some patients with microscopic involvement of the mediastinal N2 nodes.

It is not clear whether the addition of adjuvant therapy postoperatively for this group of patients results in any survival benefit, and there is potential for harm due to therapy-related toxicity. Adjuvant radiation therapy alone does appear to decrease the rate of local recurrence (316). However, in a meta-analysis of nine randomized trials of postoperative radiation therapy in Stage IIIA disease, treatment was associated with an increased risk of death and with a risk ratio of 1.2 (317). Adjuvant chemotherapy, likewise, has historically not been associated with survival benefit, though a meta-analysis reported by Le Chevalier in 1998 suggested a 5% improvement in survival with cisplatin-based adjuvant regimens (318). The combination of chemotherapy with radiation therapy postoperatively also has not been associated with improved overall survival and would be anticipated to potentially be associated with more toxicity (319,320). In sum, there is currently no evidence that adjuvant radiation therapy or chemotherapy, alone or in combination, are associated with survival benefit for patients with pathologic Stage IIIA disease diagnosed at surgical resection of the primary tumor. Any treatment of these patients with adjuvant therapies should be ideally done in the context of a clinical trial as this remains an area of controversy.

PATIENTS WITH CLINICALLY EVIDENT N2 DISEASE. The approach to patients with Stage IIIA disease and clinical evidence of mediastinal N2 involvement is an area of intense interest. The presence of N2 disease has historically rendered these patients nonresectable as surgery alone is associated with extremely poor prognosis. Because of this, there has been growing interest in a multidisciplinary approach to such patients. Several studies in the last decade have reported the benefit of neoadjuvant treatment followed by surgical resection (313,321,322–325). Rosell et al. and Roth et al. reported that patients with Stage IIIA disease randomized to receive cisplatin-based induction chemotherapy before surgical resection followed by radiation therapy (322,323) or chemotherapy (324,325) demonstrated improvement in median survival. These studies have been criticized because of small patient numbers and the nonuniformity of pathologic confirmation of mediastinal disease prior to treatment, and these were not corroborated in a neoadjuvant trial published by the French Thoracic Cooperative Group in 2002 (326). Although a neoadjuvant approach is now widely practiced, whether it should represent the standard of care for this group of patients is still unclear. It should be noted that reevaluation prior to surgery is an inherent part of this approach. Patients who have persistent biopsy-proven tumor in the mediastinal nodes after induction chemotherapy should probably not undergo surgical resection as these patients have substantially poorer survival than patients with complete pathologic clearing of nodal disease (313,327,328).

There is a further subset of patients with Stage IIIA disease with "bulky" N2 disease who are deemed unresectable because of the burden of nodal disease or because the primary tumor cannot be resected. Historically, these patients were offered radiation therapy alone as it seemed most likely to control local disease. However, long-term survival was poor, and interest has been shifted to the combination of local radiation therapy and chemotherapy to contain systemic disease. Although optimal time sequencing of the two modalities is still being

investigated, the combination of platinum-based chemotherapy with radiation therapy does appear to result in improved survival rates compared to no treatment or to radiation therapy alone (329–331).

The evaluation and treatment of patients with Stage IIIA disease clearly remains a challenge. Enrollment of these patients into larger clinical treatment trials will be necessary to delineate the best approach to Stage IIIA disease.

Stage IIIB Non–small Cell Lung Cancer

The staging classification for Stage IIIB disease includes patients with T4 primary lesions without nodal disease and patients with T1–3 primary lesions and N3 nodal involvement without distant metastases to distant sites (T4N0M0 and T1–3N3M0) (Tables 14-5 and 14-6). The N3 designation includes contralateral hilar, mediastinal, or scalene as well as supraclavicular nodal metastasis (241). An estimated 10% to 15% of patients present with Stage IIIB disease (332). Five-year survival in this group of patients is extremely poor and is estimated at 3% to 7% (241).

With two exceptions, surgical resection is not generally a part of the treatment plan for patients with IIIB disease (332). These exceptions include patients with T4N0–1M0 disease whose T4 designation is due to a satellite tumor nodule within the lobe of lung containing the primary tumor or who have tumor involving the main carina (Table 14-6). In these patients, surgical resection may be associated with 5-year survival of up to 20% (332).

The standard of care for patients with Stage IIIB disease is combined modality treatment with radiation and chemotherapy. The decision to pursue such therapy must be tempered by the individual patient's overall health, as measured by performance status. Performance status is known to be an important independent predictor of survival (333–335). Two commonly used scales of performance status are outlined in Tables 14-8 and 14-9. Assessment of performance status is useful in helping to objectively gauge a patient's ability to undergo potentially toxic treatment for the small survival benefit to be gained and to anticipate outcome.

The current American Society of Clinical Oncology guidelines recommend the combination of platinum-based chemotherapy and thoracic radiation therapy for patients with unresectable IIIA and IIIB disease and for those who have good performance status (336). Concurrent rather than sequential therapy is generally recommended on the basis of improvement in median or 5-year survival in a limited number of clinical trials (337,338). Overall, the 5-year survival rate for the subgroup of patients with Stage-IIIB disease deemed candidates

TABLE 14-8. Eastern Cooperative Oncology Group (ECOG) Performance Status Scale

Patient Description	Scale
Normal	0
Fatigue without significant decrease in activity	1
Fatigue with significant impairment of activities of daily living or bed rest <50% waking hours	2
Bed rest >50% waking hours	3
Bedridden or unable to care for self	4

TABLE 14-9. Karnofsky Performance Status Scale

Patient Description	Scale
Normal	100
Normal activity with minor symptoms	90
Normal activity with effort	80
Independent in activities of daily living but unable to perform work or usual activity	70
Requires occasional assistance but able to care for most activities of daily living	60
Requires considerable assistance but able to care for most needs	50
Disabled; requires special care and assistance	40
Severely disabled	30
Hospitalization necessary; active supportive treatment necessary	20
Moribund	10
Dead	0

for combined modality treatment is approximately 10% to 15% (332).

Stage IV Non–small Cell Lung Cancer

Patients with Stage IV NSCLC have distant metastases (any T, any N, and M1). The M1 designation includes any distant organ metastasis as well as ipsilateral metastasis in a nonprimary tumor lobe. Survival for this group of patients is poor, with 1-year survival being less than 20% (241). Although the chances of cure are dismally low, these patients should still be evaluated for treatment. It is essential that specific attention be given to supportive and palliative therapy as the vast majority will have symptomatic disease at presentation as well as through their course. Best supportive care, including such interventions as aggressive pain management, palliative radiation therapy, oxygen, and symptom management of complications such as hemoptysis, but without chemotherapy, is associated with a median survival time of 3.6 months (339). Ten randomized trials and four separate meta-analyses of those trials demonstrated that platinum-based or combination chemotherapy is associated with an improvement in median survival time to 6.5 months (312,340–342). In some, but not all, of these studies, this increase in absolute survival time was statistically significant.

The decision to pursue chemotherapy in patients with Stage IV disease should be tempered by the patient's performance status (Tables 14-8 and 14-9). As noted above, this assessment of the patient's global health is an independent prognostic factor influencing outcome. Patients with good performance status are more likely to benefit from chemotherapy. Patients with poor performance status are more likely to suffer toxicity without survival benefit. It should be noted that although the primary purpose of chemotherapy is to prolong life, it may also be helpful in palliation of symptoms related to the tumor and can improve quality of life (QOL) for patients with symptomatic disease (339).

Chemotherapy for NSCLC has evolved over the last decades. The present first-line standard of care is the administration of a platinum-based agent (typically cisplatin or carboplatin) in combination with a second agent. The choice of this second agent is variable and may include any of the newer drugs with activity against NSCLC, including paclitaxel, docetaxel, vinorelbine, gemcitabine, and irinotecan (339,343). Randomized trials of these platinum-based combinations compared to single-agent regimens have demonstrated improved 1-year survival of 30% to 40% of patients compared to 10% to 15% of patients with best supportive care alone (312,343–345). On the basis of two large randomized studies evaluating optimal duration of therapy, it appears that the duration of treatment should be relatively short, lasting three to four cycles if there is evidence of containment of disease (346,347). If disease progresses, the chemotherapeutic regimen should be reevaluated. In this latter group, second-line therapy may be reasonable as long as the patient has retained adequate performance status (339). A number of agents have been evaluated as salvage therapies, including among others docetaxel and the EGFR tyrosine kinase inhibitor gefitinib (348–352).

A great deal of interest is now focused on the potential role of molecular-targeted therapy for solid tumors, including NSCLC. A number of molecular pathways important to tumor growth, including tumor angiogenesis, signal transduction pathways, and cell cycle control, are actively being investigated as potential targets for novel therapeutic interventions. New data emerging about specific gene mutations associated with different cancers suggest that subgroups of patients with such mutations may be able to receive treatment targeted to those specific genes. The clinical relevance of such an approach has been evident in the successful treatment of chronic myeloid leukemia with the tyrosine kinase inhibitor imatinib (353). Such targeted therapy may soon be clinically relevant for lung cancer. Lynch et al. recently reported that identification of specific mutations in the EGFR gene in a subgroup of patients with NSCLC correlated with clinical responsiveness to gefitinib (83). The ability to pinpoint such molecular mutations may thus contribute to targeted antitumor therapies in the future.

Further Issues in Treatment of Non–small Cell Lung Cancer

It is beyond the capacity of this chapter to comprehensively review certain uncommon but important issues in NSCLC treatment. Specifically, these include the evaluation and treatment of patients with Pancoast tumors (tumors that occur in the lung apex, which may involve chest wall structures including the brachial plexus, sympathetic chain, and subclavian vessels), solitary metastasis to the brain, satellite nodules in the same lobe as the primary tumor, synchronous primary tumors in different lobes, or metachronous second primary lung cancers (354–356). These and other situations can present tremendous challenges in management and are probably best evaluated by physicians experienced in lung cancer care.

SMALL CELL LUNG CANCER

The current treatment of choice for patients with limited-stage small cell carcinoma is combined chemotherapy and radiation therapy (101,231,357–359). Chemotherapy is necessary as the vast majority of patients have visible or microscopic extrathoracic metastases at the time of diagnosis. Patients with extensive disease may derive local benefit from chest irradiation, but survival does not appear to improve, presumably because of the involvement of extrathoracic organs by tumor (101). However, local radiation has been combined with chemotherapy because of the high incidence of symptomatic local chest relapse in patients receiving chemotherapy alone (360).

Radiation therapy in small cell carcinoma is also beneficial in treating cranial involvement (101). CNS spread occurs in more than 50% of patients at some time during the course of their disease and may provide a sanctuary for tumor from chemotherapeutic agents because of the blood–brain barrier. Cranial irradiation reduces the development of CNS metastases but has little effect on survival because of concomitant spread of disease to other sites (361,362). Thus, prophylactic cranial irradiation is reserved for patients who are judged to have a complete response to chemotherapy. Treatment is usually given 2 to 4 months after the beginning of chemotherapy.

The role of surgery in small cell carcinoma has been undergoing reevaluation (249,363). In general, surgery has not been shown to improve outcome because of the frequent presence of extrathoracic metastasis, visible or microscopic, at the time of diagnosis. However, there is renewed enthusiasm for operating on patients with limited-stage disease because removal of the primary tumor combined with chemotherapy may limit local chest relapse. Several prospective trials of primary surgery and surgery as an adjuvant to chemotherapy for small cell lung cancer are under way. As yet, surgical removal of small cell lung tumors has not been conclusively shown to favorably alter outcome (249).

PALLIATIVE CARE

Palliation is an important part of lung cancer treatment. The vast majority of patients with lung cancer already have symptomatic disease at their initial presentation and will eventually succumb to their disease. Thus, it should be anticipated that complications of the primary lesion as well as those related to metastatic sites will require palliative treatment.

Symptoms may be related to the primary tumor itself. These may present as endobronchial complications such as postobstructive pneumonia, atelectasis, or lobar collapse. Hemoptysis may result from the primary tumor as well. Intrathoracic spread of disease can result in symptomatic pleural effusion, SVC syndrome related to mediastinal lymph node enlargement, extension of the primary tumor, or tumor-related hypercoagulability. Distant metastases may cause a wide variety of symptoms related to the organs involved. Pain is a common symptom with tremendous impact on QOL. Pain management represents a key area in palliative care for patients with advanced lung cancer.

Recognizing that most patients with lung cancer present with disease that is not surgically resectable and therefore unlikely to be cured, it is extremely important that clinicians involved in lung cancer care be prepared to include palliation in the treatment plan for their patients. In the medical effort to provide state-of-the-art treatment for patients with malignancy, the patient's comfort and QOL should remain an essential part of focus of care. The Agency for Health Care Policy and Research has provided clinical practice guidelines for management of cancer pain (364). Kvale et al. writing for the ACCP Evidence-Based Guidelines for the Diagnosis and Management of Lung Cancer have also provided recommendations for palliative care specifically for patients with cancer

of the lung (365). These two guidelines present a comprehensive overview of directed palliative management for pain control, dyspnea, and symptoms related to specific organ involvement.

REFERENCES

1. Jemal A, et al. Cancer statistics. *CA Cancer J Clin* 2004;54(1):8–29.
2. Ferlay J, et al. Cancer incidence, mortality, and prevalence worldwide. In: *Globocan 2000*. Lyon: IARC Press, 2001.
3. Alberg AJ, Samet JM. Epidemiology of lung cancer. *Chest* 2003; 123(1 Suppl):21S–49S.
4. Doll R, Hill AB. Smoking and carcinoma of the lung; preliminary report. *Br Med J* 1950;2(4682):739–748.
5. Levin ML, Goldstein H, Gerhardt PR. Cancer and tobacco smoking: a preliminary report. *JAMA* 1950;143:336–338.
6. Wynder EL, Graham EA. Tobacco smoking as a possible etiologic factor in bronchiogenic carcinoma: a study of six hundred and eighty-four proved cases. *JAMA* 1950;143:329–336.
7. Roffo A. Leucoplasia tabaquica experimental. *Bol. Institute de medicine experimental para el estud. y trat, del cancer* 1930;7:501.
8. Bilello KS, Murin S, Matthay RA. Epidemiology, etiology, and prevention of lung cancer. *Clin Chest Med* 2002;23(1):1–25.
9. The surgeon general's 1989 report on reducing the health consequences of smoking: 25 years of progress. *MMWR* 1989; 38(Suppl 2):1–32.
10. Loeb LA, et al. Smoking and lung cancer: an overview. *Cancer Res* 1984;44(12 Pt 1):5940–5958.
11. Capewell S et al. Edinburgh Lung Cancer Group. Lung cancer in lifelong non-smokers. *Thorax* 1991;46(8):565–568.
12. Peto R, et al. Smoking, smoking cessation, and lung cancer in the UK since 1950: combination of national statistics with two case-control studies. *Br Med J* 2000;321(7257):323–329.
13. Peto R. Influence of dose and duration of smoking on lung cancer rates. In: *Tobacco: a major international health hazard; proceedings of an international meeting*. Moscow, USSR: International Agency for Research on Cancer Science, 1985.
14. Hegmann KT, et al. The effect of age at smoking initiation on lung cancer risk. *Epidemiology* 1993;4(5):444–448.
15. Hecht SS. Tobacco smoke carcinogens and lung cancer. *J Natl Cancer Inst* 1999;91(14):1194–1210.
16. *Reducing tobacco use: A report of the US Surgeon General Centers for Disease Control and Prevention, Office on Smoking and Health.* US Department of Health and Human Services, 2000:33.
17. Stratton K, et al. Clearing the smoke: the science base for tobacco harm reduction—executive summary. *Tob Control* 2001;10(2): 189–195.
18. *Smoking and Health. Report of the Advisory Committee to the Surgeon General of the Public Health Services.* Washington, DC: U. S. Public Health Service, 1964.
19. Brown CC, Kessler LG. Projections of lung cancer mortality in the United States: 1985-2025. *J Natl Cancer Inst* 1988;80(1):43–51.
20. *Respiratory health effects of passive smoking: lung cancer and other disorders.* Environmental Protection Agency, 1993.
21. *Involuntary Smoking.* International Agency for Research on Cancer, 2002.
22. Hecht SS, et al. A tobacco-specific lung carcinogen in the urine of men exposed to cigarette smoke. *N Engl J Med* 1993;329(21): 1543–1546.
23. 1986 Surgeon General's report: the health consequences of involuntary smoking. *MMWR* 1986;35(50):769–770.
24. Cardenas VM, et al. Environmental tobacco smoke and lung cancer mortality in the American Cancer Society's Cancer Prevention Study. II. *Cancer Causes Control* 1997;8(1):57–64.
25. Pershagen G. Passive smoking and lung cancer. In: Sa JM, ed. *Epidemiology of Lung Cancer.* New York: Marcel Dekker Inc, 1994: 109–130.
26. *Smoking and health. A report of the Surgeon General.* Washington, DC: U.S. Department of Health and Human Services, 1980.
27. Brownson RC, Chang JC, Davis JR. Gender and histologic type variations in smoking-related risk of lung cancer. *Epidemiology* 1992;3(1):61–64.

28. Lubin JH, et al. Quantitative evaluation of the radon and lung cancer association in a case control study of Chinese tin miners. *Cancer Res* 1990;50(1):174–180.

29. McDuffie HH, Klaassen DJ, Dosman JA. Female-male differences in patients with primary lung cancer. *Cancer* 1987;59(10): 1825–1830.

30. Risch HA, et al. Are female smokers at higher risk for lung cancer than male smokers? A case-control analysis by histologic type. *Am J Epidemiol* 1993;138(5):281–293.

31. Zang EA, Wynder EL. Differences in lung cancer risk between men and women: examination of the evidence. *J Natl Cancer Inst* 1996;88(3-4):183–192.

32. Taioli E, Wynder EL. Re: Endocrine factors and adenocarcinoma of the lung in women. *J Natl Cancer Inst* 1994;86(11):869–870.

33. Dresler CM, et al. Gender differences in genetic susceptibility for lung cancer. *Lung Cancer* 2000;30(3):153–160.

34. *Surgeon General's Report: The health consequences of smoking for women.* Washington, DC: U. S. Department of Health and Human Services, Public Health Service, Office of the Assistant Secretary for Health, Office on Smoking and Health, 1980:8411.

35. Doll R, Peto R. The causes of cancer: quantitative estimates of avoidable risks of cancer in the United States today. *J Natl Cancer Inst* 1981;66(6):1191–1308.

36. Chahinian AP, Chretien J. Present incidence of lung cancer: epidemiologic data and etiologic factors. In: Israel L, ed. *Lung cancer- natural history, prognosis, and therapy.* New York: Academic Press, 1976:1–22.

37. Cohen AJ. Air pollution and lung cancer: what more do we need to know? *Thorax* 2003;58(12):1010–1012.

38. Pope CA III, et al. Lung cancer, cardiopulmonary mortality, and long-term exposure to fine particulate air pollution. *JAMA* 2002; 287(9):1132–1141.

39. Pyne S. Air pollution. Small particles add up to big disease risk. *Science* 2002;295(5562):1994.

40. Beckett WS. Epidemiology and etiology of lung cancer. *Clin Chest Med* 1993;14(1):1–15.

41. Morgan WKC, Andrews CE. Bronchogenic carcinoma. In: Morgan WNC, ed. *Textbook of Pulmonary Diseases*, 2nd ed. Boston: Little, Brown and Company, 1974:755.

42. Brown LM, Pottern LM, Blot WJ. Lung cancer in relation to environmental pollutants emitted from industrial sources. *Environ Res* 1984;34(2):250–261.

43. Samet JM, et al. Uranium mining and lung cancer in Navajo men. *N Engl J Med* 1984;310(23):1481–1484.

44. Radford EP, Renard KG. Lung cancer in Swedish iron miners exposed to low doses of radon daughters. *N Engl J Med* 1984;310(23): 1485–1494.

45. Wright ES, Couves CM. Radiation-induced carcinoma of the lung—the St. Lawrence tragedy. *J Thorac Cardiovasc Surg* 1977; 74(4):495–498.

46. Frank AL. The epidemiology and etiology of lung cancer. *Clin Chest Med* 1982;3(2):219–228.

47. Tanoue LT, Matthay RA. Lung cancer: epidemiology and carcinogenesis. In: Shields TW, ed. *General thoracic surgery*, 5th ed. Philadelphia, PA: Lippincott Williams & Wilkins, 2000:1215–1228.

48. Harting F, Hesse W. Der Lungenkrebs, die Bergkrankheit in den Schneeberger Gruben. *Gesundheitswesen* 1879;31:102–105, 313–337.

49. Hei TK, et al. Mutagenic effects of a single and an exact number of alpha particles in mammalian cells. *Proc Natl Acad Sci U S A* 1997;94(8):3765–3770.

50. Hornung RW, Meinhardt TJ. Quantitative risk assessment of lung cancer in U.S. uranium miners. *Health Phys* 1987;52(4):417–430.

51. Archer VE, Gillam JD, Wagoner JK. Respiratory disease mortality among uranium miners. *Ann N Y Acad Sci* 1976;271:280–293.

52. Archer VE, Saccomanno G, Jones JH. Frequency of different histologic types of bronchogenic carcinoma as related to radiation exposure. *Cancer* 1974;34(6):2056–2060.

53. Lubin JH, Boice JD Jr. Lung cancer risk from residential radon: meta-analysis of eight epidemiologic studies. *J Natl Cancer Inst* 1997;89(1):49–57.

54. EPA. *Technical support document for the 1992 citizen's guide to radon.* Washington, DC: US Environmental Protection Agency (EPA), 1992.

55. Selikoff IJ, Hammond EC. Asbestos-associated disease in United States shipyards. *Cancer J Clin* 1978;28(2):87–99.

56. Craighead JE, Mossman BT. The pathogenesis of asbestos-associated diseases. *N Engl J Med* 1982;306(24):1446–1455.

57. Yesner R. Pathogenesis and pathology. *Clin Chest Med* 1993;14(1): 17–30.

58. Carter D, Yesner R. Carcinomas of the lung with neuroendocrine differentiation. *Semin Diagn Pathol* 1985;2(4):235–254.

59. Steinbach G, et al. The effect of celecoxib, a cyclooxygenase-2 inhibitor, in familial adenomatous polyposis. *N Engl J Med* 2000; 342(26):1946–1952.

60. Baron JA, et al. A randomized trial of aspirin to prevent colorectal adenomas. *N Engl J Med* 2003;348(10):891–899.

61. Rahme E, et al. The cyclooxygenase-2-selective inhibitors rofecoxib and celecoxib prevent colorectal neoplasia occurrence and recurrence. *Gastroenterology* 2003;125(2):404–412.

62. Thompson IM, et al. The influence of finasteride on the development of prostate cancer. *N Engl J Med* 2003;349(3):215–224.

63. Dragnev KH, Stover D, Dmitrovsky E. Lung cancer prevention: the guidelines. *Chest* 2003;123(1 Suppl):60S–71S.

64. Shekelle RB, et al. Dietary vitamin A and risk of cancer in the Western Electric study. *Lancet* 1981;2(8257):1185–1190.

65. Hennekens CH, et al. Lack of effect of long-term supplementation with beta carotene on the incidence of malignant neoplasms and cardiovascular disease. *N Engl J Med* 1996;334(18):1145–1149.

66. Darby S, et al. Diet, smoking and lung cancer: a case-control study of 1000 cases and 1500 controls in South-West England. *Br J Cancer* 2001;84(5):728–735.

67. Samet JM, et al. Lung cancer risk and vitamin A consumption in New Mexico. *Am Rev Respir Dis* 1985;131(2):198–202.

68. The Alpha-Tocopherol, Beta Carotene Cancer Prevention Study Group. The effect of vitamin E and beta carotene on the incidence of lung cancer and other cancers in male smokers. *N Engl J Med* 1994;330(15):1029–1035.

69. Omenn GS, et al. Effects of a combination of beta carotene and vitamin A on lung cancer and cardiovascular disease. *N Engl J Med* 1996;334(18):1150–1155.

70. Sellers TA, et al. Evidence for mendelian inheritance in the pathogenesis of lung cancer. *J Natl Cancer Inst* 1990;82(15):1272–1279.

71. Kern JA, Filderman AE. Oncogenes and growth factors in human lung cancer. *Clin Chest Med* 1993;14(1):31–41.

72. Ooi WL, et al. Increased familial risk for lung cancer. *J Natl Cancer Inst* 1986;76(2):217–222.

73. Samet JM, Humble CG, Pathak DR. Personal and family history of respiratory disease and lung cancer risk. *Am Rev Respir Dis* 1986;134(3):466–470.

74. Kazazian HH Jr. A geneticist's view of lung disease. *Am Rev Respir Dis* 1976;113(3):261–266.

75. Brauch H, et al. Molecular analysis of the short arm of chromosome 3 in small cell and non-small cell carcinoma of the lung. *N Engl J Med* 1987;317(18):1109–1113.

76. Rodenhuis S, et al. Mutational activation of the K-ras oncogene. A possible pathogenetic factor in adenocarcinoma of the lung. *N Engl J Med* 1987;317(15):929–935.

77. Economou P, Lechner JF, Samet JM. Familial and genetic factors in the pathogenesis of lung cancer. In: Samet JM, ed. *Epidemiology of lung cancer.* New York: Marcel Dekker Inc, 1994:353–396.

78. Amos CI, Caporaso NE, Weston A. Host factors in lung cancer risk: a review of interdisciplinary studies. *Cancer Epidemiol Biomarkers Prev* 1992;1(6):505–513.

79. Nazar-Stewart V, et al. The glutathione S-transferase mu polymorphism as a marker for susceptibility to lung carcinoma. *Cancer Res* 1993;53(10 Suppl):2313–2318.

80. Seidegard J, et al. Isoenzyme(s) of glutathione transferase (class Mu) as a marker for the susceptibility to lung cancer: a follow up study. *Carcinogenesis* 1990;11(1):33–36.

81. Kellermann G, Shaw CR, Luyten-Kellerman M. Aryl hydrocarbon hydroxylase inducibility and bronchogenic carcinoma. *N Engl J Med* 1973;289(18):934–937.

82. Karki NT, et al. Aryl hydrocarbon hydroxylase in lymphocytes and lung tissue from lung cancer patients and controls. *Int J Cancer* 1987;39(5):565–570.

83. Lynch TJ, et al. Activating mutations in the epidermal growth factor receptor underlying responsiveness of non-small cell lung cancer to gefitinib. *N Engl J Med* 2004;350(21):2129–2139.

84. Rom WN, et al. Molecular and genetic aspects of lung cancer. *Am J Respir Crit Care Med* 2000;161(4 Pt 1):1355–1367.

85. The World Health Organization histological typing of lung tumours. Second edition. *Am J Clin Pathol* 1982;77(2):123–136.
86. Shimosato Y. Pulmonary neoplasms. In: Steinberg SS, ed. *Diagnostic surgical pathology*. Philadelphia, PA: Lippincott Williams & Wilkins, 1999:1114–1115.
87. Yesner R, Carter D. Pathology of carcinoma of the lung. Changing patterns. *Clin Chest Med* 1982;3(2):257–289.
88. Travis WD, Linder J, Mackay B. Classification, histology, cytology, and electron microscopy. In: Pass HI, Mitchell JB, Johnson DH, eds. *Lung cancer principles and practice*. Philadelphia, PA: Lippincott–Raven Publishers, 1996.
89. Matthews MJ, Mackay B, Lukeman J. The pathology of non-small cell carcinoma of the lung. *Semin Oncol* 1983;10(1):34–55.
90. Matthews MJ. Problems in morphology and behavior of bronchopulmonary malignant disease. In: Israel L, ed. *Lung cancer-natural history, prognosis, and therapy*. New York: Academic Press, 1976.
91. Matthews MJ. Panel report. Morphologic classification of bronchogenic carcinoma. *Cancer Chemother Rep 3* 1973;4(2):299–301.
92. Gail MH, et al. Prognostic factors in patients with resected stage I non-small cell lung cancer. A report from the Lung Cancer Study Group. *Cancer* 1984;54(9):1802–1813.
93. Kodama T, et al. Morphometric study of adenocarcinomas and hyperplastic epithelial lesions in the peripheral lung. *Am J Clin Pathol* 1986;85(2):146–151.
94. Kurokawa T, et al. Surgically curable "early" adenocarcinoma in the periphery of the lung. *Am J Surg Pathol* 1994;18(5):431–438.
95. Cox JD, Yesner RA. Adenocarcinoma of the lung: recent results from the Veterans Administration Lung Group. *Am Rev Respir Dis* 1979;120(5):1025–1029.
96. Ginsberg SS, et al. Giant cell carcinoma of the lung. *Cancer* 1992;70(3):606–610.
97. Razzuk MA, et al. Pulmonary giant cell carcinoma. *Ann Thorac Surg* 1976;21(6):540–545.
98. World Health Organization. In: Shimosato Y, Subin L, Spencer H, eds. *Histological typing of lung tumors*. Geneva: World Health Organization, 1981.
99. Radice PA, et al. The clinical behavior of "mixed" small cell/large cell bronchogenic carcinoma compared to "pure" small cell subtypes. *Cancer* 1982;50(12):2894–2902.
100. Aisner SC, et al. The clinical significance of variant-morphology small cell carcinoma of the lung. *J Clin Oncol* 1990;8(3):402–408.
101. Johnson BE. Management of small cell lung cancer. *Clin Chest Med* 1993;14(1):173–187.
102. Arroliga AC, Carter D, Matthay RA. Other primary neoplasms of the lung. In: Bone RC, Dantzker DR, George RB, eds. *Pulmonary and critical care medicine*. St. Louis: Mosby-Year Book, 1993:H2-H6.
103. Andrews CE, Morgan WKC. Tumors of the lung other than bronchogenic carcinoma. In: Morgan WKC, ed. *Textbook of pulmonary diseases*. Boston: Little, Brown and Company, 1974:789.
104. Kee Jr JL, Bronchial adenoma. In: Shaw RR, Paulson DL, Kee Jr JS, eds. *Treatment of bronchial neoplasms*. Springfiled: Charles C Thomas Publisher, 103–121:1955.
105. Arrigoni MG, Woolner LB, Bernatz PE. Atypical carcinoid tumors of the lung. *J Thorac Cardiovasc Surg* 1972;64(3):413–421.
106. Mills SE, et al. Atypical carcinoid tumor of the lung. A clinicopathologic study of 17 cases. *Am J Surg Pathol* 1982;6(7):643–654.
107. Travis WD, et al. Neuroendocrine tumors of the lung with proposed criteria for large-cell neuroendocrine carcinoma. An ultrastructural, immunohistochemical, and flow cytometric study of 35 cases. *Am J Surg Pathol* 1991;15(6):529–553.
108. Reid JD. Adenoid cystic carcinoma (cylindroma) of the bronchial tree. *Cancer* 1952;5(4):685–694.
109. Turnbull AD, et al. Mucoepidermoid tumors of bronchial glands. *Cancer* 1971;28(3):539–544.
110. Ashmore PG. Papilloma of the bronchus: case report. *J Thorac Surg* 1954;27(3):293–294.
111. Yousem SA, Hochholzer L. Mucoepidermoid tumors of the lung. *Cancer* 1987;60(6):1346–1352.
112. Moran CA, Suster S, Koss MN. Primary adenoid cystic carcinoma of the lung. A clinicopathologic and immunohistochemical study of 16 cases. *Cancer* 1994;73(5):1390–1397.
113. Helmuth RA, Strate RW. Squamous carcinoma of the lung in a nonirradiated, nonsmoking patient with juvenile laryngotracheal papillomatosis. *Am J Surg Pathol* 1987;11(8):643–650.
114. Miura H, et al. Asymptomatic solitary papilloma of the bronchus: review of occurrence in Japan. *Eur Respir J* 1993;6(7):1070–1073.
115. Spencer H. *Pathology of the lung*. Philadelphia: WB Saunders, 1977:773–859.
116. Bejui-Thivolet F, et al. Detection of human papillomavirus DNA in squamous bronchial metaplasia and squamous cell carcinomas of the lung by in situ hybridization using biotinylated probes in paraffin-embedded specimens. *Hum Pathol* 1990;21(1):111–116.
117. Liebow AA, Hubbell DS. Sclerosing hemangioma (histiocytoma, xanthoma) of the lung. *Cancer* 1956;9(1):53–75.
118. Hill GS, Eggleston JC. Electron microscopic study of so-called "pulmonary sclerosing hemangioma." Report of a case suggesting epithelial origin. *Cancer* 1972;30(4):1092–1106.
119. Nagata N, et al. Sclerosing hemangioma of the lung. An epithelial tumor composed of immunohistochemically heterogenous cells. *Am J Clin Pathol* 1987;88(5):552–559.
120. Sugio K, et al. Sclerosing hemangioma of the lung: radiographic and pathological study. *Ann Thorac Surg* 1992;53(2):295–300.
121. Yousem SA, Hochholzer L. Alveolar adenoma. *Hum Pathol* 1986;17(10):1066–1071.
122. Dail DH, et al. Intravascular, bronchiolar, and alveolar tumor of the lung (IVBAT). An analysis of twenty cases of a peculiar sclerosing endothelial tumor. *Cancer* 1983;51(3):452–464.
123. Corrin B, et al. Histogenesis of the so-called "intravascular bronchioloalveolar tumour." *J Pathol* 1979;128(3):163–167.
124. Liebow AA. Tumors of the lower respiratory tract. In: Liebow AA, ed. *Atlas of tumor pathology*. Washington, DC: Armed Forces Institute of Pathology, 1952.
125. Bateson EM. So-called hamartoma of the lung—a true neoplasm of fibrous connective tissue of the bronchi. *Cancer* 1973;31(6):1458–1467.
126. Hochberg LA, Schacter B. Benign tumors of the bronchus and lung. *Am J Surg* 1955;89(2):425–438.
127. Pastlethwait RW, Hagerty RF, Trent JC. Endobronchial polypoid hamartochondroma. *Surgery* 1948;24:732–738.
128. Sun CC, Kroll M, Miller JE. Primary chondrosarcoma of the lung. *Cancer* 1982;50(9):1864–1866.
129. Ma CK, et al. Benign mixed tumor of the trachea. *Cancer* 1979;44(6):2260–2266.
130. Watts CF, Clagett OT, McDonald JR. Lipoma of the bronchus: discussion of benign neoplasms and a report of endobronchial lipoma. *J Thorac Surg* 1946;15:131–144.
131. McCall RE, Harrison W. Intrabronchial lipoma; a case report. *J Thorac Surg* 1955;29(3):317–322.
132. Agnos JW, Starkey GW. Primary leiomyosarcoma and leiomyoma of the lung; review of the literature and report of two cases of leiomyosarcoma. *N Engl J Med* 1958;258(1):12–17.
133. Guccion JG, Rosen SH. Bronchopulmonary leiomyosarcoma and fibrosarcoma. A study of 32 cases and review of the literature. *Cancer* 1972;30(3):836–847.
134. Gal AA, Brooks JS, Pietra GG. Leiomyomatous neoplasms of the lung: a clinical, histologic, and immunohistochemical study. *Mod Pathol* 1989;2(3):209–216.
135. Misra DP, et al. Malignant fibrous histiocytoma in the lung masquerading as recurrent pulmonary thromboembolism. *Cancer* 1983;51(3):538–541.
136. Lee JT, Shelburne JD, Linder J. Primary malignant fibrous histiocytoma of the lung. A clinicopathologic and ultrastructural study of five cases. *Cancer* 1984;53(5):1124–1130.
137. Stuart AP. Fibrosarcoma: malignant tumor of fibroblasts. *Cancer* 1948;1:30–63.
138. McDonnell T, et al. Malignant fibrous histiocytoma of the lung. *Cancer* 1988;61(1):137–145.
139. Noehren TH, McKee FW. Sarcoma of the lung. *Dis Chest* 1954;25(6):663–678.
140. Koss MN, et al. Primary non-Hodgkin's lymphoma and pseudolymphoma of lung: a study of 161 patients. *Hum Pathol* 1983;14(12):1024–1038.
141. L'Hoste RJ Jr, et al. Primary pulmonary lymphomas. A clinicopathologic analysis of 36 cases. *Cancer* 1984;54(7):1397–1406.
142. Donner LR, et al. Angiocentric immunoproliferative lesion (lymphomatoid granulomatosis). A cytogenetic, immunophenotypic, and genotypic study. *Cancer* 1990;65(2):249–254.

143. Beckles MA, et al. Initial evaluation of the patient with lung cancer: symptoms, signs, laboratory tests, and paraneoplastic syndromes. *Chest* 2003;123(1 Suppl):97S–104S.

144. Carbone PP, Frost JK, Feinstein AR. Lung cancer: perspectives and prospects. *Ann Intern Med* 1970;73:1003–1024.

145. Shimizu N, et al. Outcome of patients with lung cancer detected via mass screening as compared to those presenting with symptoms. *J Surg Oncol* 1992;50(1):7–11.

146. Midthun DE, Jett JR. Clnical presentation of lung cancer. In: Pass HI, Mitchell JB, Johnson DH, eds. *Lung cancer principles and practice.* Philadelphia: Lippincott–Raven Publishers, 1996:421–435.

147. Darling G, Dresler CM. Clinical presentation of lung cancer. In: Shields TW, LoCicero III J, Ponn RB, eds., *General thoracic surgery.* Philadelphia: Lippincott Williams & Wilkins, 2000: 1269–1282.

148. Darling G, Dresler CM. Clinical presentation of lung cancer, In : Shields TW, LoCicero III J, Ponn RB, eds. *General Thoracic Surgery.* Philadelphia: Lippincott Williams & Wilkins, 1999: p. 1269–1282.

149. Hyde L, Hyde I. Clinical manifestations of lung cancer. *Chest* 1974;65(3):299–306. C.

150. Chute CG, et al. Presenting conditions of 1539 population-based lung cancer patients by cell type and stage in New Hampshire and Vermont. *Cancer* 1985;56(8):2107–2111.

151. Parish JM, et al. Etiologic considerations in superior vena cava syndrome. *Mayo Clin Proc* 1981;56(7):407–413.

152. Chernow B, Sahn SA. Carcinomatous involvement of the pleura: an analysis of 96 patients. *Am J Med* 1977;63(5):695–702.

153. Johnston WW. The malignant pleural effusion. A review of cytopathologic diagnoses of 584 specimens from 472 consecutive patients. *Cancer* 1985;56(4):905–909.

154. Newman SJ, Hansen HH. Proceedings: Frequency, diagnosis, and treatment of brain metastases in 247 consecutive patients with bronchogenic carcinoma. *Cancer* 1974;33(2):492–496.

155. Merchut MP. Brain metastases from undiagnosed systemic neoplasms. *Arch Intern Med* 1989;149(5):1076–1080.

156. Le Roux BT. Bronchial carcinoma. *Thorax* 1968;23(2):136–143.

157. Shields TW. Carcinoma of the lung. In: Shields TW, ed. *General thoracic surgery.* Philadelphia: Lea & Febiger, 1972:797–845.

158. Gerber RB, Mazzone P, Arroliga AC. Paraneoplastic syndromes associated with bronchogenic carcinoma. *Clin Chest Med* 2002; 23(1):257–264.

159. Merrill WW, Bondy PK. Production of biochemical marker substances by bronchogenic carcinomas. *Clin Chest Med* 1982;3(2): 307–320.

160. Patel AM, Davila DG, Peters SG. Paraneoplastic syndromes associated with lung cancer. *Mayo Clin Proc* 1993;68(3):278–287.

161. Delisle L, et al. Ectopic corticotropin syndrome and small cell carcinoma of the lung. Clinical features, outcome, and complications. *Arch Intern Med* 1993;153(6):746–752.

162. Dimopoulos MA, et al. Paraneoplastic Cushing syndrome as an adverse prognostic factor in patients who die early with small cell lung cancer. *Cancer* 1992;69(1):66–71.

163. Kovacs L, Robertson GL. Syndrome of inappropriate antidiuresis. *Endocrinol Metab Clin North Am* 1992;21(4):859–875.

164. De Troyer A, Demanet JC. Clinical, biological and pathogenic features of the syndrome of inappropriate secretion of antidiuretic hormone. A review of 26 cases with marked hyponatraemia. *Q J Med* 1976;45(180):521–531.

165. List AF, et al. The syndrome of inappropriate secretion of antidiuretic hormone (SIADH) in small cell lung cancer. *J Clin Oncol* 1986;4(8):1191–1198.

166. Rose BD, Post TW. *Clinical physiology of acid-base and electrolyte disorders,* 5th ed. New York: McGraw-Hill, 2001:729–733.

167. Decaux G, et al. Treatment of the syndrome of inappropriate secretion of antidiuretic hormone with furosemide. *N Engl J Med* 1981;304(6):329–330.

168. Forrest JN Jr, et al. Superiority of demeclocycline over lithium in the treatment of chronic syndrome of inappropriate secretion of antidiuretic hormone. *N Engl J Med* 1978;298(4):173–177.

169. Decaux G, Genette F. Urea for long-term treatment of syndrome of inappropriate secretion of antidiuretic hormone. *Br Med J (Clin Res Ed)* 1981;283(6299):1081–1083.

170. Adrogue HJ, Madias NE. Hyponatremia. *N Engl J Med* 2000; 342(21):1581–1589.

171. Ellis SJ. Severe hyponatraemia: complications and treatment. *QJM* 1995;88(12):905–909.

172. Laureno R, Karp BI. Myelinolysis after correction of hyponatremia. *Ann Intern Med* 1997;126(1):57–62.

173. Shields TW, Ritts RE. *Bronchial carcinoma.* Springfield: Charles C Thomas Publisher, 1974.

174. Bensch KG, et al. Oat-cell carcinoma of the lung. Its origin and relationship to bronchial carcinoid. *Cancer* 1968;22(6):1163–1172.

175. Gaich G, Burtis WJ. The diagnosis and treatment of malignancy associated hypercalcemia. *Endocrinologist* 1991;1:371–378.

176. Arroliga AC, Matthay RA. Paraneoplastic syndromes in bronchogenic carcinoma. *Clin Pulm Med* 1994;1:322–332.

177. Bender RA, Hansen H. Hypercalcemia in bronchogenic carcinoma. A prospective study of 200 patients. *Ann Intern Med* 1974;80(2):205–208.

178. Mundy GR, et al. The hypercalcemia of cancer. Clinical implications and pathogenic mechanisms. *N Engl J Med* 1984;310(26): 1718–1727.

179. Strewler GJ. The physiology of parathyroid hormone-related protein. *N Engl J Med* 2000;342(3):177–185.

180. Rosol TJ, Capen CC. Mechanisms of cancer-induced hypercalcemia. *Lab Invest* 1992;67(6):680–702.

181. Dalmau J, Gultekin HS, Posner JB. Paraneoplastic neurologic syndromes: pathogenesis and physiopathology. *Brain Pathol* 1999;9(2):275–284.

182. Douglas CA, Ellershaw J. Anti-Hu antibodies may indicate a positive response to chemotherapy in paraneoplastic syndrome secondary to small cell lung cancer. *Palliat Med* 2003;17(7):638–639.

183. Lucchinetti CF, Kimmel DW, Lennon VA. Paraneoplastic and oncologic profiles of patients seropositive for type 1 antineuronal nuclear autoantibodies. *Neurology* 1998;50(3):652–657.

184. Graus F, et al. Anti-Hu-associated paraneoplastic encephalomyelitis: analysis of 200 patients. *Brain* 2001;124(Pt 6): 1138–1148.

185. Lennon VA, et al. Calcium-channel antibodies in the Lambert-Eaton syndrome and other paraneoplastic syndromes. *N Engl J Med* 1995;332(22):1467–1474.

186. Viglione MP, O'Shaughnessy TJ, Kim YI. Inhibition of calcium currents and exocytosis by Lambert-Eaton syndrome antibodies in human lung cancer cells. *J Physiol* 1995;488(Pt 2):303–317.

187. Hollings HE, Brody RS, Boland HC. Pulmonary hypertrophic osteoarthropathy. *Lancet* 1961;2:1269–1273.

188. Holman CW. Osteoarthropathy in lung cancer: disappearance after section of intercostal nerves. *J Thorac Cardiovasc Surg* 1963; 45:679–681.

189. Stenseth JH, Clagett OT, Woolner LB. Hypertrophic pulmonary osteoarthropathy. *Dis Chest* 1967;52(1):62–68.

190. Fontana RS, et al. Screening for lung cancer. A critique of the Mayo Lung Project. *Cancer* 1991;67(4 Suppl):1155–1164.

191. Fontana RS, et al. Early lung cancer detection: results of the initial (prevalence) radiologic and cytologic screening in the Mayo Clinic study. *Am Rev Respir Dis* 1984;130(4):561–565.

192. Frost JK, et al. Early lung cancer detection: results of the initial (prevalence) radiologic and cytologic screening in the Johns Hopkins study. *Am Rev Respir Dis* 1984;130(4):549–554.

193. Berlin NI. Overview of the NCI Cooperative Early Lung Cancer Detection Program. *Cancer* 2000;89(11 Suppl):2349–2351.

194. Melamed MR. Lung cancer screening results in the National Cancer Institute New York study. *Cancer* 2000;89(11 Suppl):2356–2362.

195. Early lung cancer detection: summary and conclusions. *Am Rev Respir Dis* 1984;130(4):565–570.

196. Flehinger BJ, et al. Early lung cancer detection: results of the initial (prevalence) radiologic and cytologic screening in the Memorial Sloan-Kettering study. *Am Rev Respir Dis* 1984;130(4): 555–560.

197. Melamed MR, et al. Detection of true pathologic stage I lung cancer in a screening program and the effect on survival. *Cancer* 1981;47(5 Suppl):1182–1187.

198. Melamed MR, Flehinger BJ. Should asymptomatic smokers have annual chest x-rays after age 55 years? *Debates Med Yearbook* 1990;3:123–124.

199. Bach PB, Niewoehner DE, Black WC. Screening for lung cancer: the guidelines. *Chest* 2003;123(1 Suppl):83S–88S.

200. Bach PB, et al. Screening for lung cancer: a review of the current literature. *Chest* 2003;123(1 Suppl):72S–82S.

201. Prorok PC, et al. Design of the Prostate, Lung, Colorectal and Ovarian (PLCO) Cancer Screening Trial. *Control Clin Trials* 2000;21(6 Suppl):273S–309S.

202. Kaneko M, et al. Peripheral lung cancer: screening and detection with low-dose spiral CT versus radiography. *Radiology* 1996;201(3):798–802.

203. Henschke CI, et al. Early lung cancer action project: initial findings on repeat screenings. *Cancer* 2001;92(1):153–159.

204. Henschke CI, et al. Early Lung Cancer Action Project: overall design and findings from baseline screening. *Lancet* 1999;354(9173):99–105.

205. Henschke CI, et al. Early lung cancer action project: a summary of the findings on baseline screening. *Oncologist* 2001;6(2):147–152.

206. Swensen SJ, et al. Screening for lung cancer with low-dose spiral-computed tomography. *Am J Respir Crit Care Med* 2002;165(4):508–513.

207. Etzioni R, et al. The case for early detection. *Nat Rev Cancer* 2003;3(4):243–252.

208. Mahadevia PJ, et al. Lung cancer screening with helical computed tomography in older adult smokers: a decision and cost-effectiveness analysis. *JAMA* 2003;289(3):313–322.

209. Heitzman ER. Bronchogenic carcinoma: radiologic-pathologic correlations. *Semin Roentgenol* 1977;12(3):165–174.

210. Heitzman ER. *The lung: radiologic-pathologic correlations.* St. Louis: Mosby, 1984.

211. Filderman AE, Shaw C, Matthay RA. Lung cancer. Part I: Etiology, pathology, natural history, manifestations, and diagnostic techniques. *Invest Radiol* 1986;21(1):80–90.

212. Theros EG. 1976 Caldwell Lecture: varying manifestation of peripheral pulmonary neoplasms: a radiologic-pathologic correlative study. *Am J Roentgenol* 1977;128(6):893–914.

213. White CS, Templeton PA. Radiologic manifestations of bronchogenic cancer. *Clin Chest Med* 1993;14(1):55–67.

214. O'Keefe ME Jr., Good CA, McDonald JR. Calcification in solitary nodules of the lung. *Am J Roentgenol Radium Ther Nucl Med* 1957;77(6):1023–1033.

215. Savage PJ, Donovan WN, Dellinger RP. Sputum cytology in the management of patients with lung cancer. *South Med J* 1984;77(7):840–842.

216. Mehta AC, Marty JJ, Lee FY. Sputum cytology. *Clin Chest Med* 1993;14(1):69–85.

217. Shaw GL, Mulshine JL. General stagies for early detection: new ideas and future directions. In: Pass HI, Mitchell JB, Johnson DH, eds. *Lung cancer principles and practice.* Philadelphia: Lippincott–Raven Publishers, 1996:329–340.

218. The American Thoracic Society and The European Respiratory Society. Pretreatment evaluation of non-small cell lung cancer. *Am J Respir Crit Care Med* 1997;156(1):320–332.

219. Martini N, McCormick PM. Assessment of endoscopically visible bronchial carcinomas. *Chest* 1978;73(5 Suppl):718–720.

220. Shure D, Fedullo PF. Transbronchial needle aspiration in the diagnosis of submucosal and peribronchial bronchogenic carcinoma. *Chest* 1985;88(1):49–51.

221. Stringfield JT, et al. The effect of tumor size and location on diagnosis by fiberoptic bronchoscopy. *Chest* 1977;72(4):474–476.

222. Wallace JM, Deutsch AL. Flexible fiberoptic bronchoscopy and percutaneous needle lung aspiration for evaluating the solitary pulmonary nodule. *Chest* 1982;81(6):665–671.

223. Arroliga AC, Matthay RA. The role of bronchoscopy in lung cancer. *Clin Chest Med* 1993;14(1):87–98.

224. Shure D. Tissue procurement: bronchoscopic techniques for lung cancer. In: Pass HI, Mitchell JB, Johnson DH, eds. *Lung cancer principles and practice.* Philadelphia: Lippincott–Raven Publishers, 1996:471–479.

225. Zavala DC. Diagnostic fiberoptic bronchoscopy: Techniques and results of biopsy in 600 patients. *Chest* 1975;68(1):12–19.

226. Credle WF Jr., Smiddy JF, Elliott RC. Complications of fiberoptic bronchoscopy. *Am Rev Respir Dis* 1974;109(1):67–72.

227. Wang KP, Terry PB. Transbronchial needle aspiration in the diagnosis and staging of bronchogenic carcinoma. *Am Rev Respir Dis* 1983;127(3):344–347.

228. Westcott JL. Direct percutaneous needle aspiration of localized pulmonary lesions: result in 422 patients. *Radiology* 1980;137(1 Pt 1):31–35.

229. Salazar AM, Westcott JL. The role of transthoracic needle biopsy for the diagnosis and staging of lung cancer. *Clin Chest Med* 1993;14(1):99–110.

230. Khouri NF, et al. Transthoracic needle aspiration biopsy of benign and malignant lung lesions. *Am J Roentgenol* 1985;144(2):281–288.

231. Calhoun P, et al. The clinical outcome of needle aspirations of the lung when cancer is not diagnosed. *Ann Thorac Surg* 1986;41(6):592–596.

232. Poe RH, et al. Predicting risk of pneumothorax in needle biopsy of the lung. *Chest* 1984;85(2):232–235.

233. Fish GD, et al. Postbiopsy pneumothorax: estimating the risk by chest radiography and pulmonary function tests. *Am J Roentgenol* 1988;150(1):71–74.

234. Sinner WN, Zajicek J. Implantation metastasis after percutaneous transthoracic needle aspiration biopsy. *Acta Radiol Diagn (Stockh)* 1976;17(4):473–480.

235. Muller NL, et al. Seeding of malignant cells into the needle track after lung and pleural biopsy. *Can Assoc Radiol J* 1986;37(3):192–194.

236. Salyer WR, Eggleston JC, Erozan YS. Efficacy of pleural needle biopsy and pleural fluid cytopathology in the diagnosis of malignant neoplasm involving the pleura. *Chest* 1975;67(5):536–539.

237. Boutin C, Cargnino P, Viallat JR. Thoracoscopy in the early diagnosis of malignant pleural effusions. *Endoscopy* 1980;12(4):155–160.

238. Mountain CF. Lung cancer staging classification. *Clin Chest Med* 1993;14(1):43–53.

239. Mountain CF. A new international staging system for lung cancer. *Chest* 1986;89(4 Suppl):225S–233S.

240. Denoix PF. Enquete permanente dans les centres anticancereux. *Bull Inst Natl Hyg* 1946;1:70–75.

241. Mountain CF. Revisions in the International System for Staging Lung Cancer. *Chest* 1997;111(6):1710–1717.

242. Hande KR, Des Prez RM. Current perspectives in small cell lung cancer. *Chest* 1984;85(5):669–677.

243. Hansen HH, Dombernowsky P, Hirsch FR. Staging procedures and prognostic features in small cell anaplastic bronchogenic carcinoma. *Semin Oncol* 1978;5(3):280–287.

244. Filderman AE, Shaw C, Matthay RA. Lung cancer. Part II. Staging and therapy. *Invest Radiol* 1986;21(2):173–185.

245. Swett HA, Nagel JS, Sostman HD. Imaging methods in primary lung carcinoma. *Clin Chest Med* 1982;3(2):331–351.

246. Inouye SK, Sox Jr HC. Standard and computed tomography in the evaluation of neoplasms of the chest. A comparative efficacy assessment. *Ann Intern Med* 1986;105(6):906–924.

247. Silvestri GA, et al. The noninvasive staging of non-small cell lung cancer: the guidelines. *Chest* 2003;123(1 Suppl):147S–156S.

248. Toloza EM, Harpole L, McCrory DC. Noninvasive staging of non-small cell lung cancer: a review of the current evidence. *Chest* 2003;123(1 Suppl):137S–146S.

249. Shields TW. Surgical therapy for carcinoma of the lung. *Clin Chest Med* 1993;14(1):121–147.

250. Webb WR, et al. Bronchogenic carcinoma: staging with MR compared with staging with CT and surgery. *Radiology* 1985;156(1):117–124.

251. Scott WJ, Dewan NA. Use of positron emission tomography to diagnose and stage lung cancer. *Clin Pulm Med* 1999;6:198–204.

252. Vansteenkiste JF, et al. Lymph node staging in non-small cell lung cancer with FDG-PET scan: a prospective study on 690 lymph node stations from 68 patients. *J Clin Oncol* 1998;16(6):2142–2149.

253. Higashi K, et al. Fluorine-18-FDG PET imaging is negative in bronchioloalveolar lung carcinoma. *J Nucl Med* 1998;39(6):1016–1020.

254. Kim BT, et al. Localized form of bronchioloalveolar carcinoma: FDG PET findings. *Am J Roentgenol* 1998;170(4):935–939.

255. Strauss LG, Conti PS. The applications of PET in clinical oncology. *J Nucl Med* 1991. 32(4): p. 623–648; discussion 649–650.

256. Toloza EM, et al. Invasive staging of non-small cell lung cancer: a review of the current evidence. *Chest* 2003;123(1 Suppl):157S–166S.

257. Detterbeck FC, et al. Lung cancer. Invasive staging: the guidelines. *Chest* 2003;123(1 Suppl):167S–175S.

258. Hashim SW, Baue AE, Geha AS. The role of mediastinoscopy and mediastinotomy in lung cancer. *Clin Chest Med* 1982;3(2):353–359.

259. Nohl-Oser HC. In: Shields TW, ed. *Lymphatics of the lung, in General thoracic surgery.* Philadelphia: Lea & Febiger, 1972.74–85.

260. Straus MJ. *Lung cancer: clinical diagnosis and treatment.* New York: Grune & Stratton, 1977:123.

261. Bowen TE, et al. Value of anterior mediastinotomy in bronchogenic carcinoma of the left upper lobe. *J Thorac Cardiovasc Surg* 1978;76(2):269–271.

262. The Canadian Lung Oncology Group. Investigating extrathoracic metastatic disease in patients with apparently operable lung cancer. *Ann Thorac Surg* 2001;71(2):425–433; discussion 433–434.

263. Hooper RG, Beechler CR, Johnson MC. Radioisotope scanning in the initial staging of bronchogenic carcinoma. *Am Rev Respir Dis* 1978;118(2):279–286.

264. Ramsdell JW, et al. Multiorgan scans for staging lung cancer. Correlation with clinical evaluation. *J Thorac Cardiovasc Surg* 1977;73(5):653–659.

265. Silvestri GA, Littenberg B, Colice GL. The clinical evaluation for detecting metastatic lung cancer. A meta-analysis. *Am J Respir Crit Care Med* 1995;152(1):225–230.

266. Hooper RG, et al. Computed tomographic scanning of the brain in initial staging of bronchogenic carcinoma. *Chest* 1984;85(6):774–776.

267. Silvestri GA, et al. The relationship of clinical findings to CT scan evidence of adrenal gland metastases in the staging of bronchogenic carcinoma. *Chest* 1992;102(6):1748–1751.

268. Grant D, Edwards D, Goldstraw P. Computed tomography of the brain, chest, and abdomen in the preoperative assessment of non-small cell lung cancer. *Thorax* 1988;43(11):883–886.

269. Sandler MA, et al. Computed tomographic evaluation of the adrenal gland in the preoperative assessment of bronchogenic carcinoma. *Radiology* 1982;145(3):733–736.

270. Stoller JK, Ahmad M, Rice TW. Solitary pulmonary nodule. *Cleve Clin J Med* 1988;55(1):68–74.

271. Lillington GA, Caskey CI. Evaluation and management of solitary and multiple pulmonary nodules. *Clin Chest Med* 1993;14(1):111–119.

272. Steele JD. The solitary pulmonary nodule: report of a cooperative study of resected asymptomatic solitary pulmonary nodules in males. *J Thorac Cardiovasc Surg* 1963;46:21–39.

273. Mathur PN, et al. Treatment of early stage non-small cell lung cancer. *Chest* 2003;123(1 Suppl):176S–180S.

274. Imamura S, et al. Photodynamic therapy and/or external beam radiation therapy for roentgenologically occult lung cancer. *Cancer* 1994;73(6):1608–1614.

275. Furuse K et al, The Japan Lung Cancer Photodynamic Therapy Study Group. A prospective phase II study on photodynamic therapy with photofrin II for centrally located early-stage lung cancer. *J Clin Oncol* 1993;11(10):1852–1857.

276. Kato H. Photodynamic therapy for lung cancer—a review of 19 years' experience. *J Photochem Photobiol B* 1998;42(2):96–99.

277. Kato H, Okunaka T, Tsuchida T. Analysis of the cost-effectiveness of photodynamic therapy in early stage lung cancer. *Diagn Ther Endosc* 1999;6:9–16.

278. Cortese DA, Edell ES, Kinsey JH. Photodynamic therapy for early stage squamous cell carcinoma of the lung. *Mayo Clin Proc* 1997;72(7):595–602.

279. Smythe WR. Treatment of stage I non-small cell lung carcinoma. *Chest* 2003;123(1 Suppl):181S–187S.

280. Martini N, Kris MG, Ginsberg RJ. The role of multimodality therapy in locoregional non-small cell lung cancer. *Surg Oncol Clin North Am* 1997;6(4):769–791.

281. Naruke T, et al. Prognosis and survival in resected lung carcinoma based on the new international staging system. *J Thorac Cardiovasc Surg* 1988;96(3):440–447.

282. Yellin A, Benfield JR. Surgery for bronchogenic carcinoma in the elderly. *Am Rev Respir Dis* 1985;131(2):197.

283. Luketich JD, Ginsberg RJ. Limited resection versus lobectomy for Stage I non-small cell lung cancer. In: Pass HI, Mitchell JB, Johnson DH, eds. *Lung cancer principles and practice.* Philadelphia: Lippincott–Raven Publishers, 1996:561–566.

284. Martini N, et al. Prospective study of 445 lung carcinomas with mediastinal lymph node metastases. *J Thorac Cardiovasc Surg* 1980;80(3):390–399.

285. Martini N, Beattie Jr EJ. Results of surgical treatment in Stage I lung cancer. *J Thorac Cardiovasc Surg* 1977;74(4):499–505.

286. Wyser C, et al. Prospective evaluation of an algorithm for the functional assessment of lung resection candidates. *Am J Respir Crit Care Med* 1999;159(5 Pt 1):1450–1456.

287. Tanoue LT. Preoperative evaluation of the high-risk surgical patient for lung cancer resection. *Semin Respir Crit Care Med* 2000;21:421–432.

288. Beckles MA, et al. The physiologic evaluation of patients with lung cancer being considered for resectional surgery. *Chest* 2003;123(1 Suppl):105S–114S.

289. Errett LE, et al. Wedge resection as an alternative procedure for peripheral bronchogenic carcinoma in poor-risk patients. *J Thorac Cardiovasc Surg* 1985;90(5):656–661.

290. Martini N, et al. Incidence of local recurrence and second primary tumors in resected stage I lung cancer. *J Thorac Cardiovasc Surg* 1995;109(1):120–129.

291. Ginsberg R, Rubinstein LV. A randomized comparative trial of lobectomy versus limited resection for patients with TINO non-small cell lung cancer. *Lung Cancer* 1995;7:83–88.

292. Warren WH, Faber LP. Segmentectomy versus lobectomy in patients with stage I pulmonary carcinoma. Five-year survival and patterns of intrathoracic recurrence. *J Thorac Cardiovasc Surg* 1994;107(4):1087–1093; discussion1093–1094.

293. Coy P, Kennelly GM. The role of curative radiotherapy in the treatment of lung cancer. *Cancer* 1980;45(4):698–702.

294. Smart J, Hilton G. Radiotherapy of cancer of the lung; results in a selected group of cases. *Lancet* 1956;270(6928):880–881.

295. Cooper JD, et al. Radiotherapy alone for patients with operable carcinoma of the lung. *Chest* 1985;87(3):289–292.

296. Sibley GS, et al. Radiotherapy alone for medically inoperable stage I non-small cell lung cancer: the Duke experience. *Int J Radiat Oncol Biol Phys* 1998;40(1):149–154.

297. Sause WT, Turrisi AT. Principles and applications of preoperative and standard radiotherapy for regionally advanced non-small cell lung cancer. In: Pass HI, Mitchell JB, Johnson DH, eds. *Lung cancer principles and practice.* Philadelphia: Lippincott–Raven Publishers, 1996:697–710.

298. Bloedorn FG, Cowley RW, Cuccia CA. Combined therapy: irradiation and surgery in the treatment of bronchogenic carcinoma. *Am J Roentgenol* 1961;85:875–885.

299. Arriagada R, et al. Cisplatin-based adjuvant chemotherapy in patients with completely resected non-small cell lung cancer. *N Engl J Med* 2004;350(4):351–360.

300. Kato H, et al. A randomized trial of adjuvant chemotherapy with uracil-tegafur for adenocarcinoma of the lung. *N Engl J Med* 2004;350(17):1713–1721.

301. Blum RH. Adjuvant chemotherapy for lung cancer—a new standard of care. *N Engl J Med* 2004;350(4):404–405.

302. Scott WJ, Howington J, Movsas B. Treatment of stage II non-small cell lung cancer. *Chest* 2003;123(1 Suppl):188S–201S.

303. Inoue K, et al. Prognostic assessment of 1310 patients with non-small cell lung cancer who underwent complete resection from 1980 to 1993. *J Thorac Cardiovasc Surg* 1998;116(3):407–411.

304. van Rens MT, et al. Prognostic assessment of 2,361 patients who underwent pulmonary resection for non-small cell lung cancer, stage I, II, and IIIA. *Chest* 2000;117(2):374–379.

305. Adebonojo SA, et al. Impact of revised stage classification of lung cancer on survival: a military experience. *Chest* 1999;115(6):1507–1513.

306. Downey RJ, et al. Extent of chest wall invasion and survival in patients with lung cancer. *Ann Thorac Surg* 1999;68(1):188–193.

307. Piehler JM, et al. Bronchogenic carcinoma with chest wall invasion: factors affecting survival following en bloc resection. *Ann Thorac Surg* 1982;34(6):684–691.

308. Patterson GA, et al. The value of adjuvant radiotherapy in pulmonary and chest wall resection for bronchogenic carcinoma. *Ann Thorac Surg* 1982;34(6):692–697.

309. Ratto GB, et al. Chest wall involvement by lung cancer: computed tomographic detection and results of operation. *Ann Thorac Surg* 1991;51(2):182–188.

310. Dartevelle PG, et al. Tracheal sleeve pneumonectomy for bronchogenic carcinoma: report of 55 cases. *Ann Thorac Surg* 1988;46(1):68–72.

311. Martini N, et al. Management of non-small cell lung cancer with direct mediastinal involvement. *Ann Thorac Surg* 1994;58(5):1447–1451.

312. Stewart LA. Chemotherapy in non-small cell lung cancer: a meta-analysis using updated data on individual patients from 52 randomised clinical trials. *Br Med J* 1995;311:899–909.

313. Robinson LA, Wagner Jr H, Ruckdeschel JC. Treatment of stage IIIA non-small cell lung cancer. *Chest* 2003;123(1 Suppl):202S–220S.

314. Fernando HC, Goldstraw P. The accuracy of clinical evaluative intrathoracic staging in lung cancer as assessed by postsurgical pathologic staging. *Cancer* 1990;65(11):2503–2506.

315. Goldstraw P, et al. Surgical management of non-small cell lung cancer with ipsilateral mediastinal node metastasis (N2 disease). *J Thorac Cardiovasc Surg* 1994;107(1):19–27; discussion 27–28.

316. The Lung Cancer Study Group. Effects of postoperative mediastinal radiation on completely resected stage II and stage III epidermoid cancer of the lung. *N Engl J Med* 1986;315(22):1377–1381.

317. PORT Meta-analysis Trialist Group. Postoperative radiotherapy in non-small cell lung cancer: systematic review and meta-analysis of individual patient data from nine randomised controlled trials. *Lancet* 1998;352:257–263.

318. Le Chevalier T. Adjuvant chemotherapy in non-small cell lung cancer. *Semin Oncol* 1998;25(4 Suppl 9):62–65.

319. Lad T, Rubinstein L, Sadeghi A, The Lung Cancer Study Group. The benefit of adjuvant treatment for resected locally advanced non-small cell lung cancer. *J Clin Oncol* 1988;6(1):9–17.

320. Keller SM et al., Eastern Cooperative Oncology Group. A randomized trial of postoperative adjuvant therapy in patients with completely resected stage II or IIIA non-small cell lung cancer. *N Engl J Med* 2000;343(17):1217–1222.

321. Rusch VW. Surgery for stage III non-small cell lung cancer. *Cancer Control* 1994;1:455–466.

322. Rosell R, et al. A randomized trial comparing preoperative chemotherapy plus surgery with surgery alone in patients with non-small cell lung cancer. *N Engl J Med* 1994;330(3):153–158.

323. Rosell R, et al. Preresectional chemotherapy in stage IIIA non-small cell lung cancer: a 7-year assessment of a randomized controlled trial. *Lung Cancer* 1999;26(1):7–14.

324. Roth JA, et al. A randomized trial comparing perioperative chemotherapy and surgery with surgery alone in resectable stage IIIA non-small cell lung cancer. *J Natl Cancer Inst* 1994;86(9):673–680.

325. Roth JA, et al. Long-term follow-up of patients enrolled in a randomized trial comparing perioperative chemotherapy and surgery with surgery alone in resectable stage IIIA non-small cell lung cancer. *Lung Cancer* 1998;21(1):1–6.

326. Depierre A, et al. Preoperative chemotherapy followed by surgery compared with primary surgery in resectable stage I (except T1N0), II, and IIIa non-small cell lung cancer. *J Clin Oncol* 2002;20(1):247–253.

327. Albain KS, et al. Concurrent cisplatin/etoposide plus chest radiotherapy followed by surgery for stages IIIA (N2) and IIIB non-small cell lung cancer: mature results of Southwest Oncology Group phase II study 8805. *J Clin Oncol* 1995;13(8):1880–1892.

328. Bueno R, et al. Nodal stage after induction therapy for stage IIIA lung cancer determines patient survival. *Ann Thorac Surg* 2000;70(6):1826–1831.

329. Jeremic B, et al. Hyperfractionated radiation therapy with or without concurrent low-dose daily carboplatin/etoposide for stage III non-small cell lung cancer: a randomized study. *J Clin Oncol* 1996;14(4):1065–1070.

330. Dillman RO, et al. Improved survival in stage III non-small cell lung cancer: seven-year follow-up of cancer and leukemia group B (CALGB) 8433 trial. *J Natl Cancer Inst* 1996;88(17):1210–1215.

331. Schaake-Koning C, et al. Effects of concomitant cisplatin and radiotherapy on inoperable non-small cell lung cancer. *N Engl J Med* 1992;326(8):524–530.

332. Jett JR, et al. Guidelines on treatment of stage IIIB non-small cell lung cancer. *Chest* 2003;123(1 Suppl):221S–225S.

333. Lanzotti VJ, et al. Survival with inoperable lung cancer: an integration of prognostic variables based on simple clinical criteria. *Cancer* 1977;39(1):303–313.

334. Finkelstein DM, Ettinger DS, Ruckdeschel JC. Long-term survivors in metastatic non-small cell lung cancer: an Eastern Cooperative Oncology Group Study. *J Clin Oncol* 1986;4(5):702–709.

335. Albain KS, et al. Survival determinants in extensive-stage non-small cell lung cancer: the Southwest Oncology Group experience. *J Clin Oncol* 1991;9(9):1618–1626.

336. American Society of Clinical Oncology. Clinical practice guidelines for the treatment of unresectable non-small cell lung cancer. *J Clin Oncol* 1997;15:2996–3018.

337. Furuse K, et al. Phase III study of concurrent versus sequential thoracic radiotherapy in combination with mitomycin, vindesine, and cisplatin in unresectable stage III non-small cell lung cancer. *J Clin Oncol* 1999;17(9):2692–2699.

338. Pierre F, Maurice P, Gilles R. A randomized phase III trial of sequential chemoradiotherapy in locally advanced non-small cell lung cancer. *Proc Amer Soc Clin Oncol* 2001;20:312a.

339. Socinski MA, et al. Chemotherapeutic management of stage IV non-small cell lung cancer. *Chest* 2003;123(1 Suppl):226S–243S.

340. Grilli R, Oxman AD, Julian JA. Chemotherapy for advanced non-small cell lung cancer: how much benefit is enough? *J Clin Oncol* 1993;11(10):1866–1872.

341. Marino P, et al. Chemotherapy vs supportive care in advanced non-small cell lung cancer. Results of a meta-analysis of the literature. *Chest* 1994;106(3):861–865.

342. Souquet PJ, et al. Polychemotherapy in advanced non-small cell lung cancer: a meta-analysis. *Lancet* 1993;342(8862):19–21.

343. Kim TE, Murren JR. Therapy for stage IIIB and stage IV non-small cell lung cancer. *Clin Chest Med* 2002;23(1):209–224.

344. Smit EF, et al. Three-arm randomized study of two cisplatin-based regimens and paclitaxel plus gemcitabine in advanced non-small cell lung cancer: a phase III trial of the European Organization for Research and Treatment of Cancer Lung Cancer Group—EORTC 08975. *J Clin Oncol* 2003;21(21):3909–3917.

345. Scagliotti GV, et al. Phase III randomized trial comparing three platinum-based doublets in advanced non-small cell lung cancer. *J Clin Oncol* 2002;20(21):4285–4291.

346. Socinski MA, et al. Phase III trial comparing a defined duration of therapy versus continuous therapy followed by second-line therapy in advanced-stage IIIB/IV non-small cell lung cancer. *J Clin Oncol* 2002;20(5):1335–1343.

347. Smith IE, et al. Duration of chemotherapy in advanced non-small cell lung cancer: a randomized trial of three versus six courses of mitomycin, vinblastine, and cisplatin. *J Clin Oncol* 2001;19(5):1336–1343.

348. Shepherd FA, et al. Prospective randomized trial of docetaxel versus best supportive care in patients with non-small cell lung cancer previously treated with platinum-based chemotherapy. *J Clin Oncol* 2000;18(10):2095–2103.

349. Fossella FV et al. The TAX 320 Non-Small Cell Lung Cancer Study Group. Randomized phase III trial of docetaxel versus vinorelbine or ifosfamide in patients with advanced non-small cell lung cancer previously treated with platinum-containing chemotherapy regimens. *J Clin Oncol* 2000;18(12):2354–2362.

350. Johnson DH. Gefitinib (Iressa) trials in non-small cell lung cancer. *Lung Cancer* 2003;41(Suppl 1):S23–S28.

351. Herbst RS et al. Gefitinib in combination with paclitaxel and carboplatin in advanced non-small cell lung cancer: a phase III trial—INTACT 2. *J Clin Oncol* 2004;22(5):785–794.

352. Langer CJ. Emerging role of epidermal growth factor receptor inhibition in therapy for advanced malignancy: focus on NSCLC. *Int J Radiat Oncol Biol Phys* 2004;58(3):991–1002.

353. Druker BJ, et al. Efficacy and safety of a specific inhibitor of the BCR-ABL tyrosine kinase in chronic myeloid leukemia. *N Engl J Med* 2001;344(14):1031–1037.

354. Detterbeck FC, et al. Lung cancer. Special treatment issues. *Chest* 2003;123(1 Suppl):244S–258S.

355. Tanoue LT, Ponn RB. Therapy for stage I and stage II non-small cell lung cancer. *Clin Chest Med* 2002;23(1):173–190.

356. LoCicero III J, Ponn RB, Daly BDT. Surgical treatment of non-small cell lung cancer, In: Shields TW, LoCicero III J, Ponn RB, eds. *General thoracic surgery*, 5th ed. Philadelphia: Lippincott Williams & Wilkins, 2000:1311–1341.

357. Sandler AB. Current management of small cell lung cancer. *Semin Oncol* 1997;24(4):463–476.

358. Bunn PA Jr, Carney DN. Overview of chemotherapy for small cell lung cancer. *Semin Oncol* 1997;24(2 Suppl 7):S7–74.

359. Perry MC, et al. Chemotherapy with or without radiation therapy in limited small cell carcinoma of the lung. *N Engl J Med* 1987;316(15):912–918.

360. Hansen HH, Elliott JA. Patterns of failure in small cell lung cancer: implications for therapy. *Recent Results Cancer Res* 1984;92:43–57.

361. Rosen ST, et al. Role of prophylactic cranial irradiation in prevention of central nervous system metastases in small cell lung cancer. Potential benefit restricted to patients with complete response. *Am J Med* 1983;74(4):615–624.

362. Ball DL, Matthews JP. Prophylactic cranial irradiation in small cell lung cancer. In: Pass HI, Mitchell JB, Johnson DH, eds. *Lung cancer principles and practice*. Philadelphia: Lippincott–Raven Publishers, 1996:761–773.

363. Friess GG, et al. Effect of initial resection of small cell carcinoma of the lung: a review of Southwest Oncology Group Study 7628. *J Clin Oncol* 1985;3(7):964–968.

364. Jacox A, Carr DB, Payne R. *Management of cancer pain: clinical practice guideline No. 9*. Rockville: Agency for Health Care Policy and Research, U.S. Department of Health and Human Services, Public Health Service, 1994.

365. Kvale PA, Simoff M, Prakash UB. Lung cancer. Palliative care. *Chest* 2003;123(1 Suppl):284S–311S.

CHAPTER 15

Respiratory Tract Infections

Michael S. Niederman

George A. Sarosi

EPIDEMIOLOGY OF RESPIRATORY INFECTIONS

DEFINITIONS

BACTERIOLOGY OF THE RESPIRATORY TRACT
The Normal Respiratory Tract

SPECIFIC INFECTIOUS SYNDROMES—CLINICAL FEATURES AND THERAPY
The Upper Respiratory Tract
Airway Infections
Parenchymal Lung Infections
Fungal Lung Disease: Normal Host
Opportunistic Fungal Infections

In spite of the sophistication and advances in modern medicine, respiratory tract infections remain a major source of morbidity, mortality, and economic cost in our society. The availability of new and potent antibiotics, the development of rapid and elegant diagnostic methods, the emergence of effective vaccines for certain infections, and the appreciation of the role of newly recognized organisms in causing disease have not reduced the scope of the problem presented by respiratory tract infections. In fact, the current ability of modern medicine to extend life and the application of novel life-sustaining therapies have created patient populations with specific impairments in their ability to resist infection and have thereby added to the problem of one specific infection: pneumonia. The risk factors for pneumonia are always changing, and we now have individuals with novel forms of immunosuppressive illness as the result of either organ transplantation or infection with the human immunodeficiency virus (HIV). Although our therapeutic armamentarium is ever expanding, the organisms responsible for respiratory infections continue to adapt to the selective pressure of antibiotics. In the new millennium, we have multiple-drug–resistant tuberculosis (TB), penicillin-resistant pneumococci, β-lactamase–producing *Haemophilus influenzae*, methicillin-resistant *Staphylococcus aureus* (MRSA), and highly resistant gram-negative enteric bacteria. The changing epidemiology and ecology of respiratory infections make these illnesses an ongoing challenge.

EPIDEMIOLOGY OF RESPIRATORY INFECTIONS

The common cold is a viral infection of the upper respiratory tract that accounts for 20% of all acute disabling conditions and for 40% of all acute respiratory conditions annually in the United States. Adults have more than 100 million occurrences of disabling colds annually, leading to 250 million days of restricted activity and 30 million lost days of work, amounting to a staggering economic impact (1). Furthermore, more than 1 billion dollars are spent annually on over-the-counter cold remedies. In spite of these data, a preventative vaccine for the common cold is unlikely because more than 200 different viruses lead to this type of infection. Similarly, the common cold is an unavoidable annual event for most adults because, even with four colds per year, it would take at least 50 years to contract an infection with every available cold virus and to develop immunity to each one.

Pneumonia, or infection of the lung parenchyma, is also common and occurs in as many as 5.6 million Americans annually. Pneumonia can occur in the community or in the hospital, and different types of individuals have varying susceptibilities to this infection. It has been estimated that there are 1.1 million cases of community-acquired pneumonia (CAP) requiring hospitalization each year, at an estimated cost of $8 billion (2). Community-acquired infections may be viral, bacterial, or, rarely, fungal and parasitic. Nosocomial or hospital-acquired pneumonia occurs yearly in at least 275,000 individuals and is the most important hospital-acquired infection because it is associated with the highest mortality rate of nosocomial infections that contribute causally to death (3). Most nosocomial pneumonias are bacterial in origin, although hospital-acquired viral infections can also occur, particularly if personnel come to work carrying such an illness. In addition to direct patient care costs, pneumonia is responsible for over 50 million days of restricted activity from work and (in concert with influenza) is the sixth leading cause of death in this country, with a mortality rate of 13.4 per 100,000 (4,5). Each year, more than 100,000 patients are hospitalized for influenza-related complications and more than 35,000 people die as a result of influenza.

Certain patient populations have an enhanced risk for pneumonia that reflects disease-associated impairments in the host defenses of their respiratory tract. Among the elderly, pneumonia is the fourth leading cause of death, with a mortality rate of 169.7 per 100,000 (6). Similarly, 80% of the excess deaths from influenza are in individuals above the age of 65 (5). This enhanced rate of death due to respiratory infection with advancing age has been recognized for a long time, and Sir William Osler called pneumonia the "friend of the aged," but recent data have questioned just how much of a friend pneumonia really is (7). One study compared 158,960 Medicare patients with CAP to 794,333 hospitalized controls and found that the in-hospital mortality rate for CAP exceeded that of controls (11% versus 5.5%), but the differences in 1-year mortality were even more dramatic (40.9% versus 29.1%). The high mortality after patients developed a seemingly self-limited disease means that one in three survivors of CAP died in the subsequent year, following hospital discharge.

Among the elderly, the risk of pneumonia varies with an individual's general health and is often reflected by his or her place of residence. Thus, pneumonia occurs in 25 to 44 per 1,000 noninstitutionalized elderly individuals and in 68 to 114 per 1,000 residents of chronic care institutions. At any given time, as many as 3.2% of all nursing home residents will have pneumonia (8). In the setting of CAP, the elderly are hospitalized more often than younger patients and have a longer length of stay, both being a reflection of a greater frequency of comorbid illness; this may explain why the elderly make up only one-third of all CAP patients, yet account for more than 50% of the dollars spent on CAP (2). In the hospital, the elderly have a threefold greater incidence of pneumonia than younger patients do, with 1.6% of all hospital admissions in the elderly being complicated by lung infection (8). In one study, patients over the age of 60 represented only 23% of all hospitalized patients, yet they accounted for 64% of all nosocomial infections (9). In the National Nosocomial Infection Surveillance (NNIS) study, 54% of more than 100,000 nosocomial infections were seen in patients over the age of 55. Pneumonia was more common in the elderly than in younger patients and accounted for 48% of all infection-related mortality in the elderly (10).

Among critically ill patients treated with mechanical ventilation, nosocomial pneumonia develops in 20% to 55% of all patients, depending on the type of illness that has led to the need for mechanical ventilation. Patients who have had general surgery and who require mechanical ventilation in an intensive care unit (ICU) have at least a 10% incidence of pneumonia, a general medical ICU population has a 20% incidence,

and patients with the acute respiratory distress syndrome (ARDS) have a 55% incidence of secondary pneumonia (11). Particularly with ARDS, the mortality implications of this infection can be striking. In one study, when ARDS was complicated by infection, only 12% of patients survived, whereas when the ARDS patient remained free of infection, survival rate was 67% (12). In contrast, in one recent study, the mortality rate of patients with ARDS and pneumonia was high, but it was no higher than that for ARDS patients without pneumonia (11). These data raise the question of "attributable mortality," namely, whether some patients are so ill that pneumonia does not add further to their risk of dying. Although not all populations, particularly surgical trauma patients, have an attributable mortality from nosocomial pneumonia, recent data have shown that many patients do not die merely in the presence of nosocomial pneumonia but, in fact, they actually die because of nosocomial pneumonia, with up to 50% of all deaths being the direct effect of infection and not comorbid illness, particularly if effective antibiotic therapy is not provided in a timely manner (13,14).

Other groups at increased risk for pneumonia include patients with cardiac disease, alcoholism, chronic obstructive lung disease (COPD), malnutrition, head injury, cystic fibrosis or bronchiectasis, splenic dysfunction, malignancy, cirrhosis, diabetes, renal failure, sickle cell disease, and any immunosuppressive therapy or disease state. Recognition of the increased risk of infection in all of these patient groups should prompt the use of available vaccines to prevent respiratory infection.

Bronchitis—infection of the large bronchi—can be caused by either viruses or bacteria. In children, more than 40% of episodes of acute bronchitis are viral and the remainder are bacterial. Viral bronchitis in children may lead to transient or even persistent airway hyperreactivity and, thereby, may be a risk factor for subsequent adult asthma. Chronic bronchitis is an adult disease characterized by a persistent inflammatory state of the large airways, generally caused by cigarette smoking, and found in 12.5 million Americans (5,15–17). Patients with this condition frequently have acute infectious bronchitis (viral or bacterial) superimposed on their chronic condition, with such exacerbations happening three times per year on average (18). Bronchiolitis is an acute infection, usually viral, of the small airways that occurs in children usually between the ages of 1 month and 1 year, with an attack rate in this age group being six to seven cases per 100 children per year (19).

In recent years, particularly with the application of immunosuppressive therapy for a variety of illnesses, with the emergence of the acquired immunodeficiency syndrome (AIDS), and with an increasing number of institutionalized elderly individuals, TB and fungal and parasitic lung infections have emerged once again as important and common infections. Mycobacterial illnesses frequently complicate AIDS or occur in nursing homes, and fungal infections may emerge from a dormant state in patients living in endemic areas when a disease such as AIDS develops. From 1985 to 1992, the incidence of TB increased, but this trend has recently reversed, with the case rate falling below 10 per 100,000 cases. Certain populations are at increased risk for TB, particularly blacks, Hispanics, and immigrant populations. Minority groups now account for as many as 70% of all TB cases in the United States, even though they represent only one-fourth of the population (5,20). An additional concern today is the emergence of multiple-drug–resistant disease, a phenomenon that is particularly common in certain areas of the country such as large cities in the Northeast. Lastly, our world is changing, and with global travel and industrialization, we are seeing the emergence of such unusual viral illnesses as severe acute respiratory syndrome (SARS) and monkeypox. In addition, iatrogenic severe pneumonia as a consequence of bioterrorism remains a persistent and unsettling possibility.

DEFINITIONS

The respiratory tract can be anatomically divided into an upper and lower system, with the vocal cords serving as the dividing line between them. Infections of the upper respiratory tract include the common cold, sinusitis, pharyngitis, tonsillitis, and epiglottitis. Influenza is a viral infection that can involve the epithelial cells of both the upper and lower respiratory tract, and some patients have predominantly upper-respiratory infectious symptoms, whereas others have more marked lower-airway signs and symptoms.

Infections of the lower respiratory tract can involve the airways, lung parenchyma, or pleural space. When infection involves the large airways, it is termed "bronchitis," and symptoms are a reflection of this localization, with patients complaining of cough, sputum production, and, often, wheezing. If the infection involves smaller, more peripheral airways, it is termed "bronchiolitis"; this infection primarily involves children, but, recently, an adult version, possibly initiated by an infectious agent, has been recognized and is termed "bronchiolitis obliterans with organizing pneumonia" (BOOP). One chronic airways disease, bronchiectasis, is often a consequence of preceding respiratory infection and is frequently characterized by multiple episodes of infection in the areas of diseased airways. Bronchiectasis is characterized pathologically by abnormal and permanent dilation of subsegmental airways, which are inflamed and are usually filled with secretions (21). It is these areas of stagnant secretions that frequently become infected. Similarly, chronic bronchitis, a disease usually caused by cigarette smoking, is often complicated by bouts of acute infectious bronchitis.

Pneumonia is an infection of the lung parenchyma itself, involving the alveolar space with microbial invasion. In the immunocompetent individual, this type of infection is accompanied by a brisk filling of the alveolar space with inflammatory cells and fluid. When this alveolar infection involves an entire anatomic lobe of the lung, it is termed "lobar pneumonia," and more than one lobe can be involved in some instances. When the alveolar process occurs in a distribution that is patchy and is adjacent to bronchi without filling an entire lobe of the lung, it is termed a "bronchopneumonia." From a clinical perspective, pneumonias have been classified as being "typical" or "atypical," depending on their mode of clinical presentation. Although the "typical" pneumonia syndrome is characterized by sudden onset of fever, chills, pleuritic chest pain, and productive cough, this type of presentation can be expected only if the patient has an intact immune response system and if the infection is due to a bacterial pathogen such as *Streptococcus pneumoniae* (pneumococcus), *H. influenzae*, *Klebsiella pneumoniae*, *S. aureus*, aerobic gram-negative bacilli, or anaerobes. If a patient is infected by one of these organisms but has an impaired immune response, the classic pneumonia

symptoms may be absent, as can be the case with the elderly and debilitated patient. The atypical pneumonia syndrome, characterized by preceding upper respiratory symptoms, fever without chills, nonproductive cough, headache, myalgias, and mild leukocytosis, is often the result of infection with viruses, *Mycoplasma pneumoniae*, *Legionella* organisms, and other unusual infectious agents (as in psittacosis and Q fever). In clinical practice, it is often very difficult to use this type of classification to predict the microbial etiology of pneumonia. In fact, clinical features may be, at best, only 40% accurate in distinguishing *M. pneumoniae*, pneumococcus, and other pathogens (22). Another classification system that is often applied to pneumonias is their place of origin, and, thus, the infection can be community-acquired or hospital-acquired (nosocomial). In recent years, the distinction between these two populations has blurred, creating a new group of pneumonia patients, those with health care–related pneumonia, who have recently been hospitalized or those who have come from nursing homes or other complex outpatient settings such as dialysis units. Patients who develop pneumonia while receiving immunosuppressive therapy or those who have abnormal immune systems are referred to as *compromised hosts*, and the infectious possibilities will vary with the localization of the immune defect.

When a parenchymal lung infection leads to necrosis and breakdown of lung tissue and when a cavity is evident within the pneumonic area, the infection is termed a *lung abscess*. These infections are usually caused by anaerobes, but other etiologic agents include *S. aureus*, *K. pneumoniae*, *Escherichia coli*, and *Pseudomonas aeruginosa*. Empyema is an infection of the pleural space characterized by grossly purulent material and usually caused by anaerobes, gram-negative bacilli, *S. aureus*, and, occasionally, TB.

BACTERIOLOGY OF THE RESPIRATORY TRACT

THE NORMAL RESPIRATORY TRACT

Certain sites in the respiratory tract are sterile under normal conditions, and the isolation of a microorganism from these sites generally connotes infection; other sites may contain organisms because they are colonized but not infected. When organisms persist at a particular body site without evidence of a host response or without adverse effects to the host, it is termed *colonization*. When organisms lead to a host response or adverse tissue effects, then an infection is present. Respiratory tract sites that are sterile in normal individuals include the paranasal sinuses and the lower respiratory tract. Although bacteria can colonize the proximal tracheobronchial tree of smokers and of others with impaired host defenses, the more distal areas of the lung are normally sterile unless infection is present. On the other hand, the nasopharynx and oropharynx are normally colonized and have an endogenous microflora; it is the identity of these colonizing organisms that changes when disease is present.

The Upper Airway

The oropharynx is normally colonized by a mixture of aerobic and microaerophilic bacteria as well as by anaerobic organisms.

The "normal" oral flora can include *Streptococcus mitis*, *Streptococcus salivarius*, *Staphylococcus epidermidis*, *Neisseria* spp, pneumococcus, *Candida* spp, lactobacilli, and a variety of anaerobic bacteria. In spite of frequent colonization, the anaerobes that actually cause lung infection include *Peptostreptococcus* spp, *Fusobacterium nucleatum*, *Fusobacterium necorphorum*, *Prevotella melanogenicus*, and, occasionally, *Bacteroides* spp (19,23). Conspicuously absent from this group of colonizing bacteria are the enteric gram-negative bacilli. Multiple investigators have shown that normal individuals are not colonized by these gram-negative bacteria, but patients with serious illness of any type may harbor these organisms in the oropharynx. The likelihood that a given individual will have upper-airway colonization by these bacteria is directly related to the severity and duration of illness. Patients with "moderate" illness will harbor gram-negative organisms in the oropharynx 35% of the time, whereas 73% of "moribund" individuals will be colonized by the same (24). Most patients develop colonization of the oropharynx when they enter a hospital, usually by the third hospital day. Risk factors for upper-airway colonization include alcoholism, endotracheal intubation, neutropenia, prior antibiotic use, azotemia, coma, hypotension, smoking, surgery, prior viral illness, and malnutrition (23–25).

The microbial ecology of the upper airway changes with infection, and the bacteriology of infection differs depending on the site (see Table 15-1). This tendency of specific organisms to cause infection at one airway site but not at another can be

TABLE 15-1. Common Pathogens for Upper Respiratory Tract Infections

Pharyngitis
 Group A streptococci
 Viruses
  Adenovirus
  Enteroviruses
  Influenza
  Epstein–Barr virus
  Herpesvirus hominis
Laryngitis
 Viruses
Common cold
 Viruses
  Rhinovirus
  Adenovirus
  Coronavirus
  Influenza
Sinusitis
 Haemophilus influenzae
 Pneumococcus
 Anaerobes
 Rhinovirus
Epiglottitis
 H. influenzae
 Haemophilus parainfluenzae
 Staphylococcus aureus
 Group A streptococci
Croup
 Viruses
  Parainfluenza virus
  Respiratory syncytial virus
  Adenovirus
 Mycoplasma pneumoniae

described as a "tissue tropism," or preference, of certain organisms for certain epithelial locations. The reason for tissue tropisms is not fully known, but their existence would suggest that colonization and infection proceed in unique ways for each mucosal site, making some sites more susceptible to the effects of a particular organism than are others.

The Tracheobronchial Tree

The lower respiratory tract is sterile in healthy individuals but may become colonized when illness is present (26). Smokers commonly will have *H. influenzae* recovered from tracheobronchial secretions even when there is no evidence of an acute bronchitis. In patients with chronic bronchitis, tracheobronchial colonization is common and can include *H. influenzae*, pneumococci, *Moraxella catarrhalis*, and, occasionally, enteric gram-negative bacteria (23). Gram-negative colonization becomes a particularly common event if the patient has one of a variety of acute or chronic illnesses, including ciliary dysfunction (cystic fibrosis and bronchiectasis), corticosteroid therapy, immunodeficiency, tracheostomy, prior antibiotic therapy, viral infection, malnutrition, and endotracheal intubation (23,25). Most bacteria enter the lower airway via aspiration from a previously colonized oropharynx, and, thus, there is frequently a congruence of organism identity at the two respiratory tract sites. Occasionally, organisms reach the lung hematogenously from nonrespiratory sites of infection, including the tricuspid heart valve in patients with right-sided endocarditis. Inhalation is not a major route of bacterial entry to the lung, with the exception of certain organisms such as *Legionella pneumophila* viruses and *Mycobacterium tuberculosis*. More recently, the intestinal tract has been identified as another potential source of organism entry to the lung. Either by reflux or by passage along a nasogastric tube, gastric bacteria can enter the oropharynx and then be aspirated into the lung. Although many studies have documented the presence of this route of infection, controversy exists as to how commonly this route of entry actually operates in the ICU patient (27). Also, in critically ill patients treated with an endotracheal tube or tracheostomy, certain organisms, such as *P. aeruginosa*, can enter the lower airway directly from environmental sources and colonization can follow (28).

With infectious illness, as with the upper respiratory tract, the lower airway and lung parenchyma can also become infected with different organisms at different sites. These "tropisms" of specific organisms causing specific illnesses are summarized in Table 15-2.

SPECIFIC INFECTIOUS SYNDROMES—CLINICAL FEATURES AND THERAPY

THE UPPER RESPIRATORY TRACT

The Common Cold

The common cold is a complex of symptoms caused by 1 of more than 200 viral agents. The most common viral etiologic agent is a rhinovirus, of which there are at least 100 types and which is a member of the picornavirus family (29). Other common agents causing this infection are adenovirus; coronavirus; parainfluenza virus; respiratory syncytial virus; and influenza A, B, and C viruses. Less common viral pathogens

TABLE 15-2. Common Pathogens for Lower Respiratory Tract Infections

Bronchitis
  Haemophilus influenzae
  Pneumococcus
  Moraxella catarrhalis
  Mycoplasma pneumoniae
  Viruses
    Adenovirus
    Influenza
    Rhinovirus
    Respiratory syncytial virus
Bronchiolitis
  Viruses
    Respiratory syncytial virus
    Parainfluenza virus
    Adenovirus
    Rhinovirus
Pneumonia
  Pneumococcus
  Legionella pneumophilia
  M. pneumoniae
  Chlamydia pneumoniae
  H. influenzae
  Anaerobes
  Staphylococcus aureus
  Enteric gram-negatives
  Viruses
    Influenza
    Respiratory syncytial virus
    Adenovirus
  Chlamydia psittaci
  Pneumocystis carinii
Bronchiectasis
  Pseudomonas aeruginosa
  S. aureus
  Mucoid *Escherichia coli*
  H. influenzae

is person to person via the hand–nose–hand inoculation route, but there is some evidence that cold viruses can also be spread via droplet nuclei generated by sneezing (32).

Therapy is entirely symptomatic and supportive unless a secondary bacterial infection supervenes. Nasal decongestants, warm saline gargles, cough suppressants, and antipyretics are generally effective, along with bed rest. Aspirin should be used cautiously in children and adolescents because of its association with Reye syndrome, especially after influenza and varicella infection. Antibiotics should not be routinely administered unless bacterial infection is present. Therapy with vitamin C is unproven. *Echinacea* has also been studied, and compared to placebo, it was not able to decrease the incidence, duration, or severity of colds and respiratory infections (29,33). Some data have shown that zinc lozenges can reduce the duration of symptoms in adults, but this therapy has not been proven to be of benefit to children and adolescents (34). Antiviral agents have had limited success, but one agent, pleconaril, which acts by serving as a viral capsid–binding inhibitor, has been able to reduce the duration of symptoms, but it is not approved for clinical use (29). Prevention of cold transmission can be achieved by careful hand washing after contact with an infected individual. Experimental prophylactic approaches have included the use of virucidal-impregnated tissues to wipe the nose of infected individuals and the application of intranasal interferon α-2 (29).

Sinusitis

Infection of one or more of the paranasal sinuses can be a cryptogenic event (5% of cases) or can be associated with other conditions such as viral upper-respiratory infection, allergic rhinitis, or mechanical obstruction of the sinuses. There are four different paranasal sinuses; they are ordinarily sterile but they can fill with serous fluid when the ostia are obstructed as the result of inflammation or infection. The fluid-filled sinus can in turn become infected by viruses (especially rhinovirus), pneumococcus, *H. influenzae*, *M. catarrhalis*, or anaerobes. Most cases result from the common cold or from allergic rhinitis, leading to ostial obstruction, but 10% to 15% of cases can arise from a dental abscess. The maxillary sinus is most frequently infected in both adults and children; the frontal sinus is the second most commonly infected site in adults (35).

If the maxillary or frontal sinuses are affected, the patient may note facial pain and tenderness to percussion over these areas. Purulent nasal discharge and low-grade fever are common symptoms. Infection of the ethmoid sinus can result in retroorbital pain, tearing, and headache that worsen in the supine position. Sphenoidal sinusitis may lead to a vertex headache that is most severe at night.

A clinical diagnosis of sinusitis can be made with typical headache pain and other associated findings, particularly, if they arise after a viral upper-respiratory tract infection. Transillumination of the sinuses can also lead to a diagnosis. To perform this maneuver for the maxillary sinus, a light is placed over the orbital rim and transmission to the hard palate is observed. Opacity by this maneuver is highly related to bacterial infection, whereas bright transillumination indicates that sinus infection is unlikely (36). Sinus radiographs may also confirm the diagnosis. In fact, a four-view radiographic series is 72% to 96% as accurate for demonstrating maxillary

include enterovirus, Epstein–Barr, and herpes simplex viruses. Typical symptoms include nasal congestion and discharge, sneezing, sore throat, and cough. In contrast to some other viral illnesses, upper-respiratory tract symptoms predominate, whereas systemic symptoms are mild or absent, and fever is not usually high. The incubation period of the illness varies for each virus, but is generally 48 to 72 hours (30). The illness may last up to 1 week, but up to one fourth of patients will be ill for up to 2 weeks. When symptoms persist, consideration must be given to the occurrence of a secondary bacterial infection such as sinusitis (in 0.5% of cases) or pharyngitis. Other complications can include bacterial otitis media (in 2% of cases) and persistent bronchospastic cough. Physical findings are generally confined to the upper respiratory tract and include nasal mucosal swelling and exudation and pharyngeal erythema. Only a few viral "colds" will be accompanied by an exudative pharyngitis, most notably those caused by adenovirus.

Most adults develop two to four colds per year, whereas children may have six to eight such infections. Smokers have more frequent and more severe viral respiratory illnesses (31). Illness is more common in fall and winter, helping to distinguish a cold from seasonal allergies, which are more common in spring and early fall. The major route of viral transmission sinusitis as is sinus aspiration and culture (37). When sinus radiographs are used to define the illness, certain clinical findings can be elicited that correlate highly with the presence of radiographic abnormalities. In a logistic regression model (37), patients were likely to have sinusitis if they had at least four of the following signs or symptoms: maxillary toothache, poor response of symptoms to nasal decongestants, a history of colored nasal discharge, purulent nasal secretions, and an abnormal transillumination of the sinuses. Sinus tenderness is only present in about 50% of all patients with sinusitis. Acute sinusitis is best diagnosed if patients have at least two or more of the following symptoms: nasal fullness, nasal obstruction, nasal purulence, facial pain, loss of smell, and fever. The diagnosis can also be made if there is purulent drainage from the nose and multiple other features such as cough, ear pressure, fatigue, halitosis, headache, or maxillary toothache. In addition to acute sinusitis (which can last for up to 4 weeks), some patients can have resolution and then recurrent acute sinusitis, whereas others can have subacute sinusitis (lasting more than 4 but less than 12 weeks) or chronic sinusitis (lasting more than 12 weeks), usually due to chronic inflammatory changes initiated by a preceding acute infection (35).

Bacteriologic studies have shown that sinusitis is caused by *H. influenzae*, pneumococcus, and anaerobes, with viruses (rhinovirus, influenza virus, and parainfluenza virus) being found occasionally. Less common are *S. aureus*, gram-negative bacteria, and fungi (36). Patients with chronic sinusitis can have any of these organisms, with many having staphylococci, although the bacteria may be commensals and not true pathogens. On the basis of this spectrum, therapy of acute sinusitis is usually with an oral antimicrobial agent for 10 to 14 days. Some clinical improvement should be seen within 48 hours of therapy, but if the findings are not completely resolved by 2 weeks, then an additional week of therapy may be used. Appropriate therapy can be achieved with high dose amoxicillin (up to 3 g per day), amoxicillin/clavulanate, cefpodoxime, or one of the new flouroquinolones (gatifloxacin, levofloxacin, or moxifloxacin). Trimethoprim–sulfamethoxazole is a less active agent for the likely pathogens. The use of β-lactamase–resistant agents may be necessary if resistance to ampicillin is encountered, an increasingly likely possibility with many of the etiologic organisms producing β-lactamase enzymes. Adjunctive therapy can include analgesics and decongestants. When antibiotic therapy does not work, complications such as osteomyelitis, facial cellulitis, intracranial abscess, cavernous sinus thrombosis, and even meningitis must be considered.

Epiglottitis

Acute swelling and inflammation of the epiglottis and aryepiglottic folds caused by an infectious agent can be a life-threatening illness, particularly in children. This infection does not descend into the lower airway and is usually bacterial, with *H. influenzae* type B being the most common etiologic pathogen (38–41). The seriousness of this infection is related to its potential to cause sudden upper-airway obstruction and asphyxiation. The disease is more common in children than in adults, with the incidence greatest between the ages of 2 and 4 and with a peak around the age of 3.5. There is no seasonal predisposition. Adults can develop this illness, with an incidence as high as 9.7 cases per million (38).

Patients with epiglottitis fall into one of three age ranges: below the age of 2, above the age of 2, and adults. Children above the age of 2 present with "classic" epiglottitis (40), with symptoms of sore throat or mild upper-respiratory symptoms that can rapidly progress to high fever, drooling, dysphagia, and lethargy (42). The symptoms can be described as the "four Ds": dysphagia, dysphonia, dyspnea, and drooling (40). Generally, all patients have respiratory distress, and breathing can be noisy with signs of inspiratory stridor. Unlike the case with croup, there is no prominent cough, stridor is lower pitched, and patients are generally older (the peak age for croup is 2 years).

When adults develop this disease, sore throat is the most common symptom, with less than 50% of the patients having respiratory distress and approximately one-fourth having drooling. Both infants (below the age of 2) and adults have a similar form of illness that is more a supraglottitis illness than an epiglottitis one. In infants, the illness is similar to croup but with a more severe clinical course. In adults, the infection is also primarily a supraglottitis, and the disease can be either gradual or accelerated (43). Factors associated with a more accelerated illness and the need for intubation are bacteremia and tachycardia (41). The most common pathogens in adults are *H. influenzae* type b, *S. aureus*, and *Klebsiella* spp (40). In adults, abscess formation can be a complication, and the bacteriology of these lesions includes *S. aureus* and a variety of streptococci.

The diagnosis is usually made by recognition of typical signs and symptoms. An attempt at direct or indirect visualization of the epiglottis may reveal the presence of a swollen, cherry-red epiglottis projecting over the back of the tongue. The patient should never be examined with a tongue blade as this may precipitate total airway obstruction. A lateral neck radiograph can confirm the diagnosis when the "thumb sign" of an enlarged epiglottis is seen, but this technique may be negative even with life-threatening disease. In adults, the findings may be subtler, with only mild erythema or even pale edema of the epiglottis. In one series, lateral neck radiographs were abnormal in 79% of affected adults (38). Other radiographic signs of epiglottitis have been described. In one series, epiglottic width in relation to epiglottic height or in relation to the width of the third cervical vertebra has been described as a sensitive and specific diagnostic finding (44). In adults, laryngoscopy (direct, indirect, or flexible) can establish the diagnosis and, generally, can be performed safely and without complications (41). Other diseases to be considered in the differential diagnosis are angioedema, bacterial tracheitis, croup, foreign body aspiration, and peritonsillar abscess.

Management is directed at maintenance of a patent airway to minimize mortality. With the use of a prophylactic artificial airway, mortality in children has fallen below 1%. In one of the largest series, 134 children and 273 adults were evaluated, and 79% of adults and 32% of children were treated without artificial airways, with mortality rates of 2.2% and 3.2%, respectively. Factors associated with airway obstruction included symptomatic respiratory distress, stridor, drooling, short duration of symptoms, enlarged epiglottis on x-ray, and *H. influenzae* bacteremia (43). The authors concluded that in the absence of adverse clinical features, careful observation, without immediate intubation, is appropriate and safe (43).

Other adjunctive measures include humidified oxygen and antibiotics. The pediatric illness is almost always caused by *H. influenzae*, and in adults *H. influenzae* is still the predominant organism, with it being recovered in 56% of patients in one se-ries (38). Blood cultures are positive, usually for *H. influenzae*, in up to 75% of children and 23% of adults. As mentioned, other possible infecting agents include pneumococcus, *S. aureus*, *Haemophilus parainfluenzae*, *Fusobacterium* spp, and group A streptococcus. With this bacteriologic spectrum in mind, ther-apy is usually with ampicillin (200 mg/kg/day in six divided doses), ampicillin/sulbactam (if β-lactamase–resistant strains are suspected), or alternatively, a second- or third-generation cephalosporin. The use of corticosteroids in conjunction with an antibiotic is of unproven benefit but may be helpful just prior to removal of an endotracheal tube to prevent laryngeal edema after extubation.

Other Upper Respiratory Tract Infections

PHARYNGITIS. Pharyngitis may occur with or without symptoms of the common cold. Etiologic agents may be viral or bacterial, with pharyngitis due to group A β-hemolytic streptococci (GABHS) being potentially the most important type to be recognized and treated. In the first 2 years of life, in-fection by group A streptococci is uncommon, but the inci-dence rises between the ages of 5 and 10. In children, GABHS accounts for one-third of all cases of pharyngitis. In college-age students, one fourth of cases are streptococcal, but viral pharyngitis is seen in 38% of cases (45). In those over the age of 35, streptococcal infection is present in only 5% of those with pharyngitis (29). In children and adults, other common infecting agents besides streptococci include adenovirus, res-piratory syncytial virus, rhinovirus, coronavirus, influenza and parainfluenza viruses, Epstein–Barr virus, *Herpesvirus ho-minis*, and *M. pneumoniae*. Less common agents include *Neisseria gonorrhoeae* and *Neisseria meningitides*, *H. influenzae*, *Corynebac-terium diphtheriae*, and anaerobes in a mixed pattern.

It may be difficult to distinguish the responsible pathogen from clinical features, but the onset of streptococcal pharyngitis may be sudden, with high fever, pharyngeal and uvular edema, yellowish pharyngeal exudate, along with red follicular lesions, with yellow centers being found on the uvula. However, infec-tions with the Epstein–Barr virus, herpesviruses, adenoviruses, and enteroviruses may also present with similar findings.

Streptococcal pharyngitis should be treated with penicillin VK, 500 mg every 6 hours for 10 days, or another antibiotic such as a macrolide (erythromycin, azithromycin, or clar-ithromycin) if the patient is allergic. However, it is important to be sure that the diagnosis is streptococcal because, occa-sionally, exudative pharyngitis may be due to oral anaerobes and can progress to Lemierre syndrome (postanginal sepsis), with jugular vein thrombosis, if not adequately treated, and macrolides do not effectively treat oral anaerobes, whereas penicillin can. Therapy provides four benefits: reduction in illness duration, avoidance of spread of infection to others, prevention of suppurative complications (such as peritonsillar and retropharyngeal abscess), and prevention of rheumatic fever (but probably not glomerulonephritis) (46).

CROUP. Croup, or acute laryngotracheobronchitis, is a dis-ease of young children usually between the ages of 3 months and 3 years, with a peak incidence in the second year of life. The etiology is usually viral, and this complication may occur in certain individuals, whereas others infected with the same

virus develop only a mild upper-respiratory illness. Some chil-dren develop recurrent episodes whenever they acquire a viral upper-respiratory infection, and in these instances the disease is termed "spasmodic croup." Parainfluenza virus type 1 is the most common cause, but the disease may also result from in-fluenza viruses, respiratory syncytial virus, adenovirus, my-coplasma, or rhinoviruses (45). Patients with croup present with acute dyspnea following an upper-respiratory illness. A barking cough is seen, followed by symptoms of hoarseness and stridor. The stridor may be accompanied by severe dysp-nea, and the course may be fluctuating, with improvement in the daytime. Airway edema is less severe than with epiglotti-tis, and, thus, acute upper-airway obstruction is less likely. Treatment is supportive, with inhalation of moist cold air, racemic epinephrine, and, possibly, steroids, the latter being controversial. Antibiotics are not needed unless the patient has secondary bacterial infection.

AIRWAY INFECTIONS

Bronchitis

Bronchitis is acute infection and inflammation of the large conducting airways and may be viral or bacterial in origin. When this infection occurs in a previously normal host, the re-sulting acute bronchitis will present in a manner very similar to a mild form of pneumonia, and the responsible pathogens will be similar for both illnesses. In the presence of chronic res-piratory disease or chronic inflammatory bronchitis, the mani-festations and etiologic agents will differ from those seen with acute bronchitis in the normal host.

IN A PREVIOUSLY HEALTHY ADULT. Acute bronchitis in a normal host may be due to viruses in at least 40% of cases, and these include adenovirus, influenza A and B virus, coron-avirus, rhinovirus, herpes simplex, respiratory syncytial virus, and parainfluenza virus. The role of bacteria in acute bronchitis is difficult to establish, particularly in those with chronic bron-chitis, because it may be difficult to distinguish colonization from infection. Bacterial agents implicated include *H. influen-zae*, both typable and nontypable strains, and pneumococcus. *M. pneumoniae* may account for 10% of infections. Newer agents identified as causing bronchitis are *M. catarrhalis* and *Chlamydia pneumoniae* (47).

Patients with bronchitis have symptoms of cough, purulent sputum, low-grade fever, chest burning, and substernal dis-comfort. These lower-respiratory symptoms usually follow a preceding upper respiratory infection. Hemoptysis can also occur, and acute bronchitis is the most common cause of this symptom. Dyspnea is generally mild, and the physical exami-nation may demonstrate diffuse adventitious sounds such as crackles, rhonchi, and wheezes. Diagnosis is made by discov-ering appropriate clinical features in the absence of a lung infiltrate on chest film. Sputum gram stain will show numer-ous polymorphonuclear (PMN) cells and, possibly, bacterial pathogens. Therapy is supportive, with cough suppressants, liquids, and antipyretics. There is no clear role for antibiotics in this illness, and its use in this setting can be reduced with patient education, an intervention that may help prevent an-tibiotic resistance and that is not associated with any adverse patient outcomes (48). Many patients with acute bronchitis will develop the frustrating complication of postinfectious bronchospasm. This is characterized by persistent dry cough and wheezing lasting 4 to 6 weeks after the acute infection subsides. Symptoms are treated with bronchodilators and, sometimes, corticosteroids, and only rarely will the airway reactivity persist and lead to chronic asthma. Some data indicate that children who have multiple episodes of acute viral bronchitis are at risk for developing adult chronic airways disease and asthma (49).

IN A PATIENT WITH CHRONIC LUNG DISEASE. Patients with chronic bronchitis are defined as having chronic recurrent cough, with sputum production, for at least 3 months during 2 consecutive years. These patients commonly have COPD complicated by episodes of acute bronchitis, but the clinical picture and bacteriology differ from those seen in the normal host. These episodes of acute airway infection occur every 20 to 78 weeks, with most studies reporting an exacerbation of chronic bronchitis three times per year on average (18). With infection, patients may note increasing dyspnea, purulent sputum, wheezing, fever, and general malaise. The three cardinal symptoms of an exacerbation—dyspnea, increased sputum purulence, and increased sputum volume—can be counted and used to grade the severity of an exacerbation. Patients with all three symptoms have the most severe exacerbation, a type 1 exacerbation (50). It has been estimated that 80% of all exacerbations are accompanied by two or three of these cardinal symptoms (50).

Examination may reveal diffuse crackles, rhonchi, or wheezes, and the chest radiograph shows no acute infiltrate. Exacerbations in this setting may be viral or bacterial, with some investigators believing that viral causes are most common. It is very difficult to reach such a conclusion with any certainty because patients with chronic bronchitis have bacterial colonization of the tracheobronchial tree in the absence of acute infection, and, thus, the recovery of bacterial pathogens from their sputum may represent either colonization or infection. However, in one study that used quantitative bacteriologic methods in patients with severe exacerbation, nearly 50% of all patients had bacteria present in concentrations equal to that seen in the presence of pneumonia (51). Even with less severe exacerbations, bronchoscopic studies have reported that 50% of all episodes are bacterial in origin. Several recent studies have clarified how it is possible to attribute exacerbations to bacteria in a population of patients that is chronically colonized (52). Using molecular typing, investigators have found that even when patients have the same organism in the airway over time, the specific surface-exposed epitopes can change because patients are acquiring new "strains" of the same organism. When a new strain of pneumococcus, *H. influenzae*, or *M. catarrhalis* was acquired, the likelihood of exacerbation was increased more than two-fold. In addition, investigators have found that the acquisition of a new strain was associated with a strain-specific antibody response, at least for new strains of *H. influenzae*. These findings are consistent with previous serologic studies that did not demonstrate an antibody response to laboratory strains of *H. influenzae* following an exacerbation because these strains can be viewed as heterologous and not homologous.

The clinical features of exacerbation (fever, hypoxemia, and leukocytosis) are similar for bacterial and nonbacterial

episodes, making it difficult to identify the responsible pathogen on clinical grounds. Common viral pathogens are adenovirus, influenza, rhinovirus, coronavirus, herpes simplex, and respiratory syncytial virus. The most common bacterial pathogens are *H. influenzae*, pneumococcus, and *M. catarrhalis*. Other recently recognized pathogens include *C. pneumoniae* and *M. pneumoniae* (47). *Moraxella* spp are *Neisseria*-like organisms that have only recently been recognized as pathogens after being appreciated as simply being part of the "normal" flora in the past (47). More than 90% of *Moraxella* spp produce β-lactamase enzymes and are resistant to β-lactam antibiotics such as amoxicillin. Similarly, up to 40% of *H. influenzae* produce β-lactamase enzymes or are resistant to ampicillin via other mechanisms. Most patients with *Moraxella* infections have abnormal host defenses, with most being smokers and having preexisting cardiopulmonary disease.

The role of antibiotics in treating acute bronchitic exacerbations of chronic bronchitis is controversial (16,53). The benefits of such therapy are uncertain in many studies, possibly because many episodes are viral. However, a recent meta-analysis has examined nine placebo-controlled studies and has concluded that antibiotics do speed the resolution of symptoms and the return of peak flow rates, especially if the patient has at least two of the cardinal symptoms of exacerbation (increased dyspnea, increased sputum volume, and increased sputum purulence) (54). In addition, antibiotics can eradicate organisms and, thus, reduce the host inflammatory response to the presence of bacteria, thereby preventing inflammatory injury to the airway (16). In doing so, antibiotics may disrupt the "vicious cycle" of infection, inflammation, and further infection (53). In the past, amoxicillin, 500 mg three times a day for 10 days, or ampicillin were appropriate antibiotic choices, but now with the emergence of drug-resistant pneumococci, *M. catarrhalis*, and β-lactamase-producing *H. influenzae* as pathogens, amoxicillin combined with a β-lactamase inhibitor (amoxicillin/clavulanate 500 mg every 8 hours, or higher if resistant pneumococci are likely), a new cephalosporin, one of the new macrolides (azithromycin or clarithromycin), tetracycline, or a fluoroquinolone is an appropriate choice. Trimethoprim–sulfamethoxazole is no longer reliable against pneumococcus and erythromycin does not cover *H. influenzae*, and, thus, these agents should not be used. Because the bacteriology of exacerbation becomes more complex with the presence of comorbid illness, severe airway obstruction, and frequent exacerbations, these patients may need broader spectrum therapy to include coverage for enteric gram negatives and other drug-resistant pathogens than for less complicated patients with acute exacerbations. For these more complex patients, therapy should focus on the quinolones and other β-lactamase-resistant agents.

In patients treated with chronic tracheostomy or mechanical ventilation, an illness termed "febrile tracheobronchitis" may develop (55). Clinically, the disease is similar to nosocomial pneumonia with fever, leukocytosis, and purulent respiratory secretions. In some individuals, bacteremia may occur. Unlike with pneumonia, the patient has no new parenchymal lung infiltrate. The disease is diagnosed if the patient has a compatible clinical picture and no new parenchymal lung infiltrate. The etiology is usually enteric gram-negative bacteria, particularly, *P. aeruginosa* in the most seriously ill patients and, occasionally, nontypable *H. influenzae*. Therapy is usually with systemic antibiotics directed against the responsible pathogen, but aerosolized antibiotics may be effective in patients without systemic toxicity; however, the role of therapy is uncertain.

Bronchiolitis

Bronchiolitis, an infection of the small airways, is primarily a viral infection of children, seen in the first year of life. Respiratory syncytial virus, parainfluenza virus type 3, influenza virus, adenovirus, and rhinovirus are the most common causes (19). Other infectious agents leading to bronchiolitis include *M. pneumoniae, L. pneumophila, Nocardia asteroides*, and *Pneumocystis carinii* (56). Children present with fever, tachypnea, wheezing, cough, and malaise. Therapy is supportive, with hydration, oxygen, and, possibly, bronchodilators. Recently, aerosolized ribavirin has been advocated to treat respiratory syncytial virus, a common cause of bronchiolitis in the midwinter and spring.

An adult form of this infection has been recognized and termed "BOOP." Although bronchiolitis obliterans (BO) can result from any viral bronchiolitis, the adult disease may present in an indolent manner, with cough and dyspnea and no evident acute infection. Because of distal atelectasis beyond the inflamed airways, segmental infiltrates may be seen in what has been termed the "proliferative" form of bronchiolitis (56). BOOP may be of viral origin or may be the result of inhalational injury, drug effects, or inflammation from a noninfectious systemic illness such as rheumatoid arthritis (56,57). Therapy is generally with corticosteroids.

Influenza

Influenza is an acute respiratory infection that results from an RNA virus of either type A or B, with the disease from type A being generally more severe (58). Influenza A virus is the most important respiratory virus on a global scale, with the highest overall morbidity and mortality. The virus has two major surface glycoprotein antigens, hemagglutinin (H) and neuraminidase (N), which can change yearly, and, thus, the disease appears in epidemics annually. Both antigenic drift and waning immunity make this infection a yearly threat, particularly to those who have underlying cardiac or respiratory illnesses, the elderly, and pregnant women. The virus has an incubation period of 2 to 4 days and is spread via aerosol or mucosal contact with infected secretions. Epidemics occur yearly in late fall and extend into early spring. Influenza A can coexist with other viral infections including respiratory syncytial virus and parainfluenza virus, particularly in the elderly (59,60).

The virus has its main site of infection in the respiratory mucosa, leading to desquamation of the respiratory mucosa with cellular degeneration, edema, and airway inflammation with mononuclear cells (61). Although up to 50% of the infections are subclinical, the typical illness lasts 3 days and is characterized by sudden onset of fever, chills, severe myalgia, malaise, and headache. As the major symptoms recede, respiratory symptoms dominate, with dry cough and substernal burning that may persist for several weeks. Laboratory data and physical examination are not specific, and diagnosis is made by noting the presence of typical symptoms during the time of a known epidemic. Serologic evaluation, using hemagglutinating-inhibiting antibody or enzyme linked immunosorbent assay (ELISA) testing, and viral cultures can confirm the diagnosis. The illness can be more severe in smokers, the elderly, those under the age of 1, pregnant women, and patients with chronic cardiorespiratory disease.

Influenza viruses can interfere with many aspects of respiratory host defenses and, thus, may be complicated by secondary bacterial pneumonia. The virus can interfere with mucociliary clearance, can promote tracheal bacterial colonization, and can interfere with the function of PMN cells and macrophages. Respiratory complications include obliterative bronchiolitis, airway hyperreactivity, exacerbation of chronic bronchitis, primary viral pneumonia, and secondary bacterial pneumonia. When viral pneumonia develops, the disease follows the classic 3-day illness without a hiatus and is characterized by cough (dry or productive) and severe dyspnea. Chest radiograph reveals bilateral infiltrates and mortality is high. Bacterial pneumonic superinfection follows the primary influenza illness with a hiatus of patient improvement for 3 to 4 days before the pneumonia begins. In this setting, pneumonia is usually lobar, and the most common pathogens are pneumococcus, *H. influenzae*, enteric gram-negative organisms, and *S. aureus*. Other serious complications include myocarditis and pericarditis, seizures, neuritis, coma, transverse myelitis, toxic shock, and renal failure (58).

Therapy of influenza is mainly symptomatic, with antipyretics, bed rest, and fluids. Amantadine can ameliorate the illness caused by influenza A if given within the first 24 to 48 hours. This medication may also be used prophylactically during an epidemic in high-risk individuals in doses of 100 mg twice a day until the epidemic passes or for 2 weeks until vaccination can be given and can become effective. Dosage must be reduced with renal insufficiency, and confusion may occur in 3% to 7% of treated individuals. Rimantadine, a derivative of amantadine, is also effective for the therapy and prevention of influenza A infection (62). Rimantadine can be given once daily because of its long half-life, and it has fewer central nervous system (CNS) and other side effects than amantadine. A new class of influenza agents, the neuraminidase inhibitors, is effective against both influenza A and B, and these agents appear to be effective for either therapy or prophylaxis. The neuraminidase inhibitors Zanamivir and Oseltamivir can be used during acute infection and will reduce the duration of symptoms if given within 36 to 48 hours. Immunization should be given to all high-risk patients yearly with a vaccine prepared against the strains most likely to be epidemic. If an epidemic of influenza A develops in a closed environment (e.g., a nursing home) among nonimmunized patients, antiviral therapy should be given along with vaccination, and antiviral therapy should be continued for 2 weeks until the vaccine takes effect.

Bronchiectasis

Bronchiectasis is another chronic airway disease that can be complicated by intermittent bouts of airway infection. In addition, the disease itself and its progression may be the result of airway infection. The disease is characterized pathologically by an abnormal and permanent dilation of subsegmental airways (21). In this condition, the airways are dilated and inflamed, and they become obstructed by thick secretions that may intermittently become infected. The actual shape of the abnormal airways has led to a classification system that characterizes the involvement as being cylindrical, varicose, or saccular.

The causes of bronchiectasis are multiple, and in past years it was most often the result of a preceding respiratory infection such as TB or a virulent bacterial, fungal, or viral illness. A localized process can lead to focal bronchiectasis, whereas a more extensive process or a systemic illness can lead to diffuse bronchiectasis. Some of the diseases that may be complicated by bronchiectasis include cystic fibrosis, rheumatoid arthritis, influenza, lung abscess, foreign body aspiration, hypoglobulinemia, immotile cilia syndrome, and allergic bronchopulmonary aspergillosis.

The major symptom of bronchiectasis is cough, which is generally productive but may also be dry. In severe disease, patients may expectorate more than 150 mL of sputum daily. Dyspnea and hemoptysis are also common, with massive hemoptysis at times of acute infection in some patients. The disease is accompanied by chronic bacterial colonization of the lower respiratory tract. When the quantity of sputum increases and it becomes purulent, usually in association with fever and dyspnea, infection is present and requires antibiotics. In some settings, patients are given antibiotics monthly to prevent recurrent bouts of airway infection. The usual pathogens are bacterial and include pneumococcus and *H. influenzae*. Patients with cystic fibrosis may have *S. aureus*. In more advanced forms of bronchiectasis and cystic fibrosis, airway infection is with mucoid variants of *E. coli* or *P. aeruginosa*. Recovery of these mucoid variants should immediately prompt consideration of the diagnosis of bronchiectasis if it has not been previously recognized because these organisms are not ordinarily found in the absence of chronic airway infection.

Some investigators (63) have found evidence for progression of the airway damage as a result of recurrent infection episodes. When airway infection occurs, it is accompanied by a brisk inflammatory response, with the release of neutrophilic proteases that can damage the airways and lead to more bronchiectasis. Observations such as these have prompted the suggestion that airway infection be treated promptly and, possibly, in a prophylactic manner to limit disease progression. Episodes of airway infection are treated with antibiotics similar to those used in exacerbations of chronic bronchitis; it may not be necessary to treat every pathogen recovered from the sputum because some organisms may be colonizers and not infecting agents. One effective regimen is amoxicillin 500 to 1,000 mg three times a day for 14 days; but when *P. aeruginosa* is present, ciprofloxacin should be used. In cystic fibrosis and bronchiectasis, the use of aerosolized aminoglycosides in a prophylactic manner may be effective in preventing acute episodes of airway infection, and these agents may also be used for the therapy of airway infection. In cystic fibrosis patients, DNAse has been used via aerosol to help in sputum clearance and to prevent exacerbations. In addition, some data indicate that the chronic use of macrolide therapy can improve lung function and can reduce the frequency of exacerbations in patients with cystic fibrosis patients by serving as an antiinflammatory agent rather than an antibiotic. Other adjunctive therapies include chest physical therapy with percussion and postural drainage, bronchodilators, oxygen, pneumococcal vaccine, and yearly influenza vaccine. In cases of severe hemoptysis or localized recurrent infections due to bronchiectasis, surgical resection of the involved lung may be considered.

When bronchiectasis is suspected by history, it should be confirmed by high resolution computed tomography (HRCT) of the chest. Routine chest radiographs (see Fig. 15-1) may

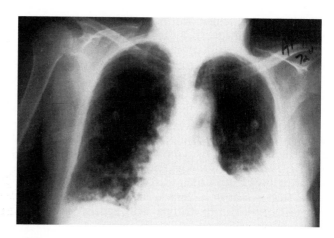

FIGURE 15-1. This patient had long-standing bronchiectasis with chronic increased markings in both lower-lung zones. The typical increased markings of this disease are seen in the right lower lobe, whereas the left lower lobe has evidence of pneumonia due to *Pseudomonas aeruginosa*.

show areas of increased airway markings, atelectasis, dilated bronchi, "tramlines," or cavities. Physical examination may show clubbing, nasal polyposis, and adventitious breath sounds (rhonchi, rales, and wheezes). If the history is appropriate, a workup for hypogammaglobulinemia (immunoglobulin quantitation), immotile cilia syndrome (electron microscopy of nasal cilia), or cystic fibrosis (sweat chloride) may be indicated. Although cystic fibrosis is an inherited disease that usually appears in childhood, recognition in adolescence and longevity into adulthood are increasingly common.

PARENCHYMAL LUNG INFECTIONS

Pathogenesis of Pneumonia

Bacteria commonly enter the lower airway and do not lead to pneumonia because of the presence of an intact, elaborate, host defense system. When pneumonia does occur, it is the result of an exceedingly virulent organism, a large inoculum, and/or an impaired host defense system. In the nonhospitalized person, bacteria reach the lung by one of four routes: inhalation from ambient air, hematogenous spread, direct inoculation from contiguous infected sites, or aspiration from a previously colonized upper airway. Critically ill patients in the hospital may acquire organisms from a colonized gastrointestinal tract (particularly if a nasogastric tube is present to direct bacteria from the stomach to the oropharynx), or bacteria may reach the lung directly through the endotracheal tube from a contaminated hospital environment (27,28). Aspiration is the major route of acquisition for most forms of pneumonia, but in fact, very few individuals who do aspirate contaminated oropharyngeal secretions actually develop pneumonia. As many as 45% of normals and 70% of obtunded patients aspirate oral secretions, and the effectiveness of the normal respiratory tract defenses prevents most from becoming ill (64).

The upper airway is normally colonized, as mentioned above, and with increasing degrees of systemic illness, the flora become dominated by enteric gram-negative bacteria. In healthy individuals, these organisms are unable to colonize the oropharynx because they are repelled by salivary proteases, lysozyme, and IgA (23). In addition, the "normal" flora of the oropharynx inhibit the growth of pathogens through a process termed "bacterial interference," whereby unfavorable growth conditions for pathogens are created. The absence of gram-negative organisms in the oral flora of normals may also reflect the fact that these organisms have a poor ability to adhere, or bind, to the surface of normal upper-airway epithelial cells. This process—bacterial adherence—is a bacterial–mucosal interaction in which organisms bind irreversibly to cell surfaces and form a nidus from which overt colonization may follow (23,65) (see Fig. 15-2). In many mucosal sites throughout the body, adherence is the first step leading to colonization. With systemic illnesses such as starvation, uremia, and surgical stress, salivary proteases are released into the oral cavity, and they act upon the mucosa to remove a glycoprotein—fibronectin—from it, thereby exposing previously covered epithelial cell receptors to gram-negative bacteria. An increase in oral mucosal cell receptivity to bacteria has been observed in individuals with acute illness and has been correlated with the clinical finding of gram-negative colonization of the oropharynx in such settings (23).

Once bacteria reach the lower airway, they encounter a variety of specific (organism directed) and nonspecific defense mechanisms. The nonspecific physical barriers include cough, reflex bronchoconstriction, angulation of the airways (favoring impaction and subsequent transport upward), and the mucociliary escalator. Immune defenses in the lower airway include bronchus-associated lymphoid tissue, phagocytosis (by PMN cells and macrophages), immunoglobulins A and G, complement, cytokines, surfactant, and cell-mediated immunity by T lymphocytes. Bacterial adherence also plays a role in colonization of the lower airway, and normal tracheal cells have the capacity to bind to gram-negative bacteria such as *P. aeruginosa*. It is likely that when bacteria have prolonged

contact with the tracheobronchial mucosa, as is the case when mucociliary clearance is reduced (bronchiectasis, cystic fibrosis, and endotracheal intubation), then the potential interaction of organisms with the tracheobronchial mucosa will occur. In the lower airway, adherence would be a particularly useful way for bacteria to "stick" to the mucosa and resist the constant flow of air and secretions. In tracheostomized patients, colonization by gram-negative organisms has been correlated with an increase in tracheal cell capacity to bind bacteria (66). In intubated patients, an increase in tracheal cell bacterial adherence has been correlated with the occurrence of ventilator-associated pneumonia (67).

Colonization of both the oropharynx and the tracheobronchial tree with gram-negative bacteria is an important harbinger of pneumonia, particularly when it arises in an ill, hospitalized individual. In one study, 23% of ICU patients with gram-negative bacteria in the oropharynx developed pneumonia, in contrast to only 3.3% of patients without this finding (68). Similarly, lower airway colonization by these organisms is a risk factor for pneumonia because bacteria gain a foothold in the tracheobronchial tree from where they can propagate downward toward the alveoli. Many clinical features have been correlated with colonization, but a general principle is that colonization is a "marker" of a patient with systemic illness who has impairments in the host defense system at multiple sites throughout the respiratory tract. Clinical risk factors for colonization of either the oropharynx or the tracheobronchial tree include antibiotic therapy, azotemia, diabetes, coma, hypotension, endotracheal intubation, malnutrition, corticosteroid therapy, smoking, chronic bronchitis, cystic fibrosis, and viral infection (see Table 15-3).

When an organism of low virulence or a small inoculum enters the lung, it is contained by phagocytosis and killing by the

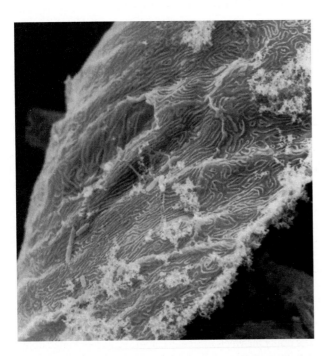

FIGURE 15-2.   This scanning electron micrograph shows the bacterial adherence interaction between *Pseudomonas aeruginosa* and the surface of tracheal cells.

TABLE 15-3.   Risk Factors for Airway Colonization by Enteric Gram-negative Bacilli

Oropharyngeal colonization
    Underlying serious illness
    Prior antibiotic therapy
    Coma
    Diabetes
    Renal failure
    Malnutrition
    Hypotension
    Advanced age
    Recent surgery
    Underlying lung disease
    Cigarette smoking
Tracheobronchial colonization
    Advanced age
    Tracheostomy
    Malnutrition
    Endotracheal intubation
    Prior antibiotics
    Neurologic disease
    Bronchiectasis, cystic fibrosis
    Acute lung injury [acute respiratory distress syndrome (ARDS)]
    Chronic bronchitis
    Corticosteroid therapy
    Prolonged hospitalization
    Recent surgery

alveolar macrophage, and lung inflammation does not result. More virulent insults are contained by a complex inflammatory response (69). This mechanism requires a variety of chemotactic factors (complement, alveolar macrophage cytokine products such as IL-8 and others) to attract PMN cells to the alveolus and to generate an inflammatory response to prevent the growth of any invading pathogens. Phagocytosis of bacteria by PMN cells and macrophages can then occur, but this step requires opsonization by immunoglobulins, complement, or surfactant. In addition, effective phagocytosis by macrophages may require activation of these cells by T helper lymphocytes. Thus, all the components of lower respiratory tract defenses can be integrated to deal with large inocula of bacteria or organisms of intrinsic virulence that reach them. When this inflammatory response has been studied in patients with unilateral pneumonia, the response has generally been contained at the site of infection and has not "spilled over" to the uninvolved lung or to the serum. This type of contained response explains why most patients with pneumonia have a focal process and only rarely develop bilateral inflammation in the form of ARDS.

An understanding of the normal host defense system will allow the clinician to understand why pneumonia results in specific patient settings. In addition, with an understanding of any specific patient's immune function, a likely guess about the responsible pathogen is possible. Thus, if a previously healthy patient develops pneumonia, it will usually be with a pathogen of intrinsic virulence such as pneumococcus, *Legionella* spp, or *M. pneumoniae*. Patients with certain specific host impairments may become infected by *H. influenzae*, *S. aureus*, TB, or gram-negative bacteria.

Certain organisms are known to predominate in specific clinical settings, and these associations should always be considered when such a patient is encountered (see Table 15-4). For example, alcoholics may develop pneumonia with *K. pneumoniae*; those with chronic bronchitis can be infected with *H. influenzae* or *M. catarrhalis*; cystic fibrosis patients may be infected by *S. aureus* or *P. aeruginosa*; cardiac patients may develop pneumococcal infection; splenectomized patients become infected by encapsulated bacteria; the elderly have enteric gram-negative bacteria causing pneumonia in 20% to 40% of all cases, and infection with *H. influenzae* and anaerobes is also possible (70); postinfluenza patients may develop infection with *S. aureus*, *H. influenzae*, or pneumococcus; leukemics have gram-negative and fungal pneumonias; and mechanically ventilated and tracheostomized patients often have gram-negative pneumonias, particularly with *P. aeruginosa*, and if a gram-positive organism is present, it is usually MRSA. Similarly, if helper T lymphocyte function is impaired, as is the case with AIDS, then macrophage activation will be abnormal, and organisms usually contained by cell-mediated immunity will predominate.

When a patient is evaluated for the risk of developing pneumonia, several factors should be considered. First, the patient's primary medical status should be evaluated so that diseases associated with an increased risk of infection can be identified. These might include cardiac disease, advanced age, ARDS, or diabetes. Other associated illnesses, in addition to the primary disease, should also be recognized. For example, hypotension, cancer, stroke, head injury, sepsis, hypophosphatemia, hypoxia, and ethanol intake have associated specific

TABLE 15-4. Pathogens Causing Pneumonia in Specific Settings

Setting	Pathogens
Cardiac disease	Pneumococcus, gram-negative bacilli
Alcoholism	*Klebsiella pneumoniae, Haemophilus influenzae, Mycobacterium tuberculosis*, anaerobes, pneumococcus (including drug-resistant organisms)
Cystic fibrosis	*Pseudomonas aeruginosa, Staphylococcus aureus*
Postinfluenza	Pneumococcus, *H. influenzae, S. aureus*, enteric gram-negatives
Mechanical ventilation, acute respiratory distress syndrome (ARDS)	*P. aeruginosa*, other enteric gram-negative bacilli
Chronic obstructive pulmonary disease (COPD)	*H. influenzae*, pneumococcus, *Moraxella catarrhalis*
Splenic dysfunction	Pneumococcus, *H. influenzae*
Neutropenia and steroid use	*Aspergillus*, gram-negative bacilli (esp. *P. aeruginosa*)
High-risk aspiration	anaerobes, enteric gram-negatives
Acquired immunodeficiency syndrome (AIDS)	Pneumococcus, *Pneumocystis carinii*, tuberculosis, *P. aeruginosa*, *Mycobacterium avium*, cytomegalovirus, *Salmonella*, *Cryptococcus*
Rabbit exposure	*Francisella tularensis*
Exposure to farm animals	*Coxiella burnetti* (Q fever)
Structural lung disease	*P. aeruginosa, Pseudomonas cepacia, S. aureus*
Rat droppings	Hantavirus
Bioterrorism	Anthrax, *Franisella tularensis*, plague
Travel to Asia	severe acute respiratory syndrome (SARS), tuberculosis, meliodosis
Nursing home, residence	*Streptococcus pneumoniae*, gram negatives, *H. influenzae, S. aureus*, tuberculosis, anaerobes

impairments in lower-airway defenses. Another factor that may increase the risk of lung infection—and one that is frequently overlooked—is the therapeutic interventions that patients undergo while receiving medical care. Many medications can interfere with the lung's handling of bacteria, including oxygen, aspirin, digoxin, calcium channel blockers, morphine, cimetidine, antacids, corticosteroids, antibiotics, and β-blockers. The last factor to be considered is the patient's nutritional status because malnutrition can interfere with cell-mediated and humoral immunity in the lung, in addition to increasing epithelial cell receptivity to bacteria. Table 15-5 shows how many of these factors can interact with the respiratory host defenses in one population of patients—the elderly—thereby partially explaining the increased incidence of pneumonia in these individuals.

Community-Acquired Pneumonia: General Clinical Features

The distinction between "typical" and "atypical" presentations of pneumonia has been referred to above. Although some clinicians have used this distinction in patterns of clinical presentation to predict the etiology of CAP, this approach does not

TABLE 15-5.   Host Defenses and Aging Features

Defense Mechanism	Impairments Related to Age, Comorbid Illness, or Drug Therapy
UPPER AIRWAY	
Nasal filtration	Bypassed by endotracheal tube, tracheostomy
Oropharyngeal bacterial adherence	Severe coexisting illness, increased oral proteases, xerostomia with a fall in intraoral pH, malnutrition, viral illness, smoking
Bacterial interference	Prior antibiotic therapy, altered colonization patterns resulting from aging
EPIGLOTTIS	Sedating medications, stroke, feeding tube, endotracheal tube, carcinoma of the upper airway
LOWER AIRWAY	
Cough	Sedating medications, stroke, neuromuscular illness, malnutrition, chronic bronchitis
Mucociliary transport	Aging, cigarette smoking, chronic bronchitis, bronchiectasis, dehydration, vitamin A deficiency, decreased airway pH, airway inflammatory proteases, morphine, atropine, hyperoxia
Immunoglobulins: IgG, IgA, IgM	Malnutrition, aging, vitamin deficiency (B₆ and folate), zinc deficiency, malignancy
Complement	Normal with aging
Polymorphonuclear cells	Aging, hypothermia, cytotoxic therapy, diabetes, corticosteroids, ethanol, salicylates, malnutrition, hypophosphatemia
T cells	Aging, zinc deficiency
Tracheal cell adherence	Malnutrition, inflammatory proteases, viral illness, endotracheal intubation, ? zinc excess
Alveolar macrophages	Viral illness, malnutrition, ? aging, corticosteroids, cytotoxic therapy, salicylates

From Niederman MS, Fein AM. Pneumonia in the elderly. *Clin Geriatr Med* 1986;2:247, with permission.

work very well in recent studies (22,71). There are two reasons why clinical features correlate poorly with the etiology of pneumonia. First, certain pathogens, such as *Legionella* and *Chlamydia pneumoniae*, can have a clinical picture that overlaps both syndromes, with high fever, chills, prodromal symptoms, dry cough, leukocytosis, and relative bradycardia (71,72). Secondly, if the host is not normal because of comorbid illness or advanced age, then the clinical features may be altered, even in the presence of a bacterial pathogen that should lead to the "typical"pneumonia syndrome. Thus, in one study, clinical features were only 40% accurate in determining the difference between pneumococcal, mycoplasmal, and other pneumonic infections (22). Similarly, in a study of 196 patients with CAP, multilobar disease, pleural effusion, lung collapse, and cavitation were so common in patients with pneumococcal pneumonia, Legionnaires' disease, mycoplasma, and psittacosis that the radiograph could not be used to determine etiology (73). Because it is usually impossible to recognize a specific pathogen

by its clinical presentation or radiographic picture, a judicious use of epidemiology, laboratory data, and clinical findings is needed in approaching therapy, and, often, more than one potential pathogen is targeted for therapy. The American Thoracic Society (ATS) has presented an approach to initial empiric therapy of CAP that is based on an assessment of disease severity, place of therapy, and the presence of cardiopulmonary disease and/or "modifying factors" that put patients at risk for infection with such specific pathogens as drug-resistant *S. pneumoniae* (pneumococcus) (DRSP) or enteric gram negatives (71). In developing this approach, the use of clinical features to predict microbial pathogens was rejected as being unhelpful. Modifying factors that put patients at risk for infection with DRSP include: age above 65 years, β-lactam therapy within the past 3 months, alcoholism, immune suppression, comorbid medical illness, and exposure to a child in day care. Risks for gram negatives include: nursing home residence, underlying cardiopulmonary disease, multiple medical comorbidities, and recent antibiotic therapy. Risks for one specific gram negative, *P. aeruginosa*, include structural lung disease (bronchiectasis), corticosteroid therapy, broad-spectrum antibiotics for more than 7 days within the previous month, and malnutrition.

As mentioned, many patient populations present with bacterial pneumonia with unusual patterns and clinical features. When the elderly develop bacterial pneumonia, fever, rigors, and pleuritic chest pain are less common than in younger patients. In the elderly, pneumonia may present with such nonspecific findings as confusion, lethargy, worsening of an underlying chronic medical condition, or raised respiratory rate. Certain medications such as aspirin and corticosteroids can mask the expected features of pneumonia. Coexisting illness such as COPD can interfere with expected physical findings, whereas congestive cardiac failure may be associated with lung infiltrates that mimic or hide pneumonia (70).

Pneumonia can be caused by a wide variety of pathogens, but the responsible agent will vary depending on the status of the patients underlying host defenses, which is often reflected in the place of patient residence. Community-acquired infection has a specific etiologic agent identified in approximately 50% of cases. The exact incidence of viral pneumonia in the community setting is unclear, but these agents may account for up to one-third of all such pneumonias. The most common bacterial pathogen for CAP is pneumococcus for all types of patients. The bacteriology varies for different populations, and one approach is to define likely pathogens on the basis of the severity of initial presentation, the need for hospitalization (and site of care), and the presence of cardiopulmonary disease and/or "modifying factors," as shown in Figure 15-3 (71). In patients with mild to moderate pneumonia treated out of the hospital, pathogens vary depending on the presence of cardiopulmonary disease and/or modifying factors. For those without these risks, after pneumococcus, the most common pathogens are *M. pneumoniae*, respiratory viruses, *C. pneumoniae*, *H. influenzae*, and *Legionella* spp. Unusual pathogens should be suspected in this setting if the patient has an unusual travel or exposure history. In these circumstances, pneumonia may be a presentation of tularemia (in hunters), plague (from exposure to small animals or bioterrorism), anthrax (in wool sorters, tanners, and with bioterrorism), cryptococcosis (from pigeon

ATS 2001: Algorithm for CAP

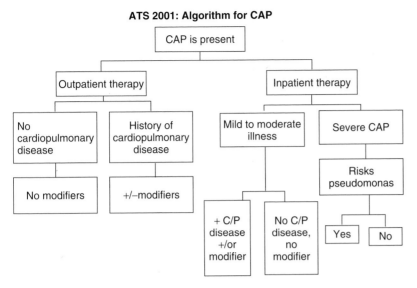

FIGURE 15-3. Shown here is an approach to stratifying patients with community-acquired pneumonia (CAP). Patients fall into one of four groups, each with its own likely pathogens and suggested therapy. The groups are defined by the need for hospitalization, severity of illness on initial presentation, and the presence of cardiopulmonary disease and/or "modifying factors." (From Niederman MS, Mandell LA, Anzueto A, et al. Guidelines for the management of adults with community-acquired lower respiratory tract infections: Diagnosis, assessment of severity, antimicrobial therapy and prevention. *Am J Respir Crit Care Med* 2001;163: 1730–1754, with permission.)

droppings), histoplasmosis (from river valleys or bat droppings), coccidioidomycosis (from travel to the southwestern United States), psittacosis (from infected birds), or parasitic infestation (from foreign travel to the tropics). If the patient has mild to moderate pneumonia but cardiopulmonary disease and/or modifying factors, then the most common pathogens are pneumococcus, respiratory viruses, *H. influenzae*, aerobic gram-negative bacilli, *S. aureus*, and other miscellaneous organisms.

When the patient is hospitalized, a distinction is made between pneumonia treated out of the ICU and severe pneumonia requiring admission to the ICU. As mentioned below, the bacteriology of severe CAP is predictable but subtly different from that for CAP in general. Criteria for severe pneumonia include the presence of two of the following three: hypoxemia defined as a PaO_2/FiO_2 ratio <250 mm Hg, bilateral or multilobar infiltrates, or systolic blood pressure under 90 mm Hg; or one of the following two: need for mechanical ventilation or septic shock (74). The mortality rate for severe CAP varies from 25% to 50% or higher, with the greatest death rates being found in populations that have the most patients treated with mechanical ventilation (71,75). Other prognostic factors indicating a poor outcome for hospitalized patients with CAP include advanced age (at least 65 years), hypotension, a respiratory rate of at least 30 per minute, the presence of comorbidity, hospitalization within the previous year, altered mental status on presentation, fever above 101°F, blood urea nitrogen (BUN) above 19.6 mg per dL, and extrapulmonary seeding of infection (71,76).

If the patient is hospitalized but not in the ICU, then the likely pathogens are pneumococcus, *H. influenzae*, polymicrobial infection (including anaerobes), *Legionella* spp, *S. aureus*, *C. pneumoniae*, viruses, and other miscellaneous pathogens. In patients with severe CAP requiring admission to the ICU, the most likely pathogens are pneumococcus, *Legionella* spp, and enteric gram-negative bacteria (including *P. aeruginosa*). It is important to consider *Legionella* as a likely pathogen in patients with severe CAP because many studies of this illness document the importance of this pathogen (75,77). In one series,

the frequency of "atypical" pathogens, over the course of time, was relatively constant, but the identity varied between *Legionella*, *Mycoplasma*, and *Chlamydia* spp. Other pathogens that can cause severe CAP include *M. pneumoniae*, respiratory viruses, and *H. influenzae*.

In the past several years, the role of atypical pathogens in all patients with CAP has been redefined. Many studies have shown that these organisms are common, being present in up to 40% of all CAP patients, often as copathogens along with bacterial organisms (78). When mixed infection is present, it can be found in patients of all ages and may lead to a more complex course than when monomicrobial infection is present. If coinfection is indeed common, routine therapy of atypical pathogens may be necessary in most patients because outcomes (mortality) have been improved with this approach.

Community-acquired Pneumonia: Specific Illnesses

STREPTOCOCCUS PNEUMONIAE. *S. pneumoniae* a gram-positive, lancet-shaped diplococcus is the most common cause of CAP and can be found in all age groups and all clinical settings. There are 84 different serotypes, each with a distinct antigenic polysaccharide capsule, but 85% to 90% of all infections are caused by 1 of 23 serotypes, which are now included in a vaccine. Type 3 pneumococcus serotype is particularly virulent and is also one of the most commonly encountered serotypes (79). Infection is most common in winter and early spring, which may relate to the finding that up to 70% of patients have a preceding viral illness (80). Spread of infection is from person to person, but the organism commonly colonizes the oropharynx of patients before it leads to pneumonia. Carriage rates vary from 5% in adults without children to 60% in infants, and rates also vary throughout the year. Pneumonia develops when colonizing organisms are aspirated into a lung that is unable to contain the aspirated inoculum. Infection is more common in the elderly; in those with asplenia, multiple myeloma, congestive heart failure, alcoholism; after influenza; and in patients with chronic lung disease. In patients with

AIDS, pneumococcal pneumonia with bacteremia is more common than in healthy populations of the same age.

Clinically, patients with an intact immune response present with the "typical" pneumonia syndrome of abrupt onset of illness accompanied by a toxic appearance, pleuritic chest pain, and rusty-colored sputum. In the past, a lobar pattern was most common, and patients with this finding had consolidation by physical examination with bronchial breath sounds, egophony, dullness to percussion, and increased tactile fremitus (see Fig. 15-4). More recently, it has been recognized that pneumococcus can cause bronchopneumonia, and in some series, this is the most common pattern (81). Bacteremia can occur in 15% to 25% of all patients and will increase the mortality rate of the illness and may delay recovery (70,79). In patients with HIV infection, the incidence of bacteremia may exceed 50% but is not associated with an enhanced mortality rate. Laboratory data are not specific but will usually show leukocytosis and slight liver function abnormalities. With overwhelming infection, neutropenia may occur. In the absence of a positive blood culture, diagnosis is often empiric and epidemiologic based on finding appropriate clinical features in a compatible setting. In many patients without a specific etiologic diagnosis of CAP, after usual diagnostic testing, pneumococcus has been identified using more sophisticated molecular diagnostic testing of respiratory tract samples. Sputum gram stain may show pneumococci, but this finding can be absent in 50% of infected patients, whereas it may be present when there is oropharyngeal colonization without infection or in patients who have pneumococcus as part of a mixed infection as the etiology of CAP. The role of sputum gram stain in guiding the diagnosis and therapy of patients with CAP remains controversial. Urinary antigen testing for pneumococcus has a high sensitivity and specificity for diagnosing pneumococcal pneumonia, especially if concentrated urine is examined, but false-positive tests can occur in patients who have had recent pneumococcal infection.

Recently, penicillin and multi-drug–resistant pneumococci have been identified with an ever-increasing frequency. Currently, at least 40% of all pneumococci may be penicillin resistant, but most of this is "intermediate" and not high-level resistance. The clinical impact of resistance is uncertain because the outcome of patients with resistant organisms is often the same as the outcome of patients who have sensitive organisms (71,82,83). One of the reasons why most studies have not shown an impact of *in vitro* resistance on mortality may be that the clinically relevant degree of resistance is quite high, and, fortunately, not commonly present in most organisms (83). However, high-level resistance to certain agents, such as cefuroxime, may be associated with a worse outcome than when resistance to this antibiotic is absent (71). Penicillin resistance may coexist with resistance to other agents including the macrolides, trimethoprim–sulfamethoxazole, and, possibly, even the quinolones. With current definitions of resistance, patients with DRSP can be successfully treated with high doses of penicillins, carbapenems, or with selected cephalosporins such as cefotaxime or ceftriaxone. The new antipneumococcal quinolones (gatifloxacin, gemifloxacin, levofloxacin, or moxifloxacin) are also highly active against these resistant organisms. If meningeal involvement with DRSP is suspected or proven, then high-dose ceftriaxone or vancomycin should be used. Although the incidence of resistance is rising, empiric therapy should be focused on these organisms mainly in patients with clinical risk factors for resistance, which include age above 65 years or less than 5 years, β-lactam therapy within the past 3 months, alcoholism, immune suppression, exposure to a child in day care, or multiple medical comorbidities (71).

With effective therapy, clinical improvement follows in 24 to 48 hours, but fever may persist for 5 to 7 days. Most patients are treated for 5 to 7 days, but patients with AIDS may need to be treated longer. Radiographic improvement may lag behind clinical response, and only about 70% of patients have a normal radiograph after 2 months (84). Mortality is age-related, with 4% below the age of 40 dying, and 26% dying if they are between ages 40 and 69 (70). More recent data have questioned these age-related mortality statistics and have suggested that mortality could well be a function of coexisting diseases seen in the aged rather than the aging process itself. Diseases that can increase the mortality of pneumococcal infection are cardiac illness, pulmonary disease, cirrhosis, malignancy, and asplenia. Mortality is also greater with bacteremia, multilobar involvement, and extrapulmonary spread of infection. In patients with advanced illness, antibiotic therapy may be of no benefit because mortality in the first 36 hours of illness is unchanged by therapy (85). Extrapulmonary involvement may be seen with meningitis, arthritis, endocarditis, brain abscess, and pericarditis and should be suspected if the patient fails to improve in the expected time period. Although pleural effusion

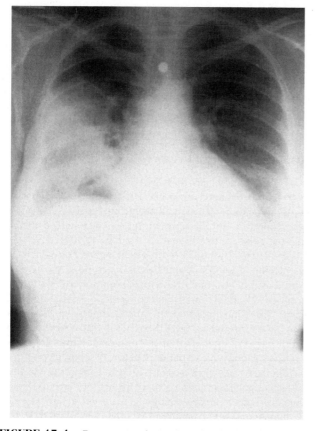

FIGURE 15-4. Pneumococcal pneumonia with lobar consolidation in the right lower lobe and a patchy bronchopneumonia in the left lower lobe.

is common and may be seen in 25% of patients, empyema is less common.

Patients at risk for pneumococcal infection should be considered for prophylaxis with the currently available pneumococcal vaccine (71,85–87). This injection is active against 23 serotypes of pneumococcus that account for 85% to 90% of all cases. At the present time, the vaccine is not being utilized in many of the at-risk population's for a variety of unsound reasons. There are no major side effects of immunization, and although the efficacy of vaccination has been questioned, the current consensus is that the vaccine is effective, particularly if the patient is immunocompetent and if the vaccine is given before the patient is ill enough to be unable to have an adequate immune response (87). In patients with an abnormal immune response (the immunocompromised patient), one revaccination after 5 years is recommended. Vaccination is recommended for all patients with CAP, once they are responding to initial therapy, and often prior to discharge from the hospital.

LEGIONELLA PNEUMOPHILA. L. pneumophila is a small, weakly staining, gram-negative bacillus that was first characterized after it led to an epidemic of pneumonia in Philadelphia in 1976 that was known as Legionnaires disease. Since this initial recognition, it has become clear that *L. pneumophila* is not a new bacterium but one that has only recently been recognized. It is one species of *Legionellae*, of which more than 30 species have been identified. *Legionellae* have been isolated since as early as 1943, and retrospective serum analysis has shown that *L. pneumophila* has caused human disease since at least 1965 (88). At present, 12 different serogroups of the species *L. pneumophila* have been described, and these account for 90% of all cases of Legionnaires disease, with serogroup 1 causing the most cases. The other species that commonly causes human illness is *Legionella micdadei.*

Infection by *Legionella* spp can be in an epidemic manner, and in the Philadelphia experience more than 200 individuals were infected, with a mortality of at least 16%. The organism is water borne and can emanate from air conditioning equipment, drinking water, lakes and riverbanks, water faucets, and showerheads. When a water system becomes infected in an institution, endemic outbreaks may occur, as has been the case in some hospitals. In addition to these patterns, *Legionella* infection can be in the form of sporadic cases and may account for 7% to 15% of all cases of CAP (89,90). In some studies, *Legionella* is the most common cause of CAP, a possible artifact of careful testing for this organism. *Legionella* has consistently emerged as a common pathogen in severe CAP.

Infection is caused by inhalation of an infected aerosol generated by a contaminated water source. Person-to-person spread has not been documented, but it is possible that infection can occur via aspiration from a colonized oropharynx or after subclinical aspiration of contaminated water. The incubation period is 2 to 10 days, and disease may occur in normal hosts as some organisms have significant virulence. Other strains are less virulent and infect impaired hosts with risk factors for infection, including renal transplantation, dialysis, malignancy, smoking, chronic lung disease, diabetes, age above 50, male sex, and alcoholism. In hospitalized patients, the most important risk factor for nosocomial *Legionella* pneumonia is the use of corticosteroids, but an environmental source is needed for

this type of nosocomial infection to occur (91). Once the organism is inhaled, it localizes intracellularly to the alveolar macrophage and multiplies, generating an inflammatory response that involves neutrophils, lymphocytes, and antibody. Because cell-mediated immunity is needed to contain infection, the disease can occur in compromised hosts and may relapse if not treated long enough.

Patients with *Legionella* pneumonia commonly have high fever, chills, headache, myalgias, and leukocytosis. Features that can suggest the diagnosis are the presence of pneumonia with preceding diarrhea, along with mental confusion, hyponatremia, relative bradycardia, and liver function abnormalities, but this syndrome is usually not present. Symptoms are rapidly progressive, and the patient may appear to be quite toxic. As mentioned, the presence of severe forms of CAP should automatically prompt consideration of *Legionella* spp. The patient may have purulent sputum, pleuritic chest pain, and dyspnea. The chest radiograph is not specific and may show bronchopneumonia, unilateral or bilateral disease, lobar consolidation, or rounded densities with cavitation. Up to 15% of patients will have pleural effusion, but empyema is uncommon. Proteinuria is common, and some patients develop glomerulonephritis and acute tubular necrosis. Myocarditis and cerebellar dysfunction have been reported as rare complications of *Legionella* pneumonia.

Diagnosis can be made serologically by detecting a serial rise in antibody titer to the organism. Using indirect immunofluorescence on samples collected 6 to 8 weeks apart during and after the illness, a four-fold rise in titer to 1:128 or >1:512 was detected. This method may not be useful clinically because it may take up to 9 weeks to make a diagnosis. When patients with proven infection are studied at the time of initial presentation, a single acute serum titer is usually not diagnostic, but testing for urinary antigen is the most sensitive test, being positive in more than 50% of all patients in this setting (92). The urinary antigen test can detect only *L. pneumophila* serotype 1 but has a high sensitivity and specificity for this organism, which causes more than 80% of clinically evident *Legionella* infections. The organism can also be identified in cultures using special medium such as buffered charcoal–yeast extract. Direct fluorescent antibody staining of sputum or bronchoscopy specimens may lead to the diagnosis by detecting *Legionella* antigen. In most clinical settings, the direct fluorescent antibody technique is available, and all appropriate clinical specimens should be tested using this, although it will not be positive in all cases. A DNA probe for the *Legionella* genome has also become available for use.

Once the diagnosis is made, therapy should be with erythromycin in doses of 500 to 1,000 mg every 6 hours intravenously until fever is absent for 2 days. Then a daily dose of 2 g orally is continued for a total of 2 weeks in immunocompetent patients and for 3 weeks in immunocompromised patients. With severe infection, rifampin should be added in doses of 600 mg every 12 hours. Alternatives to erythromycin are tetracycline and azithromycin. Clarithromycin has been reported to be effective when other agents have failed. Quinolone antibiotics, such as ciprofloxacin, levofloxacin or other newer agents, may also be effective (71,93). With therapy, decline in fever may be slow, and high spikes in temperature may continue for 1 week after starting appropriate therapy. Mortality is less than 5% in normal hosts but may be much higher in compromised hosts (89).

ASPIRATION PNEUMONIA. Pulmonary aspiration pneumonia occurs in specific patient populations who are at risk of having material enter the lung because of impaired consciousness or altered respiratory tract anatomy. Aspiration can be in one of three forms: gastric acid or other toxic fluids may enter the lung and cause a chemical pneumonitis; inert substances such as water or solid particles can reach the lung and can lead to drowning or airway obstruction, respectively; or pathogenic bacteria from the stomach or oropharynx can enter the lung and cause pneumonitis or lung abscess (94). Risk factors for aspiration include uncontrolled seizures, stroke, drug intoxication, shock, acute neurologic illness, tracheoesophageal fistula, esophageal diverticulum or dysmotility, tracheostomy, intestinal obstruction, and nasogastric tube use. When aspiration occurs, it is generally in a dependent lung segment, and in a supine, prone patient this will be the superior segment of the lower lobe or the posterior segment of the upper lobe, with the right side being affected more often than the left because of the relatively straighter takeoff of the right mainstem bronchus.

If gastric contents are aspirated and solid material obstructs the airway, patients may develop cough and atelectasis and, later on, may have secondary bacterial infection distal to the obstruction in the form of lung abscess, bronchiectasis, or even empyema. If gastric acid or other toxic material is aspirated, a chemical pneumonitis results, which may be complicated by secondary infection. Acutely, patients who inhale gastric acid with a pH below 2.4 may have dyspnea, bronchospasm, hypotension, hypoxemia, frothy sputum, and pulmonary edema. When aspiration involves primarily bacteria, acute infectious pneumonitis may follow. This process may be indolent and is characterized by fever and purulent sputum, followed by necrosis and, possibly, lung abscess 1 to 2 weeks later. When aspiration occurs out of the hospital, infection is usually with anaerobes that have colonized the mouth, including *Prevotella* (formerly *Bacteroides*) *melaninogenicus* and *Bacteroides fragilis*, *Fusobacterium* spp, peptococci, and peptostreptococci. Pneumococci and staphylococci may also be aspirated in this setting. Recent studies in elderly patients who have aspiration risks in the setting of pneumonia have documented a high frequency of enteric gram negatives as a cause of pneumonia (95). In the hospital, aspiration is usually with both anaerobes and aerobes, usually *S. aureus* and enteric gram-negative bacilli (96).

When aspiration is witnessed, the major therapy is to suction the airway, provide oxygen, and support the patient. The use of corticosteroids is of no proven value, but a 24-hour course of antibiotic therapy may be of value to kill organisms that were aspirated during an emergent intubation process, especially in patients with impaired levels of consciousness. If an infiltrate is present, it should develop within 24 hours of the aspiration event, in which case antibiotics are indicated. In cases of aspiration out of the hospital, penicillin G (up to 12 million units per day), clindamycin (600 mg every 6 hours), or even a quinolone, can be used. Nosocomial aspiration is best treated with a second- or third-generation cephalosporin or with another agent active against enteric gram negatives, combined with clindamycin. Alternatively, a β-lactam/β-lactamase inhibitor combination can be used alone. Failure to respond to therapy should prompt a search for continued aspiration conditions, airway obstruction by a foreign body or tumor, or lung abscess.

LUNG ABSCESS. Lung abscess is a necrotizing parenchymal lung infection generally caused by aspiration of anaerobic bacteria. When a lung abscess arises in this manner, it is termed a "primary or simple abscess," and it follows the anatomic distribution of aspiration discussed above. The radiograph will show a cavity of at least 2 cm. The cavity may contain an air-fluid level and may be associated with or preceded by a pneumonitis (see Fig. 15-5). The cavities may be multiple and generally average 4 to 5 cm (97). Empyema is often associated with lung abscess. The risk factors and microbiology of lung abscess are similar to those of out-of-hospital aspiration, and lung abscess is itself a complication of aspiration. Patients present with low-grade fever, weight loss, and cough with foul-smelling sputum. When lung abscess arises in the absence of a predisposing condition or in a patient without teeth (which can harbor the growth of anaerobes in the periodontal area), then lung cancer or another bronchial obstruction should be suspected. Even without these findings, many patients present with such an indolent course and with weight loss so that malignancy is part of the differential diagnosis. Therapy is with penicillin G or clindamycin, in the doses stated above, with some data to suggest that the latter is more effective (98). With therapy, the patient may improve within a week, with a decline in fever. However, it may take 1 month for the cavity to close and up to 2 months for the radiograph to clear, and therapy should be continued until the infection has cleared on chest film. Generally, therapy is intravenous until the patient improves and then is oral for 4 to 8 weeks. Complications of lung abscess include empyema, bronchopleural fistula, and brain abscess.

If lung abscess arises unrelated to aspiration, other pathogens besides anaerobes should be considered. Cavitary pneumonias can result from infection with TB, fungi, *S. aureus*, *K. pneumoniae*, *P. aeruginosa*, and group A streptococci. Another clinical situation that may be confused with lung abscess is periemphysematous infection of lung bullae. In this setting, pneumonia develops in a diseased lung with preexisting bullae due to emphysema. As these air sacs become infected, they fill with fluid and simulate a lung abscess. This type of infection can be distinguished from lung abscess if prior radiographs show bullae. In addition, the bullae are thin walled in contrast to the thick and irregular walls of a true lung abscess (see Fig. 15-6).

HAEMOPHILUS INFLUENZAE. *H. influenzae* is a gram-negative coccobacillary rod that can occur in either a typable, encapsulated form or a nontypable, unencapsulated form; either can cause pneumonia. The nontypable organisms are also a common cause of bronchitis and a frequent colonizer in patients with COPD. The encapsulated organism can be one of seven types, but type B accounts for 95% of all invasive infections. Opsonizing IgG antibody is required to phagocytose the encapsulated organisms; this may not be the case for the unencapsulated bacteria. It has been suggested that because encapsulated organisms require a more elaborate host response, they are more virulent than unencapsulated organisms. However, several studies have shown that in adults, particularly those with COPD, infection with unencapsulated bacteria is more common than infection with encapsulated organisms and that opsonizing antibody is needed to control unencapsulated bacteria as well (99). It is probably safe to assume that pneumonia from these bacteria results if there is some impairment

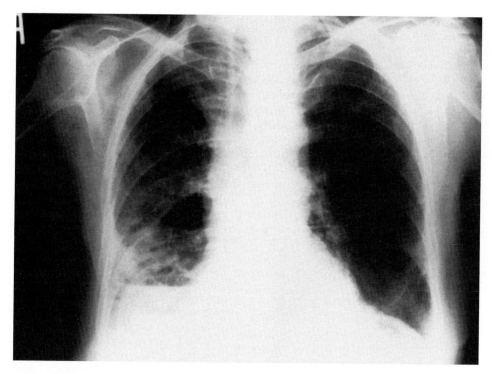

FIGURE 15-5. Aspiration pneumonia in the right lower lobe of an alcoholic with a seizure disorder. A patchy pneumonitis is evident in the right lower lobe, along with two lung abscesses and a pleural effusion due to empyema. A thick-walled cavity is present in the right perihilar area, whereas an air-fluid level—due to an abscess that has ruptured into the pleural space and has caused an empyema—is present in the lower-lung zone.

in host defense, which may include both humoral immunity and local phagocytic dysfunction.

When pneumonia is present, the organism may be bacteremic in some patients, particularly in those with segmental pneumonias as opposed to those with bronchopneumonia. It has been estimated (100) that 15% of cases are segmental but that up to 70% of these patients have bacteremia, whereas only 25% of bronchopneumonia cases are bacteremic. The encapsulated type B organism is more common in patients with segmental pneumonia than in those with bronchopneumonia. Because pneumonia with *H. influenzae* represents a host defense failure, most patients have some underlying illness and 50% may be alcoholics. In patients with COPD, bronchopneumonia is more common than segmental pneumonia.

Patients with segmental pneumonia present with a sudden onset of fever and pleuritic chest pain along with a sore throat. Those with bronchopneumonia will have a slightly lower fever, tachypnea, and constitutional symptoms. Multilobar, patchy bronchopneumonia is the most common radiographic pattern, and pleural reaction is also common, being seen in more than 50% of patients with segmental pneumonia and in approximately 20% of those with bronchopneumonia (see Fig. 15-7). Overall, the adult mortality is 30%, a reflection of the type of impaired host who develops the illness. Complications include empyema, lung abscess, meningitis, arthritis, pericarditis, epiglottitis, and otitis media, particularly in children.

Therapy had traditionally been with ampicillin, but, recently, resistance to this antibiotic has been reported in up to 40% of nontypable *H. influenzae* isolates and in up to 50% of type B organisms as a result of bacterial production of β-lactamase

enzymes. Currently, effective antibiotics are the third-generation cephalosporins, the β-lactam/β-lactamase inhibitor combinations, the newer macrolides (azithromycin is more active than clarithromycin), and the fluoroquinolones. A vaccine against type B organisms is available but its use is limited, and it is best used in young children over the age of 2 to prevent invasive infection such as meningitis (86). Adults who are chronically colonized by *H. influenzae* achieve this condition in spite of the presence of antibodies to this organism and they are often infected with an unencapsulated organism; thus, it is unlikely that the vaccine will have utility in this type of adult population.

MYCOPLASMA PNEUMONIAE. Although *M. pneumoniae* closely resembles a bacterium, it lacks a cell wall and is surrounded by a three-layer membrane. Most of the respiratory infections caused by *M. pneumoniae* are minor and are in the form of upper respiratory tract illness or bronchitis. Although pneumonia occurs in only 3% to 10% of all mycoplasma infections, this organism is still a common cause of pneumonia. In the general population, it may account for 20% of all pneumonia cases and up to 50% in certain closed populations, such as college students (101). The disease is seen year-round, with a slight increase in fall and winter. All age groups are affected, and although it is common in those younger than 20 years, it is also a common cause of CAP, even in older adults, and may be a pathogen in patients with acute exacerbations of chronic bronchitis.

Respiratory infection occurs after the organism is inhaled and then binds via neuraminic acid receptors to the airway

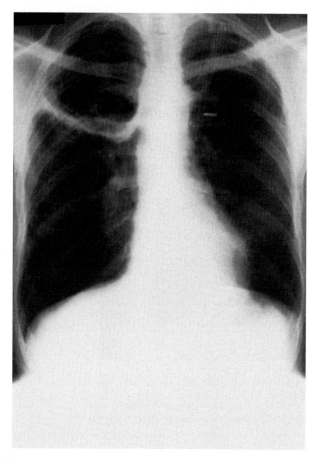

FIGURE 15-6. Periemphysematous bullous infection in a preexisting upper-lobe bulla. Unlike a lung abscess, the location is the entire upper lobe, there is no air-fluid level, and the wall of the bulla are thin, unlike the thick and irregular walls of an abscess.

epithelium. An inflammatory response with neutrophils, lymphocytes, and macrophages then follows, accompanied by the formation of IgM and then IgG antibody. Some of the observed pneumonitis may be mediated by the host response to the organism rather than by direct tissue injury by the mycoplasma. Up to 40% of infected individuals will have circulating immune complexes (102).

When pneumonia is present, it is usually in the form of an "atypical" pneumonia. Patients commonly have a dry cough, fever, chills, headache, and malaise after a 2- to 3-week incubation period. Up to 50% of patients will have upper respiratory tract symptoms, including sore throat and earache. Some of the patients with earache will have hemorrhagic or bullous myringitis. Pleural effusion is quite common, being seen in at least 20% of patients with pneumonia, although it may be small. Chest radiograph will show interstitial infiltrates, which are usually unilateral and in the lower lobe but can be bilateral and multilobar, although the patient usually does not appear as ill as suggested by the radiographic picture. Rarely, patients will have a severe illness, with respiratory failure or a necrotizing pneumonia, but most cases resolve in 7 to 10 days in an uncomplicated manner (75).

Infection with *M. pneumoniae* is often characterized by its extrapulmonary manifestations. These include neurologic illness such as meningoencephalitis, meningitis, transverse myelitis, and cranial nerve palsies, which can be seen in 7% of hospitalized patients (101). The most common extrapulmonary finding is an IgM autoantibody that is directed against the I antigen on the red blood cell and that causes cold agglutination of the erythrocyte. Although up to 75% of patients may have this antibody and a positive Coombs test, clinically significant autoimmune hemolytic anemia is uncommon. Other systemic complications include myocarditis, pericarditis, hepatitis, gastroenteritis, erythema multiforme, arthralgias, pancreatitis,

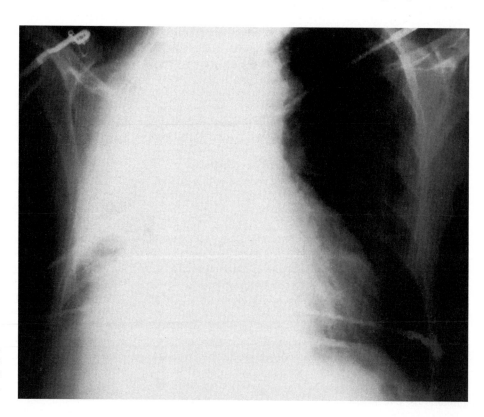

FIGURE 15-7. This patient with advanced chronic bronchitis had bacteremic *Haemophilus influenzae* from this extensive segmental pneumonia. A dense pleural reaction accompanied the pneumonia.

generalized lymphadenopathy, and glomerulonephritis. The extrapulmonary manifestations may follow the respiratory symptoms after as long as 3 weeks.

Diagnosis is made by finding a compatible clinical picture and radiograph in a host with pneumonia and, possibly, some extrapulmonary findings. Confirmation can be made by isolating the organism in culture from respiratory tract secretions. Serologic diagnosis is made by finding a four-fold rise in specific antibody to *M. pneumoniae* by complement-fixation (CF) test, although a single titer of 1:64 is suggestive of infection. If this finding is present with a cold agglutinin titer of 1:64, then the diagnosis is made. Recently, testing for IgM antibody has also been used to determine the infection. Using these methods, some investigators have found that *M. pneumoniae* can be a copathogen along with bacterial agents in patients with CAP (71). Once the diagnosis is made, therapy is given with erythromycin (2 g per day), a newer macrolide (azithromycin or clarithromycin), a quinolone, or tetracycline, which can reduce the duration and severity of the illness. Therapy is usually given for 10 to 14 days.

CHLAMYDIA SPECIES. Psittacosis is a pneumonia due to *C. psittaci*, an agent transmitted by inhaling infected excrement from avian species; the infectious bird does not need to be ill to transmit disease. Patients commonly have headache, high fever, splenomegaly, and dry cough, all showing an insidious onset after a 1- to 2-week incubation period (103). A macular rash similar to that of typhoid fever may also be seen, along with relative bradycardia. Other extrapulmonary involvement may occur, including hepatitis, encephalitis, hemolytic anemia, and renal failure. Diagnosis is based on a compatible contact history and can be confirmed serologically. Treatment is with tetracycline (2 to 3 g per day) for 14 to 21 days.

Recently, another *Chlamydia* spp, *C. pneumoniae*, (also called Chlamydophila pneumoniae) has been found to cause respiratory infection. In some series, this organism is a common cause of CAP in patients of all ages and can also be present as a coinfecting pathogen, potentiating the severity of pneumococcal pneumonia (71). This organism is not transmitted by birds and antibody has been found in 25% to 45% of adults, and the organism can cause up to 12% cases of pneumonia in a student population and 6% cases of pneumonia in an elderly population (104,105). In one report, the organism led to an epidemic of respiratory infection, including pneumonia in patients residing in nursing homes (105). The disease has no specific features but is commonly seen with laryngitis and pharyngitis. Patients have fever, chills, pleuritic chest pain, headache, and cough and can occasionally have respiratory failure. Therapy is with tetracycline (2 g per day), but erythromycin, as well as the newer macrolides and fluoroquinolones, may also be effective; duration of therapy is uncertain.

Although all the agents of atypical pneumonia have not been thoroughly discussed, the clinical features of the most important infections are summarized in Table 15-6.

KLEBSIELLA PNEUMONIAE. K. pneumoniae is an enteric gram-negative rod that can cause both CAP and nosocomial pneumonia. When it arises out of the hospital, it can be an explosive illness with up to 50% mortality, and it generally affects debilitated individuals (106). Known as Friedländer pneumonia, after the physician who first observed this illness,

it affects patients who are predominantly men and usually middle aged or older, with alcoholism being the most common coexisting condition. Other patients at risk are diabetics, the elderly in nursing homes, those with malignancy, and patients with chronic cardiopulmonary or renal disease. The onset is sudden with productive cough, pleuritic chest pain, rigors, and prostration. Sputum may be thick and purulent with blood as well, or it may be thin with a "currant jelly" appearance. Patients appear toxic, with high fever and tachycardia, and examination reveals signs of lobar consolidation. The radiographic finding that is most distinct is consolidation in the upper lobe with a fissure bulging downward because of the dense infiltrate, but this finding is not specific. Lung abscess and bronchopneumonia may also occur. Other complications include pericarditis, meningitis, and empyema. Diagnosis is suspected by finding gram-negative rods in the sputum of a patient with a compatible illness and risk factors. Therapy should be for 2 weeks, and, usually, two drugs that are active against the bacteria are used to avoid emerging resistance and to provide antibacterial synergy. There is some debate about the need for combination therapy, but if third-generation cephalosporins are used alone, resistance may emerge during therapy (107). Effective agents in addition to third-generation cephalosporins include an aminoglycoside, an antipseudomonal penicillin, aztreonam, a carbapenem, or a fluoroquinolone.

STAPHYLOCOCCUS AUREUS. S. aureus may account for up to 5% of CAPs but may also arise in the hospital. In the community setting, it is most common in the elderly and in residents of nursing homes. Pneumonia is also seen after influenza or in patients with chronic lung disease. Hematogenous pneumonia with this organism can be seen in drug addicts with right-sided endocarditis. Clinical features include sudden onset of fever, tachypnea, and cough with purulent sputum. The radiograph may show pleural effusion, cavitary bilateral infiltrates, lung abscess, or pneumatoceles (see Fig. 15-8). Empyema is common, being found in 8 of 31 patients in one series (108). In the series that included both CAP and nosocomial pneumonia, infiltrates were typically multilobar and bilateral, and involved the lower lobes. Pleural effusion was common (48%), but abscess was infrequent (16%). Therapy is with an antistaphylococcal penicillin or a first-generation cephalosporin; for MRSA, vancomycin can be used, but linezolid may be a more effective agent because it penetrates better to respiratory sites of infection. Therapy should be continued for 4 to 6 weeks in complicated infections. Reinfection can occur, and a mortality rate of 32% was reported for all infected patients in one study (108). MRSA is becoming increasingly common, especially in patients with ventilator-associated pneumonia, in the setting of late-onset infection (after day 5 of mechanical ventilation), and in patients with chronic lung disease, those on corticosteroids, and after prior antibiotic therapy. Extrapulmonary complications include endocarditis and meningitis. Although MRSA has been viewed as a nosocomial pathogen, there are now reports of CAP caused by this pathogen in two different populations: patients with recent hospitalization or other risk factors who may have carried the organism to the community from a hospital; and patients who were previously healthy and have acquired a highly virulent toxin-producing strain that is also antibiotic-resistant.

TABLE 15-6. Diagnostic Features of the Atypical Pneumonias

Key Characteristics	Mycoplasma Pneumonia	Legionnaires Disease	Psittacosis	Q Fever	Tularemia	Chlamydia Pneumoniae
SYMPTOMS						
Mental confusion	±	+	−	−	−	−
Prominent headache	−	−	+	+	−	−
Meningismus	−	−	+	−	−	−
Myalgias	+	+	+	+	−	±
Ear pain	±	−	−	−	−	−
Pleuritic pain	±	+	−	−	−	−
Abdominal pain	−	+	−	−	−	−
Diarrhea	±	+	−	−	−	−
SIGNS						
Rash	± (E. multiforme)	± (Pretibial rash)	± (Horder's spots)	−	−	−
Raynaud's phenomenon	±	−	−	−	−	−
Nonexudative pharyngitis	+	−	+	−	±	+[a]
Hemoptysis	−	+	+	−	−	−
Lobar consolidation	±	±	±	±	±	−
Cardiac involvement	± (Myocarditis/ heart block/ pericarditis)	−	± (Myocarditis)	± (Endocarditis)	−	−
Splenomegaly	−	−	+	−	−	−
Relative bradycardia	−	+	+	−	−	−
CHEST FILM INFILTRATE	Patchy	Patchy/ consolidation[b]	Patchy/ consolidation	Perihilar pattern	"Ovoid bodies"	Single "circumscribed" lesions
Bilateral hilar adenopathy	−	−	−	−	+	−
Pleural effusion	± (Small)	±	−	−	+ (Bloody)	±
LABORATORY ABNORMALITIES						
White blood cell count	↑/N	↑	↓	↑/N	↑/N	N[a]
Hyponatremia/hypophosphatemia	−	+	−	−	−	−
Increase in SGOT/SGPT		+	+	+		
Cold agglutinins	+	−	−	−		−
Microscopic hematuria	−	+	−	−		−
DIAGNOSTIC TESTS						
Direct isolation (culture)	±	±	±	−	−	+
Serology (specific)	CF	IFA	CF	CF	TA	CF
Psittacosis CF titers	−	↑	↑	−	−	↑
Legionella IFA titers	−	↑	−	−	↑	−

N, normal; SGOT, serum glutamic-oxaloacetic transaminase; SGPT, serum glutamic-pyruvic transaminase; CF, complement fixation; IFA, indirect fluorescence antibody; TA, tularemia antibody.

[a] Often associated with laryngitis.

[b] Asymmetric, rapidly progressive infiltrates are characteristic. *Legionella micdadei* pneumonia is suggested by a nodular infiltrate.

From Cotton EM, Strampfer MJ, Cunha BA. *Legionella* and mycoplasma pneumonia—a community hospital experience with atypical pneumonias. *Clin Chest Med* 1987;8:443, with permission.

VIRUSES. The exact incidence of viral pneumonia is difficult to estimate because careful serologic testing for viruses is not done in most cases of lung infection. However, viral pneumonia probably accounts for 20% or more of all cases of CAP. The common agents causing lower-respiratory infection may be spread by aerosol or via person-to-person contact through infected secretions (see Table 15-7) and include adenovirus, influenza virus, herpes group viruses (which include cytomegalovirus), parainfluenza virus, and respiratory syncytial virus. Recently, a new viral pneumonia has emerged in Asia called SARS, and this agent has proven to be highly contagious, especially to healthcare workers who have cared for infected patients.

Viral lower-respiratory infections are usually in the tracheobronchial tree or small airways, but primary pneumonia may also occur. The virus first localizes to the respiratory epithelial cell and causes destruction of the cilia and mucosal surface. The resulting loss of mucociliary function may then predispose the patient to a secondary bacterial pneumonia (109). If the infection reaches the alveoli, there may be hemorrhage, edema, and hyaline membrane formation, and the physiology of ARDS may follow. Viral lower–respiratory-tract involvement can be in the form of an airway infection with a normal chest radiograph, a primary viral pneumonia, a bacterial superinfection, or a combined viral and bacterial pneumonia. As was

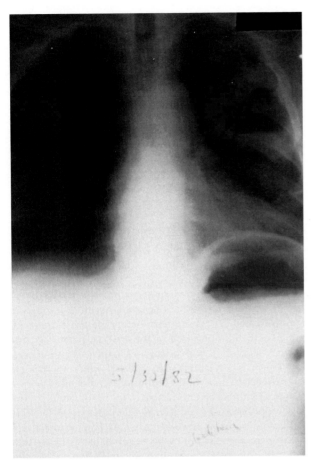

FIGURE 15-8. Multiple necrotizing lung cavities due to *Staphylococcus aureus.*

discussed with influenza, primary viral pneumonia may be a severe illness, with diffuse infiltrates and extensive parenchymal injury along with severe hypoxemia (see Fig. 15-9). This pattern is often seen in those with underlying cardiopulmonary disease, immunosuppression, or pregnancy. However, many patients with primary viral pneumonia get only a mild "atypical" pneumonia with dry cough, fever, and a radiograph that indicates a more severe infection than is actually present. When bacterial superinfection is present, the illness is biphasic, with initial improvement from the primary viral infection, followed by sudden increase in fever along with purulent sputum and lobar consolidation. Another common complication of viral lower-airway infection is bronchial hyperreactivity; asthma and chronic airflow obstruction may occur.

The newly described viral illness SARS can be a severe type of primary viral pneumonia and often leads to respiratory failure. Clinically, after a 2- to 11-day incubation period, SARS patients present with fever, rigors, chills, dry cough, dyspnea, malaise, headache, and, frequently, pneumonia and ARDS. Laboratory data show not only hypoxemia but also elevated liver function tests. In many hospitals, 15% to 20% of patients develop respiratory failure. Respiratory involvement typically begins on day 3 of the hospital stay, but respiratory failure is not until day 8. The mortality rate for ICU–admitted SARS patients has been more than 30% and when patients die, it is generally from multiple-system organ failure and sepsis. There is no specific therapy, but anecdotal reports have suggested a benefit from the use of pulse doses of steroids and from the use of ribavirin.

The major clinical distinctions between the many viral agents that can cause pneumonia involve the type of host that becomes infected and the type of extrapulmonary manifestations that accompany the pneumonia. Immunocompromised hosts (ICH)

TABLE 15-7. Characteristics of Common Respiratory Viruses Causing Lower Respiratory Tract Infection

Agent	Genetic Structure	Mode of Transmission	Epidemiology	Clinical Syndromes
Adenovirus group (41 serotypes)	Linear double-stranded DNA	Aerosol, direct person-to-person contact	Ubiquitous agent, no seasonal prevalence	Epidemic pneumonia in closed populations (e.g., military recruits), disseminated disease in immunosuppressed hosts
Coronavirus	Single-strand RNA	Presumed person-to-person contact	Common in winter and spring, clusters within families	Occasional pneumonia, exacerbation of asthma, bronchitis
Herpes group (CMV, HSV, VZV)	Double-stranded DNA	venereal route, blood products, transplanted organs, aerosol (VZV)	Immunosuppressed host	Tracheobronchitis (HSV), interstitial pneumonitis
Influenza virus (types A, B)	Seven single RNA strands	Small particle aerosol	Peak prevalence in winter and early spring, highest attack rates at extreme ages of life	Tracheobronchitis, pneumonia with or without bacterial superinfection
Parainfluenza	Single-strand RNA	Direct person-to-person spread	Late fall to early winter peaks, severe infection commonest between 6 months and 6 years	Croup (serotypes 1–3), pneumonia and bronchitis (type 1 and 2)
Respiratory syncytial virus	Single-strand RNA	Selfinoculation with fomites	Outbreaks in winter and spring, most serious infection in first 2 years of life	Pneumonia and bronchitis (infants), bronchitis and pneumonia (adults)

DNA, deoxyribonucleic acid; RNA, ribonucleic acid; CMV, cytomegalovirus; HSV, herpes-simplex virus; VZV, varicella-zoster virus.
From Rose RM, Pinkston P, O'Donnell C, et al. Viral infections of the lower respiratory tract. *Clin Chest Med* 1987;8:406, with permission.

with AIDS, malignancy, and major organ transplantation are often infected by cytomegalovirus, varicella-zoster, and herpes simplex virus. Children are most affected by respiratory syncytial virus and parainfluenza virus, which can cause both airway and parenchymal lung infections. Children and military recruits develop pneumonia with adenovirus, whereas influenza pneumonia can develop in adults, particularly the debilitated elderly. Extrapulmonary signs may suggest a specific viral agent. Rash may be seen with varicella-zoster, cytomegalovirus, measles, and enterovirus infections (Fig. 15-9). Pharyngitis may accompany infection by adenovirus, influenza, and enterovirus. Hepatitis may be seen with cytomegalovirus and infectious mononucleosis (Epstein–Barr virus).

The diagnosis of viral illness can be clinical or it can be confirmed by specific laboratory methods. Viruses can be isolated with special culture techniques if specimens are properly collected and prepared. Upper-airway swabs, sputum, bronchial washes, rectal swabs, and tissue samples should be placed in viral transport media as early in the patient's illness as possible while viral shedding is still prominent. These samples are then cultured on certain laboratory cell lines, and viral growth may be detected in 5 to 7 days. More recently, the shell vial culture method has allowed for identification of viruses within 1 to 2 days. In this method, a clinical specimen is centrifuged onto a tissue culture monolayer and then stained with virus-specific antibodies (110). Viral illness can also be rapidly diagnosed using immunofluorescence or ELISA assays to test patient samples for viral antigens. Immunofluorescent tests are available for influenza, parainfluenza, respiratory syncytial virus, adenovirus, measles, rubella, coronavirus, and herpesvirus. ELISA assays are also available for most of these agents (110). Serology can be used retrospectively to diagnose a suspected viral infection, but this technique may be a "shot in the dark" if specific viruses are not suspected and sought directly. A new technique that shows promise is the use of genetic probes to detect specific viral DNA or RNA. Such methodology is now available for cytomegalovirus, varicella-zoster virus, herpes simplex, and adenovirus.

With the current interest and understanding of viral infections, some specific therapy with antiviral agents has become available. Pneumonia from herpes simplex and varicella-zoster can be treated with acyclovir. Influenza A can be treated or prevented using amantadine 200 mg orally per day or rimantadine or the newer neuraminidase inhibitors oseltamivir and zanamivir (also active against influenza B). Ribavirin aerosol has been used to treat respiratory syncytial virus, SARS, and influenza B. Patients with cytomegalovirus infection have been successfully treated by the acyclovir analog, ganciclovir.

Hospital-Acquired Pneumonia

The epidemiology and pathogenesis of nosocomial pneumonia have been discussed above. When pneumonia arises in the hospitalized or institutionalized patient, the bacteriology shifts, and gram-negative organisms are responsible for most cases. In addition to the enteric gram-negative bacilli, other common causes of nosocomial pneumonia are *S. aureus* (including methicillin-resistant organisms), *H. influenzae*, pneumococcus, aspiration with anaerobes, *Legionella* spp in certain places (such as a hospital with infected water sources), and viruses in certain hosts or in settings of an epidemic among the staff (69). It should be emphasized that nosocomial pneumonia is an opportunistic occurrence that preys upon the sickest patients in a hospital. In one study, nosocomial infections in general were seen in 2% of all hospitalized patients but in nearly one fourth of those with an underlying fatal illness (111). In patients with ARDS, as many as 55% have secondary pneumonia, and this complication may adversely affect survival (11,12,112) (see Fig. 15-10). The responsible pathogen is usually an enteric gram-negative bacillus, particularly *P. aeruginosa* in the most ill individuals; it is the impairment of

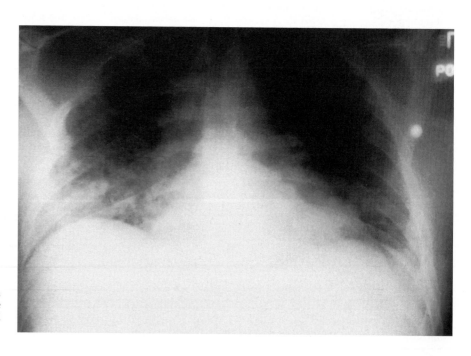

FIGURE 15-9.   Primary viral pneumonia due to varicella-zoster in a 35-year-old male with an extensive vesicular rash and a clinical syndrome of chickenpox.

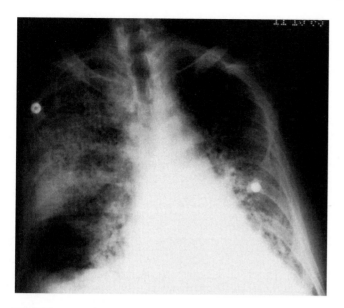

FIGURE 15-10. Acute respiratory distress syndrome (ARDS) with bilateral diffuse infiltrates and a complicating nosocomial pneumonia in the right upper lobe. Distinguishing pneumonia from the primary lung process is very difficult, although asymmetry can be a clue, as it was in this case.

the host response to bacterial challenge and not usually the intrinsic virulence of the organism that leads to this infection. Much of the current research in this field is focused on prevention, and this approach arises out of a thorough understanding of modifiable risk factors.

There is still considerable difficulty in determining whether nosocomial pneumonia is present because many noninfectious illnesses may present a similar clinical picture, particularly in the critically ill patient. An accepted definition of this infection is onset after 48 to 72 hours of hospitalization, with development of a new or progressive lung infiltrate on radiograph plus two of the following: fever, leukocytosis, and purulent tracheobronchial secretions (113,114). This diagnosis may be particularly difficult to make in the mechanically ventilated patient with coexisting ARDS or congestive heart failure because either illness is associated with lung infiltrates, and the other clinical features of infection may be the result of tracheobronchitis and not pneumonia. Conversely, the elderly and the immunocompromised patient may have pneumonia in the absence of clear-cut signs and symptoms of infection because of the absence of adequate inflammation. In these patients, fever and purulent sputum may not be present.

Risk factors for nosocomial pneumonia can be categorized as being one of four types: acute illness (such as ARDS, sepsis, and hemorrhagic shock) with its attendant alterations in a variety of lower-airway defense mechanisms; coexisting illnesses such as diabetes, smoking, chronic cardiac or pulmonary disease, recent intra-abdominal surgery, advanced age, shock, intra-abdominal infection, uremia, and other systemic illnesses; therapeutic interventions; and impaired nutritional status (112). The area of therapeutic interventions that predispose to pneumonia is particularly interesting because an appreciation of these factors will prompt the physician to minimize therapies that increase the chance of developing infection.

Such therapies include antacids, possibly H_2-blocking drugs, high oxygen concentrations, sedating drugs, corticosteroids, use of nasogastric tube, broad-spectrum antibiotics, and endotracheal intubation (112).

The diagnosis of nosocomial pneumonia is hampered by the problems cited above. It is common practice to both underdiagnose and overdiagnose this illness in certain populations. For example, in patients with ARDS, one-third of all autopsy-proven cases of pneumonia had been unrecognized, whereas one-fifth of uninfected patients were treated for pneumonia (115). It is likely that this degree of misdiagnosis is common in other settings because of the imprecision of the clinical diagnosis of this illness. Some studies have reported that only one of three mechanically ventilated patients with a clinical diagnosis of pneumonia had microbiologic confirmation of the diagnosis (116). Although this estimate may be overly pessimistic, it is likely that pneumonia is overdiagnosed in mechanically ventilated patients. Many hospitalized patients are colonized by potential pathogens, and, thus, their recovery from the lower airway does not always represent invasive infection. However, it is unlikely that if pneumonia is present, the organism responsible would not be found in the culture of a tracheal aspirate. Thus, in the ventilated patient, a sputum (tracheal aspirate) culture is sensitive but not specific for the etiologic organisms of pneumonia.

In an effort to improve the accuracy of diagnosing nosocomial pneumonia, several invasive techniques have been developed (116). With these methods, lower-respiratory secretions are sampled, either bronchoscopically or via endotracheal suction, and the recovered material is cultured quantitatively. The bacteriologic results are then used to determine whether pneumonia is present on the basis of how many organisms are recovered. Invasive methods have involved the use of special "protected" brushes or bronchoalveolar lavage (BAL) for the recovery of secretions for culture. Debate continues about the accuracy and clinical utility of invasive methods (116). Concern about invasive methods centers around the potential arbitrariness of thresholds selected to separate pneumonia from nonpneumonia. In addition, there are concerns about the reproducibility of the methods, the potential for these techniques to overlook early infection, and the limited value of the methods if the patient is on antibiotics at the time of testing. Studies of ventilator-associated pneumonia have shown that the major determinant of outcome is the timeliness and accuracy of initial therapy, and unless invasive methods add to the accuracy of initial empiric therapy, it is unlikely that they can affect outcome (117).

Therapy is with antimicrobial agents directed at the likely pathogens, which fall into a "core" group of bacteria including *Klebsiella* spp, *Enterobacter* spp, *E. coli*, *Proteus* spp, *Serratia marcescens*, *S. pneumoniae*, *H. influenzae*, and *S. aureus* (113,114). Some patients with nosocomial pneumonia have infection with a polymicrobial flora, and up to 40% of nosocomial pneumonia in mechanically ventilated patients is polymicrobial (114). Patients with certain comorbidities or therapies can be at risk for other organisms in addition to the core bacteria. *S. aureus* (including the MRSA form) is more likely in patients who are in coma as well as in those with head injury, renal failure, and recent influenza. MRSA is a particular concern in patients with pneumonia of late onset (after day 5 of mechanical ventilation) and in those on corticosteroid therapy or after a recent course of antibiotics. *Legionella* spp are more likely in patients receiving corticosteroids or cytotoxic chemotherapy who are in a hospital with Nosocomial Legionellosis, and *Aspergillus* spp are more likely if patients have received antibiotics or corticosteroids (118). Patients with recent thoracoabdominal surgery or witnessed aspiration are at risk for anaerobic organisms. *P. aeruginosa* is a concern in patients who have severe nosocomial pneumonia and in those who develop pneumonia in the setting of prolonged mechanical ventilation, prior broad-spectrum antibiotics, corticosteroid use, malnutrition, or chronic structural lung disease (such as bronchiectasis). In any patient who develops nosocomial pneumonia after at least 5 to 7 days in the hospital, at a time that they are receiving antibiotics, the risk that the infection is with a multi-drug–resistant gram-positive or gram-negative pathogen is at least 60%.

Therapy should be directed at the core bacteria for all patients, with modifications if specific other organisms are suspected or documented. The core organisms can be treated with a second-generation cephalosporin, a nonpseudomonal third-generation cephalosporin, a β-lactam/β-lactamase inhibitor combination, ertapenem, or a fluoroquinolone (levofloxacin or moxifloxacin). If MRSA is suspected and if the Gram stain of a tracheal aspirate shows gram-positive organisms, vancomycin or linezolid should be added. If *P. aeruginosa* is suspected, dual antipseudomonal therapy should be initiated because monotherapy of infection by this organism is often complicated by the emergence of resistance during therapy. The antipseudomonal antibiotics include the antipseudomonal penicillins (piperacillin, azlocillin, and mezlocillin), certain third-generation cephalosporins (ceftazidime), the fourth-generation cephalosporin cefepime, aztreonam, imipenem/cilastatin, meropenem, piperacillin/tazobactam, ticarcillin/clavulanic acid, ciprofloxacin, high-dose levofloxacin (750 mg daily), and the aminoglycosides.

PSEUDOMONAS AERUGINOSA. P. aeruginosa is an aerobic gram-negative bacillus that is the most common cause of nosocomial pneumonia, accounting for up to 15% of all cases and colonizes the airway of up to 40% of all mechanically ventilated patients (28). The bacteria reach the lung by aspiration, direct entry via the endotracheal tube, or hematogenously. Patients at maximum risk for infection are those with prior antibiotic therapy, cystic fibrosis, bronchiectasis, burns, corticosteroid therapy, neutropenia, tracheostomy, and prolonged mechanical ventilation. A necrotizing pneumonia can occur, with alveolar septal necrosis, microabscesses, and vascular thrombosis. In postoperative patients, the mortality from pseudomonal pneumonia can be as high as 70% (see Fig. 15-11). The virulence of the organism can be enhanced by production of a slime layer in its surface capsule, endotoxin lipopolysaccharide, pili, exotoxins, and proteases. Exotoxin A, phospholipase, fibrinolysin, and elastase help mediate the lung injury that accompanies infection. One virulence factor that has recently been identified is the Type III secretion system, which is commonly present in patients with severe infection and often involves the production of the Exo U effector protein (119). Patients with this infection may be quite toxic and have confusion, fever, chills, and productive cough, along with relative bradycardia, leukocytosis, and hemorrhagic pleural effusion. Bilateral bronchopneumonia, particularly in the lower lobes; nodular infiltrates; and cavitation may be seen. With bacteremia in the neutropenic patient, a characteristic skin

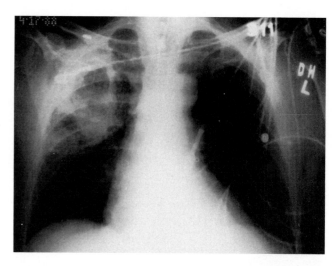

FIGURE 15-11. Nosocomial pneumonia due to *Pseudomonas aeruginosa* in a patient treated chronically with corticosteroids. Necrotization is evident, with a cavity in the right upper lobe.

lesion—ecthyma gangrenosum—may be seen. With bacteremic infection, combination therapy is associated with improved survival compared to monotherapy.

Pneumonia in Special Settings

THE IMMUNOCOMPROMISED HOST. Patients with specific immune impairments related to an underlying primary illness (often malignancy or HIV infection) or those arising as a consequence of medical therapy (most typically chemotherapy or transplant-related immunosuppression) may develop respiratory infections; these individuals are referred to as ICHs (110,120). More recently, AIDS has led to a large and important population of ICH patients who may develop pneumonia. In any ICH, a new infiltrative pulmonary process may be infectious or noninfectious (such as an adverse drug reaction). Pneumonia may be a life-threatening infection in patients with malignancy or immunosuppressive therapy, and efforts at making a specific etiologic diagnosis are often necessary. As shown in Table 15-8, the spectrum of possible infections is broad and will vary with the nature of the immune deficit.

It is often possible to narrow down the infectious possibilities with an understanding of the basic immune impairment (Table 15-8). Thus, patients who have had a splenectomy (including those with sickle cell anemia and autosplenectomy) are usually infected by encapsulated bacteria such as pneumococcus, staphylococci, *H. influenzae*, and *N. meningitides*. Patients with chemotherapy-induced neutropenia may be infected with *P. aeruginosa*, other gram-negative bacteria, and *Aspergillus* spp. Patients with abnormal T-lymphocyte function, such as those with certain lymphomas or AIDS, may be infected by bacteria such as *Listeria monocytogenes*, *Salmonella* spp, *Legionella* spp, *Mycobacterium avium*, or *M. tuberculosis*; fungi such as *Cryptococcus neoformans*, *Histoplasma capsulatum*, or *Coccidioides immitis*; viruses such as cytomegalovirus and herpes simplex; or parasites such as *P. carinii*, *Toxoplasma gondii*, or *Cryptosporidium* spp (121,122). In the HIV–infected patient, the type of infection that develops is directly related to the degree of immune dysfunction, as reflected by the patient's CD4 lymphocyte count. Those

TABLE 15-8. Type of Immunologic Defect and Associated Microorganisms

Defect or Factor	Microorganism			
	Bacteria	*Fungi*	*Viruses*	*Parasites*
Abnormal T lymphocyte function lymphoma, acquired immunodeficiency syndrome (AIDS)	*Listeria monocytogenes* *Nocardia* *Salmonella* (species other than *Salmonella typhi*) *Mycobacteria* *Legionella*	*Cryptococcus neoformans* *Histoplasma capsulatum* *Coccidioides immitis* *Candida* *Trichosporon*	Cytomegalovirus Varicella-zoster Herpes simplex	*Pneumocystis carinii* *Toxoplasma gondii* *Strongyloides stercoralis*
Abnormal B lymphocyte function myeloma, primary and acquired deficiency	*Streptococcus pneumoniae* *Haemophilus influenzae*			
Neutropenia (< 500 neutrophils/mm³): Myeloproliferative disease, lymphoma cytotoxic therapy, alcoholism, sickle cell disease	*Pseudomonas aeruginosa* *Escherichia coli* *Klebsiella* *Serratia* Other gram-negative bacilli	*Aspergillus* *Zygomycetes*		
Splenectomy	*S. pneumoniae* *H. influenzae* *E. coli* *Staphylococcus aureus* *Neisseria meningitis*			
Decreased serum complement	*S. pneumoniae*			
Primary, collagen vascular disease	*H. influenzae* *Neisseria* spp			
Use of corticosteroid therapy equivalent to >20 mg of prednisone daily or cytotoxic therapy (or both)	*S. aureus* *L. monocytogenes* Mycobacteria *P. aeruginosa* *Nocardia* Other gram-negative bacilli	*Aspergillus* *Zygomycetes* *H. capsulatum* *C. neoformans* *C. immitis*	Cytomegalovirus Varicella-zoster Herpes simplex	*P. carinii* *T. gondii* *Strongyloides stercoralis*

From Rosenow EC, Wilson WR, Cockerill FR. Pulmonary disease in the immunocompromised host. *Mayo Clin Proc* 1985;60:612, with permission.

with little immune dysfunction and a CD4 count above 500 per mm³ usually do not develop opportunistic infection, and their predominant pneumonia is bacterial, especially pneumococcal. As the CD4 count falls, the risk of opportunistic infection rises, and patients with a count below 200 per mm³ are at particular risk for such infections as *P. carinii* (122).

Immunocompromised patients should have a careful clinical examination with attention to the skin, gastrointestinal tract, CNS, optic fundi, liver, and lungs. Respiratory symptoms may be minimal, with fever as the only finding, or the patient may have cough and dyspnea. Certain extrapulmonary findings in conjunction with a specific immune defect can suggest an etiologic agent. Skin lesions are common with infections caused by *P. aeruginosa*, *Aspergillus*, *M. tuberculosis*, nocardia, varicella-zoster, herpes simplex, *Cryptococcus*, and *Blastomyces*. The CNS may be affected by *Nocardia*, pneumococcus, *H. influenzae*, *P. aeruginosa*, *M. tuberculosis*, *Legionella*, *Aspergillus*, *Cryptococcus*, *Toxoplasma*, varicella-zoster, and cytomegalovirus. Liver function abnormalities can be seen with cytomegalovirus, *Legionella* and *Nocardia* infection, tuberculosis, histoplasmosis, toxoplasmosis, and *S. aureus* and *P. aeruginosa* infection. Diarrhea can occur with *Legionella*, *Cryptosporidium*, cytomegalovirus, or herpes simplex (120).

Patients who have received organ transplants represent an expanding population of ICH individuals. Infections in this population can be related to hospitalization, the presence of

serious illness, and transplant immunosuppression. Within the first month of transplant, patients get the usual bacterial nosocomial pneumonias. In the period from 1 to 6 months after transplant, infection is related to immunosuppression and can involve cytomegalovirus, *P. carinii*, fungal agents, *L. monocytogenes*, and *Legionella* spp. After 6 months, these same pathogens may still lead to infection in patients who are heavily immunosuppressed, whereas chronic viral infection can develop in those less heavily immunosuppressed (123).

The diagnosis of pneumonia is often made by chest radiography because many patients will have only fever and no respiratory complaints or findings. Focal lung lesions can be seen with bacterial, fungal, and mycobacterial illness. Diffuse infiltrates are seen with *P. carinii*, cytomegalovirus, *Legionella* infection, miliary TB, viral pneumonia, *Aspergillus*, and *Candida*. After a careful clinical examination, samples of sputum and blood should be collected and cultured for bacteria, fungi, *M. tuberculosis*, and viruses. Special stains for *M. tuberculosis*, *Legionella*, and *P. carinii* can be applied to respiratory tract secretions. On the basis of all available data, the patient is usually given empiric antibiotic therapy directed at the most likely pathogens. If improvement occurs, therapy is continued for 2 to 3 weeks. If there is no improvement, an invasive procedure is performed. If the patient has an adequate platelet count, the procedure is either a transbronchial or an open-lung biopsy. With inadequate platelets, BAL without biopsy can be performed or transfusion and biopsy can be undertaken. The decision between bronchoscopic and surgical lung biopsy is made on the basis of how rapidly the patient is deteriorating and on the expected yield and risks of bronchoscopy. In all patients who are immunocompromised, consideration must be given to drug-induced lung disease, malignant involvement of the lung, heart failure, and pulmonary hemorrhage, in addition to the possibility of opportunistic infection (120).

LUNG INFECTION IN THE PATIENT WITH HUMAN IMMUNODEFICIENCY VIRUS INFECTION. Patients with HIV infection have impairment of T-cell function but also have humoral immune dysfunction. Thus, infections with bacteria, fungi, viruses, and parasites have all been seen in this population. The T-cell deficiency can lead to pneumonia caused by *P. carinii*, cytomegalovirus, and *Mycobacterium*, *Legionella*, and *Nocardia* spp (121). The humoral immune dysfunction has been responsible for infections by pneumococcus and *H. influenzae*. As mentioned, the degree of T-lymphocyte depletion will determine which infections the patient is most likely to develop.

The most common pneumonias in immunosuppressed patients with HIV infection are caused by *P. carinii* (now renamed *P. jerovici*) [Pneumocystis carinii pneumonia (PCP)] and pneumococcus. In early HIV infection, with profound immune suppression, PCP is quite common, but after therapy with antiretroviral agents, bacterial pathogens are a more common cause of respiratory infection (122). PCP can exist in a cyst form containing sporozoites or in free form as a trophozoite. The organism can be recognized by methenamine silver stain or by Giemsa stain, usually of lung tissue or BAL fluid. Infection may represent endogenous reactivation of latent infection present in early childhood. Most patients probably acquire *Pneumocystis* from natural sources prior to the onset of AIDS and contain it within the lung. Once AIDS develops, these latent stores of organism may become reactivated, but new primary infection or reinfection is also possible. Most patients present with a subacute course of fever, cough, dyspnea, and weight loss. Chest pain, malaise, fatigue, and night sweats may also occur, and some patients may even be asymptomatic. Chest radiograph usually shows bilateral diffuse interstitial or alveolar infiltrates (see Fig. 15-12). Asymmetric or focal infiltrates may occasionally be seen, as can predominantly upper-lobe disease and solitary pulmonary nodules (124). Less common findings include pneumothorax and pleural effusion. Upper-lobe disease and pneumothorax have been reported to be more likely in patients who have received aerosolized pentamidine for prophylaxis of *P. carinii* infection.

The diagnosis of *Pneumocystis* may be elusive because it may be the first presentation of HIV infection for many individuals. Therefore, all patients with pneumonia, particularly one that is subacute, should be questioned for HIV risk factors, and if these are present, *Pneumocystis* should be considered in the differential diagnosis. Findings that suggest the diagnosis are a compatible radiograph, leukopenia and lymphopenia, elevated serum lactic acid dehydrogenase (LDH), oral candidiasis, and a widened alveolar–arterial oxygen tension gradient. When this infection arises in an AIDS patient, it is usually associated with a more prolonged course, lower fever, less tachypnea, and less hypoxemia than when it occurs in other immunocompromised patients, such as those with

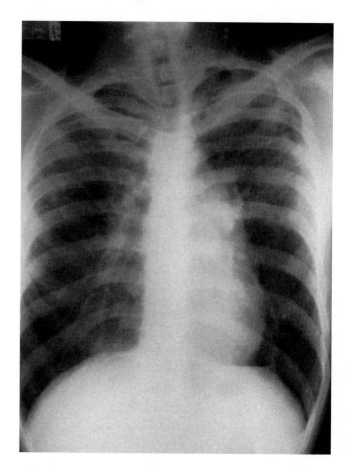

FIGURE 15-12. Diffuse bilateral interstitial infiltrates in a "ground glass" pattern in a 33-year-old intravenous drug abuser. This pattern is typical for *Pneumocystis carinii*.

lymphoma. In AIDS patients, *Pneumocystis* may coexist with cytomegalovirus, toxoplasmosis, or mycobacterial illness. Diagnosis is usually made by BAL or transbronchial biopsy, and in some centers, the induction of sputum for expectoration has led to the diagnosis in up to 50% of all patients.

With therapy, improvement can be slow, and fever may persist for 7 to 10 days, and overall survival from the infection is as high as 90%. Survival is more likely if the clinical manifestations are mild, if the organism burden is not large, and if the infection is the first episode of *P. carinii*. Therapy is begun with intravenous trimethoprim–sulfamethoxazole (15 to 20 mg/kg/day of trimethoprim and 75 to 100 mg/kg/day of sulfamethoxazole), but as many as 50% of all AIDS patients will not be able to tolerate therapy because of adverse reactions. These patients, as well as those who do not respond to trimethoprim–sulfamethoxazole, are then treated with pentamidine (4 mg/kg/day). Other effective agents are trimethoprim/dapsone or, for mild-to-moderate infections, atovaquone (750 mg orally three times daily). Trimetrexate and aerosolized pentamidine have been tried but are generally less effective than standard therapy (125,126). Therapy with most regimens is continued for 21 days. If the illness leads to hypoxemia, with a room-air arterial PO_2 below 70 mm Hg, then corticosteroids should be added to ameliorate the host inflammatory response to the killing of organisms that accompanies therapy. Corticosteroids are given in a dose of prednisone 40 mg twice daily for 5 days, followed by 20 mg twice daily for 5 days, and then 20 mg once daily for 11 days (122). After recovery from pneumonia, patients should receive chemoprophylaxis against recurrent infection, which can be done with oral trimethoprim–sulfamethoxazole or aerosolized pentamidine.

Approach to the Patient with Pneumonia

HISTORY AND PHYSICAL EXAMINATION. Although it may be impossible to identify a specific etiologic agent on clinical grounds alone, a careful evaluation can help guide initial therapy. As shown in Figure 15-3, patients with CAP should have initial empiric therapy selected by assessing three factors: the need for hospitalization, the presence of cardiopulmonary disease and/or "modifying factors," and the severity of the patient's illness (71). In addition, therapeutic selection should be made with a consideration of the presence of smoking history and risk factors for DRSP and gram negatives. On the basis of these assessments, a likely set of pathogens can be identified, and from this list therapeutic choices can follow. In the statement by the ATS, an empiric approach utilizing these determinations was endorsed; other approaches were discussed and found to have only limited value. For example, the use of clinical features to predict microbial etiology, the routine use of sputum Gram stain to guide initial therapy, and the routine use of extensive diagnostic testing were all regarded as not useful (71).

The initial history and physical examination can be used to define how ill the patient is and whether hospitalization will be needed (71). Indicators of more severe pneumonia include a respiratory rate above 30 per minute, diastolic hypotension (under 60 mm Hg), systolic hypotension, oliguria, need for vasopressors, or the presence of respiratory failure. Examination can also reveal other findings indicating a poor prognosis, including altered mental status, high fever, or evidence of extrapulmonary spread of infection. Other historical information may help in determining the probable etiologic pathogen. Thus, patients should be specifically questioned about rash, diarrhea, headache, myalgias, change in mentation, and nausea. Travel history, pets, unusual occupations, and unusual hobbies can also help raise suspicion about certain of the less common infectious agents. If aspiration pneumonia is suspected, the patient should be asked about neurologic disease, esophageal disease, and alcohol use. In addition, an allergic history should be obtained before antimicrobial therapy is prescribed. Another important historical consideration for patients with both CAP and nosocomial pneumonia is a history of recent antibiotic exposure so that empiric therapy can be initiated with a class of antibiotics that is different from what the patient has recently received. It is now known that pneumococcus is more likely to be resistant to a macrolide, quinolone, or β-lactam if one of these agents was used by the patient in the last 3 months (71,72). In addition, *P. aeruginosa* is more likely to be resistant to a quinolone or β-lactam if the patient has received this type of therapy in the past 15 days.

Physical examination can also help identify certain etiologic pathogens and disease complications. Respiratory examination can reveal consolidation, pleural effusion, and bronchopneumonia. Examination of the skin, fundi, liver, heart, and neurologic system can help point to specific etiologic diagnoses. In some patients, the examination may be the first clue to the presence of pneumonia. In the elderly, the most reliable physical finding for pneumonia, because of the abnormal inflammatory response in this population, is elevation of the respiratory rate above 25 per minute (127). Patients should also be evaluated for their ability to cough and expectorate sputum so that individuals with impaired cough can receive physical therapy to aid in tracheobronchial toilet.

When a patient has nosocomial pneumonia, the same assessments of comorbidity and severity of illness should be made, and these factors can be used to guide initial therapy (113,114). However, because many patients develop nosocomial pneumonia owing to impaired host defenses, nosocomial pneumonia is commonly present in the absence of fever or other classic respiratory features of pneumonia.

CHEST RADIOGRAPH. In many patients, the history and examination may suggest pneumonia, but the diagnosis is firmly established by finding a new parenchymal lung infiltrate. The infiltrate should be lobar, interstitial, nodular, cavitary, or bronchopneumonic. Bilaterality, pleural effusion, and multiple lobe involvement should also be noted. Multilobar infiltrates, cavitation, and rapidly expanding infiltrates (more than 50% increase in 48 hours) all predict an increased mortality from CAP (71,75). The location of the infiltrate can also be helpful—apical disease can suggest TB, disease in dependent segments is compatible with aspiration, and consolidation of the upper lobe suggests infection with *K. pneumoniae* or pneumococcus. In some patients, early in the course of infection, focal physical findings of pneumonia may be present but the chest radiograph can be normal. In addition, if a HRCT scan of the chest is obtained, it can demonstrate infiltrates in patients whose chest radiographs are normal, and the extent of computed tomography (CT) abnormalities is often greater than that suggested by the chest radiograph.

The chest film can also be used to follow the patient during therapy of pneumonia to detect any complications. Cavitation and empyema should be suspected and sought if the patient develops a new or persistent fever during treatment. Serial radiographs can also be used to determine the duration of a pneumonia and whether it is resolving appropriately. When radiographs fail to show improvement, this may suggest an unusual or unsuspected organism (*M. tuberculosis* or fungus), an antibiotic-resistant organism, a noninfectious inflammatory disease (such as Wegener's granulomatosis), an impaired host (with a normally slow response to therapy), or an unsuspected malignancy (128). Before a pneumonia is termed *unresolving*, the natural course of radiographic improvement for each infection should be appreciated. Both pneumococcal and *Legionella* infections may have radiographic deterioration in up to 50% of all patients during the initial week of a successful course of therapy. In each of these infections, radiographic clearing will begin in the first 2 weeks of treatment, but the chest film may not be entirely normal for 3 to 6 months.

DIAGNOSTIC METHODS. Many techniques are available to identify the etiologic agent in lower respiratory tract infection, including sputum Gram stain and culture, blood culture, transtracheal aspirate culture, bronchoscopic specimen culture (protected brush samples, BAL, transbronchial biopsy, and bronchial wash), open-lung biopsy, and immunologic methods (129). For most patients, collection of sputum is the primary diagnostic test, along with blood cultures (which are positive in no more than 15% of all cases of pneumonia) and a careful clinical evaluation. In spite of these assessments, many patients require empiric therapy, with modifications being made after the results of diagnostic testing become available. If there is no response or if a specific diagnosis is required (as in certain ICHs), then more invasive tests are done.

Sputum samples are not always the source of reliable data. Culture of expectorated sputum may be of no help because the sample can be contaminated by oral flora as it passes through the oropharynx, the sample may not contain the responsible pathogen, or the sample may contain pathogens that are colonizing the patient but not causing the invasive infection. A sputum sample should be assessed for quality by microscopic examination. If there are fewer than 10 squamous epithelial cells and more than 25 neutrophils per low-power field, the sample is probably a good representation of the lower-airway's secretions. Samples with more than 25 squamous epithelial cells are too contaminated by oral secretions to be useful. The value of sputum Gram stain is widely debated (71). Although Gram staining can show a dominant organism, the sensitivity and specificity vary widely depending on the criteria used to define a sample as "positive." Often, the test is performed by individuals who cannot correlate the findings with the clinical picture or it is performed by clinicians with limited technical expertise. All of these practical considerations limit the utility of a sputum Gram stain. The difficulty with sputum Gram stain data is highlighted by finding false-positive rates of up to 88% and false-negative rates of 50% (129). With pneumococcal pneumonia, up to 50% of the sputum Gram stains will be negative. Given all of these considerations, it is possible to use a Gram stain to broaden empiric therapy to include organisms seen on the stain that were not initially included in therapy, but it is probably not possible to narrow therapy on the basis of findings. Certain organisms whose presence alone is diagnostic of infection can be recovered by staining or by culture of sputum because these organisms never colonize without causing infection; they include *M. tuberculosis*, *P. carinii*, certain fungi, and *L. pneumophila*. A sputum culture should be obtained from any CAP patient who is suspected of having one of these unusual organisms or a drug-resistant organism, and the results should be correlated with the finding of the Gram stain in these situations.

Of the noninvasive techniques, immunologic methods can be applied to many patients with varying degrees of sensitivity and rapidity of receiving diagnostic information. Serologic titers for viral, fungal, *Legionella*, and certain atypical agents can be diagnostic, but there is often a delay in receiving results and, often, convalescent titers must be collected. Thus, this method is of little use in the acute management of patients and is more helpful for epidemiologic studies. Immunologic staining of respiratory secretions for bacterial or viral antigens can occasionally be useful. Urinary antigen testing for pneumococcus may have value for the rapid diagnosis of this infection. Direct fluorescent antibody staining of sputum for *L. pneumophila* can be positive in 70% of cases, and testing for urinary antigen is positive in more than 50% of all patients at the time of initial evaluation (129). Genetic probes for the nucleic acids of *Legionella* and certain viruses are increasingly available.

Of the invasive techniques, open-lung biopsy is generally reserved for the immunocompromised patient or for the patient with an unresolving pneumonia. The most commonly used invasive procedure is bronchoscopy, and it should be used only if its risks are less than the risks of empiric therapy or if empiric therapy is not successful. Transbronchial biopsy allows histologic examination and culture for mycobacteria, *Pneumocystis*, fungi, and viral agents. Bronchoscopy has its greatest utility in the ICH and (as mentioned) is controversial and of uncertain value in patients with suspected nosocomial pneumonia (130,131). In patients with CAP, it should be reserved for the nonresponding patient, and, possibly, for the patient with severe illness. One value of bronchoscopy in both CAP and nosocomial pneumonia is to help streamline and narrow therapy once culture data become available. Thus, it may be necessary to start multiple, broad-spectrum antibiotics as empiric therapy, but bronchoscopic data can be used to focus this initial therapy and simplify the regimen in some patients. BAL has been used in the ICH and has had a diagnostic yield of more than 60% (130). By wedging the bronchoscope and by instilling 210 mL of saline in 30 mL aliquots, the lavage fluid can be returned and collected for culture and staining. This method has detected ICHs with infections caused by *Pneumocystis*, viruses, fungi, and mycobacteria.

Therapy of Pneumonia

Antibiotics represent the mainstay of pneumonia therapy and may be viewed as specific in contrast to many of the other therapies, which are primarily supportive. Antibiotic therapy is organism directed, but if a specific pathogen is not identified, empiric therapy directed at the most likely pathogens is commonly used and will be selected after a careful epidemiologic assessment of the patient. The supportive measures that are not specific to any organism are classified as adjunctive therapy and include supplemental oxygen, intravenous hydration, and measures to promote tracheobronchial toilet such as mucolytic and mucokinetic agents, bronchodilators, and bronchoscopy.

INDICATIONS FOR HOSPITALIZATION OF COMMUNITY-ACQUIRED PNEUMONIA PATIENTS. Individuals who have moderate to severe illness generally require intravenous antibiotics, hydration, and supplemental oxygen (arterial oxygen tension <60 mm Hg on room air), and these therapies require admission to the hospital. In addition, those with serious coexisting illness, certain social needs (homelessness, alcoholism, or drug abuse), or multiple risk factors for a poor outcome should also be treated in an inpatient setting. Risk factors for a complicated course of illness include the presence of coexisting diseases such as congestive heart failure, obstructive lung disease, diabetes, renal failure, hospitalization within the last year, and neurologic illness; age above 65 years; certain physical findings such as tachypnea, hypotension, or high fever; hypoxemia or hypercarbia ($PaO_2 < 60$ mm Hg or $PaCO_2 > 50$ mm Hg) on room air; and evidence of sepsis or end-organ dysfunction (71). Recently, scoring systems have been developed to predict mortality from CAP, and these can be used to guide the admission decision. However, the use of such systems in place of clinical judgment has not yet been proven to be safe or cost effective and do not always provide for all the medical and social needs of patients (71, 132).

In addition to offering specific therapy that is unavailable to outpatients, hospitalization allows observation of the patient's course during therapy. Individuals with serious comorbidity may have deterioration of their underlying illness in response to infection, their pneumonia may progress rapidly, and, on initial evaluation, they may appear less ill than they actually are because of an impaired host inflammatory response. Hospitalization is also able to provide specific therapy for patients who are in respiratory failure (severe hypoxemia or hypercarbia) as well as for those with an impaired cough reflex and copious sputum (so that they may receive adequate tracheobronchial toilet), those with atelectasis, and those with systemic sepsis.

ANTIBIOTIC THERAPY. If a specific pathogen is identified, therapy should be as narrowly directed as possible, with the agents mentioned above for each organism. If no etiology can be established, empiric therapy is required, with full appreciation of the pitfalls of this approach. With empiric regimens, multiple antibiotics are often required; not all likely pathogens can be covered and some combination therapies are nephrotoxic.

Therapy for community-acquired infection is directed toward pneumococcus, *M. pneumoniae*, and *C. pneumoniae* if the patient has no host impairment, but all patients with CAP should receive an empiric therapy regimen that is active against pneumococcus and atypical pathogens (the latter as either primary infection or coinfection) (71). If the patient is elderly, has aspirated, is an alcoholic, or has serious coexisting illness, then in addition to these organisms the empiric regimen must also cover enteric gram-negative organisms, *H. influenzae*, *S. aureus*, and anaerobes. Hospitalized patients should be treated for pneumococcus, enteric gram-negative organisms, *H. influenzae*, *S. aureus*, anaerobes, and, possibly, *Legionella*. Those with severe CAP should be treated for pneumococcus, *Legionella*, enteric gram-negative organisms (including *P. aeruginosa*), and, possibly, *M. pneumoniae* and *H. influenzae*. DRSP should be covered in patients with risk factors such as age above 65 years, β-lactam therapy within the last 3 months, immunosuppressive illness, alcoholism, and multiple medical comorbidities.

When antibiotics are used, precautions are necessary in certain settings. With renal or hepatic failure, certain drugs will have their elimination interfered with; hence, dosage must be adjusted. Renally cleared drugs include the aminoglycosides, certain cephalosporins, some quinolones (not moxifloxacin), penicillins, and other β-lactams. Liver-excreted drugs include erythromycin, chloramphenicol, and nafcillin. In patients with a reduction in lean body mass and an increase in body fat, such as the elderly, there may be a rise in serum drug levels if the drugs are given on a per-kilogram basis. With a reduction in serum albumin, the free concentration of certain drugs that are ordinarily highly protein bound may rise. Some drugs, particularly the penicillins, have a high sodium content, which should be considered if the patient has coexisting heart failure.

Some antibiotics penetrate poorly into bronchial secretions, and topical antibiotics may be indicated to increase antibiotic levels in the lung. This approach is not a standard one, but it has been used successfully to treat *P. aeruginosa* airway infections in patients with cystic fibrosis, bronchiectasis, and refractory nosocomial pneumonia (especially with drug-resistant organisms). It may also be indicated in the treatment of patients with severe gram-negative infections that have not responded to parenteral antibiotics. When topical therapy is given, it may be via direct intratracheal injection or by aerosolization and should be preceded by bronchodilator treatment to avoid

reflex bronchospasm. One aerosolized aminoglycoside (inhaled tobramycin) has been specially formulated for inhaled use and is constituted in a manner that avoids bronchospasm. The drugs most commonly used in this manner are polymyxin and the aminoglycosides. Some evidence suggests that topical antibiotics can be used prophylactically in critically ill patients to prevent nosocomial pneumonia.

Once the patient has responded to initial therapy, a rapid switch to oral therapy followed by prompt hospital discharge is recommended. Criteria for switch to oral therapy include subjective improvement in cough, sputum, and dyspnea; resolution of fever (afebrile, two occasions, and 8 hours apart); improvement in leukocytosis; and ability to take oral medications. In many CAP patients, this switch can be safely achieved by the third or fourth hospital day.

OXYGENATION AND MECHANICAL VENTILATION. Endotracheal intubation and mechanical ventilation are required in patients with refractory hypoxemia (arterial oxygen tension <60 mm Hg on maximal mask oxygen) or hypercarbic respiratory failure with acute respiratory acidosis and in patients who cannot adequately clear secretions (to allow deep airway suctioning). Recently, there has been some success in treating patients with pneumonia and hypoxemic or hypercarbic respiratory failure with noninvasive positive-pressure ventilation using a mask interface with a positive-pressure ventilator, and this approach may help avoid some of the complications of endotracheal intubation. When patients have severe hypoxemia and a unilateral pneumonia, their oxygenation can be improved by positioning them with the unaffected lung in a gravity-dependent position. This maneuver increases perfusion to the normal lung relative to the diseased lung, and thereby minimizes ventilation–perfusion mismatches.

TRACHEOBRONCHIAL TOILET. Chest physiotherapy can be used to promote clearance of respiratory secretions. This therapy, which employs components of postural drainage, chest percussion, vibration, coughing, and forced expiratory breathing, is best used for patients with copious secretions (>30 mL per day) who have a reduced ability to cough. These physical methods may be no more effective than a good cough, but many patients are unable to provide this and assistance may be required (133).

Agents that reduce the viscosity and consistency of sputum are termed "mucolytic"; those that increase mucociliary clearance are termed "mucokinetic" (134). Mucolytic therapy can be achieved with hydration, aerosolized saline, and inhaled *N*-acetylcysteine. The use of mucolytic agents is best reserved for patients with retained secretions who have developed atelectasis. Mucokinetic drugs are rarely used, but some agents that may be used for other purposes have mucokinetic effects. These include β-agonist bronchodilators and theophylline. Another technique that may be helpful for some patients with mucous plugging and retained secretions is bronchoscopy. If atelectasis is present without an air bronchogram, there may be a large central airway plug, and bronchoscopy can be used for suction removal under direct vision. Bronchoscopy can also be used in patients with unresolving pneumonia to evaluate the presence of a tumor or aspirated foreign body. For patients with nosocomial pneumonia, secretions may also be mobilized by endotracheal suctioning. Another approach is to place the patient on an oscillating bed that rotates from side to side. Although it is unclear whether this approach can help resolve pneumonia more rapidly, there are data suggesting that this type of intervention can prevent pneumonia in high-risk patients, possibly by mobilizing secretions (135).

Tuberculosis

EPIDEMIOLOGY AND PATHOGENESIS. TB may be a pulmonary disease, an extrapulmonary disease, or both and is caused by Koch bacillus, *M. tuberculosis*. The organism is a nonmotile, acid-fast staining, gram-positive rod with a high lipid content. It is an obligate aerobe that is not pigmented (in contrast to some of the other mycobacterial species) and is normally contained by cell-mediated immunity. Patients with impaired cellular immune responses, such as the elderly, diabetics, patients treated with immunosuppressives, patients with renal failure, those with hematologic malignancy, and individuals with HIV infection, are thus at increased risk of illness from this organism. Patients with HIV infection have an increased risk of TB because of impaired T1 lymphocyte response and a corresponding reduction in the production of interferon-γ.(136). Disease is spread from person to person via inhalation of droplet nuclei produced by infected persons when they talk, cough, or sneeze. Casual contacts of infected persons are not usually infected, but those with prolonged and close contacts, particularly in areas of poor ventilation, are most at risk. This mode of spread, which favors disease in crowded, small spaces, may contribute to the predominance of this illness among those of lower socioeconomic status and in persons living in underdeveloped nations.

In the United States, there were about 15 new cases per 100,000 population during the 1970s, and the incidence declined at a rate of 6.7% annually until 1985. Beginning in 1986 and continuing until 1992, the incidence of new cases began to rise, which has been attributed to the frequent infection of AIDS patients with the tubercle bacillus (20,136). In 1990, it was estimated that 4.3% of HIV–infected persons had TB infection (20). With aggressive measures of disease control and directly observed therapy, this rise was reversed in 1993. In addition, TB remains an important infection in many immigrants to this country, among the homeless, and in the elderly who are confined to nursing homes. Currently, more than two thirds of TB cases occur in nonwhite racial and ethnic groups. One fourth of all cases in the United States occur in the foreign born, but still, one third of cases occur in middle- and upper-income groups (20). Among patients aged 25 to 44 years, most are nonwhites and Hispanics, whereas whites predominate in the elderly population of TB patients. One other recent change in TB epidemiology has been the emergence of organisms that are multiply resistant to traditional TB medications. Multidrug-resistant tuberculosis (MDR-TB) is a particular problem among HIV–infected individuals and those with a history of prior TB therapy. In New York City, as many as 23% of all previously untreated TB patients had primary drug resistance to at least one drug in the early 1990s (137).

Most individuals who encounter the tubercle bacillus become infected with it, contain the organism within the lung by developing an adequate immune response, and, thus, do not develop clinical illness. Those with the clinical disease "TB" are either individuals who cannot contain the primary infection or

persons who have reactivated a previously contained and dormant infection. Thus, much of the literature makes a distinction between "infection" and "disease" due to *M. tuberculosis*. Many people have had the infection, but <10% of infected individuals will develop the disease.

The initial infection with the organism, the primary infection, is usually in the middle or lower zones of the lung. Because these areas receive the most ventilation with each breath, it is not surprising that an airborne organism would localize in this manner. Over the next few weeks, the organisms multiply and spread via lymphatics to the regional lymph nodes, particularly in the hilum. The combination of a primary peripheral lung lesion with an enlarged hilar lymph node is termed a "Ghon complex." During this time, some organisms may disseminate via the bloodstream to extrapulmonary sites, where they are usually contained but may reactivate at a later date. The favored sites for secondary seeding and growth of these aerobic bacteria are ones with high tissue oxygen content such as the apex of the lung, the renal parenchyma, and the growing ends of long bones.

Within 3 to 6 weeks of primary infection, sensitized T lymphocytes release lymphokines that can attract monocytes and macrophages to the infected area in the lung to phagocytose the bacteria. Lymphocytes are also attracted, and during this time, the host develops immunity to reinfection, which becomes detectable by a positive tuberculin skin test. Once the skin test becomes positive, the host can usually kill any other organisms that are inhaled, but it may not always be able to eliminate the organisms already within the lung and lung macrophages. Thus, most cases of active TB are in patients with positive skin tests and are due to progressive primary disease or reactivation disease; they are less commonly due to reinfection after exposure to another infected patient with active disease. However, in the HIV–infected patient, superinfection with a resistant TB strain during TB therapy for infection with another strain has been reported (138).

The initial tissue response to infection involves mononuclear cells that may crowd together with their lipid-rich cytoplasm and form a tubercle made up of cells that are described as epithelioid. The tubercle may contain multinucleated giant cells, called Langhans cells, and is surrounded by fibroblasts, lymphocytes, and more monocytes to form a granuloma, which is characteristic of TB. This granulomatous reaction must be distinguished from other granulomatous tissue reactions such as those seen with sarcoidosis and fungal disease. When a host cannot contain the organism by this inflammatory response, the organism continues to multiply, and the center of the granuloma undergoes a process of liquefaction necrosis termed "caseation." The progression to this necrotizing process does not occur in most infected patients, but only in those who cannot contain the organism. The caseous material is full of living organisms that can spread within the lung. The necrotic, caseating granuloma then becomes a tuberculous cavity, which may contain up to 10^9 organisms (139). Without caseation, a granuloma has many fewer organisms. When large quantities of caseous material are spread along the bronchi from a cavity to another part of the lung, a tuberculous pneumonia may develop. When granulomas finally do heal, they often develop calcification, particularly if caseation has occurred.

About 5% of patients with primary infection will not be able to contain the organism and will develop progressive primary disease within 2 years of infection. Rates of progressive primary disease may be higher with HIV infection, reaching as high as 38% in the first year and averaging 8% per year afterwards (140) as the onset of illness is accelerated by the HIV coinfection. As primary infection usually involves the lower-lung zones, the patient with progressive primary disease may manifest with lower-lobe TB (see Fig. 15-13). Recently, with the advent of antiretroviral therapy for HIV infection, patients have had reconstitution of immune function, and reactivation tuberculosis rather than primary TB has become more common (141). The failure to contain the organism may be related to the size of inoculum and the status of the host defense system. Patients at risk for progressive primary infection are the very young, the elderly, the malnourished, blacks, diabetics, alcoholics, and those with immunosuppressive medications or illnesses (including HIV infection). An additional 5% will develop disease more than 2 years after infection, which will be due to reactivation of live bacilli that had been contained and dormant within healed granulomas. This reactivation illness usually develops in sites where the organism was hematogenously disseminated during the primary infection. The lung apex is a common site for reactivation disease, particularly in the apical posterior segment (see Fig. 15-14). Thus, on the basis of this pathogenetic schema, lower-lobe TB is usually a progressive primary disease, whereas upper-lobe disease may

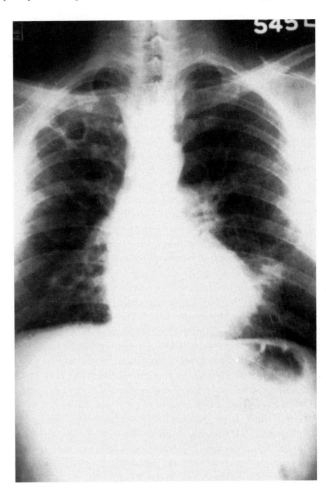

FIGURE 15-14. Reactivation tuberculosis with cavity formation and infiltrate in the upper lobe and endobronchial spread from an upper-lobe cavity to the lower lobes.

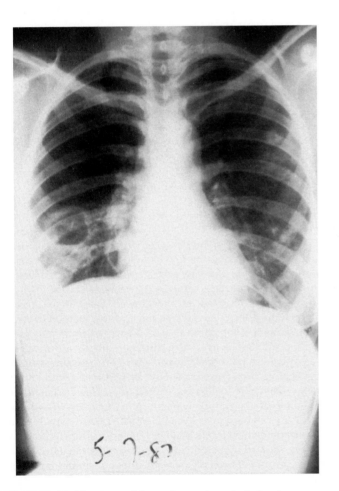

FIGURE 15-13. Lower-lobe cavitary tuberculosis due to progressive primary disease in a 46-year-old black diabetic man.

represent reactivation. In either situation, the patient with TB is unable to contain the organism, whereas most people who are infected do not develop disease because they can contain the organism. For this reason, a deficit in host defense should be sought in all patients with active TB, and HIV testing should be considered in all patients with active TB. Extrapulmonary disease may occur as a result of progressive primary infection or with reactivation.

CLINICAL FEATURES. With primary infection, most patients are asymptomatic or may have mild, nonspecific symptoms of a transient lower–respiratory-tract infection. When disease is present, symptoms are usually chronic and may cause respiratory symptoms as well as systemic manifestations. Many patients note just malaise, headache, fever, night sweats, and weight loss. Some patients may have abdominal pain and anorexia. Pulmonary symptoms are common but not specific. Persistent cough may be present, with or without mucoid sputum, and, occasionally, hemoptysis is present. Hemoptysis can be the result of tuberculous pneumonia but is more commonly due to cavitary disease or rupture of an artery in an old tuberculous cavity (Rasmussen aneurysm). Several late posttuberculous complications can cause hemoptysis, including bronchiectasis, broncholithiasis, or the presence of an aspergilloma in a prior tuberculous cavity. Another pulmonary symptom can be chest pain, particularly pleurisy-type pain, when a pleural effusion is present. Tuberculous effusions usually result when a small number of organisms from a subpleural granuloma, early in the course of the illness, rupture into the pleural cavity and the patient has a hypersensitivity response to this material. Because most of the pleural fluid is inflammatory, not many organisms are present, and culture of the pleural fluid yields the tubercle bacillus in no more than 20% to 40% of cases. Because the pleural response is hypersensitivity, it usually correlates with a positive tuberculin test. Much less commonly, a large inoculum of organisms can reach the pleural space and cause a tuberculous empyema. Dyspnea may occur as a result of extensive parenchymal disease, pneumothorax, or a large pleural effusion. Both the systemic and pulmonary symptoms are usually chronic, having been present for weeks to months prior to diagnosis, but, occasionally, an acute pneumonia presentation is seen and acute respiratory failure may result. The elderly generally have less dramatic symptoms than younger patients do (142).

Extrapulmonary disease is seen in more than 15% of TB cases in the United States. However, in patients with AIDS and severe immune suppression ($CD4^+$ counts <200 per cubic millimeter), this pattern is much more common and may occur in 60% to 70% of all TB cases in this population (143,144). When extrapulmonary involvement is present, the patient may present with a skin lesion that is slow to heal or a chronic draining cervical lymph node (scrofula or cervical lymph node TB). When genital TB is present, men may have epididymal involvement with a slightly painful scrotal mass, whereas women may have pelvic pain or infertility. Renal TB is usually without symptoms, but patients will have "sterile" pyuria or hematuria on urinalysis. Tuberculous meningitis may cause dementia, coma, cranial nerve abnormalities (because the base of the brain is involved), focal neurologic deficits, or headache. Abdominal pain, fever, ascites, and anorexia can be manifestations of tuberculous peritonitis. Chest pain, fever, and dyspnea may result from pericardial involvement. Tuberculous involvement of the skeleton may cause bone pain or spine collapse with spinal cord compression. When the disease is fulminant and hematogenously disseminated, it is termed "miliary" because of the millet seed appearance of the multiple pulmonary lesions that are seen on chest radiograph. Miliary disease may occur with progressive primary infection or reactivation but is the result of bloodstream invasion and dissemination of large numbers of bacteria that overcome host defenses at multiple sites. Miliary TB may cause fever, malaise, cough, dyspnea, weight loss, anorexia, and headache. The lungs, liver, adrenals, kidneys, and spleen are often involved, and diagnosis may require lung or bone marrow biopsy, although organisms may be recovered from BAL or urine.

Physical findings are not specific, and patients may show signs of pneumonitis (rales), pleural effusion (dullness to percussion and reduced breath sounds), or specific extrapulmonary involvement. Laboratory data may reveal anemia, leukopenia, or severe leukocytosis. Hyponatremia and hypercalcemia are also common findings. Liver function tests may be abnormal with disseminated infection. Pleural fluid is usually an exudate with lymphocytosis, low glucose, and low pH. Spinal fluid may show low glucose, high protein, and lymphocytes if meningitis is present.

DIAGNOSIS. The chest radiograph is an important clue to the presence of TB. Lower-lobe involvement with infiltrates or cavitation may occur in progressive primary disease, but most patients have evidence of apical involvement, particularly in the posterior segments. Apical scarring may indicate prior infection, and a change in a previously stable upper-lobe pattern may indicate reactivation. Cavitation is common with reactivation and may accompany a parenchymal, reticular upper-lobe infiltrate (Fig. 15-14). Some patients will have extensive nodular lung involvement in conjunction with one or multiple cavities, and this pattern of extensive parenchymal infection is the result of endobronchial dissemination of bacteria from a caseating cavitary lesion. Nodal enlargement in the hilum and mediastinum as well as nodal calcification can result from TB. Solitary nodules may occasionally represent a tuberculoma, and, sometimes, these lesions can cavitate. Other radiographic findings can include a miliary pattern with bilateral, diffuse, small densities or pleural effusion with or without an evident parenchymal lesion. In one series (145), patients with primary TB had pulmonary consolidation in the lower-lung zones or anteriorly in the upper lobe (50%), cavitation (29%), miliary disease (6%), or a normal radiograph (15%). Those with reactivation disease had a different pattern, with 91% having apical and posterior fibrous infiltrates, 45% having cavities, and 21% having bronchogenic spread of disease.

Clinical and radiographic features may be different when HIV infection is present. As mentioned, fewer HIV–infected patients in comparison to other infected individuals have only pulmonary disease. With lung involvement, HIV–infected patients with TB have lower-lobe infiltrates and adenopathy and infrequently have cavitation. Even with bacteriologically confirmed pulmonary TB, HIV–infected persons can have a normal chest radiograph (136). In general, the more classic, typical, radiographic patterns are seen in HIV–infected persons who are early in their disease or in those on active antiretroviral therapy and are relatively intact immunologically. The severely immunosuppressed HIV patient tends to have more unusual TB manifestations, and infection with *M. avium intracellulare* is also frequently present.

A definitive diagnosis of TB is made by isolating the organism from a clinical specimen such as sputum, urine, a biopsy of involved tissue, pleural fluid, bone marrow aspirate, spinal fluid, ascites fluid, or bronchoscopic lavage. Sputum is best sampled by collecting the first sample produced in the early morning. In some patients, gastric aspirates can be collected and cultured, and these samples may contain organisms that have been expectorated and swallowed. Clinical specimens can be stained for organisms by the acid-fast method or with the rhodamine fluorochrome stain. Gastric aspirates may give a false-positive stain as some gastric saprophytes are acid fast. If a patient has pulmonary involvement and sputum samples are negative, bronchoscopy should be performed with lavage as the diagnostic yield may exceed 90%. Newer diagnostic modalities are becoming available, and they have the advantage of identifying a mycobacterial organism more rapidly than more traditional methods. With radiometric culture techniques and nucleic acid probes, organisms can be identified in a week or less, and fewer bacteria are needed than with traditional diagnostic methods (136).

Latent tuberculous infection (but not disease) is diagnosed by finding a positive skin-test response to tuberculin antigen.

The standard Mantoux test uses purified protein derivative (PPD) of tuberculin, and a dose of 5 tuberculin units in 0.1 mL is administered intradermally. The degree of induration at 48 to 72 hours is measured, and a positive test is defined in relation to the individual's relative risk of being infected with the TB bacterium (20,143,146). A reaction of 5 mm or more is defined as positive for patients who are HIV positive or who have HIV risk factors and are of unknown HIV status, those who are close contacts of an active case, those with organ transplant and immune compromise (more than 15 mg prednisone daily), and those who have a chest radiograph consistent with old, healed TB. A reaction of 10 mm or more is defined as positive in patients who do not fall in any of the above categories but who are foreign born from high-prevalence countries, intravenous drug users, in minority or medically underserved groups, residents of a chronic-care facility or correctional institution, and patients with medical conditions that increase the risk of TB. Such medical conditions include silicosis, gastrectomy, ileal bypass, chronic renal failure, diabetes mellitus, high-dose corticosteroids or immunosuppressive therapy or illness, and malnutrition. All other persons who do not fit into any of these groups are defined as positive only if the skin test reaction is 15 mm or more, but in general, skin testing should not be done in this latter population (143,144,146).

More than 90% of patients with TB will have a positive skin test, and those who do not are either anergic due to overwhelming illness or are too early in the course of disease to have converted the skin test to positive. If a skin test reaction increases in size by 10 mm or more in a previously negative person a "conversion" is said to have occurred, and this indicates infection during the time between the two skin tests (143,146). In some populations, particularly the elderly, a false-negative skin test can occur because of a "loss of immunologic memory." In such patients, a second skin test will be positive because the antigenic exposure of the first skin test would have "boosted" the immune response that had been present but was suppressed. When comparing the first and second skin test, one should not conclude that these patients have converted from a negative test to a positive one, but rather that they have had their false-negative result unmasked by the so-called "booster effect." It is important in mass screening programs to account for this phenomenon by giving a second skin test to all negative reactors 1 to 2 weeks after the first test so that a boosted response will be recognized and not confused with a new conversion.

TREATMENT. Antituberculous therapy can be given to individuals with infection who are at high risk of developing active disease; this practice, which can prevent illness, is called treatment of latent disease (143). In addition, patients with active TB are treated with medications that are generally able to cure the disease effectively.

Latent disease is treated with isoniazid (INH) 10 mg/kg/day (up to a maximum of 300 mg) for 9 months (143,144). If the patient has had contact with a patient who has INH-resistant disease, then therapy should be with rifampin for 4 months, or rifampin and pyrazinamide for 2 months (143). Those with HIV may require longer therapy, but the current recommendation is treatment for 9 months (143,144). Because any person with a positive PPD skin test has been infected with the tubercle bacillus and can develop disease, treatment of latent disease should be considered for all skin-test reactors who meet the criteria for a positive test, as defined in the preceding text, but the focus is to limit skin testing to high-risk individuals. INH can cause hepatotoxicity, and the incidence of this complication rises with age, particularly above the age of 35. A positive tuberculin test (as defined above) indicates the need for therapy, but those who are at the most risk include those with (a) known or suspected HIV infection; (b) close contact with an active case; (c) recent convertor (defined in the preceding text); (d) radiographic evidence of prior TB; and (e) presence of a medical condition that increases the risk of TB (listed above).

Active TB, both pulmonary and extrapulmonary, should be treated with INH 300 mg daily along with rifampin 600 mg daily for 6 months, combined with pyrazinamide (25 mg per kg) for the first 2 months if the organism is not drug resistant, but for most patients, ethambutol is also added if there is any possibility of drug resistance (139,147). If the patient has a sensitive organism, then ethambutol is stopped, pyrazinamide continued for a total of 2 months, and the remaining therapy is continued for 4 more months, and, thus, therapy is completed in 6 months. An alternative is to use INH and rifampin together for 9 months for drug-sensitive organisms. Both INH and rifampin are bactericidal for the tubercle bacillus, and when used together, they can eliminate the organism rapidly and usually prevent relapse due to resistant bacteria. Rifampin is rapidly bactericidal to tubercle bacilli that exist in any of the three populations present in the body: actively growing extracellular organisms, slowly growing intracellular (in macrophages) organisms at acid pH, and slowly growing extracellular organisms. INH is bactericidal against the first two of these populations; streptomycin kills only actively growing extracellular bacteria; and pyrazinamide kills slowly growing intracellular bacteria. Two active drugs are needed for therapy because naturally occurring drug-resistant mutants are present in most patients. It has been estimated that one in 10^5 organisms is resistant to INH and one in 10^9 is resistant to rifampin. Because an active tuberculous cavity has no more than 10^8 to 10^9 organisms, the combination therapy will effectively kill any naturally occurring drug-resistant mutants. If drug combinations other than INH, rifampin, and pyrazinamide are used, therapy must be extended to 18 to 24 months because other drugs are not as active. These regimens are used if the patient develops toxicity to one of the standard drugs or if drug-resistant disease is documented or suspected (as is common in certain immigrant populations). Ethambutol and streptomycin are commonly used in these extended regimens; second-line drugs include capreomycin, ethionamide, cycloserine, and paraamino salicylic acid (PAS). Compliance can be improved with intermittent regimens given under direct supervision 3 to 5 times per week. In some communities, directly observed therapy has become the standard of care and can reduce the incidence of TB, especially drug-resistant disease.

The current concerns about MDR-TB have changed the initial approach to therapy in many parts of the country. When the possibility of resistance is entertained, as mentioned, the patient is usually started on a 4-drug regimen, and the therapy is often given under direct supervision (148). If susceptibility patterns reveal that the organism is not drug resistant, then the period of therapy can be as short as 6 months, as described above. If MDR-TB is identified, therapy is continued with at least two active first-line drugs. These include INH, pyrazinamide, ethambutol, and rifampin. If the organism is not sensitive to at least two of these agents, second-line drugs should be used, but at least three of these will be required (137). Some patients with MDR-TB require multiple drugs for prolonged periods of time, and, occasionally, drug therapy must be supplemented with resectional surgery. To improve the outcome of therapy of MDR-TB in certain populations, directly observed therapy has been recommended, but this approach may be valuable for all patients with active TB (148).

Mycobacteria Other Than Tuberculosis

Mycobacteria other than tuberculosis (MOTT) are generally slow-growing mycobacteria that, unlike *M. tuberculosis*, are niacin-negative (i.e., they metabolize and do not accumulate niacin) in the laboratory. Although some of the MOTT are niacin-positive and some are rapid growers, most human diseases are caused by species that do not fit this pattern. MOTT differ from the tubercle bacillus in several other important ways. They are not spread from person to person, and they are not always pathogens when isolated from human samples. In fact, most normal individuals can effectively resist infection by these organisms without the occurrence of tissue invasion, whereas others may become colonized but not infected. MOTT can cause illnesses very similar to TB, but usually only in abnormal hosts, especially those with bronchiectasis. Because of the similarities and differences that these organisms and their manifestations have to the tubercle bacillus, they are sometimes called "atypical mycobacteria." In recent years, the incidence of infection by these organisms has risen, particularly in the AIDS population, where disseminated infection with *M. avium* complex (MAC) occurs. There are multiple species of MOTT, many of which rarely cause human disease. The species that are potentially pathogenic in humans include MAC, *Mycobacterium kansasii*, *Mycobacterium chelonei*, *Mycobacterium fortuitum*, *Mycobacterium scrofulaceum*, *Mycobacterium xenopi*, *Mycobacterium szulgai*, *Mycobacterium simiae*, *Mycobacterium marinum*, *Mycobacterium ulcerans*, and *Mycobacterium haemophilum* (149).

The diseases caused by MOTT may cause findings in the lungs, in the cervical lymph nodes (lymphadenitis), in the skin (abscess or nonhealing ulcer), or, occasionally, systemically. The pulmonary disease may appear radiographically (see Fig. 15-15) similar to TB but may differ in that cavities can be thin-walled with little surrounding infiltrate. In addition, bronchogenic spread is unusual, pleural disease is uncommon, and preexisting chronic pulmonary disease is often present (150). Symptoms are more slowly progressive than in TB but may include cough, dyspnea, weight loss, and, occasionally, hemoptysis and fever. The pulmonary disease is usually indolent, and when it occurs, it commonly affects older patients with COPD. This pattern can occur with MAC, *M. kansasii*, or others of the MOTT group. A much more virulent and disseminated form of disease, caused by MAC, has been found in AIDS patients (144). Mortality from this infection is high, and symptoms are not specific and commonly include fever, weight loss, abdominal pain, malabsorption, and diarrhea. Pulmonary symptoms may also be present but not in every case. Patients may have generalized lymphadenopathy and hepatosplenomegaly. Diagnosis of disseminated MAC infection in the AIDS patient can be made by finding the organism in bone marrow, liver, urine, lymph nodes, or blood cultures.

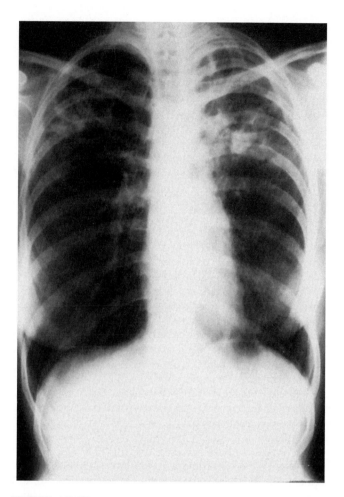

FIGURE 15-15. Chest radiograph of a patient with chronic bronchitis and slowly progressive cavitary disease in both upper lobes due to *Mycobacterium avium* complex.

In general, the diagnosis of MOTT infections is difficult because simple isolation of the organisms from sputum is not sufficient to establish infection because these bacteria may colonize diseased lungs yet not cause invasive infection. A diagnosis of pulmonary disease by MOTT is made by having a compatible clinical picture and radiograph in a patient with repeated isolation of organisms from sputum or with evidence of tissue invasion by organisms on biopsy. If cavitary disease is present, the diagnosis can be made by finding the organisms on two or more sputum samples, provided that other diagnoses have been excluded. If cavitary disease is absent, the diagnosis requires the above findings plus a failure to convert sputum samples to negative, with either bronchial hygiene or 2 weeks of specific drug therapy (151). If the sputum is nondiagnostic, the diagnosis can also be established by finding the organisms in a biopsy specimen. Skin testing is not widely available or clinically useful in diseases caused by these bacteria. In the AIDS patient, the recovery of MAC organisms from blood or stool in a patient with a compatible illness will establish the diagnosis of disseminated infection. Once the diagnosis of MOTT infection is made, therapy is started with multiple antituberculous drugs, but the success rate, particularly in the AIDS patient, may be quite low because the organisms are usually resistant to most available medications. Some newer agents that may be active against some of the MOTT organisms are clarithromycin, azithromycin, the quinolones (especially ciprofloxacin and ofloxacin), and rifabutin.

FUNGAL LUNG DISEASE: NORMAL HOST

The dimorphic fungi *Histoplasma capsulatum*, *Blastomyces dermatitides*, *Coccidioides immitis*, *Paracoccidioides brasiliensis*, and *Sporothrix schenckii* are all soil-growing organisms. With the exception of *Sporothrix*, they have sharply defined endemic areas. Again with the exception of *S. schenckii*, their primary mechanisms of infection are via the lungs; *S. schenckii* may also invade the host via the lungs but the usual manifestation of the illness is lymphocutaneous. Moreover, most primary infections are asymptomatic, and only a certain percentage of infected individuals go on to develop clinically recognizable illness. Occasionally, following the acute illness, chronic or disseminated disease may develop.

After the infecting spores are inhaled, these organisms convert at body temperature to their pathogenic forms, which for all but *C. immitis* is a yeast. At body temperature, *C. immitis* converts to giant spherules. Whereas the yeasts multiply by binary fission, giant spherules multiply by endosporulation.

The underlying state of immunity of the host will determine the extent and nature of human illness. Normal hosts are usually able to localize the illness to the lungs, and spontaneous recovery is the rule. However, when the disease occurs in patients who are immunocompromised, either by another underlying illness or because of the administration of cytotoxic agents or glucocorticoids, dissemination to multiple organs is the rule.

Histoplasmosis

The endemic area for *H. capsulatum* includes most of the Midwestern and South-Central United States, extending down to the Gulf Coast in Texas and to the St. Lawrence Valley in Canada (152). The organism occurs in microfoci in nature and grows in soil enhanced by organic nitrogen, usually by droppings of birds or bats. In nature, the organism grows as a mold, and when the sites are disturbed, an infecting aerosol is produced, leading to inhalation of the spores.

Following inhalation, the spores produce an area of pneumonitis in the lung after conversion to the yeast form. After spread to the hilar nodes, the organism gains access to the bloodstream and disseminates throughout the body. Cells of the reticuloendothelial (RE) system remove the organism from circulation, and once specific delayed hypersensitivity develops, the "armed" macrophages will destroy the organisms, leading to granuloma formation. Frequently, healing causes necrosis, which may undergo calcification over the years.

In abnormal hosts such as infants, the very old, or in patients who are immunosuppressed by underlying disease or by administration of various agents, progressive disseminated disease occurs frequently (153). In these individuals, adequate cell-mediated immunity fails to develop, and the organism begins to replicate within cells of the RE system.

The vast majority of primary infections with *H. capsulatum* are either asymptomatic or minimally symptomatic. Only a

small fraction of patients will ever visit a physician because of the onset of acute histoplasmosis. Those who are symptomatic usually have a "flu-like" illness, with arthralgias and myalgias as well as a non-productive cough. Fever is usually low grade. Chest roentgenograms may be normal or show extensive bilateral nodular disease with hilar adenopathy. In addition, erythema nodosum and erythema multiforme may accompany the onset of clinical illness (154).

The primary infection in patients with altered lung anatomy, such as that seen with centrilobular emphysema of smokers, looks different from that seen in normal hosts. In these patients, the acute infection may surround these abnormal air spaces, giving the roentgenographic appearance of cavity formation. It is important to remember that the vast majority of these patients will also recover spontaneously, and only in rare instances will the upper-lobe disease become progressive and require treatment (155).

Symptoms of progressive upper-zone histoplasmosis are chronic illness with low-grade fever, weight loss, anorexia, and a cough productive of mucopurulent sputum. Because of the great similarity between the symptoms and the chest roentgenogram of upper-zone histoplasmosis and TB, many of these patients are initially thought to have TB (see Fig. 15-16) (156). Among the other residuals following primary infection, the most common is the "coin lesion" caused by rounding off and hardening of the area of previous pneumonitis. The main significance of these lesions is that they frequently occur in patients at high risk for bronchogenic neoplasms.

An unusual complication of acute histoplasmosis is the development of mediastinal fibrosis, which is probably an abnormal host response rather than an unusual effect of the parasite (see Fig. 15-17) (157).

In patients in whom the original dissemination of *Histoplasma* becomes progressive, a life-threatening illness occurs. As a rule, cell-mediated immunity is either weak or does not develop at all (153). In patients with the most severe form of immunodeficiency, such as those with AIDS or with Hodgkin disease, progressive disseminated histoplasmosis (PDH) follows a fulminant course. Manifestations include fever, weight loss, and hepatosplenomegaly, as well as the appearance of severe bone marrow involvement with anemia, leukopenia, and thrombocytopenia. Histopathologic examination of affected tissues reveals complete absence of granulomata, and all one sees is macrophages containing multiple organisms (153,158).

In patients in whom partial cell-mediated immunity still remains, PDH follows a much more subacute or chronic course. Histopathologically, the disease is characterized by the appearance of granulomata with a relative scarcity of organisms. Clinical symptoms in these patients are primarily those of a chronic illness; special areas of *Histoplasma* involvement include oropharyngeal, rectal, and genital ulcers as well as hepatosplenomegaly (153). Adrenal gland involvement may occur, which, occasionally, may lead to frank Addison disease (159).

With the emergence of the AIDS epidemic, PDH has become recognized as a frequent opportunistic infection in individuals infected by HIV. The nearly total deficiency of T-lymphocyte–mediated immune function (the hallmark of AIDS) renders every HIV–positive individual uniquely susceptible to developing PDH. Two potential pathogenic mechanisms exist. First

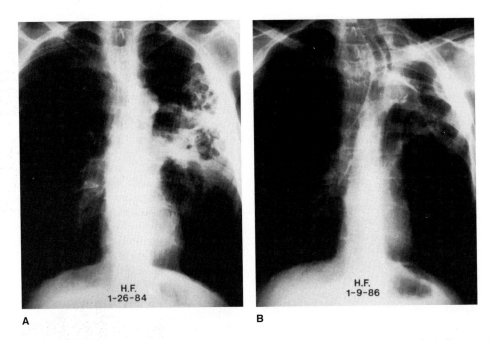

FIGURE 15-16. **A**: Chronic pulmonary histoplasmosis. Note the extensive left upper-lobe infiltrate with apparent cavitation. This patient received 400 mg ketoconazole daily for 9 months. **B**: Follow-up chest roentgenogram shows clearing 15 months after completion of successful drug therapy. Note extensive retraction of the lobe with marked tracheal shift.

is the progression from primary infection. When immunocompromised individuals become infected with *H. capsulatum*, progressive dissemination will develop in most of them (160). Thus, it is to be anticipated that when patients with AIDS become exposed to the fungus, the outcome will be the development of PDH. The second mechanism is reactivation of previously dormant foci of infection. Following recovery

from the primary infection, after development of specific cell-mediated immunity has successfully localized the fungus, healing with granuloma formation takes place. Resected specimens of such granulomas frequently show persisting organisms. Such dormant foci may reactivate when immunosuppressive treatment is given (161). During progression of HIV infection, most T-cell–mediated immunity wanes, and when an individual

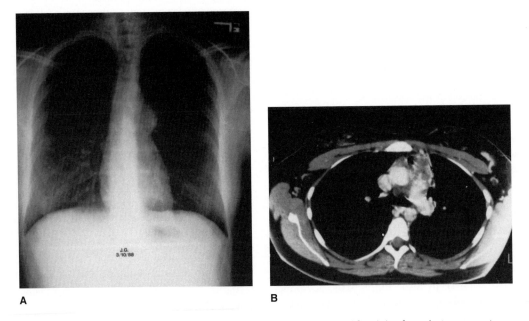

FIGURE 15-17. **A**: Chest roentgenogram of a 33-year-old woman with minimal respiratory symptoms. There is a large left-sided anterior mediastinal mass. **B**: Computed tomographic (CT) scan showing the full extent of the mass. Open biopsy showed healing granulomatous lesions. Histopathologic examination confirmed histoplasmosis.

harboring dormant foci of histoplasmosis reaches the critical level of waning immunity, the fungus begins to multiply and PDH develops. Most likely, both mechanisms are operative in HIV–infected patients.

The second mechanism is probably the more important consideration for physicians who reside outside the usual endemic area for histoplasmosis. The first mechanism (as well as reactivation disease) is more likely to occur in the endemic area. As Wheat et al. have pointed out, the diagnosis of PDH should prompt one to evaluate the patient's HIV status (160).

In Houston, which is on the fringe of the endemic area, 5% of patients with AIDS have developed PDH (162). However, in more endemic areas, the risk is far greater. In Indianapolis, almost 27% of HIV–infected patients have developed PDH (163). Experience during the early years of the HIV pandemic from both the East Coast and the West Coast have documented a rapidly increasing incidence of PDH among HIV–infected individuals, most of whom had resided in endemic areas for histoplasmosis prior to moving to either New York (164) or California. Remember that in addition to Central United States, both Central America and the Caribbean are endemic areas. Since the advent of highly active antiretroviral therapy (HAART), the incidence of PDH among HIV–infected patients has decreased rapidly.

The clinical manifestation of PDH in AIDS is a severe febrile illness. More than 50% of patients would not have had the diagnosis of AIDS established prior to the onset of PDH. Symptoms are those of a febrile illness with anorexia and weight loss. Physical examination is often normal, but hepatosplenomegaly may be present in up to one-third of patients. The chest roentgenogram may show diffuse interstitial changes with multiple small nodules, but is often negative (see Fig. 15-18) (162). Pancytopenia is frequently present, but it is a non-specific finding because HIV–infected patients receiving zidovudine or other similar agents may have bone marrow suppression.

Rapid diagnosis is facilitated by remembering that any febrile individual at high risk for HIV infection may have PDH. Blood cultures and bone marrow examination and culture are the best tests (see Fig. 15-19), and the fungus may be seen on examination of the buffy coat, where circulating phagocytes may be parasitized (165).

Isolation of the fungus from biologic material or visualization of the organism in histopathologic sections remains the gold standard. Proper handling of biologic specimens will yield a high frequency of positive cultures. Depending on inoculum size, a tentative diagnosis may be offered as early as 5 days, but, usually, this takes much longer—up to 4 to 6 weeks. When PDH is suspected, the best organ to sample is the bone marrow. Multiple blood cultures are frequently useful, especially when they are processed with the lysis-centrifugation system, or by a radiometric fungal culture system.

Skin testing for the diagnosis of histoplasmosis no longer has any role. Although the skin test is still an outstanding epidemiologic tool, it simply cannot be used for the diagnosis of acute histoplasmosis. It is also no longer available commercially.

In acute illness, serodiagnosis is the mainstay of diagnosis. Of the currently available serologic tests, the CF test remains the best. Unfortunately, it suffers from the fact that it is seldom timely enough because it frequently takes 2 to 6 weeks or more before a four-fold rise can be demonstrated. The immunodiffusion (ID) test, although highly specific, is relatively insensitive. In a recent outbreak, it was positive in only 50% of the proven cases even after 6 weeks.(166). The best available test is the measurement of the *Histoplasma* polysaccharide antigen, especially in AIDS patients (167). The test is also helpful in following the course of treatment and in detecting relapses (168).

Acute histoplasmosis, unless it results in significant interference with gas exchange, does not require treatment. Patients with severe, life-threatening, acute histoplasmosis will

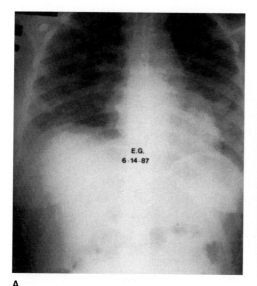

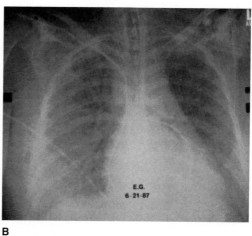

A   B

FIGURE 15-18. **A:** Admission chest radiograph of a 26-year-old, human immunodeficiency virus (HIV)–positive pregnant woman showing interstitial infiltrates bilaterally. The main complaint was shortness of breath and fever. Bronchial washings showed small, 2 to 4 μm round organisms thought to be *Pneumocystis carinii*. **B:** One week later, in spite of aggressive therapy, infiltrates have progressed. Blood cultures obtained on the day of admission yielded *Histoplasma capsulatum*.

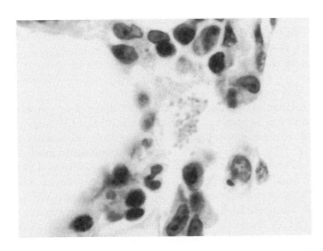

FIGURE 15-19. Bone marrow biopsy of an acquired immunodeficiency syndrome (AIDS) patient with progressive disseminated histoplasmosis. Note the large number of organisms inside a macrophage (hematoxylin and eosin stain × 1,000).

respond readily to intravenous administration of amphotericin B (AMB) (152).

Upper-lobe cavitary disease should be treated with itraconazole, 200 mg twice daily (169). Treatment failures may occur with oral agents, and in these patients, AMB in a total dose of 35 mg per kg is effective (170). PDH is best treated with full courses of AMB until the patient's clinical condition has stabilized. This stabilization occurs somewhere between 500 and 1,000 mg of AMB. Following stabilization, it is usually reasonable to switch to itraconazole. This form of combination therapy was worked out carefully in HIV–infected patients with PDH and is extremely effective. Itraconazole should be continued for life in HIV–infected patients. Although its use makes excellent sense, this form of combination therapy has not been tested in HIV–negative patients with PDH (170a). Itraconazole may be used as primary therapy for patients with PDH if the tempo of the illness is slow and if the patient is clinically stable.

Patients need no treatment after resection of solitary pulmonary nodules containing *Histoplasma*.

Blastomycosis

The endemic area of blastomycosis overlaps that of histoplasmosis but extends farther north. The endemic areas are the states and provinces bordering on the Great Lakes as well as large areas of the Southeast United States. Besides humans, dogs are frequent victims of the disease, and veterinary practitioners are usually quite knowledgeable about blastomycosis (171). Much less is known about the epidemiology of blastomycosis than about that of histoplasmosis. It appears that the organism exists in microfoci in nature, usually in areas well watered by streams (172). Disturbance of the mycelial growth results in the formation of the infecting aerosol, following which the infecting particles are inhaled into the lung. Once in the lung, conversion to the yeast phase takes place, and propagation begins by binary fission.

The portal of entry is the lung. In the original area of pneumonitis, the initial cellular exudate is primarily PMN. Once delayed hypersensitivity develops, macrophages move in, but the PMN component of the infiltrate never disappears completely. The organism is frequently restricted to the lungs by the establishment of cell-mediated immunity, but in some instances blood-borne dissemination may occur. The organs most commonly involved are the skin, bone, prostate, and meninges (171).

Acute pulmonary blastomycosis may be a severe, febrile illness, with cough productive of mucopurulent sputum. Frequently, it is accompanied by arthralgia and myalgia. Chest roentgenogram usually reveals single or multiple areas of pneumonitis. Pleural involvement is more common in blastomycosis than in histoplasmosis. Acute blastomycosis is frequently self limited (173) (see Fig. 15-20). Progressive pulmonary disease, as well as dissemination outside the confines of the lung, may occur (see Fig. 15-21). Frequently, the original pulmonary infiltrate may resolve spontaneously while the extrapulmonary components of the disseminated disease progress. Recently, a number of HIV–infected patients with blastomycosis have been described. The illness is usually rapidly progressive and is frequently widely disseminated, including frequent involvement of the meninges (174).

Visualization of the organism, either on histopathologic sections or in sputum, as well as culture of the organism, is the only means of diagnosing blastomycosis reliably. The simplest and most effective diagnostic test is the examination of sputum (or aspirated pus) after digestion with 10% potassium hydroxide (KOH) (175). Under reduced light, the characteristic large, double-refractile, thick-walled yeasts are readily identifiable. The daughter cell is attached by a broad neck. On histopathologic sections, the organism is readily seen either by the periodic acid–Schiff (PAS) stain or by one of the silver stains. Culture identification is not difficult but may take time. A small inoculum usually takes up to 30 days before positive identification is possible. There is no commercially available skin test.

The serodiagnosis of blastomycosis is not well developed. Of the currently available serologic tests, CF and ID tests are more specific but far less sensitive; the recently introduced enzyme immunoassay (EIA) is far more sensitive but much less specific (176). At the present time, a positive serodiagnostic test for blastomycosis does not establish the diagnosis of the disease. Nevertheless, a positive serologic test should serve as a strong indicator that the disease might be present (177). The recently developed *Blastomyces* urinary antigen may represent a step forward.

In most instances, acute pulmonary blastomycosis resolves spontaneously (178). In rapidly progressive disease or in patients coinfected with HIV, especially when air exchange problems develop, AMB to a total of 2 g is the agent of choice (171). Similarly, meningeal involvement requires prompt intravenous AMB treatment. In more chronic or subacute forms of the illness, both pulmonary and disseminated, itraconazole with a dose of 200 mg twice daily has proved to be an excellent drug, replacing ketoconazole (179,180). Itraconazole is highly effective and is far less difficult to administer than ketoconazole (169, 180a).

Coccidioidomycosis

The endemic area in the United States for coccidioidomycosis includes the Southwestern states of Texas, New Mexico, Arizona,

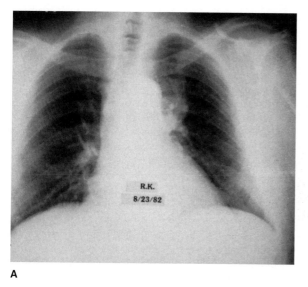

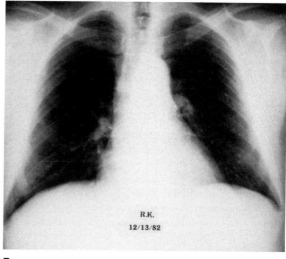

A   B

FIGURE 15-20.   **A:** Active self-limited blastomycosis with left upper-lobe infiltrate. Sputum digestion with 10% potassium hydroxide was positive for *Blastomyces dermatitidis*. **B:** Four months later, the infiltrate had diminished in size. Sputum examination no longer showed the fungus.

Nevada, and California and the adjacent areas of Mexico. In addition, the disease is also found in Central and South America. The organism usually resides several inches below the surface, and following the brief rainy season, rapid growth occurs. Disruption of these microfoci results in the production of the infecting aerosol (181). Because much of the endemic area is dry, dusty desert, wind-borne outbreaks of coccidioidomycosis have been noted (182,183).

Although primary cutaneous inoculations may occur, the usual portal of entry for most patients is the lung. Following inhalation of the arthrospores, germination occurs in the alveoli, leading to the production of giant spherules. Following maturity of the giant spherule, it bursts and releases a large number of endospores that in turn lead to the formation of new giant

spherules. Histopathologically, the inflammatory exudate involves PMN cells as well as macrophages, and the PMN component seldom disappears completely even after the development of cell-mediated immunity (181).

Following the successful development of cell-mediated immunity, the infection is contained. In certain high-risk groups, this localization is not successful, leading to either progressive pulmonary or extrapulmonary disease. Diabetics, immunosuppressed individuals, members of the dark-skinned races—especially African Americans—and men, in general, localize the disease poorly, and these "high-risk" groups contain most patients in whom progressive extrapulmonary spread occurs.

The primary infection is very similar to that seen in other soil-dwelling fungal infections. It is usually an influenzalike

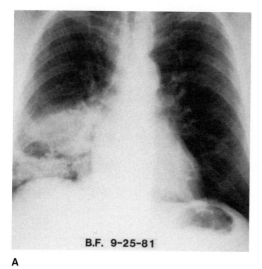

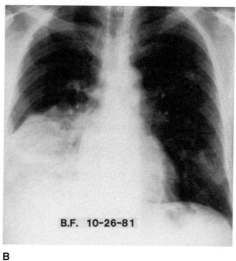

A   B

FIGURE 15-21.   **A:** Extensive right lower-lobe pneumonia due to *Blastomyces dermatitidis*. **B:** One month later, cultures are reported growing the fungus. Note worsening right lower-lobe consolidation and spread of the infection to the left.

illness with a dry cough. Pleuritic chest pain is often severe. Arthralgias and myalgias are common. Erythema nodosum is a frequent accompaniment to these symptoms, leading to the characteristic "valley fever" or "desert rheumatism." Chest roentgenogram may show single or multiple densities with involvement of the hilar nodes.

Resolution of the primary symptoms with clearing of the chest roentgenogram is the most common fate of acute infection. Occasionally, especially in members of the high-risk groups, resolution is slow or incomplete, and progressive pulmonary or extrapulmonary illness may develop. Extrapulmonary spread involves the skin, bones, and visceral organs. In about one third of these patients, the meninges are also involved. Dissemination, when it occurs, is usually a relatively early event. It is uncommon to see stable disease that leads to dissemination after 1 year. Coccidioidomycosis occurring in HIV–positive individuals produces a severe, relentlessly progressive disease with widespread dissemination (184,185).

In an occasional patient, the pulmonary lesions may persist. The characteristic lesion is a thin-walled cavity (see Fig. 15-22). Under observation, the vast majority of these cavities will close. Occasionally, however, the cavities grow and may reach the pleural surface, where they may rupture, leading to a bronchopleural fistula (186). Rarely, progressive pulmonary coccidioidomycosis involves the upper zones, mimicking TB (187).

Although cultural identification is not difficult, extreme care must be taken when working with biologic material suspected of harboring *C. immitis*. In most laboratories, cultural identification no longer takes place, but cultures are processed for the presence of the characteristic exoantigen. In any event, clinicians suspecting coccidioidomycosis should alert the laboratory, to prevent laboratory-borne infections.

Although excellent skin-test antigens exist, skin tests are seldom used to establish the diagnosis of coccidioidomycosis. In disseminated disease, the skin test is frequently negative, whereas in endemic areas, a positive skin test could easily have been acquired prior to the onset of the clinical illness in question.

Unlike the other fungal illnesses, serodiagnostic tests are not only diagnostic but also frequently produce excellent prognostic information (188). Early on, determination of IgM antibodies, either by the tube precipitation or by the latex-agglutination method, is extremely helpful. CF antibodies are readily measured, and a rising titer frequently signifies impending dissemination. The CF test is extremely useful in suspected meningitis, and any CF activity in cerebrospinal fluid (CSF) should be considered proof of disease (186).

Most recently, the more easily performed ID test has replaced the time-honored but cumbersome tests for IgM and IgG antibody. Our common practice is to screen patients with the ID test and then follow up the positive test by CF testing performed at a reference laboratory for prognostic purposes.

Regrettably, coccidioidal infections are much more difficult to deal with than either histoplasmosis or blastomycosis. Some authorities recommend treating stable pulmonary disease in members of the high-risk group. It is thought that a brief course of 0.5 to 1.5 g of AMB might prevent subsequent dissemination. Even though this is common clinical practice, proof of efficacy is lacking. Disseminated disease not involving the meninges can usually be treated with large doses of AMB intravenously (186). Treatment courses of up to 3.5 g are not uncommon. Because AMB is far less effective in the treatment of coccidioidomycosis than it is in either histoplasmosis or blastomycosis, alternative treatments are needed. Ketoconazole, although originally thought to be effective, produces lasting benefit in less than one third of the patients (189). The recently introduced oral triazoles, fluconazole and itraconazole, appear to be a significant improvement over ketoconazole, both in reported lower toxicity and in increased efficacy (190). In a recently completed study, fluconazole and itraconazole were compared in patients with stable, nonmeningeal coccidioidomycosis. Both drugs performed well, with itraconazole showing a slight edge over fluconazole in some subgroups of patients.

The treatment of coccidioidomycosis in HIV–infected patients has been difficult and generally not successful. Most patients are treated initially with AMB until stabilization occurs. Fluconazole has been used successfully in several patients, especially in those who are not critically ill initially, and it is especially helpful in meningeal coccidioidomycosis (191).

Coccidioidal meningitis requires both intravenous and intrathecal administration of AMB. Most authorities recommend

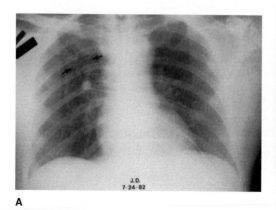
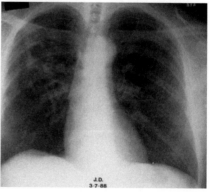

A   B

FIGURE 15-22.   **A**: Residual thin-walled cavity in right upper lobe (*arrows*). Sputum was positive for *Coccidioides immitis*. **B**: After almost 6 years and several courses of therapy with both amphotericin B (AMB) and ketoconazole, the cavity still persisted, and sputum was still intermittently positive for the organism. This patient declined surgery.

long-term intrathecal therapy even after all apparent disease activity has ceased in the CNS. Fluconazole is highly effective in the treatment of meningeal coccidioidomycosis and is now the treatment of choice for stable patients (191). It is important to remember that fluconazole should not be discontinued after apparently successful resolution of coccidioidomycotic meningitis. The risk of relapse, even in not obviously immunocompromised patients, is very high, necessitating lifelong suppressive therapy with fluconazole (192,192a). In the event that surgery is attempted for an enlarging coccidioidal granuloma, some surgeons prefer to perform the surgery with pre- and postoperative administration of AMB. Although this is common practice, proof of efficacy is lacking.

Paracoccidioidomycosis

Paracoccidioides brasiliensis is the most common dimorphic fungus in Latin America. The endemic area stretches from Mexico to Argentina. Occupational exposure to the soil is common, and men are most commonly affected. Interestingly, point-source epidemics have not been reported, perhaps because of the rudimentary health care system in the endemic area.

As with all the other dimorphic fungi, the lung is probably the portal of entry. Inhalation of the infecting particles leads to the production of an area of pneumonitis, with granuloma formation occurring later. The organism may remain localized to the lung or may disseminate to the skin, mucous membranes, or organs with RE cells (193). Commonly, disseminated paracoccidioidomycosis occurs in younger patients in whom the major manifestations of the disease involve the RE system, leading to hepatosplenomegaly and hilar adenopathy. This form of the disease is referred to as the juvenile type. The adult form may present many years after the primary infection. Chronic pulmonary manifestations may still be present, and symptoms are those of low-grade chronic illness. Characteristic lesions involve the oropharynx, lips, and gums and frequently involve the skin, leading to ulcerations. Draining lymph nodes are frequent, and adrenal involvement may occur in up to 50% of the patients.

Recovery of the organism from culture or visualization in KOH–digested specimens is relatively easy. The characteristic "pilot-wheel" appearance of the yeast is diagnostic in sputum or pus.

Ketoconazole in 200 mg doses is currently one of the drugs of choice (194). In cases that are difficult to treat, AMB or sulfadiazine may be used. Itraconazole is also highly effective at doses of 100 mg daily for 6 months (195).

Sporotrichosis

By far, the most common form of sporotrichosis is lymphocutaneous disease. Pulmonary involvement is rare, with perhaps less than 50 cases reported in the literature. The disease appears as a chronic pulmonary infection indistinguishable by symptoms or by roentgen appearance from TB.

Diagnosis is usually by recovery of the fungus from sputum, although a serologic test is also available.

Although many authors recommend AMB as the initial treatment, it is far from certain that it is as effective as in the other fungal illnesses (196,197). The other treatment modality is oral administration of saturated solution of potassium iodide.

There have been numerous patients in whom drug therapy is reported to have failed, but resection of the involved tissues has proved to be curative. The recently introduced oral agent itraconazole has shown considerable success in treating this infection (198).

Cryptococcosis

The encapsulated yeast *Cryptococcus neoformans* is the one truly cosmopolitan fungus. The disease has been reported from all continents, and the fungus is easily recovered from pigeon droppings. Disturbance of the dried pigeon guano produces the infecting aerosol (199).

The portal of entry is the lung. Following inhalation, the yeasts begin to germinate and form large capsules. This polysaccharide capsule is antiphagocytic. Histopathologic examination of tissue confirms the antiphagocytic nature of encapsulated cryptococci: large clumps of the yeast are surrounded by essentially no inflammatory exudate. Despite the ability of the organism to resist phagocytosis and killing by PMN cells, cell-mediated immunity figures prominently in the normal host defenses for dealing with cryptococcal infection. Long before cytotoxic chemotherapy or glucocorticoid administration produced large numbers of ICH, the literature was replete with instances of cryptococcal disease complicating such naturally occurring immunocompromised states as Hodgkin disease. To further emphasize the role of T-cell–mediated protection against the cryptococci, AIDS patients have an unusually high incidence of cryptococcal disease (200,201).

In normal hosts, cryptococcal pulmonary disease is rapidly dealt with by the development of granulomatous inflammatory response and by the clearing of the infiltrate. It appears that the natural history of cryptococcal pulmonary disease in normal hosts is usually completely resolved.

Occasionally, however, even in immunologically competent hosts, the organism gains access to the bloodstream and establishes itself in extrapulmonary tissues, most commonly in the meninges. There is, as yet, no clear understanding of the remarkable tropism of cryptococci for the CNS.

Cryptococcal pulmonary infection in immunocompromised patients, on the other hand, is a severe, potentially life-threatening and almost always disseminated illness. The general rule of thumb should be that anyone who is immunocompromised will develop disseminated disease following pulmonary infection by the fungus (202).

The acute pulmonary infection is relatively uncommon. Symptoms include acute onset of fever followed by chest pain and cough. Frequently, however, patients present with cryptococcal meningitis. In these instances, the inference is that an asymptomatic pulmonary infection has preceded the obvious meningeal disease. Chest radiographic findings are variable but usually consist of patchy areas of consolidation involving the lower lung fields, often bilateral. Some lesions appear as nodules with associated areas of infiltration. Pleural effusions are uncommon.

The cornerstone of diagnosis in pulmonary cryptococcosis is the recovery of the fungus from respiratory secretions. A confounding variable is the frequent presence of cryptococci in patients with other, unrelated pulmonary diseases in whom *Cryptococcus* in respiratory secretions frequently represents colonization only.

Immunodiagnosis of cryptococcal disease is highly refined. Determination of cryptococcal antigen by the latex-agglutination method is highly reproducible, and when the results are corrected for the possible presence of rheumatoid factor, false positives are remarkably infrequent.

The diagnosis of cryptococcal meningitis may be established by visualization of the large encapsulated yeasts on India ink preparation. Moreover, determination of the cryptococcal antigen on all CSF samples will further hasten diagnosis. Cultural recovery of the organism is also relatively simple, and the organism grows in 3 to 5 days.

It is uncertain whether occasional isolates of *Cryptococcus* from sputum in patients with chronic pulmonary disease merit treatment. It was previously thought that acute cryptococcal disease in immunocompetent hosts could be observed with relative safety once the absence of CNS involvement has been documented by a negative lumbar puncture. The reason for this belief was that at the time the original manuscript of Kerkering et al. was published (202), the only available treatment for cryptococcal disease was AMB. Given this option, it seemed reasonable to observe patients because a large majority of immunocompetent patients would likely have recovered without antifungal treatment. Today, with the availability of both fluconazole and itraconazole, it makes more sense to treat such patients to prevent the occasional deterioration or dissemination (203). In the unlikely event that treatment is deemed necessary, AMB 0.7 mg/kg/day should be administered along with 5-fluorocytosine (5-FC), 100 mg/kg/day in four divided doses, for a total of 4 weeks. Meningeal disease should also be treated with a combination of AMB and 5-FC in the same doses for a minimum of 4 weeks in nonimmunocompromised patients, and for 6 weeks or longer in non–HIV–infected immunocompromised individuals (204).

Since the advent of the HIV endemic, cryptococcal meningitis has increased 20-fold in frequency to become the most common fungal complication of HIV infection. It usually occurs late during the course of the HIV infection. With the availability of fluconazole, with its excellent penetration into the CSF, AIDS–related cryptococcal meningitis has frequently been treated with this agent. In a carefully randomized, controlled study, fluconazole performed about as well (but both with a high failure rate) as AMB, making fluconazole appear attractive due to the presence of fewer side effects. Subsequent review of this study, however, identified the fact that one of the reasons for the unacceptably high failure rate was that the dose of AMB used was smaller than it should have been (205). In a second, smaller study from a single institution, larger doses of AMB clearly outperformed fluconazole (206). The observations led to the last multicenter study, which established the new standard for the treatment of cryptococcal meningitis (207). On the basis of these studies, the recent recommendations are to use 0.7 mg/kg/day of AMB with 5-FC at 100 mg/kg/day until the CSF is sterile, followed by 400 mg of fluconazole. In the above-mentioned study, fluconazole was compared with itraconazole after CSF sterilization, not only showing fluconazole to be more effective but also showing that itraconazole may be used in the case of intolerance to fluconazole (207a).

OPPORTUNISTIC FUNGAL INFECTIONS

The preceding subsections describe the normally pathogenic fungi, which, although frequently infecting immunocompromised individuals, are also capable of infecting immunologically normal hosts. The following subsections deal with infections due to opportunistic fungi: *Aspergillus* spp, *Mucorales*, and *Pseudallescheria boydii*.

Aspergillosis

Members of the genus *Aspergillus* are widespread in nature. They are readily recoverable from decomposing organic matter, and the fungi are capable of withstanding extreme environmental conditions. Although well over 100 species of this genus have been identified in human illness, the vast majority of human illness is caused by *Aspergillus fumigatus*. Other *Aspergillus* spp that occasionally cause human disease are *Aspergillus niger*, *Aspergillus terreus*, *Aspergillus flavus*, and *Aspergillus nidulans*. It is thought that initiation of the illness follows inhalation of spores from the fruiting head of the fungus into the lungs.

Aspergillus causes a vast array of human illness, and thus a unitary hypothesis for its pathogenesis is difficult, if not impossible. A form of aspergillosis usually seen in asthmatics, allergic bronchopulmonary aspergillosis, is discussed in Chapter 8, Asthma.

Aspergillomas, or fungus balls, occur in air spaces in the lungs. These air spaces may be the residua of healed TB, other fungal diseases, sarcoidosis, or tumor. The fungi grow within these epithelialized cavities as a mycelial mat, deriving their nourishment from the wall of the cavity. The most frequent symptom is hemoptysis, with occasional life-threatening results (208).

The other major form of aspergillosis involves granulocytopenic hosts. This illness is most frequently seen in patients with hematologic malignancies and leukemias who are undergoing intense cytotoxic chemotherapy. Aspergillosis has also emerged as the most feared complication of organ transplantation, especially bone marrow transplantation.

It appears that in these individuals, the organism gains access to the lungs where, following multiplication in the alveolar spaces, the fungus invades blood vessels. The hallmark of this disease is the appearance of rapidly progressive, large pulmonary infiltrates accompanied by high fever and pleuritic chest pain. Frequently, a great deal of confusion exists because of the appearance of these infiltrates, which closely mimic pulmonary emboli with infarction. Indeed, histopathologically, these lesions are pulmonary infarctions secondary to the growth of the organism within vascular channels. In the vast majority of patients, invasive aspergillosis restricted to the lungs alone is capable of killing the host. Occasionally, however, apparent blood-borne dissemination takes place with dissemination of the organism. The most common sites of dissemination include the brain, the myocardium, and the thyroid gland (209).

Recent reports have described an admixture of the fungus ball and invasive aspergillosis. Most affected patients, in addition to underlying chronic lung disease, had mild immunosuppression, resulting from either diabetes or administration of chronic glucocorticoid therapy. The disease appears as a chronic, low-grade infection in which most of the symptoms are those of the underlying lung disease. Radiographically, there is an aspergilloma with a slowly progressive infiltrate surrounding it. Treatment with AMB appears to slow down the progression of the illness, but it is not yet certain whether the process can be arrested or cured (210). Itraconazole also appears to be effective (211).

Diagnosis of aspergillomas is relatively easy. The chest roentgenogram is characteristic, showing a round, freely movable density within a previously existing cavity. Sputum culture is frequently positive for the fungus, and serologic diagnosis is very helpful because the vast majority of patients with aspergillomas have positive serum precipitins against *Aspergillus.* One must remember, however, that precipitins are species-specific, which accounts for the occasionally negative precipitin tests observed in patients with an obvious aspergilloma.

Disseminated aspergillosis or acute invasive aspergillosis is usually a difficult diagnosis. Although the disease is frequently suspected on clinical grounds alone, attempts to recover the organism from respiratory secretions or bronchoscopic material frequently fail. Occasionally, however, positive cultures can be obtained from respiratory secretions. Although these positive cultures do not definitely establish the etiology of the infection, they frequently serve to point it in the right direction.

Although aspergillosis was originally listed among the agents causing opportunistic infections complicating HIV infection, this fungus was removed from the list soon after because of the paucity of reported patients. Recently, however, an increasing number of patients have been reported with various forms of aspergillosis complicating the late course of HIV infection. Although most reported patients had the usual predisposing conditions to aspergillosis, such as drug-induced neutropenia or glucocorticoid administration, a sizable number of patients did not (212,213). All previously reported forms of aspergillosis have been seen in HIV–infected individuals, and two new forms have been added. These new forms are obstructing endobronchial aspergillosis and pseudomembranous aspergillosis.

Most authorities consider the diagnosis of aspergillosis definite only when the organism is seen invading host tissues. This usually requires either bronchoscopic biopsy or open-lung biopsy. Blood cultures are usually sterile.

Clinical and roentgenographic features of the infection are relatively nondiagnostic. The roentgenogram may show single or multiple areas of rapidly advancing pulmonary infiltrates, which do not cavitate until the granulocyte count begins to return toward normal. Since the availability of HRCT scans, the appearance of the "halo" sign may be seen early during the infection.

Drug therapy is not indicated for the treatment of aspergillomas because it universally fails. In patients with life-threatening hemoptysis, surgery is the only reasonable choice of therapy. Unfortunately, the majority of such patients have severely compromised pulmonary function, rendering surgery difficult if not impossible (208).

Treatment of acute invasive aspergillosis is difficult. AMB is the drug of choice, and the recommendation is that early and large doses of the agent be used. Recently, especially in institutions dealing with large numbers of patients with hematologic malignancies, the custom has been to begin AMB treatment after 3 to 7 days of a febrile course not responding to routine antibiotic treatment (214). Although definite proof of the success of this regimen is still lacking, it appears to have significantly reduced the incidence of invasive aspergillosis at postmortem examination. More recently, the role of liposomal AMB has been better defined. These preparations are as effective as AMB but far less toxic and are now the treatment of choice.

The recently introduced triazole, itraconazole, has been used in some patients with different forms of aspergillosis with good results. Although it is uncertain whether rapidly progressive invasive disease is likely to improve, it appears that the more chronic indolent forms of aspergillosis infections can be treated with itraconazole and can be expected to respond (211). More recently, voriconazole has been introduced, which shows great promise. It is easy to administer and may be used orally. Its effect appears similar to liposomal AMB.

Mucormycosis

Members of the genus *Mucorales,* like *Aspergillus,* are widespread in nature. Although much less is known and understood about mucormycosis than about aspergillosis, it appears to be quite similar to aspergillosis. The organism has a high affinity for invasion of blood vessels and will frequently produce extensive tissue necrosis because of occlusion of blood vessels.

Clinical manifestations are very similar to those of aspergillosis, as is the chest roentgenogram, which usually shows multiple, large pulmonary infiltrates extending to the pleura, mimicking pulmonary embolization with infarction. The diagnosis requires identifying the invading broad, nonseptate fungus either in histopathologic material or by culture. There are no immunologic tests available. Blood culture and sputum culture are seldom, if ever, positive.

Treatment of mucormycosis is similar to that of aspergillosis and requires large doses of AMB. Early starting of the treatment is essential, and the best results have been in patients in whom treatment was started very early in the course of the illness.

Pseudallescheriasis

The organism *P. boydii* is an occasionally identified saprophyte. Clinically and histopathologically, the illness is indistinguishable from invasive aspergillosis. Cultural identification is extremely important because it appears that miconazole, rather than AMB, is the drug of choice in this illness.

REFERENCES

1. Couch RB. The common cold: control? *J Infect Dis* 1984;150: 167–173.
2. Niederman MS, McCombs J, Unger A, et al. The cost of treating community-acquired pneumonia. *Clin Ther* 1998;20:820–837.
3. Vincent JL, Behari DJ, Sueter PM, et al. The prevalence of nosocomial infection in intensive care units in Europe. *JAMA* 1995; 274:634–644.
4. Garibaldi RA. Epidemiology of community-acquired respiratory tract infections in adults: incidence, etiology, and impact. *Am J Med* 1985;78[Suppl 6B]:32–37.
5. American Lung Association. *Lung disease data 1994.* New York: American Lung Association, 1994:37–42.
6. Schneider EL. Infectious diseases in the elderly. *Ann Intern Med* 1983;98:395–400.
7. Kaplan V, Clermont G, Griffin MF, et al. Pneumonia: still the old man's friend? *Arch Intern Med* 2003;163:317–323.
8. Niederman MS. Nosocomial pneumonia in the elderly patient: chronic care facility and hospital considerations. *Clin Chest Med* 1993;14:479–490.
9. Gross PA, Van Antwerpen C. Nosocomial infections and hospital deaths: a case-control study. *Am J Med* 1983;75:658–662.
10. Emori TG, Banerjee SN, Culver DH, et al. Nosocomial infections in elderly patients in the United States, 1986–1990. *Am J Med* 1991;91(3):289S–293S.

11. Chastre J, Trouillet JL, Vuagnat A, et al. Nosocomial pneumonia in patients with acute respiratory distress syndrome. *Am J Respir Crit Care Med* 1998;157:1165–1172.

12. Seidenfeld JJ, Pohl DF, Bell RD, et al. Incidence, site, and outcome of infections in patients with the adult respiratory distress syndrome. *Am Rev Respir Dis* 1986;134:12–16.

13. Heyland DK, Cook DJ, Griffith L, Brun-Buisson SP, et al., the Canadian Critical Trials Group. The attributable morbidity and mortality of ventilator-associated pneumonia in the critically ill patient. *Am J Respir Crit Care Med* 1999;159:1249–1256.

14. Fagon JY, Chastre J, Vaugnat A, et al. Nosocomial pneumonia and mortality among patients in intensive care units. *JAMA* 1996;275:866–869.

15. Kronenberg RS. Chronic bronchitis: significant infection or social annoyance? *Semin Respir Infect* 1988;3:1–4.

16. Niederman MS. Antibiotic therapy of exacerbations of chronic bronchitis. *Semin respir Infect* 2000;15:59–70.

17. Niederman MS. Chronic obstructive pulmonary disease (COPD): The role of infection. *Chest* 1997;112(6):301S–302S.

18. Ball P, Harris JM, Lowson D, et al. Acute infective exacerbations of chronic bronchitis. *Q J Med* 1995;88:61–68.

19. Penn RL, George RB. Respiratory infections. In: Matthay RA, Light RM, George RB, eds. *Chest medicine*, 1st ed. New York: Churchill Livingstone, 1983:403–479.

20. American Thoracic Society. Control of tuberculosis in the United States. *Am Rev Respir Dis* 1992;146:1623–1633.

21. Barker AF, Bardana EJ. Bronchiectasis: update of an orphan disease. *Am Rev Respir Dis* 1988;137:969–978.

22. Farr BM, Kaiser DL, Harrison BDW, et al. Prediction of microbial aetiology at admission to hospital for pneumonia from presenting clinical features. *Thorax* 1989;44:1031–1035.

23. Niederman MS. Gram-negative colonization of the respiratory tract: pathogenesis and clinical consequences. *Semin Respir Infect* 1990;5:173–184.

24. Johanson WG, Pierce AK, Sanford JP. Changing pharyngeal flora of hospitalized patients: emergence of gram-negative bacilli. *N Engl J Med* 1969;281:1137–1140.

25. Palmer LB. Bacterial colonization: pathogenesis and clinical significance. *Clin Chest Med* 1987;8:455–466.

26. Laurenzi GA, Potter RT, Kass EH. Bacteriologic flora of the lower respiratory tract. *N Engl J Med* 1961;265:1273–1278.

27. Niederman MS, Craven D. Devising strategies for nosocomial pneumonia prevention: should we ignore the stomach? *Clin Infect Dis* 1997;24:320–323.

28. Niederman MS, Mantovani R, Schoch P, et al. Patterns and routes of tracheobronchial colonization in mechanically ventilated patients: the role of nutritional status in colonization of the lower airway by *Pseudomonas* species. *Chest* 1989;95:155–161.

29. Anzueto A, Niederman MS. Diagnosis and treatment of rhinovirus respiratory infections. *Chest* 2003;123:1664–1672.

30. Gwaltney JM. The common cold: epidemiology and strategies for prevention. In: Sande MA, Hudson LD, Root RK, eds. *Respiratory infections*. New York: Churchill Livingstone, 1986:139–147.

31. Blake GH, Abell TD, Stanley WG. Cigarette smoking and upper respiratory infection among recruits in basic combat training. *Ann Intern Med* 1988;109:198–202.

32. Dick EC, Jennings LC, Mink KA. Aerosol transmission of colds. *J Infect Dis* 1987;156:442–448.

33. Grimm W, Muller HH. A randomized controlled trial of the effect of fluid extract of Echinacea purpurea on the incidence and severity of colds and respiratory infections. *Am J Med* 1999;106:138–143.

34. Macknin ML, Piedmonte M, Claendine C, et al. Zinc gluconate lozenges for treating the common cold in children: a randomized controlled trial. *JAMA* 1998;279:1962–1967.

35. Benninger MS, Ferguson BJ, Hadley JA, et al. Adult chronic rhinosinusitis: definitions, diagnosis, epidemiology and pathophysiology. *Otolaryngol Head Neck Surg* 2003;129(3 Suppl):S1–32.

36. Evans FO, Syndor JB, Moore WEC, et al. Sinusitis of the maxillary antrum. *N Engl J Med* 1975;293:735–739.

37. Williams JW, Simel DL. Does this patient have sinusitis? Diagnosing acute sinusitis by history and physical examination. *JAMA* 1993;270:1242–1246.

38. MayoSmith MF, Hirsch PJ, Wodzinski SF, et al. Acute epiglottitis in adults: an eight-year experience in the state of Rhode Island. *N Engl J Med* 1986;314:1133–1139.

39. Baker AS, Eavey RD. Adult supraglottitis (epiglottitis). *N Engl J Med* 1986;314:1185–1186.

40. Loos GD. Pharyngitis, croup and epiglottitis. *Prim Care* 1990;17:335–345.

41. Solomon P, Weisbrod M, Irish JC, et al. Adult epiglottitis: the Toronto Hospital experience. *J Otolaryngol* 1998;27:332–336.

42. Ashcraft CK, Steele RW. Epiglottitis: a pediatric emergency. *J Respir Dis* 1988;9(7):48–60.

43. Mayo-Smith MF, Spinale JW, Donsky CJ, et al. Acute epiglottitis: An 18-year experience in Rhode Island. *Chest* 1995;108:1640–1647.

44. Rothrock SG, Pignatiello GA, Howard RA. Radiologic diagnosis of epiglottitis: objective criteria for all ages. *Ann Emerg Med* 1990;19:978–982.

45. Hall CB, McBride JT. Upper respiratory tract infections: the common cold, pharyngitis, croup, bacterial tracheitis and epiglottitis. In: Pennington JE, ed. *Respiratory infections: diagnosis and management*. New York: Raven Press, 1988:97–118.

46. Centor RM, Meier FA. Throat cultures and rapid tests for diagnosis of group A streptococcal pharyngitis. *Ann Intern Med* 1986;105:892–899.

47. Balter MS, LaForge J, Low DE, Mandell L, Grossman RF, and the Chronic Bronchitis Working Group. Canadian guidelines for the management of acute exacerbations of chronic bronchits. *Can Respir J* 2003; 10[Suppl B]:3B–32B.

48. Gonzales R, Steiner JF, Lum A, et al. Decreasing antibiotic use in ambulatory practice: impact of a multidimensional intervention on the treatment of uncomplicated bronchitis in adults. *JAMA* 1999;281:1512–1519.

49. Schroeckenstein DC, Busse WW. Viral bronchitis in childhood: relationship to asthma and obstructive lung disease. *Semin Respir Infect* 1988;3:40–48.

50. Anthonisen NR, Manfreda J, Warren CPW, et al. Antibiotic therapy in exacerbations of chronic obstructive pulmonary disease. *Ann Intern Med* 1987;106:196–204.

51. Fagon JY, Chastre J, Trouillet JL, et al. Characterization of distal bronchial microflora during acute exacerbation of chronic bronchitis: use of the protected specimen brush technique in 54 mechanically ventilated patients. *Am Rev Respir Dis* 1990;142:1004–1008.

52. Niederman MS. Does the presence of antibodies justify the use of antibiotics in exacerbations of chronic bronchitis? *Am J Respir Crit Care Med* 2004;169:434–435.

53. Murphy T, Sethi S, Niederman M. The role of bacteria in exacerbations of COPD (a constructive View). *Chest* 2000;118:204–209.

54. Saint S, Bent S, Vittinghoff E, et al. Antibiotics in chronic obstructive pulmonary disease exacerbations: a meta-analysis. *JAMA* 1995;273:957–960.

55. Nseir S, Di Pompeo C, Pronnier P, et al. Nosocomial tracheobronchitis in mechanically ventilated patients: incidence, aetiology and outcome. *Eur Respir J* 2002;20:1483–1489.

56. Ryu JH, Myers JL, Swensen SJ. Bronchiolar disorders. *Am J Respir Crit Care Med.* 2003;168:1277–1292.

57. Epler GR, Colby TV, McLoud TC, et al. Bronchiolitis obliterans organizing pneumonia. *N Engl J Med* 1985;312:152–158.

58. Cox NJ, Fukuda K. Influenza. *Infect Dis Clin North Am* 1998;12:27–38.

59. Mathur U, Bentley DW, Hall CB. Concurrent respiratory syncytial virus and influenza A infections in the institutionalized elderly and chronically ill. *Ann Intern Med* 1980;93:49–52.

60. Gross PA, Rodstein M, LaMontagne JR, et al. Epidemiology of acute respiratory illness during an influenza outbreak in a nursing home: a prospective study. *Arch Intern Med* 1988;148:559–561.

61. Hayden FG, Gwaltney JM. Viral infections. In: Murray JF, Nadel JA, eds. *Textbook of respiratory medicine*. Philadelphia: WB Saunders, 1988:769–778.

62. Van Voris LP, Newell PM. Antivirals for the chemoprophylaxis and treatment of influenza. *Semin Respir Infect* 1992;7:61–70.

63. Stockley RA. Bronchiectasis—new therapeutic approaches based on pathogenesis. *Clin Chest Med* 1987;8:481–494.

64. Huxley EJ, Viroslav J, Gray WR, et al. Pharyngeal aspiration in normal subjects and patients with depressed consciousness. *Am J Med* 1978;64:565–568.

65. Beachey EH. Bacterial adherence: adhesin-receptor interactions mediating the attachment of bacteria to mucosal surfaces. *J Infect Dis* 1981;143:325–345.

66. Niederman MS, Merrill WW, Ferranti RD, et al. Nutritional status and bacterial binding in the lower respiratory tract in patients with chronic tracheostomy. *Ann Intern Med* 1984;100:795–800.

67. Todd TRJ, Franklin A, Mankinen-Irvin P, et al. Augmented bacterial adherence to tracheal epithelial cells is associated with gram-negative pneumonia in an intensive care unit population. *Am Rev Respir Dis* 1989;140:1585–1589.

68. Johanson WG Jr, Pierce AK, Sanford JP, et al. Nosocomial respiratory infections with gram-negative bacilli: the significance of colonization of the respiratory tract. *Ann Intern Med* 1972;77:701–706.

69. Toews GB. Nosocomial pneumonia. *Clin Chest Med* 1987;8:467–479.

70. Niederman MS, Ahmed QA. Community-acquired pneumonia in elderly patients. *Clin Geriatr Med.* 2003;19:101–120.

71. Niederman MS, Mandell LA, Anzueto A, et al. Guidelines for the management of adults with community-acquired lower respiratory tract infections: Diagnosis, assessment of severity, antimicrobial therapy and prevention. *Am J Respir Crit Care Med* 2001;163:1730–1754.

72. Mandell LA, Bartlett JG, Dowell SF, et al, Infectious Diseases Society of America. Update of practice guidelines for the management of community-acquired pneumonia in immunocompetent adults. *Clin Infect Dis* 2003;37:1405–1433.

73. MacFarlane JT, Miller AC, Smith WH, et al. Comparative radiographic features of community-acquired Legionnaires' disease, pneumococcal pneumonia, mycoplasma pneumonia, and psittacosis. *Thorax* 1984;39:28–33.

74. Ewig S, Ruiz M, Mensa J, et al. Severe community-acquired pneumonia: assessment of severity criteria. *Am J Respir Crit Care Med* 1998;158:1102–1108.

75. Ruiz M, Ewig S, Marcos MA, et al. Etiology of community-acquired pneumonia: impact of age, comorbidity, and severity. *Am J Respir Crit Care Med* 1999;160:397–405.

76. Farr BM, Sloman AJ, Fisch MJ. Predicting death in patients hospitalized for community-acquired pneumonia. *Ann Intern Med* 1991;115:428–436.

77. Pachon J, Prados MD, Capote F, et al. Severe community-acquired pneumonia. Etiology, prognosis, and treatment. *Am Rev Respir Dis* 1990;142:369–373.

78. Porath A, Schlaeffer F, Lieberman D. The epidemiology of community-acquired pneumonia among hospitalized adults. *J Infect* 1997;34:41–48.

79. Ramirez JA, Bordon J. Earlly switch from intravenous to oral antibiotics in hospitalized patients with bacteremic community-acquired *Streptococcus pneumoniae* pneumonia. *Arch Intern Med* 2001;161:848–850.

80. Johnson CC, Finegold SM. Pyogenic bacterial pneumonia, lung abscess, and empyema. In: Murray JF, Nadel JA, eds. *Textbook of respiratory medicine.* Philadelphia: WB Saunders, 1988: 803–841.

81. Ort S, Ryan JL, Barden G, et al. Pneumococcal pneumonia in hospitalized patients: clinical and radiological presentations. *JAMA* 1983;249:214–218.

82. Plouffe JF, Breiman RF, Facklam RR, Franklin County Pneumonia Study Group. Bacteremia with *Streptococcus pneumoniae.* Implications for therapy and prevention. *JAMA* 1996;275:194–198.

83. Feikin DR, Schuchat A, Kolczak M, et al. Mortality from invasive pneumococcal pneumonia in the era of antibiotic resistance, 1995–1997. *Am J Public Health* 2000;90:223–229.

84. Jay SJ, Johanson WG, Pierce AK. The radiographic resolution of *Streptococcus pneumoniae* pneumonia. *N Engl J Med* 1975;293: 798–801.

85. Austrian R. A reassessment of pneumococcal vaccine. *N Engl J Med* 1984;310:651–653.

86. Bassin A, Niederman MS. Strategies for prevention of community-acquired pneumonia. *Semin Respir Infect* 1998;13: 68–78.

87. Centers for Disease Control and Prevention. Prevention of pneumococcal disease: recommendations of the Advisory Committee on Immunization Practice. *MMWR* 1997;46(RR-8):1–24.

88. Brenner DJ. Classification of the legionellae. *Semin Respir Infect* 1987;4:190–205.

89. Stout JE, Yu VL. Legionellosis. *N Engl J Med* 1997;337:682–687.

90. Yu VL, Kroboth FJ, Shonnard J. Legionnaires' disease: new clinical perspective from a prospective pneumonia study. *Am J Med* 1982;73:357–361.

91. Carratala J, Gudiol F, Pallares R, et al. Risk factors for nosocomial *Legionella pneumophila* pneumonia. *Am J Respir Crit Care Med* 1994;149:625–629.

92. Plouffe JF, File TM Jr, Breiman RF, et al, Community Based Pneumonia Incidence Study Group. Reevaluation of the definition of Legionnaires' disease: use of the urinary antigen assay. *Clin Infect Dis* 1995;20:1286–1291.

93. Edelstein PH. Antimicrobial chemotherapy for Legionnaires disease: time for a change. *Ann Intern Med* 1998;129:328–330.

94. Bartlett JG, Gorbach SL. The triple threat of aspiration pneumonia. *Chest* 1975;68:560–566.

95. El –Solh AA, Pietrantoni C, Bhat A, et al. Microbiology of severe aspiration pneumonia in institutionalized elderly. *Am J Respir Crit Care Med* 2003;167:1650–1654.

96. Mier L, Dreyfuss D, Darchy B, et al. Is penicillin G an adequate initial treatment for aspiration pneumonia? A prospective evaluation using a protected specimen brush and quantitative cultures. *Intensive Care Med* 1993;19:279–284.

97. Bartlett JG, Finegold SM. Anaerobic infections of the lung and pleural space. *Am Rev Respir Dis* 1974;110:56–77.

98. Levison ME, Mangura CT, Lorber B, et al. Clindamycin compared with penicillin for the treatment of anaerobic lung abscess. *Ann Intern Med* 1983;98:466–471.

99. Musher DM, Kubitschek KR, Crennan J, et al. Pneumonia and acute febrile tracheobronchitis due to *Haemophilus influenzae.* *Ann Intern Med* 1983;99:444–450.

100. Smith AL. *Haemophilus influenzae* pneumonia. In: Pennington JE, ed. *Respiratory infections: diagnosis and management.* New York: Raven Press, 1988:364–380.

101. Cassell GH, Cole BC. Mycoplasmas as agents of human disease. *N Engl J Med* 1981;304:80–89.

102. Tuazon CU, Murray HW. Atypical pneumonias. In: Pennington JE, ed. *Respiratory infections: diagnosis and management.* New York: Raven Press, 1988:341–363.

103. Cotton EM, Strampfer MJ, Cunha BA. *Legionella* and mycoplasma pneumonias—a community hospital experience with atypical pneumonias. *Clin Chest Med* 1987;8:441–453.

104. Grayston JT, Kuo CC, Wang SP, et al. A new *Chlamydia psittaci* strain, TWAR, isolated in acute respiratory tract infections. *N Engl J Med* 1986;315:161–168.

105. Troy CJ, Peeling RW, Ellis AG, et al. *Chlamydia pneumoniae* as a new source of infectious outbreaks in nursing homes. *JAMA* 1997;277:1214–1218.

106. Pierce AK, Sanford JP. Aerobic gram-negative bacillary pneumonias. *Am Rev Respir Dis* 1974;110:647–658.

107. Meyer KS, Urban C, Eagan JA, et al. Nosocomial outbreak of *Klebsiella* infection resistant to late-generation cephalosporins. *Ann Intern Med* 1993;119:353–358.

108. Kaye MG, Fox MJ, Bartlett JG, et al. The clinical spectrum of *Staphylococcus aureus* pulmonary infection. *Chest* 1990;97: 788–792.

109. Rose RM, Pinkston P, O'Donnell C, et al. Viral infections of the lower respiratory tract. *Clin Chest Med* 1987;8:405–418.

110. Shellhammer J, Gill VJ, Quinn TC, et al. The laboratory evaluation of opportunistic pulmonary infections. *Ann Intern Med* 1996;124:585–599.

111. Britt MR, Schleupner CJ, Matsumiya S. Severity of underlying disease as a predictor of nosocomial infection. *JAMA* 1978;239: 1047–1051.

112. Niederman MS, Fein AM. Sepsis syndrome, the adult respiratory distress syndrome, and nosocomial pneumonia: a common clinical sequence. *Clin Chest Med* 1990;11:633–656.

113. Mandell LA, Marrie TJ, Niederman MS. Initial antimicrobial treatment of hospital acquired pneumonia in adults: a conference report. *Can J Infect Dis* 1993;4:317–321.

114. Campbell GD, Niederman MS, Broughton WA, et al. Hospital-acquired pneumonia in adults: diagnosis, assessment of severity, initial antimicrobial therapy, and preventative strategies: A consensus statement. *Am J Respir Crit Care Med* 1996;153:1711–1725.

115. Andrews CP, Coalson JJ, Johanson WG Jr. Diagnosis of nosocomial bacterial pneumonia in acute diffuse lung injury. *Chest* 1981;80:254–258.

116. Niederman MS, Torres A, Summer W. Invasive diagnostic testing is not needed routinely to manage suspected VAP. *Am J Respir Crit Care Med* 1994;150:565–569.

117. Luna CM, Vujacich P, Niederman M, et al. Impact of bronchoalveolar lavage data on the therapy and outcome of ventilator-associated pneumonia. *Chest* 1997;111:676–685.

118. Rodrigues J, Niederman MS, Fein AM, et al. Nonresolving pneumonia in steroid-treated patients with obstructive lung disease. *Am J Med* 1992;93:29–34.

119. Schulert GS, Feltman H, Rabin SD, et al. Secretion of the toxin ExoU is a marker for highly virulent *Pseudomonas aeruginosa* isolates obtained from patients with hospital-acquired pneumonia. *J Infect Dis* 2003;188:1695–1706.

120. Rosenow EC, Wilson WR, Cockerill FR. Pulmonary disease in the immunocompromised host. *Mayo Clin Proc* 1985;60:473–487.

121. Beck JM, Rosen MJ, Peavy HH. Pulmonary complications of HIV infection. Report of the Fourth NHLBI Workshop. *Am J Respir Crit Care Med* 2001;164:2120–2126.

122. Wolff AJ, O'Donnell AE. Pulmonary manifestations of HIV infection in the era of highly active antiretroviral therapy. *Chest* 2001;120:1888–1893.

123. Hibberd PL, Rubin RH. Renal transplantation and related infections. *Semin Respir Infect* 1993;8:216–224.

124. Levine SJ, White DA. *Pneumocystis carinii*. *Clin Chest Med* 1988; 9:395–423.

125. Conte JE, Hollander H, Golden JA. Inhaled or reduced-dose intravenous pentamidine for *Pneumocystis carinii* pneumonia: a pilot study. *Ann Intern Med* 1987;107:495–498.

126. Allegra CJ, Chabner BA, Tuazon CU, et al. Trimetrexate for the treatment of *Pneumocystis carinii* pneumonia in patients with the acquired immunodeficiency syndrome. *N Engl J Med* 1987; 317:978–985.

127. McFadden JP, Price RC, Eastwood HD, et al. Raised respiratory rate in elderly patients: a valuable physical sign. *Br Med J* 1982; 1:626–627.

128. Fein AM, Feinsilver SH, Niederman MS, et al. When pneumonia doesn't get better. *Clin Chest Med* 1987;8:529–541.

129. Tobin MJ. Diagnosis of pneumonia: techniques and problems. *Clin Chest Med* 1987;8:513–527.

130. Stover DE, Zaman MB, Hajdu SI, et al. Bronchoalveolar lavage in the diagnosis of diffuse pulmonary infiltrates in the immunosuppressed host. *Ann Intern Med* 1984;101:1–7.

131. Chastre J, Fagon JY, Bornet M, et al. Diagnosis of nosocomial bacterial pneumonia in intubated patients undergoing ventilation: comparison of the usefulness of bronchoalveolar lavage and the protected specimen brush. *Am J Med* 1988;85:499–506.

132. Atlas SJ, Benzer TI, Borowsky LH, et al. Safely increasing the proportion of patients with community-acquired pneumonia treated as outpatients: an interventional trial. *Arch Intern Med* 1998;158:1350–1356.

133. Graham WGB, Bradley DA. Efficacy of chest physiotherapy and intermittent positive-pressure breathing in the resolution of pneumonia. *N Engl J Med* 1978;299:624–627.

134. Wanner A, Rao A. Clinical indications for and effects of bland, mucolytic and antimicrobial aerosols. *Am Rev Respir Dis* 1980; 122:79–87.

135. de Boisblanc BP, Castro M, Everret B, et al. Effect of air-supported, continuous, postural oscillation on the risk of early ICU pneumonia in nontraumatic critical illness. *Chest* 1993;103:1543–1547.

136. Havlir DV, Barnes PF. Tuberculosis in patients with human immunodeficiency virus infection. *N Engl J Med* 1999;340:367–373.

137. Hirschtick RE, Glassroth J. Multidrug-resistant tuberculosis: epidemiology, treatment, and prevention. *Clin Pulm Med* 1994;1: 78–83.

138. Small PM, Shafer RW, Hopewell PC, et al. Exogenous reinfection with multidrug-resistant *Mycobacterium tuberculosis* in patients with advanced HIV infection. *N Engl J Med* 1993;328: 1137–1144.

139. Small PM, Fujiwara PI. Management of tuberculosis in the United States. *N Engl J Med* 2001;345:189–200.

140. Daley CL, Small PM, Schecter GM, et al. An outbreak of tuberculosis with accelerated progression among persons infected with human immunodeficiency virus: an analysis using restriction-fragment-length polymorphisms. *N Engl J Med* 1992;326: 231–235.

141. Rizzi EB, Schinina V, Palmieri F, et al. Radiological patterns in HIV-associated pulmonary tuberculosis: Comparison between HAART-treated and non-HAART–treated patients. *Clin Radiol* 2003;58:469–473.

142. Alvarez S, Shell C, Berk SL. Pulmonary tuberculosis in elderly men. *Am J Med* 1987;82:602–606.

143. American Thoracic Society. Targeted tuberculin testing and treatment of latent tuberculosis infection. *Am J Respir Crit Care Med.* 2000;161:S221–S247.

144. American Thoracic Society. Mycobacteriosis and the acquired immunodeficiency syndrome. *Am Rev Respir Dis* 1987;136:492–496.

145. Woodring JH, Vandiviere HM, Fried AM, et al. Update: the radiographic features of pulmonary tuberculosis. *Am J Roentgenol* 1986;497–506.

146. American Thoracic Society. Diagnostic standards and classification of tuberculosis. *Am Rev Respir Dis* 1990;142:725–735.

147. Grosset J. Bacteriologic basis of short-course chemotherapy for tuberculosis. *Clin Chest Med* 1980;1:231–241.

148. Nardell EA. Beyond four drugs: public health policy and the treatment of the individual patient with tuberculosis. *Am Rev Respir Dis* 1993;148:2–5.

149. Woods GL, Washington JA. Mycobacteria other than *Mycobacterium tuberculosis*: review of microbiologic and clinical aspects. *Rev Infect Dis* 1987;9:275–294.

150. Tellis CJ. Bombenger. Pulmonary disease caused by nontuberculous mycobacteria. In: Pennington JE, ed. *Respiratory infections: diagnosis and management*. New York: Raven Press, 1988:544–569.

151. American Thoracic Society. Diagnosis and treatment of disease caused by nontuberculous mycobacteria. *Am J Respir Crit Care Med* 1997;156:S1–S25.

152. Goodwin RA, DesPrez RM. Histoplasmosis: state of the art. *Am Rev Respir Dis* 1978;117:929–956.

153. Goodwin RA, Shapiro JL, Thurman GH, et al. Disseminated histoplasmosis: clinical and pathologic correlations. *Medicine* 1980;59:1–33.

154. Goodwin RA, Loyd JE, DesPrez RM. Histoplasmosis in normal hosts. *Medicine* 1981;60:231–266.

155. Davies SF, Sarosi GA. Acute cavitary histoplasmosis. *Chest* 1978; 73:103–105.

156. Goodwin RA, Owens FT, Snell JD, et al. Chronic pulmonary histoplasmosis. *Medicine* 1976;55:413–452.

157. Loyd JE, Tillman BF, Atkinson JB, et al. Mediastinal fibrosis complicating histoplasmosis. *Medicine* 1988;67:295–310.

158. Davies SF, McKenna RW, Sarosi GA. Trephine biopsy of the bone marrow in disseminated histoplasmosis. *Am J Med* 1979;67: 617–622.

159. Sarosi GA, Voth DW, Dahl BA, et al, A Center for Disease Control Cooperative Mycose Study. Disseminated histoplasmosis: results of long term follow-up. *Ann Intern Med* 1971;75:511–516.

160. Wheat LJ, Slama TG, Norton JA, et al. Risk factors for disseminated or fatal histoplasmosis. *Ann Intern Med* 1982;96:159–163.

161. Davies SF, Khan M, Sarosi GA. Disseminated histoplasmosis in immunologically suppressed patients. *Am J Med* 1978;64:94–100.

162. Johnson PC, Khardori N, Najjar AF, et al. Progressive disseminated histoplasmosis in patients with acquired immunodeficiency syndrome. *Am J Med* 1988;85:152–158.

163. Wheat LJ, Connolly-Stringfield PA, Baker RL, et al. Disseminated histoplasmosis in the acquired immune deficiency syndrome: clinical findings, diagnosis and review of the literature. *Medicine (Baltimore)* 1990;69:361–374.

164. Mandell W, Goldberg DM, Neu HC. Histoplasmosis in patients with the acquired immune deficiency syndrome. *Am J Med* 1986; 81:974–978.

165. Sarosi GA, Johnson PC. Disseminated histoplasmosis in patients infected with human immunodeficiency virus. *Clin Infect Dis* 1992;14[Suppl 1]:60–67.

166. Davies SF. Serodiagnosis of histoplasmosis. *Semin Respir Infect* 1986;1:9–15.

167. Wheat LJ, Kohler RB, Tewari RP. Diagnosis of disseminated histoplasmosis by detection of *Histoplasma capsulatum* antigen in serum and urine specimens. *N Engl J Med* 1986;314:83–88.

168. Wheat LJ, Connolly-Stringfield P, Kohler RB, et al. *Histoplasma capsulatum* polysaccharide antigen detection in diagnosis and management of disseminated histoplasmosis in patients with acquired immunodeficiency syndrome. *Am J Med* 1989;87: 396–400.

169. Dismukes WE, Bradsher RW Jr, Cloud GC, et al. Itraconazole therapy for blastomycosis and histoplasmosis: NIAID Mycosis Study Group. *Am J Med* 1992;93:489–497.

170. Parker JD, Sarosi GA, Doto IL, et al. A National Communicable Disease Center Cooperative Mycoses Study. Treatment of chronic pulmonary histoplasmosis. *N Engl J Med* 1970;283:225–229.

170a. Wheat LJ, Sarosi GA, McKinsey D, et al. Practice guidelines for the management of patients with histoplasmosis. *Clin Infect Dis* 2000;30:688–695.

171. Sarosi GA, Davies SF. Blastomycosis: state of the art. *Am Rev Respir Dis* 1979;120:911–938.

172. Klein BS, Vergeront JM, Weeks RJ, et al. Isolation of *Blastomyces dermatitidis* in soil associated with a large outbreak of blastomycosis in Wisconsin. *N Engl J Med* 1986;314:529–534.

173. Sarosi GA, Hammerman KJ, Tosh FE, et al. Clinical features of acute pulmonary blastomycosis. *N Engl J Med* 1974;290:540–543.

174. Pappas PG, Pottage JC, Powderly WG, et al. Blastomycosis in patients with the acquired immunodeficiency syndrome. *Ann Intern Med* 1992;116:847–853.

175. Sanders JS, Sarosi GA, Nollet DJ, et al. Exfoliative cytology in the rapid diagnosis of pulmonary blastomycosis. *Chest* 1977;72:193–196.

176. Klein BS, Vergeront JM, Kaufman L, et al. Serological tests for blastomycosis: assessments during a large point source outbreak in Wisconsin. *J Infect Dis* 1987;155:262–268.

177. Bradsher RW, Pappas PG. Detection of specific antibodies in human blastomycosis by enzyme immunoassay. *South Med J* 1995;88(12):1256–1259.

178. Sarosi GA, Davies SF, Phillips JR. Self-limited blastomycosis: a report of 39 cases. *Semin Respir Infect* 1986;1:40–44.

179. National Institute of Allergy and Infectious Diseases Mycoses Study Group. Treatment of blastomycosis and histoplasmosis with ketoconazole. *Ann Intern Med* 1985;103:861–872.

180. Bradsher RW, Rice DC, Abernathy RS. Ketoconazole therapy for endemic blastomycosis. *Ann Intern Med* 1985;103:872–879.

180a. Chapman SW, Bradsher RW Jr, Campbell GD Jr, et al. Practice guidelines for the management of patients with blastomycosis. *Clin Infect Dis* 2000;30:679–683.

181. Drutz DJ, Catanzaro A. Coccidioidomycosis: state of the art. Part I. *Am Rev Respir Dis* 1978;117:559–585.

182. Galgiani JN. Coccidioidomycosis. *West J Med* 1993;159:153–171.

183. Stevens DA. Coccidioidomycosis. *N Engl J Med* 1995;332:1077–1082.

184. Fish DG, Ampel NM, Galgiani JN, et al. Coccidioidomycosis during human immunodeficiency virus infection. A review of 77 patients. *Medicine* 1990;69:384–391.

185. Singh VR, Smith DK, Lawrence J, et al. Coccidioidomycosis in patients infected with human immunodeficiency virus: review of 91 cases from a single institution. *Clin Infect Dis* 1996;23:563–568.

186. Drutz DJ, Catanzaro A. Coccidioidomycosis: state of the art. Part II. *Am Rev Respir Dis* 1978;117:727–771.

187. Sarosi GA, Parker JD, Doto IL, et al. Chronic pulmonary coccidioidomycosis. *N Engl J Med* 1970;283:325–329.

188. Smith CD, Saito MT, Beard RR, et al. Serologic tests in the diagnosis and prognosis of coccidioidomycosis. *Am J Hyg* 1950;52:1–21.

189. Galgiani JN, Stevens DA, Graybill JR, et al. Ketoconazole therapy of progressive coccidioidomycosis. *Am J Med* 1988;84:603–610.

190. Graybill JR, Stevens DA, Galgiani JN, et al. Itraconazole treatment of coccidioidomycosis. *Am J Med* 1990;89:282–290.

191. Galgiani JN, Catanzaro A, Cloud GA, et al. Fluconazole therapy for coccidioidal meningitis. *Ann Intern Med* 1993;119:28–35.

192. Dewsnup DH, Galgiani JN, Greybill JR. Is it ever safe to stop azole therapy for coccidioides immitis meningitis? *Ann Intern Med* 1996;124:305–310.

192a. Galgiani JN, Ampel NM, Catanzaro A, et al. Practice guidelines for the treatment of coccidioidomycosis. *Clin Infect Dis* 2000;30:658–661.

193. Restrepo A, Robledo M, Giraldo R, et al. The gamut of paracoccidioidomycosis. *Am J Med* 1976;61:33–42.

194. Cuce LC, Wroclawski EL, Sampaio SAP. Treatment of paracoccidioidomycosis with ketoconazole. *Rev Inst Med Trop Sao Paulo* 1981;23(2):82–85.

195. Restrepo A, Gomez I, Robledo J, et al. Itraconazole in the treatment of paracoccidioidomycosis: a preliminary report. *Rev Infect Dis* 1987;9[Suppl 1]:551–553.

196. Gerding DN. Treatment of pulmonary sporotrichosis. *Semin Respir Infect* 1986;1:61–65.

197. Pluss JL, Opal SM. Pulmonary sporotrichosis: review of treatment and outcome. *Medicine* 1986;65:143–153.

198. Sharkey-Mathis PK, Kauffman CA, Graybill JR, et al. Treatment of sporotrichosis with itraconazole: NIAID Mycoses Study Group. *Am J Med* 1993;95:279–285.

199. Powell KE, Dahl BA, Weeks RJ, et al. Airborne *Cryptococcus neoformans*: particles from pigeon excreta compatible with alveolar deposition. *J Infect Dis* 1972;125:412–415.

200. Kovacs JA, Kovacs AA, Polis M, et al. *Cryptococcus* in the acquired immunodeficiency syndrome. *Ann Intern Med* 1985;103:533–538.

201. Zuger A, Louie E, Holzman RS, et al. Cryptococcal disease in patients with the acquired immunodeficiency syndrome. *Ann Intern Med* 1986;104:234–240.

202. Kerkering TM, Duma RD, Shadmy S. The evolution of pulmonary cryptococcosis. *Ann Intern Med* 1981;794:611–616.

203. Sarosi GA. Cryptococcal lung disease in patients without HIV infection. *Chest* 199;115(3):610–611.

204. Dismukes WE, Cloud G, Gallis HA, et al. Treatment of cryptococcal meningitis with combination amphotericin B and flucytosine for four as compared with six weeks. *N Engl J Med* 1987;317:334–341.

205. Saag MS, Powderly WG, Cloud GA, et al. Comparison of amphotericin B with fluconazole in the treatment of acute AIDS-associated cryptococcal meningitis. *N Engl J Med* 1992;326:83–9.

206. Larsen RA, Leal MAE, Chan LS. Fluconazole compared with amphotericin B plus Flucytosine for cryptococcal meningitis in AIDS. A randomized trial. *Ann Intern Med* 1990;113:183–87.

207. Van der Horst CM, Saag MS, Cloud GA, et al. Treatment of cryptococcal meningitis associated with acquired immunodeficiency syndrome. *N Engl J Med* 1997;337:15–21.

207a. Saag MS, Graybill RJ, Larsen RA, et al. Practice guidelines for the management of cryptococcal disease. *Clin Infect Dis* 2000;30:710–718.

208. Varkey B, Rose HD. Pulmonary aspergilloma—a rational approach to treatment. *Am J Med* 1976;61:626–631.

209. Young RC, Bennett JE, Vogal CL, et al. Aspergillosis: the spectrum of the disease in 98 patients. *Medicine* 1970;49:147–173.

210. Binder RE, Faling LJ, Pugatch RD, et al. Chronic necrotizing pulmonary aspergillosis: a discrete clinical entity. *Medicine* 1982;60:109–124.

211. Denning DW, Tucker RM, Hanson LH, et al. Treatment of invasive aspergillosis with itraconazole. *Am J Med* 1989;86:791–800.

212. Denning DW, Follansbee SE, Scolaro M, et al. Pulmonary aspergillosis in the acquired immunodeficiency syndrome. *N Engl J Med* 1991;324:654–662.

213. Minamoto GY, Barlam TF, Vander Els NJ. Invasive aspergillosis in patients with AIDS. *Clin Infect Dis* 1992;14:66–74.

214. Pizzo PA, Robichaud KJ, Gill FA, et al. Empiric antibiotic and antifungal therapy for cancer patients with prolonged fever and granulocytopenia. *Am J Med* 1982;72:101–111.

CHAPTER 16

Pulmonary Complications in the Immunosuppressed Patient

Boaz A. Markewitz

G. Douglas Campbell

INTRODUCTION
Neutrophil Dysfunction
Defects in Humoral Immunity
Defects in Cell-Mediated Immunity
Workup of the Patient

IMMUNOCOMPROMISED STATES
Bone Marrow
Human Immunodeficiency Virus

INTRODUCTION

The immunosuppressed patient is an individual with increased susceptibility to organisms with minimal virulence. The number of immunosuppressed patients continues to increase with wider usage of immunosuppressive agents for treatment of malignancy, autoimmune diseases, and inflammatory conditions and for prevention of rejection of transplanted organs, and the number increases as the population infected with human immunodeficiency virus-1 (HIV-1) increases. Infection is a common complication with the likely spectrum of pathogens, affected by the type, severity and duration of immunosuppression, prior exposure to certain pathogens [i.e., *Mycobacterium tuberculosis*, endemic fungi, cytomegalovirus (CMV), varicella-zoster virus (VZV), etc.], use of prophylactic regimens, and prior or ongoing antibiotic therapy. Noninfectious events are also frequently encountered among the immunosuppressed, accounting for up to 50% of all complications in some settings. Broadly, immunosuppression results from three conditions: neutrophil dysfunction, defects in humoral immunity, or defects in cell-mediated immunity (see Table 16-1).

NEUTROPHIL DYSFUNCTION

Neutrophil dysfunction may be due to either qualitative defects that are mainly limited to the pediatric population or quantitative defects resulting in neutropenia. Neutropenia is defined as less than 1,000 granulocytes per cubic millimeter, and absolute neutropenia is defined as less than 500 cells per cubic millimeter. Neutropenia is most commonly seen in the setting of myelogenous leukemias, myeloproliferative disorders, aplastic anemia, neoplastic replacement of the bone marrow, postadministration of chemotherapy toxic to the bone marrow, splenic sequestration, and other rare causes.

The incidence of infection is dependent upon both the duration and the depth of neutropenia. The risk of bacterial infection is high if neutropenia lasts for more than 10 days, and after 3 weeks, the risk of opportunistic fungal infections usually due to *Aspergillus* or *Candida* spp. increases (1,2). The most commonly encountered bacterial pathogens include gram-positive bacteria, especially *Staphylococcus aureus*; coagulase-negative *Staphylococcus*; enterococci; *Streptococcus viridans*; gram-negative bacilli, especially *Enterobacter* spp. and *Pseudomonas* spp.; and anaerobic organisms. The presence of bilateral pulmonary

TABLE 16-1. Relationship among Host Defect, Disease State, and Infection for the Immunocompromised Host

	Defect	*Disease State*	*Pulmonary Infection*
Neutrophil defects	Neutropenic Qualitative defect	Myelogenous leukemias Myeloproliferative disorders Aplastic anemia Neoplastic replacement of the bone marrow Use of chemotherapy toxic to the bone marrow Splenic sequestration	*Staphylococcus aureus* *Staphylococcus epidermidis* *Streptococcus veridans* *Enterobacter* spp. *Pseudomonas aeruginosa* *Aspergillus* spp. *Candida* spp.
Defects in humoral immunity	Disorders in Ig production	Congenital or acquired hypo- or agammaglobulinemias Multiple myeloma Waldenström macroglobulinemia Chronic lymphocytic leukemia B-cell lymphomas Postsurgery Sickle cell	*Streptococcus pneumoniae* *Hemophilus influenzae* *Salmonella* spp.
Defects in cell-mediated immunity	Hypo- or asplenia Hypocomplementemia	Acquired immuno deficiency syndrome (AIDS) Radiation immunosuppressive therapy Antirejection therapy (AIDS and transplantation) Corticosteroids Lymphomas Solid tumors T-cell malignancies	Bacteria (*Listeria, Legionella*) *Mycobacterium* spp. Human herpes viruses (HSV, CMV, EBV, VZV) Fungal (*Aspergillus, Candida* spp., *Cryptococcus neoformans, Histoplasma, Coccidioides, Pneumocystis jiroveci*) *Strongyloides*

cavities in different stages of progression with predominant location in the dependent lungs should prompt an evaluation for bacteremia either from infected intravenous catheters or from endocarditis. Initial empiric therapy including vancomycin or linezolid should be considered if there is concern of methicillin-resistant *S. aureus*.

Febrile neutropenia, commonly seen with myeloablative therapy, is associated with both neutropenia and mucositis, which results in gram-negative and gram-positive bacteremia frequently arising from the gastrointestinal (GI) tract, but may also result from colonization of long-term intravascular (IV) devices. Because the immune response is impaired, traditional signs of inflammation are uncommon. In this setting, empiric monotherapy with a broad-spectrum agent along with extensive culturing has been shown to be effective in reducing mortality (3). When choosing antimicrobial therapy, it is important to know the local hospital sensitivity rates.

Aspergillus infections are most commonly encountered in the setting of prolonged neutropenia, predominantly infect the lung, and have a radiographic presentation that ranges from pulmonary opacities to cavitary lesions. Empiric antifungal therapy should be considered in any neutropenic patient who remains febrile for more than 5 to 7 days despite the use of broad-spectrum antibacterial therapy.

DEFECTS IN HUMORAL IMMUNITY

The primary function of humoral immunity is the production of antibodies and complement to opsonize and clear potential pathogens. Defects in humoral immunity include disorders in immunoglobulin production, hyposplenism or asplenia (either postsurgical or from diseases like sickle cell disease),

and hypocomplementemia. Disorders of immunoglobulin production include congenital or acquired hypo- or agammaglobulinemias, multiple myeloma, Waldenström macroglobulinemia, chronic lymphocytic leukemia, and B-cell lymphomas. Encapsulated organisms are most commonly encountered, including *Streptococcus pneumoniae* and *Hemophilus influenzae*. The individual with asplenia, whether functional or anatomic, is at particular risk for severe pneumonia including community-acquired pneumonia, and the potential for being infected by drug resistant-pathogens should always be considered. Because of the high mortality associated with infection, use of the pneumococcal vaccine is recommended, and revaccination should be considered every 5 years.

DEFECTS IN CELL-MEDIATED IMMUNITY

Cell-mediated immunity is important in defending against viruses, mycobacterial species, certain bacteria (i.e., *Listeria* spp.), protozoans (i.e., *Strongyloides*) and most fungi, and, especially, intracellular pathogens. Cell-mediated immunity requires functional macrophages and T cells, which, in concert, result in the production of cytokines, lymphokines, and chemotactic agents. Disorders that may result in impaired cell-mediated immunity include HIV infection, radiation, immunosuppressive therapy, antirejection therapy for transplantation, corticosteroids, lymphomas, solid tumors, and T-cell malignancies.

WORKUP OF THE PATIENT

The clinical recognition of infection may be subtle in immunocompromised patients as many typical signs and/or symptoms of infection are blunted or absent. The patient may only present with minimal constitutional symptoms like fever or shortness of breath. The physical examination, though important, is frequently unrewarding. Skin lesions, neurologic defects, and ocular findings can point to a likely organism or can at least provide an additional site for obtaining culture material.

While evaluating the patient, it is important to consider the type, degree, and duration of immunosuppression and to review recent antimicrobial and prophylactic therapy because this will affect the potential spectrum of etiologies and result in increased risk of antibiotic resistance. Also, knowledge of prior exposure to members of the herpes virus family [CMV, VZV, and herpes simplex virus (HSV)], tuberculosis, and zoonotic pathogens, and knowledge of residence in areas of endemic fungi can alert the physician to possible reactivation. With specific types of immunosuppression like bone marrow transplantation (BMT), evaluation for the presence of graft-versus-host disease (GVHD), the time after engraftment, and the types of prophylactic therapies that have been used are important in anticipating various complications. The presence of noninfectious processes should be considered. Following surgery or BMT, pulmonary edema secondary to high fluid requirements is a frequent cause of pulmonary opacities that can often be recognized by reviewing fluid input and output or daily weights.

The chest radiograph and clinical history may be helpful in narrowing the differential in the management and treatment of the patient (see Table 16-2). Rapidly progressive illness is more common with bacterial or viral infections, pulmonary edema, pulmonary emboli, or alveolar hemorrhage; if there are cavitary lesions, septic emboli should be considered. A subacute picture, developing over a few days to a few weeks, is more consistent with fungal (including *Pneumocystis jiroveci* formerly *P. carinii*), nocardial, viral or mycobacterial processes, drug-induced lung disease, or radiation fibrosis. A computed tomography (CT) scan of the thorax may show early cavitation or subtle findings that might help direct lower–respiratory tract sampling.

Fiber-optic bronchoscopy (FOB) with bronchoalveolar lavage (BAL) and, when possible, transbronchial biopsy (TBB) may be helpful when coagulation parameters permit. BAL is particularly helpful in detecting infectious etiologies, with a reported sensitivity in the 60% to 95% range. TBB may increase the yield, especially when looking for invasive infections like *Aspergillus* pneumonia (4). Open lung biopsy is usually reserved for extreme cases but rarely alters the patient's course.

This chapter reviews both infectious and noninfectious processes that result in pulmonary complications in various immunocompromised states. Most of the chapter deals with

BMT and HIV disease because of the frequent severity of the immunosuppression and their very frequent pulmonary involvement.

IMMUNOCOMPROMISED STATES

The lung is the most frequently involved site of serious infection and injury in the immunocompromised patient. Pulmonary complications occur not only because of immunosuppression and resultant infection but also as a consequence of treatment or response to cancer. All chemotherapeutic agents have the potential to cause lung injury either directly by affecting the lung parenchyma or indirectly through immunosuppression. The incidence of toxicity varies. A comprehensive list of drugs and their related toxicity along with clinical and radiographic patterns of involvement of the respiratory system is listed at the internet site www.pneumotox.com. Chemotherapeutic agents can affect surfactant production, which results in an increased risk of atelectasis, lung injury, and infection (5). The lung can also respond to malignancy with a sarcoidlike reaction and with the development of noncaseating granulomas in the lymph nodes and in parenchymal nodules (6).

BONE MARROW

BMT is increasingly used for management of malignant as well as nonmalignant conditions including hematologic diseases, solid tumors, and metabolic and genetic diseases. Worldwide estimates of the number of BMTs performed annually exceed 45,000 events. The post-BMT course is complicated by both infectious and noninfectious pulmonary events. Such events have been reported in as many as 50% of cases with overall mortality of up to 40%. The incidence of pulmonary complications is affected by coexisting disease, the type and intensity of induction agents and radiation employed, the duration of immunosuppression, the type of transplantation performed (allogenic, autologous, or stem cell), the prophylactic agents used, and the development of GVHD (7).

Mortality from pulmonary complications is highest among patients requiring mechanical ventilation. Between 12% and 21% of BMT patients require mechanical ventilation, and of those extubated following their initial event, only 27% were alive after 6 months (8–10). In one study of mechanically ventilated BMT patients, patients with severe lung injury [F_{IO_2} greater than 0.6 or positive end-expiratory pressure (PEEP) >5 cm H_2O after 24 hours of support], hepatic–renal dysfunction (bilirubin more than 4 mg per dL and creatinine more than 2 mg per dL), or hypotension (more than 4 hours of 5 μg/kg/minute of dopamine) had a 30-day survival rate of less than 2% (11). A more recent study has noted a slightly higher survival rate of 16% (12).

Historically, BMT pulmonary complications have been divided into early (less than 100 days following transplantation) or late (more than 100 days following transplantation) events (13). However, with the use of prophylactic regimens and with careful monitoring for viral replication, certain complications may be prevented or their occurrence delayed; this is especially true for *P. jiroveci*, CMV, HSV, and *Candida albicans* or *tropicalis*. In general, allogenic BMTs are associated with a higher incidence of pulmonary complications than are autologous BMTs and stem-cell transfers.

TABLE 16-2. Common Radiographic Presentations of Lung Disease in the Immunocompromised Patient

Consolidation	Nodular	Interstitial
Bacterial	Fungal	Viral
Fungal	*Nocardia*	Diffuse alveolar hemorrhage
Hemorrhage	Mycobacteria	Pulmonary edema[a]
	Tumor	Radiation
	Septic emboli	Drug toxicity

[a]Cardiogenic or noncardiogenic pulmonary edema

Noninfectious Complications

Extensive reviews have been published on noninfectious complications (14).

UPPER AIRWAY COMPLICATIONS. Upper airway complications are the earliest complications noted following BMT, occurring within the first 2 months and caused by the conditioning regimen. The resultant mucosal damage can be severe and lead to mucositis, upper airway inflammation, laryngeal edema, dysphagia, or aspiration pneumonitis. Treatment varies depending upon severity and ranges from local symptomatic care to intubation for laryngeal edema.

PULMONARY EDEMA. Pulmonary edema is reported in up to 50% of patients and is usually seen in the second or third week following BMT. Its onset is acute with a presentation that includes dyspnea, weight gain, bibasilar crackles, and hypoxemia. Chest radiographic findings are similar to typical pulmonary edema, and pleural effusions may also be noted. The causes of pulmonary edema can be increased hydrostatic pressure and/or increased capillary permeability. Increased hydrostatic pressure results from aggressive hydration employed to limit chemotherapeutic toxicity, need for blood products, total parenteral nutrition, and the presence of cardiac or renal dysfunction either as an underlying condition or resulting from use of certain chemotherapeutic agents (i.e., cisplatin, cyclosporin, cyclophosphamide, and doxorubicin). Increased capillary permeability can result from total body radiation, chemotherapy, or sepsis. Treatment is similar to that for pulmonary edema due to other causes.

IDIOPATHIC PNEUMONIA SYNDROME. Acute lung injury following BMT for which no other infectious or noninfectious etiology can be found is defined as idiopathic pneumonia syndrome (IPS). It has been reported as early as day 14 following BMT and as late as 5 months following the procedure but with a mean occurrence at 35 to 49 days (15,16). It accounts for almost 50% of all cases of interstitial pneumonitis following BMT, and several mechanisms for its development have been proposed (17). Its incidence is higher among allogenic than autologous BMT patients (12% and 2%, respectively). Mortality is as high as 71%, with most patients succumbing to secondary complications such as fungal infections without resolution of IPS. Clinical presentation includes fever, dyspnea, dry cough, hypoxemia, and a radiographic picture of nonlobar opacities. The diagnosis is one of exclusion. A National Institutes of Health (NIH) consensus workshop developed the following four criteria to help diagnose IPS (11): (a) signs and symptoms of pneumonia; (b) abnormal pulmonary physiology as manifested by worsening alveolar to arterial oxygen gradient or pulmonary function testing usually restrictive in nature; (c) radiographic evidence of bilateral alveolar or interstitial opacities; and (d) no evidence of lower–respiratory tract infection. Many authors suggest FOB with BAL and, possibly, TBB to rule out infectious etiologies (4). Interestingly, high-dose total body radiation (>1,200 rad) and the presence of GVHD are associated with increased resolution. Treatment is nonspecific, and use of steroids has not been proven to be efficacious (16). In one report, disease severity for GVHD was reduced with use of cyclosporin or intravenous immunoglobulin prophylaxis (18).

DIFFUSE ALVEOLAR HEMORRHAGE. Diffuse alveolar hemorrhage (DAH) occurs at the time of engraftment—not during the nadir of suppression—and is felt to be caused by the influx of neutrophils, which result in inflammation. It is more common among autologous BMT recipients, where it is reported to occur in 7% to 14% of patients. DAH usually occurs during the second or third week following BMT, with a range of 5 to 34 days following transplantation. The etiology of DAH is unknown but may be related to epithelial injury occurring at the time of neutrophil recovery. There is controversy over risk factors. Clinical features appear suddenly and include fever, dry cough, dyspnea, hypoxemia, and, rarely, hemoptysis. Chest radiographic findings are nonspecific and include mild central- to lower-lung alveolar opacities, which occur rapidly, with significant changes seen in less than 24 hours. A decline in hemoglobin and hematocrit may be noted. Diagnosis is usually made by FOB and BAL where the lavage is noted to become progressively bloodier. Early diagnosis is important because the rapid institution of high-dose corticosteroids has been shown to improve survival and prevent subsequent respiratory failure.

GRAFT-VERSUS-HOST DISEASE. GVHD appears both as an acute and a chronic disease. GVHD is a complex event but appears to result from activation of the donor T cells against the recipient due to minor human leukocyte antigen (HLA) incompatibilities (19). It can be severe and is significantly more common following allogeneic BMT than autologous BMT. Acute GVHD occurs within the first 100 days in 25% to 75% of recipients and mainly affects the skin, liver, and GI tract. The lung is usually spared but, if affected, results in symptoms of a mild bronchiolitis-like infection clinical presentation. The incidence of chronic GVHD ranges from 20% to 45% of patients who survive at least 6 months following BMT and is more common among patients who, previously, were diagnosed with acute GVHD. Its median time of onset is 5 months with a range of 1 to 13 months. Dyspnea, dry cough, crackles, and/or wheezes are common clinical findings and the chest radiograph may be normal or may show diffuse bilateral disease. Chronic GVHD is associated with an increased risk for spontaneous pneumothorax. If the patient presents with fever or productive sputum, then other or additional causes should be considered. Pulmonary function testing initially may show a decline in vital capacity (VC) and in forced expiratory volume in 1 second (FEV_1), but as the disease progresses, a dramatic decline in FEV_1/VC ratio consistent with airflow obstruction may be witnessed. Along with the pulmonary involvement, more generalized findings frequently seen include skin rash, sicca syndrome, scleroderma-like skin findings, liver function abnormalities, serositis, and malabsorption. The histologic picture of GVHD is lymphocytic interstitial pneumonitis with diffuse alveolar damage, lymphocytic bronchitis, and bronchiolitis obliterans (BO). The initiation of high-dose steroids (prednisolone 1 to 2 mg per kg) gradually tapering over a 3- to 12-month period frequently results in a complete response. If the approach is not successful or if the GVHD is severe, then the addition of cyclosporin A, azathioprine, or thalidomide should be considered.

BRONCHIOLITIS OBLITERANS. Following allogeneic BMT, BO is reported in 2% to 14% of patients with at least 3 months survival but is rarely described following autologous BMT (20). The time of onset for BO is usually 6 to 12 months post-BMT, and is rare in the first 3 months. Risk factors include low immunoglobulin levels (especially IgA and IgG) following transplantation, use of methotrexate, and chronic GVHD. The etiology of BO is unknown; however, viral agents, autoimmune processes, and GVHD have been postulated (21). The clinical presentation can be subtle and includes symptoms of upper–respiratory tract infection, with gradually increasing dyspnea, persistent cough, and an expiratory wheeze. The chest radiograph may be unchanged from prior exams or may reveal hyperinflation. A mosaic pattern and/or evidence of bronchial dilatation may be seen on CT scan of the thorax. Pulmonary function testing shows early airflow obstruction followed by reductions in the diffusing capacity; occasionally, there is evidence for a restrictive ventilatory component. The diagnosis of BO can be made by the clinical, radiographic, and pulmonary function findings, but if there is doubt, TBB or open lung biopsy should be considered. Unfortunately, the prognosis is dismal, with 65% of patients dying within 3 years of diagnosis, and though frequently used, high-dose immunosuppressive agents are of uncertain benefit in treating this disorder.

MISCELLANEOUS NONINFECTIOUS PROCESSES. There are a number of additional noninfectious processes to consider when evaluating BMT patients with pulmonary involvement. Symptomatic radiation pneumonitis is reported to occur in up to 7% of patients, but the incidence of radiation fibrosis is higher if asymptomatic radiographic changes are included. Symptoms, especially dyspnea and fever, usually do not occur for several weeks following radiation therapy. The chest radiograph is helpful because the radiographic abnormalities can have sharp borders that do not follow pulmonary anatomy.

Obstructive airways disease (FEV_1/FVC less than 70% and FEV_1 less than 80%) is reported to occur in up to 17% of patients. Symptoms of dyspnea, cough, and wheezing in the setting of a normal chest radiograph are first reported 6 to 12 months following transplantation. The mortality is high, and in a small subset of patients, the process is rapid.

Approximately 20% of patients at 12 months are noted to have mild to moderate restrictive lung disease and a decreased diffusing capacity [Diffusing Capacity of Carbon Monoxide (D_{LCO})] frequently with an associated cough, fever, chest tightness, and dyspnea. The restriction usually does not progress. The etiology for this appears to be multifactorial and includes the cytotoxic effects of chemotherapy and radiation, recurrent lung infections, and limitation to chest wall mechanics due to GVHD–induced sclerodermal changes of the skin on the chest wall, and muscle weakness.

Pleural effusion can be related to fluid overload, infection, venoocclusive disease, or pulmonary thromboemboli. The risk of venous thromboembolism is increased in BMT patients because of limited mobility, the presence of central catheters, and, possibly, the underlying condition. Additional complications include transfusion-related acute lung injury, secondary pulmonary alveolar proteinosis, recurrent or secondary malignancies, and pulmonary cytolytic thrombi (22–24).

Infectious Complications

Infectious complications occur in 60% to 80% of BMT recipients, and the risk is greatest within the first month following transplantation (25). The incidence of infectious complications has decreased with the adoption of guidelines for the prevention of opportunistic infections (26). One of the first prophylaxis approaches was the use of trimethoprim–sulfamethoxazole (TMP/SMX) to prevent *P. jiroveci* pneumonia (PCP). The regimen has the added benefit of decreasing the incidence of infections caused by encapsulated bacteria. Prophylaxis regimens now frequently also include acyclovir and fluconazole.

BACTERIAL INFECTIONS. Bacterial infections occur in the early phase following BMT prior to engraftment, when the patient is profoundly neutropenic and when mucositis is common. Despite antibiotic prophylaxis, it is estimated that 20% to 50% of patients develop infection and that the lung is involved in 4% to 30% of patients. The most common bacteria are gram-negative bacilli that originate from the GI tract or oropharynx and arrive in the lung following translocation or aspiration. Gram-positive pathogens are increasingly identified as a complication of long-term intravascular catheters. When bacteremia or septicemia is documented or suspected, there is often concern that these catheters may be the source. Decision as to whether to remove the catheter depends upon clinical judgment. One study looked at criteria for determining whether the catheter was the source of bacteremia or candidemia. In this study, quantitative blood cultures drawn from a catheter, which yielded more than 100 cfu per mL and that had a differential growth time of more than 2 hours compared to cultures of blood drawn through a peripheral stick, were predictive of catheter-associated infection (27). Aspiration pneumonia also occurs in heavily sedated patients or in patients having difficulty swallowing because of severe mucositis. Finally, *Legionella* and *Nocardia* infections are also seen. Nosocomial *Legionella* infections often occur in outbreaks, and if one patient is diagnosed with *Legionella* infection, a careful evaluation of other patients residing in the BMT facility should be considered.

FUNGAL INFECTIONS. Infections by a wide spectrum of fungi are particularly common within the first 30 days following BMT, reported in up to 40% of patients. Risk factors for fungal infections include neutropenia, corticosteroid use, and the use of broad-spectrum antibacterial agents. The most commonly encountered fungi are *Candida* spp. and *Aspergillus* spp. *P. jiroveci* is less common now because of the wide use of prophylactic TMP/SMX. In the BMT patient, candidal colonization of the GI tract, skin, and oropharynx is common, especially if the patient has been exposed to broad-spectrum antibacterial agents. Prophylactic use of fluconazole has dramatically reduced the incidence of *C. albicans* infections, but *Candida glabrata* and *Candida krusei* are frequently resistant to fluconazole. Treatment of candidemia or deep-seated candidal infections in patients who have been on prophylactic triazoles should include some formulation of amphotericin B. Caspofungin, an echinocandin that is effective against most species of *Candida* with the possible exception of *Candida parapsilosis*, is an alternative agent and has been reported to be as effective as amphotericin B, with fewer drug-related side effects (28).

Fluconazole is also not effective against invasive molds like *Aspergillus* spp., *Fusarium* spp., and *Mucorales* spp. including the Zygomycetes. These fungi are reported to cause infections in more than 10% of allogeneic stem-cell BMT patients and appear to be increasing with increased use of anticandidal prophylaxis with fluconazole 400 mg daily (29). More worrisome is that amphotericin B resistance has increased over the past decade. *Aspergillus* spp. infections are the most common and may occur early while the patient is neutropenic or later with the occurrence of chronic GVHD, with corticosteroid usage, or in association with viral infections. Mortality from *Aspergillus* infections is high, approaching 90% in some studies. Clinically, the patient presents with fever that does not improve with antimicrobial therapy, dry cough, dyspnea, pleuritic chest pain, and rarely, hemoptysis. In this setting, the presence of sinusitis is suggestive of aspergillosis. Radiographic presentation is variable, with opacities and/or nodules seen with occasional necrosis on chest radiograph, and on CT scan of the thorax, the "halo sign" may be noted. The halo sign is most often present during periods of neutropenia, may be seen less frequently with other pathogens, and appears as a perinodular zone of lower density surrounding a denser center. In addition, the CT scan may reveal perivascular necroses and peripheral parenchymal infarctions. Delays in initiating therapy can be fatal. Thus, though a definitive diagnosis requires the demonstration of tissue invasion, the presence of *Aspergillus* in the sputum or BAL culture is considered enough evidence to initiate therapy. Voriconazole monotherapy has been shown to substantially improve both clinical response and outcome when compared to amphotericin B (30). Under *in vitro* conditions, Caspofungin has been shown to improve the efficacy of either voriconazole or amphotericin B therapy when used in combination (31,32).

VIRAL INFECTIONS. Viruses may cause severe infections among BMT recipients, and the potential spectrum includes members of the human herpes viruses (HHV) family and community-acquired viruses. The most common members of the HHV family that cause pneumonias in BMT patients are CMV, HSV, and HHV-6. Infection may be a consequence of either reactivation, especially during periods of profound immunosuppression, or primary infection. The more common community-acquired viruses include influenza viruses A and B, respiratory syncytial virus (RSV), and parainfluenza viruses. CMV is the most common viral pathogen, and infection usually develops from 6 to 16 weeks following transplantation. Historically, 10% to 40% of transplant recipients developed CMV infection, and of the approximately one-third who developed pneumonia, 85% died. With preemptive serial screening of blood for CMV antigenemia or DNA and prompt initiation of antiviral therapy, the incidence of CMV disease has been reduced to less than 5% during the first 100 days following BMT (33). Because of prophylaxis and screening, CMV is being seen in later stages following transplantation. CMV pneumonia presents as a dry cough, fever, dyspnea, hypoxemia, myalgias, and, often, GI disease. Chest radiograph shows bilateral interstitial opacities. FOB with biopsy often leads to a diagnosis. The classic histopathologic feature is the "owl eye" inclusion body. There is controversy as to whether CMV isolated in BAL should be treated without evidence of active disease, but in at least one report, 50% of patients with CMV colonization eventually developed CMV pneumonia. Treatment includes antiviral agents (ganciclovir) and polyclonal immunoglobulin with an induction phase of 2 to 3 weeks followed by 3 to 4 weeks of maintenance. Despite this, mortality from CMV pneumonia remains at more than 50% (34). HSV usually results in stomatitis, but, rarely, can cause pneumonia.

HHV-6 reactivation is noted in up to 75% of BMT patients usually during the first 30 to 40 days following transplantation. Its significance remains to be determined.

Community-acquired viruses are common; they result from primary infection, not reactivation, and their incidence mirrors that of the community at large. Transmission is usually by large droplet except for influenza virus, which can be spread by small aerosol droplets. With large droplets, hand washing can serve as an effective deterrent to viral spread. Influenza virus A and B and RSV are seasonal, usually occurring in winter and early spring. In the general population, early initiation of neuraminidase inhibitors appears to be effective in treating influenza, whereas aerosolized ribavirin alone or in combination with RSV-specific antibodies may have efficacy in RSV infections. To date, there are no well-controlled trials of efficacy with any agent in the setting of BMT. RSV presents with coryza and may have associated symptoms of sinusitis, bronchiolitis, and pneumonia. It may appear in epidemics or nosocomial spread. Parainfluenza has a presentation similar to RSV except that it occurs year-round. All three of these community-acquired viruses can be deadly. Adenoviruses consist of more than 50 serotypes and may present as an upper–respiratory tract infection, pneumonia, hemorrhagic cystitis, hepatitis, or gastroenteritis. The incidence of serious adenovirus infections may be increasing because of the increased use of broad immunosuppressive therapy. Risk factors for serious infections include younger age, allogeneic BMT, total body radiation, and isolation of adenovirus from more than one site of the patient. There are no controlled trials for treatment; however, decreasing the level of immunosuppression may be helpful.

HUMAN IMMUNODEFICIENCY VIRUS

More than 40,000 people are newly infected with HIV in the United States each year. Nearly 50% of all new infections occur in people under the age of 25. Unfortunately, the downward trend in new HIV infections has leveled off and in certain populations has, in fact, increased. More than 800,000 people have developed the acquired immunodeficiency syndrome (AIDS) in this country since first reported, with slightly less than 50% of that number living with AIDS today. Though development of highly active antiretroviral therapy (HAART) in 1996 has altered the natural history of HIV infection, infectious and noninfectious disorders of the respiratory tract continue to be common complications in this population (see Table 16-3). The risk of developing HIV-related respiratory complications is linked to the degree of immunocompromise, as assessed by the circulating $CD4^+$ lymphocyte count (see Table 16-4), patient demographics, and whether patients are using prophylaxis regimens against common infections. The radiographic presentations of these disorders are outlined in Table 16-5 (35–42).

Noninfectious Complications

MALIGNANCIES

Kaposi sarcoma. Kaposi sarcoma (KS) is the most common tumor in HIV-infected patients and is an AIDS-defining illness; its incidence, however, is decreasing since the introduction of HAART. HHV-8 is associated with the development of

TABLE 16-3. Respiratory Complications in Patients with Human Immunodeficiency Virus (HIV) Infection (35–40)

Noninfectious Complications	Infectious Complications
Malignancies	Bacteria
Kaposi sarcoma	*Streptococcus pneumoniae*
Lymphoma	*Haemophilus influenzae*
Bronchogenic carcinoma	*Staphylococcus aureus*
Cardiovascular disorders	*Pseudomonas aeruginosa*
Dilated cardiomyopathy	*Legionella* spp.
Pericardial effusions	*Nocardia* spp.
Pulmonary arterial hypertension	*Rhodococcus equi*
Interstitial lung disease	*Mycobacterium*
Nonspecific interstitial	*tuberculosis*
pneumonitis	Atypical mycobacterial
Lymphocytic interstitial	infections
pneumonitis	Fungi
Bronchiolitis obliterans	*Pneumocystis jiroveci*
organizing pneumonia	*Cryptococcus neoformans*
Emphysema	*Aspergillus* spp.
Airway inflammation	*Histoplasma capsulatum*
Chronic bronchitis	*Coccidioides immitis*
Bronchiolitis	Viruses
	Cytomegalovirus
	Parasites
	Toxoplasmosis gondii
	Strongyloides stercoralis

From Hirschtick RE, Glassroth J, Jordan M, et al. Bacterial pneumonia in persons infected with the Human Immunodeficiency Virus. *N Engl J Med* 1995;333:845–851; Boiselle PM, Aviram G, Fishman JE. Update on lung disease in AIDS. *Semin Roentgenol* 2002;37:54–71; Bartlett JG. Pneumonia in the patient with HIV infection. *Infect Dis Clin North Am* 1998;12:807–820; Maki DD. Pulmonary infections in HIV/AIDS. *Semin Roentgenol* 2000;35:124–139; Rosen MJ. Epidemiology and risk of pulmonary disease. *Semin Respir Infect* 1999;14:301–308; and Barbaro G. Cardiovascular manifestations of HIV infection. *Circulation* 2002;106:1420–1425, with permission.

this malignancy. Although HHV-8 is necessary, additional factors not yet fully delineated have to be present for a person to develop KS (43,44). HHV-8 infection has also been linked to the development of primary effusion lymphoma and multicentric Castleman disease in patients with HIV infection and has been associated with idiopathic pulmonary arterial hypertension (IPAH) (45,46).

KS typically involves the skin over the lower extremities, face, and genitalia; it may be associated with considerable lymphedema. Extracutaneous spread of KS to the oral cavity, GI tract, lungs, and lymph nodes is common. Approximately one-third of patients have oral lesions. The lesions are red to purple in color and can be macular or nodular in appearance. The most common site is the palate (especially the hard palate), followed by the gingiva and tongue (43,46). Pulmonary involvement by KS can be a challenge to distinguish from other malignancies and opportunistic infections. Nearly all patients present with cough and dyspnea; fever and night sweats are frequent as well but may indicate a concomitant infection (43,47). Hemoptysis and significant airway narrowing have been reported in 29% and 2% of patients, respectively (47). Although patients with pulmonary KS characteristically have mucocutaneous involvement, in one study 15% of patients with bronchoscopically confirmed KS had disease limited to the lungs (47). The airways, parenchyma, pleura, and

lymph nodes can be involved, and on autopsy, pulmonary spread is found to be higher than what is clinically suspected.

Chest radiographic findings of KS include focal or linear opacities, consolidation, bronchial wall thickening, nodules, and/or adenopathy. At times, the radiograph appears normal (Table 16-5). Opacities are typically in the mid- and lower-lung zones with central predominance, and patients with more extensive airway disease tend to have more diffuse parenchymal involvement (47,48). Bronchoscopic inspection with recognition of characteristic red to purple macules or papules appears to be the most sensitive diagnostic technique for pulmonary KS. Transbronchial biopsies have a diagnostic yield of less than 60%, and cytologic examination of the exudative pleural fluid is not diagnostic. Thus, the diagnosis of parenchymal, pleural, and lymphatic disease is made clinically in patients with mucocutaneous or tracheobronchial KS in whom opportunistic infections have been excluded.

Patients with KS are divided into high-risk and low-risk groups on the basis of the NIH AIDS-related KS staging classification according to the tumor extent (T), immune status (I), and presence of systemic illness (S). The TIS staging system, however, was developed in the pre-HAART era and may not be an accurate predictor of outcome today (49). The use of systemic steroids and presence of opportunistic infections may exacerbate KS. The goal of treatment is palliation and involves HAART, local therapy (e.g., altiretinoin gel, vinblastine, and radiation/laser therapy), chemotherapy (e.g., liposomal doxorubicin, liposomal daunorubicin, and paclitaxel), and possible biologic response modifiers (e.g., interferon).

Lymphoma. The risk for developing non-Hodgkin's lymphoma (NHL) and Hodgkin disease (HD) are both significantly increased in HIV patients compared with the general

TABLE 16-4. Respiratory Complications and Level of Immunocompromise (36, 38, 42)

CD4$^+$ count >500 cells/μL
  Infections of the upper airway
  Bronchitis
  Bronchogenic carcinoma
CD4$^+$ count 200–499 cells/μL
  Bacterial pneumonia
  Mycobacterial infections
  Thrush
  Lymphocytic interstitial pneumonitis
  Lymphoma
CD4$^+$ count 100–199 cells/μL
  Bacterial sepsis
  Disseminated *Mycobacterium tuberculosis*
  Pneumocystis jiroveci pneumonia
  Kaposi sarcoma
  Burkitt lymphoma
CD4$^+$ count <100 cells/μL
  Disseminated mycobacterial species
  Disseminated fungal infections
  Cytomegalovirus

From Boiselle PM, Aviram G, Fishman JE. Update on lung disease in AIDS. *Semin Roentgenol* 2002;37:54–71; Maki DD. Pulmonary infections in HIV/AIDS. *Semin Roentgenol* 2000;35:124–139; and Hanson DL, Chu SY, Farizo KM, et al. Distribution of CD4+ lymphocytes at diagnosis of acquired immunodeficiency syndrome-defining and other human immunodeficiency virus-related illnesses. *Arch Intern Med* 1995;155:1537–1542, with permission.

TABLE 16-5. Chest Radiographic Patterns and Etiologies in Patients with Human Immunodeficiency Virus (HIV) Infection (38, 41)

Chest radiograph within normal limits	Nodules
Kaposi sarcoma	Lymphoma
Pneumocystis jiroveci	Kaposi sarcoma
Mycobacteria	Bronchogenic carcinoma
Fungi	Mycobacteria
Focal opacities	Fungi
Bacteria	*Nocardia*
Mycobacteria	LIP/NSIP
Fungi	Septic emboli
Pneumocystis carinii	Pleural effusions
Kaposi sarcoma	Kaposi sarcoma
Lymphoma	Lymphoma
Cavitary lesions	Congestive heart failure
Pneumocystis jiroveci	Bacterial empyema
Fungi	Parapneumonic
Mycobacteria	Mycobacteria
Septic emboli/bacterial abscesses	Fungi
Rhodococcus equii	*Nocardia*
Nocardia	Hypoproteinemia
Bronchogenic carcinoma	Lymphadenopathy
Linear opacities	Lymphoma
Pneumocystis jiroveci	Kaposi sarcoma
Kaposi sarcoma	Mycobacteria
Lymphoma	Fungi
Bacteria	Pneumothorax
Mycobacteria	*Pneumocystis jiroveci*
Virus	Cavitary lung diseases
Fungi	
LIP/NSIP	

LIP, lymphocytic interstitial pneumonitis; NSIP, nonspecific interstitial pneumonitis.
From Maki DD. Pulmonary infections in HIV/AIDS. *Semin Roentgenol* 2000;35:124–139; and Schneider RF. Screening and noninvasive testing for pulmonary disease. *Semin Respir Infect* 1999;14:309–317, with permission.

population, though only the former is considered an AIDS-defining illness. The incidence is twice as high in whites and in men compared with African Americans and women; the relative risk increases with the increasing duration of HIV infection and decreasing immune status (36,38,50,51). HAART appears to have decreased the incidence of NHL but not HD; however, in a single-center retrospective review conducted between July 1997 and June 2000, patients on HAART had an increased rate of NHL compared with patients not on an aggressive antiviral regimen (50,52). AIDS-related NHL is of B-cell origin, high grade, and aggressive. Epstein–Barr virus genome is detected in more than 50% of the cases (36,51).

Intrathoracic NHL occurs in approximately 10% of patients and is typically extranodal. Symptoms are nonspecific, and the disease can involve the pleura, parenchyma, or lymph nodes. Radiographic abnormalities include pleural effusions (most common), nodules, linear opacities, focal opacities, and lymphadenopathy; pericardial involvement has also been noted (Table 16-5) (36,38). The diagnosis is usually made by lung biopsy or cytopathologic review of pleural fluid; BAL has a low diagnostic yield. In the HIV population, HD occurs most commonly in the intravenous drug use group and presents prior to the development of severe immune depression.

Systemic symptoms are common at diagnosis, though thoracic adenopathy is less common in this case than in the general population (36).

Bronchogenic carcinoma. Bronchogenic carcinoma is becoming one of the more frequent non–AIDS-defining malignancies with a median age of onset being below 40 (53). It is unclear if HIV infection is an independent risk factor for the development of lung cancer. The incidence of cigarette smoking may be higher in this population, and HIV patients appear more susceptible to the effects of cigarette smoke (54,55). In addition, microsatellite alterations occur more commonly in HIV patients with lung cancer (56). There is also a suggestion of an association between a history of *M. tuberculosis* and/or *P. jiroveci* pneumonia and development of peripheral upper-lobe malignancies; whether this represents a "scar" carcinoma is not known (57). Though HIV-infected patients with bronchogenic carcinoma are younger than their noninfected counterparts, the malignancy is typically more advanced at diagnosis, demonstrates rapid growth, and is associated with a poorer prognosis. The clinical presentation of lung cancer in HIV patients is no different than in the general population. The radiographic presentation is also the same (Table 16-5).

CARDIOVASCULAR DISORDERS

Cardiomyopathy and pericardial effusions. Prior to the introduction of HAART, the estimated annual incidence of HIV-associated dilated cardiomyopathy was 16 per 1,000 patients; this is noteworthy because survival is decreased in patients with left ventricular dysfunction (40). The effect of HAART on this incidence is unclear; however, protease inhibitors may contribute to the development of coronary artery disease. Potential causes for cardiomyopathy in the HIV-infected patient include direct myocardial injury from HIV, opportunistic infections, an autoimmune response to infection, nutritional deficiencies, drug toxicities, recreational drug use, and endocrinopathies. In addition to the usual therapies for dilated cardiomyopathy, intravenous immunoglobulin may be beneficial for patients whose cardiac injury is autoimmune in origin (40). The incidence of pericardial effusions in the preHAART era in AIDS patients was 11% per year (58). The effusions are typically small, not hemodynamically significant, resolve spontaneously, and are most often of undetermined etiology (though opportunistic infections and malignancies are known causes of pericardial disease). AIDS patients with pericardial effusions have increased mortality even if the effusions resolve (40,58).

Pulmonary arterial hypertension. Pulmonary arterial hypertension (PAH), defined as a mean pulmonary artery pressure >25 mm Hg at rest (or >30 mm Hg during exercise), is a rare disorder that may be of unknown cause (i.e., IPAH) or may be related to various conditions including HIV infection. IPAH may be sporadic or familial. A mutation in the BMPR2 gene, which codes for bone morphogenetic receptor II, is a cause of familial IPAH (approximately 50% of families affected by IPAH have recognized mutations in BMPR2) as well as sporadic IPAH. Investigators, however, have not found BMPR2 mutations in patients with PAH related to HIV disease (59,60).

The incidence of HIV-associated PAH is not well defined and it has no relationship to the CD4$^+$ count. The pathophysiology leading to PAH in this population is not known but is not believed to be a direct effect of HIV on the pulmonary circulation. Cellular mediators released by endothelial or smooth muscle cells, such as endothelin-1, may be involved. It is not clear if there is a causal role for HHV-8 or another infectious agent in the HIV population (45).

The clinical presentation of PAH in patients with and without HIV is similar; dyspnea, particularly with activity, is the most common feature. The physical findings are those of pulmonary hypertension and right ventricular failure. Although the development of PAH is not related to the immune status, patients with decreased CD4$^+$ counts have reduced survival. Therapy is similar to that of the non–HIV-infected population, namely, anticoagulation and vasodilators. The effect of HAART on PAH is not known (60,61).

INTERSTITIAL LUNG DISEASE

Nonspecific interstitial pneumonitis. Nonspecific interstitial pneumonitis is a condition characterized by chronic interstitial inflammation of uncertain etiology. Histologic findings also include type II pneumocyte hyperplasia, a mild alveolitis, interstitial edema, and bronchial inflammation. Radiographic findings include linear, reticulonodular, and ground-glass opacities. In one study, it was the most common mimic of *P. jiroveci* pneumonia (62). Symptoms are nonspecific and typically mild. The most important consideration is to rule out other treatable conditions. Symptomatic patients are treated with systemic steroids.

Lymphocytic interstitial pneumonitis. Lymphocytic interstitial pneumonitis is a lymphoproliferative disorder more commonly affecting children than adults with HIV infection. It is characterized by infiltration of the interstitium by lymphocytes, plasma cells, and histiocytes; linear or reticulonodular opacities are usually present on chest radiograph. Its course is chronic and indolent and does not typically progress to a frank lymphoma; in fact, it can resolve spontaneously (36,38).

OTHER NONINFECTIOUS CONDITIONS

Bronchiolitis obliterans with organizing pneumonia. Bronchiolitis obliterans with organizing pneumonia (BOOP) has been described in patients with HIV infection (63,64). It is not an uncommon finding at autopsy, and its relationship to opportunistic infections is not known (36). It can be associated with respiratory failure and may respond dramatically to systemic steroids (63,64).

Emphysema. As previously noted, HIV patients may be particularly sensitive to the effects of cigarette smoke (54,55). An accelerated form of emphysema and an emphysema-like pulmonary disease (i.e., increased lung volume, increased residual volume, decreased diffusion capacity but minimal airway obstruction) have been described in HIV-infected patients (55,65). A pathologic role for cytotoxic lymphocytes has been postulated (55).

Airway inflammation. HIV patients with advanced disease are at risk for developing chronic airway inflammation even if they do not smoke, which is not related to increased nonspecific airway hyperresponsiveness.

Infectious Complications

BACTERIA

Bacterial pneumonia. The presence of impaired humoral immunity, in addition to cell-mediated immunity, places HIV-infected patients at increased risk for developing bacterial infections, particularly by encapsulated organisms (35,66). A multicenter 5-year longitudinal study conducted prior to the HAART era reported a significantly greater incidence of upper– and lower–respiratory tract infections (LRTI) in HIV-infected individuals compared with uninfected persons. The most common LRTI was acute bronchitis with nearly twice the incidence in patients with HIV infection. Bacterial pneumonia was also more common in the HIV group with an incidence of 5.5 episodes per 100 person years (py) compared with 0.9 episodes per 100 py in the HIV seronegative population (67). The incidence of bacterial pneumonia in the HIV group increased over the course of the study and was higher than that of PCP. The rate of bacterial pneumonia increased with lower CD4$^+$ counts and was higher in patients who contracted HIV through intravenous drug use (as opposed to sexual transmission), had a history of PCP, and were cigarette smokers (see Table 16-6). Prophylaxis with TMP/SMX reduced the risk of developing bacterial pneumonia (35,67). Recurrent bacterial pneumonia is now an AIDS-defining condition and may accelerate the course of HIV.

The clinical presentation of bacterial pneumonia in the HIV group is similar to the general population. Patients typically present with fever, chills, productive cough, dyspnea, and parenchymal opacities on chest radiograph. The most common radiographic abnormality is focal consolidation (36,38,68, 69). In up to 50% of the HIV patients with bacterial pneumonia, however, the radiographic findings are atypical and may mimic opportunistic infections; diffuse bilateral alveolar opacities, interstitial opacities, nodules, and cavities have been described in bacterial pneumonia (38,69–71). HIV patients with

TABLE 16-6. Incidence of Respiratory Tract Infections in Human Immunodeficiency Virus (HIV) Patients (Number of Episodes per 100 Person Years Unless Otherwise Noted) (67)

	Year 1	Year 5
Patients (*n*)	1,143	721
CD4$^+$ count <200 cells/μL at start of year (%)	19	34
Any respiratory illness	69	87
Upper–respiratory tract	47	52
Lower–respiratory tract	21	34
Bronchitis	13	14
Bacterial pneumonia	3.9	7.3
Pneumocystis jiroveci	2.8	9.5
Mycobacterium tuberculosis	0.5	1.0
Other opportunistic organisms	0.6	1.8

From Boeckh M. Current antiviral strategies for controlling cytomegalovirus in hematopoietic stem cell transplant recipients: prevention and therapy. *Transpl Infect Dis* 1999;1:165–178, with permission.

abnormal chest radiographs without respiratory symptoms, however, are unlikely to have bacterial pneumonia (72). Encapsulated organisms are most commonly identified, especially *S. pneumoniae* and *H. influenzae*. Intravenous drug users can present with septic emboli caused by *S. aureus* and gram-negative bacilli. *Pseudomonas aeruginosa* pneumonia is seen in patients with advanced disease (i.e., CD4$^+$ count less than 50 cells per μL). *Legionella*, *Chlamydia*, and *Mycoplasma* are uncommon causes of pneumonia in HIV patients. Unusual pathogens that occasionally cause pneumonia include the organisms causing zoonotic diseases (e.g., *Rhodococcus equi* and *Bartonella* spp.) and *Nocardia asteroides* (36,38,68,69).

The treatment of bacterial pneumonia in HIV patients is the same as that for HIV seronegative persons. In HIV patients, however, bacterial pneumonia may progress more rapidly and lead to more complications. Most studies report that HAART has decreased the incidence of pneumonia, but its effect on clinical outcome is not clear (52,73,74). All patients should receive pneumococcal and influenza vaccination.

MYCOBACTERIUM TUBERCULOSIS AND ATYPICAL MYCOBACTERIAL INFECTIONS. People with HIV infection are at dramatically increased risk for having tuberculosis (primary or reactivation) compared with the general population (75–78). Active tuberculosis develops in 8% of patients with positive tuberculin skin tests per year (75). Worldwide, tuberculosis is one of the foremost infectious causes of death in the AIDS population (79). The susceptibility of the HIV population to *Mycobacterium* appears to be due to an altered response of lymphocytes to this organism (i.e., decreased Th1 lymphocyte response) (80). In addition, pulmonary tuberculosis enhances HIV replication in the lung and can accelerate the clinical course of HIV infection (81,82).

The symptoms and radiographic presentation of tuberculosis are linked to the patient's degree of immunosuppression. In patients in whom the CD4$^+$ count is more than 200 cells per μL, the clinical features are similar to those in the non-HIV population. They present with fever, night sweats, weight loss, and cough and have upper-lobe opacities on chest radiograph, which may be cavitary. Pleural effusions are more common in this group. More severely immunosuppressed patients are more likely to have disseminated disease; nearly three-fourths of AIDS patients with CD4$^+$ count of less than 100 cells per μL develop extrathoracic disease (36,38,77). The chest radiograph from this subset of HIV patients may be unremarkable (up to 20% of patients) or may show features not typical of reactivation including diffuse or lower lobe consolidation, miliary patterns, adenopathy, and rapid progression. These patients may also present with endobronchial disease. HIV patients with tuberculosis on HAART are more likely to have a radiographic appearance consistent with reactivation (36,38,77,83).

The atypical chest radiograph features and anergic response to skin tests in HIV patients with advanced disease makes diagnosis more complex. Whereas the sensitivity of sputum acid-fast smears in HIV patients with only mild immunosuppression and a cavitary lesion is similar to that of immunocompetent persons with reactivation disease, patients with advanced AIDS frequently have negative sputum cultures when infected (38). If the clinical suspicion is present, molecular techniques [e.g., amplified *M. tuberculosis* direct test for detection of ribosomal ribonucleic acid (rRNA)] or FOB should be performed. In addition, patients with very low CD4$^+$ counts at high risk for dissemination may be mycobacteremic.

Therapy for susceptible tuberculosis in the HIV–infected patient generally follows the standard recommendations of the American Thoracic Society/Center for Disease Control/Infectious Disease Society of America (ATS/CDC/IDSA) (two *caveats* to this statement are that once weekly isoniazid–rifapentine is not to be used in the continuation phase and that twice weekly isoniazid–rifampin is not to be used in patients with CD4$^+$ counts less than 100 cells per μL). For patients with a slow or suboptimal clinical or bacterial response, the duration of therapy could be continued beyond the normal 6 months. Other important issues include potential interactions between rifamycins and antiretroviral drugs, timing of initiation of antiretroviral agents in previously untreated patients, development of a paradoxical reaction (i.e., immune reconstitution syndrome), and emergence of multidrug resistant strains (84). Chemoprophylaxis in anergic HIV patients at high risk for tuberculosis is no longer uniformly recommended (78). For patients with a positive tuberculin skin test, 3-month regimens with more than one drug may be superior to 6 months of isoniazid (79).

Atypical mycobacterial infections, most often due to *Mycobacterium avium-intracellulare*, are severe complications in patients with advanced disease. Pulmonary involvement occurs in the setting of dissemination. The chest radiograph may be within normal limits or may show air space disease, nodules, and/or adenopathy. HIV patients with acid-fast bacilli in respiratory samples, however, should be treated for *M. tuberculosis* until culture results are obtained (36,38).

FUNGI

Pneumocystis jiroveci. P. carinii has been renamed *P. jiroveci* (85). PCP in adults is a disease of immunocompromised persons. Its incidence has decreased dramatically in the HIV population with the introduction of primary prophylaxis and HAART. Between 1996 and 1998 its incidence declined 21.5% per year; nonetheless, it remains one of the most common opportunistic infections in this population (86). Currently, it develops primarily in HIV patients not previously receiving medical care; not being prescribed prophylaxis, though they meet criteria; or not being compliant with recommended therapies (86). Up to 30% of patients are infected with multiple strains (suggesting that recurrence may be a consequence of reinfection with a different strain, as opposed to reactivation), and analysis of *Pneumocystis* gene mutations suggests that person-to-person transmission is likely (87).

PCP usually presents with fever, nonproductive cough, and progressive dyspnea over several weeks. The classic radiographic presentation is bilateral interstitial opacities, which have been described as granular, reticular, or ground glass. In approximately 10% of cases, the chest x-ray is unremarkable; however, in that setting, ground-glass opacities are present on the high-resolution CT scan of the thorax (87,88). Other radiographic patterns include cystic lung disease, upper-lobe parenchymal opacities, lung nodules, and spontaneous pneumothoraces (seen more commonly in patients with cystic disease); pleural effusions and lymphadenopathy remain uncommon (38,88). An apparent chronic form of PCP with lung fibrosis has also been described (36,38).

The majority of patients with PCP will have an elevated lactate dehydrogenase level and hypoxemia, but these findings are not specific. As the organism cannot consistently be grown in culture, the diagnosis is made by microscopic evaluation of respiratory secretions obtained by induced sputum or by FOB and BAL with special stains (e.g., methenamine silver, Giemsa, and monoclonal antibodies with immunofluorescence); transbronchial biopsies or open lung biopsies are rarely necessary (87,89). Molecular techniques to diagnose PCP without need for respiratory specimens are also being developed (87). It should be noted that the absolute need for establishing a diagnosis versus empiric therapy in the proper clinical setting is an area of controversy.

The treatment regimen for PCP depends upon the severity of illness and on the patient's ability to take oral medications. The first line treatment for PCP remains a 2- or 3-week course of TMP/SMX followed by secondary prophylaxis. Patients with severe disease should be treated with systemic steroids concomitantly (see Table 16-7 for various treatment regimens) (87,90,91). As discussed with *M. tuberculosis*, the development of the immune reconstitution syndrome can occur with treatment of PCP (92). Though mortality remains high in patients with PCP and respiratory failure, survival rate is now approximately 40%, and post-discharge survival and quality of life are improved (93,94).

HIV patients are most susceptible to PCP when $CD4^+$ counts are less than 200 cells per μL. Thus, chemoprophylaxis is recommended when patients are moderate to severely immunosuppressed (i.e., $CD4^+$ less than 200 cells per μL or a history of thrush). Primary or secondary prophylaxis, however, may be discontinued if antiretroviral therapy leads to a sustained elevation in the $CD4^+$ cell count above this threshold (95). Preferred and alternative prophylaxis options are listed in Table 16-7 (95–97).

Other fungi. Other fungal infections are much less common than PCP. *Cryptococcus neoformans* is the most common cause of pulmonary disease after *Pneumocystis*. Other causes of pneumonia include the endemic mycoses (depending on patient geography), *Candida* (quite rare), and *Aspergillus* spp. *C. neoformans* is an encapsulated organism with worldwide distribution and is found in soil and bird droppings. The primary manifestation of cryptococcosis in HIV-infected patients is meningitis; however, the rate has decreased in the HAART era (98,99). It is present in up to 10% of AIDS patients with severe immunosuppression (i.e., $CD4^+$ count less than 100 cells per μL). Its clinical presentation is nonspecific and radiographic findings are typically diffuse parenchymal opacities similar to PCP. Other roentgenographic presentations include single or multiple nodules, cavitary lesions, lymphadenopathy, pleural effusions, and rarely, a miliary pattern. The diagnosis is made by culturing the organism from respiratory fluids; the serum cryptococcal antigen is usually positive. If pulmonary cryptococcosis is diagnosed, lumbar puncture should be performed. For patients with isolated pulmonary disease, the treatment of choice is fluconazole with lifelong maintenance therapy (100).

In endemic regions, *Histoplasma capsulatum* is a more common fungal infection than *Cryptococcus*. It occurs in approximately 5% of patients with AIDS who live in these regions. Risks for disseminated disease (typically a consequence of reactivation) include $CD4^+$ counts less than 100 cells per μL and working with soil contaminated with bird or bat droppings. Treatment with antiretroviral agents, history of PCP, and therapy with a triazole drug decrease the risk of disease (101). The presentation is typically subacute or chronic with fever and weight loss being common symptoms. Diffuse small nodules are usually seen on chest radiograph, and calcified granulomas and lymphadenopathy are frequently noted; as with PCP and disseminated mycobacteria, an unremarkable chest radiograph is reported in a minority of patients (38,98). Histoplasmosis is diagnosed by culture (often blood), by positive polysaccharide antigen test (not widely available), or histologically. For severe disease, the treatment of choice is liposomal amphotericin B followed by suppressive therapy with itraconazole (102). *Coccidiomycosis* and *Blastomycosis* are less common infections in patients with AIDS. Fever and dyspnea are usually present, and diffuse bilateral reticulonodules are typically seen on chest radiograph.

Aspergillus is an uncommon infection in patients with HIV. When it occurs, it is usually in the setting of advanced disease (median $CD4^+$ count less than 30 cells per μL) with concomitant neutropenia, neutrophil dysfunction, or systemic steroid therapy (37,103). The clinical presentation is broad, and massive (even fatal) hemoptysis can occur. The most common radiographic findings are upper-lobe masses with cavities (i.e., angioinvasion with infarction) (38,103). Although histologic evidence of invasive disease is the classic diagnostic strategy, the presence of organisms in BAL fluid in the proper setting is probably sufficient for the diagnosis. Therapeutic options include voriconazole, amphotericin B, or caspofungin; the role of combination chemotherapy is not clear.

VIRAL INFECTIONS

Cytomegalovirus. CMV is commonly isolated from the lungs of HIV patients but is much less frequently a cause of pulmonary disease. CMV pneumonia also presents in patients with very advanced disease (median $CD4^+$ count of 20 cells per μL) usually with extrathoracic infection. Ground-glass opacities are the most common findings on chest imaging studies; pulmonary nodules, masses, and airway abnormalities are also reported (36–38). Pneumonia is diagnosed by excluding other pathogens with histologic evidence of disease; the BAL is not diagnostic (104). HAART is effective in controlling viremia in HIV patients without end-organ disease (105). Pneumonia is treated with intravenous ganciclovir (or foscarnet) and, possibly, with IV immunoglobulin (106).

PARASITES

Toxoplasmosis gondii and Strongyloides stercoralis. T. gondii and S. stercoralis are uncommon causes of pneumonia in the HIV population. T. gondii is primarily a pathogen of the central nervous system in patients with HIV infection; select PCP prophylaxis regimens are active in preventing T. gondii infections as well (Table 16-7). S. stercoralis is most likely to be seen in patients from countries where nematode infection is endemic.

TABLE 16-7. *Pneumocystis jiroveci* Prophylaxis and Treatment Regimens (87, 90, 91, 95–97)

Prophylaxis

Primary	Dose	Comments
TMP/SMX[a]	1 DS (preferred) or 1 SS by mouth daily	Cross protection against toxoplasmosis and select bacterial infections; side effects are common.

Alternatives	Dose	Comments
TMP/SMX	1 DS 3 times per wk by mouth	
Dapsone	100 mg by mouth daily	
Dapsone +	50 mg ([b]200 mg) by mouth daily	May confer protection against toxoplasmosis
Pyrimethamine +	50 mg ([b]75 mg) by mouth weekly	
Leucovorin	25 mg ([b]25 mg) by mouth weekly	
Pentamidine	300 mg aerosolized monthly	Respirgard II nebulizer
Atovaquone	1,500 mg by mouth daily	May confer protection against toxoplasmosis

Treatment

Primary	Dose	Comments
Mild		$PaO_2 > 70$ mm Hg or $PAO_2 - PaO_2 < 35$ mm Hg
TMP/SMX	2 DS by mouth 3x/d	
Severe[c]		$PaO_2 < 70$ mm Hg or $PAO_2 - PaO_2 > 35$ mm Hg
TMP/SMX	TMP 15 mg/kg/d IV every 8 h	

Alternatives	Dose	Comments
Mild		
Dapsone +	100 mg by mouth daily	Nearly as effective as TMP/SMX (97)
TMP	5 mg/kg by mouth 3x/d	—
Clindamycin +	300–450 mg by mouth 4x/d	As effective as TMP/SMX (91)
Primaquine	15 mg base by mouth daily	—
Atovaquone	750 mg by mouth 2x/d	—
Severe		—
Clindamycin +	600 mg IV every 8 h	—
Primaquine	30 mg by mouth daily	—
Pentamidine	4 mg/kg IV each day	—
Trimetrexate +	45 mg/m² IV each day	—
Leucovorin	20 mg/m² IV or by mouth every 6 h	—

[a]TMP/SMX, trimethoprim–sulfamethoxazole; DS, double strength; SS, single strength; PaO_2, arterial pressure of oxygen; PAO_2, alveolar pressure of oxygen; IV, intravenous

[b]alternative dapsone + pyrimethamine + leucovorin regimen

[c]Patients with severe PCP should be treated with systemic steroids using the following regimen: Day 1 to 5 prednisone 40 mg by mouth twice per day; day 6 to 10 prednisone 40 mg by mouth once per day; day 11 to 21 prednisone 20 mg by mouth once per day (or IV methylprednisolone at 75% of above dose).

From Kovacs JA, Gill VJ, Meshnick S, et al. New insights into transmission, diagnosis, and drug treatment of *Pneumocystis carinii* pneumonia. *JAMA* 2001;286:2450–2460; Masur H, Meier P, McCutchan JA, et al. Consensus statement on the use of corticosteroids as adjunctive therapy for *Pneumocystis* pneumonia in the acquired immunodeficiency syndrome. *N Engl J Med* 1990;323:1500–1504; Toma E, Thorne A, Singer J, et al. Clindamycin with primaquine vs. trimethoprim-sulfamethoxazole therapy for mild and moderately severe *Pneumocystis carinii* pneumonia in patients with AIDS: a multicenter, double-blind, randomized trial (CTN 004). *Clin Infect Dis* 1998;27:524–530; Furrer H, Egger M, Opravil M, et al. Discontinuation of primary prophylaxis against *Pneumocystis carinii* pneumonia in HIV-1-infected adults treated with combination antiretroviral therapy. *N Engl J Med* 1999;340:1301–1306; Kaplan JE, Masur H, Holmes KK. Guidelines for preventing opportunistic infections among HIV-infected persons—2002: recommendations of the U.S. Public Health Service and the Infectious Diseases Society of America. *MMWR* 2002;51(RR08):1–46; and Hughes WT. Use of Dapsone in the prevention and treatment of *Pneumocystis carinii* pneumonia: a review. *Clin Infect Dis* 1998;27:191–204, with permission.

REFERENCES

1. Pizzo PA. Management of fever in patients with cancer and treatment-induced neutropenia. *N Engl J Med* 1993;328:1323–1332.
2. Gerson SL, Talbot GH, Hurwitz S, et al. Prolonged granulocytopenia: the major risk factor for invasive pulmonary aspergillosis in patients with acute leukemia. *Ann Intern Med* 1984;100:345–351.
3. Ramphal R. Is monotherapy for febrile neutropenia still a viable alternative? *Clin Infect Dis* 1999;29:508–514.
4. Jain P, Sandur S, Meli Y, et al. Role of flexible bronchoscopy in immunocompromised patients with lung infiltrates. *Chest* 2004;125:712–722.
5. Yang S, Milla C, Panoskaltsis-Mortari A, et al. Human surfactant protein a suppresses T cell-dependent inflammation and attenuates the manifestations of idiopathic pneumonia syndrome in mice. *Am J Respir Cell Mol Biol* 2001;24:527–536.
6. Hunsaker AR, Munden RF, Pugatch RD, et al. Sarcoidlike reaction in patient with malignancy. *Radiology* 1996;200:255–261.
7. Folz RJ. Mechanisms of lung injury after bone marrow transplantation. *Am J Respir Cell Mol Biol* 1999;20:1097–1099.
8. Crawford SW, Schwartz DA, Peterson FB, et al. Mechanical ventilation after marrow transplantation: risk factors and clinical outcomes. *Am Rev Respir Dis* 1988;137:682–687.
9. Paz HL, Crilley P, Weinar M, et al. Outcome of patients requiring medical ICU admission following bone marrow transplantation. *Chest* 1993;104:527–531.
10. Crawford SW. Using outcomes research to improve the management of blood and marrow transplant recipients in the intensive care unit. *New Horiz* 1998;6:69–74.
11. Clark JG, Hansen JA, Hertz MI, et al. Idiopathic pneumonia syndrome after bone marrow transplantation. *Am Rev Respir Dis* 1993;147:1601–1606.
12. Rubenfeld GD, Crawford SW. Withdrawing life support from mechanical ventilated recipients of bone marrow transplants: a case for evidence-based guidelines. *Ann Intern Med* 1996;125:625–633.
13. Krowka MJ, Rosenow EC, Hoagland HC. Pulmonary complications of bone marrow transplantation. *Chest* 1985;87:237–246.
14. Khurshid I, Anderson LC. Non-infectious pulmonary complications after bone marrow transplantation. *Postgrad Med J* 2002;78:257–262.
15. Clark JF, Hansen JA, Hertz MI, et al. Idiopathic pneumonia syndrome after bone marrow transplantation. *Am Rev Respir Dis* 1993;147:1601–1606.
16. Crawford SW, Hackman RC. Clinical course of idiopathic pneumonia syndrome after bone marrow transplantation. *Am Rev Respir Dis* 1993;147:1393–1400.
17. Shankar G, Cohen DA. Idiopathic pneumonia syndrome after bone marrow transplantation: the role of pre-transplant radiation conditioning and local cytokine dysregulation in promoting lung inflammation and fibrosis. *Int J Exp Pathol* 2001;82:101–113.
18. Wingard Jr, Mellitis Ed, Sostrin MB, et al. Interstitial pneumonias after allogenic bone marrow transplantation. *Medicine* 1988;67:175–186.
19. Ferrara Jl. Pathogenesis of acute graft-versus-host disease: cytokines and cellular effectors. *J Hematother Stem Cell Res* 2000;9:299–306.
20. Chan CK, Hyland RH, Hutcheon MA. Pulmonary complications following bone marrow transplantation. *Clin Chest Med* 1990;11:323–332.
21. Paz HL, Crilley P, Patchefsky A, et al. Bronchiolitis obliterans after autologous bone marrow transplantation. *Chest* 1992;102:775–778.
22. Cordonnier C, Fleury-Feith J, Escudier E, et al. Secondary alveolar proteinosis in a reversible cause of respiratory failure in leukemic patients. *Am J Respir Crit Care Med* 1994;149:788–794.
23. Witherspoon RP, Fisher LD, Schoch G, et al. Secondary cancers after bone marrow transplantation for leukemic or aplastic anemia. *N Engl J Med* 1989;321:784–789.
24. Woodard JP, Gulbahce E, Shreve M, et al. Pulmonary cytolytic thrombi: a newly recognized complication of stem cell transplantation. *Bone Marrow Transplant* 2000;25:293–300.
25. Nichols WG. Management of infectious complications in the hematopoietic stem cell transplant recipient. *J Intensive Care Med* 2003;18:295–312.
26. Sullivan KM, Dykewicz CA, Longworth DL, et al. Preventing opportunistic infections after hematopoietic stem cell transplantation: the Centers for Disease Control and Prevention, Infectious Diseases Society of America, and American Society for Blood and Marrow Transplantation Practice Guidelines and beyond. *Hematology* 2001;392–421.
27. Mermel LA, Farr BM, Sherertz RJ, et al. Guidelines for the management of intravascular catheter-related infections. *Clin Infect Dis* 2001;32:1249–1272.
28. Mora-Duarte J, Betts R, Rotstein C, et al. Comparison of caspofungin and amphotericin B for invasive candidiasis. *N Engl J Med* 2002;347:2020–2029.
29. Marr KA, Carter RA, Crippa F, et al. Epidemiology and outcome of mould infections in hematopoietic stem cell transplant recipients. *Clin Infect Dis* 2002;34:909–917.
30. Herbrecht R, Denning DW, Patterson TF, et al. Voriconazole versus amphotericin B for primary therapy of invasive aspergillosus. *N Engl J Med* 2002;347:408–415.
31. Perea S, Gonzalez G, Fothergill AW, et al. In vitro interaction of caspofungin acetate with voriconazole against clinical isolates of *Aspergillus* spp. *Antimicrob Agents Chemother* 2002;46:3039–3041.
32. Arikan S, Lozano-chiu M, Paetznick B, et al. In vitro synergy of caspofungin and amphotericin B against *Aspergillus* and *Fusarium* spp. *Antimicrob Agents Chemother* 2002;46:245–247.
33. Boeckh M, Ljungman P. Cytomegalovirus infection after BMT. In: Bowden RA, Ljungman P, Paya CV, eds. *Transplant infections.* Philadelphia: Lippincott–Raven Publishers, 1998:215–227.
34. Boeckh M. Current antiviral strategies for controlling cytomegalovirus in hematopoietic stem cell transplant recipients: prevention and therapy. *Transpl Infect Dis* 1999;1:165–178.
35. Hirschtick RE, Glassroth J, Jordan M, et al. Bacterial pneumonia in persons infected with the Human Immunodeficiency Virus. *N Engl J Med* 1995;333:845–851.
36. Boiselle PM, Aviram G, Fishman JE. Update on lung disease in AIDS. *Semin Roentgenol* 2002;37:54–71.
37. Bartlett JG. Pneumonia in the patient with HIV infection. *Infect Dis Clin North Am* 1998;12:807–820.
38. Maki DD. Pulmonary infections in HIV/AIDS. *Semin Roentgenol* 2000;35:124–139.
39. Rosen MJ. Epidemiology and risk of pulmonary disease. *Semin Respir Infect* 1999;14:301–308.
40. Barbaro G. Cardiovascular manifestations of HIV infection. *Circulation* 2002;106:1420–1425.
41. Schneider RF. Screening and noninvasive testing for pulmonary disease. *Semin Respir Infect* 1999;14:309–317.
42. Hanson DL, Chu SY, Farizo KM, et al. Distribution of CD4+ lymphocytes at diagnosis of Acquired Immunodeficiency Syndrome-defining and other Human Immunodeficiency Virus-related illnesses. *Arch Intern Med* 1995;155:1537–1542.
43. Aboulafia DM. The epidemiologic, pathologic, and clinical features of AIDS-associated pulmonary Kaposi's sarcoma. *Chest* 2000;117:1128–1145.
44. Bubman D, Cesarman E. Pathogenesis of Kaposi's sarcoma. *Hematol Oncol Clin North Am* 2003;17:717–745.
45. Cool CD, Rai PR, Yeager ME, et al. Expression of human herpesvirus 8 in primary pulmonary hypertension. *N Engl J Med* 2003;349:1113–1122.
46. Nichols CM, Flaitz CM, Hicks MJ. Treating Kaposi's lesions in the HIV-infected patient. *J Am Dent Assoc* 1993;124:78–84.
47. Huang L, Schnapp LM, Gruden JF, et al. Presentation of AIDS-related pulmonary Kaposi's sarcoma diagnosed by bronchoscopy. *Am J Respir Crit Care Med* 1996;153:1385–1390.
48. Gruden JF, Huang L, Webb WR, et al. AIDS-related Kaposi's sarcoma of the lung: radiographic findings and staging system with bronchoscopic correlation. *Radiology* 1995;195:545–552.
49. Dezube BJ. Acquired immunodeficiency syndrome-related Kaposi's sarcoma: clinical features, staging and treatment. *Semin Oncol* 2000;27:424–430.
50. Sparano JA. Human immunodeficiency virus associated lymphoma. *Curr Opin Oncol* 2003;15:372–378.

51. Mbulaiteye SM, Parkin DM, Rabkin CS. Epidemiology of AIDS-related malignancies: an international perspective. *Hematol Oncol Clin North Am* 2003;17:673–696.

52. Wolf AJ, O'Donnell AE. Pulmonary manifestations of HIV infection in the era of highly active antiretroviral therapy. *Chest* 2001; 120:1888–1893.

53. Cooley TP. Non-AIDS-defining cancer in HIV-infected people. *Hematol Oncol Clin North Am* 2003;17:889–895.

54. Elssner A, Carter JE, Yunger TM, et al. HIV-1 infection does not impair human alveolar macrophage phagocytic function unless combined with cigarette smoking. *Chest* 2004;125:1071–1076.

55. Diaz PT, King MA, Pacht ER, et al. Increased susceptibility to pulmonary emphysema among HIV-seropositive smokers. *Ann Intern Med* 2000;132:369–372.

56. Wistuba II, Behrens C, Milchgrub S, et al. Comparison of molecular changes in lung cancers in HIV-positive and HIV-indeterminate subjects. *JAMA* 1998;279:1554–1559.

57. Fishman JE, Schwartz DS, Sais GJ, et al. Bronchogenic carcinoma in HIV-positive patients: findings on chest radiographs and CT scans. *Am J Roentgenol* 1995;164:57–61.

58. Heidenreich PA, Eisenberg MJ, Kee LL, et al. Pericardial effusion in AIDS: incidence and survival. *Circulation* 1995;92:3229–3234.

59. Elliott CG, Markewitz BA. Genetics of primary pulmonary hypertension. Harrison's Online 2004 (www.harrisonsonline.com).

60. Nunes H, Humbert M, Sitbon O, et al. Prognostic factors for survival in human immunodeficiency virus-associated pulmonary arterial hypertension. *Am J Respir Crit Care Med* 2003;167: 1433–1439.

61. Aguilar RV, Farber HW. Epoprostenol (prostacyclin) therapy in HIV-associated pulmonary hypertension. *Am J Respir Crit Care Med* 2000;162:1846–1850.

62. Sattler F, Nichols L, Hirano L, et al. Nonspecific interstitial pneumonitis mimicking *Pneumocystis carinii* pneumonia. *Am J Respir Crit Care Med* 1997;156:912–917.

63. Allen JN, Wewers MD. HIV-associated bronchiolitis obliterans organizing pneumonia. *Chest* 1989;96:197–198.

64. Joseph J, Harley RA, Frye MD. Bronchiolitis obliterans with organizing pneumonia in AIDS. *N Eng J Med* 1995;332:273.

65. Diaz PT, Clanton TL, Pacht ER. Emphysema-like pulmonary disease associated with human immunodeficiency virus infection. *Ann Intern Med* 1992;116:124–128.

66. Ammann AJ, Schiffman G, Abrams D, et al. B-cell immunodeficiency in acquired immune deficiency syndrome. *JAMA* 1984;251: 1447–1449.

67. Wallace JM, Hansen MI, Lavange L, et al. Respiratory disease trends in the pulmonary complications of HIV infection study cohort. *Am J Respir Crit Care Med* 1997;155:72–80.

68. Schneider RF. Bacterial pneumonia. *Semin Respir Infect* 1999;14: 327–332.

69. Brecher CW, Aviram G, Boiselle PM. CT and radiography of bacterial respiratory infections in AIDS patients. *Am J Roentgenol* 2003;180:1203–1209.

70. Jasmer RM, Edinburgh KJ, Thompson A, et al. Clinical and radiographic predictors of the etiology of pulmonary nodules in HIV-infected patients. *Chest* 2000;117:1023–1030.

71. Aviram G, Fishman JE, Sagar M. Cavitary lung disease in AIDS: etiologies and correlation with immune status. *AIDS Patient Care STDS* 2001;15:353–361.

72. Gold JA, Rom WN, Harkin TJ. Significance of abnormal chest radiograph findings in patients with HIV-1 infection without respiratory symptoms. *Chest* 2002;121:1472–1477.

73. Sullivan JH, Moore RD, Deruly JC, et al. Effect of antiretroviral therapy on the incidence of bacterial pneumonia in patients with advanced HIV infection. *Am J Respir Crit Care Med* 2000;162: 64–67.

74. Wolf AJ, O'Donnell AE. HIV-related pulmonary infections: a review of the recent literature. *Curr Opin Pulm Med* 2003;9:10–214.

75. Selwyn PA, Hartel D, Lewis VA, et al. A prospective study of the risk of tuberculosis among intravenous drug users with human immunodeficiency virus infection. *N Engl J Med* 1989;320: 545–550.

76. Markowitz N, Hansen NI, Hopewell PC, et al. Incidence of tuberculosis in the United States among HIV-infected persons. *Ann Intern Med* 1997;126:123–132.

77. Havlir DV, Barnes PF. Tuberculosis in patients with human immunodeficiency virus infection. *N Engl J Med* 1999;340:367–373.

78. Gordin FM, Matts JP, Miller C, et al. A controlled trial of isoniazid in persons with anergy and human immunodeficiency virus infection who are at high risk for tuberculosis. *N Engl J Med* 1997; 337:315–320.

79. Johnson JL, Odwera A, Hom DL, et al. Duration of efficacy of treatment of latent tuberculosis infection in HIV-infected adults. *AIDS* 2001;15:2137–2147.

80. Zhang M, Gong J, Iyer DV, et al. T cell cytokine responses in persons with tuberculosis and human immunodeficiency virus infection. *J Clin Invest* 1994;94:2435–2442.

81. Nakata K, Rom WN, Condos R, et al. Mycobacterium tuberculosis enhances human immunodeficiency virus-1 replication in the lung. *Am J Respir Crit Care Med* 1997;155:996–1003.

82. Whalen C, Horsburgh CR, Hom D, et al. Accelerated course of human immunodeficiency virus infection after tuberculosis. *Am J Respir Crit Care Med* 1995;151:129–135.

83. Busi Rizzi E, Schinina V, Palmieri F, et al. Radiological patterns in HIV-associated pulmonary tuberculosis: comparison between HAART-treated and non-HAART-treated patients. *Clin Radiol* 2003;58:469–473.

84. Centers for Disease Control and Prevention. Treatment of tuberculosis. American Thoracic Society, CDC, and Infectious Diseases Society of America. *MMWR* 2003;52(RR-11):1–77.

85. Stringer JR, Beard CB, Miller RF, et al. A new name (*Pneumocystis jiroveci*) for *Pneumocystis* from humans. *Emerg Infect Dis* 2002;8:891–896.

86. Kaplan JE, Hanson D, Dworkin MS, et al. Epidemiology of human immunodeficiency virus-associated opportunistic infections in the United States in the era of highly active antiretroviral therapy. *Clin Infect Dis* 2000;30:S5–S14.

87. Kovacs JA, Gill VJ, Meshnick S, et al. New insights into transmission, diagnosis, and drug treatment of *Pneumocystis carinii* pneumonia. *JAMA* 2001;286:2450–2460.

88. Boiselle PM, Crans CA, Kaplan MA. The changing face of *Pneumocystis carinii* pneumonia in AIDS patients. *Am J Roentgenol* 1999;172:1301–1309.

89. Cruciani M, Marcati P, Malena M, et al. Meta-analysis of diagnostic procedures for *Pneumocystis carinii* pneumonia in HIV-1-infected patients. *Eur Respir J* 2002;20:982–989.

90. Masur H, Meier P, McCutchan JA, et al. Consensus statement on the use of corticosteroids as adjunctive therapy for pneumocystis pneumonia in the acquired immunodeficiency syndrome. *N Engl J Med* 1990;323:1500–1504.

91. Toma E, Thorne A, Singer J, et al. Clindamycin with primaquine vs. trimethoprim-sulfamethoxazole therapy for mild and moderately severe *Pneumocystis carinii* pneumonia in patients with AIDS: a multicenter, double-blind, randomized trial (CTN 004). *Clin Infect Dis* 1998;27:524–530.

92. Hirsch HH, Kaufmann G, Sendi P, et al. Immune reconstitution in HIV-infected patients. *Clin Infect Dis* 2004;38:1159–1166.

93. Randall Curtis J, Yarnold PR, Schwartz DN, et al. Improvements in outcomes of acute respiratory failure for patients with human immunodeficiency virus-related *Pneumocystis carinii* pneumonia. *Am J Respir Crit Care med* 2000;162:393–398.

94. Franklin C, Friedman Y, Wong T, et al. Improving long-term prognosis for survivors of mechanical ventilation in patients with AIDS with PCP and acute respiratory failure: five-year follow-up of intensive care unit discharges. *Arch Int Med* 1995; 155:91–95.

95. Furrer H, Egger M, Opravil M, et al. Discontinuation of primary prophylaxis against *Pneumocystis carinii* pneumonia in HIV-1-infected adults treated with combination antiretroviral therapy. *N Engl J Med* 1999;340:1301–1306.

96. Kaplan JE, Masur H, Holmes KK. Guidelines for preventing opportunistic infections among HIV-infected persons—2002: recommendations of the U.S. Public Health Service and the Infectious Diseases Society of America. *MMWR* 2002;51(RR08): 1–46.

97. Hughes WT. Use of Dapsone in the prevention and treatment of *Pneumocystis carinii* pneumonia: a review. *Clin Infect Dis* 1998; 27:191–204.

98. Sarosi GA, Ampel N, Cohn DL, et al. Fungal infection in HIV-infected persons. *Am J Respir Crit Care Med* 1995;152:816–822.

99. Sacktor N, Lyles RH, Skolasky R, et al. HIV-associated neurologic disease incidence changes: multicenter AIDS cohort study, 1990–1998. *Neurology* 2001;56:257–260.

100. Saag MS, Graybill RJ, Larsen RA, et al. Practice guidelines for the management of cryptococcal disease. *Clin Infect Dis* 2000;30:710–718.

101. Hajjeh RA, Pappas PG, Henderson, et al. Multicenter case-control study of risk factors for histoplasmosis in human immunodeficiency virus-infected persons. *Clin Infect Dis* 2001; 32:1215–1220.

102. Johnson PC, Wheat LJ, Cloud GA, et al. Safety and efficacy of liposomal amphotericin B compared with conventional amphotericin B for induction therapy of histoplasmosis in patients with AIDS. *Ann Intern Med* 2002;137:105–109.

103. Denning DW. Invasive aspergillosis. *Clin Infect Dis* 1998;26:781–805.

104. Mann M, Shelhamer JH, Masur H, et al. Lack of utility of bronchoalveolar lavage cultures for cytomegalovirus in HIV infection. *Am J Respir Crit Care Med* 1997;155:1723–1728.

105. Deayton J, Mocroft AA, Wilson PB, et al. Loss of cytomegalovirus (CMV) viraemia following highly active antiretroviral therapy in the absence of specific anti-CMV therapy. *AIDS* 1999;13:1203–1206.

106. Whitley RJ, Jacobson MA, Friedberg DN, et al. Guidelines for the treatment of cytomegalovirus diseases in patients with AIDS in the era of potent antiretroviral therapy. *Arch Int Med* 1998;158:957–969.

107. Soubani AO, Miller KB, Hassoun PM. Pulmonary complications of bone marrow transplantation. *Chest* 1996;109:1066–1077.

CHAPTER 17

Diseases of the Pleura, Mediastinum, Chest Wall, and Diaphragm

Richard W. Light

DISEASES OF THE PLEURA

The pleural space is not really a space but rather a potential space between the lung and chest wall. It is a crucial feature of the breathing apparatus because it serves as a coupling system between the lung and chest wall. There is normally a very thin layer of fluid (from 2 to 10 μm thick) between the two pleural surfaces. The pleural space and the fluid within it are not under static conditions. During each respiratory cycle, the pleural pressures and the geometry of the pleural space fluctuate widely. Fluid constantly enters and leaves the pleural space. In this section are discussed the anatomy and physiology of the pleural space, as well as the etiology, diagnosis, and treatment of various diseases that affect it.

ANATOMY OF THE PLEURAL SPACE

The serous membrane covering the lung parenchyma is called the *visceral pleura*. The remainder of the lining of the pleural cavity is designated the *parietal pleura*. The parietal pleura includes the diaphragmatic pleura, the mediastinal pleura, and the costal pleura, which cover the diaphragm, mediastinum, and thoracic skeleton, respectively. The visceral pleura and the parietal pleura meet at the lung root at the hilum.

The parietal pleura receives its blood supply from the systemic capillaries. The branches of the bronchial artery predominantly supply the visceral pleura in humans and the thick visceral pleura in large animals such as sheep or horses (1). The lymphatic vessels in the parietal pleura are in direct communication with the pleural space by means of stomata (2). These stomata are the only route through which cells and large particles can leave the pleural space and are the primary route through which liquid exits the pleural space. Although there are abundant lymphatics in the visceral pleura, these lymphatics do not appear to participate in the removal of particulate matter or fluid from the pleural space.

PHYSIOLOGY OF THE PLEURAL SPACE

Fluid can enter the pleural space from the capillaries in the parietal or visceral pleura or from the interstitial spaces or lymphatics in either pleural surface. The passage of protein-free liquid across the pleural capillaries is dependent on the hydrostatic and oncotic pressures across them (see Fig. 17-1). When the capillaries in the parietal pleura are considered, the net hydrostatic pressure favoring the movement of fluid from these capillaries to the pleural space is the difference between the systemic capillary pressure (28 cm H_2O) minus the negative pleural pressure (5 cm H_2O), that is, 33 cm H_2O. Opposing this is the difference between the oncotic pressure in the blood (30 cm H_2O) minus the oncotic pressure in the pleural fluid (4 cm H_2O), that is, 26 cm H_2O. The resulting net pressure difference of 7 cm H_2O (33–26) favors movement of fluid from the parietal pleura into the pleural space.

The only difference between the visceral and the parietal pleura in the scheme outlined in Figure 17-1 is that the capillaries of the visceral pleura have a slightly lower hydrostatic pressure because they drain into the low-pressure pulmonary veins. The net force across the visceral pleura is 2 cm H_2O, again favoring the movement of fluid into the pleural space.

In recent years, it has become apparent that the origin of much pleural fluid is the interstitial spaces of the lung. The pleural membranes are leaky to both liquid and protein (3). The pleural pressure is lower than the interstitial pressure, and this pressure difference produces a gradient for fluid to move from the interstitium to the pleural space (4). When the acute respiratory

distress syndrome (ARDS) is induced in sheep with the intravenous (IV) injection of oleic acid, 20% of the edema fluid exits the lung via the pleural space (5). When high-pressure pulmonary edema is induced in sheep with fluid overload, again about 20% of the edema fluid is cleared via the pleural space (6). Patients with heart failure are much more likely to have pleural effusions if there is radiologic evidence of pulmonary edema (7).

The rate of pleural fluid formation in each pleural space in normal animals with a thick visceral pleura is approximately 0.01 mL/kg/hour or 15 mL per 24 hours for a 60-kg individual (8). There is a small amount of protein in this fluid. Normally, the pleural space is maintained nearly fluid-free because the filtered fluid is removed from the pleural space by the pleural lymphatics, which can remove more than 0.20 mL/kg/hour from each pleural space (8). Pleural fluid will accumulate, producing a pleural effusion, when the rate of pleural fluid formation exceeds the capacity of the lymphatics in the parietal pleura to remove the fluid. Pleural effusions can also develop when chyle escapes from the thoracic duct (i.e., chylothorax), when blood vessels are disrupted (i.e., hemothorax), or when there is free fluid in the peritoneal cavity if there are holes in the diaphragm.

PLEURAL EFFUSIONS

Pathophysiology

Pleural fluid will accumulate when the rate of pleural fluid formation is greater than the rate of pleural fluid removal by the lymphatics. Pleural fluid will continue to accumulate until another equilibrium is reached. Pleural effusions have classically been divided into transudative and exudative pleural effusions. A transudative pleural effusion occurs when alterations in the *systemic* factors that influence pleural fluid movement result in a pleural effusion (e.g., increased pulmonary interstitial fluid and elevated visceral pleural capillary pressure with left ventricular failure, elevated parietal pleural capillary pressure with right ventricular failure, and elevated portal pressures with cirrhosis, leading to ascites and a pleural effusion in some cases). In contrast, exudative pleural effusions occur when *local* factors are altered in such a way that pleural fluid accumulates. Inflammation of the lung or the pleura leading to increased flux of fluid from the capillaries of the lung or the pleura into the pleural space is the most common cause of exudative pleural effusions. However, exudative effusions can also occur with decreased lymphatic flow or with a more negative pleural pressure, as with atelectasis.

Clinical Manifestations

The symptoms of a patient with a pleural effusion are to a large extent dictated by the underlying process causing the effusion. Many patients have no symptoms referable to the effusion. When symptoms are related to the effusion, they arise either from inflammation of the pleura or from compromise of pulmonary mechanics. Pleuritic chest pain is the usual symptom of pleural inflammation. Because there are pain fibers only in the parietal pleura, pleuritic chest pain indicates inflammation of the parietal pleura. Some patients with pleural effusion experience dull, aching chest pain. This symptom is particularly common if the underlying process directly involves the parietal pleura, as with metastatic tumor or lung abscess. Irritation of the pleural surfaces may also result in a dry, nonproductive cough.

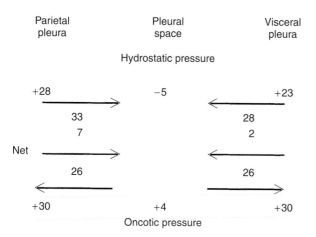

FIGURE 17-1. Diagrammatic representation of the pressures involved in the formation and absorption of pleural fluid.

The presence of a large effusion can compromise pulmonary mechanics and cause dyspnea.

Physical examination of a patient with pleural effusion reveals decreased or absent tactile fremitus, dullness to percussion, and diminished breath sounds over the site of the effusion. Bronchial breath sounds and egophony are frequently present immediately above the effusion.

A pleural effusion acts as a space-occupying process in the thoracic cavity and therefore reduces all subdivisions of lung volumes. However, the increase in lung volumes after a therapeutic thoracentesis is much less than the volume of fluid removed (9). With larger effusions, dyspnea results from lung compression and diaphragmatic flattening or inversion (10). Even though an entire lung may be compressed when the pleural effusion occupies a complete hemithorax, blood gases usually remain nearly normal owing to a reflex reduction in perfusion to the unventilated lung.

Radiographic Appearance

Because pleural fluid is denser than the lung, the fluid tends to go to the lowermost parts of the thoracic cavity as the lung floats in the fluid. In contrast, with pneumothorax the air is lighter than the lung, so it tends to rise to the uppermost part of the thoracic cavity. The other factor governing the radiologic appearance of a pleural effusion is the inherent tendency of the lung to maintain its usual shape at all stages of collapse.

The first fluid accumulates in the most dependent portion of the thoracic cavity, which is the posterior costophrenic angle. Therefore, the earliest radiologic sign of a pleural effusion is blunting of the posterior costophrenic angle on the lateral chest radiograph. After several hundred milliliters of fluid accumulate, the fluid spills out into the costophrenic sinuses laterally and anteriorly. At this time, the lateral costophrenic angle on the posteroanterior radiograph is obliterated. Blunting of the posterior and lateral costophrenic angles also occurs as a result of previous inflammation or chronic obstructive pulmonary disease (COPD). Pleural fluid can be differentiated from these entities by obtaining lateral decubitus radiographs. If a posteroanterior radiograph is obtained with the patient lying on the affected side, free pleural fluid will gravitate inferiorly and a pleural fluid line (see Fig. 7-1 in Chapter 7) will be visible. If the film is obtained with the patient lying on the contralateral side, the angle will clear if the blunting is caused by fluid. Alternatively, if the blunting is not due to free-flowing fluid, neither a pleural fluid line nor clearing of the blunted angle will be observed.

Pleural fluid is said to be *loculated* when it does not shift freely in the pleural space as the patient's position is changed. Loculated pleural effusions occur when there are adhesions between the visceral and parietal pleurae. Such adhesions result from marked inflammation of the pleura. It follows that loculated pleural effusions are more common with empyema or hemothorax. At times, the differentiation of loculated pleural fluid from pleural thickening or parenchymal disease is quite difficult. Both ultrasound and computed tomography (CT) have proved useful in making this differentiation (11).

Approach to the Patient with Pleural Effusion

There are many different diseases that can be associated with pleural effusion (see Table 17-1). When a pleural effusion is

TABLE 17-1. Differential Diagnosis of Pleural Effusion

Transudative pleural effusions
- Congestive heart failure
- Cirrhosis
- Pericardial disease
- Nephrotic syndrome
- Myxedema
- Peritoneal dialysis
- Urinary tract obstruction

Exudative pleural effusions
- Infectious diseases
  - Bacterial infections
  - Tuberculosis
  - Fungal infections
  - Viral infections
  - Parasitic infections
- Neoplastic diseases
  - Metastatic disease
  - Mesotheliomas
- Collagen vascular diseases
  - Systemic lupus erythematosus
  - Rheumatoid pleuritis
- Pulmonary embolism
- Gastrointestinal diseases
  - Acute pancreatitis
  - Pancreatic pseudocyst
  - Esophageal perforations
  - Intraabdominal abscess
- Postsurgical pleural effusions
  - Post–coronary artery bypass surgery
  - Post–abdominal surgery
  - Post–lung transplant
  - Post–liver transplant
  - Post–endoscopic esophageal sclerotherapy
- Drug hypersensitivity
  - Nitrofurantoin
  - Methysergide
  - Dantrolene
  - Ergot alkaloids
  - Procarbazine
  - Amiodarone
- Miscellaneous diseases
  - Asbestos exposure
  - Meigs syndrome
  - Uremia
  - Post–cardiac injury syndrome
  - Trapped lung
  - Yellow nail syndrome
  - Sarcoidosis
- Hemothorax
- Chylothorax
  - Traumatic
  - Nontraumatic
  - Pulmonary and lymphangioleiomyomatosis

discovered, two questions need to be answered: (a) Is the effusion a transudate (i.e., is it due to systemic factors) or is it an exudate (i.e., is it due to disease of the pleura itself)? (b) If the effusion is an exudate, what is the disease responsible for its production? Answers to these two questions can be obtained only by examining the pleural fluid.

Nearly every patient with a pleural effusion should have a diagnostic thoracentesis. No difficulty should be encountered in obtaining fluid if the pleural fluid is more than 10 mm in thickness on the lateral decubitus roentgenogram. The performance of the diagnostic thoracentesis, the separation of transudates from exudates, and the utility of various diagnostic tests on the pleural fluid are discussed in Chapter 7, Invasive Diagnostic Procedures.

TRANSUDATIVE PLEURAL EFFUSIONS

Congestive Heart Failure

Congestive heart failure is probably responsible for more pleural effusions than any other disease entity. The accumulation of pleural fluid can be secondary to increases in the hydrostatic pressures in either the systemic or the pulmonary circulation. Clinically, however, pleural effusion due to congestive heart failure usually occurs only when the pulmonary wedge pressure is elevated (7). It is thought that the origin of the increased pleural fluid is the interstitial spaces of the lung. The pleural effusion is usually bilateral, but if it is unilateral it is more commonly on the right (12). A large unilateral effusion is uncommon in uncomplicated congestive heart failure and suggests malignancy, pulmonary emboli, or other complicating disease.

The diagnosis is usually suggested by the clinical picture of congestive heart failure. With appropriate treatment of the heart failure, the effusion will resolve rapidly in most cases. When the patient is first evaluated, a thoracentesis is indicated if the effusions are not bilateral and comparable in size, if the patient has pleuritic chest pain, or if the patient is febrile. If an initial thoracentesis is not performed and the pleural effusion persists after treatment, a diagnostic thoracentesis can be performed subsequently. When pleural fluid accumulates because of congestive heart failure, it is a transudate by definition. However, with diuresis, the protein and lactic acid dehydrogenase (LDH) levels in the pleural fluid may increase such that they meet Light's exudative criteria (13). However, if the serum level of protein is more than 3.1 gm per dL higher than the pleural fluid protein level, the fluid can be said to be transudative (13).

Cirrhosis

The incidence of pleural effusion with cirrhosis is approximately 5%. The predominant mechanism leading to a pleural effusion in a patient with cirrhosis and ascites appears to be the movement of the ascitic fluid from the peritoneal cavity through a diaphragmatic defect into the pleural space (14). The decreased plasma oncotic pressure is only a secondary factor.

The clinical picture is of cirrhosis and ascites, although at times, the ascites may be minimal. The effusions are most commonly on the right side but may be bilateral or left sided. At times, the effusions may be very large, occupying almost an entire hemithorax. These large effusions may induce respiratory symptoms. Therapeutic thoracentesis is of virtually no use because the fluid reaccumulates very rapidly as it flows from the peritoneal cavity into the pleural cavity.

The initial management of the pleural effusion associated with cirrhosis and ascites should be directed toward treatment

of the ascites with a low-salt diet and diuretics. If the ascites cannot be controlled with conservative measures, more aggressive measures are indicated. The optimal treatment is liver transplantation, but the implantation of a transjugular intrahepatic portal systemic shunt (TIPS) usually controls the ascites and the effusion (14). If neither TIPS nor liver transplantation is feasible, the best alternative is probably videothoracoscopy with closure of the diaphragmatic defects and pleurodesis (15), but this approach is associated with significant morbidity and mortality (15).

Other Causes of Transudative Pleural Effusions

PERICARDIAL DISEASE. The incidence of pleural effusion in patients with pericardial disease is about 30% (16). Most of the effusions are left sided or bilateral and are small to moderate in size. The pleural effusion is usually transudative and results from either elevated capillary pressures or pericardial inflammation.

NEPHROTIC SYNDROME. Patients with the nephrotic syndrome commonly have an associated pleural effusion. The mechanism responsible for the effusion is probably decreased plasma oncotic pressure secondary to the hypoproteinemia in combination with the increased hydrostatic pressure because of salt retention producing hypervolemia (17). The fluid is a typical transudate. Treatment is aimed at the nephrotic syndrome in an attempt to increase the serum proteins.

MYXEDEMA. A pleural effusion sometimes occurs as a complication of myxedema. Most patients with myxedema and pleural effusion have a concomitant pericardial effusion, in which case the pleural effusion is a transudate. The rare isolated pleural effusion seen in conjunction with myxedema can be either a transudate or an exudate (18).

PERITONEAL DIALYSIS. Approximately 1% to 2% of patients on continuous ambulatory peritoneal dialysis will develop a pleural effusion. The mechanism is probably the same as that with cirrhosis and ascites. The peritoneal dialysis increases the intraabdominal pressure, and the dialysate flows from the peritoneal cavity into the pleural cavity through pores in the diaphragm. The pleural fluid in such instances is similar to the dialysate. The treatment of choice is thoracoscopy with closure of the diaphragmatic defects, followed by pleurodesis (19).

URINARY TRACT OBSTRUCTION. Obstruction of the urinary tract, with its associated retroperitoneal urine collection, can lead to a pleural effusion. It is believed that the urine moves directly retroperitoneally into the pleural space. The diagnosis is established by the demonstration that the pleural fluid creatinine level is higher than the serum creatinine level. The pleural effusion will rapidly disappear when the urinary tract obstruction is relieved (20).

EXUDATIVE PLEURAL EFFUSIONS

Parapneumonic Effusion

Any pleural effusion associated with bacterial pneumonia, lung abscess, or bronchiectasis is a parapneumonic effusion.

Parapneumonic effusions are common because more than one million patients are hospitalized annually in the United States, and 40% of these have an associated parapneumonic effusion (21). The amount of fluid varies from a few milliliters, in which case the fluid is usually not detected, to several liters. The character of the fluid varies from a clear, straw-colored fluid with a few hundred white blood cells (WBC) per cubic millimeter to frank pus. Parapneumonic effusions that require tube thoracostomy or which are culture positive are designated *complicated parapneumonic effusions*.

NATURAL HISTORY OF PARAPNEUMONIC EFFUSIONS. The evolution of a parapneumonic effusion can be divided into three stages (18). The first stage is the *exudative* stage, in which a focus of parenchymal infection leads to increased pulmonary interstitial fluid. This fluid traverses the visceral pleura and results in the accumulation of pleural fluid. In this stage, the pleural fluid is characterized by a relatively low LDH level and a normal glucose and pH.

The second stage is the *fibropurulent* stage, which is characterized by the invasion of the pleural fluid by bacteria. As this stage progresses, the pleural fluid becomes increasingly cloudy and viscous because it contains large amounts of fibrin, cellular debris, and WBCs. In this stage, there is a progressive tendency toward loculation of the fluid and the formation of limiting membranes. Although the loculation prevents extension of the pleural infection, it makes drainage of the pleural space difficult.

The third stage is the *organization* stage, in which fibroblasts grow into the exudate from both the visceral and parietal pleural surfaces to produce an inelastic membrane called the *pleural peel*. This peel encases the lung and prevents it from expanding to obliterate the pleural space. At this stage, the exudate is very thick, and if the patient has remained untreated, the fluid may drain spontaneously through the chest wall (*empyema necessitatis*) or into the lung, in which case a bronchopleural fistula will be produced.

INITIAL MANAGEMENT OF PATIENTS WITH PARAPNEUMONIC EFFUSION. When a patient with acute bacterial pneumonia is initially evaluated, the physician should determine whether a parapneumonic effusion is present. If the posterior costophrenic angles are not blunted on the lateral chest radiograph, one can assume that there is not a clinically significant pleural effusion unless the chest radiograph reveals loculated fluid elsewhere in the chest. If the posterior costophrenic angles are blunted or if the diaphragm is obscured by the infiltrate, then an ultrasonic examination or a lateral decubitus chest roentgenogram should be obtained with the suspicious side down (22). The amount of pleural fluid can be semiquantitated on the decubitus film by measuring the distance between the inside of the chest wall and the bottom of the lung. If this measurement is <10 mm, it can be assumed that the effusion is not clinically significant and thoracentesis is not indicated (22).

If the thickness of the fluid is >10 mm on the decubitus x-ray film, a therapeutic thoracentesis should be performed with an attempt to remove all the pleural fluid. If the fluid is removed completely with the therapeutic thoracentesis and does not reaccumulate, no additional therapy needs to be directed toward the effusion. At the time of the initial therapeutic thoracentesis, the pleural fluid should be Gram stained and cultured and analyzed for leukocyte count, LDH, glucose, and pH levels. Indicators of a poor prognosis, in order of decreasing seriousness, are the presence of pus, a glucose level <60 mg per dL, a pH <7.00, and an LDH level more than three times the upper limit of normal (23).

If the therapeutic thoracentesis removes all the pleural fluid and the fluid recurs, the next step is guided by the initial pleural fluid findings. If none of the poor prognostic indicators listed above are present, no invasive procedures are indicated if the patient is doing well clinically. If any of the poor prognostic indicators were present at the initial thoracentesis, a second therapeutic thoracentesis should be performed and the pleural fluid reanalyzed. If the pleural fluid accumulates a third time, a small (8 to 13 French) chest tube should be inserted into the pleural space unless none of the poor prognostic factors were present at the time of the second thoracentesis (23).

The presence of a pleural effusion affects the choice of antibiotics because aminoglycosides do not enter the pleural space well and anaerobic organisms frequently are the causative organisms for complicated parapneumonic effusions (22). For patients hospitalized with community-acquired pneumonias (CAP) that are not severe, the recommended agents are a fluoroquinolone alone or a β-lactam combined with a macrolide. For patients with severe CAP, the recommended agents are an IV β-lactam plus a macrolide or an IV fluoroquinolone (24).

LOCULATED PLEURAL FLUID. If the pleural fluid cannot be removed completely with a therapeutic thoracentesis or with a small chest tube, it is probably loculated. The loculation indicates a high level of inflammation in the pleural space. Most loculated pleural effusions require drainage. If the pleural fluid is loculated and if any of the poor prognostic factors listed above are present, efforts should be made to break down the loculations in order to obtain complete drainage of the pleural space.

The two primary means by which the loculations can be broken down are with fibrinolytics or with thoracoscopy. However, intrapleural streptokinase was no more effective than saline in promoting drainage in loculated parapneumonic effusions in a recently completed multicenter study with more than 350 patients (25). Alternative fibrinolytics to use in this situation are tissue plasminogen activator (TPA) 10 mg or urokinase 250,000 units once or twice daily.

The alternative approach to the patient with loculated pleural effusions is thoracoscopy with the breakdown of adhesions. Most patients who undergo thoracoscopy need no additional therapy. When four recent studies with a total of 232 patients are combined, thoracoscopy was the definitive procedure in 77% of the patients (18). Postthoracoscopy, the median hospital stay ranged from 5.3 to 12.3 days, the median time for chest tube drainage postprocedure ranged from 3.3 to 7.1 days, and the overall mortality was 3% (18). One study (26) concluded that proceeding directly to thoracoscopy was more cost effective than using an intermediate step with fibrinolytics. One advantage of thoracoscopy is that the chest tube can be positioned in the most dependent part of the empyema cavity. Before thoracoscopy is performed, a CT scan should be obtained. This examination will provide information about the size and extent of the empyema cavity that will guide the planned procedure.

A thickened visceral pleural peel without septations suggests that the empyema may be chronic and probably will not be amenable to thoracoscopic debridement alone (27).

When faced with a patient with a loculated parapneumonic effusion, should fibrinolytics be administered intrapleurally or should thoracoscopy be performed? It is recommended that patients with loculated parapneumonic effusions and poor prognostic indicators in the pleural fluid be treated initially with thoracoscopy if the expertise for this procedure is available locally. If the expertise is not available locally, then a trial of fibrinolytics is warranted. If there is not substantial improvement with the fibrinolytics within a few days, one should proceed to more invasive procedures.

THORACOTOMY WITH DECORTICATION. This is the most invasive procedure for the treatment of parapneumonic effusions and empyema. With decortication, all the fibrous tissue is removed from the visceral pleura and all pus is evacuated from the pleural space (28). The primary indication for decortication is a trapped lung; loculations are better treated with thoracoscopy. This procedure allows the underlying lung to reexpand and obliterate the pleural space. Some thoracic surgeons recommend decortication in all cases in which a thick pleural peel remains after either closed or open drainage of a pleural infection. However, because the pleural peel frequently improves substantially in the months after the drainage, it is recommended that decortication be delayed for at least 6 months if the infection has been controlled and if the lung has reexpanded. After this time, decortication should be performed only if the patient has limited exercise capacity and if close evaluation of the patient's pulmonary status suggests that the procedure will improve pulmonary function.

Tuberculous Pleural Effusions

In many parts of the world, the most common cause of an exudative pleural effusion is tuberculosis (TB). However, in the United States, the annual incidence of tuberculous pleural effusion is only about 1,000 cases. Of all the patients with TB in the United States, approximately 1 in every 30 has pleural TB, which is also known as *tuberculous pleuritis* (29). In some countries, however, the percentage of patients with TB who have a pleural effusion exceeds 30% (30).

PATHOGENESIS. The exudative pleural effusion associated with pleural TB appears to be predominantly a manifestation of delayed hypersensitivity to tuberculous protein. Frequently, it is difficult to demonstrate the tubercle bacillus in either the pleural fluid or the pleural tissue. It is probable that granulomatous pleuritis results any time a patient with a positive tuberculin purified protein derivative (PPD) skin test gets tubercle bacillus protein into their pleural space. It should be emphasized that many patients with tuberculous pleuritis have a negative PPD test when first seen. The possible explanations for the negative PPD test in these individuals are that there are circulating adherent cells that suppress the delayed hypersensitivity reaction to the PPD in the skin or that the specifically sensitized lymphocytes are sequestered in the pleural space (31).

CLINICAL MANIFESTATIONS. A pleural effusion as a manifestation of TB has been likened to a primary chancre as a manifestation of syphilis. Both are self-limited and of little immediate concern, but both may lead to serious disease at a later date. Most cases of isolated tuberculous effusion will resolve spontaneously without treatment, but active TB will subsequently develop in a large percentage of these patients. Patiala (32) followed 2,816 members of the Finnish armed forces who developed pleural effusion during World War II before antituberculous drugs were available. More than 40% of these individuals developed active TB during the 7-year follow-up period. Accordingly, when managing a patient with a pleural effusion, it is the physician's obligation either to treat the patient for tuberculous pleuritis or to exclude this diagnosis.

At the onset of tuberculous pleuritis, most patients have symptoms of an upper respiratory tract infection and many also have pleuritic chest pain. Most, but not all, patients also have a temperature elevation commonly in the 103° to 105°F range. Subsequently, the patient develops a chronic illness characterized by anorexia, weight loss, and a low-grade fever. Without treatment, most patients will recover completely, only to develop active TB at another site later. Most patients with tuberculous pleuritis do not have radiologically evident parenchymal infiltrates. In those without parenchymal infiltrates, the effusion is almost always unilateral.

DIAGNOSIS. The diagnosis of tuberculous pleuritis should be considered in every patient with an exudative pleural effusion. The diagnosis of tuberculous pleuritis depends on the demonstration of a positive marker for TB in the pleural fluid, tubercle bacilli in the sputum, pleural fluid, or pleura, or of granulomas in the pleura. A negative PPD test when the patient is first seen certainly does not rule out the diagnosis. Sputum should be examined for acid-fast bacilli because it is positive for acid-fast bacilli in up to 50% of patients with tuberculous pleuritis whether or not there are parenchymal infiltrates (33).

Pleural fluid analysis in tuberculous pleuritis is useful. The fluid is invariably an exudate. Frequently, the pleural fluid protein is more than 5.0 g per 100 mL, and this finding is very suggestive of tuberculous pleuritis. In most cases, the differential white cell count reveals more than 80% lymphocytes, but if symptoms have been present for less than 1 week, neutrophils at times predominate. A pleural effusion that contains more than 10% eosinophils at the time of the initial thoracentesis is seldom, if ever, tuberculous. The pleural fluid glucose level may be reduced with tuberculous pleuritis, but most patients have a pleural fluid glucose level above 60 mg per dL (18). Cultures of the pleural fluid for tubercle bacilli are positive in less than 20% of cases (34).

As discussed in detail in Chapter 7, Invasive Diagnostic Procedures, in the last few years three tests on pleural fluid have been developed that can establish the diagnosis of tuberculous pleuritis, namely, adenosine deaminase (ADA), γ interferon, and polymerase chain reaction (PCR) for tuberculous DNA. A pleural fluid ADA level that exceeds 40 IU per L is seen in virtually all patients with tuberculous pleuritis (35). The pleural fluid ADA is elevated in patients with tuberculous pleuritis who are immunosuppressed (36). The other two diseases associated with an elevated pleural fluid ADA are rheumatoid pleuritis and empyema, and these should be easy to differentiate from tuberculous pleuritis clinically (34). A pleural fluid ADA less than 40 IU per L is highly suggestive of nontuberculous disease because a pleural fluid ADA level above 40 IU per L is seen in less than 5% of other lymphocyte-predominant pleural effusions (37). The level of γ interferon is higher in patients with tuberculous pleuritis than it is in pleural fluids due to other etiologies. In one recent study, a pleural fluid γ interferon level of 3.7 U per mL had a sensitivity of 0.99 and a specificity of 0.98 in a series of 388 pleural effusions (38). Pleural fluid PCR analysis holds promise for the diagnosis of tuberculous pleuritis, but ADA levels are just as good, less expensive, and less difficult technically (39). In patients with lymphocytic pleural effusions, an elevated level of one of the pleural fluid TB markers is sufficient for the diagnosis of tuberculous pleuritis.

For the past 50 years, pleural biopsy has been the most common way to establish the diagnosis of tuberculous pleuritis. However, the pleural fluid tests for TB markers, as discussed above, are at least as sensitive as the needle biopsy of the pleura and are less invasive. Hence, needle biopsy of the pleura is being used less and less frequently to establish the diagnosis of tuberculous pleuritis (34).

TREATMENT. Patients with tuberculous pleuritis should be treated with the same antituberculous treatment regimens as are patients with pulmonary TB, as discussed in Chapter 15, Respiratory Tract Infections. With treatment, patients generally become afebrile within about 2 weeks, and the pleural effusion resolves within 6 weeks. Repeated pleural fluid aspiration has not been shown to be beneficial in preventing chronic pleural thickening (40). The administration of corticosteroids will rapidly relieve the patient's symptoms of pleuritic chest pain, malaise, and fever and does not lead to dissemination of the TB. Markedly symptomatic patients should be started on prednisone 40 mg per day and then gradually tapered over several weeks.

Actinomycosis

More than 50% of patients with thoracic actinomycosis have pleural involvement. The characteristic chest radiographic finding is a localized lung lesion extending to the chest wall, with pleural thickening or effusion. The presence of chest wall abscesses or draining sinus tracts suggests the diagnosis, as do bone changes consisting of periosteal proliferation or bone destruction. The definitive diagnosis is established with the demonstration of *Actinomyces israelii* by anaerobic cultures. The appropriate treatment is high doses of penicillin or another suitable antimicrobial agent for prolonged periods.

Nocardiosis

Pleural effusions develop in nearly 50% of patients with pulmonary nocardiosis. When pleural involvement does occur, grossly purulent pleural fluid and draining sinuses are common. The diagnosis is established by demonstrating the organism on aerobic culture. Because the organism is slow growing, cultures should be maintained for 4 weeks to exclude the diagnosis. Frequently with pleural nocardiosis, TB is wrongly diagnosed because the nocardia organisms are acid fast. The drug treatment of choice is the combination of trimethoprim and sulfamethoxazole (Bactrim), two double strength tablets twice daily for at least 2 months.

Fungal Diseases of the Pleura

ASPERGILLOSIS. Pleural aspergillosis usually occurs in one of two settings. Pleural aspergillosis may complicate lobectomy or pneumonectomy, in which situation a bronchopleural fistula is almost always present. Once the diagnosis is established, a chest tube should be inserted, and the pleural space should be irrigated daily with amphotericin B 25 mg or nystatin 75,000 units. The diagnosis of pleural aspergillosis should also be suspected in any patient with a history of artificial pneumothorax therapy for TB who has signs and symptoms of chronic infection. The diagnosis is established by demonstrating the organisms on stains or cultures of the pleural fluid. The optimal treatment for pleural aspergillosis in this situation is surgical removal of the involved pleura and resection of the involved lobe or the entire ipsilateral lung if necessary (41).

BLASTOMYCOSIS. Approximately 10% of patients with blastomycosis will have a pleural effusion. The clinical picture with pleural blastomycosis is identical to that of pleural TB. The diagnosis is established by demonstrating the organism in the pleural fluid or histologic sections. The treatment of choice is an azole, such as iatraconazole, or amphotericin B if the patient is immunosuppressed or has central nervous system blastomycosis.

COCCIDIOIDOMYCOSIS. Pleural effusions of two types occur in association with coccidioidomycosis. The incidence of pleural effusion with symptomatic primary coccidioidomycosis is about 7%, and 50% of the patients with pleural effusion will also have a coexisting parenchymal infiltrate. Most patients are febrile and have pleuritic chest pain, and nearly 50% have either erythema nodosum or erythema multiforme. The pleural effusion is a lymphocyte-predominant exudate. Pleural fluid cultures are positive in about 20%, whereas cultures of pleural biopsy specimens are almost always positive. Most patients with primary coccidioidal pleural effusion require no systemic antifungal therapy. Only patients who are immunosuppressed, have a negative skin test, or have other evidence of dissemination need to be treated with antifungal therapy (42).

The other type of coccidioidomycosis-associated pleural effusion is hydropneumothorax, which develops in 1% to 5% of patients with chronic cavitary coccidioidomycosis. These patients should undergo tube thoracostomy immediately to drain the air and fluid from the pleural space. Most patients will require a thoracotomy with a partial or total lobectomy, as well as some degree of decortication. The administration of antifungal drugs does not appear to be required (43).

CRYPTOCOCCOSIS. Pleural involvement with cryptococcosis appears to result from extension of a primary subpleural cryptococcal nodule into the pleural space (44). Most patients who have a cryptococcal pleural effusion are immunosuppressed, in many cases secondary to human immunodeficiency virus (HIV) infection. The pleural fluid is usually a lymphocyte-predominant exudate. Immunosuppressed patients should be treated with a combination of amphotericin B (0.4 mg per kg) and 5-flucytosine (100 mg per kg) daily for 6 weeks, as should patients with cryptococcal antigen in either their blood or their cerebrospinal fluid. If none of these criteria is met, the patient probably does not need to be treated. However, if the effusion increases in size, if the LDH levels in the effusion increase with serial sampling, or if antigens appear in the blood or cerebrospinal fluid, treatment should be initiated (18).

HISTOPLASMOSIS. On rare occasions, patients with histoplasmosis will have a lymphocyte-predominant exudative pleural effusion. The pleural biopsy will reveal noncaseating granulomas. No systemic treatment is necessary unless the patient is immunosuppressed or the effusion persists for more than 4 weeks.

Viral Diseases of the Pleura

Viral infections are probably responsible for a sizable percentage of undiagnosed exudative pleural effusions. However, the diagnosis is rarely established because it depends on isolation of the virus or the demonstration of a significant increase in the antibodies to the virus. The incidence of pleural effusion with primary atypical pneumonia is as high as 20% (45).

Parasitic Diseases of the Pleura

AMEBIASIS. Pleural involvement with the parasite *Entamoeba histolytica* is invariably secondary to a liver abscess. Most patients present with fever and right upper-quadrant tenderness. Right-sided pleuritic chest pain is common and is frequently referred to the right shoulder as a manifestation of diaphragmatic irritation. Thoracentesis can yield either "chocolate-sauce" fluid or "anchovy paste" fluid or a serous exudate that develops in response to the diaphragmatic irritation. The expectoration of "chocolate-sauce" sputum is nearly pathognomonic and indicates that a bronchohepatic fistula has developed. The discovery of "chocolate sauce" in either the sputum or the pleural space serves as an indication for therapy with metronidazole, 750 mg three times a day for 5 to 10 days (46). Tube thoracostomy should be performed if "chocolate sauce" is found on thoracentesis.

PARAGONIMIASIS. This diagnosis should be suspected in patients with undiagnosed pleural effusion who have recently been to East Asia because the oriental lung fluke, *Paragonimus westermani*, at times produces pleural disease. Patients with pleural paragonimiasis present with a chronic illness. The pleural fluid in patients with pleural paragonimiasis is quite characteristic in that it is an exudate with a glucose level <10 mg per dL, an LDH level more than three times the upper limit of normal for serum, a pH below 7.10, and a differential revealing a high percentage of eosinophils (47). The pleural fluid findings are virtually pathognomonic, but the diagnosis is established by demonstrating the typical operculated eggs in the sputum, pleural fluid, or stool. The treatment of choice is praziquantel, 25 mg per kg three times a day for 3 days (46). At times, thoracotomy with decortication is necessary for resolution of the process.

ECHINOCOCCOSIS. Pleural disease from *Echinococcus granulosus* usually results from rupture of either a pulmonary or a hepatic hydatid cyst into the pleural space. When the cyst ruptures, the patient often experiences the abrupt onset of chest pain, fever, and systemic toxicity. Diagnosis is dependent on the demonstration of hooklets from scolices in the sputum or pleural fluid. The treatment of choice is surgical excision of the

cyst combined with tube drainage of the pleural space. After surgery, patients should be treated with albendazole 400 mg twice a day for several weeks (48).

Pleural Effusions Secondary to Neoplasms

PATHOGENESIS. Neoplasms are responsible for a high percentage of pleural effusions. Along with congestive heart failure, they account for most pleural effusions in patients above the age of 50. Pleural effusions associated with neoplasms arise through at least five different mechanisms:

1. The pleural surfaces may be involved by the tumor, which leads to increased permeability of the pleural membranes, possibly due to vascular endothelial growth factor (VEGF) (49).
2. The neoplasm may obstruct the lymphatics or veins draining the pleural space, leading to the accumulation of pleural fluid.
3. An endobronchial tumor may completely obstruct a bronchus, leading to atelectasis and decreasing the pleural pressure.
4. A pneumonitis distal to a partially obstructed bronchus may lead to a parapneumonic effusion.
5. The neoplasm may disrupt the thoracic duct, leading to a chylothorax.

Pleural effusions in patients with known malignancy may not be related to the malignancy itself; these patients may also develop heart failure, pulmonary emboli, pneumonia, hypoproteinemia, pericardial disease, or TB, any of which may be responsible for the effusion. It should be noted that not all patients with metastases to the pleura develop pleural effusions. Meyer (50) reviewed 52 cases of metastatic carcinoma to the pleura and found that only 14 of these patients had recognized pleural effusions during their lifetime. He found that the development of an effusion is closely related to neoplastic infiltration of the mediastinal lymph nodes and that in all types of tumors the visceral pleura is involved much sooner and more extensively than is the parietal pleura. Pleural involvement with most bronchogenic tumors arises from pulmonary arterial emboli, but pleural involvement with nonbronchogenic tumors usually represents tertiary spread from established hepatic metastases.

Bronchogenic carcinomas in men and breast carcinomas in women are the leading types of tumors causing neoplastic effusions. The lymphomas and leukemias are the third leading type of malignancy with secondary effusions. However, many other tumors, predominantly carcinomas, are associated with metastases to the pleura and pleural effusions.

DIAGNOSIS. The diagnosis of a malignant effusion should be considered in all patients with exudative pleural effusions. The diagnosis is established by demonstrating malignant cells by cytopathologic studies or by pleural biopsy. Although there is nothing absolutely characteristic about the pleural fluid secondary to malignancy, several generalizations can be made.

The pleural fluid is almost always an exudate. A grossly bloody pleural fluid is suggestive of malignancy, but nearly 50% of malignant effusions have pleural fluid red blood cell counts of less than 10,000. The pleural fluid WBC count is usually between 500 and 25,000, and the differential can be characterized by a predominance of polymorphonuclear leukocytes, small lymphocytes, or other mononuclear cells. The pleural fluid glucose level is usually similar to the corresponding serum level, but is occasionally <50 mg per dL. The pleural fluid amylase level is elevated in approximately 10% of malignant pleural effusions. In such cases, the primary tumor is usually not in the pancreas and the amylase has a salivary rather than a pancreatic isoenzyme pattern. The pleural fluid pH may be normal or reduced. A low pleural fluid pH usually occurs in conjunction with a low pleural fluid glucose. This combination indicates a poor prognosis because it is due to a large tumor burden in the pleural space. Measurement of tumor marker levels in the pleural fluid has proved disappointing in establishing the diagnosis of malignant pleural effusion. If the cutoff level is set sufficiently high so that there are no false positives, the sensitivity of the test is less than 50% (51).

The diagnosis of a malignant pleural effusion is most commonly established by cytologic examination of the pleural fluid. When specimens from three separate thoracenteses are submitted for cytologic examination, the diagnosis can be established in approximately 80% of individuals who have pleural metastases (52). Almost all adenocarcinomas will be diagnosed with cytology, but the yield is less with mesothelioma, squamous cell carcinoma, Hodgkin disease, and sarcomas.

At times, no diagnosis will be made despite at least two cytologic examinations of the pleural fluid. How aggressive should one be in attempting to establish the diagnosis of malignancy in these patients? Most patients who have a malignant pleural effusion will have a clinical picture suggestive of malignancy with a history of a malignancy or chronic symptoms suggestive of malignancy (53). If it is felt likely that the patient has a malignancy, the best next step is thoracoscopy. If thoracoscopy is unavailable, needle biopsy of the pleura or an open thoracotomy with biopsy can be considered (18). If thoracoscopy is performed, a procedure such as pleural abrasion should also be performed at the same time to effect a pleurodesis (18).

In a patient with a known neoplasm and pleural effusion, the key questions are whether the pleural effusion is secondary to the malignancy and, if so, by what mechanism. Again, cytologic studies can demonstrate direct involvement of the pleura. The chest x-ray is useful in delineating the responsible mechanisms. If the mediastinum is shifted toward the contralateral side, the pleural surfaces are probably involved. If the mediastinum is shifted toward the ipsilateral side and the bronchi are not outlined by air on the routine chest radiograph, total bronchial obstruction with resulting atelectasis and effusion is the probable explanation. A parapneumonic effusion is suggested by a high white cell count, predominantly neutrophils, in the pleural fluid. A mediastinal mass on the chest x-ray film suggests lymphatic obstruction or disruption. Protein analysis of peripheral blood demonstrates hypoproteinemia. A globular cardiac shadow suggests pericardial involvement and pericardial effusion. Commonly, a combination of these mechanisms is responsible.

TREATMENT. The initial step in the management of a patient with a malignant pleural effusion is to attempt to identify the site of the primary tumor in order to decide whether to administer systemic chemotherapy. Patients who have primary tumors that are responsive to systemic chemotherapy, such as small cell carcinoma of the lung, breast carcinoma, and lymphoma, should be given chemotherapy to treat the primary disease. Prior to chemotherapy, it is best to drain the pleural effusion.

The proper therapy for a pleural effusion associated with malignancy depends on the mechanism responsible for it. If an endobronchial tumor is responsible for complete bronchial obstruction, the obstruction should be treated with a stent or laser therapy. If pneumonitis behind a partial obstruction is present, the patient should be treated with appropriate antibiotics and postural drainage in combination with therapy for the obstruction. If the pleural effusion is due to lymphatic blockage in the mediastinum, radiotherapy to the mediastinum may be effective in controlling the effusion. This is particularly true for lymphomas.

When the effusion is due to pleural metastases, consideration should be given to performing a procedure that will prevent the pleural fluid from reaccumulating. Candidates for such a procedure should meet two criteria. First, the quality of the patient's life should be diminished by dyspnea. Second, the dyspnea should improve after a therapeutic thoracentesis. Many patients with malignant pleural effusions do not meet both of these criteria.

If the above two conditions are met, the two primary means to prevent reaccumulation of the pleural fluid are to insert an indwelling catheter or to inject a material intrapleurally to produce a pleurodesis. The catheter that is most commonly used is a 15.5 Fr silicone rubber catheter (Pleurx catheter, Denver Biomaterials, Golden, Colorado) that can be inserted on an outpatient basis (54,55) by pulmonologists, interventional radiologists, or surgeons. The catheter is tunneled and has a valve on the distal end that prevents fluid or air from passing in either direction through the catheter unless the catheter is accessed with the matched drainage line. The pleural fluid is drained at 24- to 48-hour intervals by inserting the access tip of the drainage line into the valve of the catheter and then draining the fluid via an external tube into vacuum bottles (56). Interestingly, a spontaneous pleurodesis will occur in approximately 50% of patients in whom the catheter is inserted at a median of 25 days after insertion (56). The biggest advantage of the indwelling catheter is that it can be inserted in an outpatient. The biggest disadvantage is that the patients who do not experience a pleurodesis must continue to drain their pleural fluid for the remainder of their lives. Studies are presently under way to determine if pleurodesis can be done as an outpatient by the injection of sclerosing agents through this catheter.

With chemical pleurodesis, an irritant (e.g., doxycycline) is injected into the pleural space, creating an intense pleural inflammation leading to fusion of the visceral and parietal pleura. Many different agents have been used as pleural sclerosants, but doxycycline 500 mg is the agent recommended by the author at the present time. The only two agents approved for pleurodesis by the Food and Drug Administration (FDA) are talc and bleomycin. Talc is the agent most commonly used (57), but it is not recommended because it causes a fatal ARDS in about 1% of patients and nonfatal ARDS in an additional 5% (58,59). Bleomycin is not recommended because it is less effective than doxycycline (60), is more expensive, and does not effect a pleurodesis in animals (61).

The following procedure is recommended for pleurodesis. A chest tube is inserted into the pleural space to drain the fluid. Before the sclerosant is injected, the patient should be given systemic medications such as lorazepam or midazolam to produce conscious sedation because the procedure can be very painful (62). As soon as the underlying lung has reexpanded, doxycycline 500 mg in 50 mL saline is injected through the chest tube into the pleural space. After the injection, the chest tube is clamped for the next 60 to 90 minutes. There appears to be no need to place the patient into various positions after the injection (63). The chest tube is then unclamped and negative pressure is applied through the chest tube for 48 to 72 hours or until the drainage becomes <15 mL per hour. At this time, the chest tube is removed. The intense inflammation induced by the sclerosant results in fusion of the visceral and parietal pleural surfaces when they are brought into close approximation by the negative pressure applied by the chest tubes. Pleurodesis performed in this manner is effective in obliterating the pleural space and in controlling the pleural effusion about 80% of the time (64).

Mesothelioma

Malignant mesothelioma is an uncommon disease that is highly malignant and has been shown to be associated with exposure to asbestos. It is thought that asbestos exposure is responsible for most mesotheliomas, but no history of significant asbestos exposure can be obtained in approximately 30% of patients with mesothelioma (65). Mesotheliomas are thought to arise from the cells that line the pleural cavity.

Once the tumor is present, it spreads rapidly along the pleural surfaces. Eventually, the entire visceral and parietal pleural surfaces become infiltrated by a continuous layer of tumor encasing the entire lung. Metastases to regional lymph nodes are common, but distant metastases are rare. Histologically, diffuse mesotheliomas frequently contain large amounts of fibrous tissue. The predominant cellular type may be either mesenchymal or epithelial, and most of these tumors have both cell types.

Most patients with malignant mesothelioma present with either chest pain or dyspnea. The chest pain is nonpleuritic, aching, and frequently referred to the upper abdomen or shoulder. When the patient initially presents, the chest film invariably reveals a unilateral pleural effusion. The prognosis of patients with mesothelioma is poor, with a median survival time of slightly more than 12 months after diagnosis (66). It should be noted that this is significantly better than the survival with other malignant pleural effusions.

It is sometimes difficult to establish the diagnosis of malignant mesothelioma. Although cytologic smears, needle biopsies, and sections from cell blocks of pleural fluid can establish the diagnosis of malignancy, they usually cannot distinguish between a metastatic adenocarcinoma and a mesothelioma. Thoracoscopy is probably the best procedure with which to establish the diagnosis of mesothelioma (65). At thoracoscopy, a small portion of the specimen should be placed in glutaraldehyde for electron microscopy in any patient suspected of having mesothelioma (67). In addition, during thoracoscopy, attempts should be made to create a pleurodesis using pleural abrasion or some other procedure.

Three techniques are available to help establish the diagnosis of mesothelioma with greater certainty. Most adenocarcinomas are positive with the periodic acid–Schiff (PAS) stain after diastase digestion, whereas all mesotheliomas are negative. Electron microscopy is also useful in differentiating mesothelioma from metastatic adenocarcinoma in that mesotheliomas are characterized by long, lush microvilli. Lastly, immunohistochemical studies can be used to distinguish adenocarcinoma that is positive with the monoclonal antibodies CEA and MOC-31 and mesotheliomas that are positive with calretinin and cytokeratin 5/6 (68).

There has been no satisfactory treatment for malignant mesothelioma, and it was unclear whether any of the available treatments prolonged life (69). Although there are reports of prolonged survival with radical pneumonectomy followed by radiotherapy and chemotherapy, the percentage of mesothelioma patients eligible for this treatment is less than 2% (69) and there are no controlled studies demonstrating that it improves survival (70). It has recently been shown, however, that chemotherapy may prolong life in patients with mesothelioma (71). In a recent study, 456 patients were randomized to the single-agent cisplatin or combination therapy with pemetrexed plus the same dose of cisplatin. The combination chemotherapy was superior with respect to median survival time (12.1 versus 9.3 months), 1-year survival rates (50% versus 38%), and tumor response rates (16.7% versus 4.3%). Chemical pleurodesis should be attempted if the patient is dyspneic from a large pleural effusion. Analgesics, including opiates, should be given in sufficient quantities to alleviate pain and dyspnea.

Solitary Fibrous Tumors of the Pleura

Solitary fibrous tumors of the pleura, also referred to as *benign mesotheliomas*, are localized pleural tumors with an excellent prognosis. Their occurrence does not appear to be related to previous asbestos exposure. These tumors appear radiologically as solitary, sharply defined, discrete masses located at the periphery of the lung or related to a fissure. The most frequent symptoms are cough, chest pain, and dyspnea, but approximately 50% of patients are asymptomatic. Hypertrophic pulmonary osteoarthropathy occurs in approximately 20% of patients with solitary fibrous tumors, and in such instances the tumor is usually greater than 7 cm in diameter. The association of hypertrophic osteoarthropathy and a large pleural-based intrathoracic mass should strongly suggest the possibility of a solitary fibrous tumor of the pleura. Symptomatic hypoglycemia occurs in about 4% of patients with solitary fibrous tumors of the pleura. The treatment is surgical excision and the prognosis is excellent (72).

Primary Effusion Lymphoma

Primary effusion lymphomas grow in body cavities and present as malignant lymphomatous effusions without an identifiable contiguous tumor mass (73). These tumors usually occur in homosexual patients with acquired immune deficiency syndrome (AIDS) and contain the Kaposi sarcoma–associated herpes virus (KSHV or HHV-8); most are also characterized by the presence of the Epstein–Barr virus. The primary effusion lymphoma has a distinctive morphology bridging large-cell immunoblastic lymphoma and anaplastic large-cell lymphoma. The pleural fluid is a lymphocytic exudate characterized by a very high LDH level. No effective treatment is known.

Pyothorax-associated Lymphoma

Pyothorax-associated lymphoma occurs almost exclusively in patients who received artificial pneumothorax several decades previously for the treatment of pulmonary TB (74). Accordingly, these lymphomas should actually be named *pneumothorax-associated lymphoma*. These lymphomas are of B-cell lineage, and the Epstein–Barr virus genome has been detected in all of the tumors tested. CT scans reveal pleural masses without effusions in most patients.

Pleural Effusions Secondary to Collagen Vascular Disease

SYSTEMIC LUPUS ERYTHEMATOSUS. The pleura is frequently involved in systemic lupus erythematosus (SLE). Pleurisy without effusion is more common than pleurisy with effusion. In one series of patients observed for a prolonged period, 72% had pleuritic chest pain and 40% had pleural effusions at some time during their course (75). The effusions are frequently bilateral but may be unilateral and change from one side to the other (76). Pericardial effusions are frequently present concomitantly with the pleural effusions.

The diagnosis of SLE should be considered in all patients with undiagnosed pleurisy or pleural effusion. The pleural fluid is typically a serous exudate, and the differential may reveal predominantly lymphocytes, neutrophils, or mesothelial cells. The pleural fluid in most cases is characterized by a normal pH and glucose level and an LDH below 500 IU per L (77). Measurement of the pleural fluid antinuclear antibody does not appear to be useful in diagnosing lupus pleuritis (76). The diagnosis of lupus pleuritis is established by using the diagnostic criteria published by the American Rheumatism Association for SLE.

Patients with lupus pleuritis should be treated with oral prednisone, 80 mg every alternate day, with rapid tapering once the symptoms are controlled.

RHEUMATOID PLEURITIS. Approximately 20% of patients with rheumatoid arthritis will at some time have pleuritic chest pain and about 4% will have a pleural effusion. The pleuritic chest pain may occur before, be coincident with, or occur after the onset of arthritis. The pleural effusion usually occurs after the onset of the arthritis, frequently in conjunction with an arthritic flare. Most rheumatoid pleural effusions occur in men, and most patients with rheumatoid effusions also have subcutaneous rheumatoid nodules. The effusion may be on either side and is sometimes bilateral. It is usually small to moderate in size and only occasionally produces symptoms, including fever and pleuritic chest pain (77).

The diagnosis is suggested by the clinical picture of rheumatoid arthritis and the presence of a pleural effusion. The pleural fluid with rheumatoid pleuritis is very distinctive in that it is characterized by a glucose level <30 mg per dL, an LDH level above two times the upper limit of normal, a pH <7.20, low levels of complement, and the presence of immune complexes (77). The other condition that is likely to yield similar pleural fluid findings is a complicated parapneumonic effusion. Because patients with rheumatoid disease tend to have a high incidence of complicated parapneumonic effusion, the differentiation of the two entities is important and is dependent on the Gram stain and on the culture of the pleural fluid.

The optimal therapy for rheumatoid pleural effusions remains unclear. Most such effusions resolve spontaneously over several months; in some, however, the effusion persists, leading to the development of a thick peel covering the visceral pleura and producing a severe restrictive ventilatory defect. No studies have demonstrated that systemic antiinflammatory therapy has any influence on the course of rheumatoid pleuritis, and the results after intrapleural corticosteroids have not been conclusive (78).

OTHER COLLAGEN VASCULAR DISEASES. An eosinophilic pleural effusion with a very high LDH level, a low glucose level, and a low pH may occur with Churg–Strauss syndrome, which is characterized by hypereosinophilia and systemic vasculitis in the patient with asthma. Patients with Wegener's granulomatosis, familial Mediterranean fever, and immunoblastic lymphadenopathy also get pleural effusions. The effusions in these situations rarely dominate the clinical picture (18).

Pleural Effusions Secondary to Pulmonary Embolism

The diagnosis of pulmonary embolism should almost always be considered in every patient with an undiagnosed pleural effusion. At least 30% of patients with pulmonary emboli have a pleural effusion (79). The pleural effusions secondary to pulmonary emboli are mostly exudative (80). The ischemia and release of the vasoactive amines secondary to the embolus increase the permeability of the capillaries in the lung, leading to an increased amount of interstitial fluid and the exudative pleural effusion. Transudative effusions, if they occur, probably result from increased pressure in the central veins.

Most pleural effusions associated with pulmonary emboli are small; in one recent study, 48 of 56 patients (86%) had only blunting of the costophrenic angle, and no patient had an effusion that occupied more than one third of a hemithorax (79). The effusions are usually unilateral, but a recent study with chest CT scan demonstrated bilateral pleural fluid in 6 of 13 patients with pulmonary emboli (81). The pleural fluid is almost always an exudate (80). The fluid is frequently not bloody. Patients with undiagnosed pleural effusions should have the possibility of pulmonary embolism investigated with a spiral CT scan (82). The spiral CT will not only identify vascular filling defects that are highly suggestive of pulmonary embolism but it will also demonstrate concomitant parenchymal abnormalities and mediastinal lymphadenopathy.

The treatment of choice for the patient with pleural effusions secondary to pulmonary embolism is adequate anticoagulation (see Chapter 11, Pulmonary Thromboembolism and Other Pulmonary Vascular Diseases). The presence of blood in the pleural fluid does not serve as a contraindication for anticoagulation. Tube thoracostomy for a bloody pleural effusion secondary to pulmonary emboli should be performed only if the hematocrit of the pleural fluid is above 20%.

Pleural Effusions Secondary to Gastrointestinal Conditions

ACUTE PANCREATITIS. In one study of 133 patients with acute pancreatitis who had a chest CT scan, the prevalence of pleural effusion was 66% (83). In this study, the effusion was bilateral in 51 (77%), unilateral left sided in 10 (15%), and unilateral right sided in 5 (8%). The mechanism responsible for the pleural effusion associated with pancreatitis appears to be inflammation of the diaphragmatic pleura secondary to the transdiaphragmatic transfer of pancreatic enzymes. The clinical picture is usually dominated by abdominal symptoms; however, at times respiratory symptoms consisting of pleuritic chest pain and dyspnea may predominate. In addition to the small- to moderate-sized pleural effusion, the chest radiograph may reveal an elevated diaphragm and basilar infiltrates. The diagnosis is confirmed with demonstration of an elevated pleural fluid amylase level. Patients with pancreatitis and a pleural effusion should be treated for their pancreatitis in the usual manner, but it should be noted that patients with acute pancreatitis and a pleural effusion tend to have more severe disease and are more likely to subsequently develop a pseudocyst (83).

CHRONIC PANCREATIC PLEURAL EFFUSION. Patients with a pancreatic pseudocyst at times develop a large chronic pleural effusion. The pathogenesis of the pleural effusion is a sinus tract that runs from the pancreas retroperitoneally into the mediastinum and then into the pleural space. The clinical picture is usually dominated by chest symptoms. Most patients do not have abdominal symptoms because the pancreaticopleural fistula decompresses the pseudocyst. The pleural effusion is usually massive and recurs rapidly after thoracentesis. It most commonly is left sided but it may be right sided or bilateral. The diagnosis is supported by a markedly elevated pleural fluid amylase level. This is an important diagnosis to consider because most patients with this entity appear to have malignancy. Accordingly, the pleural fluid amylase level should be measured in all patients with large, unexplained, chronic pleural effusions. The diagnosis is established with CT scan of the abdomen. Treatment consists of total parenteral nutrition plus drainage of the pleural space. Some patients also require surgical drainage of the pancreas or decortication (84).

ESOPHAGEAL PERFORATIONS. Most esophageal perforations are associated with either a pleural effusion or a hydropneumothorax. Because the mortality associated with this condition approaches 100% if it remains undiagnosed for several days, it should be considered in every patient with a pleural effusion who appears acutely ill. Esophageal perforations occur in three different settings: (a) as a complication of endoscopy, esophageal dilation, thoracic surgery, or the insertion of a Blakemore–Sengstaken tube; (b) spontaneously (Boerhaave syndrome) when there is a sudden explosive rise in intraabdominal pressure, usually in association with vomiting; and (c) as a complication of esophageal carcinoma.

The clinical picture associated with esophageal rupture is impressive and is highly suggestive of the diagnosis. Pain is the most striking symptom and is characteristically excruciating, unremitting, and unrelieved by opiates. Thirst is a prominent symptom, and most patients show at least some degree of circulatory collapse. A pathognomonic triad of physical signs consists of rapid respiration, abdominal rigidity, and subcutaneous emphysema in the suprasternal notch. The chest radiograph usually reveals a pleural effusion or hydropneumothorax.

The diagnosis is not difficult if it is considered. The pleural fluid amylase level is usually very high (>2,500 units). The

amylase in this condition has a salivary origin, and the high pleural fluid amylase level is due to the saliva leaking from the esophagus into the pleural space (85). The pleural fluid pH is usually low (below 7.00) because of the mediastinal and pleural infection. Both Gram stain and culture of the pleural fluid usually reveal organisms. If there is any doubt as to the diagnosis, it can be substantiated by having the patient swallow methylene blue, in which case the pleural fluid will turn blue if there is an esophageal perforation. Immediate thoracotomy with drainage of the mediastinum and pleural space is indicated once the diagnosis is made. A delay of only several hours is associated with a much higher mortality than if treatment is initiated promptly. The tear in the esophagus should be repaired and high doses of systemic broad-spectrum antibiotics should be administered (86).

INTRAABDOMINAL ABSCESS. Pleural effusions frequently occur with intraabdominal abscesses. The incidence of pleural effusion is approximately 80% with subphrenic, 40% with pancreatic, 33% with splenic, and 20% with intrahepatic abscess (18). The possibility of intraabdominal abscess should be considered in any patient with an undiagnosed exudative pleural effusion containing predominantly polymorphonuclear leukocytes, particularly when there are no pulmonary parenchymal infiltrates. The diagnosis of intraabdominal abscess is best established with abdominal CT scanning or ultrasound. The appropriate treatment is drainage of the abscess combined with parenteral antibiotics (87).

Postsurgical Procedures

POST–CORONARY ARTERY BYPASS SURGERY. More than 600,000 patients undergo coronary artery bypass graft (CABG) surgery in the United States each year. Because approximately 10% of patients who undergo CABG surgery will develop a pleural effusion that occupies more than 25% of their hemithorax in the subsequent month (88), CABG surgery is one of the more common causes of pleural effusions in the United States. The prevalence of small pleural effusions is high following CABG surgery. In a recent study of 349 patients, the prevalence of pleural effusion on chest radiograph 30 days postoperatively was 62%; 40 of the 349 patients (11%) had an effusion that occupied more than 25% of the hemithorax (88). The pleural effusions after CABG surgery tend to be left sided or bilateral, and when bilateral, the effusion is usually larger on the left (88).

The primary symptom of a patient with a pleural effusion post-CABG is dyspnea, which usually occurs only when the effusion is large (88). The presence of either chest pain or fever should alert the physician to an alternative diagnosis. When all patients with larger pleural effusions post-CABG surgery are considered, the effusions can be divided into those that are bloody and those that are serous. The bloody effusions are probably secondary to bleeding into the pleural space. They reach their maximal size within 30 days of surgery, are frequently associated with pleural fluid or peripheral eosinophilia or both, have a high pleural fluid LDH level, and respond to one or two therapeutic thoracenteses (89). In contrast, the serous effusions tend to reach their maximal size more than 30 days after surgery, have more than 50% small lymphocytes, and have a relatively low pleural fluid LDH level (89). Most of these late effusions can also be managed with one or two therapeutic thoracenteses (88), but some are very refractory. It is unknown whether antiinflammatory agents or diuretics are beneficial in the treatment of these effusions. An occasional patient will require thoracoscopy with decortication because of a lung trapped by a thin fibrous membrane (90).

POST–ABDOMINAL SURGERY. Nearly 50% of patients who have undergone abdominal surgery will develop a pleural effusion postoperatively (91). The incidence of pleural effusion is higher after upper abdominal surgery, in patients with postoperative atelectasis, and in patients with free abdominal fluid at surgery. Most of the effusions are exudates and are thought to be due to diaphragmatic irritation or atelectasis. Nevertheless, a diagnostic thoracentesis should be performed if the effusion is more than minimal in size to rule out a complicated parapneumonic effusion. Pleural effusions developing several days after abdominal surgery suggest either pulmonary embolism or subphrenic abscess.

POST–LUNG TRANSPLANTATION. With lung transplantation, the lymphatics that normally drain the lung are severed. As a result, all the fluid that enters the interstitial spaces of the lung exits via the pleural space, and the amount of pleural drainage is increased. The amount of pleural fluid does slow dramatically during the first postoperative week. The incidence of pleural effusion 3 months posttransplant varies from 30% to 60% (92,93), but the incidence at 12 months is less than 10% (93). The effusions are characteristically a lymphocyte-predominant exudate with a benign course (92). Nevertheless, patients who develop complications post–lung transplantation frequently have a pleural effusion. Pleural effusions occurred in 14 of 19 (74%) episodes of acute rejection, 7 of 8 (88%) instances of chronic rejection, 6 of 11 (55%) episodes of infection, and 3 of 4 (75%) instances of lymphoproliferative disease in one study (94).

POST–LIVER TRANSPLANTATION. Most patients who undergo orthotopic liver transplantation develop a pleural effusion (95). In one study, 68% of 300 patients undergoing liver transplantation developed a pleural effusion, and the effusion occupied more than 25% of the hemithorax in 21 patients (7%) (95). The effusion was unilateral right sided in 153 patients and bilateral in 53 patients. The effusions are large enough to require therapeutic thoracentesis or tube thoracostomy in approximately 10%. These effusions tend to increase in size over the first few postoperative days and then gradually resolve over several weeks to months. These effusions are probably due to injury or irritation of the right hemidiaphragm caused by the extensive right upper-quadrant dissection. If a fibrin sealant is sprayed on the undersurface of the diaphragm around the insertion of the liver ligaments at the time of the transplantation, the development of the effusions can largely be prevented (96).

POST–ENDOSCOPIC VARICEAL SCLEROTHERAPY. Small pleural effusions complicate this procedure approximately 50% of the time. The effusion is thought to result from extravasation of the sclerosant into the esophageal mucosa, which results in an intense inflammatory reaction in the mediastinum and pleura. If the effusion persists for more than 24 to 48 hours and is accompanied by fever, or if the effusion occupies more than 25% of the hemithorax, a thoracentesis should be done to rule out an infection or an esophagopleural fistula (97).

Pleural Effusions Due to Drug Reactions

Pleural effusions have been reported definitely to occur as a complication of the administration of seven different drugs, namely, nitrofurantoin, methysergide, dantrolene, ergot alkaloids, procarbazine, amiodarone, and interleukin-2 (18). Other drugs have been reported to cause pleural effusion, but the association is less definite (18). In addition, many other drugs may cause drug-induced lupus erythematosus, which frequently has an associated pleural effusion.

NITROFURANTOIN. The administration of nitrofurantoin is occasionally associated with the development of a syndrome characterized by chills, fever, and cough, soon followed by dyspnea, malaise, and pleuritic chest pain. The chest x-ray is characterized by bilateral interstitial infiltrates, and a pleural effusion is present in about 25% of the cases. This diagnosis should be suspected in any patient taking nitrofurantoin who has a pleural effusion associated with bilateral pulmonary infiltrates. If the drug is discontinued, the symptoms and radiologic abnormalities resolve within a few days.

METHYSERGIDE. The administration of methysergide for migraine headaches can be complicated by the development of pleuritis with effusion without parenchymal infiltrates. The pleural effusions are bilateral in nearly 50% of the patients. They develop within 3 weeks to 3 years after starting the drug. Discontinuation of the drug early in the course results in complete resolution. However, if the pleuritis has been present for several months, pleural thickening may remain after the drug is discontinued.

DANTROLENE. Dantrolene sodium is a long-acting skeletal muscle relaxant used in treating patients with spastic neurologic disorders. It is structurally similar to nitrofurantoin. Its administration is at times associated with the development of sterile exudative pleural effusions without parenchymal infiltrates. Patients with this syndrome have both peripheral and pleural eosinophilia. The syndrome develops only after at least 2 months of therapy with dantrolene and may be complicated by the presence of pericardial effusion. The pleural effusion and eosinophilia typically take several months to resolve after the drug is discontinued.

ERGOT ALKALOIDS. The long-term administration of ergot alkaloid drugs such as bromocriptine, ergotamine, dihydroergotamin, nicergoline, pergolide, and dopergine, which are sometimes used in the long-term treatment of Parkinson disease, can lead to pleuropulmonary changes (98). The incidence of pleural disease is higher if the patient has previous exposure to asbestos (99). Patients who have taken the drugs for more than 6 months may develop pleural thickening or a pleural effusion or both. The natural history of pleuropulmonary disease during ergot alkaloid therapy is unclear as the disease progresses only in some of the patients who continue taking the drug (18).

PROCARBAZINE. There have been two detailed case reports in which pleuropulmonary reactions consisting of chills, cough, dyspnea, and bilateral pulmonary infiltrates with pleural effusion occurred after treatment with procarbazine. In both cases, symptoms redeveloped within hours of rechallenge (18).

AMIODARONE. Amiodarone is an antiarrhythmic that may produce severe pulmonary toxicity. Pleural effusions occur as a complication of amiodarone administration, but pulmonary infiltrates are much more common. Most cases with pleural effusion have concomitant parenchymal involvement (18).

Exudative Pleural Effusions Due to Other Diseases

ASBESTOS PLEURAL EFFUSION. Asbestos exposure that may have been brief, intermittent, and in the immediate or distant past may lead to a pleural effusion. Epler et al. (100) reviewed the medical histories of 1,135 asbestos workers whom they had observed for several years and found that 35 of the workers (3%) had pleural effusions for which there was no other explanation. The heavier the asbestos exposure, the likelier the patient is to develop a pleural effusion. The pleural effusion sometimes develops within 5 years of the initial exposure but sometimes may not develop until more than 30 years after the initial exposure (101). Most patients with benign asbestos pleural effusions are asymptomatic. The pleural fluid is an exudate and frequently has more than 10% eosinophils (18).

The diagnosis of benign asbestos pleural effusion is one of exclusion and requires the following: (a) a history of exposure to asbestos; (b) exclusion of other causes, especially mesothelioma and other malignancies, infection, and pulmonary embolism; and (c) a follow-up of at least 3 years to verify that the effusion is benign. There is no known treatment for benign asbestos pleural effusion but it does resolve spontaneously with time.

MEIGS SYNDROME. By definition, Meigs syndrome is the presence of a pleural effusion and ascites in association with an ovarian tumor that is solid, benign, and characteristically a fibroma. Resection of the tumor must effect resolution of the ascites and pleural effusion with no recurrence. The basic abnormality with Meigs syndrome appears to be fluid loss from the benign tumor into the peritoneum (18). At laparotomy, these tumors are frequently noted to be oozing serous fluid. It is thought that VEGF plays an important role in the pathogenesis of the ascites and pleural fluid because VEGF levels are high in both the ascites and the pleural fluid (102). The pleural effusion results from the ascitic fluid passing through defects in the diaphragm into the pleural space. The effusion is usually on the right side but may be bilateral or left sided. The size of the pleural effusion is largely independent of the amount of ascites. The pleural fluid is usually an exudate with a relatively low WBC count (<1,000 per mL). The diagnosis is made at laparotomy with the demonstration of the benign tumor and is confirmed when the ascites and pleural fluid disappear postoperatively. Although Meigs syndrome is uncommon, it is important to consider it in patients with a pelvic mass, pleural effusion, and ascites so that they are not labeled as having disseminated ovarian malignancy without histologic proof.

PULMONARY LYMPHANGIOLEIOMYOMATOSIS. This rare condition (103) is characterized by the widespread proliferation of smooth muscle in the lymph nodes and lungs, resulting in a honeycomb lung and, frequently, a chylothorax. All the cases have been in women, and most of the patients present with dyspnea or pneumothorax (103). The patients may also present with a chylothorax resulting from obstruction of the lymphatics by the smooth muscle proliferation. In one recent series of 50 patients from the United Kingdom, 30 (60%) had pneumothorax and 11 (22%) had chylothorax (103). The chest radiograph reveals bilateral pulmonary infiltrates with hyperinflation. The diagnosis is strongly suggested by the high-resolution CT scan, which reveals numerous air-filled cysts surrounded by normal lung parenchyma. However, the diagnosis is made by lung biopsy. Treatment in general is unsatisfactory; most patients die within 10 years of onset. There is some evidence that the smooth muscle proliferation is hormonally dependent. It is therefore recommended that patients be treated with medroxyprogesterone intramuscularly at a dose of 400 to 800 mg per month for at least 1 year. Other therapies that may be attempted if the medroxyprogesterone fails are oophorectomy or tamoxifen (104). In general, these therapies are at best marginally effective. Accordingly, many patients have been subject to lung transplantation. However, the disease has recurred in the transplanted lung in some of the recipients (105).

UREMIA. A fibrinous pleurisy occasionally occurs in the course of uremia (106). The pathogenesis of this pleuritis is probably similar to that of the pericarditis seen with uremia. More than 50% of the patients with uremic pleuritis also have uremic pericarditis. The blood urea nitrogen concentration has borne little relationship to the occurrence of the pleuritis. The prevalence of pleural abnormalities in patients undergoing hemodialysis is high. In a recent study of 117 patients who had been receiving hemodialysis for a mean of 48 months and had had a CT scan for pulmonary symptoms, the prevalence of pleural effusion was 51% (more than 50% bilateral) and the prevalence of pleural thickening was 22% (107). Patients with uremia frequently have pleural effusions because of other causes. In one series of 100 hospitalized patients with uremia and pleural effusion, the etiologies of the pleural effusions were as follows: heart failure in 46 patients, uremia in 16 patients, parapneumonic in 15 patients, atelectasis in 11 patients, and miscellaneous etiologies in 12 patients (108). The pleural fluid with uremic pleuritis is an exudate, which is frequently bloody with many eosinophils. The diagnosis is made by excluding other causes of exudative pleural effusions in patients with uremia.

TRAPPED LUNG. As a result of inflammation, a fibrous peel may form over the visceral pleura. The peel can prevent the underlying lung from expanding and can lead to a chronic decrease in the pleural pressure. From Figure 17-1, it is easily seen how a more negative pleural pressure can lead to pleural fluid accumulation. The effusion usually becomes evident several months after the initial insult, which can be pneumonitis, thoracic surgery, pneumothorax, trauma, or any other condition producing intense inflammation of the pleura. The pleural fluid associated with trapped lung usually meets the criteria for an exudate, but the values tend to be borderline. The diagnosis of trapped lung is best made by measuring the pleural pressures as fluid is withdrawn during a therapeutic thoracentesis (109). If the pleural pressure drops more than 2 cm H_2O for each 100 mL of pleural fluid withdrawn, the patient in all probability has a trapped lung. If the patient is asymptomatic, no therapy is necessary. If the patient is symptomatic from the effusion, a decortication should be considered.

POST–CARDIAC INJURY SYNDROME. The post–cardiac injury syndrome (PCIS or Dressler syndrome) is characterized by pericarditis with pericardial effusion, pleuritis, and pneumonitis following myocardial infarction, cardiac surgery, or cardiac trauma (110). This syndrome occurs between 1 and 12 weeks following the initiating event and complicates about 1% of myocardial infarctions. The two primary symptoms with the PCIS are chest pain and fever. Noncomplicated PCIS is defined as the presence of temperature greater than 100.5°F, patient irritability, pericardial friction rub, and a small pericardial effusion with or without pleural effusion following cardiac injury (111). A complicated PCIS is defined as a noncomplicated PCIS plus the need for hospital readmission with or without the need for pericardiocentesis or thoracentesis (111). The pleural effusions may be either unilateral or bilateral and are usually small to moderate in size. The pleural fluid is an exudate that is often bloody. The diagnosis is established by excluding other causes of pleural effusion in the patient with a recent history of myocardial insult. The treatment of choice is nonsteroidal antiinflammatory drugs (NSAIDS) if the patient is not excessively symptomatic because the syndrome is self-limiting. If the patient is distressed, corticosteroids are rapidly effective in relieving symptoms.

YELLOW NAIL SYNDROME. Pleural effusions are frequently associated with congenital abnormalities of the lymphatics. The most common syndrome is characterized by yellow nails, lymphedema, and chronic pleural effusion (112). Often, the pleural effusion does not appear until the patient reaches middle age. Examination of the pleural fluid reveals an exudate that is not chylous with a relatively low LDH. The diagnosis can be made by examining the fingernails. When the patient is symptomatic from a large effusion, pleurodesis with a sclerosing agent such as doxycycline should be considered.

SARCOIDOSIS. The incidence of pleural effusion with sarcoidosis is probably below 1% (113). Patients with pleural effusion due to sarcoid usually have extensive parenchymal sarcoidosis and, frequently, extrathoracic sarcoidosis (113). The pleural effusions are usually small, and the pleural fluid is an exudate with predominantly small lymphocytes. The pleural biopsy with sarcoid pleural effusion may reveal noncaseating granulomas. The pleural effusion secondary to sarcoidosis may resolve spontaneously, or corticosteroid therapy may be required for its resolution. It is important to rule out the diagnosis of tuberculous pleuritis in patients with known sarcoid and an exudative pleural effusion, especially if they have been on immunosuppressive therapy (113).

CHYLOTHORAX AND PSEUDOCHYLOTHORAX

Pleural fluid is occasionally found to be milky or turbid. When this cloudiness persists after centrifugation, it is almost always due to a high lipid content in the pleural fluid. Two different situations bring about the accumulation of high levels of lipid in the pleural fluid. In the first, chyle enters the pleural space as a result of disruption of the thoracic duct, producing a *chylothorax* or a *chylous* effusion. In the second, large amounts of cholesterol or lecithin–globulin complexes accumulate in a long-standing pleural effusion to produce a *pseudochylothorax* or a *chyliform* pleural effusion.

Chylothoraces can be traumatic or nontraumatic in origin. The most common traumatic cause is a cardiovascular surgical procedure, but penetrating injuries or nonpenetrating injuries in which the spine is hyperextended can lead to chylothorax. Tumors, most commonly lymphomas, are the most common cause of nontraumatic chylothorax. Other diseases associated with chylothorax include pulmonary lymphangioleiomyomatosis (discussed earlier in this chapter), abnormalities of the lymphatic vessels such as intestinal lymphangiectasis, filariasis, lymph node enlargement, lymphangitis of the thoracic duct, and tuberous sclerosis (18). If no etiology can be found for the chylothorax, it is labeled as *idiopathic*. Before attaching this label, however, lymphoma should be excluded.

Patients with chylothorax present with large pleural effusions. Pleuritic chest pain is very rare because chyle is not irritating to the pleura. The pleural fluid with chylothorax is distinctive in that it looks like milk and has no odor. At times, the pleural fluid may be blood tinged or frankly bloody. Patients who have a chylothorax usually have a pleural fluid triglyceride level above 110 mg per dL (1.24 mmol per L), a ratio of the pleural fluid to the serum triglyceride of greater than 1.0, and a ratio of the pleural fluid to the serum cholesterol of less than 1.0 (114). If doubt remains as to whether a patient has a chylothorax, lipoprotein analysis of the pleural fluid should be obtained. The demonstration of chylomicrons in the pleural fluid by lipoprotein analysis establishes the diagnosis of chylothorax.

The primary danger to the patient with chylothorax is malnutrition and a compromised immunologic status caused by the removal of large amounts of chyle, with its high levels of protein, fat, electrolytes, and lymphocytes, with repeated thoracenteses or chest tube drainage. Therefore, it is important to undertake definitive treatment for the chylothorax before the patient becomes too cachectic to tolerate the treatment. Most patients with traumatic or idiopathic chylothorax should initially be treated with a pleuroperitoneal shunt (115) unless they also have chylous ascites. The shunt takes the chyle with its nutrients and leukocytes from the pleural space to the peritoneal cavity, where it is absorbed. This treatment keeps the patient from becoming malnourished and allows time for the thoracic duct to heal, which it will do spontaneously in most patients. If the chylothorax persists for more than 4 weeks, consideration should be given to surgical exploration with ligation of the thoracic duct (18). Patients with nontraumatic chylothorax can also be treated with the pleuroperitoneal shunt, and this is probably the treatment of choice if the patient's life expectancy is limited. If the patient has mediastinal lymphoma, the chylothorax will usually resolve after radiotherapy or effective chemotherapy. If the patient has benign disease, consideration should be given to chemical pleurodesis or surgical exploration with ligation of the thoracic duct.

There are two new approaches to the management of chylothorax. Octreotide, a somatostatin analog, has been reported in uncontrolled studies to decrease the amount of chyle drainage with chylothorax (116). The mechanism of its action is not clear, but it is believed to be related to the reduction of intestinal fat absorption, particularly triglycerides (116). Cope has developed a method by which the thoracic duct is canulated transthoracically and then embolized with platinum microcoils or microparticles. She has reported that this procedure is successful in 65% of 50 patients, with no side effects (117).

The diagnosis of pseudochylothorax is usually easy. The patient usually has had a pleural effusion for 5 years or longer, and the pleura is thickened or calcified. Most patients with pseudochylothorax either have rheumatoid pleuritis or have been treated by artificial pneumothorax therapy for TB (118). Chemical analysis of the pleural fluid usually reveals cholesterol crystals or pleural fluid cholesterol levels above 250 mg per dL. If the patient's exercise capacity is limited by shortness of breath, a therapeutic thoracentesis should be performed because some patients will improve markedly (118). If the patient is symptomatic and the underlying lung is believed to be functional, a decortication should be considered (118).

HEMOTHORAX

A hemothorax is said to be present when the hematocrit of the pleural fluid is greater than 50% of the peripheral hematocrit. Most hemothoraces are due to trauma. A spontaneous hemothorax occasionally occurs with malignancy. Other causes of a spontaneous hemothorax include a leaking aortic aneurysm or pulmonary arteriovenous malformations, a complication of overzealous anticoagulation, or as a complication of splenoportography. There are several other rare causes of hemothorax, and at times, the etiology of the hemothorax remains unknown despite exploratory thoracotomy.

One would think that the diagnosis of a hemothorax is simple. However, frequently pleural fluid will appear to be pure blood when in fact the hematocrit of the fluid is less than 5%. Accordingly, when bloody pleural fluid is obtained by thoracentesis, a hematocrit should be obtained. The diagnosis of hemothorax should be made only when the pleural fluid hematocrit is more than 50% that of the peripheral blood. At times, it may be difficult to determine whether the bloody fluid obtained is venous or arterial blood or pleural fluid. However, blood that has been present in the pleural space for more than a few minutes will not clot, but both venous and arterial blood will clot.

Patients with traumatic hemothoraces should be managed initially by inserting a chest tube (119). Not only can the blood be removed by the chest tube, diminishing the likelihood of a subsequent fibrothorax, but also the amount of the drainage from the chest tube indicates whether a thoracoscopy or thoracotomy is necessary for controlling the bleeding. If persistent bleeding is not observed but more than one third of the hemithorax is occupied by a blood clot, thoracoscopy should probably be performed to remove the retained blood (120).

PLEURAL DISEASES NOT ASSOCIATED WITH EFFUSION

Fibrothorax

A dense layer of fibrous tissue may be deposited over the pleural surface when there is intense inflammation in the pleural space. This occurs most commonly following empyema or hemothorax. The fibrous tissue creates a cast around the lung rendering it immobile and essentially unavailable for air exchange. Recent studies suggest that profibrotic cytokines, especially transforming growth factor β, play an important role in generating the fibrosis (121). On physical examination, the affected side is fixed and does not move with respiration. Breath sounds are absent and the percussion note is dull. It should be emphasized that patients who have marked pleural thickening due to a recent episode of empyema, hemothorax, or tuberculous pleuritis frequently show marked spontaneous improvement in their symptoms and in the degree of pleural thickening in the 3 to 6 months following the acute episode. If the patient's lifestyle is compromised by exertional dyspnea after this period, decortication should be considered. However, the degree of improvement after decortication varies with many series showing disappointing results. If the underlying lung is intact, decortication may result in spectacular improvement subjectively and in the patient's pulmonary function test results. This improvement can occur even if the fibrothorax has been present 10 or more years.

Pleural Thickening Associated with Asbestos Exposure

The pleura of patients exposed to asbestos may develop plaques or diffuse thickening. The pleural disease is thought to be the result of short, submicroscopic asbestos fibers entering the pleural space. The small asbestos fibers lodge in the pleural lymphatics and, in conjunction with appropriate inflammatory cells, create inflammation that eventually leads to plaque formation or diffuse fibrosis (122). Pleural calcification usually occurs only 20 or more years after the initial exposure to asbestos. Patients with pleural thickening or calcification are usually asymptomatic. The pleural involvement with asbestos exposure is usually bilateral, but if it is unilateral, the left hemithorax is more frequently involved. The detection of pleural plaques or calcification is significant primarily as an indication of previous exposure to asbestos. The pleural plaques themselves do not affect pulmonary function to such a degree as to produce exertional dyspnea (123). However, because it is known that heavy asbestos exposure is associated with a markedly higher incidence of bronchogenic carcinomas and mesotheliomas, the presence of these abnormalities should alert the clinician to these possibilities. At times, patients with a history of asbestos exposure will develop extensive bilateral pleural fibrosis. Results with decortication in these patients have been disappointing (123).

PNEUMOTHORAX

Pneumothorax is the presence of gas in the pleural space. A *spontaneous* pneumothorax is one that occurs without antecedent trauma to the thorax. These pneumothoraces can be subdivided into *primary* spontaneous pneumothorax, for which there is no underlying predisposing disease, and *secondary* spontaneous pneumothorax, for which there is an underlying disease such as COPD or cystic fibrosis. A *traumatic* pneumothorax occurs as a result of penetrating or nonpenetrating chest injuries. An *iatrogenic* pneumothorax occurs as a consequence of a diagnostic or therapeutic maneuver. A *tension* pneumothorax is a pneumothorax in which the pressure in the pleural space is positive throughout the respiratory cycle.

Pathogenesis

The pressure in the pleural space is negative with respect to the atmospheric pressure and the alveolar pressure. Therefore, if there is a communication either between the alveoli and the pleural space or between the outside of the thoracic cavity and the pleural space, air will continue to enter the pleural space until the pleural pressure becomes atmospheric or the communication is closed. The increase in the pleural pressure will result in both a hyperexpanded hemithorax and a collapsed lung. Occasionally, when the communication is between the alveoli and the pleural space, a "ball-valve" effect is present, resulting in a one-way flow of air into the pleural space. Because the alveolar pressure becomes very positive with respect to atmospheric pressure during expiration, especially when there is coughing, the pleural pressure may become very positive, producing a tension pneumothorax.

Primary Spontaneous Pneumothorax

Approximately 8,600 individuals in the United States develop a primary spontaneous pneumothorax each year (18). Tall, thin individuals are more susceptible to this entity, and almost all affected individuals are smokers. Primary spontaneous pneumothoraces are usually due to the rupture of apical pleural blebs. These are small cystic spaces, seldom exceeding 1 to 2 cm in diameter, which lie within or immediately under the visceral pleura. The main symptoms associated with a spontaneous pneumothorax are chest pain and dyspnea, which begin abruptly in about two thirds of the cases and insidiously in the remainder. In most cases, the symptoms start while the patient is sedentary. The diagnosis is established with the demonstration of a visceral pleural line on the chest radiograph.

If the pneumothorax is small and if the patient has only mild symptoms, the recommended treatment is observation (124,125). Otherwise, the recommended initial treatment for primary spontaneous pneumothorax is simple aspiration (125,126). A 16-gauge needle with an overlying polyethylene catheter is inserted into the second or third anterior intercostal space at the midclavicular line after local anesthesia. After the needle is inserted, it is extracted from the cannula. Then a three-way stopcock and a 60-mL syringe are attached to the catheter and air is manually withdrawn until no more can be aspirated. If the total volume of air aspirated exceeds 4 L and no resistance has been felt, it can be assumed that no expansion has occurred and a chest tube should be inserted or an immediate thoracoscopy should be performed (125,126).

The recurrence rate for primary spontaneous pneumothorax after the initial occurrence is between 30% and 50% over 5 years if no attempts are made to produce a pleurodesis (18). Once a patient has one recurrence, subsequent recurrences are even more common. Patients who have a recurrent primary spontaneous pneumothorax and those in whom the initial aspiration is unsuccessful are best managed by thoracoscopy with stapling of blebs and pleural abrasion (127). If thoracoscopy is not available, one can attempt to induce a pleurodesis by the intrapleural injection of doxycycline (10 mg per kg) (18). The intrapleural injection of a tetracycline derivative will decrease the subsequent risk of a pneumothorax by about 50% (62). Talc slurry is not recommended because of its propensity to induce ARDS (59), and bleomycin is not recommended because it does not induce a pleurodesis when the pleural space is normal (61). Another alternative is open thoracotomy with stapling of blebs and abrasion of the parietal pleura, but this is a bigger surgical procedure.

Secondary Spontaneous Pneumothorax

COPD is responsible for most secondary spontaneous pneumothoraces, although almost every lung disease has also been associated with this entity. In one series of 505 patients with secondary spontaneous pneumothoraces from Israel, 348 patients had COPD, 93 had tumors, 26 had sarcoidosis, 9 had TB, 16 had other pulmonary infections and 13 had miscellaneous diseases (128). The occurrence of a pneumothorax in these patients is more life threatening than it is in a normal individual on account of their limited pulmonary reserve. Owing to the diminished breath sounds and lung hyperinflation of these patients, the diagnosis, both by physical examination and by chest radiograph, is much more difficult than it is in the normal individual. The possibility of a pneumothorax should be considered in all patients with an exacerbation of their COPD, and the chest radiograph should be closely examined for a pleural line. Because small pneumothoraces can lead to marked respiratory embarrassment, all patients should be treated with tube thoracostomy. We routinely recommend thoracoscopy with the stapling of blebs and pleural abrasion or instillation of doxycycline into the pleural space of such patients in an attempt to prevent a recurrence. If after 4 days of tube thoracostomy the lung remains collapsed or a bronchopleural fistula persists, thoracoscopy should be considered (18).

Secondary spontaneous pneumothoraces complicate about 1% of cases of parenchymal TB. Such cases should be treated with tube thoracostomy. Frequently, multiple tubes are necessary for long periods to effect resolution of the process. Bacterial pneumonia, particularly that due to *Staphylococcus aureus*, may be complicated by pneumothorax. In this situation, there is usually a complicating empyema. Such cases should have two chest tubes inserted: one high to drain the air and the other low to drain the pus. Secondary spontaneous pneumothoraces have also been reported in association with AIDS and *Pneumocystis carinii* pneumonia, asthma, cystic fibrosis, lymphangioleiomyomatosis, scleroderma, histiocytosis X, tuberous sclerosis, interstitial pneumonitis, sarcoidosis, pulmonary embolism, rheumatoid disease, hydatid disease, silicosis, metastatic malignancy, and primary carcinoma of the lung.

Tension Pneumothorax

A tension pneumothorax is present when the intrapleural pressure exceeds the atmospheric pressure throughout the respiratory cycle. The positive pleural pressure is life threatening, not only because ventilation is severely compromised but also because the positive pressure is transmitted to the mediastinum, resulting in decreased venous return to the heart and reduced cardiac output (129). In addition, patients with tension pneumothorax are usually markedly hypoxemic. Tension pneumothorax most commonly occurs in patients who are receiving positive pressure to their airways (mechanical ventilation or resuscitation). In patients not receiving positive airway pressure, the positive pressure in the pleural space is sustained by a "ball-valve" mechanism. Strong inspiratory efforts promote the entry of air into the pleural space, but the check valve prevents its egress, so the pressure continues to increase in the pleural space.

Patients with tension pneumothorax are acutely ill with dyspnea, tachycardia, and tachypnea. The neck veins are distended and the decreased venous return results in a thready pulse and hypotension. The trachea is deviated toward the side contralateral to the pneumothorax. The side with the tension pneumothorax is hyperexpanded and moves poorly with respiration. Tactile fremitus and breath sounds are absent, and the percussion note is hyperresonant on the side with the pneumothorax.

The treatment of a tension pneumothorax is a medical emergency (18). If the tension in the pleural space is not relieved, the patient is likely to die from inadequate cardiac output or marked hypoxemia. The diagnosis is made by physical examination. In the acutely ill patient, valuable time should not be wasted in obtaining radiologic confirmation. If the diagnosis is suspected, a large-bore needle should be inserted immediately into the pleural space through the second anterior intercostal space. If large amounts of gas come forth through the needle after its insertion, the diagnosis is confirmed. Observation of this phenomenon is facilitated by attaching the needle to a syringe containing sterile saline. With the plunger removed from the syringe, bubbling of air through the saline will establish the diagnosis. If a tension pneumothorax is present, the needle should be left in place until a thoracostomy tube can be inserted. In contrast, if air passes from the atmosphere into the pleural space, a tension pneumothorax is not present and the needle should be immediately withdrawn.

DISEASES OF THE MEDIASTINUM

The mediastinum is the region between the pleural sacs. It is bounded laterally by the mediastinal pleura and extends from the thoracic inlet superiorly to the diaphragm inferiorly and from the sternum anteriorly to the spine posteriorly. The mediastinum contains the heart, the thoracic aorta, and its proximal branches, the venae cavae, the azygos and proximal innominate veins, the thoracic duct, the lymph nodes and lymphatics, the esophagus, the trachea, the thymus, and the vagus, phrenic, posterior intercostal, and sympathetic nerves. Anatomically, the mediastinum is divided into three compartments (see Fig. 17-2). The anatomical boundaries, the normal contents, and the lesions that occur in the three compartments are shown in Table 17-2.

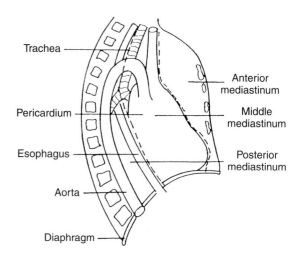

FIGURE 17-2. Subdivisions of the mediastinum. The *dashed lines* separate the middle mediastinum from the anterior and the posterior mediastinum.

MEDIASTINAL MASSES

Mediastinal masses may be discovered as a result of routine chest radiographs or in the evaluation of symptoms suggestive of mediastinal disease. Regardless, the differential diagnosis involves an abnormal shadow in the mediastinum on a radiograph. Because a given mediastinal lesion tends to be located in one mediastinal compartment, the first step in evaluating a mediastinal lesion is to place it in one of the three mediastinal compartments. Lesions that tend to appear in each of the three compartments are listed in Table 17-2. The following discussion of mediastinal masses is organized according to the three compartments. It should be emphasized that the locations listed in Table 17-2 are those in which the various masses are most likely to occur. For example, lymph node involvement in lymphoma occurs almost as frequently in the anterior as in the middle compartment. Aortic aneurysms may be situated in any of the three compartments.

TABLE 17-2. The Anatomical Boundaries, the Normal Contents, and the Lesions That Occur Predominantly in the Three Different Mediastinal Compartments

	Anterior Compartment	*Middle Compartment*	*Posterior Compartment*
Anatomical boundaries	Manubrium and sternum anteriorly; pericardium, aorta, and brachiocephalic vessels posteriorly	Anterior mediastinum anteriorly; posterior mediastinum posteriorly	Pericardium and trachea anteriorly; vertebral column posteriorly
Contents	Thymus gland, anterior mediastinal lymph nodes, internal mammary arteries and veins	Pericardium, heart, ascending and transverse arch of aorta, superior and inferior vena cavae, brachiocephalic arteries and veins, phrenic nerves, trachea, and main bronchi and their contiguous lymph nodes, pulmonary arteries, and veins	Descending thoracic aorta, esophagus, thoracic duct, azygos and hemizygos veins, sympathetic chains, and the posterior group of mediastinal lymph nodes
Common abnormalities	Thymoma, lymphomas, teratomatous neoplasms, thyroid masses, parathyroid masses, mesenchymal tumors, giant lymph node hyperplasia, hernia through foramen of Morgagni	Metastatic lymph node enlargement, granulomatous lymph node enlargement, pleuropericardial cysts, bronchogenic cysts, masses of vascular origin	Neurogenic tumors, meningocele, meningomyelocele, gastroenteric cysts, esophageal diverticula, hernia through foramen of Bochdalek, extramedullary hematopoiesis

TABLE 17-3. Relative Frequency of Various Primary Mediastinal Tumors and Cysts in Adults and Children

Tumor or Cyst	Adults Number	%	Children Number	%
Neurogenic tumor	384	21	135	39
Thymoma	387	21	0	0
Lymphoma	242	13	68	19
Teratomatous neoplasm	201	11	42	12
Primary carcinoma	65	4	16	5
Mesenchymal tumor	134	7	35	10
Endocrine tumor	115	6	0	0
Pleuropericardial cysts	126	7	0	0
Bronchogenic cysts	126	7	28	8
Enteric cysts	57	3	24	7
	1832	100	349	100

From Jones KW, Pietra GG, Sabiston DC Jr. Primary neoplasms and cysts of the mediastinum. In: Fishman AP, ed. *Pulmonary diseases and disorders.* New York: McGraw-Hill, 1980, with permission of McGraw-Hill Book Co.

It is evident from Table 17-2 that there are many different abnormalities that can produce abnormal mediastinal shadows. The relative incidence of the more common primary mediastinal tumors and cysts is outlined in Table 17-3. This table was compiled by combining nine series of adult patients and five series of pediatric patients (130). The incidence is heavily dependent on the patient's age. Thymomas are the most common abnormality in adults but are rare in children. Neurogenic tumors occur very frequently in children, but mesothelial cysts and endocrine (thyroid and parathyroid) tumors are very uncommon in children. When only primary mediastinal malignancies are considered, most are lymphoproliferative diseases (55%), followed by germ cell tumors (18%) and thymomas (14%) (131).

It should be emphasized that many abnormal mediastinal shadows do not represent primary mediastinal cysts or tumors.

In a review of 782 cases of mediastinal masses, Lyonset et al. (132) found that the most common cause of mediastinal masses was tumors (41.6%), followed closely by inflammatory diseases (35.7%), such as sarcoidosis, histoplasmosis, and TB, and then by vascular abnormalities (10.6%), hernias, diverticula, and achalasia (5.4%), cysts (2.8%), and miscellaneous disorders (3.9%).

The diagnostic approach to disorders of the mediastinum may be divided into imaging techniques [CT and magnetic resonance imaging (MRI), radionuclide studies, and barium studies] and procedures for obtaining tissue samples (needle aspiration and biopsy, thoracoscopy, and mediastinoscopy). CT imaging of the mediastinum is the most valuable imaging technique. The accurate cross-sectional information provided by CT scan can be very useful when a mediastinal mass cannot be accurately delineated by conventional radiographic methods, as illustrated in Figure 17-3. With a thoracic CT scan, normal variations and benign neoplasms such as fat and fluid-filled cysts can be distinguished from other processes, and the site of origin of masses can be better identified. MRI is usually reserved for clarifying problems encountered on CT scan or to examine patients who cannot tolerate IV administration of contrast material (133). At times, barium studies of the gastrointestinal tract are indicated because hernias, diverticula, and achalasia are readily diagnosed in this manner.

In many patients with mediastinal masses, a definitive diagnosis can be obtained with radiologically guided percutaneous needle biopsy of the mass. In one series of 95 patients, the diagnosis of malignancy was established with greater than 90% sensitivity and 100% specificity (134). Fine needle aspiration techniques usually suffice for carcinomatous lesions, but a cutting-needle biopsy should be performed whenever possible when lymphoma, thymoma, or neural masses are suspected in order to obtain larger specimens for more accurate histologic diagnosis. At times, endoscopic ultrasound-guided fine needle aspiration (135), mediastinoscopy (136), thoracoscopy (137), or anterior mediastinotomy is necessary to establish the diagnosis.

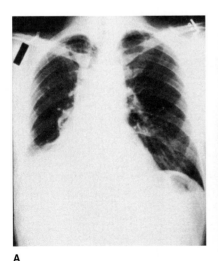
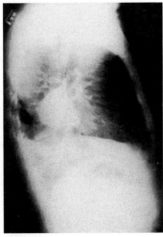
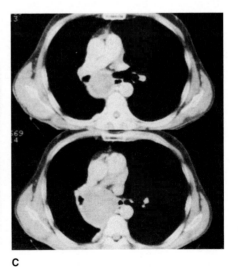

A **B** **C**

FIGURE 17-3. The value of CT scanning of the mediastinum in delineating mediastinal masses. Posteroanterior **(A)** and lateral **(B)** radiographs of a patient demonstrating a mediastinal mass or a right lower-lobe mass. Mediastinal CT scan **(C)** reveals that the mass is in the middle and posterior mediastinum and is separate from the right lower lobe. The patient had a bronchogenic cyst.

Mediastinal Masses Located Primarily in the Anterior Compartment

THYMOMA. Thymic tumors are the most common tumors in the anterior mediastinum and account for about 20% of all primary mediastinal tumors. Thymomas are slowly progressing tumors. Fifty percent are located within a capsule and do not infiltrate the adjacent tissue. However, all thymomas are potentially invasive and should be treated as a malignant disease (138).

The peak incidence of thymomas occurs between the ages of 40 and 60; they are rare in children. Thymomas are detected by chance on a chest x-ray in about 50% of the cases. In the other 50%, thymomas lead to coughing, dyspnea, chest pain, the superior vena cava (SVC) syndrome, or myasthenia gravis (138).

There are several paraneoplastic syndromes that occur in patients with thymomas (139). The most common is myasthenia gravis. Approximately 40% of patients with thymic tumors have myasthenia gravis, but 15% of patients with myasthenia have thymomas. Because thymectomy will lead to improvement of the myasthenia gravis in approximately two-thirds of patients with myasthenia and thymoma, mediastinal CT is indicated in all patients with myasthenia gravis. Patients with thymoma should have a serum antiacetylcholine receptor antibody level test preoperatively to exclude myasthenia gravis even if they are asymptomatic (139). Thymomas have also been linked to the occurrence of hypogammaglobulinemia, red cell aplasia, and various other autoimmune disorders and tumors.

Radiologically, thymomas present as well-defined, rounded, or lobulated anterior–superior mediastinal masses on one or both sides of the superior mediastinal shadow (see Fig. 17-4). At times, they are visible only in the lateral views, where they appear as a rounded or elongated shadow in the anterior part of the upper mediastinum. The upper pole of a thymoma can usually be seen clearly in the posteroanterior (PA) film, and this differentiates it from retrosternal goiter.

All thymomas should be treated surgically, but surgery is not always curative. In one series of 70 patients who had their thymomas surgically removed, 25 patients subsequently died from progression of their thymoma, and four other patients had evidence of recurrence (140). Radiotherapy is usually recommended for invasive or incompletely excised tumors (138). Postoperative chemotherapy should also be administered to patients in whom the tumor cannot be resected completely (138,139).

LYMPHOMATOUS TUMORS. Lymphomas as a group are one of the most common causes of mediastinal abnormalities. It has been estimated that lymphomas account for approximately 20% of all mediastinal neoplasms in adults and 50% of those in children (141). Mediastinal involvement with lymphoma usually occurs in conjunction with extrathoracic lymphoma, but in about 5% of instances, the mediastinum is the sole site of abnormality (141). Lymph node enlargement with lymphomas is most common in the anterior mediastinum but occurs frequently in the middle mediastinum and sometimes in the posterior mediastinum (see Fig. 17-5). Of patients with peripheral lymphoma and mediastinal involvement, 50% to 70% have Hodgkin lymphoma, and 15% to 25% have non-Hodgkin lymphoma. Nodular sclerosing Hodgkin lymphoma, the most common subtype of Hodgkin lymphoma in women, has a unique predilection for the anterior mediastinum, especially the thymus (142). Two variants of non-Hodgkin lymphoma, large B-cell lymphoma and lymphoblastic lymphoma, also primarily involve the anterior mediastinum and are the most frequent primary mediastinal non-Hodgkin lymphomas (142).

Patients with lymphomatous involvement of the mediastinum rarely present with isolated asymptomatic mediastinal disease. Usually, they also have enlargement of peripheral lymph nodes, hepatosplenomegaly, constitutional symptoms, or cutaneous or retroperitoneal disease. The mediastinal lymph node enlargement secondary to lymphoma is usually bilateral but asymmetric. In most cases, the mass has a nodular contour that suggests lymph node enlargement. If the diagnosis cannot be made by biopsy of a peripheral or scalene node, then mediastinoscopy is recommended. Although the treatment in the past has included attempted surgical excision, radiotherapy and chemotherapy now appear to be the treatments of choice (142).

GERM CELL TUMORS. These neoplasms, which include teratoma, seminoma, embryonal cell carcinoma, and choriocarcinoma, constitute the third most common tumors (following

FIGURE 17-4. Thymoma. Posteroanterior **(A)** and lateral **(B)** radiographs from a 23-year-old woman with a malignant thymoma. On the posteroanterior view, the superior mediastinum is widened, whereas on the lateral view, the retrosternal air space is obliterated.

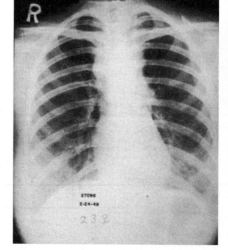

A

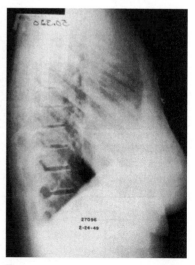

B

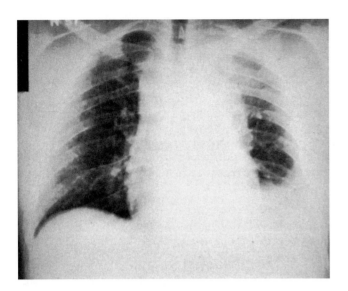

FIGURE 17-5. Mediastinal lymphoma. Posteroanterior radiograph from a patient with lymphocytic lymphoma demonstrating marked widening of the entire mediastinum.

thymomas and lymphomas) occurring in the anterior mediastinum. These tumors develop from residual embryonal tissues that migrated from the branchial clefts. *Dermoid cysts* are germ cell tumors that consist of only epidermis and its appendages, but *teratomas* contain ectodermal, mesodermal, and endodermal derivatives. Although they are presumably present from birth, they are discovered only in adolescence or early adulthood in most cases. About 20% of mediastinal teratomatous neoplasms are malignant, with malignancy occurring much more frequently in men. More than 90% of these neoplasms are located in the anterior mediastinum, but a few are located in the middle or posterior mediastinum (143). Adenocarcinoma is the most common malignancy found in these tissues, but seminomas, choriocarcinomas, and embryonal carcinomas are also found. Mixed histologic patterns are common.

It is unusual for symptoms to be associated with these tumors if they are benign, but symptoms are common with malignant tumors (143). Tumors that grow large may give rise to shortness of breath, cough, or a sensation of pressure in the retrosternal area. Rarely, a cystic tumor becomes infected and spills its contents into the mediastinum or pleural cavity.

Radiographically, most teratodermoid tumors are in the anterior mediastinum close to the origin of the major vessels from the heart. Benign lesions tend to be oval and smooth in contour, but malignant lesions tend to be lobulated. In rare cases, a bone or tooth is visible radiographically in the mass, and this establishes the diagnosis.

Measurement of serum tumor markers, β-subunit human chorionic gonadotropin (β-HCG) and α-fetoprotein (AFP), is indispensable in the management of mediastinal germ cell tumors. Patients with benign teratoma are marker negative; a significant elevation of HCG or AFP implies a malignant component of the tumor (143). The AFP is elevated in approximately 80% of malignant nonseminomatous germ cell tumors, whereas the β-HCG is elevated in 30%. Between 50% and 70% of patients with mediastinal testicular germ cell tumors will have elevated β-HCG but not AFP (144). The diagnosis of malignant germ cell tumors can be made with fine needle aspiration or cutting-needle biopsy of the mass, but many oncologists would treat a mediastinal mass on the basis of elevated levels of the serum tumor markers.

Benign teratomatous tumors should be removed surgically because they have a tendency toward malignant transformation, and infection is common in cystic lesions. The recommended management of malignant teratomatous tumors is cisplatin-based chemotherapy followed by surgical removal of the residual tumor. Long-term survival with seminomas is now 60% to 80%, and long-term survival with nonseminomatous tumors is 60% (142).

THYROID MASSES. Intrathoracic goiter (see Fig. 17-6) is the fourth most frequently seen anterior mediastinal mass, even though fewer than 3% of goiters are noted to extend into the thorax at thyroidectomy (132). Most intrathoracic thyroid

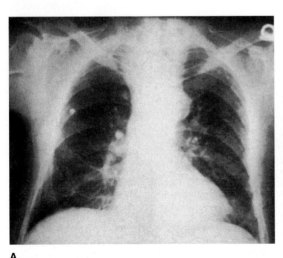
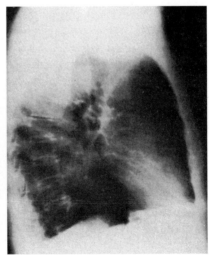

A **B**

FIGURE 17-6. Intrathoracic goiter. Posteroanterior **(A)** and lateral **(B)** radiographs from a patient with intrathoracic goiter. The goiter is evident as a right paratracheal mass in the posteroanterior view and as an anterior–superior mediastinal mass in the lateral view.

masses arise from a lower pole or from the isthmus of the thyroid and extend into the anterior mediastinum in front of the trachea. Patients are usually asymptomatic, but if the trachea becomes compressed, stridor and respiratory distress may occur. More than 50% of the patients will have associated thyromegaly with a nodular goiter, but hyperthyroidism is uncommon. The diagnosis may be made noninvasively with a CT or MRI of the mediastinum that demonstrates the thyroidal origin of the mass (145). The treatment should be surgical if symptoms are present and in most other cases (146). However, if the ^{131}I scan is positive and the patient is asymptomatic, observation may be reasonable if the patient is a poor surgical candidate.

PARATHYROID MASSES. Parathyroid tumors are a rare cause of anterior mediastinal masses. They are usually small, encapsulated, benign lesions situated in the upper or middle portion of the anterior mediastinum. Because most of these tumors produce parathyroid hormone (PTH), the presence of signs and symptoms of hyperparathyroidism allows one to make the diagnosis preoperatively. It is difficult to identify the tumor preoperatively, but CT will demonstrate the lesion about 50% of the time, as will MRI. The best way to identify the location of this tumor is with ^{99m}Tc-sestamibi scintigraphy, which has a sensitivity of 88% to 100% (139). The treatment of choice is surgical excision.

MESENCHYMAL TUMORS. The mesenchymal tumors (lipomas, fibromas, leiomyomas, lymphangiomas, hemangiomas, and mesotheliomas) account for less than 5% of mediastinal masses. Each tumor type has its malignant counterpart, and malignant changes occur in about 50% of these tumors (141). Most of these tumors occur in the anterior mediastinum, with the exception of fibrosarcoma, which occurs primarily in the posterior mediastinum. The recommended treatment for all these tumors is surgical removal. Despite treatment, malignant mesenchymal tumors are almost universally fatal.

HERNIA THROUGH FORAMEN OF MORGAGNI. The foramina of Morgagni are small triangular deficiencies in the diaphragm between the muscle fibers originating from the sternum and the seventh rib. They are a few centimeters from the midline on each side. When the foramina of Morgagni are larger than normal, abdominal contents may herniate into the thorax. This herniation is into the anterior mediastinum and is usually right sided because the left foramen is protected by the pericardium. The diagnosis is easily established with thoracic CT. To avoid the possibility of obstruction or incarceration, these hernias should be repaired surgically if they are large or if the bowel has herniated (147).

Mediastinal Masses Occurring Predominantly in the Middle Compartment

GIANT LYMPH NODE HYPERPLASIA. This unusual condition, also known as *Castleman disease*, usually presents as a solitary mass in the middle mediastinum, although it can occur in the anterior or posterior mediastinum. It has a distinctive microscopic appearance, with lymphoid follicles scattered widely throughout the mass instead of being confined to the peripheral cortical zones as in normal lymph nodes (148). Radiographically, there is a solitary mass up to 10 cm in diameter with a smooth or lobulated contour. Giant lymph node hyperplasia itself is a benign condition, but it has the potential to evolve into frank lymphoma. Some patients with Castleman disease also have associated immune defects. The treatment of choice is surgical excision.

LYMPH NODE INVOLVEMENT IN GRANULOMATOUS MEDIASTINITIS. Granulomatous inflammation of the mediastinal lymph nodes (see Fig. 17-7) is the most common cause of a middle mediastinal mass. This entity is discussed later in this chapter.

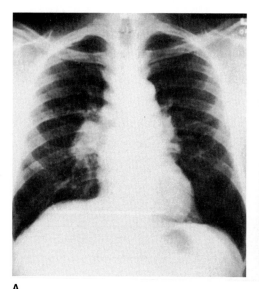
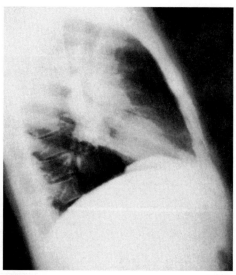

A   **B**

FIGURE 17-7. Mediastinal sarcoidosis. Posteroanterior **(A)** and lateral **(B)** radiographs from a 54-year-old patient with mediastinal sarcoidosis. Note that the lymph node enlargement is relatively symmetric and involves both the bronchopulmonary and mediastinal lymph nodes.

METASTATIC LYMPH NODE ENLARGEMENT. Nearly 90% of tumors that develop in the middle mediastinum are malignant. Metastatic disease from the lungs, upper gastrointestinal tract, prostate, or kidney is the most common middle mediastinal neoplasm (see Fig. 17-8). With metastatic disease, the bronchopulmonary nodes as well as the mediastinal nodes are almost invariably enlarged. When the primary lesion is in the lung, node enlargement is usually unilateral in the early stage. Most patients with metastatic disease to the mediastinum are symptomatic with weight loss, retrosternal pain, fever, cough, or dyspnea. Symptoms secondary to involvement of other mediastinal structures, including the SVC, phrenic nerve, recurrent laryngeal nerve, and pericardium, are common. Treatment is dependent on the site of the primary tumor, but the prognosis is, in general, dismal.

MESOTHELIAL CYSTS. Mesothelial cysts, also called *pericardial* or *pleuropericardial cysts*, have a developmental origin and appear to result from sequestration of part of the pleuroperitoneal cavity by the developing diaphragm. They rarely cause symptoms and are usually discovered on screening chest radiographs. Their most common location by far is anteriorly in the right cardiophrenic angle (149). They may also occur in the left cardiophrenic angle, in the hilar region, and in the anterior mediastinum. Mesothelial cysts contain crystalclear fluid and are at times called *spring water cysts* because of their contents. The diagnosis is strongly suggested by the CT scan and ultrasound. Aspiration of the lesion with demonstration of the clear fluid will establish the diagnosis. Once the diagnosis is established, resection is unnecessary because these cysts virtually never produce symptoms (149).

BRONCHOGENIC CYSTS. Bronchogenic cysts represent pinched-off buds of the primitive foregut or trachea and are lined with pseudostratified columnar epithelium. They occur paratracheally or adjacent to the main carina and project into the posterior part of the middle mediastinum. Because they contain fluid, they have a relatively uniform density, a smooth border, and a round or teardrop configuration (as do pleuropericardial cysts). Esophageal endoscopic ultrasound is now the preferred imaging technique (150). Bronchogenic cysts frequently become symptomatic, and for this reason surgical removal is recommended (150).

MEDIASTINAL MASSES OF VASCULAR ORIGIN. Mediastinal masses of vascular origin are most frequently found in the middle mediastinum. However, it is important to consider this diagnosis with all mediastinal masses because invasive procedures such as needle aspiration, needle biopsy, or mediastinoscopy may have disastrous consequences if the lesion is vascular (see Figs. 17-9 and 17-10). CT scan with contrast effectively demonstrates the vascular nature of the apparent mass.

Mediastinal Masses Situated Predominantly in the Posterior Compartment

NEUROGENIC TUMORS. Neurogenic tumors are the most common cause of a posterior mediastinal mass (142). They are characteristically situated in the posterior mediastinum because they arise from the paravertebral sympathetic nerve trunk and the spinal nerves. Approximately 20% of neural tumors are malignant.

Neurogenic tumors may be divided into three groups: (a) tumors that arise from peripheral nerves (neurofibroma, neurofibrosarcoma, and neurilemoma); (b) tumors that arise from sympathetic ganglia (ganglioneuroma, neuroblastoma, and sympathicoblastoma); and (c) tumors that arise from paraganglionic cells (pheochromocytoma and chemodectoma). Chemodectoma is the only neurogenic tumor that shows no strong tendency to be located in the posterior mediastinum.

The highest incidence of neurogenic neoplasms is in the younger age group, but they may develop at any age. In von Recklinghausen disease, mediastinal neurofibromas are associated with neurofibromas elsewhere in the body. Most patients with neurogenic tumors are asymptomatic, the tumors being discovered on screening radiographs. When symptoms are present, the most common is pain, presumably resulting from bony erosion. Radiographically, the tumors typically appear as round, dense, well-demarcated, solid-appearing masses in the posterior mediastinum in close association with a vertebral body. At times, the ribs or vertebrae are eroded, with either

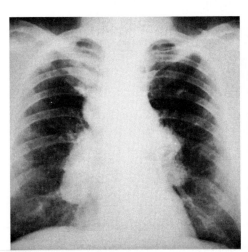

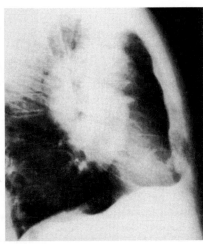

A   B

FIGURE 17-8. Metastatic lymph node enlargement. Posteroanterior **(A)** and lateral **(B)** radiographs from a patient with metastatic kidney carcinoma, demonstrating marked enlargement of both the mediastinal and bronchopulmonary nodes.

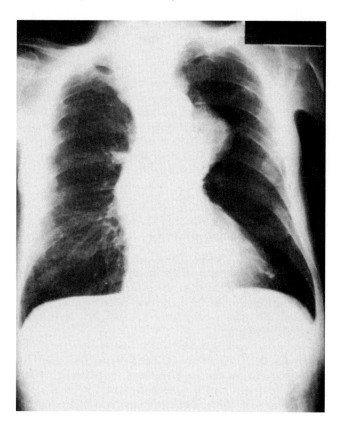

FIGURE 17-9. Aneurysm of ascending aorta. Posteroanterior radiograph demonstrating a mass in the superior left mediastinum. At aortography, the mass proved to be an aneurysm of the ascending aorta. This case illustrates how deceiving vascular masses may be at times. In fact, this patient underwent needle aspiration of the mass before the correct diagnosis was established.

benign or malignant lesions. A neurofibroma that originates in a nerve root within the spinal canal may be shaped like a dumbbell or an hourglass, one part being inside and another part being outside the spinal canal, with enlargement of the intervertebral foramen. Neurogenic tumors should be surgically removed because of their propensity to undergo malignant change (142). MRI should be performed preoperatively in all patients with suspected neurogenic tumors to definitely exclude intraspinal tumor extension.

MENINGOCELE AND MENINGOMYELOCELE

These are rare anomalies of the spinal canal in which the leptomeninges herniate through an intervertebral foramen. They are therefore located in the posterior mediastinum and are difficult to distinguish from neurogenic tumors. A meningocele contains only cerebrospinal fluid; a meningomyelocele contains nerve elements also. Many patients have kyphoscoliosis. Myelography may be diagnostic; treatment is by excision.

DISEASES OF THE ESOPHAGUS. The esophageal diseases described below produce masses in the posterior mediastinum.

Gastroenteric cysts. These cysts are identical to bronchogenic cysts except that they are lined with esophageal, gastric, or small intestinal mucosa. They are located adjacent to the esophagus at any level in the posterior mediastinum. Most are found in infants less than 1 year, in whom they produce

symptoms from tracheal or esophageal compression. Esophageal endoscopic ultrasound is now the preferred imaging technique (150). Because most are attached to the esophagus, the diagnosis is strongly suggested by a barium swallow that discloses a localized defect in the esophageal lumen covered with intact mucosa. Treatment is by surgical excision (149).

Esophageal diverticula. Zenker's diverticulum originates between the transverse and oblique fibers of the inferior pharyngeal constrictor muscle (148). It may become large enough to be visible on a plain radiograph of the superior mediastinum. Frequently, there is an air-fluid level. The diagnosis can be made with a barium swallow, and treatment is surgical. Diverticula arising from the lower third of the esophagus are almost always congenital. They present as round, cystlike structures to the right of the midline and just above the diaphragm (148). An air-fluid level is present in most cases. The diagnosis is established with a barium swallow, and surgical treatment is definitive.

Hiatal hernia. In patients with hiatal hernia, the chest radiograph often shows abnormalities behind the heart and slightly to the right of the midline. Many times, an air-fluid level is present. A barium swallow should be obtained in all patients with radiographic abnormalities in this area to rule out hiatal hernia (148).

Dilation. When the esophagus becomes dilated, it is apparent as a shadow projecting entirely to the right side of the mediastinum. Depending on the underlying cause of the dilation, an air-fluid level may be present or the entire esophagus may contain air. The diagnosis is made with a barium swallow.

HERNIA THROUGH THE FORAMEN OF BOCHDALEK. The Bochdalek hernia is the most common congenital diaphragmatic hernia, and at times it presents as a posterior mediastinal

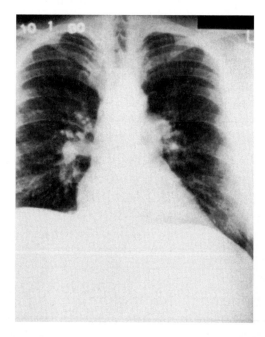

FIGURE 17-10. Enlarged pulmonary arteries. Posteroanterior radiograph from a 37-year-old man with primary pulmonary hypertension, demonstrating markedly enlarged pulmonary arteries that could be confused with a mediastinal mass.

mass. Although any portion of the diaphragm may be absent, most defects are posterolateral on the left side and result from failure of the fetal pleuroperitoneal membrane to fuse. Because the defects are congenital, herniation is identified most frequently in children and only occasionally in adults. Any intraabdominal organ may herniate through these foramina. A definitive diagnosis can be established with CT scan. Only symptomatic hernias require surgical intervention (151).

DISEASES OF THE THORACIC SPINE. A wide variety of primary neoplasms of bone and cartilage may involve the thoracic spine and posterior rib cage. Most of these lesions do not produce an extraosseous mass, but occasionally, the major radiographic finding is a posterior mediastinal mass. Tuberculous and nontuberculous spondylitis are often associated with a paraspinal mass. This is most commonly manifested as a bilateral fusiform mass in the paravertebral zone, with its maximal diameter at the point of major bone destruction. Fractures of thoracic vertebral bodies may result in extraosseous hemorrhage and in the development of unilateral or bilateral paraspinal masses (148).

EXTRAMEDULLARY HEMATOPOIESIS. This is a rare entity but should be kept in mind in any case of a paravertebral mass in a patient with severe anemia. Characteristically, extramedullary hematopoiesis is manifested as multiple paravertebral masses, being smooth or lobulated in contour, and having homogeneous density, either unilaterally or bilaterally. A presumptive diagnosis can usually be made on the basis of the radiographic appearance in patients with severe anemia and splenomegaly.

MEDIASTINITIS

Acute Mediastinitis

Most cases of acute mediastinitis are either due to esophageal perforation or occur after median sternotomy for cardiac surgery. The diagnosis and management of patients with esophageal perforation have been discussed earlier in this chapter. Rupture or perforation of the trachea or bronchi can also lead to acute mediastinitis. Occasionally, acute mediastinitis results from direct extension of infection from adjacent soft tissues. Prognosis in acute mediastinitis is inversely related to how long it takes to establish the diagnosis. Therapy in all cases consists of immediate surgical drainage in conjunction with high doses of systemic broad-spectrum antibiotics.

Mediastinitis after Cardiac Surgery

The incidence of mediastinitis following median sternotomy is approximately 0.5% to 3% (152). The incidence appears to be higher in obese patients and in patients with COPD. Patients who have blood cultures positive for *S. aureus* postoperatively are much more likely to develop mediastinitis (152). Most commonly, the mediastinitis manifests itself between 4 and 36 days postoperatively. The most common presentation of patients with mediastinitis is wound drainage, sternal pain, or sternal drainage (152). Sternal dehiscence is seen in most patients (153). Some will have a widened mediastinum on the chest radiograph; at times, the patients may present with occult sepsis. The primary diagnostic procedure has been mediastinal

needle aspiration, although CT scan, indium-111 leukocyte scanning, and epicardial pacer wire cultures also appear to be useful (154). Treatment requires immediate drainage, debridement, and parenteral antibiotic therapy. Mortality is in the range of 20% (154).

Granulomatous Mediastinitis and Fibrosing Mediastinitis

These two conditions represent separate ends of a spectrum of chronic granulomatous inflammation of the mediastinum. The mediastinal lymph nodes participate in the primary phase of certain granulomatous infections of the lung. Mediastinal granulomatous disease is most commonly due to TB or histoplasmosis, but it can also be due to sarcoidosis (Fig. 17-7), silicosis, and other fungal diseases. In most patients, the primary infections are relatively asymptomatic, and the adenitis subsides spontaneously over a period of weeks to months without untoward incident. However, in some instances there may be considerable periadenitis. In these, a mediastinal granuloma may eventually form when a cluster of caseating lymph nodes breaks down into a single mass. This conglomeration then heals by fibrous encapsulation. The diameter of these mediastinal granulomas ranges from 4 to 10 cm. The thickness of the fibrous capsule, rather than the size of the mass, is the major determinant of structural and functional damage to contiguous organs. The reason inflammation and fibrosis progress in some individuals but not in others is unknown (148).

In the spectrum from active granulomatous mediastinitis to burned-out mediastinal fibrosis, the former tends to be asymptomatic and to be discovered incidentally on chest roentgenography, and the latter is symptomatic either from a localized mass effect or because of the fibrotic process invading or compressing mediastinal structures. Clinical presentations are (a) the SVC syndrome; (b) traction diverticula, disturbances of esophageal motility, or dysphagia from esophageal involvement; (c) obstruction of the trachea or major bronchi; (d) obstruction of the pulmonary artery or proximal pulmonary veins; or (e) involvement of the mediastinal nerves producing hoarseness because of compression of the recurrent laryngeal nerve, diaphragmatic paralysis because of phrenic nerve involvement, or Horner syndrome from involvement of autonomic ganglia or nerves.

Although most cases of mediastinal fibrosis are thought to represent end stages of chronic granulomatous mediastinitis, there appear to be a few other situations in which this entity occurs. A small percentage of patients have an associated similar fibrotic process elsewhere, such as retroperitoneal fibrosis, pseudotumor of the orbit, Riedel struma of the thyroid, or ligneous perityphlitis of the cecum. In more than 40 cases, sclerosing mediastinitis has occurred during treatment with methysergide, an antiseritonin drug used for the relief of migraine headaches. In all cases but one, regression occurred when the drug was withdrawn (155).

In most instances, surgical exploration is necessary to distinguish between benign and malignant causes for these clinical manifestations. Occasionally, dense calcification within the mass allows a definite diagnosis without operation. The chest radiograph with granulomatous mediastinitis usually demonstrates a localized mass, usually in the right paratracheal area. Subsequently, with the development of fibrosing mediastinitis, there is generalized widening of the superior portion of the mediastinum. CT scan may be helpful in demonstrating areas of impingement on mediastinal structures or other abnormalities not evident on plain radiographs (156). MRI is superior in assessing vascular patency without the need for contrast media (148).

Specific therapy for granulomatous mediastinitis or mediastinal fibrosis is generally not indicated. Antituberculous therapy should be initiated if smears or cultures are positive for TB. If histoplasmosis is demonstrated, amphotericin B need not be administered. Corticosteroids and radiotherapy do not appear to be useful in the treatment of mediastinal fibrosis (157). At the time of exploration for diagnosis, some surgeons advise removal of as much of the inflammatory or fibrous mass as possible, but the efficacy of this practice has not been demonstrated by a controlled clinical trial. Surgery to relieve the obstruction of an airway or a blood vessel is difficult technically but successful at times (157).

MEDIASTINAL EMPHYSEMA

Mediastinal emphysema (pneumomediastinum) is the presence of gas in the interstices of the mediastinum. The primary causes are (a) alveolar rupture with dissection of air into the mediastinum; (b) perforation or rupture of the esophagus, trachea, or main bronchi; and (c) dissection of air from the neck or the abdomen into the mediastinum.

If there is a local increase in alveolar pressure, the alveolus may rupture. Air then enters the interstitial space of the lungs, and if air dissects along interstitial spaces to the hilum and mediastinum, mediastinal emphysema is produced (158). If the air dissects peripherally and the visceral pleura ruptures, a pneumothorax is produced. With mediastinal emphysema, a pneumothorax can also be produced if the mediastinal pleura ruptures.

To produce the local increase in alveolar pressure, there usually needs to be airway disease plus some maneuver such as coughing, vomiting, sneezing, mechanical ventilation, or repeated Valsalva maneuvers to increase alveolar pressure. It follows that mediastinal emphysema is seen in asthmatics and in patients with diabetic ketoacidosis with hyperventilation and pernicious vomiting, and it may also occur during childbirth (repeated Valsalva maneuvers), mechanical ventilation, scuba diving, and rapid ascents in airplanes. Pneumomediastinum has been reported in an individual who inhaled cocaine while his partner was applying positive ventilatory pressure (159).

The symptoms associated with pneumomediastinum range from none to severe. Typically, there is dyspnea or substernal chest pain with or without radiation into the neck and arms (160). The pain may be aggravated by respiration or swallowing. Physical examination usually reveals subcutaneous emphysema in the suprasternal notch. The *Hamman sign*, a crunching or clicking noise synchronous with the heartbeat and best heard in the left lateral decubitus position, is present in less than 50% of cases. The diagnosis is confirmed by the radiographic demonstration of gas within the mediastinal tissues. In the posteroanterior projection, the mediastinal pleura is displaced laterally, creating a longitudinal line shadow parallel to the heart border and separated from the heart by gas (148).

Usually no treatment is required, but the mediastinal air will be absorbed faster if the patient inspires high concentrations of oxygen. On rare occasions, the mediastinal air can compress the veins in the mediastinum, impeding venous return and leading to hypotension. In such cases, surgical decompression of the mediastinum should be performed, usually through needle aspiration or mediastinotomy just above the suprasternal notch (161).

DISEASES OF THE CHEST WALL

KYPHOSCOLIOSIS

Kyphoscoliosis is a combination of excessive anteroposterior and lateral curvature of the thoracic spine. The abnormal curvature may be predominantly lateral (scoliosis) or posterior (kyphosis). Abnormalities of curvature are common, occurring in about 3% of the population. However, deformity of a sufficient degree leading to symptoms and signs referable to the heart and lungs is rare, occurring in less than 3% of those with abnormal curvature.

Etiology

About 85% of the cases of scoliosis are idiopathic, that is, of no clear origin. Idiopathic scoliosis is classified into one of three types—infantile, juvenile, or adolescent—depending on the age at onset (162). Most cases fall into the adolescent class, in which the onset is between ages 10 and 14. In these patients, the curvature increases rapidly in the fast-growth period. The ratio of females to males is 4:1. The second category of kyphoscoliosis is congenital. These cases are related either to abnormalities of the thoracic spine, such as hemivertebrae, or to various hereditary diseases in which deformity of the thoracic spine constitutes only a part of the clinical picture—neurofibromatosis, muscular dystrophy, Friedreich ataxia, and several others. The third category is neuromuscular, in which kyphoscoliosis develops in response to asymmetric neuromuscular diseases such as poliomyelitis.

Pathophysiology

The major pathophysiologic effects of severe kyphoscoliosis are restrictive lung disease and ventilation–perfusion imbalances that result in chronic alveolar hypoventilation, hypoxic vasoconstriction, and, eventually, pulmonary arterial hypertension and cor pulmonale. Pathologic studies of the lungs of patients with kyphoscoliosis and cor pulmonale reveal severe muscular hypertrophy of the pulmonary arteries (163). The genesis of the pulmonary artery hypertension is thought to be chronic hypoxia secondary to regional inhomogeneity of ventilation and perfusion. Arterial hypoxemia may be present in some adolescents with severe kyphoscoliosis, but it becomes more prevalent as the age of the patient increases (164). Older patients with kyphoscoliosis also tend to develop an elevated $PaCO_2$. This elevation is thought to be related to the combination of the increased work of breathing secondary to the skeletal abnormality and the decreased functional capacity of the inspiratory muscles. Indeed, the PaO_2 and the $PaCO_2$ are much more closely correlated with the maximal transdiaphragmatic pressure than with the forced vital capacity (FVC) or the degree of scoliosis (165).

As would be expected from the deformity of the chest wall, pulmonary function tests reveal a decrease in vital capacity and total lung capacity and an increase in residual volume. Flow is reduced only in proportion to the reduction in vital capacity. In addition, the inspiratory muscle function is markedly impaired in patients with severe kyphoscoliosis, presumably from the mechanical disadvantages from the thoracoabdominal deformity.

In general, the degree of scoliosis correlates with the severity of the cardiopulmonary disease. The degree of scoliosis is best quantitated by using the Cobb method to calculate the angle of curvature (see Fig. 17-11). In subjects with an angle of curvature less than 60 degrees , there is seldom severe ventilatory impairment or significant alteration of blood gases. Individuals with curvatures between 60 and 90 degrees have an increased frequency of severe ventilatory abnormalities, and most patients with curvatures exceeding 90 degrees develop marked ventilatory abnormalities.

It should be emphasized that there are other factors in addition to the degree of scoliosis that are correlated with the reduction in the vital capacity. Patients with a greater number of vertebrae associated with the scoliosis, with a more cephalad location of the curve, and with loss of the normal thoracic kyphosis will have a greater reduction in the FVC for a given degree of scoliosis (166). Patients with kyphoscoliosis have a reduced work capacity. In one study of 79 patients with a mean Cobb angle of 45 $\pm$ 18.5 degrees, the mean work capacity was 86% of predicted. The work capacity correlated better with the vital capacity than with the angle of scoliosis (167).

Clinical Picture

Patients with severe spinal deformity generally present with increasing exertional dyspnea and exercise intolerance.

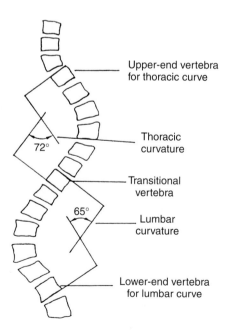

FIGURE 17-11. Cobb method of measuring scoliosis curves. First the "end vertebrae" of the curve are identified. These are the vertebrae that have the maximum tilting toward the curve to be measured. Then horizontal lines are drawn at the superior border of the superior-end vertebra and at the inferior border of the inferior-end vertebra. Then perpendicular lines are erected from each of the horizontal lines. The angle between the intersecting perpendicular lines is the angle of curvature.

Eventually, they may develop a rapidly deteriorating course characterized by recurrent respiratory infections, hypoxia, hypercapnia, and the development of pulmonary hypertension and right heart failure. There may be associated polycythemia secondary to hypoxemia. Respiratory failure rarely appears before the fourth decade. Some adults with severe kyphoscoliosis remain asymptomatic.

Treatment

Much effort has been devoted to restoring the normal curvature of the spine by either internal or external devices. In general, these manipulations result in improvement of the cosmetic appearance of the patients rather than their pulmonary function. Indeed, in one report of 14 patients with a mean age of 26 who underwent surgery, the mean vital capacity actually decreased by 0.21 L postoperatively (168). However, one report of 15 teenagers studied 1 year after corrective therapy demonstrated that the maximal inspiratory pressure increased by 14 cm H_2O and the peak expiratory flow rate increased by 32% (169). The earlier the corrective actions are undertaken, the better the results. Once cardiorespiratory failure has developed, there is a high mortality from operative intervention.

It appears that patients with kyphoscoliosis and recurrent episodes of respiratory failure benefit from chronic nocturnal mechanical ventilation. Studies with substantial follow-up have demonstrated that chronic nocturnal ventilation with positive-pressure ventilators can significantly diminish the symptoms of dyspnea on exertion and the signs of cor pulmonale. In addition, the arterial P_{CO_2} falls, the arterial P_{O_2} increases, the maximum inspiratory pressures increase, and the pulmonary artery pressures fall (170,171). Therefore, consideration of nocturnal ventilation should be given to all patients with kyphoscoliosis who have significant daytime symptoms and hypercapnia, a maximal inspiratory pressure below 60 cm H_2O, or nocturnal hypoxemia. Recent studies have suggested that nasal continuous positive airway pressure (CPAP) is probably the initial therapy of choice (170,171).

ANKYLOSING SPONDYLITIS

Ankylosing spondylitis is an inherited arthritic condition that ultimately immobilizes the spine. Ankylosis of the posterior intervertebral, costovertebral, and sacroiliac joints and ossification of the spinal ligaments and the margins of the intervertebral discs result in fixation of the thoracic cage. Accordingly, ventilation becomes almost entirely dependent on diaphragmatic movement. Because the diaphragm is the major contributor to ventilation normally, the fixation of the chest wall results in only minimal disability, and respiratory symptoms are uncommon. Patients with ankylosing spondylitis have a mild restrictive ventilatory dysfunction and a normal exercise capacity (172).

PECTUS EXCAVATUM (FUNNEL CHEST) AND PECTUS CARINATUM (PIGEON BREAST)

With pectus excavatum, the lower portion of the sternum is displaced posteriorly. The anterior ribs are markedly bowed, which results in a depressed panel in the anterior chest. The intrathoracic structures may be displaced laterally, and this may cause the heart to appear enlarged when actually it is not. Pectus carinatum is the opposite of pectus excavatum, with the sternum protruding anteriorly. The most common cause of acquired pectus carinatum (pigeon breast) is congenital atrial or ventricular septal defects. Approximately 50% of individuals with these cardiac defects have a pigeon breast. Severe prolonged childhood asthma is also associated with pectus carinatum.

Symptoms with pectus excavatum are infrequent during early childhood but become increasingly severe during adolescent years with easy fatigability, dyspnea with mild exertion, decreased endurance, pain in the anterior chest, and tachycardia (173). Repair is recommended for patients who are symptomatic and who have a markedly elevated pectus severity index. The optimal age for repair is between 12 and 16 years (173). After surgery, cardiorespiratory function is significantly improved (174). Symptoms are similar with pectus carinatum and the optimal age for repair appears to be about the same (175).

FRACTURES OF SINGLE RIBS

Trauma to the chest is responsible for most rib fractures. Nevertheless, minimal stress can result in fracture of a single rib if the rib is diseased. Ribs affected with bone cysts or metastatic neoplasms may fracture during stresses so slight that they have been unrecognized by the patient. An apparently normal rib may be fractured with modest stress such as from coughing or a passionate embrace. Cough fractures of the ribs occur more often in women than in men and almost invariably involve the sixth to ninth ribs, most often the seventh, and usually in the posterior axillary line.

Typically, the patient with a fractured rib will complain of severe, well-localized chest pain with deep breathing, coughing, stooping, and lifting. Physical examination usually reveals point tenderness over the fractured rib and localization of the pain when pressure is applied over the sternum. Chest radiographs may demonstrate the fracture; however, with nondisplaced fractures, the chest x-ray film is frequently positive only after 3 to 6 weeks, when callus formation is established. Therefore, the diagnosis should be made on the basis of the history and physical examination.

The treatment of fractured ribs has two goals—to alleviate the chest pain and to prevent secondary disease. The chest pain is probably best treated with systemic analgesics, although these must be administered carefully to patients with COPD. Local relief may be provided by a local anesthetic injected at the fracture site or by an intercostal nerve block. Chest strapping to immobilize the ribs may be used, but in general, it is not recommended because it is not very effective. The pain and tenderness tend to improve markedly within 10 days regardless of treatment, although some pain on inspiration or cough may persist for up to 6 months.

FRACTURES OF MULTIPLE RIBS

When multiple rib fractures are present, the chest wall may become unstable, a condition termed *flail chest*. With inspiration, when the thorax normally expands in all directions, the negative intrapleural pressure will cause the unstable portion of the chest wall to draw in. Similarly, on expiration the unstable portion of the chest wall will move outward with the positive pleural pressure. Frequently, the flail chest is not apparent within the first few hours of the injury on account of splinting. Flail chest generally results from fractures of three or more ribs in at least two locations. The major result of flail chest is to diminish the effectiveness of ventilation. The pain from the rib fractures, with the resultant splinting of the chest wall, further impairs ventilation. The major determinant of survival of patients with flail chest is the extent of the associated injuries.

The management of patients with flail chest is difficult and requires a great deal of skill and judgment. Patients with minimal degrees of instability require no ventilatory assistance but should be observed carefully for the development of atelectasis or pulmonary infections. In patients with larger degrees of chest wall instability, mechanical ventilation must be considered. Hypoxia can usually be managed with increased concentrations of inspired oxygen. However, if a PaO_2 of 60 mm Hg cannot be maintained or if the $PaCO_2$ starts to increase, intubation and mechanical ventilation should be initiated (176). The mechanical ventilation provides internal fixation of the unstable chest wall. For optimal care, the patient should not be permitted to make an inspiratory effort because the resulting negative intrapleural pressure would result in retraction of the mobile panel. Although one would expect that controlled ventilation would be necessary until the chest wall becomes fixed, mechanical ventilation can usually be discontinued within 14 days (176). This is probably related to the recovery of the underlying lung from its acute injuries. An alternative approach is to perform a thoracotomy and internally fixate the ribs. Patients treated in the latter manner tend to have less time on the ventilator (3.9 versus 14 days) and less time in the hospital than do patients treated with intubation and ventilation (177).

DISEASES OF THE DIAPHRAGM

UNILATERAL PARALYSIS OF THE DIAPHRAGM

Diaphragmatic paralysis results from interruption of the nerve supply (the phrenic nerve) to the diaphragm. The most common cause is nerve invasion from malignancy, usually a bronchogenic carcinoma. The second most common category of diaphragmatic paralysis is that for which no etiology can be detected. An increasingly common cause is open heart surgery. Injury to the phrenic nerve, almost always the left, occurs in approximately 20% of open heart surgery patients and is attributed to the use of cold cardioplegic solutions or to the stretching of the nerve particularly when the internal mammary artery is harvested. The paralysis resolves within 12 months in approximately two thirds of patients (178). Benign causes of diaphragmatic paralysis are poliomyelitis, herpes zoster, Huntington chorea, injuries or diseases of the cervical vertebrae, diphtheria, lead poisoning, tetanus antitoxin, measles, pulmonary infarction, pneumonia, mediastinitis, and pericarditis (179).

The diagnosis of unilateral paralysis of the diaphragm is suggested by finding an elevated hemidiaphragm on the chest roentgenogram. With diaphragmatic paralysis, the negative pleural pressure tends to pull the paralyzed diaphragm upward. Normally, the right diaphragmatic dome is on a plane approximately half an interspace above the left. In a review of

500 normal subjects by Felson (180), the right diaphragm was more than 3 cm higher than the left in 2% of subjects. However, the left diaphragm was at the same height or higher than the right in 9% of subjects. Confirmation of diaphragmatic paralysis is best established with the "sniff test." In this test, the diaphragm is observed fluoroscopically as the patient sniffs. The normal diaphragm will move downward during the sniff maneuver as the diaphragmatic muscles contract. A paralyzed diaphragm will move paradoxically upward because of the negative pleural pressure (179). With a normal large breath, a paralyzed diaphragm may move downward because of the change in the configuration of the chest wall. The diagnosis of a paralyzed diaphragm can also be made with ultrasonography (181).

Patients with a paralyzed diaphragm may be asymptomatic or may complain of dyspnea on effort. Pulmonary function testing reveals that the vital capacity and the total lung capacity are reduced by about 25%. In addition, the maximal transdiaphragmatic pressure is reduced by about 50%, and the maximal inspiratory pressure is reduced by about 40% (182).

The management of patients with diaphragmatic paralysis depends on the likely diagnosis. For example, a hilar mass in conjunction with diaphragmatic paralysis suggests bronchogenic carcinoma and serves as an indication for bronchoscopy. In patients post-CABG, the paralysis will usually resolve within 1 year. In asymptomatic patients with normal chest roentgenograms save for the diaphragmatic paralysis, probably no invasive procedures are warranted. In one report of 142 such patients, the diaphragmatic paralysis persisted in more than 90%, but over a mean follow-up period of nearly 10 years, only 4% of patients developed intrathoracic malignancy (183).

BILATERAL PARALYSIS OR PARESIS OF THE DIAPHRAGM

The presence of bilateral diaphragmatic paralysis or severe paresis almost always causes severe morbidity in adults. The most common causes are high spinal cord injury, thoracic trauma (including cardiac surgery), multiple sclerosis, anterior horn cell disease, and muscular dystrophy.

Most patients with severe diaphragmatic weakness will present with hypercapnic respiratory failure, frequently complicated by cor pulmonale and right ventricular failure, atelectasis, and pneumonia. Most will have dyspnea at rest that is worse in the supine position. Anxiety, insomnia, and excessive daytime somnolence are common, as is morning headache. The characteristic physical finding is the Hoover sign, which is a paradoxical inward motion of the anterior abdominal wall on inspiration that is most readily detectable in the supine position. The chest roentgenogram usually shows elevation of both hemidiaphragms, and the respiratory excursion of the diaphragm is usually minimal or absent.

The degree of diaphragmatic weakness is best quantitated by measuring transdiaphragmatic pressures. Probably the best measure is the transdiaphragmatic pressure generated during a sniff maneuver. Normally, this pressure is >98 cm H_2O, but in patients with diaphragmatic weakness the pressure may be <20 cm H_2O. The transdiaphragmatic pressures generated during the sniff maneuver appear to be more reproducible than the maximal transdiaphragmatic

pressure at total lung capacity or functional residual capacity. In patients with severe diaphragmatic weakness, the FVC diminishes from the seated to the supine position. A decrease of more than 30% is suggestive of severe diaphragmatic weakness (184). The maximal inspiratory pressure at the mouth is also reduced proportional to the diaphragmatic weakness (184).

The clinical course and treatment of patients with bilateral diaphragmatic weakness depend on the underlying disease. There can be recovery of diaphragmatic function when the nerve injury is not permanent. A good example of such recovery is that which occurs in patients who have bilateral diaphragmatic paralysis after cardiac surgery (184). In such patients, it may take 6 or more months for recovery to occur. In such cases, nasal intermittent positive airway pressure at night may be helpful until recovery (184). Most patients with progressive neuromuscular disease eventually require mechanical ventilation to maintain adequate ventilation.

Diaphragmatic Plication

Paralysis of the diaphragm may produce severe respiratory difficulties owing in part to the paradoxical motion of the affected diaphragm. One treatment that has been advocated to prevent the paradoxical motion is diaphragmatic plication (185). This treatment appears to be more effective in children than in adults. Ventilator-dependent children can often be weaned from the ventilator postplication. Even though ventilator-dependent adults usually cannot be weaned from the ventilator postplication, the pulmonary function and dyspnea of adults with diaphragmatic paralysis improve significantly (185).

Diaphragmatic Pacing

This is one alternative that can be considered in patients in whom the primary problem is above the anterior horn cell and the phrenic nerve is intact (e.g., a patient with a high cervical spinal cord lesion). Before pacing is seriously considered, the functional integrity of the phrenic nerve must be documented. This can be done by measuring the velocity of conduction of an electric pulse delivered percutaneously in the neck and recorded as the diaphragmatic action potential. This is best done by recording the diaphragmatic electromyelogram with an esophageal electrode and measuring the transdiaphragmatic pressure (186).

Once the functional integrity of the phrenic nerve has been demonstrated, consideration can be given to implanting a permanent diaphragmatic pacer. There are three different systems currently available, and each costs approximately $30,000. If continuous ventilation is required, bilateral pacers must be implanted because each phrenic nerve can be stimulated for only about 12 hours. It should be emphasized that even in centers with much experience with diaphragmatic pacing, the outcome is not always successful. However, if careful attention is paid to patient selection, patients can be maintained ventilator free with diaphragmatic pacing for more than 10 years (187).

EVENTRATION

Eventration is a congenital anomaly resulting from faulty muscular development of part or all of one or both diaphragms.

The eventrated diaphragm consists of a thin membranous sheet attached peripherally to normal muscle at points of origin from the rib cage. Radiologically, eventration cannot be distinguished from diaphragmatic paralysis. However, a previously normal chest x-ray will rule out eventration. If the eventration is complete, consideration should be given to diaphragmatic plication. With this procedure, the redundant fibrous tissue is folded on itself and stitched laterally to the chest wall so that the dome becomes almost flat.

HICCUP

A hiccup is an involuntary spasm of the inspiratory muscles followed by an abrupt closure of the glottis, which is responsible for the characteristic sound. Hiccups are usually precipitated by irritation of the diaphragm. This is most commonly due to gastric distention or inflammation following rapid or excessive eating or drinking. Hiccups also occur in other conditions in which the vagus nerve is stimulated, such as inferior wall myocardial infarction, peritonitis, pleurisy, pericarditis, and mediastinitis. Hiccups may be troublesome in uremia, in which instance they are thought to have a central origin.

Although hiccups are usually of short duration and resolve spontaneously, long-continued hiccups can be a serious symptom and a manifestation of important disease. Interestingly, Engleman's treatment is very effective and consists of having the patient rapidly swallow one teaspoon of ordinary white, granulated, dry sugar (188). If this does not work, the stomach can be decompressed with a nasogastric tube in conjunction with pharyngeal irritation. The next step is to administer chlorpromazine, 25 to 50 mg IV. If this works, the drug should be administered orally 10 to 20 mg every 4 to 6 hours for 10 days. In cases of intractable hiccups (daily hiccup present for at least 6 months), the administration of baclofen, an analogue of γ-aminobutyric acid at a dose of 10 mg t.i.d. will significantly reduce the severity of the hiccup and increase the percentage of the hiccup-free periods (189).

REFERENCES

1. Albertine KH, Wiener-Kronish JP, Roos RJ, et al. Structure, blood supply, and lymphatic vessels of the sheep's visceral pleura. *Am J Anat* 1982;165:277–294.
2. Albertine KH, Wiener-Kronish JP, Staub NC. The structure of the parietal pleura and its relationship to pleural liquid dynamics in sheep. *Anat Rec* 1984;208:401–409.
3. Negrini D, Townsley MI, Taylor AE. Hydraulic conductivity of the canine parietal pleura in vivo. *J Appl Physiol* 1990;69:438–442.
4. Bhattacharya J, Gropper MA, Staub NC. Interstitial fluid pressure gradient measured by micropuncture in excised dog lung. *J Appl Physiol* 1984;56:271–277.
5. Wiener-Kronish JP, Broaddus VC, Albertine KH, et al. Relationship of pleural effusions to increased permeability pulmonary edema in anesthetized sheep. *J Clin Invest* 1988;82:1422–1429.
6. Broaddus VC, Wiener-Kronish JP, Staub NC. Clearance of lung edema into the pleural space of volume-loaded, anesthetized sheep. *J Appl Physiol* 1990;68:2623–2630.
7. Wiener-Kronish JP, Matthay MA, Callen PW, et al. Relationship of pleural effusions to pulmonary hemodynamics in patients with congestive heart failure. *Am Rev Respir Dis* 1985;132:1253–1256.
8. Nahid P, Broadus VC. Liquid and protein exchange. In: Light RW, Lee YC, eds. *Textbook of pleural diseases*. London: Arnold Publishers, 2003:35–44.
9. Light RW, Stansbury DW, Brown SE. The relationship between pleural pressures and changes in pulmonary function following therapeutic thoracentesis. *Am Rev Respir Dis* 1986;133:658–661.
10. Light RW. Physiological effects of pleural air or fluid. In: Light RW, Lee YC, eds. *Textbook of pleural diseases*. London: Arnold Publishers, 2003:45–55.
11. McLoud TC, Flower CD. Imaging the pleura: sonography, CT, and MR imaging. *Am J Roentgenol* 1991;156:1145–1153.
12. Kataoka H, Takada S. The role of thoracic ultrasonography for evaluation of patients with decompensated chronic heart failure. *J Am Coll Cardiol* 2000;35:1638–1646.
13. Romero-Candeira S, Fernandez C, Martin C, et al. Influence of diuretics on the concentration of proteins and other components of pleural transudates in patients with heart failure. *Am J Med* 2001;110:681–686.
14. Kinasewitz GT, Keddissi JI. Hepatic hydrothorax. *Curr Opin Pulm Med* 2003;9:261–265.
15. De Campos JRM, Filho LOA, Werebe EC, et al. Thoracoscopy and talc poudrage in the management of hepatic hydrothorax. *Chest* 2000;118:13–17.
16. Weiss JM, Spodick DH. Association of left pleural effusion with pericardial disease. *N Engl J Med* 1983;308:696–697.
17. Kinasewitz GT. Transudative effusions. *Eur Respir J* 1997;10:714–718.
18. Light RW. *Pleural diseases*, 4th ed. Philadelphia: Lippincott Williams & Wilkins, 2000.
19. Tang S, Chui WH, Tang AW, et al. Video-assisted thoracoscopic talc pleurodesis is effective for maintenance of peritoneal dialysis in acute hydrothorax complicating peritoneal dialysis. *Nephrol Dial Transplant* 2003;18:804–808.
20. Baron RL, Stark DD, McClennan BL, et al. Intrathoracic extension of retroperitoneal urine collections. *Am J Roentgenol* 1981;137:37–41.
21. Light RW, Girard WM, Jenkinson SG, et al. Parapneumonic effusions. *Am J Med* 1980;69:507–511.
22. Light RW. Update: management of parapneumonic effusions. *Clin Pulm Med* 2003;10:336–342.
23. Light RW. The management of parapneumonic effusion and empyema. *Curr Opin Pulm Med* 1998;4:227–229.
24. American Thoracic Society. Guidelines for the management of adults with community-acquired pneumonia: diagnosis, assessment of severity, antimicrobial therapy and prevention. *Am J Respir Crit Care Med* 2001;163:1730–1754.
25. Davies RJO, Maskell NA, Nunn AJ. Primary result from the UK MRC/BTS randomised trial of streptokinase v placebo in pleural infection *Am J Respir Crit Care Med* 2004;160.
26. Wait MA, Sharma S, Hohn J, et al. A randomized trial of empyema therapy. *Chest* 1997;111:1548–1551.
27. Silen ML, Naunheim KS. Thoracoscopic approach to the management of empyema thoracis. Indications and results. *Chest Surg Clin North Am* 1996;6:491–499.
28. Thurer RJ. Decortication in thoracic empyema: indications and surgical technique. *Chest Surg Clin North Am* 1996;6:461–490.
29. Mehta JB, Dutt A, Harvill L, et al. Epidemiology of extrapulmonary tuberculosis. *Chest* 1991;99:1134–1138.
30. Mlika-Cabanne N, Brauner M, Mugusi F, et al. Radiographic abnormalities in tuberculosis and risk of coexisting human immunodeficiency virus infection. *Am J Respir Crit Care Med* 1995;152:786–793.
31. Rossi GA, Balbi B, Manca FP. Tuberculous pleural effusions: evidence for selective presence of PPD-specific T-lymphocytes at site of inflammation in the early phase of the infection. *Am Rev Respir Dis* 1987;136:575–579.
32. Patiala J. Initial tuberculous pleuritis in the Finnish armed forces in 1939–1945 with special reference to eventual post-pleuritic tuberculosis. *Acta Tuberc Scand Suppl* 1957;36:1–57.
33. Conde MB, Loivos AC, Rezende VM, et al. Yield of sputum induction in the diagnosis of pleural tuberculosis. *Am J Respir Crit Care Med* 2003;167:723–725.
34. Light RW. Closed needle biopsy of the pleura was important in its time, but should be relegated to the archives of medical history. *J Bronchol* 1998;5:332–336.
35. Valdes L, Alvarez D, San Jose E, et al. Tuberculous pleurisy: a study of 254 patients. *Arch Intern Med* 1998;158:2017–2021.

36. Riantawan P, Chaowalit P, Wongsangiem M, et al. Diagnostic value of pleural fluid adenosine deaminase in tuberculous pleuritis with reference to HIV coinfection and a Bayesian analysis. *Chest* 1999;116:97–103.

37. Lee YCG, Rogers JT, Rodriguez RM, et al. Adenosine deaminase levels in nontuberculous lymphocytic pleural effusions. *Chest* 2001;120:356–361.

38. Villena V, Lopez-Encuentra A, Pozo F, et al. Interferon gamma levels in pleural fluid for the diagnosis of tuberculosis. *Am J Med* 2003;115:365–370.

39. Querol JM, Minguez J, Garcia-Sanchez E, et al. Rapid diagnosis of pleural tuberculosis by polymerase chain reaction. *Am J Respir Crit Care Med* 1995;152:1977–1981.

40. Lai YF, Chao TY, Wang YH, et al. Pigtail drainage in the treatment of tuberculous pleural effusions: a randomised study. *Thorax* 2003;58:149–151.

41. Hillerdal G. Pulmonary aspergillus infection invading the pleura. *Thorax* 1981;36:745–751.

42. Lonky SA, Catanzaro A, Moser KM, et al. Acute coccidioidal pleural effusion. *Am Rev Respir Dis* 1976;114:681–688.

43. Cunningham RT, Einstein H. Coccidioidal pulmonary cavities with rupture. *J Thorac Cardiovasc Surg* 1982;84:172–177.

44. Conces DJ Jr, Vix VA, Tarver RD. Pleural cryptococcosis. *J Thorac Imaging* 1990;5:84–86.

45. Fine NL, Smith LR, Sheedy PF. Frequency of pleural effusions in mycoplasma and viral pneumonias. *N Engl J Med* 1970;282:790–793.

46. Drugs for parasitic infections. *Med Lett Drugs Ther* 1998;40:1–12.

47. Johnson RJ, Johnson JR. Paragonimiasis in Indochinese refugees. *Am Rev Respir Dis* 1983;128:534–538.

48. Aribas OK, Kanat F, Gormus N, et al. Pleural complications of hydatid disease. *J Thorac Cardiovasc Surg* 2002;123:492–497.

49. Cheng D-S, Rodriguez RM, Perkett EA, et al. Vascular endothelial growth factor in pleural fluid. *Chest* 1999;115:760–765.

50. Meyer P. Metastatic carcinoma of the pleura. *Thorax* 1966;21:437–443.

51. Light RW. Pleural effusion. *N Engl J Med* 2002;346:1971–1977.

52. Light RW, Erozan Y, Ball WC Jr. Cells in pleural fluid. *Arch Intern Med* 1973;132:854–860.

53. Poe RW, Israel RH, Utell MJ, et al. Sensitivity, specificity, and predictive values of closed pleural biopsy. *Arch Intern Med* 1984;144:325–328.

54. Putnam JB Jr, Walsh GL, Swisher SG, et al. Outpatient management of malignant pleural effusion by a chronic indwelling pleural catheter. *Ann Thorac Surg* 2000;69:369–375.

55. Pollak JS, Burdge CM, Rosenblatt M, et al. Treatment of malignant pleural effusions with tunneled long-term drainage catheters. *J Vasc Interv Radiol* 2001;12:201–208.

56. Putnam JB, Light RW, Rodriguez MR, et al. A randomized comparison of indwelling pleural catheter and doxycycline pleurodesis in the management of malignant pleural effusions. *Cancer* 1999;86:1992–1999.

57. Lee YC, Baumann MH, Maskell NA, et al. Pleurodesis practice for malignant pleural effusions in five English-speaking countries: survey of pulmonologists. *Chest* 2003;124:2229–2238.

58. Milanez Campos JR, Werebe EC, Vargas FS, et al. Respiratory failure due to insufflated talc. *Lancet* 1997;349:251–252.

59. Rehse DH, Aye RW, Florence MG. Respiratory failure following talc pleurodesis. *Am J Surg* 1999;177:437–440.

60. Walker-Renard PB, Vaughan LM, Sahn SA. Chemical pleurodesis for malignant pleural effusions. *Ann Intern Med* 1994;120:56–64.

61. Vargas FS, Wang N-S, Lee HM, et al. Effectiveness of bleomycin in comparison to tetracycline as pleural sclerosing agent in rabbits. *Chest* 1993;104:1582–1584.

62. Light RW, O'Hara VS, Moritz TE, et al. Intrapleural tetracycline for the prevention of recurrent spontaneous pneumothorax. *JAMA* 1990;264:2224–2230.

63. Vargas FS, Teixeira LR, Coelho IJC, et al. Distribution of pleural injectate: effect of volume of injectate and animal rotation. *Chest* 1994;106:2146–2149.

64. Heffner JE, Nietert PJ, Barbieri C. Pleural Fluid pH as a predictor of pleurodesis failure: analysis of primary data. *Chest* 2000;117:87–95.

65. Astoul P. Malignant mesothelioma. In: Light RW, Lee YC, eds. *Textbook of pleural diseases*. London: Arnold Publishers, 2003:35–44.

66. De Pangher Manzini V, Brollo A, Franceschi S, et al. Prognostic factors of malignant mesothelioma of the pleura. *Cancer* 1993;72:410–417.

67. Antman KH. Natural history and epidemiology of malignant mesothelioma. *Chest* 1993;103(Suppl. 4):373S–376S.

68. Ordonez NG. The immunohistochemical diagnosis of mesothelioma: a comparative study of epithelioid mesothelioma and lung adenocarcinoma. *Am J Surg Pathol* 2003;27:1031–1051.

69. Lee YCG, Light RW, Musk AW. Management of malignant pleural mesothelioma: a critical review. *Curr Opin Pulm Med* 2000;6:267–274.

70. Sugarbaker DJ, Flores RM, Jakiltsch MT, et al. Resection margins, extrapleural nodal status, and cell type determine postoperative long-term survival in trimodality therapy of malignant pleural mesothelioma: Results in 183 patients. *J Thorac Cardiovasc Surg* 1999;117:54–65.

71. Vogelzang NJ, Rusthoven JJ, Symanowski J, et al. Phase III study of pemetrexed in combination with cisplatin versus cisplatin alone in patients with malignant pleural mesothelioma. *J Clin Oncol* 2003;21:2636–2644.

72. Mitchell JD. Solitary fibrous tumor of the pleura. *Semin Thorac Cardiovasc Surg* 2003;15:305–309.

73. Nador RG, Cesarman E, Chadburn A, et al. Primary effusion lymphoma: a distinct clinicopathologic entity associated with the Kaposi's sarcoma-associated herpes virus. *Blood* 1996;88:645–656.

74. Taniere P, Manai A, Charpentier R, et al. Pyothorax-associated lymphoma: relationship with Epstein-Barr virus, human herpes virus-8 and body cavity-based high grade lymphomas. *Eur Respir J* 1998;11:779–783.

75. Winslow WA, Ploss LN, Loitman B. Pleuritis in systemic lupus erythematosus: its importance as an early manifestation in diagnosis. *Ann Intern Med* 1958;49:70–88.

76. Wang DY, Yang PC, Yu WL, et al. Comparison of different diagnostic methods for lupus pleuritis and pericarditis: a prospective three-year study. *J Formos Med Assoc* 2000;99:375–380.

77. Halla JT, Schrohenloher RE, Volanakis JE. Immune complexes and other laboratory features of pleural effusions. A comparison of rheumatoid arthritis, systemic lupus erythematosus and other disease. *Ann Intern Med* 1980;92:748–752.

78. Chapman PT, O'Donnell JL, Moller PW. Rheumatoid pleural effusion: response to intrapleural corticosteroid. *J Rheumatol* 1992;19:478–480.

79. Stein PD, Henry JW. Clinical characteristics of patients with acute pulmonary embolism stratified according to their presenting syndromes. *Chest* 1997;112:974–979.

80. Romero-Candeira S, Hernandez Blasco L, Soler MJ, et al. Biochemical and cytologic characteristics of pleural effusions secondary to pulmonary embolism. *Chest* 2002;121:465–469.

81. Coche EE, Muller NL, Kim KI, et al. Acute pulmonary embolism: ancillary findings at spiral CT. *Radiology* 1998;207:753–758.

82. Coche E, Verschuren F, Keyeux A, et al. Diagnosis of acute pulmonary embolism in outpatients: comparison of thin-collimation multi-detector row spiral CT and planar ventilation-perfusion scintigraphy. *Radiology* 2003;229:757–765.

83. Lankisch PG, Groge M, Becher R. Pleural effusions: a new negative prognostic parameter for acute pancreatitis. *Am J Gastroenterol* 1994;89:1849–1851.

84. Rockey DC, Cello JP. Pancreaticopleural fistula. Report of 7 patients and review of the literature. *Medicine* 1990;69:332–344.

85. Sherr HP, Light RW, Merson MH, et al. Origin of pleural fluid amylase in esophageal rupture. *Ann Intern Med* 1972;76:985–986.

86. Bufkin BL, Miller JI Jr, Mansour KA. Esophageal perforation: emphasis on management. *Ann Thorac Surg* 1996;61:1447–1451.

87. Voros D, Gouliamos A, Kotoulas G, et al. Percutaneous drainage of intra-abdominal abscesses using large lumen tubes under computed tomographic control. *Eur J Surg* 1996;162:895–898.

88. Light RW, Rogers JT, Moyers JP, et al. Prevalence and clinical course of pleural effusions at 30 days after coronary artery and cardiac surgery. *Am J Respir Crit Care Med* 2002;166:1563–1566.

89. Sadikot RT, Rogers JT, Cheng DS, et al. Pleural fluid characteristics of patients with symptomatic pleural effusion after coronary artery bypass graft surgery. *Arch Intern Med* 2000;160:2665–2668.

90. Lee YCG, Vaz MA, Ely KA, et al. Symptomatic persistent post-coronary artery bypass graft pleural effusions requiring operative treatment: clinical and histologic features. *Chest* 2001;119:795–800.
91. Light RW, George RB. Incidence and significance of pleural effusion after abdominal surgery. *Chest* 1976;69:621–626.
92. Shitrit D, Izbicki G, Fink G, et al. Late postoperative pleural effusion following lung transplantation: characteristics and clinical implications. *Eur J Cardiothorac Surg* 2003;23:494–496.
93. Ferrer JS, Roldan J, Roman A, et al. Acute and chronic pleural complications in lung transplantation. *J Heart Lung Transplant* 2003;22:1217–1225.
94. Medina LS, Siegel MJ, Bejarano PA, et al. Pediatric lung transplantation: radiographic-histologic correlation. *Radiology* 1993;187:807–810.
95. Golfieri R, Giampalma E, Morselli Labate AM, et al. Pulmonary complications of liver transplantation: radiological appearance and statistical evaluation of risk factors in 300 cases. *Eur Radiol* 2000;10:1169–1183.
96. Uetsuji S, Komada Y, Kwon AH, et al. Prevention of pleural effusion after hepatectomy using fibrin sealant. *Int Surg* 1994;79:135–137.
97. Edling JE, Bacon BR. Pleuropulmonary complications of endoscopic variceal sclerotherapy. *Chest* 1991;99:1252–1257.
98. Kalomenidis IT. Effusions due to drugs. In: Light RW, Lee YC, eds. *Textbook of pleural diseases*. London: Arnold Publishers, 2003:382–393.
99. Hillerdal G, Lee J, Blomkvist A, et al. Pleural disease during treatment with bromocriptine in patients previously exposed to asbestos. *Eur Respir J* 1997;10:2711–2715.
100. Epler GR, McLoud TC, Gaensler EA. Prevalence and incidence of benign asbestos pleural effusion in a working population. *JAMA* 1982;247:617–622.
101. Hillerdal G, Ozesmi M. Benign asbestos pleural effusion: 73 exudates in 60 patients. *Eur J Respir Dis* 1987;71:113–121.
102. Ishiko O, Yoshida H, Sumi T, et al. Vascular endothelial growth factor levels in pleural and peritoneal fluid in Meigs' syndrome. *Eur J Obstet Gynecol Reprod Biol* 2001;98:129–130.
103. Johnson SR, Tattersfield AE. Clinical experience of lymphangioleiomyomatosis in the UK. *Thorax* 2000;55:1052–1057.
104. Taylor JR, Ryu J, Colby TV, et al. Lymphangioleiomyomatosis: clinical course in 32 patients. *N Engl J Med* 1990;323:1254–1260.
105. Kalassian KG, Doyle R, Kao P, et al. Lymphangioleiomyomatosis: new insights. *Am J Respir Crit Care Med* 1997;155:1183–1186.
106. Berger HW, Rammohan G, Neff MS, et al. Uremic pleural effusion: study in 14 patients on chronic dialysis. *Ann Intern Med* 1975;82:362–364.
107. Coskun M, Boyvat F, Bozkurt B, et al. Thoracic CT findings in long-term hemodialysis patients. *Acta Radiol* 1998;40:181–186.
108. Jarratt MJ, Sahn SA. Pleural effusions in hospitalized patients receiving long-term hemodialysis. *Chest* 1995;108:470–474.
109. Light RW, Jenkinson SG, Minh VD, et al. Observations on pleural fluid pressures as fluid is withdrawn during thoracentesis. *Am Rev Respir Dis* 1980;121:799–804.
110. Light RW. Pleural effusions following cardiac injury and coronary artery bypass graft surgery. *Sem Respir Crit Care Med* 2001;22:657–664.
111. Mott AR, Fraser CDJ, Kusnoor AV, et al. The effect of short-term prophylactic methylprednisolone on the incidence and severity of postpericardiotomy syndrome in children undergoing cardiac surgery with cardiopulmonary bypass. *J Am Coll Cardiol* 2001;37:1700–1706.
112. Nordkild P, Kromann-Andersen H, Stuve-Christensen E. Yellow nail syndrome—the triad of yellow nails, lymphedema and pleural effusions. *Acta Med Scand* 1986;219:221–227.
113. Soskel NT, Sharma OP. Pleural involvement in sarcoidosis. *Curr Opin Pulm Med* 2000;6:455–468.
114. Romero S, Martin C, Hernandez L, et al. Chylothorax in cirrhosis of the liver: analysis of its frequency and clinical characteristics. *Chest* 1998;114:154–159.
115. Murphy MC, Newman BM, Rodgers BM. Pleuroperitoneal shunts in the management of persistent chylothorax. *Ann Thorac Surg* 1989;48:195–200.
116. Al-Zubairy SA, Al-Jazairi AS. Octreotide as a therapeutic option for management of chylothorax. *Ann Pharmacother* 2003;37:679–682.
117. Cope C. Management of chylothorax via percutaneous embolization. *Curr Opin Pulm Med* 2004;10:311–314.
118. Hillerdal G. Effusions from lymphatic disruptions. In: Light RW, Lee YC, eds. *Textbook of pleural diseases*. London: Arnold Press, 2003:362–369.
119. Wilson JM, Boren CH Jr, Peterson SR, et al. Traumatic hemothorax: is decortication necessary? *J Thorac Cardiovasc Surg* 1979;77:489–495.
120. Carrillo EH, Richardson JD. Thoracoscopy in the management of hemothorax and retained blood after trauma. *Curr Opin Pulm Med* 1998;4:243–246.
121. Lee YCG, Lane KB. The many faces of transforming growth factor beta in pleural diseases. *Curr Opin Pulm Med* 2001;7:173–179.
122. Hillerdal G. The pathogenesis of pleural plaques and pulmonary asbestosis: possibilities and impossibilities. *Eur J Respir Dis* 1980;61:129–138.
123. Musk AW, De Klerk NH. Benign asbestos pleural diseases. In: Light RW, Lee YC, eds. *Textbook of pleural diseases*. London: Arnold Publishers, 2003:428–434.
124. Baumann MH, Strange C, Heffner JE, et al. Management of spontaneous pneumothorax: an American College of Chest Physicians Delphi Consensus Statement. *Chest* 2001;119:590–602.
125. Henry M, Arnold T, Harvey J. BTS guidelines for the management of spontaneous pneumothorax. *Thorax* 2003;58(Suppl. 2):II39–II52.
126. Light RW. Manual aspiration: the preferred method for managing primary spontaneous pneumothorax? *Am J Respir Crit Care Med* 2002;165:1202–1203.
127. Casadio C, Rena O, Giobbe R, et al. Stapler blebectomy and pleural abrasion by video-assisted thoracoscopy for spontaneous pneumothorax. *J Cardiovasc Surg (Torino)* 2002;43:259–262.
128. Weissberg D, Refaely Y. Pneumothorax. *Chest* 2000;117:1279–1285.
129. Barton ED, Rhee P, Hutton KC, et al. The pathophysiology of tension pneumothorax in ventilated swine. *J Emerg Med* 1997;15:147–153.
130. Jones KW, Pietra GG, Sabiston DC Jr. Primary neoplasms and cysts of the mediastinum. In: Fishman AP, ed. *Pulmonary diseases and disorders*. New York: McGraw-Hill, 1980:1490.
131. Temes R, Chavez T, Mapel D, et al. Primary mediastinal malignancies: findings in 219 patients. *West J Med* 1999;170:161–166.
132. Lyons HA, Calvy GL, Sammons BP. The diagnosis and classification of mediastinal masses. A study of 782 cases. *Ann Intern Med* 1959;51:897–932.
133. Brown LR, Aughenbaugh GL. Masses of the anterior mediastinum. CT and MR imaging. *Am J Roentgenol* 1991;157:1171–1180.
134. Morrissey B, Adams H, Gibbs AR, et al. Percutaneous needle biopsy of the mediastinum: review of 94 procedures. *Thorax* 1993;48:632–637.
135. Larsen SS, Krasnik M, Vilmann P, et al. Endoscopic ultrasound guided biopsy of mediastinal lesions has a major impact on patient management. *Thorax* 2002;57:98–103.
136. Hoerbelt R, Keunecke L, Grimm H, et al. The value of a noninvasive diagnostic approach to mediastinal masses. *Ann Thorac Surg* 2003;75:1086–1090.
137. Kitami A, Suzuki T, Usuda K, et al. Diagnostic and therapeutic thoracoscopy for mediastinal disease. *Ann Thorac Cardiovasc Surg* 2004;10:14–18.
138. Schmidt-Wolf IG, Rockstroh JK, Schuller H, et al. Malignant thymoma: current status of classification and multimodality treatment. *Ann Hematol* 2003;82:69–76.
139. Strollo DDC, Rosado de Christenson ML, Jett JR. Primary mediastinal tumors. Part 1. Tumors of the anterior mediastinum. *Chest* 1997;112:511–522.
140. Gripp S, Hilgers K, Wurm R, et al. Thymoma. Prognostic factors and treatment outcome. *Cancer* 1998;83:1495–1503.
141. Fraser RS, Colman N, Muller NL, et al. Masses situated predominantly in the anterior mediastinal compartment. *Diagnosis of diseases of the chest*, 4th ed. Philadelphia: WB Saunders, 1999:2875–2937.
142. Strollo DC, Rosado de Christenson ML, Jett JR. Primary mediastinal tumors. Part II. Tumors of the middle and posterior mediastinum. *Chest* 1997;112:1344–1357.
143. Nichols CR. Mediastinal germ cell tumors. Clinical features and biologic correlate. *Chest* 1991;99:472–479.

144. Strollo DC, Rosado-de-Christenson ML. Primary mediastinal malignant germ cell neoplasms: imaging features. *Chest Surg Clin North Am* 2002;12:645–658.

145. Jennings A. Evaluation of substernal goiters using computed tomography and MR imaging. *Endocrinol Metab Clin North Am* 2001;30:401–414.

146. Wax MK, Briant TDR. The management of substernal goiter. *J Otolaryngol* 1992;21:165–170.

147. Angrisani L, Lorenzo M, Santoro T, et al. Hernia of foramen of Morgagni in adult: case report of laparoscopic repair. *JSLS* 1000;4: 177–181.

148. Fraser RS, Muller NL, Colman N, et al. Masses situated predominantly in the middle-posterior mediastinal compartment. *Diagnosis of diseases of the chest*, 4th ed. Philadelphia: WB Saunders, 1999: 2938–2972.

149. Salyer DC, Salyer WR, Eggleston JC. Benign developmental cysts of the mediastinum. *Arch Pathol Lab Med* 1977;101:136–139.

150. Cioffi U, Bonavina L, De Simone M, et al. Presentation and surgical management of bronchogenic and esophageal duplication cysts in adults. *Chest* 1998;113:1492–1496.

151. Shin MS, Mulligan SA, Baxley WA, et al. Bochdalek hernia of diaphragm in the adult. Diagnosis by computed tomography. *Chest* 1987;92:1098–1101.

152. Fowler VG Jr, Kaye KS, Simel DL, et al. *Staphylococcus aureus* bacteremia after median sternotomy: clinical utility of blood culture results in the identification of postoperative mediastinitis. *Circulation* 2003;108:73–78.

153. Gardlund B, Bitkover CY, Vaage J. Postoperative mediastinitis in cardiac surgery—microbiology and pathogenesis. *Eur J Cardiothorac Surg* 2002;21:825–830.

154. Browdie DA, Bernstein RW, Agnew R, et al. Diagnosis of poststernotomy infection: comparison of three means of assessment. *Ann Thorac Surg* 1991;51:290–292.

155. DuPont HL, Varco RL, Winchell CP. Chronic fibrous mediastinitis simulating pulmonic stenosis, associated with inflammatory pseudotumor of the orbit. *Am J Med* 1968;44:447–452.

156. Loyd JE, Tillman BF, Atkinson JB, et al. Mediastinal fibrosis complicating histoplasmosis. *Medicine* 1988;67:295–310.

157. Kalweit G, Huwer H, Straub U, et al. Mediastinal compression syndromes due to idiopathic fibrosing mediastinitis—report of three cases and review of the literature. *Thorac Cardiovasc Surg* 1996;44:105–109.

158. Macklin MT, Macklin CC. Malignant interstitial emphysema of the lungs and mediastinum as an important occult complication in many respiratory diseases and other conditions: an interpretation of the clinical literature in the light of laboratory experiment. *Medicine* 1944;23:281–352.

159. Adrouny A, Magnusson P. Pneumopericardium from cocaine inhalation. *N Engl J Med* 1985;313:48–49.

160. Niura H, Taira O, Hiraguri S, et al. Clinical features of medical pneumomediastinum. *Ann Thorac Cardiovasc Surg* 2003;9:188–191.

161. Maunder RJ, Pierson DJ, Hudson LD. Subcutaneous and mediastinal emphysema. *Arch Intern Med* 1984;144:1447–1453.

162. Bergofsky EH, Turino GM, Fishman AP. Cardiorespiratory failure in kyphoscoliosis. *Medicine* 1959;38:263–317.

163. Fraser RS, Muller NL, Colman N, et al. Diseases of the diaphragm and chest wall. *Diagnosis of diseases of the chest*, 4th ed. Philadelphia: WB Saunders, 1999:2985–3042.

164. Kafer ER. Idiopathic scoliosis. Gas exchange and the age dependence of arterial blood gases. *J Clin Invest* 1976;58:825–833.

165. Lisboa C, Moreno R, Fava M, et al. Inspiratory muscle function in patients with severe kyphoscoliosis. *Am Rev Respir Dis* 1985; 132:48–52.

166. Kearon C, Viviani G, Kirkley A, et al. Factors determining pulmonary function in adolescent idiopathic thoracic scoliosis. *Am Rev Respir Dis* 1993;148:288–294.

167. Kearon C, Viviani GR, Killian KJ. Factors influencing work capacity in adolescent idiopathic thoracic scoliosis. *Am Rev Respir Dis* 1993;148:295–303.

168. Wong CA, Cole AA, Watson L, et al. Pulmonary function before and after anterior spinal surgery in adult idiopathic scoliosis. *Thorax* 1999;51:534–536.

169. Cooper D, Rojas J, Mellins R, et al. Respiratory mechanics in adolescents with idiopathic scoliosis. *Am Rev Respir Dis* 1984;130:16–22.

170. Buyse B, Meersseman W, Demedts M. Treatment of chronic respiratory failure in kyphoscoliosis: oxygen or ventilation? *Eur Respir J* 2003;22:525–528.

171. Gonzalez C, Ferris G, Diaz J, et al. Kyphoscoliotic ventilatory insufficiency: effects of long-term intermittent positive-pressure ventilation. *Chest* 2003;124:857–862.

172. Seckin U, Bolukbasi N, Gursel G, et al. Relationship between pulmonary function and exercise tolerance in patients with ankylosing spondylitis. *Clin Exp Rheumatol* 2000;18:503–506.

173. Fonkalsrud EW. Current management of pectus excavatum. *World J Surg* 2003;27:502–508.

174. Haller JA, Loughlin GM. Cardiorespiratory function is significantly improved following corrective surgery for severe pectus excavatum. Proposed treatment guidelines. *J Cardiovasc Surg (Torino)* 2000;41:125–130.

175. Fonkalsrud EW. Management of pectus chest deformities in female patients. *Am J Surg* 2004;187:192–197.

176. Sirmali M, Turut H, Topcu S, et al. A comprehensive analysis of traumatic rib fractures: morbidity, mortality and management. *Eur J Cardiothorac Surg* 2003;24:133–138.

177. Ahmed Z, Mohyuddin Z. Management of flail chest injury: internal fixation versus endotracheal intubation and ventilation. *J Thorac Cardiovasc Surg* 1995;110:1676–1680.

178. Tripp HF, Bolton JWR. Phrenic nerve injury following cardiac surgery: a review. *J Card Surg* 1998;13:218–223.

179. Gierada DS, Slone RM, Fleishman MJ. Imaging evaluation of the diaphragm. *Chest Surg Clin North Am* 1998;6:237–280.

180. Felson B. *Chest roentgenology*. Philadelphia: WB Saunders, 1973.

181. Gottesman E, McCool FD. Ultrasound evaluation of the paralyzed diaphragm. *Am J Respir Crit Care Med* 1997;155:1570–1574.

182. Lisboa C, Paré PD, Pertuze J, et al. Inspiratory muscle function in unilateral diaphragmatic paralysis. *Am Rev Respir Dis* 1986;134: 488–492.

183. Piehler JM, Pairolero PC, Gracey DR, et al. Unexplained diaphragmatic paralysis: a harbinger of malignant disease? *J Thorac Cardiovasc Surg* 1982;84:861–864.

184. Efthimious J, Butler J, Benson MK, et al. Bilateral diaphragm paralysis after cardiac surgery with topical hypothermia. *Thorax* 1991;46:351–354.

185. Simansky DA, Paley M, Refaely Y, et al. Diaphragm plication following phrenic nerve injury: a comparison of pediatric and adult patients. *Thorax* 2002;57:613–616.

186. Moxham J, Shneerson JM. Diaphragmatic pacing. *Am Rev Respir Dis* 1993;148:533–536.

187. Elefteriades JA, Quin JA, Hogan JF, et al. Long-term follow-up of pacing of the conditioned diaphragm in quadriplegia. *Pacing Clin Electrophysiol* 2002;25(6):897–906.

188. Engleman EG, Lankton J, Lankton B. Granulated sugar as treatment for hiccups in conscious patients. *N Engl J Med* 1971;285:1489.

189. Ramirez FC, Graham DY. Treatment of intractable hiccup with baclofen. Results of a double-blind randomized, controlled, cross-over study. *Am J Gastroenterol* 1992;87:1789–1791.

CHAPTER 18

Sleep-Related Breathing Disorders

Richard B. Berry

The topic of sleep disorders is much too broad to be covered in any detail in a single chapter. Therefore, the goal of this chapter is to present the elements of sleep physiology and monitoring that are relevant to sleep-related breathing disorders and to discuss these disorders with an emphasis on the sleep apnea syndromes. The other most common sleep disorders causing excessive daytime sleepiness (EDS) are also briefly mentioned.

SLEEP ARCHITECTURE

Sleep is not a homogeneous state and, therefore, has been divided into sleep stages. This is relevant for the study of

breathing during sleep because each stage has a characteristic impact on respiration. Furthermore, disease processes frequently alter not only the total sleep time (TST) but also the relative amount of time spent in the various sleep stages.

Sleep is composed of non–rapid eye movement (NREM) sleep and rapid eye movement (REM) sleep. NREM sleep is further divided into stages 1 to 4. Stages 1 and 2 are referred to as light sleep and stages 3 and 4 as deep or slow-wave sleep. A given night of sleep is divided into periods of time called *epochs* (usually 30 seconds in duration). The predominant stage in a given epoch names that epoch. Staging is based on electroencephalographic (EEG), electrooculographic (EOG), that is, eye movement, and electromyographic (EMG) criteria (1–5).

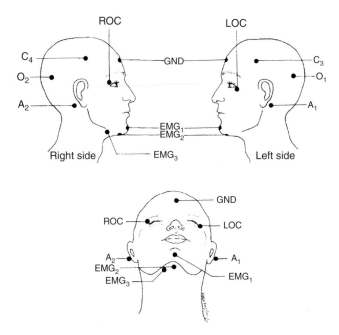

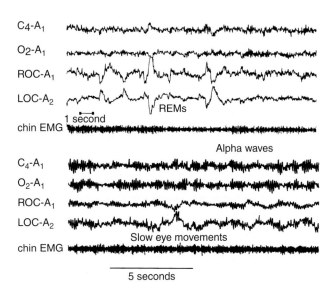

FIGURE 18-1. Electrode placement for electroencephalographic (EEG), electrooculographic (EOG), and electromyographic (EMG) leads. C_4 and C_3 are the central EEG electrodes, O_2 and O_1 are the occipital EEG electrodes, and A_2 and A_1 are the mastoid electrodes. Even indices refer to the right side of the body, whereas odd indices refer to the left side of the body. ROC and LOC are the right and left outer canthus electrodes. EMG_1, EMG_2, and EMG_3 are the electrodes used to record chin EMG. Only two of the electrodes are used at one time (EMG_1-EMG_2), and the other is reserved as a backup electrode.

FIGURE 18-2. **A:** Wakefulness (stage wake) with the eyes open is characterized by low-voltage, high-frequency electroencephalographic (EEG) activity, rapid eye movements (REMs), and relatively high electromyographic (EMG) activity. C_4-A_1 and O_2-A_1 are central and occipital EEG tracings, and ROC-A_1 and LOC-A_2 are right and left electrooculographic (EOG) tracings. **B:** Drowsy (eyes closed) wakefulness is illustrated. Prominent alpha activity is present throughout the EEG tracing, and slow eye movements are also seen.

Whereas only central EEG electrodes (C_3 and C_4) are required to stage sleep, occipital leads (O_1 and O_2) are also commonly used (see Fig. 18-1). The odd and even numbers refer to the left and right sides of the head, respectively. In sleep monitoring, the voltage difference between a central or occipital electrode and a mastoid electrode (usually on the opposite side) is recorded. The left and right mastoid electrodes are A_1 and A_2, respectively. The term *derivation* refers to the signal obtained from a pair of electrodes (e.g., C_4-A_1) amplified with a differential amplifier. In EEG and EOG monitoring the polarity of the differential amplifiers is set so that the tracing from a derivation A-B shows an upward deflection if electrode A is negative with respect to electrode B.

The EOG electrodes are positioned near the eyes. Because a potential difference exists across each eyeball (positive anterior and negative posterior), eye movements result in voltage changes that are detected in the EOG leads. Two EOG derivations are usually monitored on separate tracings (ROC-A_1 and LOC-A_2), where ROC and LOC are right and left outer canthus electrodes (Fig. 18-1). One of the eye electrodes is placed slightly above the eye and the other is placed below so that vertical as well as horizontal movement may be detected. As eye movements are conjugate, both eyes move toward one electrode and away from the other. This causes out-of-phase deflections (one up and one down) in the two eye channels. In contrast, when high-voltage EEG activity is detected in the eye channels, the deflections are in phase. Surface EMG leads, usually in the chin area, detect electric activity whose amplitude reflects the relative amount of muscle tone.

The awake EEG (see Fig. 18-2) is characterized by low-amplitude, high-frequency activity, and REMs may occur. With the onset of drowsiness, the EEG reveals alpha waves (8 to 13 Hz), which are associated with eye closure and are best detected by electrodes in the occipital area. Slow eye movements (slow rolling eye movements) may also be present in the EOG tracings. The stage 1 EEG (see Fig. 18-3) is characterized by low-voltage, mixed-frequency activity (3 to 7 Hz). Stage 1 is scored when less than 50% of an epoch contains alpha waves. Slow eye movements may also be present in stage 1 sleep. Stage 2 is characterized by the presence of either sleep spindles, which are bursts of 12- to 14-Hz activity, or K complexes, which are large-amplitude biphasic EEG deflections (Fig. 18-3). To qualify as stage 2, less than 20% of an epoch may contain slow (delta) wave activity. Slow (delta) waves are high-amplitude broad waves. Delta (slow-wave) EEG activity is usually defined as having a frequency less than 4 Hz. However, in human sleep staging, the criteria for scoring slow (delta) wave activity are a frequency of 2 Hz or less (more than 0.5 second duration) and a peak-to-peak amplitude more than 75 μV. An epoch is scored as stage 3 when it contains 20% to 50% slow-wave EEG activity and as stage 4 when it consists of more than 50% slow-wave activity (see Fig. 18-4). The chin EMG usually falls progressively on transition from wakefulness (stage wake) to stage 4, but this is somewhat variable and depends on the amplifier gain. Stage REM is defined by the presence of REMs, which are relatively sharp deflections in the EOG tracings; low-voltage, mixed-frequency EEG activity (which may contain sawtooth waves) but with no spindles or K complexes; and relatively reduced muscle tone (Fig. 18-4). "Relatively reduced" means that the EMG amplitude in REM is always equal to or lower than the lowest level recorded in NREM sleep. Note that a low-amplitude EEG

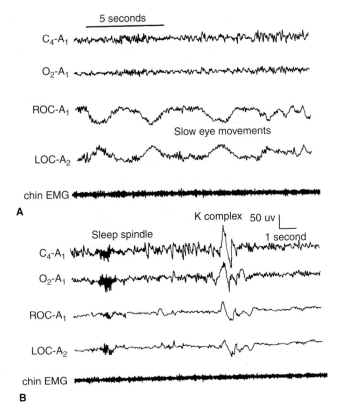

FIGURE 18-3. A: Stage 1 sleep is characterized by low-voltage, mixed-frequency electroencephalographic (EEG) activity. Alpha-wave activity is present in <50% of the EEG tracings. Slow eye movements are present in the right and left electrooculographic (EOG) tracings (ROC-A₁ and LOC-A₁). No sleep spindles or K complexes are present. **B:** Stage 2 sleep is characterized by the presence of either sleep spindles or K complexes. Note that the K-complex activity results in deflections in the EOG leads that are in phase.

pattern with EOG tracings showing REMs can occur with eyes-open wakefulness, but the muscle tone is higher in this case than in REM sleep. REMs may not occur during every epoch of REM sleep, but the EEG and chin EMG must meet criteria for REM sleep. More detailed discussions of the rules of sleep staging with examples are available (1–5).

There is a normal progression of sleep stages during the night (1–3), with sleep cycles composed of NREM followed by REM sleep. Periods of wakefulness may also be present during the night. Usually, two to four cycles of stages 1 → 2 → 3 → 4 → 3 → 2 → REM of 70 to 120 minutes duration are present in the first portion of the night. The NREM cycles in the remainder of the night mainly contain stages 1 and 2. Thus, most of the stage 3 to 4 sleep occurs in the early part of the night. In contrast, episodes of REM sleep increase in duration in the later parts of the night, as does the REM density (the number of REMs per unit time).

TST is the total minutes of REM and NREM sleep. *Sleep period time* (SPT) equals TST plus any stage wake that occurs after sleep onset but before the final awakening [wake after sleep onset (WASO)]. The *sleep latency* is the time from lights-out (beginning of monitoring) to the onset of sleep. A sleep latency of more than 30 minutes is typical of patients complaining of difficulty falling asleep (insomnia). The *REM latency* is defined as the time from sleep onset until the first epoch of stage REM. A normal REM latency is around 90 minutes (70 to 120 minutes). *Sleep onset rapid eye movement (SOREM)* refers to the appearance of REM sleep within 20 minutes of sleep onset. The time in bed (TIB) is the time from lights-out to lights-on. *Sleep efficiency* is defined as TST divided by TIB. It is customary to express the time spent in each stage (including the stage wake present during the SPT) as a percentage of SPT. A young adult typically spends less than 5% of SPT in stage wake, 5% to 10% in stage 1, 50% in stage 2, 20% to 30% in stages 3 and 4, and

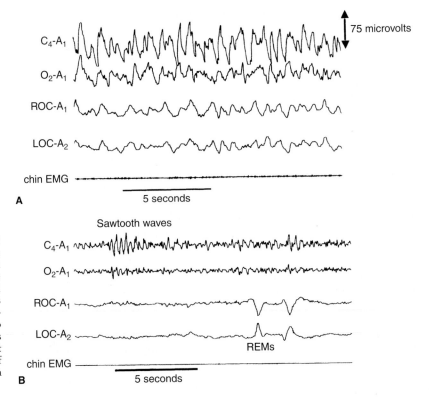

FIGURE 18-4. A: Stage 4 sleep. More than 50% of the electroencephalographic (EEG) tracings contain high-voltage, slow-wave activity that is also present in the electrooculographic (EOG) tracings. Note that the electromyographic (EMG) activity has also decreased in this example. **B:** Stage rapid eye movement (REM) is characterized by low-voltage, mixed-frequency activity that may contain bursts of sawtooth waves. No sleep spindles or K complexes are present. The REMs result in out-of-phase deflections in the right and left EOG leads (ROC-A₁ and LOC-A₂). The EMG level of activity is relatively reduced [at or below the lowest in non–rapid eye movement (NREM) sleep].

20% to 25% in stage REM. A normal 60-year-old person has a greater percentage of stage wake and stage 1 sleep and a reduced percentage of stage 3 and 4 sleep (<10%), but about the same percentage of stage REM (2).

An arousal is usually defined as an abrupt shift to a lighter stage of sleep or to an awakening that may be brief or may result in prolonged wakefulness. A task force of the American Sleep Disorders Association [now the American Academy of Sleep Medicine (AASM)] proposed a set of rules for scoring arousals that have been widely accepted (6). An arousal is characterized by an abrupt shift in EEG frequency that may include theta (4 to 8 Hz), alpha (8 to 13 Hz), and/or frequencies >16 Hz (but not spindles) lasting 3 seconds or longer. In NREM sleep, an arousal can be scored without an increase in EMG amplitude. However, in REM sleep, an increase in EMG amplitude and an EEG frequency shift are required. The rationale for this rule is that bursts of alpha waves are common in REM sleep. This definition of arousal is somewhat restrictive, and the task force recognized that some EEG changes not meeting these criteria likely represent events of physiologic significance. When sleep is filled with many brief arousals, it is not restorative. Thus, daytime sleepiness can occur even if the TST (as scored by standard criteria) is not markedly shortened (7). Sleep interrupted by frequent arousals and stage shifts is said to be fragmented. One can define the *arousal index* as the number of arousals divided by the TST in hours. The upper limit of normal for the arousal index is not well defined. In one study, the mean arousal index was 21 arousals per hour, and the 95% confidence limits were very large because of a high arousal frequency in older individuals (8). However, a respiratory arousal index >10 per hour (arousals per hour associated with respiratory events) can be associated with daytime sleepiness (9).

VENTILATION AND SLEEP

There is reduction in respiratory drive during NREM sleep because of loss of the stimulatory effect of wakefulness ("the wakefulness stimulus") and owing to decreases in chemosensitivity (10–12). There is a decrease in the ventilatory responses to hypoxia and hypercapnia. In most studies, a further decrease in the ventilatory responses has been present in stage REM. Stages 1 and 2 are often characterized by a periodic waxing and waning of tidal volume and respiratory rate. This is thought to be due to transition between the awake set point for partial pressure of carbon dioxide (PCO_2) and the sleep set point for the same, which is somewhat higher (10–13). Stages 3 and 4 are characterized by a regular pattern of tidal volume and respiratory rate. Compared to awake values, ventilation is reduced by 1 to 2 L per minute, PCO_2 is increased by 2 to 8 mm Hg, and partial pressure of oxygen (PO_2) is decreased by 5 to 10 mm Hg during sleep. Whereas animal studies have consistently shown a fall in tidal volume and an increase in respiratory rate during NREM sleep, studies in humans are less consistent. Most studies have shown a reduction in minute ventilation associated with a decrease in tidal volume and either a decrease in respiratory rate or an increase not large enough to compensate for the fall in tidal volume (11–13). Upper-airway resistance increases during NREM sleep, and this acts as a resistive load on the ventilatory system (14). Functional residual capacity decreases during NREM sleep compared to wakefulness (15).

Ventilation during REM sleep is characterized by an irregular pattern of varying tidal volume and respiratory rate; short periods of central apnea may be seen. Skeletal muscle activity (e.g., intercostal muscles) is generally inhibited during all portions of REM sleep, and inspiration is dependent on persistent diaphragmatic activity. REM sleep is often characterized by a decrease in respiratory rib cage movement (16). Those portions of REM sleep containing bursts of REMs are referred to as phasic REMs (as opposed to tonic REMs). During phasic REM, ventilation is irregular, with increases and decreases in tidal volume (17–19). Episodic decrements in inspiratory diaphragmatic and upper-airway muscle activity often occur during bursts of REMs and result in transient reductions in ventilation (17–19). As REM episodes are longer and as the REM density is higher during the early morning hours, these REM periods are usually associated with the largest reductions in ventilation. The reduction in intercostal muscle activity during REM sleep is especially important in patients with diaphragmatic weakness or with a mechanical disadvantage due to hyperinflation [chronic obstructive pulmonary disease (COPD) or asthma]. Indeed, stage REM is usually the stage of sleep associated with the most severe hypoventilation and oxygen desaturation in patients with sleep-related respiratory disorders. For the reasons mentioned above, the early morning REM episodes are usually associated with the most severe arterial oxygen desaturation.

THE UPPER AIRWAY AND SLEEP

During awake breathing, upper-airway muscle activity maintains upper-airway patency despite negative intraluminal pressure and positive extraluminal pressure (e.g., the effects of gravity on the tissue surrounding the airway) (20–21). Upper-airway muscle activity is augmented by chemical stimuli (hypoxia and hypercapnia), mechanoreceptor stimuli (negative upper-airway pressure), and brainstem activation associated with wakefulness (the "wakefulness stimulus"). Negative intraluminal pressure augments the activity of upper-airway muscles via a brainstem reflex when mucosal receptors in the upper airway are stimulated by negative pressure (22). Upper-airway muscles exhibit resting tone, referred to as tonic activity, and some muscles also exhibit inspiratory increases in activity, referred to as phasic activity. For example, the genioglossus (tongue protruder) usually displays prominent phasic (inspiratory) activity, whereas the tensor palatini (a palate muscle) does not (23).

With sleep onset, the wakefulness stimulus is lost and the negative pressure reflex is diminished (23,24). Thus, within one or two breaths after sleep onset, upper-airway muscle activity generally decreases (25) and upper-airway resistance increases, even in normal subjects (15). With sustained sleep, the activity of the genioglossus may return to waking levels, but the activity of the palate muscles often remains below that during wakefulness (25). Of note, recent studies suggest that during sleep the activity of the genioglossus appears to be determined primarily by negative pressure stimuli rather than by increases in PCO_2 or hypoxemia (26–28). The major site of upper-airway narrowing in normal subjects appears to be in the retropalatal area (29).

The patency of the upper airway depends on extraluminal tissue or gravitation factors (i.e., the supine posture predisposes to narrowing), anatomic factors (i.e., airway size and shape), the

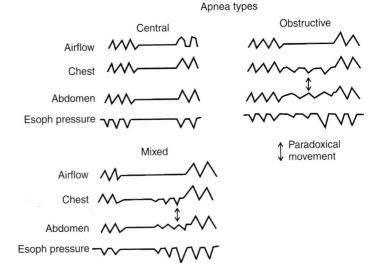

FIGURE 18-5. Schematic illustrations of apnea types (obstructive, central, and mixed). In the mixed apnea, *C* is the central portion. Esoph press is esophageal pressure. Paradoxical movement of chest and abdominal tracings may be seen in obstructive events. (From Berry RB. *Sleep Medicine Pearls.* Philadelphia: Hanley & Belfus, 2003, with permission.)

amount of negative intraluminal pressure, and the amount of upper-airway muscle activity. An additional important factor is tracheal traction, which describes the downward pull on upper-airway structures during inspiratory chest-wall expansion and the resulting passive dilation of the upper airway (30).

The upper airway size depends on lung volume, with its largest size being at total lung capacity and the smallest size being at residual volume (31). During inspiration, the phasic activation of upper-airway muscles and the effects of tracheal traction help maintain upper-airway patency despite negative intraluminal pressure. In fact, upper-airway size is actually the smallest at end expiration when muscle activity and tracheal traction are minimal (32).

One might expect that upper-airway resistance might be higher in REM than in NREM sleep because of skeletal muscle hypotonia, but the mean upper-airway resistances are similar in normal subjects (15). Although tonic activity in the upper-airway muscles is very low during all REM sleep, phasic inspiratory activity of some muscles such as the genioglossus is still present during tonic REM. However, during bursts of eye movements (phasic REM), the inspiratory activity of the genioglossus falls dramatically in parallel with the activity of the diaphragm (19).

RESPIRATORY DEFINITIONS

An apnea is defined as the cessation of airflow in the nose and mouth for 10 seconds or longer (33). Obstructive apnea (see Fig. 18-5) is present when there is continued respiratory effort (evidence of central respiratory drive such as chest and abdominal movement) during the absence of airflow. Obstructive apnea is caused by upper-airway closure during sleep. Central apneas are characterized by absence of both airflow and respiratory effort. Mixed apneas are those in which the initial portion of the apnea is central (no respiratory effort) and the remaining portion is obstructive (respiratory effort present). Arterial oxygen desaturation is usually defined as a fall in arterial oxygen saturation (SaO_2) of 4% or more from baseline. It is important to remember that the change in PO_2 associated with a 4% change in saturation depends critically on the initial PO_2 value (position on the oxyhemoglobin saturation curve). The above definitions are arbitrary but are widely used (4,33).

Periods of reduced tidal volume or airflow may also be associated with desaturations or sleep disturbance (33–34). These events are called *hypopneas* (see Fig. 18-6). Patients having primarily hypopneas have the same manifestations as those with obstructive apneas (34). In fact, some prefer the term

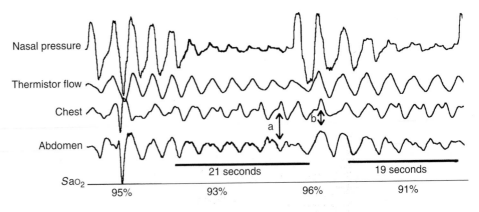

FIGURE 18-6. Two obstructive hypopneas of 21- and 19-second duration are shown. The nasal pressure signal shows a reduction in magnitude and flattening. The chest and abdominal signals show paradoxical motion *(a)* during the event but not after event termination *(b)*. An arterial oxygen desaturation follows the first event to 91%. Note that although the thermistor flow signal is also diminished during the event, the change is less obvious than the change in the nasal pressure signal.

obstructive sleep apnea hypopnea syndrome (OSAHS). Definitions of hypopnea vary among clinicians (4,33–40) and are a source of controversy (36). A task force of the AASM defined a hypopnea as either (a) a 50% or greater reduction in airflow lasting 10 seconds or longer or (b) any appreciable reduction in airflow for 10 seconds or longer that is associated with either a 3% or greater drop in the SaO_2 or an arousal (37). A respiratory effort–related arousal (RERA) is defined as an event lasting 10 seconds or longer associated with an esophageal pressure that is progressively negative (increased inspiratory effort) and that is terminated by an arousal but that would not qualify as a hypopnea (see Fig. 18-7). This definition acknowledges that respiratory events associated with increased respiratory effort can cause arousal even in the absence of a significant fall in airflow or a drop in the SaO_2. Subsequently, the Clinical Practice Committee of the AASM recommended a hypopnea definition requiring a 30% or greater reduction in airflow for 10 seconds or longer associated with a 4% or greater drop in the SaO_2 (38). Arousals are not considered in this definition. The logic behind this more restrictive definition is that the scoring of hypopnea on the basis of airflow and desaturation has good intra- and interscoring reliability, whereas the scoring of arousals does not (39,40). In addition, using this definition of hypopnea, the Sleep Heart Health Study was able to show that even mild elevations of the apnea-plus-hypopnea index (AHI) (more than 5 per hour) are associated with an increased risk of cardiovascular disease (41).

Hypopneas could be due to a fall in central drive without a change in upper-airway resistance (central hypopneas), upper-airway narrowing with increased upper airway resistance (obstructive hypopneas), or a combination of these factors (mixed hypopnea) (42). However, such a separation is not always possible from routine measurements, and most sleep centers simply report the total number of hypopneas. Obstructive hypopneas are often associated with paradoxical movements of the chest and abdomen, although in some patients, only subtler changes in phase between chest and abdominal movements can be detected. If airflow is detected with a pneumotachograph or by measuring nasal pressure, the airflow profile shows flattening consistent with airflow limitation (constant airflow with increasing driving pressure) (42,43). Esophageal pressure monitoring will usually shows progressively more negative deflections during the hypopnea. More details about esophageal and nasal pressure monitoring are given in the next section.

One can also define a RERA based on flow limitation as an event with a flattened airflow profile (pneumotachograph or nasal pressure) for 10 seconds or longer terminated by an arousal and an abrupt restoration of a rounded airflow shape. Of note, airflow limitation or flattening (increased upper-airway resistance) can occur without an increase in inspiratory effort (esophageal pressure) and vice versa. However, generally, the presence of airflow flattening (limitation) means that increased respiratory effort is present (42,43). One study suggested that the RERA index based on esophageal pressure monitoring and the one based on nasal pressure monitoring (flow limitation preceding arousal) are similar (44). As esophageal pressure is rarely used clinically; sleep centers reporting RERAs usually define them on the basis of nasal pressure monitoring. From the above discussion, one can see that an event with reduced airflow and airflow limitation followed by an arousal without an associated 4% or greater desaturation could be either a hypopnea or a RERA depending on the definition of hypopnea that is used.

The apnea and hypopnea index (AHI) is the number of apneas and hypopneas per hour of sleep (total number/TST in hours). The term respiratory disturbance index (RDI) in some sleep centers is synonymous with the AHI. In others, RDI is the sum of the AHI and the RERA index (number of RERAs per hour of sleep) (45). This is especially useful if hypopneas are required to have a 4% or greater desaturation.

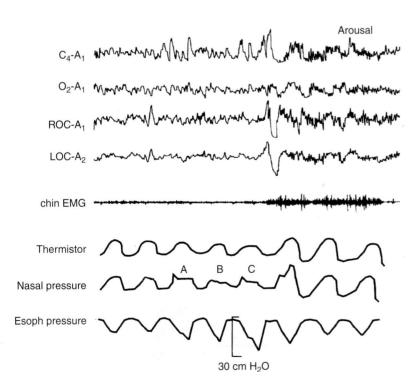

FIGURE 18-7. An example of a respiratory-effort–related arousal (RERA) in the upper-airway resistance syndrome is shown here. Note that airflow by nasal pressure shows a flattened profile prior to arousal (*A,B,* and *C*), whereas the thermocouple shows only a subtle decrease in amplitude. This event was not associated with an arterial oxygen desaturation. A crescendo increase in respiratory effort (esophageal pressure) precedes arousal. Note that this event might also be considered an obstructive hypopnea using some definitions of hypopnea [if a 4% or greater drop in the arterial oxygen saturation (SaO_2) was not required]. (From Berry RB. *Sleep Medicine Pearls.* Philadelphia: Hanley & Belfus, 2003, with permission.)

SLEEP MONITORING

POLYSOMNOGRAPHY

The detailed monitoring of sleep is called *polysomnography*. All of the electrodes illustrated in Figure 18-1 are usually put in place, although sleep staging requires only a single central EEG derivation (C_4-A_1) as well as eye movement and chin EMG tracings. Redundant electrodes are used in case of electrode failure. In modern digital sleep recording systems, a combination of AC referential, AC bipolar, and DC recording is typically utilized. EEG (C_4, C_3, O_2, O_1, A_1, and A_2), EOG (ROC and LOC), and EMG (chin EMG_1, chin EMG_2, and chin EMG_3) electrodes are usually recorded against a common reference (referential) electrode. Any combination may be displayed using electronic subtraction (C_4-ref) − (A_1-ref) = C_4-A_1. This allows multiple displays or a change in referencing during review. For example, a tracing showing C_4-A_1 can be changed to C_4-A_2 if the electrode A_1 goes bad during the night and is not replaced. A minimal display view might include all the following (C_4-A_1, C_3-A_2, O_2-A_1, O_1-A_2, ROC-A_1, LOC-A_2, or EMG_1-EMG_2). This montage uses a common mastoid electrode (A_1) as the reference. Others prefer a more extensive display using all EEG electrodes (C_4-A_1, O_2-A_1, ROC-A_1, LOC-A_1, and EMG_1-EMG_2). An alternate method used the contralateral mastoid as the reference for both EOG electrodes (ROC-A_1 or LOC-A_2). An ECG lead is also monitored to detect changes in cardiac rhythm. (For more information on the technical aspects of recording EEG and EOG, the reader is referred to references 1–5.)

In the past, airflow during sleep has been detected qualitatively using thermal-sensitive devices (thermistors or thermocouples) in the nose and mouth (4). Airflow across these devices changes their temperature and, hence, their resistance (thermistor) or voltage output (thermocouple). Unfortunately, these devices do not accurately reflect changes in either the magnitude or the time profile (shape) of airflow. Accurate measurements of airflow are possible with a pneumotachograph inserted into a face mask. Airflow is determined by measuring the pressure drop across this device (a fixed linear resistance). A more comfortable alternative that is gaining popularity is to measure nasal pressure using a small nasal cannula connected to a sensitive pressure transducer (42–44,46). This measures the pressure drop across the resistance of the nasal inlet. The nasal pressure = constant × (flow)^2 (43,47). Change in the size of the nasal pressure signal is more sensitive than change in the signal size of thermal devices for detecting a drop in airflow; the change in shape (flattening) reflects airflow limitation (narrowing of the airway) (46). Nasal pressure monitoring may not work well in patients with mainly mouth breathing. Therefore, many sleep centers use a combination of a nasal–oral thermal device and nasal pressure monitoring.

Respiratory effort is commonly monitored by devices that detect chest and abdominal movement. Such devices include impedance plethysmography, strain gauges, piezoelectric sensors, or respiratory inductance plethysmography (RIP) (48,49). In RIP, the sum of signals from rib cage and abdominal bands can be calibrated to estimate tidal volume (48,49). In some obese individuals, respiratory effort during obstructive apnea does not result in easily discernible motion of the chest wall or abdomen. A more sensitive method for detecting respiratory effort employs measurement of esophageal pressure changes, which reflect changes in pleural pressure because of

inspiratory muscle contraction (42,48). This method is not routinely used, although a small percentage of apneas can be misclassified as being central on the basis of surface measurements of respiratory effort. Recently, many laboratories have been using small, fluid-filled catheters connected to a pressure transducer to detect esophageal pressure changes, rather than the more uncomfortable esophageal balloons.

Sa_{O_2} is continuously measured by pulse oximetry using ear or finger probes. One should note that the nadir of a desaturation associated with a respiratory event usually occurs after the event has ended. The delay is due to the circulation time to the sensing device as well as due to instrumental delay. The averaging time used should not be excessive or else short arterial oxygen desaturations may not be detected. Leg movements (LMs) are detected by monitoring leg electromyograms using surface electrodes placed over both the anterior tibialis muscles (leg EMGs) (50). Periodic LMs during sleep can cause sleep disturbance and can result in symptoms.

All of the parameters described above are traditionally recorded on a polygraph, which usually runs at a paper speed of 10 mm per second. Today, most clinical sleep laboratories record directly on computer-based systems. This allows digital archiving of studies, thereby solving the costly problem of storing bulky paper sleep recordings. Although sleep staging may be somewhat more difficult on a monitor screen compared to paper, tracings can be viewed using multiple timescales (virtual paper speeds), which facilitate identification of longer events or trends. Sleep is usually staged in a 30-second window (equivalent to a paper speed of 10 mm per second), but respiratory events are often viewed on 60- to 120-second windows. Traditional EEG monitoring uses a 30-mm per second paper speed or a 10-second window.

MULTIPLE SLEEP LATENCY TEST

In addition to nocturnal polysomnography, daytime tests are used to document the degree of daytime sleepiness and to detect SOREM episodes (51,52). The multiple sleep latency test (MSLT) consists of four or five short naps, usually spaced across the day in 2-hour intervals (for example, 8:00 AM, 10:00 AM, noon, 2:00 PM, and 4:00 PM). Patients are given 20 minutes to fall asleep. If sleep occurs within the 20 minutes, patients are monitored for another 15 minutes to detect the early onset of REM sleep. The subject then gets out of bed until the next nap. The sleep latency (time from lights-out to initial sleep) and the presence or absence of REM sleep are determined. The standard MSLT criteria are shown in Table 18-1. It is important

TABLE 18-1.   Multiple Sleep Latency Criteria

Mean Sleep Latency (min)	Severity of Sleepiness	Number of REM Periods in 5 Naps
<5	Severe	0–1 Normal
5 to <10	Moderate	2 or more Abnormal*
10–15	Mild (some normal subjects)	
>15	Normal	

*Causes include Narcolepsy, Obstructive Sleep Apnea (OSA), prior REM deprivation, withdrawal of REM suppressant medications, psychiatric diseases

REM, rapid eye movement.

not to confuse the significance of a short *nocturnal* sleep latency (which is normal) with a short mean daytime sleep latency. For correct interpretation, the MSLT should always follow an all-night polysomnogram. A sleep diary documenting the pattern of sleep for 1 or 2 weeks before the test may also be useful. A modest self-imposed reduction in nocturnal sleep from 8 to 6 hours can shorten the mean daytime sleep latency into the abnormal range (under 10 minutes) (53). Medications that affect sleep (especially REM sleep) such as stimulants, sedatives (ethanol), and antidepressants that increase the REM latency should be withdrawn for 2 weeks before testing.

Sleep apnea can result in two or more SOREM periods (54). If significant sleep apnea is present during the sleep study preceding the planned MSLT, the latter test should be delayed until after the sleep apnea is adequately treated. This recommendation assumes that the primary goal of the MSLT is to diagnose narcolepsy and not to simply quantify the severity of daytime sleepiness. The MSLT is probably the most incorrectly used test in sleep medicine because of the many factors that can alter the results and lead to erroneous conclusions.

MAINTENANCE OF WAKEFULNESS TEST

In the *maintenance of wakefulness test* (MWT), subjects are requested to stay awake in a dark, quiet room during multiple 20- or 40-minute periods in a semirecumbent state and are monitored for sleep (55,56). Certain patients will have a short sleep latency on the MSLT but are able to stay awake for 20 or 40 minutes during the MWT. Whereas the MSLT is considered the standard test for assessing daytime sleepiness, the MWT may be more sensitive for demonstrating an effect of treatment or for evaluating a given patient's ability to perform the tasks of daily living. If the sleep latency on a 20-minute MWT is less than 11 minutes or is less than 19 minutes on the 40-minute MWT, the test result is considered abnormal (55).

SLEEP DISORDERS CAUSING EXCESSIVE DAYTIME SLEEPINESS

Although the sleep apnea syndromes are the most common cause of EDS, pulmonary physicians must be familiar with the other causes of this complaint (see Table 18-2) (57). A recent survey of 19 regional sleep disorders centers found that the top three reported diagnoses were obstructive sleep apnea (OSA) (67.8%), narcolepsy (4.9%), and restless legs syndrome (RLS) (3.2%) (58). One should not assume that every sleepy, snoring patient has sleep apnea. In addition, patients with sleep apnea can also have other sleep disorders. Therefore, the evaluation of every sleepy patient should include questions relevant to narcolepsy, RLS, insufficient sleep syndrome, and depression. A careful history of medications and the use of ethanol, stimulants (including caffeine), and sedatives must be obtained. Recording of the patient's usual amount and pattern of sleep may also be instructive. Most sleep centers use a sleep log (diary) that the patient completes before coming for evaluation. The Epworth sleepiness scale (ESS) is commonly used to quantify subjective propensity to fall asleep in eight familiar situations (59). The patient chooses an answer based on the likelihood of falling asleep in each situation (0—never, 1—rarely, 2—sometimes, and 3—often). The score ranges from 0 to 24 (most sleepy) (59). A score of 10 or

TABLE 18-2. Conditions Presenting with Excessive Daytime Sleepiness (EDS)

Sleep apnea syndromes (including upper airway resistance syndrome)
Narcolepsy
Idiopathic hypersomnia
Insufficient sleep syndrome
Restless legs syndrome or periodic limb movements in sleep
Posttraumatic hypersomnia
Psychiatric disorders (depression)
Drug and alcohol dependency
Circadian disorders (jet lag or shift work)

less is usually considered normal. Severe sleepiness is usually associated with scores of 16 or higher. A brief discussion of narcolepsy, periodic limb movements in sleep or RLS, idiopathic hypersomnia (IH), and insufficient sleep syndrome precedes a discussion of sleep apnea.

NARCOLEPSY

Narcolepsy (60,61) is a syndrome associated with the tetrad of sleep attacks, cataplexy, hypnagogic hallucinations, and sleep paralysis. Cataplexy refers to the sudden loss of muscle tone or strength following a period of high emotion such as surprise, laughter, or anger. The cataplectic attacks may vary from subtle weakness of an isolated muscle group (loss of facial or neck muscle tone) to sudden paralysis of all skeletal muscles and postural collapse. The affected patient maintains consciousness at least at the start of the event. Some episodes of cataplexy are associated with hallucinations and the onset of sleep. Cataplexy rarely lasts more than a few minutes. Sleep paralysis is the partial or complete inability to move at sleep onset or on awakening that lasts from a few seconds to 20 minutes. Fortunately, respiration is usually not affected, although some patients complain of dyspnea during the paralysis episodes. The hallucinations of narcolepsy are vivid dreamlike visual images or auditory sensations that occur at sleep onset (hypnagogic) or on awakening (hypnopompic). All four components of the narcolepsy tetrad are present in only 11% to 25% of cases. Of note, sleep paralysis, hypnagogic hallucinations, and cataplexy at inappropriate times can be viewed as abnormal manifestations of REM sleep (muscle hypotonia and dreaming). Unfortunately, sleep attacks, sleep paralysis, and hypnagogic hallucinations can occur in other sleep disorders. Cataplexy is the only symptom virtually specific to narcolepsy. Cataplexy without narcolepsy can occur in a few rare disorders associated with mental retardation. Only when both daytime sleepiness and unequivocal cataplexy are present can a *clinical* diagnosis of narcolepsy be made with confidence. Unfortunately, the sleep attacks may be present for many years before cataplexy. In addition, cataplexy is often subtle and difficult to document. About 60% to 70% of patients with narcolepsy develop cataplexy. Narcolepsy without cataplexy can be diagnosed using the MSLT to demonstrate SOREM. However, the MSLT can be interpreted correctly only with the results of the preceding nocturnal polysomnogram and with the clinical history in mind. The majority of patients with narcolepsy have the onset of symptoms during the teenage years and early adulthood.

However, narcolepsy can begin at any age, although it is rarely noted in children less than 5 years.

Narcolepsy occurs in about 4 of 10,000 people. The etiology of human narcolepsy with cataplexy appears to be the loss of cells in the lateral hypothalamus that secrete the neuropeptides hypocretin 1 and 2 (62). Hypocretins enhance the activity of several brain centers maintaining wakefulness. This action is believed to prevent inappropriate transitions from wake to sleep and from wake to REM sleep (63). The cause of the loss of hypocretin cells is unclear, but it could be an autoimmune phenomenon. About 90% of all patients with narcolepsy and cataplexy have no hypocretin in the cerebrospinal fluid (CSF) (64) and are positive for the human leukocyte antigen (HLA) DQB1*0602 (65,66). Unfortunately, 25% to 36% of persons in the general population are positive for this antigen. There appears to be a genetic predisposition for the development of narcolepsy, and familial narcolepsy has been described (67). However, developmental or environmental factors are also important. For example, if one patient in a pair of identical twins has narcolepsy with cataplexy, the other twin will have the disorder only about 40% of the time (67). Patients with *narcolepsy without cataplexy* have normal CSF levels of hypocretin, and only 40% to 60% are positive for DQB1*0602. More subtle abnormalities of the hypocretin system could be the cause of disease in these patients. However, this remains to be documented.

The polysomnographic hallmark of narcolepsy is a short REM latency. Whereas the normal REM latency is about 90 minutes, patients with narcolepsy often have a REM latency of less than 20 minutes. However, only around 40% to 50% of patients with narcolepsy will have a short *nocturnal* REM latency on any given sleep study. The MSLT is very useful for supporting the diagnosis of narcolepsy because it allows for more opportunities to detect SOREM as well as to document daytime sleepiness. The standard criteria are a mean sleep latency of less than 5 minutes (some recommend using 8 minutes for improved sensitivity) and two or more REM onsets in five nap opportunities (51,52,61). Of patients with known narcolepsy–cataplexy, only about 70% to 80% will meet these diagnostic criteria on a given MSLT (52). Hence, a negative MSLT does not rule out narcolepsy. In such cases, a firm diagnosis of narcolepsy would require that unequivocal cataplexy be present or that a repeat MSLT meets diagnostic criteria for narcolepsy. The MSLT should follow a night of polysomnography to document that the SOREM is not due to preceding REM deprivation (and to rule out other sleep pathologies). SOREM may also be seen in some patients with sleep apnea (which can reduce the amount of REM sleep) (51,54), depression, schizophrenia, and following withdrawal of REM-suppressing medications. If sleep apnea is found on nocturnal polysomnography, the MSLT should be delayed until after the patient has been adequately treated for this problem for several weeks. About 4% of untreated OSA patients will have an MSLT meeting narcolepsy criteria (54). If narcolepsy as well as OSA is suspected, the MSLT is delayed until the OSA is adequately treated. For example, after treatment of OSA with nasal continuous positive airway pressure (CPAP), a repeat sleep study is ordered with the patient sleeping on CPAP (this documents treatment efficacy). An MSLT is then performed with the patient on CPAP. If the results of the MSLT meet the criteria for narcolepsy, a diagnosis of the combination of narcolepsy and OSA would be supported.

The treatment of EDS in narcolepsy usually includes the use of stimulants such as methylphenidate (Ritalin) or dextroamphetamine (68). Methylphenidate is started at a dose of 15 to 20 mg per day, divided into three or four doses (total daily dose of 20 to 100 mg daily). The drug is most effective if given before sleep attacks characteristically occur. Once a sleep attack is in progress, the best treatment is a short nap. Recently, sustained-action forms of methylphenidate are gaining popularity (60). One approach is to use a long-acting form in the morning supplemented with an additional dose of short-acting medication in the afternoon. Modafinil, a new nonstimulant (alerting) medication, is the only Food and Drug Authority (FDA) approved drug for the treatment of sleepiness in narcolepsy (67). Modafinil is used in a once-daily dose of 200 to 400 mg. Although never directly compared to stimulants, modafinil is believed to have fewer side effects. A slow dose escalation will decrease the incidence of headache, the most common side effect. Unlike stimulants, modafinil is not a schedule II medication, has minimal abuse potential, and does not disturb sleep. It may be less effective than methylphenidate (69) but because of its other advantages is generally the drug of choice. Some patients require both modafinil and a smaller dose of stimulants.

The attacks of cataplexy are effectively suppressed by tricyclic antidepressants in doses less than those used for depression or by selective serotonin reuptake inhibitors in the usual antidepressant doses. Protriptyline (Vivactil) (15 to 30 mg per day in three divided doses) and imipramine (Tofranil) (75 mg per day) are the most commonly used agents. Selective serotonin reuptake inhibitors (e.g., fluoxetine) in antidepressant doses are also effective (fluoxetine 20 mg per day).

Venlafaxine, a blocker of both serotonin and norepinephrine reuptake, has also been effective in treating cataplexy. However, none of these medications is FDA approved for cataplexy treatment.

Recently, γ-hydroxybutyrate (GHB), also known as sodium oxybate (Xyrem), was approved by the FDA for treatment of cataplexy (70). The medicine has a short half-life and must be given at bedtime and repeated 2.5 to 4 hours later. The drug has been abused (the date-rape drug) and can be fatal in overdose. A single central pharmacy dispenses the medication. The drug is effective in preventing cataplexy, and by consolidating sleep, sodium oxybate may also improve daytime sleepiness. Sodium oxybate may be especially useful in patients whose cataplexy is not controlled by antidepressants or in those who do not tolerate their side effects.

IDIOPATHIC HYPERSOMNIA

IH is essentially a diagnosis of exclusion (71–74). It is characterized by daytime somnolence without cataplexy or sufficient SOREM periods to meet the diagnostic criteria for narcolepsy (71). Unlike narcolepsy, the daytime naps are typically not refreshing, and the night sleep period can be unusually long in some patients. Hypnagogic hallucinations or sleep paralysis may occur. These patients do not have reduced CSF levels of hypocretin (64). Polysomnography reveals no explanation for daytime sleepiness. The MSLT shows a short sleep latency (less than 10 minutes) but less than two SOREM periods. A sleep diary of 2 weeks before the MSLT should rule out insufficient sleep as an explanation for the short sleep latency.

Some patients previously given this diagnosis actually had upper-airway resistance syndrome (UARS) or mild OSA, which is discussed below. Sleepiness secondary to medical disease, chronic pain syndromes, and medication side effects should be ruled out. In the past, treatment with CNS stimulants was said to be less satisfactory in IH than in narcolepsy. In more recent studies, up to 75% of patients improved with stimulants or modafinil (72,73).

INSUFFICIENT SLEEP SYNDROME

Surprisingly, some patients have EDS simply due to an inadequate sleep period that is often self-enforced for societal reasons. The sleep need is genetic and cannot be shortened without impairment in daytime functioning. These patients typically sleep longer on weekends and report less daytime sleepiness (75). A sleep diary (sleep history) is essential in making this diagnosis. In addition, insufficient sleep will aggravate symptoms in other disorders such as narcolepsy.

PERIODIC LIMB MOVEMENT DISORDER AND RESTLESS LEGS SYNDROME

Periodic limb movements of sleep (PLMS), also known as periodic LMs of sleep, is a *finding on polysomnography* consisting of stereotypic periodic leg (or arm) movements during sleep that may or may not be associated with arousals (50). The LMs usually consist of dorsiflexion of the foot at the ankle, extension of the big toe, and partial flexion of the knee and hip. Patients with PLMS may or may not remember the awakenings during the night but almost never remember the LMs. Detection of PLMS requires monitoring of leg EMGs. LMs may occur in one or both legs, and therefore, monitoring of both legs is suggested (they can be monitored using a single tracing: right leg EMG-left leg EMG). Guidelines for monitoring and scoring LMs have been published (50). To be scored as a periodic leg movement (PLM) (or part of a PLM sequence), an LM must occur during sleep, must not follow an arousal due to other events, and must occur in a group of four or more LMs separated by more than 5 seconds and less than 90 seconds (event onset to onset). The number of these events per hour of sleep (PLM index) and the number of instances of sleep followed by an arousal per hour (PLM-arousal index) are used to diagnose PLMS. A PLM index ≥5 is considered abnormal; 5 to 24 is mild; 25 to 49 is moderate; and 50 or more is considered severe (76). The true impact of this disorder is probably more accurately assessed by looking at the PLM-arousal index. If enough arousals occur, sleep may be so fragmented that insomnia or daytime sleepiness results. The *periodic limb movement disorder* (PLMD) is defined as the finding of PLMS accompanied by symptoms (insomnia or daytime sleepiness) that are not explained by other disorders. Current thinking is that whereas PLMS is a very common finding, the PLMD is uncommon (77). PLMS can be seen in patients with sleep apnea, narcolepsy, and asymptomatic individuals (especially the elderly). Most patients with a finding of PLMS do not require specific treatment for this problem. PLMS has been associated with the use of antidepressants or withdrawal of antidepressants, barbiturates, and anticonvulsants. Patients with sleep apnea, on occasion, exhibit a large increase in PLMS during CPAP titration (78).

RLS is defined on the basis of clinical history as (a) a desire to move the limbs usually associated with paresthesias or dysesthesias (abnormal or unpleasant sensations), (b) motor restlessness—being compelled to move the limbs, (c) symptoms precipitated by rest or inactivity and relieved by activity (temporary relief), and (d) symptoms that are worse in the evening or at night (79). The unpleasant sensations in the limbs are often described as "creepy crawly" or "electric" but can be described as cramping. Some patients simply have an urge to move the limbs. About 80% of patients with RLS will have PLMS on a given sleep study. In contrast, a small percentage of patients with PLMS have RLS. RLS can be a significant problem for patients and can cause sleep onset insomnia. RLS is believed to be much more common than PLMD. Many patients with RLS have the idiopathic form but other common causes are iron deficiency, dopamine blockers, renal failure (with or without dialysis), and pregnancy. The diagnosis of RLS is by clinical history and not by sleep study. However, patients with OSA commonly have body movements during sleep, and a sleep study is often indicated if there is a clinical suspicion of OSA.

A number of medications have been used to treat RLS including benzodiazepines (clonazepam), dopaminergic medications (dopamine precursors or dopamine agonists), anticonvulsants (neurontin), and opioids (80). The newer nonergotamine dopamine agonists (pramipexole or ropinirole) are considered the drugs of choice for patients with moderate to severe RLS symptoms. For example, starting with pramipexole 0.125 mg 1 to 2 hours before symptoms occur, the dose is slowly increased until adequate control of symptoms occurs. Side effects include nausea, headache, sedation (not a problem at bedtime), and peripheral edema. One can treat mild forms of RLS with carbidopa/levodopa using the short-acting or sustained-release forms of the medication. However, a phenomenon called *augmentation* is common if higher doses are used. Augmentation consists of earlier RLS symptoms (e.g., 7:00 PM instead of 11:00 PM) or symptoms in the arms as well as legs. Treatment of PLMD uses similar medications except for the anticonvulsants. Most physicians would use dopaminergic drugs, but mild PLMD can be treated with benzodiazepines if sleep apnea is not present. The reader is referred to an excellent reference on treatment of RLS (80).

SLEEP APNEA SYNDROMES

The sleep apnea syndromes may be divided into the obstructive sleep apnea syndromes (OSAS) and the central sleep apnea syndromes (CSAS). Although patients with OSA may have some central apneas, the diagnosis of central sleep apnea (CSA) requires that a majority of apneas be central in nature. The CSAS is much less common than the OSAS, which composes more than 85% to 90% of all sleep apnea patients evaluated at most sleep centers. Patients with predominantly mixed apneas or repetitive hypopneas due to partial airway obstruction (34) are considered to have the OSAS as these events have the same clinical impact as obstructive apneas. Other associated disorders that can be considered subtypes of the OSAS include the obesity hypoventilation syndrome (OHS), the overlap syndrome (OSA and COPD), and the UARS. These syndromes are discussed in the following sections.

Obstructive Sleep Apnea

The true incidence of OSA is unknown, but estimates of 1% to 4% have been quoted (81–83). A large cohort study suggested that an AHI >5 per hour along with the symptoms was present in 2% of women and 4% of men (83). Patients with the OSAS usually present with a complaint of excessive daytime sleepiness or behaviors during sleep such as snoring, gasping, or breathing pauses. They typically have a long history of loud habitual snoring, and bedmates frequently report pauses in breathing terminated by snorts. A history of chronic nasal obstruction or congestion, hypertension, or recent weight gain preceding an exacerbation of daytime sleepiness is common. Other manifestations or associations include impotence, enuresis, and morning headaches (82,83). A frequently overlooked fact is that patients with OSA may actually present with prominent complaints of insomnia rather than daytime sleepiness (84). This is because of the frequent arousals and the difficulty in attaining consolidated sleep. Conditions known to predispose patients to sleep apnea include the male gender (83,85), increasing age (83), alcohol use (86,87), obesity (83,88), hypothyroidism (89), acromegaly (90), the postmenopausal state (91), and use of hypnotics (92,93).

Symptoms and signs of right heart failure are present in a minority (10% to 15%) of cases (94). Physical examination frequently reveals nasal obstruction, a large tongue, retrognathia (posterior displacement of the mandible), a dependent soft palate, or a hypertrophied uvula. Many patients have a short, thick neck. In fact, neck circumference correlates better with the AHI than body weight. Up to 40% of patients in some sleep centers are not obese. Thyroid studies should be ordered if symptoms or signs of hypothyroidism are present. The majority of patients with OSAS do not have either polycythemia or evidence of CO_2 retention on arterial blood gas analysis. We reserve arterial blood gas analysis for patients who have low awake oxygen saturations or unexplained elevations in serum bicarbonate. In one study, the best clinical predictors of the presence of the OSAS were a history of snoring, a history of apnea or gasping, a large neck circumference (>17 inches), and the presence of hypertension (95). Interestingly, the presence of daytime sleepiness (a cardinal manifestation of OSA) was not a reliable predictor. It appears that many patients minimize or underestimate the severity of this symptom. In addition, many patients with severe OSA have minimal daytime sleepiness. The correlation of measures of sleepiness with the AHI despite being statistically significant is low (96). This is probably because there is considerable variation in the degree of susceptibility to sleep fragmentation.

POLYSOMNOGRAPHY IN THE OBSTRUCTIVE SLEEP APNEA SYNDROMES. Polysomnography of patients with OSAS reveals repetitive obstructive and mixed apneas and hypopneas (see Fig. 18-8). Apneas are followed by resumption of airflow, which usually coincides with evidence of arousal and often movement. The nadir of oxygen saturation usually occurs after apnea termination. During the apnea, the chest and abdomen often move in a paradoxical manner. The heart rate usually slows at the onset of apnea and then speeds up at apnea termination or arousal (97).

Because many totally asymptomatic elderly persons may have a small amount of obstructive apnea, defining exact criteria

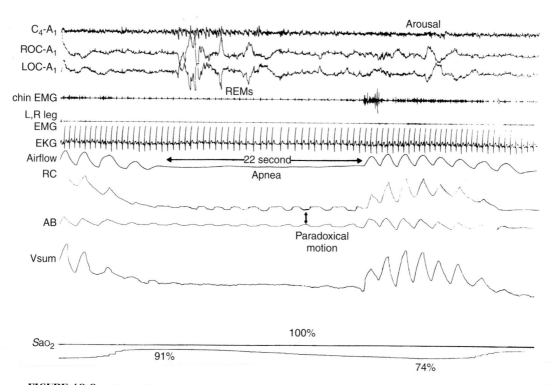

FIGURE 18-8.   A complete polysomnographic tracing of an obstructive apnea during rapid eye movement (REM) sleep. Note that the electroencephalographic (EEG) and electromyographic (EMG) change at apnea termination, signifying an arousal, and that the nadir of arterial oxygen saturation (SaO_2) occurs after the apnea has terminated.

for normality on the basis of the AHI is difficult (41,83). A widely accepted definition is an AHI >5 per hour along with symptoms or AHI >15 per hour with or without symptoms. A retrospective study (98) found an increase in mortality when the apnea index exceeded 20 per hour. The Sleep Heart Health Study found an increased risk of developing cardiovascular disease with an AHI >5 per hour (41). This provides some evidence for use of this value to define OSA. An arbitrary but useful scheme is to consider an AHI <15 as mild, 15 to 30 as moderate, and >30 as severe (37,45).

Occasionally, a sleepy, snoring patient will have surprisingly fewer apneas or hypopneas when studied. In such cases, one must consider the effects of ethanol intake, sleep stage, and posture. If a patient abstains from his or her usual ethanol intake, this could reduce the severity of apnea. Patients with mild to moderate apnea may also have positional apnea (AHI much greater in the supine position) (99) or REM-related apnea (AHI much greater or present only in REM sleep) (100). In these cases, the severity of OSA may be underestimated if small amounts of sleep in the supine position or REM sleep were recorded. Many sleep centers compute a separate AHI for NREM and REM sleep as well as for the supine and lateral sleep positions to help identify patients with sleep-stage–specific or positional sleep apnea. If airflow monitoring is performed with thermal devices only, one may underdiagnose RERAs or hypopneas. Finally, the presence of other sleep disorders including insufficient sleep must all be considered as possible explanations of the patient's sleepiness.

The gold standard for the diagnosis of OSA has been attended polysomnography including EEG, EOG, and EMG to stage sleep. Alternatives include unattended portable polysomnography, attended or unattended cardiopulmonary studies [airflow, respiratory effort, Sa_{O_2}, heart rate, or electrocardiogram (ECG)], and single or dual bioparameter studies (oximetry). After a systematic review of the evidence, a recent set of practice parameters was published concerning portable monitoring. Only attended cardiopulmonary studies could be recommended for routine use (101) as an alternative to traditional attended polysomnography. In selected circumstances (no local sleep center or long wait for a study), other types of portable monitoring can be useful on an individual case basis.

The degree of arterial oxygen desaturation in patients with OSA is not necessarily correlated with the AHI index and must also be considered in assessing the severity of disease. A study of the factors determining the severity of desaturation found that (a) a lower baseline P_{O_2}, (b) a greater percentage of sleep time spent in apnea, and (c) a smaller expiratory reserve volume (functional residual capacity minus residual volume) tended to produce more severe desaturation (102). This is consistent with the observation that patients with baseline hypoxemia due to obesity (with or without CO_2 retention) or superimposed COPD tend to desaturate more rapidly during apnea.

UPPER-AIRWAY OBSTRUCTION—PATHOPHYSIOLOGY. As outlined in a previous section, there are many factors that determine airway patency. If the forces tending to close the airway exceed those maintaining airway patency, the upper airway narrows or closes. In patients with OSA, an obstruction to airflow (extreme narrowing or closure) occurs during sleep at one or several locations in the upper airway (103,104).

Studies of the upper airway in awake patients with OSA by cephalometric radiographs, computed tomography, acoustic reflection techniques, and magnetic resonance imaging have usually shown smaller than normal upper airways (32). These patients have an increased supraglottic resistance (105) and, unlike normal subjects, require a positive intraluminal pressure to prevent airway closure during sleep (106). Some patients have a bony abnormality, whereas in others a long soft palate, a large posteriorly placed tongue, increased fat deposition, or tissue edema may all play a role in narrowing the airway. The shape of the upper airway also differs, with the airway being most narrowed in the lateral dimension in OSA patients versus anterior-posteriorly in normal subjects (32). The lateral pharyngeal walls appear to be increased in thickness, although this is not explained by fat deposition. There is considerable overlap in *awake* airway size between normal persons and patients with OSA. However, airway size during wakefulness is influenced by both anatomy and upper-airway muscle activity. Studies have shown that during wakefulness, a higher than normal percentage of the maximal upper-airway muscle activity is required to preserve upper-airway patency in OSA patients compared to normal subjects (107). This appears secondary to a higher than normal amount of tonic activity and a more negative pressure during tidal breathing (108). In addition, OSA patients may have a higher genioglossus response to negative pressure (109), although the response of the palatal muscles may be impaired (110). The higher activity is thought to be a compensation for a smaller and more collapsible (111) upper airway. There also appears to be a greater than normal upper airway dependence on lung volume in patients with OSA (31). At sleep onset, there is an abrupt and often a greater than normal fall in upper-airway muscle activity (112). However, again, considerable overlap between normal subjects and patients with OSA exists. In any case, upper-airway muscle activity is insufficient to maintain upper-airway patency. Whereas early theories of airway collapse focused on the balance between negative intraluminal pressure and dilating forces, recent studies have shown that negative intraluminal pressure is not required for airway closure. Airway collapse has been demonstrated endoscopically during central apnea (113). Indeed, upper-airway obstruction in patients with OSA usually begins when both ventilatory drive and upper-airway muscle activity are relatively reduced or are falling (114). Upper-airway size falls progressively at end expiration along with lung volume in the breaths preceding apnea (115). Thus, our current understanding emphasizes susceptible upper-airway anatomy and a loss of upper-airway muscle activity as the key elements in upper-airway obstruction.

The postapnea ventilatory period may have consequences if the patient returns to sleep quickly. If the P_{CO_2} falls below a point called the "apneic threshold" (usually 0 to 2 mm Hg above the stable awake P_{CO_2} or 4 to 6 mm Hg below the sleeping P_{CO_2} set point), then respiratory drive ceases, resulting in central apnea (116). This is thought to be the origin of the central portion of mixed apnea (117). When the upper airway is stabilized using nasal CPAP, both the central and obstructive components of mixed apnea are usually abolished.

APNEA TERMINATION AND AROUSAL. During obstructive apnea, the phasic activity of the genioglossus (and many other upper-airway muscles) and respiratory muscles progressively increases as the apneic period continues (29,103). However, the upper airway does not open, in part, because increasingly negative intraluminal pressure maintains airway collapse. Upper-airway opening appears to occur only after arousal and a preferentially large increase in upper-airway activity (103). The fact that arousal does not occur despite prolonged periods of apnea and arterial oxygen desaturation suggests that a defect in arousal mechanisms is present. The magnitude of the stimulus inducing respiratory arousal from NREM sleep appears to be related to the level of inspiratory effort (esophageal or supraglottic pressure) rather than the individual levels of P_{O_2} or P_{CO_2} stimulating ventilatory drive (118,119). Normal subjects arouse from mask occlusion at suction pressures of 20 to 30 cm H_2O, whereas patients with OSA may exert esophageal pressures more negative than 60 cm H_2O before awakening. The causes of impaired arousal in patients with OSA are unknown but are probably explained at least in part by the effects of chronic sleep fragmentation on arousal mechanisms. Of note, apnea or hypopnea termination is associated with cortical EEG changes meeting standard criteria for arousal definition only about 60% to 80% of the time. However, there is believed to be a change of state in the brainstem regardless of the cortical EEG changes. A recent study found that if frontal EEG electrodes are used, then arousal could be detected at event termination most of the time (120). Respiratory-related arousal from REM sleep is even less well understood. Normal subjects arouse much more quickly from mask occlusion during REM than NREM sleep. In contrast, the longest apneas occur during REM sleep in patients with OSA.

IMPAIRED SLEEP, DAYTIME SLEEPINESS, AND COGNITIVE PERFORMANCE IN THE OBSTRUCTIVE SLEEP APNEA SYNDROMES. The sleep architecture of patients with OSAS is impaired, with reduced amounts of REM and stage 3 and 4 sleep as well as frequent arousals and a reduced sleep efficiency. On daytime MSLT testing, a shortened sleep latency is usually noted. Two or more naps may contain REM sleep, suggesting REM deprivation (54). The first night of effective treatment of OSA with tracheostomy or nasal CPAP frequently results in long periods of stages 3, 4, and REM (deep sleep and REM rebound). A rapid improvement in daytime alertness is noted in many patients (121). The sleep latency on the MSLT after tracheostomy or nasal CPAP treatment usually improves but not always to the normal range. In one study, the MWT sleep latency improved from 18 to 32 minutes after treatment with nasal CPAP (122).

The exact causes of the excessive daytime somnolence in the OSAS are still under investigation. Sleep fragmentation is probably the most important factor, although hypoxemia may also play a role. In one study, the AHI did not differ between a group of hypersomnolent and nonhypersomnolent patients with OSA (123). In another study, the respiratory arousal index (arousals related to respiratory events per hour of sleep) correlated best with the sleep latency on the MSLT (124). However, the arousal index, a body movement index, or a neural network model of sleep state correlated with daytime sleepiness only slightly better than the AHI (96). Measures of sleep fragmentation, such as the arousal frequency or alterations in sleep architecture (increased stage 1 and decreased stages 3 and 4), appear to be more abnormal in sleepy OSA patients (125). Cheshire et al. found that a higher

AHI, more sleep disruption, and worse nocturnal hypoxemia were all associated with worsening daytime performance (126). Another study found that cognitive impairment appears to be more severe in patients with sleep apnea who have hypoxemia (127).

OBSTRUCTIVE SLEEP APNEA SYNDROMES AND DAYTIME HYPERCAPNIA. Most patients with OSA do not exhibit daytime hypoventilation. Patients with sleep apnea who have a normal daytime P_{CO_2} and P_{O_2} have normal ventilatory responses to hypercapnia and hypoxemia (128,129), although their responses to resistive loads may be reduced (129). Two groups of OSA patients with daytime hypercapnia are patients with the OHS and the overlap syndrome (OSA and COPD). Both groups tend to have severe arterial oxygen desaturation at night and often have right heart failure. Those patients with obesity and daytime hypoventilation not secondary to lung disease are said to have the OHS. These patients were formerly called *Pickwickian*. Most also have severe OSA and daytime sleepiness but some simply have a worsening of hypoventilation during sleep with few discrete apneas or hypopneas. The OHS group is somewhat heterogeneous with variable amounts of upper-airway obstruction, abnormal ventilatory control, and reduced respiratory system compliance secondary to obesity. Abnormal ventilatory control in OHS patients includes reduced ventilatory responses to hypoxemia (130) and hypercapnia (131,132). OHS patients also have a lower compliance of the respiratory system compared to nonhypercapnic patients with equivalent obesity (131). With adequate treatment of sleep apnea, the daytime CO_2 retention will improve in some but not all OHS patients (132–134). This implies both acquired (reversible) and intrinsic dysfunction of ventilatory control.

The other group of OSAS patients that commonly have daytime CO_2 retention is the group with the overlap syndrome (COPD and OSA). Whereas most patients with COPD do not retain CO_2 until the forced expiratory volume in one second (FEV_1) falls below 1 L, patients with the overlap syndrome develop hypercarbia at less severe levels of airflow obstruction (135). The CO_2 retention in this group may also improve with effective treatment of their OSA.

"UPPER-AIRWAY RESISTANCE SYNDROME" AND RESPIRATORY EFFORT—RELATED AROUSALS. Guilleminault et al. (9) reported on a group of patients with daytime sleepiness (short sleep latency on an MSLT) who had neither an AHI >5 per hour using thermal devices to measure airflow nor arterial oxygen desaturation. When esophageal pressure and accurate airflow monitoring were performed, the group had more than 10 arousals per hour following periods of increased respiratory effort. The events were also associated with a flattened airflow profile but did not qualify as hypopneas. After arousal, there was a rapid reduction in respiratory effort and a rounding of the airflow shape. The mean respiratory arousal index was 31.3 per hour with a mean nadir in esophageal pressure preceding arousal being −33 cm H_2O (9). The daytime sleepiness improved after CPAP treatment. It is controversial whether patients with the "UARS" are really a separate group or simply have a mild form of OSA (136,137). In any case, this publication focused attention on sleep disturbance from respiratory events as well as arterial oxygen desaturation. Because of these findings, a task force of the AASM introduced the term RERA, as previously discussed. Definitive diagnosis of RERAs requires demonstration of a high or a progressive increase in supraglottic or esophageal pressure defections preceding the brief arousal (Fig. 18-7). The events should not qualify as a hypopnea. Currently, there are no definitive guidelines by which RERA rate should be considered abnormal. In the original description of the UARS using esophageal pressure monitoring, a respiratory arousal rate >10 per hour was used to define the syndrome. Individual persons without daytime sleepiness may have a RERA index >10 per hour, although the mean RERA for a group of persons without symptoms is usually <10 per hour (138). In clinical practice, RERAs are usually detected by arousals preceded by flow limitation. Patients usually have combinations of apnea, hypopneas, and RERAs. One can define a respiratory arousal index as equal to the arousals per hour from apneas, hypopneas, and RERAs. Do arousals from RERAs have the same impact as those from apneas and hypopneas? The answer to this question is not known.

CARDIOVASCULAR CONSEQUENCES OF OBSTRUCTIVE SLEEP APNEA SYNDROME. The cardiovascular consequences of OSAS include episodic nocturnal pulmonary and systemic hypertension, cyclic variation in heart rate, and the potential for worsening coronary and cerebral ischemia (41,139). Recently, there has also been information suggesting that untreated OSA may increase atherosclerosis. It is likely that much of the increase in mortality associated with OSA is due to the cardiovascular consequences of OSAS. Ongoing and future studies will hopefully better define these consequences.

Pulmonary arterial blood pressure rises during episodes of arterial oxygen desaturation and then falls when the oxygen saturation returns to baseline (139). Both hypoxemia and acidosis cause pulmonary vasoconstriction. Early studies have suggested that right heart failure (94) and moderate *daytime* pulmonary hypertension (140) are generally confined to OSA patients with daytime hypoxemia. Patients with OSA and daytime hypoxemia usually have either the OHS or a mixture of OSA and COPD. Therefore, it is these groups that usually show evidence of cor pulmonale. However, more recent investigations have found that mild daytime pulmonary hypertension can occur in OSA patients without daytime hypoxia (141). This suggests that remodeling of the pulmonary vessels may have taken place. Effective treatment with positive airway pressure (PAP) can reduce daytime pulmonary pressures as well as prevent the nocturnal increases in pulmonary pressure (142).

Systemic arterial blood pressure falls during sleep in *both* normal individuals and patients with essential hypertension. In contrast, an increase in systemic blood pressure is associated with each obstructive apnea or hypopnea in patients with OSA. There is a slow rise in blood pressure during the apnea and a steeper increase in the same at the time of arousal (97,143). A significant portion of OSA patients may fail to have a mean fall in blood pressure during the night—"nondippers" (144). Studies have found that a large proportion of patients with sleep apnea have *daytime* hypertension (95) and that a significant proportion of hypertensive patients have OSA (145). Does the association between hypertension and sleep apnea indicate causality or simply that both entities are due to

other factors such as obesity? This question remains unanswered. Studies have found that there is an association between hypertension and the OSAS after controlling for obesity (146,147). The Sleep Heart Health Study found an increased risk of developing hypertension even if low levels of sleep apnea were present (41). However, even if the OSAS does not cause daytime hypertension, it may worsen the *consequences*. The lack of the normal nocturnal dip in blood pressure in hypertensive OSAS patients may predispose them to a greater degree of left ventricular hypertrophy (148). Generally, adequate treatment of OSAS patients with hypertension does not eliminate the necessity of medical treatment of daytime hypertension. However, in many patients, daytime systemic hypertension is more easily and effectively controlled. A recent study found that good adherence to effective CPAP treatment of OSA for 9 weeks resulted in a drop of 10 mm Hg in both daytime and nocturnal blood pressure in a group of patients with OSA (149). Such a drop in blood pressure should significantly lower the risk for heart disease and stroke.

The most common change in cardiac rhythm in OSA is an exaggerated sinus arrhythmia often called a *bradycardia–tachycardia pattern*. However, in many patients the heart rate remains between 60 and 100 beats per minute. The heart rate usually slows during the initial part of apnea or hypopnea and then speeds up during the arousal at event termination. The increase in heart rate at arousal appears to be secondary to a combination of an increase in sympathetic tone and a reduction in vagal tone, with the reverse occurring on the return to sleep and on the start of the next respiratory event (139,97). Sinus bradycardia, sinus pauses, heart block (all types), and atrial and ventricular arrhythmias may also be associated with sleep apnea (150). Although many OSA patients have frequent PVCs during sleep, 24-hour monitoring often shows a reduction in PVC rate during sleep. Therefore, the presence of ventricular arrhythmias during sleep apnea does not necessarily imply causality. One study found little relationship between the PVC frequency and SaO_2 until the saturation fell below 60% (151). The presence of sleep apnea can complicate control of atrial arrhythmias. A recent study of patients undergoing cardioversion for atrial fibrillation found an increased incidence of relapse if untreated OSA was present (152). OSA patients treated with CPAP had the same rate of recurrence as those without OSA.

The Sleep Heart Health Study of a large prospective cohort of patients found evidence of a modest increase in risk of having self-reported coronary artery disease at even low levels of sleep apnea (41). Peker et al. found an increase in mortality in patients with coronary artery disease who had untreated OSA (153). There have also been a growing number of studies showing changes in blood components or indicators of inflammation in OSAHS that may be associated with an increased risk of atherosclerosis or thrombosis. In OSAHS, there is an increase in the early morning hematocrit (154) and fibrinogen levels (155) that decreases after CPAP treatment. The levels of vascular endothelial growth factor (VEGF) (156), amount of neutrophil (157,158), and platelet activation (159) are also reduced with CPAP treatment of patients with OSAHS. Inflammation is now believed to play a role in atherosclerosis or plaque rupture. The level of C-reactive protein (a marker of inflammation) is elevated in patients with OSA (160,161) and is reduced with CPAP treatment (161).

PROGNOSIS AND MORTALITY IN OBSTRUCTIVE SLEEP APNEA SYNDROME AND RISK OF AUTOMOBILE ACCIDENTS. Limited information has been available concerning the natural history of the OSAS or the effect of therapy. This is an important issue as some patients with substantial sleep apnea have relatively few symptoms. It may be difficult to insist that they undergo treatment if they lack evidence of apnea-induced arrhythmias or heart failure when the consequences of untreated sleep apnea are still unclear. One retrospective study found an increase in mortality in patients with moderate to severe OSA (apnea index >20 per hour) and that both tracheostomy and nasal CPAP increased survival (98). Another study found that patients with OSA in the 30- to 50-years age range had excessive mortality (162). Most deaths were from cardiovascular causes. The Sleep Heart Health Study found evidence that even mild degrees of sleep-disordered breathing are associated with an increased risk of developing cardiovascular disease including hypertension, coronary artery disease, and cerebrovascular disease (41). However, the survival benefit of treating OSA has not been demonstrated in a large study.

Another difficult issue facing physicians is whether patients with OSA are fit to drive an automobile. Patients with OSA are at increased risk for automobile accidents (163,164,165). Those patients with a history of a recent automobile accident or episodes of falling asleep at the wheel are the group with the highest risk. State laws vary on the physician's responsibility to report patients with "impaired consciousness." The physician must balance such responsibilities with the patient's right for confidentiality. It seems prudent to instruct patients with OSA and severe sleepiness not to drive until adequate treatment has begun (and to document this in writing). A reasonable approach is to report only those patients with severe daytime sleepiness (especially with a history of falling asleep while driving) who do not adequately comply with therapy. The American Thoracic Society has published a helpful official statement on this subject (164). However, the physician treating patients with OSA should consult his or her local physician organizations for standard-of-practice guidelines. Adequate treatment with CPAP has been shown to decrease the incidence of traffic accidents (165,166). There have been efforts to develop simulated driving performance tests for patients with OSA (167). Although these are useful in demonstrating impairment, they have not been proven to have predictive value about a given patient's risk for being involved in an automobile accident.

TREATMENT OF OBSTRUCTIVE SLEEP APNEA. Treatment decisions should consider patient preference, the severity of disease (frequency of events and desaturation), the severity of the patient's symptoms, and comorbid disease likely to be affected by untreated OSA. Possible treatment options are listed in Table 18-3.

Conservative treatments and medications. The treatment of OSA begins with identification and elimination of exacerbating factors such as hypothyroidism and ethanol ingestion, as well as an examination of the patient's upper-airway anatomy for abnormalities. Weight loss of only 10% to 15% may significantly improve OSA in some cases (168). Patients having significant events only in the supine position may improve with sleep in the lateral decubitus position or with elevation of the head of the bed (169,170). Treatment of nasal congestion

TABLE 18-3. Treatments for Obstructive Sleep Apnea

Mild OSA	Moderate OSA	Severe OSA
Weight loss	Positive airway pressure	Positive airway pressure Tracheostomy
Position therapy	UPPP[a]	
UPPP	Oral appliances	Maxillofacial surgery
Oral appliances	Maxillofacial surgery	Oral appliances[a]
	Weight loss (adjunctive)	Weight loss (adjunctive)

OSA, Obstructive Sleep Apnea Syndrome; UPPP, uvulopalatopharyngoplasty.
Positive Airway Pressure = continuous positive airway pressure CPAP, bilevel PAP, auto-adjusting PAP (APAP).
[a] May be successful in some cases.

may also be of benefit in some cases. The use of medications that increase serotonin (5HT) or norepinephrine (NE) have been tried as treatments of OSA (171,172). The rationale is that an increase in 5HT or NE could augment upper-airway muscle activity and reduce airway obstruction. To date, the treatment trials have been disappointing, with only modest reductions in the AHI during NREM sleep (172). Some benefit may occur from a decrease in the amount of REM sleep that is induced by these medications. However, in general, these medications do not improve sleep quality. Medroxyprogesterone, a respiratory stimulant, does lower the daytime P_{CO_2} in patients with OHS but does not reduce the AHI (173,174). Side effects include impotence, hair loss, and hyperglycemia. In general, PAP (or tracheostomy) rather than medroxyprogesterone is the treatment of choice for patients with OHS.

Surgical treatments. The gold standard of surgical therapy for OSA has been tracheostomy (175). This bypasses the upper-airway obstruction and results in almost uniform abolition of obstructive apneas and symptoms. However, in addition to the psychological morbidity, the procedure has frequent complications, especially in patients with fat necks. Now that PAP is available, tracheostomy is usually reserved for severe cases that do not tolerate PAP. A less drastic surgical procedure is uvulopalatopharyngoplasty (UPPP). The uvula, portions of the soft palate, and redundant pharyngeal tissue are removed (176). If nasal obstruction is present, this is often repaired. Unfortunately, UPPP significantly reduces the severity of apnea and desaturation in only about 40% to 50% of the patients (177–179). Often, the AHI remains above 20 events per hour. UPPP is an effective procedure for snoring. Several methods of evaluation of the upper airway while patients are awake or asleep have suggested that patients who have significant airway narrowing mainly in the retropalatal area are more likely to improve after UPPP (104). Of note, some patients actually have an increased AHI following UPPP (180). Even those with initial improvement may have a recurrence of OSA, especially if they gain weight. Laser-assisted uvulopalatoplasty (LAUP) and radiofrequency ablation (somnoplasty) are new methods of increasing the retropalatal airway (177,179). LAUP may be performed without general anesthesia but is recommended only for treatment of snoring (181). All patients undergoing palatal surgery for OSA should have a repeat sleep study within 3 to 6 months even if a symptomatic improvement occurs. The return of apnea or hypopnea can occur even if snoring is absent or less noisy. Because of dissatisfaction with UPPP, several new surgical procedures have been developed to treat obstruction behind the tongue or in the lower pharynx (177–179,182). With anterior mandibular osteotomy, a window of bone where the genioglossus inserts into the mandible is cut and pulled anteriorly, which results in the tongue moving forward. This procedure is usually combined with a hyoid suspension in which the hyoid bone is freed of some muscular attachments and is suspended either from the mandible or from the thyroid cartilage. This procedure is known as *genioglossal advancement and hyoid myotomy* (GAHM). If this fails, the next step is maxillary mandibular osteotomy (MMO). In this procedure, the maxilla and mandible are moved forward and the orthodontic occlusion is preserved. Either tracheotomy or nasal CPAP is needed in the immediate postoperative period (182). This extensive procedure appears to be effective but is available only at specialized centers.

Oral appliances. Recently, there has been considerable interest in the use of oral appliances (OAs) as a treatment for OSA (183,184). These devices include tongue retaining devices (TRDs), which position the tongue anteriorly using a suction bulb, and mandibular advancing devices (MADs) (see Fig. 18-9), which work by moving the lower jaw (and hence the tongue) forward (183,184). Additional effects of MADs may be a downward rotation of the mandible and traction on the palate via the palatoglossal muscle. One problem to date has been a lack of standardization of a large number of devices. Mandibular advancing devices require the involvement of a qualified dentist to ensure that occlusal or temporomandibular joint problems do not occur. To date, OAs appear to be most effective in patients with mild to moderate sleep apnea. In one study of patients successfully treated with both nasal CPAP and an OA, the latter device was preferred (185). OAs may also be tried in UPPP failures when nasal CPAP is refused (186). They may work in some cases of severe OSA (187) or in patients with obstruction mainly at the palatal area (187). To be considered for a mandibular advancing device, a patient must have good teeth and no history of temporomandibular joint (TMJ) problems. The total cost for custom OAs may be up to $1,000, and unfortunately, many insurance plans will not cover this treatment. Another concern is that chronic use of an OA use may cause a shift in the teeth. To date, this has not been a major problem in most patients.

Nocturnal oxygen. Nocturnal oxygen therapy has also been tried in patients with OSA (188). Acute and chronic studies using continuous low-flow oxygen have usually found improved oxygenation and small to moderate increases in event duration. The frequency of respiratory events usually decreases only slightly or remains unchanged. Therefore, it is not surprising that oxygen therapy does not improve the sleep latency on MSLT testing (189). No long-term studies have shown improvements in morbidity or mortality with oxygen therapy for OSA. However, if the patient refuses or cannot tolerate more effective therapy, oxygen therapy may be tried to improve nocturnal oxygenation. Performing nocturnal oximetry on oxygen treatment is warranted to determine if desaturation is satisfactorily improved with supplemental oxygen. Some patients with severe OSA can have significant increases in event length during REM sleep on supplemental oxygen with persistent severe drops in the oxygen saturation. Oxygen therapy can dramatically increase the amount of CO_2 retention during sleep in patients with both hypercapnic COPD and sleep apnea (190). The development of morning headaches or increasing somnolence should alert the physician that progressive daytime hypercapnia may also be developing.

Positive airway pressure. Medical therapy for OSA was revolutionized by the introduction of nasal CPAP by Sullivan et al. (191). PAP is considered the treatment of choice for patients with moderate to severe OSA (45) and may also be effective in symptomatic patients with mild sleep apnea (192). With this method, a flow of pressurized room air via the nose maintains a positive pressure in the upper airway. Therefore, airway closure is prevented by a "pneumatic splint." Although a nasal mask is most commonly used, a number of alternative interfaces are available. These include nasal pillows or nasal prong interfaces that fit into the nostrils providing a seal without touching the face or the bridge of the nose (193). Patients with claustrophobia may benefit from these devices. A mask fitting over the nose and mouth (full face mask) can be used in patients with severe nasal congestion or in those that develop a leak from the mouth with a nasal mask (194). There are also several methods to deliver PAP including traditional CPAP, bilevel PAP (195,196), auto-adjusting or auto-titrating positive airway pressure (APAP) devices (197), and CPAP with expiratory pressure relief (Cflex). In bilevel devices, a higher inspiratory positive airway pressure (IPAP) is administered during inspiration and a lower expiratory positive airway pressure (EPAP) is administered during exhalation. This may allow maintenance of an open airway with lower expiratory pressure. In addition, the

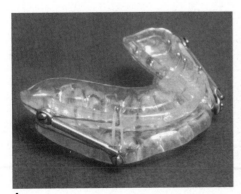

A

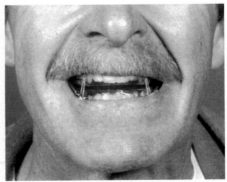

B

FIGURE 18-9. **A:** A typical oral appliance (OA) (Herbst) used to treat obstructive sleep apnea (OSA) is illustrated. **B:** This appliance fits snugly over the upper and lower teeth. (From Berry RB. *Sleep Medicine Pearls,* 2nd edition. Philadelphia: Hanley & Belfus, 2003, with permission.)

IPAP–EPAP pressure difference provides pressure support that can help augment tidal volume. For example, if IPAP is at 15 cm H_2O and EPAP is at 5 cm H_2O, the system provides a pressure support of 10 cm H_2O. One study found no improvement in compliance with bilevel devices compared to CPAP (196). However, bilevel PAP devices are very useful in patients with pressure intolerance ("can't breathe out"), COPD, expiratory muscle weakness, and hypoventilation. APAP devices have built-in algorithms that monitor variables such as airflow (apnea or hypopnea), airway vibration (snoring), and airflow limitation (flattening) to determine whether pressure should be slowly increased or decreased. The lowest effective pressure in a given circumstance is administered. Information stored in the device memory can be analyzed and a fixed pressure (CPAP) can be chosen (see Fig. 18-10). This is often the ninety-fifth percentile pressure (P95), which is exceeded only 5% of the time. Alternatively, the devices can be used for chronic treatment. The rationale is that a lower mean night pressure may improve acceptance and adherence (197). To date, not all studies have shown an increase in adherence. However, patients with large postural differences in required pressure, those on high pressures, and pressure-sensitive patients may benefit from chronic treatment with APAP. CPAP with expiratory pressure relief are devices that allow a fall in pressure during exhalation that is proportional to flow with a return to the preset pressure at end exhalation. This feature may also be useful in pressure-sensitive patients.

The traditional method of determining the amount of pressure needed to maintain airway patency is determined by a sleep study (nasal PAP trial or titration) in which the level of PAP is increased until apnea, hypopnea, desaturation, snoring, and respiratory effort arousals are prevented (198,199).

As pressure is increased, apneas, followed by obstructive hypopneas, and finally RERAs or snoring are eliminated (200). Today, most sleep centers monitor the flow signal using the positive-pressure device's accurate internal flow sensor (machine flow) to titrate PAP. Using an accurate measure of airflow, one can detect residual high upper-airway resistance by a significant flattening in the airflow profile (201). Pressures in the range of 5 to 20 cm H_2O are commonly used. Usually, higher CPAP pressures are needed during REM sleep or when the patient is supine (169,202,203). In patients with awake hypoxemia or severe obesity, hypoxemia may persist during sleep despite the reversal of upper-airway obstruction with nasal CPAP. This can be especially severe during the prolonged REM episodes (REM rebound) that occur on the first night of CPAP (204). In such cases, one may try a further increase in pressure (to decrease residual upper-airway resistance), convert to bilevel pressure, or add supplemental oxygen. Titration of bilevel PAP is similar to CPAP. One can start with bilevel pressure (IPAP/EPAP) of 8/4 cm H_2O and sequentially increase the EPAP to eliminate apnea and the IPAP to eliminate hypopnea or snoring. Another approach is to use IPAP equal to EPAP until apnea is eliminated and then start increasing the IPAP to eliminate hypopnea or snoring.

Because of economic constraints, many sleep laboratories use partial night or "split" studies (205,206). In such studies, the initial part of the night is used to document the presence and severity of sleep apnea and the second part of the night is used as a nasal CPAP trial. Such a strategy may be satisfactory in patients with clear-cut moderate to severe OSA, provided that the patients receive adequate education about PAP before bedtime, have mask fitting, and are allowed to become familiar with the equipment. Of note, split studies may result

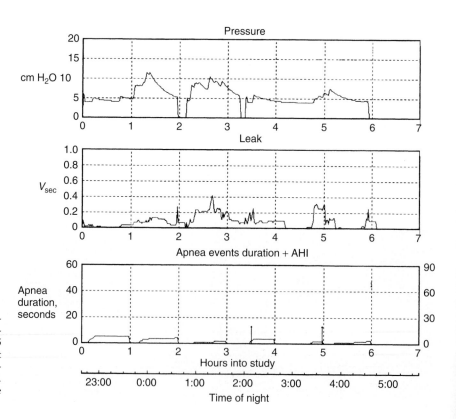

FIGURE 18-10.   A single night profile of pressure, leak, and residual AHI in a patient undergoing an auto-titration study. In this patient, the P95 was 10.1 cm H_2O and the leak was low for most of the night. In the bottom tracings, the small lollipops represent single apnea event durations. The patient was prescribed continuous positive airway pressure (CPAP) at 10 cm H_2O.

in an underestimation of the severity of sleep apnea because the diagnostic portion of the study may not contain much REM or supine sleep. There is also a limited time for the positive-pressure titration. It has been estimated that 60% to 80% of patients can have an adequate titration on a partial night study (205,206). Suggested patient criteria for a split study are an AHI >40 per hour or >20 per hour with severe desaturation for at least 2 hours of sleep during the diagnostic portion and with 3 hours remaining for the PAP titration (199). If an adequate pressure is not demonstrated that is effective in both supine and REM sleep, a repeat full-night PAP titration may be needed.

The main difficulty with PAP therapy is the problem with patient acceptance and adherence. Long-term adherence has ranged from 40% to 80% depending on the level of support and the definition of adherence (207,208). Comprehensive programs that provide close follow-up, education, objective monitoring of compliance, and involvement of the spouse report superior success (209,210). Some have suggested that a systematic organized follow-up is as important as technological improvements in improving treatment success (211). Even simple interventions such as having a CPAP-help telephone number for the patient to call can improve compliance (212).

Common PAP treatment complaints include noise, inconvenience, dryness of the nose or mouth, nasal congestion, difficulty with the mask seal (or mask discomfort), claustrophobia, mouth leak, and difficulty in tolerating the pressure (see Table 18-4). Improvements in mask and machine design have been made in an attempt to reduce these problems (211). Excellent masks will not help if they are not properly fitted and if patients are not

properly instructed in how to apply them. It has become clear that objective monitoring of adherence is essential to really know how patients are doing with treatment. Many patients "overestimate" their use in an effort to appease the physician. Objective monitoring has suggested that the pattern of use is determined within the first few weeks of starting PAP (208). Early intervention for problems is essential. Most PAP machines can give mean use from run-time meter readings, and more sophisticated machines provide time at pressure and an electronic diary provides the pattern of use. Although neither bilevel pressure (196) nor APAP (197) has consistently increased adherence, these devices can be very useful in individual cases. They can often make the difference between failure and success in pressure-sensitive patients. Another option to improve CPAP acceptance in pressure-sensitive patients is the "ramp" system. Positive pressure slowly increases to the preset goal over a set time interval. This allows patients to fall asleep on lower pressures and increases their tolerance to higher pressures. Of note, humidification systems have also been introduced to reduce complaints of a dry upper airway and nasal congestion (213). Prevention of airway drying is also essential to reduce nasal congestion. Mouth leaks are a major cause of dryness in patients using nasal masks. A flow of air out the mouth causes a loss of humidity from the nose-mask system. This can result in increases in nasal resistance (214). Heated humidification is much more effective at delivering moisture to the airway than cold humidity units. Many PAP devices now have integrated heated humidifiers to improve convenience and portability. Significant nasal congestion should be aggressively treated with nasal steroids, nonsedating antihistamines, or decongestants as indicated. Many sleep centers begin treatment of nasal congestion before patients undergo the PAP titration. If nasal congestion is intractable, a full face mask can be used.

Treatment with PAP is very effective in rapidly reversing symptoms of EDS. A placebo-controlled study (ineffective versus effective CPAP) definitively proved that CPAP results in both subjective and objective improvements in EDS (215). The minimum nightly amount of time the device must be used to obtain benefit varies between patients. Some patients may benefit from as little as 4 hours, whereas others may require 6 more hours of sleep on treatment. One study suggested that patients receive little benefit from CPAP treatment unless they have symptoms (216). However, most have recommended treatment for moderate to severe OSA even if the patient is without significant symptoms to prevent potential cardiovascular complications. Current Medicare guidelines for CPAP reimbursement are an AHI of 5 to 14 per hour with associated symptoms (sleepiness, insomnia, impaired cognition, and mood disorders) or cardiovascular disease (hypertension, coronary artery disease, and previous cerebrovascular accident) or AHI of 15 or greater regardless of whether symptoms or associated diseases are present.

Persistent daytime sleepiness on positive airway pressure treatment. The practicing sleep physician is often presented with the difficult problem of how to evaluate a patient continuing to complain of daytime sleepiness after treatment with PAP. One must first consider problems with PAP treatment. These include lack of adherence, inadequate pressure, poor mask seal (therefore, inadequate pressure), mouth leak, or an inadequate sleep period (insufficient sleep). Objective adherence should be determined.

TABLE 18-4. Common Problems with Positive Airway Pressure (PAP) Treatment and Interventions

Problem	Intervention
Questionable adherence	Objective monitoring of compliance
	Education
	Involvement of spouse
	PAP telephone help line
Mask leak or discomfort	Change mask size or type
	Educate about proper mask placement
Claustrophobia	Nasal prongs or pillow mask
Nasal congestion	Heated humidity
	Medical treatment of nose (nasal steroids and decongestants)
Mouth leak	Heated humidity
	Chin strap
	Full face mask
	Lower pressure, bilevel PAP, APAP, CPAP with Cflex
Pressure intolerance	Ramp option
	Bilevel PAP
	APAP
	CPAP with Cflex
	Reduce pressure temporarily

PAP, positive airway pressure; APAP, auto-adjusting/auto-titrating positive airway pressure; CPAP, continuous positive airway pressure.

A history of snoring while on CPAP or recent weight gain suggests that a higher prescription pressure may be needed. The symptom of severe dryness especially while using heated humidity suggests a significant mouth leak. If none of the above explanations is likely, one must consider other sleep pathology including narcolepsy, the periodic limb movement disorder, or depression.

If narcolepsy is suspected, an all-night polysomnogram using CPAP and an MSLT (also using CPAP) should be performed. The polysomnogram would determine whether the prescribed level of CPAP was adequate. The MSLT will document that persistent daytime sleepiness is present and will allow a diagnosis of other disorders. For example, a diagnosis of narcolepsy would be supported if the polysomnogram documents adequate sleep (including a normal amount of REM sleep), but the MSLT meets the criteria for narcolepsy. In such cases, stimulant medications as well as nasal CPAP may be indicated.

In cases where the MSLT is not practical (patient does not want to stop taking antidepressant medicines) and when PAP treatment has been optimized (including documentation of good objective adherence), one might empirically add the alerting medication modafinil. Studies have indicated that the addition of modafinil 200 to 400 mg daily to PAP can improve daytime sleepiness (217,218) in patients on CPAP with persistent sleepiness. The major concern about this approach is that some patients may use their CPAP less and may therefore risk cardiovascular complications.

Central Sleep Apnea Syndromes and Cheyne-Stokes Breathing

A diagnosis of the CSA syndrome requires that a majority of apneas be central in nature (219,220). Usually, only 10% to 15% of sleep apnea patients in large series are classified as having CSA. One complicating factor is that CSA is a heterogeneous group of disorders, each having different clinical presentations and pathophysiology and requiring different therapy. In fact, the only common characteristic is apnea due to a loss of central respiratory drive during sleep. A convenient classification is to divide patients with CSA into groups with and without daytime CO_2 retention (219). The nonhypercapnic group is further divided into patients with idiopathic CSA and those with central sleep apnea and Cheyne-Stokes breathing (CSA–CSB).

HYPERCAPNIC CENTRAL SLEEP APNEA. Those patients with CSA and daytime hypoventilation usually have evidence of abnormalities in awake ventilatory control, neuromuscular weakness, or an abnormality in chest-wall compliance (kyphoscoliosis) (220). Defects in ventilatory control (central alveolar hypoventilation) may be primary (congenital) or secondary to brain-stem dysfunction (cerebrovascular infarction, neoplasm, or infection). Idiopathic congenital central hypoventilation ("Ondine curse") usually presents in infancy and usually requires life-long ventilatory support (221) during sleep. The patients can voluntarily increase alveolar ventilation but have reduced or absent ventilatory responses to hypercapnia and hypoxia. They are dependent on the wakefulness stimulus for respiration. Neuromuscular diseases include poliomyelitis (222), amyotrophic lateral sclerosis (223), diaphragmatic paralysis, and myopathies. These patients with CSA usually present with episodes of hypercapnic respiratory failure and cor pulmonale. Morning headaches and daytime sleepiness are common. Polysomnography reveals worsening hypoventilation during sleep and periods of central hypopnea and apnea. The degree of arterial oxygen desaturation tends to be rather severe, especially during REM sleep. In contrast, stages 3 and 4 of NREM sleep may be the time when the hypoventilation and oxygen desaturation are the most severe in patients with idiopathic congenital central hypoventilation and absent or defective metabolic control of ventilation.

The treatment of patients with hypercapnic CSA (see Table 18-5) depends on the underlying disease. In those with decreased ventilatory drive, respiratory stimulants can be tried but are rarely effective. Supplemental oxygen may prevent nocturnal desaturation and improve symptoms (224). A sleep study is required to demonstrate efficacy and to rule out a worsening of hypoventilation with oxygen therapy. If the respiratory muscles are intact, diaphragmatic pacing is effective in some patients with abnormal ventilatory drive. Negative-pressure ventilation (225) can also be attempted in patients with intact respiratory drive. Unfortunately, these last two modes of therapy frequently tend to induce OSA because respiratory efforts are not coordinated with increases in upper-airway tone.

Nocturnal positive-pressure ventilation (PPV) via a nasal or full face mask, oral interface, or tracheostomy is probably the most effective therapy (226,227) for hypercapnic CSA. If a mask is used, some positive end-expiratory pressure may be needed to maintain airway patency. In milder cases, mask bilevel PAP providing noninvasive pressure support ventilation may prove effective. Bilevel devices with backup rates are usually used because feeble efforts may not adequately trigger the devices, especially during REM sleep. In more severe cases, volume-cycled ventilation with a backup rate is usually required to ensure minimum minute ventilation. Mask ventilation requires that the patient should be alert, be able to mobilize secretions, and have intact reflexes to prevent aspiration. The current trend in management of patients with restrictive lung

TABLE 18-5. Possible Treatments for Central Sleep Apnea

1. Hypercapnic CSA
  Oxygen (selected cases)
  Diaphragmatic pacing (selected cases)
  Negative pressure ventilation
    Cuirass
    Body wrap
  Mask bilevel positive airway pressure
  Volume-cycled ventilation (via mask or tracheostomy)

2. Nonhypercapnic CSA
  A. Idiopathic CSA
    Hypnotics (possibly)
    Acetazolamide
    Nasal CPAP
  B. CSA with Cheyne-Stokes Breathing (CHF)
    Optimize CHF therapy
    Nasal CPAP
    Oxygen

CSA, central sleep apnea; CHF, congestive heart failure; CPAP, continuous positive airway pressure.

diseases is to intervene earlier with the hope of avoiding emergent tracheostomy. Acute worsening of respiratory failure is common with pneumonia. A consensus conference (228) listed the following indications for initiation of nocturnal PAP treatment: (a) symptoms including nocturnal dyspnea and a morning headache, (b) a daytime P_{CO_2} ≥45 mm Hg, or nocturnal oximetry demonstrating 5 consecutive minutes with an arterial oxygen saturation 88%, or (c) progressive neuromuscular disease (maximal inspiratory pressure <60 cm H_2O or forced vital capacity (FVC) <50% of predicted).

NONHYPERCAPNIC CENTRAL SLEEP APNEA. The second group of patients with CSA has a normal or low daytime P_{CO_2}. They manifest central apnea when their P_{CO_2} level falls below a level required to trigger ventilation during sleep. This "apneic threshold" varies between individuals but is usually 0 to 2 mm Hg above the resting *awake* P_{CO_2} level (116). These patients may present with complaints of disturbed sleep (awakenings and choking), insomnia, or EDS. Cor pulmonale and polycythemia are usually not present. This group can be further divided into those with idiopathic CSA and those with CSA associated with CSB (CSA–CSB).

In CSB, there is a crescendo–decrescendo pattern of breathing (tidal volume and ventilatory drive), with central hypopnea or apnea at the nadir in ventilatory drive (see Fig. 18-11). If arousal occurs after apnea in CSB, it is usually several breaths after event termination during maximal ventilatory effort. The delay in the nadir in SaO_2 following apnea termination is quite long in CSA–CSB associated with congestive heart failure (CHF). In addition, the ventilatory period between apneas tends to be long and correlates with the circulation time. In idiopathic CSA, there is an abrupt resumption of ventilatory effort at apnea termination, usually associated with an arousal. If repetitive central apneas occur, the periods of ventilation between the apneas tend to be much shorter than in CSA–CSB.

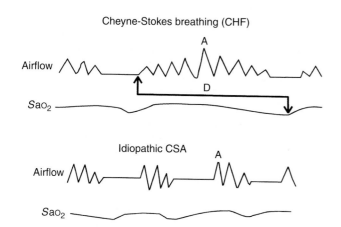

FIGURE 18-11. A schematic illustrating differences in the patterns of idiopathic central sleep apnea and central apnea associated with Cheyne-Stokes breathing (CSB) secondary to congestive heart failure. (*A*) marks the typical position of arousal and (*D*) illustrates the long delay between apnea termination and the nadir in arterial oxygen saturation (SaO_2) that occurs in CSB associated with heart failure. (From Berry RB. *Sleep Medicine Pearls*, 2nd edition. Philadelphia: Hanley & Belfus, 2003, with permission.)

IDIOPATHIC CENTRAL SLEEP APNEA. Patients with this uncommon disorder are usually men (219) and are generally less obese than patients with OSA. Complaints of insomnia may be more prominent in these cases than in typical OSA. Polysomnography shows central apnea usually in stage 1 or 2 sleep, often following arousals and awakenings. The associated desaturations are usually modest in severity, but the frequent arousals can cause severe sleep fragmentation. This group tends to have daytime hypocapnia and increased hypercapnic ventilatory responses (229). The sleeping P_{CO_2} also tends to be low and is believed to be close to the apneic threshold. Therefore, even slight increases in ventilation (and reductions in P_{CO_2}) may result in central apnea. Arousal plays an important role in initiating or perpetuating central apnea in these patients (230). Arousals precipitating apnea are typically associated with one or more large tidal volumes that lower the P_{CO_2} and increase the tendency for central apnea on the subsequent return to sleep. Indeed, arousal due to any cause may trigger a subsequent series of central apnea–arousal–central apnea events.

Several treatments have been tried for idiopathic CSA (Table 18-5). Some have suggested that sedatives might be efficacious in this specific group of CSA patients by reducing arousal or minimizing the increase in ventilation associated with arousal. In fact, a small study found that the benzodiazepine hypnotic triazolam was of modest benefit (231). Acetazolamide (Diamox) 250 mg given 1 hour before bedtime also proved effective in a group of patients with nonhypercapnic CSA, presumably by inducing metabolic acidosis (232). Application of a high flow of gas with increased CO_2 or increasing dead space also prevented central apnea in another study of patients with idiopathic CSA, presumably by raising the waking or sleeping P_{CO_2} (233). However, neither of these measures is clinically feasible. Two studies found that nasal CPAP was efficacious in groups of patients with idiopathic CSA (234,235). There are two explanations for the efficacy of nasal CPAP in this disorder: (a) CPAP prevents airway collapse and subsequent reflex central apnea and (b) nasal CPAP is an expiratory load and induces mild increases in P_{CO_2}. Further evidence for the concept that upper-airway collapse may be triggering central apnea in these patients is the observation that some patients develop central apnea only in the supine sleeping position. At present, there is little data about the long-term efficacy of any of the treatments listed above for this relatively rare group of patients. Treatment must be individualized. If medication is prescribed, a sleep study should document efficacy.

CENTRAL SLEEP APNEA WITH CHEYNE-STOKES BREATHING. The causes of CSA associated with CSB include CHF (236) and neurologic insults (237). Indeed, CSB secondary to CHF is the most common cause of CSA, with up to 40% of CHF patients having significant sleep-disordered breathing. CSB is more common during sleep stages 1 and 2. Patients with CSB have an underlying instability in ventilatory control, with oscillations in ventilation. Central hypopnea or apnea occurs when the P_{CO_2} approaches or falls below the apneic threshold. Instability is more likely with high controller gain (high ventilatory drive), feedback delay (increased circulation time), or an underdamped system (238). The traditional explanation for CSB in patients with heart failure was an increase in circulation time (low cardiac output) producing feedback delay in ventilatory control. However, one study found no difference in left ventricular ejection fraction or circulation time between groups of CHF patients with and without CSB (239). The major difference between the groups was that the patients with CSB had a lower daytime and sleeping P_{CO_2}. Patients with CSB associated with CHF also have a lower than normal increase in their arterial P_{CO_2} during NREM sleep (240) and a smaller difference between the apneic threshold and the sleeping P_{CO_2}. Having a sleeping arterial P_{CO_2} near the apneic threshold causes an instability in ventilatory control (241). Patients with CSA–CSB also tend to have higher central (242,243) and peripheral (243) ventilatory responses to CO_2. The higher ventilatory responses also tend to destabilize breathing. The reason for the lower sleeping P_{CO_2} and the higher ventilatory responses is not known but could be related to pulmonary congestion, with stimulation of breathing by reflex mechanisms. Lorenzi-Filho et al. (244) found that there was a significant and inverse correlation between the pulmonary wedge pressure and the P_{CO_2} (higher wedge associated with a lower P_{CO_2}) in heart failure patients. In another study, Solin et al. found that a higher wedge pressure was associated with a higher frequency of central apneas (245).

Several studies have looked at groups of patients with CHF to determine predictors of the presence of CSA–CSB. Blackshear et al. found that the presence of symptoms of nocturnal dyspnea or the presence of atrial fibrillation made CSB more likely (246). Sin et al. found that the risk for CSA–CSB was increased by the male gender, atrial fibrillation, and hypocapnia (247). CSA–CSB usually results in periodic desaturations during sleep and sleep disturbance (arousals). Patients may complain of daytime sleepiness, and the hypoxemia and arousals associated with CSB may cause recurrent activation of the sympathetic nervous system. Thus, CSB may have long-term adverse effects on cardiac function (248,249). Indeed, if CSA–CSB is present in a patient with CHF this implies a worse prognosis (248,249).

A number of treatments have been tried for CSA–CSB, with most studies performed in patients with heart failure. In CSA–CSB secondary to neurologic insults, supplemental oxygen or theophylline has been reported to be effective (237). Possible treatments for CSA–CSB secondary to CHF are listed in Table 18-5. Optimizing medical treatment of heart failure is the first and an important initial step. If cardiac function improves, this alone may reduce the amount of CSB (245). Studies have also shown that the amount of CSB can be reduced and oxygenation can be improved in patients with CHF using theophylline (250), supplemental oxygen (251,252), and nasal CPAP (252,254). However, the potential for exacerbating arrhythmias has limited the use of theophylline. Although oxygen can usually prevent desaturation, some patients will continue to have some CSB and sleep disturbance. The acute application of nasal CPAP may abolish CSB in a few patients; however, most will continue to have CSB. The full benefits of nasal CPAP treatment may take several weeks. Thus, a single night of pressure titration will usually not identify an "optimal level" of CPAP. One approach is to increase the level of nasal CPAP to around 10 to 12 cm H_2O as tolerated over several nights if necessary. When a group of patients with CSB secondary to heart failure was studied for 3 months comparing CPAP using this approach with standard medical therapy, the frequency of central apnea and hypopnea fell from 43 to 15 events per hour, and both the left ventricular ejection fraction

and symptoms of heart failure improved in the treatment group (253). Nasal CPAP is believed to improve CSB by reducing hypoxemia, inducing an increase in P_{CO_2}, and improving cardiac function. The improvement in cardiac function is thought to be secondary to reductions in nocturnal sympathetic activity, improvements in oxygenation, and afterload reduction during nightly CPAP use (236). Unfortunately, not all patients with CSB and CHF may benefit or tolerate nasal CPAP long enough for it to improve CSA–CSB (254). Adaptive pressure support servoventilation (ASV) is a new treatment modality that "adapts" to CSB by providing low levels of pressure support when ventilation is high and high levels of pressure support when ventilation is low. A recent study compared one night of treatment with ASV, CPAP, and bilevel PAP with a backup rate with a control night. The AHI was lowered from a baseline of 44.5 per hour to 6.3 per hour on ASV, to 28.2 per hour on oxygen, to 26.8 per hour on CPAP, and to 14.8 per hour on bilevel pressure (252). ASV appears to lower the AHI more rapidly and effectively than the other treatments do. However, ASV is currently not available for routine clinical use.

Sin et al. conducted a randomized controlled trial of CPAP versus standard therapy in a group of patients with severe CHF (with and without CSA–CSB). Nasal CPAP improved the cardiac function only in those with CSA–CSB. In addition, transplant-free survival was improved in those who complied with CPAP treatment (255). A larger trial is under way to determine whether the survival benefits can be confirmed (256). In the absence of long-term studies showing the superiority of any one treatment for CSB, the physician should treat each case on an individual basis, with a sleep study to document efficacy. Most physicians would use PAP as the first-line treatment, with oxygen for those not tolerating positive pressure.

SLEEP AND CONGESTIVE HEART FAILURE

It is important for physicians to recognize that patients with CHF may have significant sleep-disordered breathing and arterial oxygen desaturations during sleep in the absence of daytime hypoxemia. One study found that almost 50% of patients with stable CHF had an AHI of more than 20 per hour (257). Complaints of poor nocturnal sleep, frequent awakening, and daytime sleepiness may be erroneously assumed to be due to CHF alone. Sleep-disordered breathing may occur in CHF patients as (a) OSA, (b) CSA with CSB, and (c) a combination of OSA and CSB (258).

Patients with heart failure and CSB may sometimes be mistakenly thought to have typical OSA. They may complain of daytime sleepiness and exhibit mixed obstructive apnea. If underlying CSB is not recognized, the sudden appearance of central apnea of the Cheyne-Stokes type during CPAP titration may be quite confusing. These patients have upper-airway closure during the waxing period of respiratory effort in CSB. When nasal CPAP prevents upper-airway closure, a traditional pattern of CSA–CSB may emerge (see Fig. 18-12). However, unlike typical mixed obstructive apnea, repetitive central apneas usually persist once upper-airway obstruction has been prevented. Four clues for the presence of CSB in the setting of mixed apnea (see Fig. 18-13) are that the (a) maximal breaths tend to occur several breaths after the apnea is terminated, (b) the ventilatory phase between apneas may be

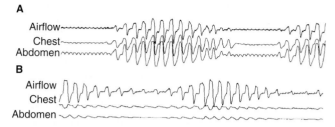

A

Airflow
Chest
Abdomen

B

Airflow
Chest
Abdomen

FIGURE 18-12. Two 90-second tracings of different patients during a continuous positive airway pressure (CPAP) titration for what was assumed to be obstructive sleep apnea (OSA). In tracing **(A)**, Cheyne-Stokes breathing with central apneas is noted. The small deflections in the chest and abdomen tracings are from cardiac pulsations. In tracing **(B)**, central hypopnea rather than central apnea is noted. The reduction in flow is proportional to changes in chest or abdominal movements, and the flow profile is rounded, as is typical of a central hypopnea. In neither case did the patient desaturate from these events. Higher levels of CPAP did not abolish these events. However, breathing stabilized once both patients entered stage 3 and 4 sleep.

long and have a crescendo–decrescendo pattern, (c) the central portion of the mixed apnea is long, and (d) the nadir in oxygen saturation is markedly delayed (increased circulation time). Recognition that CSB (as well as obstructive apnea) is present may direct attention to better treatment of CHF. In addition, the end point of nasal CPAP treatment may be unclear as central apnea typically persists even with further increases in CPAP. In such cases, an empiric approach is to treat with nasal CPAP at a level around 10 to 12 cm H_2O (as outlined above) unless a higher CPAP level is needed to prevent airway obstruction.

One uncontrolled (259) and one controlled (260) study of patients with systolic heart failure and typical OSA demonstrated improvements in sleep quality, nocturnal oxygen saturation, and left ventricular function ejection during wakefulness. In the controlled study, there was also a reduction in daytime blood pressure and heart rate. The mechanisms by which nighttime nasal CPAP improves daytime cardiac function may include decreased activation of the sympathetic nervous system and decreased cardiac work during sleep (261). Thus, treatment of obstructive apnea as well as CSA–CSB in patients with CHF many benefit cardiac function as well as improve sleep quality.

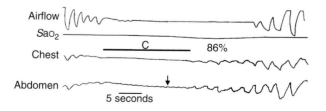

Airflow
Sao_2
Chest
Abdomen

C   86%

5 seconds

FIGURE 18-13. A mixed apnea in a patient with a cardiomyopathy and Cheyne-Stokes breathing (CSB). The nadir in arterial oxygen saturation shown here *precedes* apnea termination. This desaturation was actually related to the previous event. The long delay in the nadir in saturation is caused by a long circulation time. The central portion of the mixed apnea is marked by C. The small deflections in this portion (*arrow*) are secondary to cardiac pulsations.

SLEEP AND ASTHMA

Nocturnal asthma is a significant problem for both asthmatic patients and their physicians. In a large survey of asthmatics, 74% responded that they awoke from sleep at least one night each week with symptoms of asthma, and 40% reported symptoms every night (262). There is controversy about whether nocturnal asthma is a distinct entity or simply a marker for more severe asthma. Even in normal persons, there is a circadian rhythm in airway function, with the best pulmonary function at 4:00 PM and the worst at 4:00 AM (5% to 10% fluctuation in the FEV_1). This fluctuation in airway function is even more dramatic (>15%) in many asthmatics. In patients with nocturnal asthma, the FEV_1 or peak flow can fall by as much as 20% to 40% in the morning hours ("morning dippers"). Studies of the effects of sleep on asthma must also consider the effects of the 24-hour clock as well as those of recumbency. However, it appears that sleep induces an independent worsening of lung function, although no sleep stage–specific effects have been documented (263). Arterial oxygen desaturation is usually mild and is most severe during REM sleep. Polysomnography is not indicated unless sleep apnea is suspected. The simplest way to document a patient's predisposition for nocturnal asthma is to have the patient record a peak expiratory flow rate (PEFR) at bedtime, during nocturnal awakening, and in the morning.

The etiology of the nocturnal worsening of asthma is multifactorial (264) and may include nocturnal falls in circulating epinephrine and corticosteroids and increases in histamine, vagal tone, and, possibly, increased leukotriene synthesis. In patients with nocturnal asthma, the β-adrenergic receptor function decreases at night. Studies have found a significant increase in neutrophils and eosinophils in the bronchoalveolar lavage (BAL) fluid (265) and increased eosinophils and macrophages in alveolar tissue by transbronchial biopsy (266) in patients with nocturnal asthma at 4:00 AM compared to 4:00 PM but not in asthmatics without nocturnal asthma. In contrast, Oosterhoff et al. did not find a circadian variation in lymphocytes in BAL fluid in asthmatics with a nocturnal worsening of lung function (267). Systemic steroids will reduce the nocturnal fall in lung function in asthmatics with nocturnal worsening but may not normalize the circadian variation in lung function (268). Oral prednisone at 3:00 PM was more effective at preventing the fall in the FEV_1 in nocturnal asthma than doses at 8:00 AM or 8:00 PM (269). In addition, only oral steroids dosed at 3:00 PM reduced eosinophils and macrophages cells in the BAL fluid (269).

Treatment of patients with nocturnal asthma should begin with inhaled corticosteroids (270). This medication has been shown to reduce the circadian fluctuation in airway tone. Patients with continued nocturnal symptoms despite an adequate dose of inhaled corticosteroids can then be treated with a long-acting bronchodilator. The ideal long-term bronchodilator would be one that does not disturb sleep. Salmeterol or formoterol, long-acting inhaled β-agonists, may be particularly useful in patients with nocturnal asthma. These medications could conceivably cause less central nervous system stimulation than oral sustained-action theophylline does. However, Selby et al. (271) found only a slight advantage for salmeterol compared to theophylline in sleep quality (fewer arousals). The falls in morning flow rates were similar but awakenings were less frequent on salmeterol. There was no difference in patient preference. Wiegand et al. (272) found salmeterol to be more effective than theophylline in preventing the morning drop in flow rates. The drugs did not differ in polysomnographic findings but patients perceived better sleep with salmeterol than with theophylline. Whereas tolerance to the side effects of theophylline may develop in many patients, others may sleep better with salmeterol. If theophylline is used, the dosing should be arranged so that maximum serum levels occur at night (264). Long-acting oral β-agonists are also of potential benefit but also have the potential for sleep disturbance (273). Although asthmatics generally have a greater response to β-agonists than to anticholinergic medications, vagal tone is increased at night. Therefore, anticholinergics such as ipratropium bromide are of potential benefit in nocturnal asthma (274). There is also some preliminary evidence that medications blocking the synthesis or action of leukotrienes may benefit many patients with nocturnal asthma (275,276).

If an asthmatic patient has OSA, nasal CPAP may actually reduce asthmatic attacks (277). Snoring and recurrent upper-airway obstruction may be the triggering mechanisms in these patients. There has also been evidence that nocturnal gastroesophageal reflux (GER) may play a role in worsening of asthma in some patients (278,279). Some uncontrolled studies have shown that aggressive treatment of GER can be of benefit in asthma (280). However, a systematic review of published studies did not find enough evidence to conclude that treatment of GER definitely improves asthma in unselected patients (281). A 2- to 3-month trial of aggressive treatment of GER in individual symptomatic patients with uncontrolled nocturnal asthma and GER could be considered.

SLEEP AND CHRONIC OBSTRUCTIVE PULMONARY DISEASE

Some patients with COPD may have nocturnal desaturation without the cyclic apnea–desaturation–arousal pattern common in OSA. In contrast to the "sawtooth" pattern of desaturations on oximetry in OSA patients, a typical pattern of nocturnal SaO_2 in a COPD patient (282) includes (a) a fall in the baseline SaO_2 on transition from wakefulness to sleep, (b) small transient fluctuations in oxygen saturation (3% to 5%) during NREM sleep, and (c) larger drops in saturation during REM sleep (10% to 50%) that may last from several minutes to a half hour or more. One should recall that even normal persons have a small fall in PO_2 during sleep but, due to their position on the flat portion of the oxyhemoglobin saturation curve, little desaturation occurs. Conversely, patients with an awake PO_2 in the 55 to 60 mm Hg range (the steep portion of the curve) will have significant desaturation from small falls in PO_2. It appears that in some COPD patients, the fall in PO_2 with sleep is within the normal range (283), but desaturation is worse because of a lower baseline PO_2. Patients with CO_2 retention or low awake PO_2 are more likely to exhibit severe desaturation (283,284).

The episodes of profound desaturation during stage REM are usually associated with periods of hypopnea in which tidal volume is reduced but respiratory rate is essentially unchanged

(285). There is a reduction in pleural pressure swings in most cases, implying a reduction in central drive. The reduction in minute ventilation during hypopneas is thought to lead to alveolar hypoventilation, with a resulting increase in PCO_2 and fall in PO_2. Some evidence (286) suggests that increases in ventilation–perfusion mismatch may also contribute to the dramatic REM-associated falls in the oxygen saturation.

The benefits of chronic 24-hour oxygen therapy in patients with COPD have been well documented by the Nocturnal Oxygen Treatment Trial (NOTT) (287) and other studies of patients breathing room air and meeting the standard criteria of a daytime PO_2 <55 mm Hg. The value of 55 mm Hg was chosen because below this point pulmonary arterial pressure starts to increase significantly secondary to hypoxic vasoconstriction. In the NOTT study, patients also received oxygen if the PO_2 was 55 to 59 mm Hg and if evidence of end-organ damage was present (pedal edema, hematocrit >55%, or P pulmonale on ECG). The indication for nocturnal oxygen in patients with a daytime PO_2 >60 mm Hg but with nocturnal arterial oxygen desaturation has not been established (288). In such patients, nocturnal desaturation occurs most commonly in REM sleep. Although REM sleep desaturation may be severe, the total duration of this type of desaturation typically lasts less than an hour per night. Is treatment of this type of desaturation beneficial?

Nocturnal supplemental oxygen or room air was administered in a double-blind manner to a group of COPD patients with daytime PO_2 above 60 mm Hg and with documented REM sleep desaturation. At 3 years, the oxygen group showed nearly a 4 mm Hg decrease in daytime mean pulmonary pressure, whereas the room air group showed about a 4 mm Hg rise (288). However, no study has documented that supplemental nocturnal oxygen will decrease mortality or morbidity in the group of patients with nocturnal desaturations confined to REM sleep (289).

Until the clinical importance of isolated nocturnal desaturation in patients with COPD is clarified, widespread sleep monitoring in COPD patients cannot be justified unless OSA is suspected. Nocturnal oximetry should be considered if a patient with COPD has (a) unexplained daytime PCO_2 retention (FEV_1 >40% of predicted) or (b) when significant cor pulmonale is not explained by daytime arterial blood gas analysis (PO_2 >60 mm Hg). If a sawtooth pattern is present, a full sleep study should be ordered. Even if greater than expected nocturnal desaturation is found without evidence of OSA, no firm guidelines exist concerning the amount of desaturation required to justify nocturnal administration of oxygen. One might consider nocturnal oxygen treatment of patients with evidence of cor pulmonale and a sleeping SaO_2 below 85% for most of the night (low SaO_2 in NREM as well as REM sleep). This recommendation assumes that the other medical treatment for COPD has been optimized and that significant sleep apnea is not present. Nocturnal low-flow oxygen therapy prevents the episodes of nonapneic desaturation associated with COPD without markedly increasing the PCO_2 (190). The exception is COPD patients with significant OSA in whom large increases in PCO_2 may occur. Giving such patients oxygen alone may increase apnea duration, incompletely reverse desaturation, and may result in large increases in nocturnal PCO_2. The treatment of the overlap syndrome is discussed below.

Patients with COPD often have multiple sleep complaints such as insomnia (difficulty in initiating or maintaining sleep) and frequent awakenings with shortness of breath or cough. The sleep quality in patients with significant COPD is frequently poor. A shortened TST, low sleep efficiency, and frequent arousals are common. Like asthmatics, the diurnal variation in pulmonary function may be exaggerated in these patients, and many patients have the greatest difficulty breathing in the early morning hours. There are conflicting data on whether the sleep quality of patients with COPD is improved by oxygen therapy (290,291). As with asthmatics, bronchodilators, while improving lung function, could potentially worsen sleep quality due to central stimulation. However, in one study, sustained-action theophylline improved early-morning spirometry and the oxygen saturation in NREM sleep without impairing sleep quality (292). If patients do complain of sleep disturbance with theophylline, the long-acting inhaled β-agonist salmeterol may be better tolerated. Inhaled ipratropium bromide at bedtime has also been shown to be useful in COPD (293), and the only problem with this medication is its relatively short duration of action. The new long-acting anticholinergic medication tiotropium may be especially helpful.

Many patients with COPD request hypnotics to improve sleep quality. The benzodiazepine triazolam (294) and the non-benzodiazepine zolpidem (295) both appear to increase sleep length without significantly worsening oxygenation. Caution is still advised. Sedatives of any type are contraindicated in hypercapnic or unstable patients.

The group of patients with both COPD and OSA (overlap syndrome) tend to have more severe cardiopulmonary sequelae than those with equivalent amounts of sleep apnea (296). Furthermore, these patients may continue to have impressive nocturnal desaturation during REM sleep even after treatment of obstructive apnea with tracheostomy or nasal CPAP (297). Alternatively, oxygen alone rarely completely reverses the hypoxemia and may lead to considerable CO_2 retention and morning headache, as noted above (190). The best approach is to treat the OSA with nasal bilevel pressure or CPAP and then add oxygen as needed if nocturnal desaturation persists even though airway patency during sleep is restored (298).

REFERENCES

1. Rechtschaffen A, Kales A, eds. *A manual of standardized terminology techniques and scoring system for sleep stages of human sleep.* Los Angeles: Brain Information Service/Brain Research Institute, UCLA, 1968.
2. Williams RL, Karacan I, Hursch CJ. *Electroencephalography (EEG) of human sleep: clinical applications.* New York: John Wiley and Sons, 1974.
3. Carskadon MA, Rechtschaffen A. Monitoring and staging human sleep. In: Kryger MH, Roth T, Dement WC, eds. *Principles and practice of sleep medicine,* 3rd ed. Philadelphia: WB Saunders, 2000:1197–1215.
4. West P, Kryger MH. Sleep and respiration: terminology and methodology. *Clin Chest Med* 1985;4:691–712.
5. Berry RB. *Sleep medicine pearls,* 2nd ed. Philadelphia: Hanley & Belfus, 2003.
6. ASDA Task Force. EEG arousals: Scoring rules and examples. *Sleep* 1992;15:173–184.
7. Downey R, Bonnet MH. Performance during frequent sleep disruption. *Sleep* 1987;10:354–363.
8. Mathur R, Douglas NJ. Frequency of EEG arousals from nocturnal sleep in normal subjects. *Sleep* 1995;18:330–333.
9. Guilleminault C, Stoohs R, Clerk A, et al. Cause of excessive daytime sleepiness: the upper airway resistance syndrome. *Chest* 1993;104:781–787.
10. Phillipson EA. Control of breathing during sleep. *Am Rev Respir Dis* 1978;118:909–937.
11. Douglas NJ. Control of ventilation during sleep. *Clin Chest Med* 1985;6:563–575.
12. Phillipson EA. Sleep disorders. In: Murray JF, Nadel JA, eds. *Textbook of respiratory medicine.* Philadelphia: WB Saunders, 1994: 2301–2324.
13. Krieger J. Breathing during sleep in normal subjects. *Clin Chest Med* 1985;6:577–594.
14. Hudgel DW, Martin RJ, Johnson B, et al. Mechanics of the respiratory system and breathing pattern during sleep in normal humans. *J Appl Physiol* 1984;56:1–137.
15. Hudgel DW, Devadatta P. Decrease in functional residual capacity during sleep in normal humans. *J Appl Physiol* 1984;57: 1319–1322.
16. Tabachnik E, Muller NL, Bryan AC, et al. Changes in ventilation and chest wall mechanics during sleep in normal adolescents. *J Appl Physiol* 1981;51:557–564.
17. Neilly JB, Gaipa EA, Maislin G, et al. Ventilation during early and late rapid-eye-movement sleep in normal humans. *J Appl Physiol* 1991;71:1201–1215.
18. Gould GA, Gugger M, Molloy J, et al. Breathing pattern and eye movement density during REM sleep in humans. *Am Rev Respir Dis* 1988;138:874–877.
19. Wiegand L, Zwillich CW, Wiegand D, et al. Changes in upper airway muscle activation and ventilation during phasic REM sleep in normal men. *J Appl Physiol* 1991;71:488–497.
20. Horner RL. Motor control of pharyngeal musculature and implications for the pathogenesis of obstructive sleep apnea. *Sleep* 1996;19:827–853.
21. Badr MS. Pathophysiology of upper airway obstruction during sleep. *Clin Chest Med* 1998;19:21–32.
22. Horner RL, Innes JA, Murphy K, et al. Evidence for reflex upper airway dilatory muscle activation by sudden negative airway pressure in man. *J Physiol (London)* 1991;436:15–29.
23. Horner RL, Innes JA, Morrell MJ, et al. The effect of sleep on reflex genioglossus muscle activation by stimuli of negative airway pressure in humans. *J Physiol (London)* 1994;476:141–151.
24. Wheatley JR, Tangel DJ, Mezzanotte WS, et al. Influence of sleep on response to negative airway pressure of tensor palatini muscle and retropalatal airway. *J Appl Physiol* 1993;75:2117–2124.
25. Tangel DJ, Mezzanotte WS, Sandberg EJ, et al. Influences of NREM sleep on the activity of tonic versus inspiratory phasic muscles in normal men. *J Appl Physiol* 1992;73:1058–1066.
26. Malhotra A, Pillar G, Fogel RB, et al. Genioglossal but not palatal muscle activity relates closely to pharyngeal pressure. *Am J Respir Crit Care Med* 2000;162:1058–1062.
27. Pillar G, Malhotra A, Fogel RB, et al. Upper airway muscle responsiveness to rising P_{CO_2} during NREM sleep. *J Appl Physiol* 2000;89:1275–1282.
28. Berry RB, McNellis M, Kouchi K, et al. Upper airway anesthesia reduces genioglossus activity during sleep apnea. *Am J Respir Crit Care Med* 1997;156:127–132.
29. Schwab RJ. Upper airway imaging. *Clin Chest Med* 1998;19:33–54.
30. Van de Graaff WB. Thoracic influence on upper airway patency. *J Appl Physiol* 1988;65:2124–2131.
31. Hoffstein V, Zamel N, Phillipson EA. Lung volume dependence of cross-sectional area in patients with obstructive sleep apnea. *Am Rev Respir Dis* 1984;130:175–178.
32. Schwab RJ, Gefter WB, Hoffman EA, et al. Dynamic upper airway imaging during wake respiration in normal subjects and patients with sleep disordered breathing. *Am Rev Respir Dis* 1993; 148:1385–1400.
33. Block AJ, Boysen PG, Wynne JW, et al. Sleep apnea, hypopnea, and oxygen desaturation in normal subjects. A strong male predominance. *N Engl J Med* 1979;300:513–517.

34. Gould GA, Whyte KF, Rhind GB, et al. The sleep hypopnea syndrome. *Am Rev Respir Dis* 1988;137:895–898.
35. Redline S, Kapur VK, Sanders MH, et al. Effects of varying approaches for identifying respiratory disturbances on sleep apnea assessment. *Am J Respir Crit Care Med* 2000;161:369–374.
36. Redline S, Sander M. Hypopnea, a floating metric: implications for prevalence, morbidity estimates, and case finding. *Sleep* 1997; 20:1209–1217.
37. American Academy of Sleep Medicine Task Force. Sleep-related breathing disorders in adults: Recommendation for syndrome definition and measurement techniques in clinical research. *Sleep* 1999;22:667–689,
38. Meoli AL, Casey KR, Clark RW, Clinical Practice Review Committee-AASM. Hypopnea in sleep disordered breathing in adults. *Sleep* 2001;24:469–470.
39. Whitney C, Gottleib DJ, Redline S, et al. Reliability of scoring respiratory disturbance indices and sleep staging. *Sleep* 1998;21: 749–757.
40. Drinnan MJ, Murray A, Griffiths CJ, et al. Interobserver variability in recognizing arousal in respiratory sleep disorders. *Am J Respir Crit Care Med* 1998;15:358–362.
41. Shahar E, Whitney CW, Redline S, et al. Sleep-disordered breathing and cardiovascular disease: cross-sectional results of the Sleep Heart Health Study. *Am J Respir Crit Care Med* 2001;163: 19–25.
42. Berry RB. Nasal and esophageal pressure monitoring. In: Lee-Chiong TL, Sateia MJ, Caraskadon MA, eds. *Sleep medicine.* Philadelphia: Hanley and Belfus, 2002:661–671.
43. Hosselet J, Norman RC, Ayappa I, et al. Detection of flow limitation with nasal cannula/pressure transducer system. *Am J Respir Crit Care Med* 1998;157:1461–1467.
44. Aappa I, Norman RG, Krieger AC, et al. Non-invasive detection of respiratory effort related arousals (RERAs) by a nasal cannula/pressure transducer system. *Sleep* 2000;23:763–771.
45. Loube DI, Gay PC, Strohl KP, et al. Indications for positive airway pressure treatment of adult obstructive sleep apnea patients. A consensus statement. *Chest* 1999;115:863–866.
46. Norman RG, Ahmed MM, Walsleben JA, et al. Detection of respiratory events during NPSG: Nasal cannula/pressure sensor versus thermistor. *Sleep* 1997;20:1175–1184.
47. Monserrat JP, Farré R, Ballester E, et al. Evaluation of nasal prongs for estimating nasal flow. *Am J Respir Crit Care Med* 1997; 155:211–215.
48. Staats BA, Bonekat HW, Harris CD, et al. Chest wall motion in sleep apnea. *Am Rev Respir Dis* 1984;130:59–63.
49. Tobin MJ, Cohn MA, Sackner MA. Breathing abnormalities during sleep. *Arch Intern Med* 1983;143:1221–1228.
50. ASDA Atlas Task Force. Recording and scoring leg movements. *Sleep* 1993;16:749–759.
51. American Sleep Disorders Association. The clinical use of the multiple sleep latency test. *Sleep* 1992;15:268–276.
52. Aldrich MS, Chervin RD, Malow BA. Value of the multiple sleep latency test for the diagnosis of narcolepsy. *Sleep* 1997;20:620–629.
53. Rosenthal L, Roehrs TA, Rosen A, et al. Level of sleepiness and total sleep time following various time in bed conditions. *Sleep* 1993;16:226–232.
54. Chervin RD, Aldrich MS. Sleep onset REM periods during multiple sleep latency tests in patients evaluated for sleep apnea. *Am J Respir Crit Care Med* 2000;161:426–431.
55. Doghramji K, Mitler MM, Sangal RB, et al. A normative study of the maintenance of wakefulness test (MWT). *Electroencephalogr Clin Neurophysiol* 1997;103:554–562.
56. Sangal RB, Thomas L, Mitler MM. Maintenance of wakefulness test and multiple sleep latency test. *Chest* 1992;101:898–902.
57. Douglas NJ. "Why am I sleepy": sorting the somnolent. *Am J Respir Crit Care Med* 2001;163:1310–1313.
58. Punjabi NM, Welch D, Strohl K. Sleep disorders in regional sleep centers: a national cooperative study. Coleman II Study Investigators. *Sleep* 2000;23:471–480.
59. Johns MW. Daytime sleepiness, snoring, and obstructive sleep apnea. The Epworth Sleepiness Scale. *Chest* 1993;103:30–36.
60. Scammel TE. The neurobiology, diagnosis, and treatment of narcolepsy. *Ann Neurol* 2003;53:154–166.
61. Aldrich MS. The clinical spectrum of narcolepsy and idiopathic hypersomnia. *Neurology* 1996;46:383–401.
62. Thannickal T, Moore RY, Nienbus R, et al. Reduced number of hypocretin neurons in human narcolepsy. *Neuron* 2000;27:469–474.
63. Taheri S, Zeitzer JM, Mignot E. The role of hypocretins (orexins) in sleep regulation and narcolepsy. *Annu Rev Neurosci* 2002; 25:283–313.
64. Mignot E, Lammers GJ, Ripley MS, et al. The role of cerebrospinal fluid hypocretin measurement in the diagnosis of narcolepsy and other hypersomnias. *Arch Neurol* 2002;59:1553–1562.
65. Mignot E, Hayduk R, Black J, et al. HLA DQB1*0602 is associated with cataplexy in 509 narcoleptic patients. *Sleep* 1997;20: 1012–1020.
66. Mignot E, Lin X, Arrigoni J, et al. DQB1*0602 and DQA1*0102 are better markers than DR2 for narcolepsy in Caucasians and African-Americans. *Sleep* 1994;17:60–67.
67. Mignot E. Genetic and familial aspects of narcolepsy. *Neurology* 1998;50(Suppl.1):S16–S22.
68. Mitler M, Aldrich MS, Koob GF, et al. ASDA standards of practice: narcolepsy and its treatment with stimulants. *Sleep* 1994;17:352–371.
69. US Modafinil in Narcolepsy Study Group. Randomized trial of modafinil as a treatment for the excessive daytime somnolence of narcolepsy. *Neurology* 2000; 53:1166–1175.
70. The US Xyrem Multicenter Study Group. A randomized, double-blind, placebo-controlled multicenter trial comparing the effects of three doses of orally administered sodium oxybate with placebo for the treatment of narcolepsy (cataplexy). *Sleep* 2003;25:42–49.
71. American Sleep Disorders Association. *International classification of sleep disorders: diagnostic and coding manual.* Rochester: American Sleep Disorders Association, 1997:46–49.
72. Bassetti C, Aldrich MS. Idiopathic hypersomnia. *Brain* 1997;120: 1423–1435.
73. Billiard M. Idiopathic hypersomnia. *Neurol Clin* 1996;14:573–582.
74. Roth B, Nevsimalova S, Rechtschaffen A. Hypersomnia with sleep "drunkenness." *Arch Gen Psychiatry* 1972;26:456–462.
75. Roehrs T, Zorick F, Sicklesteel J, et al. Excessive daytime sleepiness associated with insufficient sleep. *Sleep* 1983;6:319–325.
76. American Sleep Disorders Association. *International classification of sleep disorders: diagnostic and coding manual.* Rochester: American Sleep Disorders Association, 1997:65–71.
77. Mahowald MW. Assessment of periodic leg movements is not an essential component of an overnight sleep study. *Am J Respir Crit Care Med* 2001;164:1340–1341.
78. Fry JM, Diphillip MA, Pressman MR. Periodic leg movements in sleep following treatment of obstructive sleep apnea with nasal CPAP. *Chest* 1989;96:89–91.
79. Waters AS, The International Restless Leg Syndrome Study Group. Toward a better definition of the restless leg syndrome. *Mov Disord* 1995;10:634–632.
80. Early CJ. Clinical practice. Restless legs syndrome. *N Engl J Med* 2003;348:2103–2309.
81. Young T, Palta M, Dempsey J, et al. The occurrence of sleep-disordered breathing among middle-aged adults. *N Engl J Med* 1993;328:1230–1235.
82. Strollo PJ Jr, Rogers RM. Obstructive sleep apnea. *N Engl J Med* 1996;334:99–104.
83. Young T, Peppard PE, Gottlieb DJ. Epidemiology of obstructive sleep apnea. *Am J Respir Crit Care Med* 2002;165:1271–1239.
84. Krakow B, Melendez D, Ferreira E, et al. Prevalence of insomnia symptoms in patients with sleep-disordered breathing. *Chest* 2001;120:1923–1929.
85. Sandbloom RE, Matsumoto AM, Schoene RB, et al. Obstructive sleep apnea syndrome induced by testosterone administration. *N Engl J Med* 1983;308:508–510.
86. Block AJ, Hellard DW, Slayton PC. Effect of alcohol ingestion on breathing and oxygenation during sleep. *Am J Med* 1986;80: 595–600.
87. Issa FG, Sullivan CE. Alcohol, snoring and sleep apnea. *J Neurol Neurosurg Psychiatry* 1982;45:353–359.
88. Harman E, Wynne JW, Block AJ, et al. Sleep-disordered breathing and oxygen desaturation in obese patients. *Chest* 1981;79:256–260.
89. Rajagopal KR, Abbrecht PH, Derderian SS, et al. Obstructive sleep apnea in hypothyroidism. *Ann Intern Med* 1984;101:491–494.

90. Grunstein RR, Ho KY, Sullivan CE. Sleep apnea in acromegaly. *Ann Intern Med* 1991;115:527–532.

91. Shahar E, Redline S, Young T, et al. for the Sleep Heart Health Study Research Group. Hormone replacement therapy and sleep disordered breathing. *Am J Respir Crit Care Med* 2003;167:1186–1192.

92. Dolly FR, Block AJ. Effect of flurazepam on sleep-disordered breathing and nocturnal oxygen desaturation in asymptomatic subjects. *Am J Med* 1982;73:239–243.

93. Berry RB, Kouchi K, Bower J, et al. Triazolam in patients with obstructive sleep apnea. *Am J Respir Crit Care Med* 1995;151:450–454.

94. Bradley TD, Rutherford R, Grossman R, et al. Role of daytime hypoxemia in the pathogenesis of right heart failure in obstructive sleep apnea syndrome. *Am Rev Respir Dis* 1985;131:835–839.

95. Flemons WW, Whitelaw WA, Brant R, et al. Likelihood ratios for a sleep apnea clinical prediction rule. *Am J Respir Crit Care Med* 1994;150:1279–1285.

96. Bennett LS, Langford BA, Stradling JR. Sleep fragmentation indices as predictors of daytime sleepiness and nCPAP response in obstructive sleep apnea. *Am J Respir Crit Care Med* 1998;158:778–786.

97. Weiss JW, Remsburg S, Garpestad E, et al. Hemodynamic consequences of obstructive sleep apnea. *Sleep* 1996;19:388–397.

98. He J, Kryger MH, Zorick FJ, et al. Mortality and apnea index in obstructive sleep apnea. *Chest* 1988;94:9–14.

99. Oksenberg A, Silverberg DS, Arons E, et al. Positional versus nonpositional obstructive sleep apnea patients. *Chest* 1997;112:629–639.

100. Kass JE, Akers SM, Bartter TC, et al. Rapid-eye-movement-specific sleep-disordered breathing. A possible cause of excessive daytime sleepiness. *Am J Respir Crit Care Med* 1996;154:167–169.

101. Chesson AL, Berry RB, Pack A. Practice parameters for the use of portable monitoring devices in the investigation of suspected obstructive sleep apnea in adults. *Sleep* 2003;26(7):907–913.

102. Bradley TD, Martinez D, Rutherford R. Physiological determinants of nocturnal arterial oxygenation in patients with obstructive sleep apnea. *J Appl Physiol* 1985;59:1364–1368.

103. Remmers JE, Degroot WJ, Sauerland EK, et al. Pathogenesis of upper airway occlusion during sleep. *J Appl Physiol* 1978;44:931–938.

104. Launois SH, Feroah TR, Campbell WN, et al. Site of pharyngeal narrowing predicts outcome of surgery for obstructive sleep apnea. *Am Rev Respir Dis* 1993;147:182–189.

105. Anch AM, Remmers JE, Bunce H III. Supraglottic resistance in normal subjects and patients with occlusive sleep apnea. *J Appl Physiol* 1982;53:1158–1163.

106. Gold AR, Schwartz AR. The pharyngeal critical pressure. *Chest* 1996;110:1077–1088.

107. Mezzanotte WS, Tangel DJ, White DP. Waking genioglossal electromyogram in sleep apnea patient versus normal controls (a neuromuscular compensatory mechanism). *J Clin Invest* 1992;89(5):1571–1579.

108. Fogel RB, Malhotra A, Pillar G, et al. Genioglossal activation in patients with obstructive sleep apnea versus control subjects. *Am J Respir Crit Care Med* 2001;164:2025–2030.

109. Berry RB, White DP, Roper J, et al. Awake negative pressure reflex response of the genioglossus in OSA patients and normal subjects. *J Appl Physiol* 2003;94:1875–1882.

110. Mortimore IL, Douglas NJ. Palatal muscle EMG response to negative pressure in awake sleep apneic and control subjects. *Am J Respir Crit Care Med* 1997;156:867–873.

111. Malhotra A, Pillar G, Edwards J, et al. Upper airway collapsibility: measurement and sleep effects. *Chest* 2001;120:156–161.

112. Mezzanotte WS, Tangel DJ, White DP. Influence of sleep onset on upper-airway muscle activity in apnea patients versus normal controls. *Am J Respir Crit Care Med* 1996;153:1880–1887.

113. Badr MS, Toiber F, Skatrud JB, et al. Pharyngeal narrowing/occlusion during central apnea. *J Appl Physiol* 1995;78:1806–1815.

114. Onal E, Lopata M, O'Connor T. Pathogenesis of apneas in hypersomnia–sleep apnea syndrome. *Am Rev Respir Dis* 1982;125:167–174.

115. Morrell MJ, Arabi Y, Zahn B, et al. Progressive retropalatal narrowing preceding obstructive apnea. *Am J Respir Crit Care Med* 1998;158:1974–1981.

116. Dempsey JA, Skatrud JB. A sleep induced apneic threshold and its consequences. *Am Rev Respir Dis* 1986;133:1163–1170.

117. Iber C, Davies SF, Chapman RC, et al. A possible mechanism for mixed apnea in obstructive sleep apnea. *Chest* 1986;89:800–805.

118. Berry RB, Gleeson K. Respiratory arousal from sleep: mechanisms and significance. *Sleep* 1997;20:654–675.

119. Kimoff RJ, Cheong TH, Olha AE, et al. Mechanisms of apnea termination in obstructive sleep apnea. Role of chemoreceptor and mechanoreceptor stimuli. *Am J Respir Crit Care Med* 1994;149:707–714.

120. O'Malley EB, Norman RG, Farkas DF, et al. The addition of frontal EEG leads improves detection of cortical arousal following obstructive respiratory events. *Sleep* 2003;26:435–439.

121. Rajagopal KR, Bennett LL, Dillard TA. Overnight nasal CPAP improves hypersomnolence in sleep apnea. *Chest* 1986;90:172–176.

122. Poceta JS, Timms RM, Jeong D, et al. Maintenance of wakefulness test in obstructive sleep apnea syndrome. *Chest* 1992;101:893–897.

123. Orr WC, Martin RJ, Imes NK, et al. Hypersomnolent and nonhypersomnolent patients with upper airway obstruction during sleep. *Chest* 1979;75:418–422.

124. Roehrs T, Zorick F, Wittig R, et al. Predictors of objective level of daytime sleepiness in patients with sleep-related breathing disorders. *Chest* 1989;95:1202–1206.

125. Guilleminault C, Partinen M, Quera-Salva MA, et al. Determinants of daytime sleepiness in obstructive sleep apnea. *Chest* 1988;94:32–37.

126. Cheshire K, Engleman H, Deary I, et al. Factors impairing daytime performance in patients with sleep apnea/hypopnea syndrome. *Arch Intern Med* 1992;152:538–541.

127. Findley LJ, Barth JT, Powers DC, et al. Cognitive impairment in patients with obstructive sleep apnea and associated hypoxemia. *Chest* 1986;90:686–690.

128. Garay SM, Rapoport D, Sorkin B, et al. Regulation of ventilation in the obstructive sleep apnea syndrome. *Am Rev Respir Dis* 1981;124:451–457.

129. Rajagopal KR, Abbrecht PH, Tellis CJ. Control of breathing in obstructive sleep apnea. *Chest* 1984;85:174–180.

130. Zwillich CW, Sutton FD, Pierson DJ, et al. Decreased hypoxic ventilatory drive in the obesity-hypoventilation syndrome. *Am J Med* 1975;59:343–348.

131. Rochester DF, Enson Y. Current concepts in the pathogenesis of the obesity hypoventilation syndrome. *Am J Med* 1974;57:402–420.

132. Rapoport DM, Garay SM, Epstein H, et al. Hypercapnia in the obstructive sleep apnea syndrome. *Chest* 1986;89:627–635.

133. Sullivan CE, Berthon-Jones M, Issa FG. Remission of severe obesity-hypoventilation syndrome after short-term treatment during sleep with nasal continuous positive airway pressure. *Am Rev Respir Dis* 1983;128:177–181.

134. Berthon-Jones M, Sullivan CE. Time course of change in ventilatory response to CO_2 with long-term CPAP therapy for obstructive sleep apnea. *Am Rev Respir Dis* 1987;135:144–147.

135. Bradley TD, Rutherford R, Lue F, et al. Role of diffuse airway obstruction in the hypercapnia of obstructive sleep apnea. *Am Rev Respir Dis* 1986;134:920–924.

136. Douglas NJ. Upper airway resistance syndrome is not a distinct syndrome. *Am J Respir Crit Care Med* 2000;161:1410–1415.

137. Guilleminault C, Chowdhuri S. Upper airway resistance syndrome is a distinct syndrome. *Am J Respir Crit Care Med* 2001;161:1413–1416.

138. Rees K, Kingshott RN, Wraith PK, et al. Frequency and significance of increased upper airway resistance during sleep. *Am J Respir Crit Care Med* 2000;162:1210–1214.

139. Leung RST, Bradley TD. Sleep apnea and cardiovascular disease. State of the art. *Am J Respir Crit Care Med* 2001;164:2147–2165.

140. Weitzenblum E, Krieger J, Apprill M, et al. Daytime pulmonary hypertension in patients with obstructive sleep apnea syndrome. *Am Rev Respir Dis* 1988;138:345–349.

141. Sajkov D, Cowie RJ, Thornton AT, et al. Pulmonary hypertension and hypoxemia in obstructive sleep apnea syndrome. *Am J Respir Crit Care Med* 1994;149:416–422.

142. Sajkov D, Wang T, Saunders NA, et al. Continuous positive airway pressure treatment improves pulmonary hemodynamics in patients with obstructive sleep apnea. *Am J Respir Crit Care Med* 2002;165:152–158.

143. Shephard JW Jr. Hypertension, cardiac arrhythmias, myocardial infarction, and stroke in relation to obstructive sleep apnea. *Clin Chest Med* 1992;13:437–458.

144. Suzuki M, Guilleminault G, Otsuka K, et al. Blood pressure "dipping" and "non-dipping" in obstructive sleep apnea syndrome patients. *Sleep* 1996;19:382–387.

145. Kales A, Bixler EO, Cadieux RJ, et al. Sleep apnea in a hypertensive population. *Lancet* 1984;2:1005–1008.

146. Carlson JT, Hedner JA, Ejnell H, et al. High prevalence of hypertension in sleep apnea patients independent of obesity. *Am J Respir Crit Care Med* 1994;150:72–77.

147. Peppard PE, Young T, Palta M, et al. Prospective study of the association between sleep-disordered breathing and hypertension. *N Engl J Med* 2000;342:1378–1384.

148. Verdecchia P, Schiallica G, Guerrier M, et al. Circadian blood pressure changes and left ventricular hypertrophy in essential hypertension. *Circulation* 1990;81:528–536.

149. Becker HF, Jerrentrup A, Ploch T, et al. Effect of nasal continuous positive airway pressure treatment on blood pressure in patients with obstructive sleep apnea. *Circulation* 2003;107:68–73.

150. Tilkian AG, Guilleminault C, Schroeder JS, et al. Sleep-induced apnea syndrome. Prevalence of cardiac arrhythmias and their reversal after tracheostomy. *Am J Med* 1977;63:348–358.

151. Shephard JW Jr, Garrison MW, Grither DA, et al.. Relationship of ventricular ectopy to oxyhemoglobin desaturation in patients with obstructive sleep apnea. *Chest* 1985;88:335–340.

152. Kanagala R, Murali NS, Friedman PA, et al. Obstructive sleep apnea and the recurrence of atrial fibrillation. *Circulation* 2003; 107:2589–2594.

153. Peker Y, Hender J, Kraiczi H, et al. Respiratory disturbance index: an independent predictor of mortality in coronary artery disease. *Am J Respir Crit Care Med* 2000;162:81–86.

154. Kreiger J, Sforza E, Barthelmebs M, et al. Overnight decreases in hematocrit after nasal CPAP with patients with OSA. *Chest* 1990; 97:729–730.

155. Chin K, Ohi M, Kita H, et al. Effects of NCPAP therapy on fibrinogen levels in obstructive sleep apnea syndrome. *Am J Respir Crit Care Med* 1996;153:1972–1976.

156. Lavie L, Kraiczi H, Hefetz A, et al. Plasma vascular endothelial growth factor in sleep apnea syndrome: effects of nasal continuous positive air pressure treatment. *Am J Respir Crit Care Med* 2002;165(12):1624–1628.

157. Dyugovskaya L, Lavie P, Lavie L. Increased adhesion molecules expression and production of reactive oxygen species in leukocytes of sleep apnea patients. *Am J Respir Crit Care Med* 2002;165: 934–939.

158. Schulz R, Mahmoudi S, Hattar K, et al. Enhanced release of superoxide from polymorphonuclear neutrophils in obstructive sleep apnea. Impact of continuous positive airway pressure therapy. *Am J Respir Crit Care Med* 2000;162:566–570.

159. Bokinsky G, Miller M, Ault K, et al. Spontaneous platelet activation and aggregation during obstructive sleep apnea and its response to therapy with nasal continuous positive airway pressure. A preliminary investigation. *Chest* 1995;108(3):625–630.

160. Shamsuzzaman AS, Winnicki M, Lanfranchi P, et al. Elevated C-reactive protein in patients with obstructive sleep apnea. *Circulation* 2002;105:2462–2464.

161. Yokoe T, Minoguchi K, Matsuo H, et al. Elevated levels of C-reactive protein and interleukin-6 in patients with obstructive sleep apnea syndrome are decreased by nasal continuous positive airway pressure. *Circulation* 2003;107(8):1129–1134.

162. Lavie P, Herer P, Peled R, et al. Mortality in sleep apnea patients: a multivariate analysis of risk factors. *Sleep* 1995;18:149–157.

163. Findley LJ, Unverzagt ME, Suratt PM. Automobile accidents involving patients with obstructive sleep apnea. *Am Rev Respir Dis* 1988;138:337–340.

164. American Thoracic Society. Official statement. Sleep apnea, sleepiness, and driving risk. *Am J Respir Crit Care Med* 1994;150: 1463–1473.

165. Cassel W, Ploch C, Becker D, et al. Risk of traffic accidents in patients with sleep disordered breathing: reduction with nasal CPAP. *Eur Respir J* 1996;9:2602–2611.

166. George CF. Reduction in motor-vehicle collisions following treatment of sleep apnea with nasal CPAP. *Thorax* 2001;56:508–512.

167. George CFP, Boudreau AC, Smiley A. Simulated driving performance in patients with obstructive sleep apnea. *Am J Respir Crit Care Med* 1996;154:175–181.

168. Smith PL, Gold AR, Moyers DA, et al. Weight loss in mildly to moderately obese patients with obstructive sleep apnea. *Ann Intern Med* 1985;103:850–855.

169. Neill AM, Angus SM, Sajkov K, et al. Effects of sleep posture on upper airway stability in patients with obstructive sleep apnea. *Am J Respir Crit Care Med* 1997;155:199–204.

170. Jokic R, Klimaszewski A, Crossley M, et al. Positional treatment vs continuous positive airway pressure in patients with positional obstructive sleep apnea syndrome. *Chest* 1999;115: 771–781.

171. Veasey SC. Serotonin: culprit or promising therapy for obstructive sleep apnea? *Am J Respir Crit Care Med* 2001;163(5):1045–1047.

172. Kraiczi H, Hedner J, Dalof P, et al. Effect of serotonin uptake inhibition on breathing during sleep and daytime symptoms in obstructive sleep apnea. *Sleep* 1999;22:61–67.

173. Sutton FD, Zwillich CW, Creagh CE, et al. Progesterone for outpatient treatment of the Pickwickian syndrome. *Ann Intern Med* 1975;83:476–479.

174. Rajagopal KR, Abbrecht PH, Jabbari B. Effects of medroxyprogesterone acetate in obstructive sleep apnea. *Chest* 1996;90:815–821.

175. Guilleminault C, Simmons FB, Motta J, et al. Obstructive sleep apnea syndrome and tracheostomy—long term follow up and experience. *Arch Intern Med* 1982;126:14–20.

176. Fujita S, Conway W, Zorick F, et al. Surgical correction of anatomic abnormalities in obstructive sleep apnea syndrome: uvulopalatopharyngoplasty. *Otolaryngol Head Neck Surg* 1981;89: 923–934.

177. Sher AE, Schechtman KB, Piccirillo JF. The efficacy of surgical modification of the upper airway in adults with obstructive sleep apnea syndrome. *Sleep* 1996;19:156–177.

178. American Sleep Disorders Association. Practice parameters for the treatment of obstructive sleep apnea in adults: the efficacy of surgical modifications of the upper airway. *Sleep* 1996;19: 152–155.

179. Li KK, Powell NB, Riley RW. Surgical management of obstructive sleep apnea. In: Lee-Chiong TL, Sateia MJ, Caraskadon MA. *Sleep Medicine*. Philadelphia: Hanley and Belfus, 435– 446.

180. Sasse SA, Mahutte CK, Dickel M, et al. The characteristics of five patients with obstructive sleep apnea whose apnea-hypopnea index deteriorated after uvulopalatopharyngoplasty. *Sleep Breath* 2002;6:77–84.

181. Littner M, Kushida CA, Hartse K, et al. Practice parameters for the use of laser-assisted uvulopalatoplasty: an update for 2000. *Sleep* 2001;24:603–618.

182. Riley RW, Powell NB, Guilleminault C. Maxillary, mandibular, and hyoid advancement for treatment of obstructive sleep apnea. *J Oral Maxillofac Surg* 1990;48:20–26.

183. Schmidt-Nowara W, Lowe A, Wiegand L, et al. Oral appliances for the treatment of snoring and obstructive sleep apnea. A review. *Sleep* 1995;18:501–510.

184. Lowe AA. Dental devices for treatment of snoring and obstructive sleep apnea. In: Kryger M, Roth T, Dement W, eds. *Principles and practice of sleep medicine,* 2nd ed. Philadelphia: WB Saunders, 1994:722–735.

185. Ferguson KA, Ono T, Lowe AA, et al. A randomized crossover study of oral appliance vs nasal-continuous positive airway pressure in treatment of mild-moderate sleep apnea. *Chest* 1996;109: 1269–1275.

186. Millman RP, Rosenberg CL, Carlisle CC, et al. The efficacy of oral appliances in treatment of persistent sleep apnea after uvulopalatopharyngoplasty. *Chest* 1998;113:992–996.

187. Henke KG, Frantz DE, Kuna ST. An oral elastic mandibular advancement device of obstructive sleep apnea. *Am J Respir Crit Care Med* 2000;161:420–425.

188. Fletcher EC, Munafo D. Role of nocturnal oxygen therapy in obstructive sleep apnea. *Chest* 1990;98:1497–1504.

189. Smith PL, Haponik EF, Bleecker ER. The effects of oxygen in patients with sleep apnea. *Am Rev Respir Dis* 1984;130:957–963.

190. Goldstein RS, Ramcharan V, Bowes G, et al. Effect of supplemental nocturnal oxygen on gas exchange in patients with severe obstructive lung disease. *N Engl J Med* 1984;310:425–429.

191. Sullivan CE, Issa FG, Berthon-Jones M, et al. Reversal of obstructive sleep apnoea by continuous positive airway pressure applied through the nares. *Lancet* 1981;1:862–865.

192. Redline S, Adams N, Strauss ME, et al. Improvement of mild sleep-disordered breathing with CPAP compared with conservative therapy. *Am J Respir Crit Care Med* 1998;157:858–865.

193. Massie CA, Hart RW. Clinical outcomes related to interface type in patients with obstructive sleep apnea/hypopnea syndrome who are using continuous positive airway pressure. *Chest* 2003;123:1112–1118.

194. Prosise GL, Berry RB. Oral-nasal continuous positive airway pressure as a treatment for obstructive sleep apnea. *Chest* 1994; 106:180–186.

195. Sanders MH, Kern N. Obstructive sleep apnea treated by independently adjusted inspiratory and expiratory positive airway pressures via nasal mask. *Chest* 1990;98:317–324.

196. Reeves-Hoché MK, Hudgel DW, Meck R, et al. Continuous versus bilevel positive airway pressure for obstructive sleep apnea. *Am J Respir Crit Care Med* 1995;151:443–449.

197. Berry RB, Parish JM, Hartse KM. The use of auto-titrating CPAP for treatment of adults with obstructive sleep apnea. *Sleep* 2002; 25:148–173.

198. ATS Statement. Indications and standards of use of nasal continuous positive airway pressure (CPAP) in sleep apnea syndromes. *Am J Respir Crit Care Med* 1994;150:1738–1745.

199. American Sleep Disorders Association Report. Standards of Practice Committee. Practice parameters for the indications for polysomnography and related procedures. *Sleep* 1997;20:406–422.

200. Montserrat JM, Ballester E, Olivi H. Time course of stepwise CPAP titration. *Am J Respir Crit Care Med* 1995;152:1854–1859.

201. Condos R, Norman RG, Krishnasamy I, et al. Flow limitation as a noninvasive assessment of residual upper-airway resistance during continuous positive airway pressure therapy of obstructive sleep apnea. *Am J Respir Crit Care Med.* 1994;150: 475–480.

202. Pevernagie DA, Sheard JW Jr. Relations between sleep stage, posture and effective nasal CPAP levels in OSA. *Sleep* 1992;15:162–167.

203. Oksenberg A, Silverberg DS, Arons E, et al. The sleep supine position has a major effect on optimal nasal continuous positive airway pressure. *Chest* 1999;116:1000–1006.

204. Krieger J, Weitzenblum E, Monassier JP, et al. Dangerous hypoxemia during continuous positive airway pressure treatment of obstructive sleep apnea. *Lancet* 1983;2:1429–1430.

205. Sanders MH, Kern NB, Costantino JP, et al. Adequacy of prescribing positive airway pressure therapy by mask for sleep apnea on the basis of a partial-night trial. *Am Rev Respir Dis* 1993;147: 1169–1174.

206. Yamashiro Y, Kryger MH. CPAP titration for sleep apnea using a split night protocol. *Chest* 1995;107:62–66.

207. Engleman HM, Wild MR. Improving CPAP use by patients with the sleep apnea/hypopnea syndrome. *Sleep Med Rev* 2003;7:81–99.

208. Weaver TE, Kribbs NB, Pack AI, et al. Night to night variability in CPAP use over the first three months of treatment. *Sleep* 1997;20: 278–283.

209. Pépin JL, Krieger J, Rodenstein D, et al. Effective compliance during the first 3 months of continuous positive airway pressure. A European prospective study of 121 patients. *Am J Respir Crit Care Med* 1999;160:1124–1129.

210. Hoy CJ, Vennelle M, Kingshott RN, et al. Can intensive support improve continuous positive airway pressure use in patients with the sleep apnea/hypopnea syndrome? *Am J Respir Crit Care Med* 1999;159:1096–1100.

211. Berry RB. Improving CPAP compliance. Man more than machine. *Sleep Med* 2000;1:175–178.

212. Chervin RD, Theut S, Bassetti C, et al. Compliance of nasal CPAP can be improved by simple interventions. *Sleep* 1997;20:284–289.

213. Massie CA, Hart RW, Peralez K, et al. Effects of humidification on nasal symptoms and compliance in sleep apnea patients using continuous positive airway pressure. *Chest* 1999;116:403–408.

214. Richards GN, Cistulli PA, Ungar RG, et al. Mouth leak with nasal continuous positive airway pressure increases nasal airway resistance. *Am J Respir Crit Care Med* 1996;154:182–186.

215. Jenkinson C, Davies RJO, Mullins R, et al. Comparison of therapeutic and subtherapeutic nasal continuous positive airway pressure for obstructive sleep apnea: a randomized prospective parallel trial. *Lancet* 1999;353:2100–2105.

216. Barbe F, Mayoralas LR, Duran J, et al. Treatment with continuous positive airway pressure is not effective in patients with sleep apnea but no daytime sleepiness. *Ann Intern Med* 2001;134: 1015–1023.

217. Pack AI, Black JE, Schwartz JR, et al. Modafinil as adjunct therapy for daytime sleepiness in obstructive sleep apnea. *Am J Respir Crit Care Med* 2001;164:1675–1681.

218. Kingshott RN, Vennelle M, Coleman EL, et al. Randomized, double-blind, placebo-controlled crossover trial of modafinil in the treatment of residual excessive daytime sleepiness in the sleep apnea/hypopnea syndrome. *Am J Respir Crit Care Med* 2001;163:918–923.

219. Bradley TD, McNicholas WT, Rutherford R, et al. Clinical and physiologic heterogeneity of the central sleep apnea syndrome. *Am Rev Respir Dis* 1986;134:217–221.

220. Phillipson EA. Hypoventilation syndromes. In: Murray JF, Nadel JA, eds. *Textbook of respiratory medicine.* Philadelphia: WB Saunders, 1994:2291–2300.

221. American Thoracic Society. Idiopathic congenital central hypoventilation syndrome. Diagnosis and management. *Am J Respir Crit Care Med* 1999;160:368–373.

222. Hill R, Robbins AW, Messing R, et al. Sleep apnea syndrome after poliomyelitis. *Am Rev Respir Dis* 1983;127:129–131.

223. Elman LB, Siderowf AD, McCluskedy LF. Nocturnal oximetry: utility in respiratory management of amyotrophic lateral sclerosis. *Am J Phys Med Rehabil* 2003;82:866–870.

224. McNicholas WT, Carter JL, Rutherford R, et al. Beneficial effect of oxygen in primary alveolar hypoventilation with central sleep apnea. *Am Rev Respir Dis* 1982;125:773–775.

225. Hill NS. Clinical applications of body ventilators. *Chest* 1986;90: 897–905.

226. Unterborn JN, Hill NS. Options for mechanical ventilation in neuromuscular diseases. *Clin Chest Med* 1994;15:765–781.

227. Calman DM, Piper A, Sanders MH, et al. Nocturnal noninvasive positive pressure ventilatory assistance. *Chest* 1996;110:1581–1588.

228. American College of Chest Physicians. Clinical indicators for noninvasive positive pressure ventilation in chronic respiratory failure due to restrictive lung disease, COPD, and nocturnal hypoventilation—A consensus conference report. *Chest* 1999;116: 521–534.

229. Xie A, Rutherford R, Rankin F, et al. Hypocapnia and increased ventilatory responsiveness in patients with idiopathic central sleep apnea. *Am J Respir Crit Care Med* 1995;152:1950–1955.

230. Xie A, Wong B, Phillipson EA, et al. Interaction of hyperventilation and arousals in the pathogenesis of idiopathic central sleep apnea. *Am J Respir Crit Care Med* 1994;250:489–495.

231. Bonnet MH, Dexter JR, Arand DL. The effect of triazolam on arousal and respiration in central sleep apnea patients. *Sleep* 1990;13:31–41.

232. Debacker WA, Verbracken J, Willemen M, et al. Central apnea index decreases after prolonged treatment with acetazolamide. *Am J Respir Crit Care Med* 1995;151:87–91.

233. Xie A, Rankin F, Rutherford R, et al. Effects of inhaled CO_2 and added dead space of idiopathic central sleep apnea. *J Appl Physiol* 1997;82:918–926.

234. Issa FG, Sullivan CE. Reversal of central sleep apnea using nasal CPAP. *Chest* 1986;90:165–171.

235. Hoffstein V, Slutsky AS. Central sleep apnea reversed by continuous positive airway pressure. *Am Rev Respir Dis* 1987;135: 1210–1212.

236. Bradley TD, Floras JS. Sleep apnea and heart failure. Part II: Central sleep apnea. *Circulation* 2003;107:1822–1826.

237. Nachtman A, Siebler M, Rose G, et al. Cheyne-Stokes respiration in ischemic stroke. *Neurology* 1995;45:820–821.

238. Khoo MC. Periodic breathing. In: Crystal RB, West JB, eds. *The lung.* New York: Raven Press, 1991:1419–1431.

239. Naughton M, Benard D, Tam A, et al. Role of hyperventilation in the pathogenesis of central sleep apneas in patients with congestive heart failure. *Am Rev Respir Dis* 1993;1498:330–338.

240. Xie A, Skatrud JB, Puleo DS, et al. Apnea-hypopnea threshold for CO_2 in patients with congestive heart failure. *Am J Respir Crit Care Med* 2002;165(9):1245–1250.

241. Bradley TD. Crossing the threshold: implications for central sleep apnea. *Am J Respir Crit Care Med* 2002;165(9):1203–1204.
242. Javaheri S. A mechanism of central sleep apnea in patients with heart failure. *N Engl J Med* 1999;341:949–954.
243. Solin P, Roebuck T, Johns DP, et al. Peripheral and central ventilatory responses in central sleep apnea with and without congestive heart failure. *Am J Respir Crit Care Med* 2000;162:2194–2200.
244. Lorenzi-Filho G, Azevedo ER, Parker JD, et al. Relationship of carbon dioxide tension in arterial blood to pulmonary wedge pressure in heart failure. *Eur Respir J* 2002;19:37–40.
245. Solin P, Bergin P, Richardson M, et al. Influence of pulmonary capillary wedge pressure on central apnea in heart failure. *Circulation* 1999;99(12):1574–1579.
246. Blackshear JL, Kaplan J, Thompson RC, et al. Nocturnal dyspnea and atrial fibrillation predict Cheyne-Stokes respiration in patients with congestive heart failure. *Arch Intern Med* 1995;155:1297–1302.
247. Sin DD, Fitzgerald F, Parker JD, et al. Risk Factors of central and obstructive sleep apnea in 450 men and women with congestive heart failure. *Am J Respir Crit Care Med* 1999;160:110–106.
248. Hanly PJ, Zuberi-Khokar NS. Increased mortality associated with Cheyne-Stokes respiration in patients with congestive heart failure. *Am J Respir Crit Care Med* 1996;153:272–276.
249. Lanfranchi P, Braghiroli A, Bosimini E, et al. Prognostic value of nocturnal Cheyne-Stokes respiration in chronic heart failure. *Circulation* 1999;99:1435–1440.
250. Javaheri S, Parker TJ, Wexler L, et al. Effect of theophylline on sleep disordered breathing in heart failure. *N Engl J Med* 1996;335:562–567.
251. Hanly PJ, Millar TW, Steljes DG, et al. The effect of oxygen of respiration and sleep in patients with congestive heart failure. *Ann Intern Med* 1989;111:777–782.
252. Teschler H, Dohring J, Wang YM, et al. Adaptive pressure support servo-ventilation: a novel treatment for Cheyne-Stokes respiration in heart failure. *Am J Respir Crit Care Med* 2001;164(4):614–619.
253. Naughton MT, Liu PP, Benard DC, et al. Treatment of congestive heart failure and Cheyne-Stokes respiration during sleep by continuous positive airway pressure. *Am J Respir Crit Care Med* 1995;151:92–97.
254. Davies RJ, Harrington KJ, Ormedrod OJM, et al. Nasal continuous positive airway pressure in chronic heart failure with sleep-disordered breathing. *Am Rev Respir Dis* 1993;147:630–634.
255. Sin DD, Logan AG, Fitzgerald FS, et al. Effects of continuous positive airway pressure on cardiovascular outcomes in heart failure patients with and without Cheyne-Stokes respiration. *Circulation* 2000;102:61–66.
256. Bradley TD, Logan AG, Floras JS, CANPAP Investigators. Rationale and design of the Canadian Continuous Positive Airway Pressure Trial for congestive heart failure patients with central sleep apnea—CANPAP. *Can J Cardiol* 2001;17:677–684.
257. Javaheri S, Parker TJ, Wexler L, et al. Occult sleep-disordered breathing in stable congestive heart failure. *Ann Intern Med* 1995;122:487–492.
258. Dowdell WT, Javaheri S, McGinnis W. Cheyne-Stokes respiration presenting as sleep apnea syndrome. *Am Rev Respir Dis* 1990;141:871–879.
259. Malone S, Liu PP, Holloway R, et al. Obstructive sleep apnea in patients with dilated cardiomyopathy: effects of continuous positive airway pressure. *Lancet* 1991;338:1480–1484.
260. Kaneko Y, Floras JS, Usui K, et al. Cardiovascular consequences of continuous positive airway pressure in patients with heart failure and obstructive sleep apnea. *N Engl J Med* 2003;348:1233–1241.
261. Bradley TD, Floras JS. Sleep apnea and heart failure. Part I: Obstructive sleep apnea. *Circulation* 2003;107:1671–1678.
262. Turner-Warwick M. Epidemiology of nocturnal asthma. *Am J Med* 1988;85:6–8.
263. Ballard RD, Saathoff MC, Patel DK, et al. Effect of sleep on nocturnal bronchoconstriction and ventilatory patterns in asthmatics. *J Appl Physiol* 1989;67:243–249.
264. Martin RJ, Banks-Schlegel S. Chronobiology of asthma. *Am J Respir Crit Care Med* 1998;158:1002–1007.
265. Martin RJ, Cicutto LC, Smith HR, et al. Airways inflammation in nocturnal asthma. *Am Rev Respir Dis* 1991;143:351–357.
266. Kraft M, Djukanovic R, Wilson S, et al. Alveolar tissue inflammation in asthma. *Am J Respir Crit Care Med* 1996;154:1505–1510.
267. Oosterhoff Y, Hoogsteden HC, Rutgers B, et al. Lymphocyte and macrophage activation in bronchoalveolar lavage fluid in nocturnal asthma. *Am J Respir Crit Care Med* 1995;151:75–81.
268. Beam WR, Ballard RD, Martin RJ. Spectrum of corticosteroid sensitivity in nocturnal asthma. *Am Rev Respir Dis* 1992;145:1082–1086.
269. Beam WR, Weiner DE, Martin RJ. Timing of prednisone and alterations of airways inflammation in nocturnal asthma. *Am Rev Respir Dis* 1992;146:1524–1536.
270. Weersink EJM, Douma RR, Postma DS, et al. Fluticasone propionate, salmeterol xinafoate, and their combination in the treatment of nocturnal asthma. *Am J Resp Crit Care Med* 1997;155:1241–1246.
271. Selby C, Engleman HM, Fitzpatrick MF, et al. Inhaled salmeterol or oral theophylline in nocturnal asthma? *Am J Respir Crit Care Med* 1997;155:104–108.
272. Wiegand L, Mende CN, Zaidel G, et al. Salmeterol vs theophylline. Sleep and efficacy outcomes in patients with nocturnal asthma. *Chest* 1999;115:1525–1532.
273. Stewart IC, Rhind GB, Power JT, et al. Effect of sustained release terbutaline on symptoms and sleep quality in patients with nocturnal asthma. *Thorax* 1987;42:797–800.
274. Coe CI, Barnes PJ. Reduction of nocturnal asthma by an inhaled anticholinergic drug. *Chest* 1986;90:485–488.
275. Wenzel SE, Trudeau JB, Kaminsky DA, et al. Effect of 5-lipoxygenase inhibition on bronchoconstriction and airways inflammation in nocturnal asthma. *Am J Respir Crit Care Med* 1995;152:897–905.
276. Spector SL, Smith LJ, Glass M, et al. Effects of 6 weeks of therapy with oral doses of ICI204.219 a leukotriene D4 receptor antagonist in subjects with bronchial asthma. *Am J Respir Crit Care Med* 1994;150:618–623.
277. Chan CS, Woolcock AJ, Sullivan CE. Nocturnal asthma: role of snoring and obstructive sleep apnea. *Am Rev Respir Dis* 1988;137:1502–1504.
278. Harding SM. Recent clinical investigations examining the association of asthma and gastroesophageal reflux. *Am J Med* 2003;115(Suppl 3A):39S–44S.
279. Cuttitta G, Cibella F, Visconti A. Spontaneous gastroesophageal reflux and airway patency during the night in adult asthmatics. *Am J Respir Crit Care Med* 2000;151:177–181.
280. Harding SM, Richter JE, Guzzo MR, et al. Asthma and gastroesophageal reflux: acid suppressive therapy improves asthma outcome. *Am J Med* 1996;100:395–405.
281. Gibson PG, Henry RL, Coughlan JL. Gastro-oesophageal reflux treatment for asthma in adults and children. *Cochrane Database Syst Rev* 2003;CD001496.
282. Douglas NJ. Sleep in patients with chronic obstructive pulmonary disease. *Clin Chest Med* 1998;19:115–125.
283. Catterall JR, Douglas NJ, Calverley PMA, et al. Transient hypoxemia during sleep is not a sleep apnea syndrome. *Am Rev Respir Dis* 1983;128:24–29.
284. Connaughton JJ, Catterall JR, Elton RA, et al. Do sleep studies contribute to the management of patients with severe chronic obstructive pulmonary disease? *Am Rev Respir Dis* 1988;138:341–344.
285. Hudgel DW, Martin RJ, Capehart M, et al. Contribution of hypoventilation to sleep oxygen desaturation in chronic obstructive pulmonary disease. *J Appl Physiol* 1983;55:669–677.
286. Fletcher EC, Gray BA, Levin DC. Nonapneic mechanisms of arterial oxygen desaturation during rapid-eye-movements sleep. *J Appl Physiol* 1983;54:632–639.
287. Nocturnal Oxygen Therapy Trial Group. Continuous or nocturnal oxygen therapy in hypoxemic chronic obstructive lung disease. *Ann Intern Med* 1980;93:391–398.
288. Fletcher EC, Luckett RA, Goodnight-White S, et al. A double blind trial of nocturnal supplemental oxygen for sleep desaturation in patients with chronic obstructive pulmonary disease and a daytime PO_2 above 60 mm Hg. *Am Rev Respir Dis* 1992;145:1070–1076.
289. Chaouat A, Weitzenblum E, Kessler R, et al. Outcome of COPD patients with mild daytime hypoxemia with or without sleep-related oxygen desaturation. *Eur Resp J* 2001;17:848–855.
290. Calverley PMA, Brezinova V, Douglas NJ, et al. The effect of oxygenation on sleep quality in chronic bronchitis and emphysema. *Am Rev Respir Dis* 1982;126:206–210.
291. Fleetham J, West P, Mezon B, et al. Sleep, arousals, and oxygen desaturation in chronic obstructive pulmonary disease. The effect of oxygen therapy. *Am Rev Respir Dis* 1982;125:429–433.

292. Berry RB, Desa MM, Branum JP, et al. Effect of theophylline on sleep and sleep-disordered breathing in patients with chronic obstructive pulmonary disease. *Am Rev Respir Dis* 1991;143: 245–250.

293. Martin RJ, Bartelson BL, Smith P, et al. Effect of ipratropium bromide treatment on oxygen saturation and sleep quality in COPD. *Chest* 1999;115:1338–1345.

294. Timms RM, Dawson A, Hajdukovic R, et al. Effect of triazolam on sleep and arterial oxygen saturation in patients with chronic obstructive pulmonary disease. *Arch Intern Med* 1988;148: 2159–2163.

295. Girault C, Muir JF, Mihaltan F, et al. Effects of repeated administration of zolpidem on sleep, diurnal and nocturnal respiratory function, vigilance, and physical performance in patients with COPD. *Chest* 1996;110:1203–1211.

296. Fletcher EC, Schaaf JW, Miller J, et al. Long-term cardiopulmonary sequelae in patients with sleep apnea and chronic lung disease. *Am Rev Respir Dis* 1987;135:525–533.

297. Fletcher EC, Brown DL. Nocturnal oxyhemoglobin desaturation following tracheostomy for obstructive sleep apnea. *Am J Med* 1985;79:35–42.

298. Sampol G, Sagales MT, Rocca A, et al. Nasal continuous positive airway pressure with supplemental oxygen in coexistent sleep apnea–hypopnea syndrome and severe chronic obstructive pulmonary disease. *Eur Resp J* 1996;9:111–116.

CHAPTER 19

Pulmonary and Critical Care Among Elderly Patients Admitted to the Intensive Care Unit

Cari R. Levy

Margaret A. Pisani

E. Wesley Ely

"Pulmonary and Critical Care Among Elderly Patients Admitted to the Intensive Care Unit" represents a recent addition to this textbook that informs practitioners about outcomes in the elderly population and facilitates evidence-based discussions with patients, families, and other providers. This chapter addresses some of the most commonly encountered medical and ethical dilemmas facing physicians when their elderly patients are admitted to an intensive care unit (ICU). On developing a potentially life-threatening condition, the possibility of an ICU admission mandates reexamination of a patient's preferences for medical care, and as advocates for our elderly patients who become critically ill, we must be able to respond

to such reexamination with information about whether certain treatments may be overly burdensome or potentially beneficial.

The elderly are the most rapidly growing segment of the ICU population. Approximately two-thirds of all ICU beds are occupied by patients more than 65 years old, and the number of days spent in the ICU is seven times greater for those more than 75 years old compared to those younger than 65 years old (1). There is evidence that physicians use age as a factor in the decision to admit an elderly patient to the ICU (2), and data from the Study to Understand Prognosis and Preferences for Outcomes and Risks of Treatment (SUPPORT) also suggests that older age is associated with lower intensity of care (see Fig. 19-1)

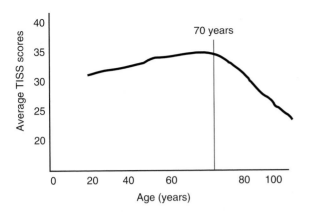

FIGURE 19-1. The relationship between patient age and the intensity of care delivered to patients enrolled in the Study to Understand Prognosis and Preferences for Outcomes and Risks of Treatment (SUPPORT) trial is depicted as patient age (*x*-axis) versus average Therapeutic Intervention Scoring System (TISS) on days 1 and 3 (*y*-axis). TISS is a valid and reliable method of measuring resource use in cohorts of patients. The solid line represents the TISS scores after adjustment for severity of illness and functional status and shows that intensity of care was lower for older patients even after these adjustments (4). (From Hamel MB, Teno JM, Goldman L, et al. Patient age and decisions to withhold life-sustaining treatments from seriously ill, hospitalized adults. *Ann Intern Med* 1999; 130:116–125, with permission.)

(3) and a greater likelihood of withholding life-sustaining treatments (see Fig. 19-2). Should age alone be used as a foundation for determining aggressiveness of care? If not, what evidence is there to help frame such decisions? This chapter reviews outcomes among the elderly after admission to an ICU in an attempt to answer these questions.

This review is prefaced by acknowledging that there are many ethical and social factors that affect the decision to admit elderly patients to an ICU, and the literature of outcomes we report

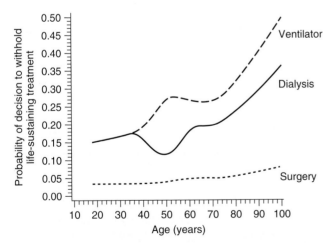

FIGURE 19-2. Relation between patient age and the adjusted probability of a decision to withhold each life-sustaining treatment by study day 30. Results are calculated on the basis of Cox proportional hazard models representing age as cubic spline functions and are adjusted for sex, income, education, insurance, prognosis, comorbid conditions, baseline function, study site, and preferences for cardiopulmonary resuscitation (CPR) and life-extending care (4). (From Hamel MB, Teno JM, Goldman L, et al. Patient age and decisions to withhold life-sustaining treatments from seriously ill, hospitalized adults. *Ann Intern Med* 1999;130:116–125, with permission.)

must be viewed in light of the fact that the data likely represent a highly selected group of older individuals. Although a thorough discussion of critical care is beyond the scope of this chapter, the following information is presented to assist health care professionals as they make decisions about aggressiveness of care for critically ill elderly patients. These topics include:

1. ICU mortality and estimating prognosis
2. Functional outcomes and quality of life (QOL)
3. Cardiopulmonary resuscitation (CPR) outcomes
4. Mechanical ventilation
5. Cognitive outcomes
6. Advance directives
7. Limiting care and futile care
8. Preoperative pulmonary evaluation of the elderly.

INTENSIVE CARE UNIT MORTALITY AND ESTIMATING PROGNOSIS

The mortality rate of elderly patients admitted to an ICU ranges widely across studies (5) (see Table 19-1). Investigators report ICU mortality as low as 8% among patients aged 65 to 74, 10% for those older than 74, and 20% mortality for those more than 80 years (6,7). Survival of those more than 80 years at 2 months is 59%, at 2 years is 33%, and at 3 years is 29% (7). Most investigators, however, report overall ICU mortality rates of 20% to 30% for patients more than 65 years. As one would anticipate, in-hospital mortality after an ICU stay is higher than ICU mortality, but these rates also vary widely across studies. In-hospital mortality has been reported to be as low as 16% for patients older than 74 years, whereas most investigators report rates ranging from 30% to 50%. In one retrospective analysis, in-hospital mortality was only 38% among patients older than 85 years. Mortality is found to increase when intubation and mechanical ventilation (MV) is required for support of respiratory failure (see Table 19-2). According to recent trials involving older patients on MV, approximately 33% to 50% of elderly do not survive to hospital discharge. Despite this overall increase in mortality, there is no consistent evidence indicating uniformly poor survival even in the oldest patients, and some investigators argue that severity of illness is a better predictor of mortality than is age (8,9).

In summary, approximately two thirds of elderly patients will survive to hospital discharge after an ICU stay. If MV is utilized during the ICU stay, survival does decrease but approximately one in two patients still survive to hospital discharge.

ESTIMATING PROGNOSIS

Estimating prognosis is difficult even for practitioners with extensive ICU experience. In the SUPPORT investigation, only 7 days before death of a patient, physicians who were experienced in the care of seriously ill adults prospectively estimated that 50% of patients with congestive heart failure (CHF), chronic obstructive pulmonary disease (COPD), and cirrhosis would live for 6 months. For patients with acute respiratory failure and multiple organ dysfunction syndrome, the same physicians estimated that 20% of the patients would live for 6 months, when in actuality, they lived for only 7 days (32).

TABLE 19-1.   Mortality of Elderly Patients Admitted to an Intensive Care Unit (5)

Reference/Year/Country	Intensive Care Unit (ICU)	Age Range (years)	Elderly Patients (n)	ICU (%)	In-hospital (%)	Postdischarge (%)
Campion et al., 1981 (6) USA	MICU/CCU	65–74	624	8	14	33 (6–18 mo)
		≥75	560	10	16	43 (6–18 mo)
Le GJ et al., 1982 (10) France	Multi	≥70	40	—	—	69 (1 yr)
Fedullo and Swinburne, 1983 (11) USA	MICU	70–79	61	26	41	—
	—	80–89	23	30	34	—
Nicolas et al., 1987 (12) France	Med/Surg 7 hospitals	>65	191	37	—	—
Sage et al., 1987 (13) USA	Med/Surg	>65	134	—	12	28 (18 mo)
		—	—	—	—	—
Chalfin et al., 1990 (14) USA	Med/Surg (cancer hospital)	65–74	324	27	36	—
		≥75	163	17	30	—
Ridley et al., 1991 (15) Scotland	MICU	65–74	102	29	—	38 (18–42 mo)
		75–84	39	21	—	—
		≥85	3	0	—	—
Wu et al., 1990 (16) USA	MICU	≥75	130	17	51	—
Mahul et al., 1991 (17) France	Med/Surg 4 hospitals	>70	295	20–29 (4 hospitals)	—	49 (1 yr)
Mayer-Oaks et al., 1991 (18) USA	MICU's, 3 hospitals	65–74	104	—	30	45 (6 mo)
		≥75	153	—	38	49
Chelluri et al., 1992 (19) USA	ICU	≥85	34	26	38	—
Heuser et al., 1992 (20) USA	ICU, 78 hospitals	≥65	2,208	—	8	—
Kass et al., 1992 (21) USA	Med/Surg	≥85	105	30	—	64 (1 yr)
Chelluri et al., 1993 (8) USA	ICU (excluded cancer patients with "poor prognosis")	65–74	43	21	40	58 (1 yr)
		≥75	54	31	39	63
Rockwood et al., 1993 (22) Canada	Multi, 2 hospitals	>65	406	16	—	49 (1 yr)
Cohen and Lambrinos, 1995 (23) USA	All beds for patients on MV, 243 NY hospitals	70–74	5,613	—	51	—
		75–79	5,874	—	56	—
		80–84	4,910	—	62	—
		85–89	3,145	—	67	—
		90+	1,812	—	75	—
Djaini and Ridley, 1997 (24) England	ICU	>70	474	19	—	47 (1 yr)
		70–74	—	12	—	—
		75–79	—	17	—	—
		80–84	—	26	—	—
		≥85	—	34	—	—

ICU, intensive care unit; MICU, medical ICU; CCU, cardiac care unit; Multi, multidisciplinary ICU; Med/Surg, medical/surgical ICU; MV, mechanical ventilation; NY, New York.

From Nelson JE, Nierman DM. Special Concerns for the Very Old. In: Curtis JR, Rubenfeld GD, editors. Managing Death in the Intensive Care Unit: The Transition from Cure to Comfort. New York: Oxford University Press, 2001: 349–367, with permission.

In an effort to assist the difficult task of providing family with prognostic information and in deciding when aggressive therapy is indicated, investigators have designed and validated prognostic models. Walter et al. used six independent risk factors including gender, number of dependent activities of daily learning (ADL), CHF, cancer, elevated creatinine, and low albumin to estimate the likelihood of 1-year mortality after hospitalization (33). The SUPPORT investigators developed a model to estimate survival of seriously ill hospitalized adults over a 180-day period (34). Predictor variables included diagnosis, age, number of days in the hospital before study entry, presence of cancer, neurologic function, and 11 physiologic measures on day 3 following study entry. The model was as accurate as physician estimates, and accuracy improved when the model was combined with physician estimates of survival. However, caring for critically ill or dying patients is emotionally challenging, and although prediction tools may assist physicians in avoiding serious errors in clinical judgment, they are difficult to apply at the bedside. Interestingly, even when prognostic information is available to physicians, practice behavior is not altered by such information (32).

TABLE 19-2. Functional Outcomes and Quality of Life of the Elderly after Intensive Care (5)

Reference/Year/Country	Intensive Care Unit (ICU)	Age Range (years)	Elderly Patients (n)	Measures/ Follow-up Period	Results
Campion et al., 1981 (6) USA	MICU/CCU	65—74 ≥75	624 560	Physical activity at 6–18 mo vs. pre-ICU	In both elderly groups, no change in % at home at f/u vs. baseline. Lifestyle with mild or more exertion: 65–74 yr, 76% (baseline) 70% (f/u) ≥75 yr, 68% (baseline); 50% (f/u) Sedentary lifestyle: 65–74 yr, 11% (baseline); 26% (f/u) ≥75 yr, 18% (baseline); 43% (f/u)
LeGall et al., 1982 (10) France	Med/Surg	≥50 ≥70	67 18	Functional status at 3 mo pre-ICU, 1 yr post-ICU	49% of survivors ≥50 yrs; no change at 1 yr; 51% had worse function; functional outcome influenced by age + number of organ failures
McLean et al., 1985 (25) Canada	Multi-RICU	≥75	14	Functional status, attitudes regarding QOL and ICU, 12–24 mo post-ICU	43% with activity level at f/u ≥baseline 85% QOL worthwhile; 77% would repeat ICU if indicated
Sage et al., 1987 (13) USA	Med/Surg	>65	59	SIP-uniscale, at 18 mo post-ICU	90% self-rated as "acceptably" or "extremely" healthy; slightly (not significant) lower adjusted SIP and uniscale for ICU survivors vs. elderly controls
Zaren and Hedstrand, 1987 (26) Sweden	Med/Surg	≥65	199	Functional status at 1 yr post-ICU vs. 3 yr post-ICU	80% of patients independent at home vs. 90% at baseline Poor baseline function, ICU LOS ≥1 wk, MV, predicted worse functional outcome
Zaren and Bergstorm, 1989 (27) Sweden	Med/Surg	≥65	350	Functional status at 1 yr post-ICU vs. 3 yr post-ICU	73% of patients' functional status at 1 yr ≥baseline MV but not ICU LOS associated with worse functional outcome
Mundt et al., 1989 (28) USA	Med/surg	≥70	262	Functional status in physical, psychologic, and social domains at 6 mo post-ICU	Most had worse functional status, but more contact with family 72% of previously working patients still working
Ridley and Wallace, 1990 (29) Scotland	Multi	≥60	40	PQOL, Katz's ADL, other functional capacity 1–3 yr post-ICU	82% of patients had same or improved status; 7% deteriorated
Mahul et al., 1991 (17) France	Med/Surg (4 hospitals)	≥70	106	Residence and functional status at 1 yr post-ICU	88% at home, 70% independent at 1 yr; 80% functional status ≥baseline; no clinical parameters at ICU admission predicted functional outcome
Chelluri et al., 1992 (19) USA	Med/Surg	≥85	21	Residence and level of activity, attitudes re: QOL and ICU	86% of patients from home; 43% independent; 62% discharged to home, 5% to rehab hospital; 80% QOL was good or fair; 90% would receive ICU care again
Vasquez et al., 1992 (30) Spain	Med/Surg	≥65	188	Function and PQOL at ICU admission and 1 yr post-ICU	50% worse function, 50% same or better function vs. baseline; lower function not mirrored by lower subjective perception of QOL; 1-yr QOL influenced by baseline QOL age, illness severity

(Continued)

TABLE 19-2. *(Continued)*

Reference/Year/Country	Intensive Care Unit (ICU)	Age Range (years)	Elderly Patients (n)	Measures/ Follow-up Period	Results
Chelluri et al., 1993 (8) USA	ICU	≥65	38	Kat's ADL, PQOL, Center of Epidemiologic Studies-Depression Score (CES-D) at 1 yr post-ICU	All 65–74-yr olds from home back at home at 1 yr; 85% pts ≥75 yr at home at 1 yr; 84% independent ADL's at 1 yr vs. 94% at baseline; no decline in PQOL from baseline; no difference in PQOL compared to community elderly controls; CES-D same as controls; 71% willing to repeat ICU if indicated
Rockwood et al., 1993 (22) Canada	Multi, 2 hospitals	>65	175	Health status, functional capacity, attitudes regarding ICU at 1 yr post-ICU	Majority independent in ADL; compared to control in community, same proportion perceived health as good to very good despite worse function; 70% satisfied with health status; 54% had health status ≥5 yr before ICU; 66% had health status ≥ contemporaries
Konopad et al., 1995 (31) Canada	Med/Surg	66–76 >75	46 175	Spitzer's QOL at ICU admission and 1 yr post-ICU	Activity level abd ADL worse for all age groups; patients >75 yr perceived health status as better; 82% of 66–75 yr olds, 71% of patients >75 yr home at 1 yr

MICU, medical ICU; CCU, cardiac care unit; ICU, intensive care unit; f/u, follow-up; Med/Surg, medical/surgical ICU; Multi, multidisciplinary ICU; RICU, respiratory ICU; QOL, quality of life; SIP, sickness impact profile; MV, mechanical ventilation; LOS, length of stay; PQOL, perceived quality of life; ADL, activities of daily living; CES-D, Center of Epidemiologic Studies-Depression Score.

From Nelson JE, Nierman DM. Special Concerns for the Very Old. In: Curtis JR, Rubenfeld GD, editors. Managing Death in the Intensive Care Unit: The Transition from Cure to Comfort. New York: Oxford University Press, 2001: 349–367, with permission.

FUNCTIONAL OUTCOMES AND QUALITY OF LIFE AFTER AN INTENSIVE CARE UNIT STAY

Although as many as one in three elderly patients will be alive 1 year after an ICU stay (Table 19-1), survival rates are meaningless without information on functional outcomes. Many studies on functional outcomes are limited by methodological flaws and small sample size (5) (Table 19-2), but consistent findings across studies include some decline in function but indicate a return to prior living situation and preservation of perceived quality of life (PQOL). For example, Chelluri et al. found that 100% of patients aged 65 to 74 and 80% of those older than 75 returned to their homes in the year following their ICU stay (8). There was no change in PQOL at 1 year, and 84% of patients were independent in ADL compared to 94% of those at baseline. Ninety percent of the survivors were independent in ADL prior to the hospitalization and 84% of them remained independent at 1 year.

Predictors of worse functional outcomes include older age, poor baseline function, the need for MV, and dysfunction of more than one organ system. Longer length of stay (LOS) and Acute Physiology and Chronic Health Evaluation (APACHE II) scores do not consistently predict functional decline (Table 19-2). Predictors of PQOL include age, baseline QOL, and illness severity. Despite worse functional outcomes, patients surviving an ICU stay frequently perceive their health as being good or better than before their critical illness and as being superior to the health of their contemporaries.

Although functional status and health-related quality of life (HRQOL) are often used interchangeably, elderly patients are more frequently satisfied with their lives in spite of chronic illness and functional impairment. It is important not to assume that patients with an impaired QOL want less aggressive treatment. Elderly patients are more likely to consider burdens of treatment than are younger adults, but they are also more likely to value living longer in suboptimal health versus living less time in excellent health (35).

In summary, most elderly survivors return to normal or near normal function after discharge from the hospital. Furthermore, when asked if they would be admitted to the ICU again, 71% to 90% of the elderly surveyed said that they would be willing if such an admission were indicated (Table 19-2).

CARDIOPULMONARY RESUSCITATION OUTCOMES

Although some have described CPR in the elderly as "an exercise in futility," age alone is not the most significant determinant of survival in patients who receive CPR. In elderly patients, survival on hospital discharge after CPR ranges from 0% to 39% (36) (see Table 19-3). Some studies have reported very poor outcomes, whereas more recent studies demonstrate improved survival that is similar to survival among young patients. If a patient survives the event that requires CPR, survival after discharge from the hospital is not uniformly dismal. Furthermore,

TABLE 19-3. Survival Rates After In-hospital Cardiac Arrest (36)

Reference	Cardiac Rhythm	Number of Patients (n)	Survival to Hospital Discharge (%)	Age Influences Outcome Unfavorably	Comments
Gulati RS et al., 1983 (37)	All	52	17	No	Of those alive at 1 mo, none had neurologic injury or physical dependence
Bedell SE et al., 1983 (38)	All	294	14	No	75% of survivors alive at 6 mo
	VF		24		
Taffet GI et al., 1988 (39)	All	77 (≥70)	0	Yes	
	VF	322 (<70)	0		
George AL et al., 1989 (40)	All	140	24	Yes	No absolute predictor of mortality
	VF		36		
Murphy DJ et al., 1989 (41)	All	259 (≥70)	3	Yes	Unwitnessed arrest survival <1%
	VF		21		
Peterson MW et al., 1991 (42)				No	Poor outcome: hypotension, sepsis, and elevated APACHE 2
Rosenberg M et al., 1993 (43)	All	178 (>70)	22	No	Survival similar in age <50
Schneider AP et al., 1993 (44)		meta-analysis	12		For age ≥90, 0% survived to discharge; community vs. teaching hospitals (19% vs. 14%)
Schwenzer KJ et al., 1993 (45)	All	137 (≥70 and <80)	22	No	Age ≥70 less likely to receive CPR but when CPR was performed, survival same as in younger pts.
Tresch DD et al., 1994 (46)	All	50	24	No	86% of survivors alive at 1 year; outcomes were similar to younger patients; 76% of arrests were witnessed; most were functionally active before admission; cardiac disease predicted success
	VF	28 (Age≥70)	39		
Di Bari M et al., 2000 (47)	All	245 (Mean age 70)	33	No	At 2-yr f/u, 60% of patients still alive and survival curve similar in older and younger patients

VF, ventricular fibrillation; APACHE, acute physiology and chronic health evaluation; CPR, cardiopulmonary resuscitation; f/u, follow-up.

From Tresch DD, Thakur RK. Cardiopulmonary resuscitation in the elderly. *Emerg Med Clin North Am* 1998; 16:649–663, with permission.

many elderly patients remain highly functional after CPR, especially if their primary illness is cardiac. Data in this area are somewhat conflicting and it is important to have a full understanding of the evidence both in support of and against CPR in older patients.

Two studies published in 1988 and 1989 reported very poor outcomes among hospitalized elderly who received CPR. These studies received much attention and led to pessimism regarding CPR. In one study, immediate survival of older (>70 years) patients was 31% versus 43% in the younger cohort, but none of the elderly patients survived to hospital discharge compared to 16% of patients younger than age 70 surviving to hospital discharge. In another retrospective study, the survival of 259 elderly patients (≥70 years) who were resuscitated between 1977 and 1987 was analyzed. Only 6.5% of those resuscitated while hospitalized survived to hospital discharge. Fifty percent of the survivors required placement in a long-term care facility or a rehabilitation unit, and 50% of the survivors had significant

functional or neurologic impairment. The conclusion from these two authors was that CPR is rarely beneficial to hospitalized elderly patients.

In contrast, recent studies have demonstrated better outcomes than those that were observed in these earlier investigations and outcomes among older patients that are similar to those for younger patients (38). Bedell et al. found 75% of survivors to be alive 6 months after having CPR performed, and Di Bari reported 60% survival at 2 years (Table 19-3) (47). Di Bari et al. studied 245 patients who received CPR in an ICU (*n* = 221) or in a general medical ward (*n* = 24). Patients older than 70 had an immediate survival of 39.4%, and in a multiple logistic analysis model, advancing age was *not* a predictor of immediate or long-term survival. Tresch et al. evaluated survival after resuscitations performed in the 1990s and noted no significant difference between those patients who were 70 years or older and those below 70 years (36). There were no significant differences in functional status pre- and postarrest. Survival at 1, 2, and 3 years in elderly and young survivors was 86% versus 80%, 76% versus 67%, and 71% versus 61%, respectively.

Age is not a consistent predictor of mortality across studies. The two most consistent predictors of survival after CPR are having a witnessed arrest and presenting with a cardiac rhythm of ventricular fibrillation or ventricular tachycardia. Patients presenting with ventricular fibrillation or ventricular tachycardia have markedly improved survival compared to those with asystole or pulseless electric activity. Most investigators also concur that a diagnosis of metastatic cancer portends a poor prognosis (48,49). Other factors variably associated with increased mortality include respiratory failure, increased number of comorbidities, greater severity of illness, very advanced age (>89 years), poor functional status, sepsis, creatinine level >2.0, albumin level <3, hypotension, CPR lasting longer than 15 minutes, and a Hct <35 mg per dL (36).

Included in Table 19-3 are frequently cited references on CPR survival among the elderly. For a detailed discussion of CPR survival rates over the past 30 years, we refer the reader to a meta-analysis by Schneider et al. (44). This meta-analysis included 98 studies of in-hospital CPR success rates. In this meta-analysis, patients younger than 70 had a success rate of 16.2%, patients older than 70 had a success rate of 12.4%, and 0% of those older than 89 survived. Community hospitals had a higher success rate than teaching hospitals (18.5% vs. 13.6%) and most deaths after CPR occurred within 72 hours. Only 1.6% of successfully resuscitated patients had a permanent neurologic deficit. The rate of successful CPR did not change over the 30 years, but the authors did note a decline in the optimism regarding its value and concluded that pessimism about CPR in the elderly was unfounded on the basis of the results of this review.

MECHANICAL VENTILATION IN THE ELDERLY PATIENT

As patients age, clinicians have more difficulty accurately predicting their preferences for MV, yet the probability of withholding MV increases with advancing age (see Fig. 19-3) (4). Physician error rates in approximating patients' preferences for MV increase from 36% at less than 50 years up to 79% at more than 80 years (4).

Many prior investigations of MV in the elderly have been limited by their retrospective design and by the absence of adjustment for severity of illness (50) (see Table 19-4). In a review of 21 published reports with data on MV in elderly patients, the author's conclusions were divided regarding the effect of age on the outcome. Another limiting factor is the inability to know how many elderly patients choose to forgo MV even though it may have been "indicated." Three recent cohort investigations have advanced the understanding of outcomes among older persons receiving MV.

The first report in this series was from a medical ICU and showed that patients more than 75 years actually passed a daily screen of weaning at a faster rate than younger patients did. This study also found that in cases of older persons on MV (with respiratory failure of various etiologies *not* confined to acute lung injury), their lengths of stay on the ventilator and

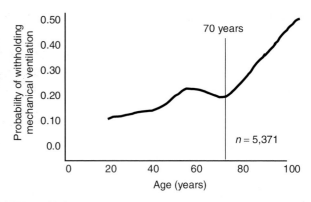

FIGURE 19-3. The relationship between patient age and the adjusted probability of a decision to withhold mechanical ventilation (MV) by study day 30 in the Study to Understand Prognosis and Preferences for Outcomes and Risks of Treatment (SUPPORT) investigation. At 70 to 79 years, relative risk is 1.5 (1.2 to 1.9), and for more than 80 years, the relative risk is 2.1 (1.6 to 2.7) (4). (From Hamel MB, Teno JM, Goldman L, et al. Patient age and decisions to withhold life-sustaining treatments from seriously ill, hospitalized adults. *Ann Intern Med* 1999;130:116–125, with permission.)

survival rates were comparable to their younger counterparts. However, this cohort was from a single center and selection bias must be taken into consideration (50).

The second cohort from an international study of respiratory failure demonstrated that 1,038 patients 75 years and older had lengths of stay and time on MV that were comparable to 4,118 patients less than 75 years (P >0.2 in both cases). The older patients did, however, have higher ICU mortality (38% vs. 30%, P <0.001) and higher in-hospital mortality (52% vs. 37%, P <0.001) than did younger patients (69).

The third report, an analysis of 902 patients from the Acute Respiratory Distress Syndrome (ARDS) network's acute lung injury investigations in the United States was the largest prospectively collected cohort to date (70). This investigation provided important insight into the outcomes of older patients with acute lung injury or ARDS. Patients aged 70 and older had 28-day and 180-day mortality rates that were nearly twice those of patients less than 70 years, with steady reductions in survival by deciles. Even after adjusting for covariates, it was determined that age was a strong predictor of mortality. Interestingly, older persons who did survive achieved initial recovery landmarks at the same rate as their younger counterparts (i.e., they passed conventional weaning criteria and were able to sustain spontaneous breathing without mechanical support) yet were delayed in their further progression through convalescence and were much more likely to be reconnected to the ventilator (70).

In summary, the duration of MV has been shown to be an independent predictor of mortality even after adjusting for covariates such as severity of illness. Older patients have comparable rates of initial physiologic recovery (i.e., ability to breathe spontaneously) to their younger counterparts but have a delayed successful liberation from the ventilator and are reintubated twice as often. Reintubation independently increases the risk of adverse outcomes including nosocomial pneumonia and mortality. Further study is warranted to determine why older patients, although exhibiting initial recovery that is comparable to younger patients, ultimately have more difficulty being liberated from the ventilator and the ICU.

TABLE 19-4. Outcomes After Mechanical Ventilation (MV) in Older Patients (50)

Author/Year/Source	Elderly (N) and Definition		Design of Study	Inclusion Criteria	Hospital Mortality (%)	Multivariate Analysis	Severity Adjustment	Age Influences Outcome[a]
Nunn et al., 1979 (51)	15	>75	Prospective	ICU[b]	73	No	No	Yes
Campion et al., 1981 (6)	565	≥75	Retrospective	ICU/CCU	16	No	No	No
Fedullo et al., 1983 (11)	84	≥70	Retrospective	MICU only	39	No	No	No
Witek et al., 1985 (52)	51	>70	Prospective	ICU	51	No	No	Yes
McLean et al., 1985 (25)	49	≥75	Prospective	ICU	43	No	No	No
Elpern et al., 1989 (53)	95	≥60	Retrospective	ICU ≥3 d	66	No	No	Yes
Tran et al., 1990 (54)	92	>70	Retrospective	MICU only	46	No	No	Yes
O'Donnell and Bohner, 1991 (55)	17	>70	Retrospective	ICU	59	No	No	No
Pesau et al., 1992 (56)	99	≥70	Retrospective	ICU	60	Yes	Yes	No
Gracey et al., 1992 (57)	496	>65	Retrospective	ICU	46	No	No	Yes
Chelluri et al., 1992 (19)	34	≥85	Retrospective	MICU only	38	No	No	No
Stauffer et al., 1993 (58)	118	>70	Retrospective	ICU	62	Yes	No	Yes
Swinburne, 1993 (59)	282	≥80	Retrospective	ICU	69	No	No	No
Cohen et al., 1993 (60)	109	≥80	Retrospective	ICU >3 d	62	No	No	Yes
Papadakis et al., 1993 (61)	138	≥70	Retrospective	ICU	76	Yes	Yes	Yes
Dardaine et al., 1995 (62)	110	≥70	Retrospective	ICU	38	No	No	No
Cohen et al., 1995 (23)	21,342	≥70	Retrospective	ICU	59	No	No	Yes
Steiner et al., 1997 (63)	40	>65	Prospective	ICU/Stroke patients	32 at 2 mo	Yes	No	Yes
Kurek et al., 1997 (64)	3,256	≥70	Retrospective	Tracheostomy	64	No	No	Yes
Zilberberg and Epstein, 1998 (65)	31	>65	Prospective	MICU	74	Yes	Yes	Yes
Kurek et al., 1998 (66)	4,101	≥75	Retrospective	ICU	55	No	No	Yes
Ely et al., 1999 (67)	63	≥75	Prospective	MICU/CCU	39	Yes	Yes	No
Ely et al., 2002 (68)	173	≥70	Prospective	ARDS/ALI	50 at 28 d	Yes	Yes	Yes

ICU, intensive care unit; CCU, cardiac care unit; MICU, medical ICU; Pts, patients; ARDS, acute respiratory distress syndrome; ALI, acute lung injury.

[a] Indicates the predominant conclusion of the authors as to whether age is independently important

[b] Investigations including only mechanically ventilated patients

From Ely EW, Evans GW, Haponik EF. Mechanical ventilation in a cohort of elderly patients admitted to an intensive care unit. *Ann Intern Med* 1999;131:96–104, with permission.

DELIRIUM AND PERSISTENT COGNITIVE IMPAIRMENT IN OLDER INTENSIVE CARE UNIT PATIENTS

Dementia, an acquired persistent form of cognitive impairment, is an increasingly common and devastating problem for the aging population. The prevalence of dementia in community samples of older persons ranges from 10% to 19% (71,72). Knowledge of a patient's preexisting cognitive status provides important information that can have an impact on ICU care, which includes (a) assessing decision-making capacity; (b) providing a baseline for evaluating changes in mental status, such as delirium, that occur during an ICU stay; (c) choosing treatment options, such as psychoactive medications, that have the potential for mental status effects; and (d) identifying patients who are at high risk for decline in mental status and who may benefit from preventive measures for delirium (73,74).

A recent study estimated the prevalence of preexisting cognitive impairment in older patients who were admitted to a medical ICU to be between 31% and 42% (75). In 40% of these patients, the cognitive impairment was severe. The term "preexisting cognitive impairment" was used to refer to either dementia or mild cognitive impairment that was present in chronic form before admission. This preexisting cognitive impairment in older ICU patients is often unrecognized by physicians caring for them. In a study of 165 older ICU patients, attending physicians were unaware of 53% of cases of preexisting cognitive impairment, and intern physicians were unaware of 59% of cases (76). Both attending and intern recognition of preexisting cognitive impairment significantly increased as the severity of cognitive impairment increased.

Delirium has been described as the brain's form of "organ dysfunction." According to the National Research Council, "For many people in good physical condition who succumb to an acute illness, cognitive decline is the main threat to their ability to recover and enjoy their favorite activities; for those whose physical activities were already limited, cognitive decline is a major additional threat to quality of life." Delirium is frequently not recognized by clinicians, and when recognized, it is often considered an inevitable outcome of critical illness (77). Recognizing delirium in the ICU is important because the medical literature has shown that delirium impacts adversely on health outcomes. Delirium has been associated with increased LOS, institutionalization, and higher mortality rates (78,79).

In a study of 48 critically ill patients, 60% developed delirium while in the ICU and 81% developed delirium at any time during hospitalization (80). In multivariate analysis, delirium was the strongest predictor of LOS in the hospital ($p = 0.006$), even after adjusting for severity of illness, age, gender, race, and days of benzodiazepine and narcotic drug administration.

Formal cognitive assessment in the ICU can be performed using the Confusion Assessment Method–Intensive Care Unit (CAM–ICU). The CAM–ICU is a 2-minute assessment instrument that can be used in intubated nonverbal patients (see Fig. 19-4). In validation studies, the CAM–ICU demonstrated a sensitivity of 93% to 100%, a specificity of 98% to 100%, and high interrater reliability ($\kappa = 0.96$) in the detection of delirium. In 48 and then 96 consecutive patients on MV, delirium occurred in more than 80% of patients in the ICU. In the subgroups expected to pose the greatest challenges for the CAM–ICU (i.e., those 65 years and older, those with suspected dementia, and those with the highest severity of illness), the instrument retained excellent sensitivity, specificity, and interrater reliability (81).

1. Acute Onset or Fluctuating Course	Absent	Present

A. Is there evidence of an acute change in mental status from the baseline?

OR

B. Did the (abnormal) behavior fluctuate during the past 24 hours, that is, tend to come and go, or increase and decrease in severity as evidenced by fluctuation on a sedation scale (e.g. RASS), GCS, or previous delirium assessment?

2. Inattention	Absent	Present

Did the patient have difficulty focusing attention as evidenced by **scores *less than 8*** on either the auditory or visual component of the **Attention Screening Examination (ASE)**? (Instructions on next page).

3. Disorganized Thinking	Absent	Present

Is there evidence of disorganized or incoherent thinking as evidenced by **incorrect answers to 2 or more of the 4 questions and/or inability to follow the commands**?

Questions (Alternate Set A and Set B):

Set A	**Set B**
1. Will a stone float on water?	1. Will a leaf float on water?
2. Are there fish in the sea?	2. Are there elephants in the sea?
3. Does one pound weigh more than two pounds?	3. Do two pounds weigh more than one pound?
4. Can you use a hammer to pound a nail?	4. Can you use a hammer to cut wood?

Other:
1. Are you having any unclear thinking?
2. Hold up this many fingers. (Examiner holds two fingers in front of patient)
3. Now do the same thing with the other hand. (Not repeating the number of fingers)

4. Altered Level of Consciousness	Absent	Present

Is the patient's level of consciousness anything *other than alert* such as vigilant, lethargic, or stuporors (e.g., RASS other than "0" at time of assessment)

Alert   spontaneously fully aware of environment and interacts appropriately

Vigilant   hyperalert

Lethargic drowsy but easily aroused, unaware of some elements in the environment, or not spontaneously interacting appropriately with the interviewer; becomes fully aware and appropriately interactive when prodded minimally

Stupor   becomes incompletely aware when prodded strongly; can be aroused only by vigorous and repeated stimuli, and as soon as the stimulus ceases, stuporous subject lapse back into the unresponsive state

Overall CAM-ICU (Features 1 and 2 and either Feature 3 or 4):	Yes	No

FIGURE 19-4. This figure represents the features and descriptions of the Confusion Assessment Method–Intensive Care Unit (CAM-ICU) instrument (81). [From Ely EW, Inouye SK, Bernard GR, et al. Delirium in mechanically ventilated patients: validity and reliability of the confusion assessment method for the intensive care unit (CAM-ICU). *JAMA* 2001;286:2703–2710, with permission.]

Sepsis, ARDS, and other covariates result in profound neurologic injury during the course of a patient's illness. Hopkins et al. demonstrated in a prospective outcome study that some degree of cognitive abnormality was present in 100% of ARDS patients at hospital discharge and in 80% of these patients at 1 year (82). In a general ICU population not restricted to ARDS, it is remarkable that neuropsychological abnormalities were found to be present in more than 50% of survivors following MV at hospital discharge. Furthermore, one in three patients have clinically relevant abnormalities in psychomotor speed, executive function and visuoconstruction abilities, memory, and verbal fluency at 6 months (83). Figure 19-5 shows a range of deficits among survivors of critical care (83). The Rey-O Copy, a test of visuoconstruction in which the patient is asked to copy a complex geometric design, was administered to all patients 6 months after hospital discharge as a component of the neuropsychological battery. Figure 19-5 shows the original Rey-O and the examples of three patients (all of whom had no detectable baseline cognitive deficits) as a visual depiction of the character of deficits found in the study cohort. It has recently been shown that neuropsychological sequelae of coronary artery bypass graft surgery have an important effect on outcomes up to 5 years later, and in another cohort, up to 25% of ICU survivors had deficits 6 years following their ICU stay.

Cognitive impairment in the ICU may be independently related to prolonged neuropsychological deficits. It is also true that evidence of baseline dementia is an independent risk factor for developing delirium while in the hospital (84). A significant percentage of individuals developing delirium in the hospital

continue to demonstrate symptoms of delirium after discharge (see Fig. 19-6). The patients who survived an ICU stay were subjected to a study conducted within 24 hours of leaving the hospital that showed that one in two patients exhibited significant impairment on the Folstein Mini-Mental State Examination (MMSE), one in five patients had some features of delirium, and one in ten patients met full delirium criteria at the time of hospital discharge. Such patients demonstrate decreased cerebral activity and increased cognitive deterioration and are more likely to develop dementia than are patients without delirium. Finally, patients who develop delirium have a greater rate of decline on cognitive tests than nondelirious patients do (85).

COGNITIVE OUTCOMES AFTER CARDIOPULMONARY RESUSCITATION

In a meta-analysis of successful CPR (defined as being discharged alive from the hospital) in 2,994 patients, central nervous system impairment was noted in only 1.6% of patients (44). In another literature review including 19 studies, only 16 of 7,324 patients (0.2%) remained in a vegetative state for up to 6 weeks until death, but up to 14% of patients in some series were in a chronic vegetative state. Rogove et al. studied a total of 774 patients who were initially comatose after successful resuscitation from cardiac arrest (86). The analyses included both in-hospital and out-of-hospital cardiac arrests. Mortality rate was 94% for the oldest group (>80 years) compared with 68% for the youngest group (≤45 years) ($p < 0.01$). Recovery of good neurologic function was

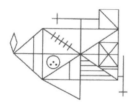

Three patients were asked to copy the picture above. Results are given below:

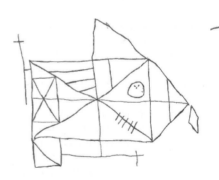 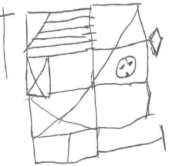 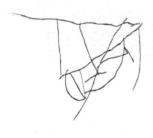

Near normal rendition by nonimpaired 69 y/o pulmonary embolus survivor

Moderate to severely impaired 89 y/o pneumonia survivor

Severely impaired 72 y/o ARDS survivor

FIGURE 19-5. Examples of Neuropsychological Deficits following ICU Care. Rey-O Copy is a test of Visuo-Construction in which the patient is asked to copy an abstract picture that is right in front of them: (each of these was completed 6 months after hospital discharge in patients with no detectable baseline cognitive deficits). (From Jackson JC, Hart RP, Gordon SM, et al. Six-month neuropsychological outcome of medical intensive care unit patients. *Crit Care Med* 2003;31:1226–1234, with permission.)

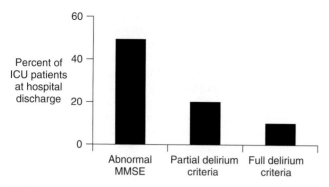

FIGURE 19-6. Rate of ongoing cognitive deficits and delirium at hospital discharge following MV. These data from survivors of ICU studied within 24 hours of leaving the hospital show that 1 in 2 patients were significantly impaired by MMSE, 1 in 5 had partial delirium, and 1 in 10 met full delirium criteria at the time of hospital discharge (81). [From Ely EW, Inouye SK, Bernard GR, et al. Delirium in mechanically ventilated patients: validity and reliability of the confusion assessment method for the intensive care unit (CAM-ICU). *JAMA* 2001;286:2703–2710, with permission.]

seen in 27% of the 774 patients. There was no statistically significant difference in neurologic recovery rates by age. Multivariate analysis showed that predictors of a good neurologic outcome were a cardiac cause of arrest, short arrest time, short CPR time, and no history of diabetes mellitus. Importantly, increasing age was *not* an independent predictor of poor neurologic outcome on either univariate or multivariate analyses.

ADVANCE DIRECTIVES

Elderly patients do want to discuss advance directives, and despite the importance of establishing preferences for care, the vast majority of patients report not having had a discussion with their physician about advance directives. Some authors suggest that while patients prefer to participate actively in determining their "code status," during periods of cognitive impairment, they are frequently asked questions associated with their acute illness and become confused by the precise treatment options and implications of such decisions (87). This quandary emphasizes the importance of having advance care planning discussions in the outpatient setting or early in the course of an illness.

In the SUPPORT investigation, the presence of an advance directive did result in limited interventions at the end of life (88). Elderly patients who presented with an advance directive upon ICU admission and for whom an order was written to limit resuscitation had the highest mortality. Patients without an advance directive but for whom an order was written to limit resuscitation during their ICU stay had the longest LOS, the most interventions, and highest mortality. Most patients died in the ICU shortly after orders were written to limit resuscitative efforts.

Unfortunately, surrogates and primary care providers are not good at predicting the preferences of elderly patients. The SUPPORT study demonstrated that less than 40% of patients recalled discussing prognosis or their preferences for life-sustaining treatments with their physician, and even when patients preferred palliative care, only 29% of them felt that

their care reflected that preference (89). Only 47% of physicians knew that their patient did not want resuscitation and 46% of the "do not resuscitate (DNR) orders" were written within 2 days of death. In another investigation, when patients and physicians were presented with medical vignettes, 40% of physicians chose a level of care different from that requested by the patient. In fact, 10% of physicians would have done CPR on a patient with a DNR request (90). Interestingly, whereas this study was utilizing hypothetical examples, the SUPPORT investigation revealed that CPR was performed on 11% of patients who had requested not to be resuscitated.

Some authors contend that patients are able to incorporate probabilistic thinking into advance care planning, and these authors suggest that rather than focusing on specific interventions, these discussions should focus on potential outcomes and burdens of treatment (91). In this investigation, seriously ill patients were asked if they wanted to receive a given treatment depending on the burden of treatment and the outcome. Patients were willing to accept high treatment burdens if they would return to their current, albeit impaired, health status. However, if the outcome was severe functional or cognitive impairment, most patients (74.4% and 88.8%, respectively) declined treatment even if the alternative was death (91).

Although there was initial enthusiasm about cost savings due to establishing advance directives, substantial cost savings are unlikely to result (92). As an illustration, if every American who died had elected hospice care, the estimated reduction in health care expenditures would only be 3.3%. This is likely attributable to lower daily and total hospital costs among older patients because less aggressive care is preferred overall by this group of patients (93). Clearly, the merit of establishing advanced directives is not to reduce medical expenditures but to spare patients the unwanted aggressive care.

MEDICAL FUTILITY AND LIMITATION OF SUPPORT

The probability of limiting life-sustaining treatment increases with advancing age (Fig. 19-2) (4). Futility is often invoked as a justification for such limitation of care but it is an inherently difficult term to define in medical care. Quantitative futility has been defined as an intervention where the estimate of success is less than or equal to 1% (94). Very few medical conditions are known to have a survival of less than 1%; hence, there is rarely an opportunity to apply the principle of quantitative futility when deciding whether to limit care. Qualitative futility has been defined as an intervention that merely preserves permanent unconsciousness or fails to end total dependence on intensive medical care. Again, it is difficult to know how long patients will need intensive care and what interventions will or will not assist in liberating them from the need for ICU care. Given these definitions, it is not surprising that futile care has been described as being uncommon in the ICU (95).

To aid in this complicated ethical dilemma, the reader is referred to a report of the Council on Ethical and Judicial Affairs of the American Medical Association (AMA) (96). The AMA recommends a standardized "fair process" rather than a strict definition of futility. The process includes deliberation and resolution among all involved parties, securing alternatives in the case of irreconcilable differences, and a final step focused on providing closure when all alternatives have been considered. Physicians should base futility decisions on factors such as clinical efficacy of treatments, likelihood of mortality, and subsequent QOL considerations rather than on chronologic age alone.

Although futility as a means of justifying the limitation of care can be onerous, limitation of life support prior to death is common in the ICU setting (97) and is independently associated with death after adjusting for severity of illness and comorbidity (14). The circumstances of withdrawal or withholding treatments vary widely from one institution to another and from one country to another (97,98). The active withdrawal of life-sustaining therapy occurs more often in patients without access to a private attending physician (29.9% vs. 80.8%; $p<0.001$), and death due to withholding life support occurs more frequently in community hospitals than in teaching hospitals (11.9% vs. 3.8%, respectively, $p = 0.004$) (99).

A national survey of all American postgraduate training programs with significant clinical exposure to critical care medicine recently examined 6,303 ICU-related deaths. Standard ICU care including failed CPR occurred in 26% of patients (range 4% to 79%); 24% (range 0% to 83%) of them received standard ICU care without CPR; 14% (range 0% to 67%) of patients had life support withheld; and 36% (range 0% to 79%) of them had life support actively withdrawn (97). Clearly, the treatments are commonly withheld and/or withdrawn in the ICU, but the basis for such decisions is complex and cannot be ascribed to a standard set of criteria that defines futility.

In the process of limiting therapy and transitioning to comfort care, health care professionals must continue to provide quality end-of-life care and must meet the needs of the patients' family members (100). Seven end-of-life domains have been identified by the Robert Wood Johnson Foundation Critical Care End-of-Life Peer Workgroup (101):

1. Patient and family-centered decision making
2. Communication within the team and with patients and families
3. Continuity of care
4. Emotional and practical support for patients and families
5. Symptom management and comfort care
6. Spiritual support for patients and families
7. Emotional and organizational support for ICU clinicians.

Each domain addresses the organizational and behavioral changes necessary to improve the quality of end-of-life care in the ICU. To date, most of the domains have not been tested in randomized trials and represent expert clinical opinion.

PREOPERATIVE PULMONARY EVALUATION IN THE ELDERLY

Physicians are commonly asked to perform "preoperative evaluations" on elderly patients scheduled for either elective or emergent surgical procedures. Furthermore, they are further asked to comment on the likelihood of postoperative pulmonary complications. Although there are well-defined assessment tools to determine the perioperative risk factors for cardiac complications (102), the development of pulmonary complications has been studied less extensively. In reality, the development of

pulmonary complications is at least as common (if not more so) as cardiac complications (103). Elderly patients tend to have more surgical procedures. More than 50% of all malignancies occur in patients above 65 years, and the primary treatment of many of these is surgery (104,105). In addition, there are an increasing number of elderly patients receiving coronary artery bypass grafting surgery (106). This section of the chapter focuses on the preoperative pulmonary evaluation, with special focus on the role of age in these assessments.

Postoperative pulmonary complications have been reported to prolong the hospital stay by an average of 1 to 2 weeks (103). One inherent difficulty in interpreting these data is that studies vary widely in their criteria for postoperative pulmonary complications—including definitions ranging from atelectasis or bronchospasm to postoperative pneumonia or ARDS (103). Postoperative "respiratory failure" may be defined as the inability to be extubated 48 hours after surgery, but some have considered it only if the patients were not liberated by day 5 (107). The in-hospital mortality rate for those with postoperative respiratory failure is around 40%, versus 5% for those without respiratory failure (107).

Potential patient-related risk factors for the development of postoperative pulmonary complications include smoking, general health status, age, obesity, COPD, neurologic status, cardiovascular status, and fluid or intravascular volume status. Procedure-related risk factors include the site of the incision (i.e., thorax vs. upper or lower abdomen), length of surgery, and the type of anesthesia. The risk of pulmonary complications increases as the incision approaches the diaphragm, with upper abdominal and thoracic procedures carrying the greatest risk (10% to 40%) (103). With the exceptions of neurologic (108,109) and head and neck procedures (108), pulmonary complications are rare following procedures outside the thorax and abdomen.

The independent importance of age in the development of postoperative pulmonary complications has not been studied in a manner that would control coexisting conditions. In fact, according to the American Society of Anesthesia (ASA) class stratification scheme, the preoperative mortality for ASA classes II through V is the same for all ages (110). In an investigation of patients above 80 years ($n = 500$), ASA Class II had a 30-day mortality rate of less than 1%, and for the entire cohort, the 30-day mortality rate was only 6.2% (111). There are no data to support the notion that age-related changes in lung function increase postoperative pulmonary complications in those without chronic pulmonary disease. Even among those with severe COPD, age was not shown to be an independent risk factor for pulmonary complications (112,113). Much like the situation with MV discussed previously, chronologic age is less predictive of pulmonary complications following surgery than coexisting conditions are. Therefore, advanced age alone is not a reason to withhold surgery.

A carefully performed history and physical examination are the most important aspects of preoperative consultations. Asking the patient about his or her ability to ambulate, details regarding the presence and character of a cough, and any recent changes in the level of dyspnea are key factors to be included in the history. The presence of COPD increases the risk of postoperative pulmonary complications by about three to five times. Many patients who have significant obstruction remain undiagnosed at the time of preoperative evaluation. Guidelines for using the clinical examination to diagnose airflow limitation could be summarized as follows (114–116):

- No single item or combination of items from the clinical examination rules out airflow limitation.
- The best finding associated with decreased likelihood of airflow limitation is a history of never having smoked cigarettes (especially in patients without a history of wheezing and without wheezing on examination).
- Wheezing noted on physical examination is the most potent predictor of airflow limitation, and patients with obstructive airflow limitation are 36 times more likely to have wheezing than are patients without this problem (i.e., likelihood ratio of 36) (114,116).
- Other findings associated with increased likelihood of airflow limitation are barrel chest, a positive match test (116,117), hyperresonance, a forced expiratory time (FET) ≥9 seconds (115,118), and a subxyphoid apical impulse.

Considering that the presence of underlying COPD is probably the largest risk factor for the development of postoperative pulmonary complication (103), it would be prudent for physicians to detect this disease in patients not yet diagnosed for the same. Two validated bedside maneuvers, which can be performed to detect unrecognized pulmonary dysfunction, include the match test and the FET. To perform the match test, the clinician holds a burning match at a distance of 10 cm from the patient's widely opened mouth. If the match is still burning after the forced expiration, the test result is positive. The inability to extinguish a match held 10 cm from the open mouth is associated with a moderate increase in the likelihood of airway obstruction (likelihood ratio = 7.1) (116,117). The FET (115,118) is performed by asking the patient to take a deep breath and *forcefully* exhale until no more air can be expelled. During this maneuver, the patient must keep his or her mouth and glottis fully open as if the patient is yawning. While the patient is performing the FET, the clinician listens over the larynx or lower trachea with a stethoscope and records the duration of audible airflow. When the longest expiratory time of a patient is chosen, a result <6 seconds is associated with a modest decrease in the likelihood of airflow limitation (likelihood ratio = 0.45); a result >9 seconds is associated with an increase in the likelihood of having a forced expiratory volume in 1 second divided by the forced vital capacity (FEV_1/FVC) of ≤70%, a level suggesting the diagnosis of airflow limitation (likelihood ratio = 4.8). The FET provides less diagnostic information in patients younger than 60 years (e.g., in those <60 years, the likelihood ratio for FET to be ≥8 seconds was 2.3) (119). Because the peak expiratory flow rate may add to other helpful predictors, such as the years of cigarette smoking and wheezing, some may choose to have the patient perform a peak expiratory flow measurement with a Wright peak flow meter. Clinicians' ability to diagnose airflow limitation clinically is variable, but it seems to improve as the severity of the disorder increases.

The utility of routine preoperative pulmonary function tests (PFTs) remains controversial. Not all candidates for lung resection or other surgical procedures need to undergo PFTs. Rather, these tests should be performed selectively in patients who demonstrate significant risks for adverse outcome (as outlined above). The position paper of the American College

of Physicians (120) recommends spirometry in the following groups of patients: those with a history of tobacco use or dyspnea who are undergoing coronary artery or upper abdominal surgery; patients with unexplained shortness of breath undergoing head and neck, orthopedic, or lower abdominal surgery; and all patients who are to receive lung resection. Although these may be prudent recommendations, it is worth noting that many of the 22 early studies of preoperative spirometry are felt to be methodologically flawed (121) and that more recent investigations have shown variable predictive results of PFTs (122). In the several studies including both clinical findings and PFTs, the history and physical examination have been found to be better predictors of pulmonary complications than are PFTs (122).

With regard to risk indexes developed to predict postoperative pulmonary complications, Epstein et al. (123) developed a cardiopulmonary risk index for lung resection patients, which included pulmonary risk factors including obesity, smoking, productive cough, diffuse wheezing or rhonchi, an FEV_1/FVC ratio of less than 70%, and an arterial partial pressure of carbon dioxide ($PaCO_2$) >45 mm Hg (also known as a modified Goldman index). Those with half of these risk factors were more than 10 times more likely to develop pulmonary complications than were those with fewer risk factors. Although potentially helpful, this index has not been validated by other investigators and has not been studied in patients undergoing abdominal surgery. It also requires the incorporation of routine preoperative arterial blood gas and PFT analysis. In general, it is not necessary to perform arterial blood gas analysis unless the patient's pulse oximetry readings are borderline to low and/or the clinician suspects significant obstructive lung disease of acid–base disturbances. In the future, other investigators will need to devise schemes for preoperative risk assessment for pulmonary complications, which might not require preoperative PFTs (124). Both thoracic and abdominal surgical procedures will also need to be incorporated into these investigations. On the other hand, risk stratification, which does not incorporate PFTs and arterial blood gas analysis, might be greatly hampered by the inability to appropriately stratify the degree of chronic pulmonary disease.

CONCLUSIONS

The elderly will continue to represent a large percentage of patients treated in the ICU. Although an ICU admission serves as a catalyst for discussions about preferences for care, such discussions should be occurring in the outpatient setting when patients are able to fully consider their treatment options, seek a better understanding of the implications of their decisions, and ultimately articulate their choices regarding health care. All too often, decisions about life-sustaining care fall to surrogates and clinicians who are frequently inaccurate in their assessment of the patient's preferences for care. Despite older age, many scenarios result in outcomes that are acceptable and valued by our older patients. Decisions about the aggressiveness of care must be carefully considered on a case-by-case basis. Regardless of the degree to which a seriously ill patient desires aggressive care, health care providers must attend to all aspects of care and keep the patient, whenever possible, free of pain, anxiety, and dyspnea.

REFERENCES

1. Angus DC, Kelly MA, et al, for the Committee on Manpower for Pulmonary and Critical Care Societies (COMPACCS). Current and projected workforce requirements for care of the critically ill and patients with pulmonary disease: Can we meet the requirements of an aging population? *JAMA* 2000;284:2762–2770.
2. Nuckton TJ, List ND. Age as a factor in critical care unit admissions. *Arch Intern Med* 1995;155:1087–1092.
3. Hamel MB, Philips RS, Teno JM, et al. Seriously ill hospitalized adults: do we spend less on older patients? *J Am Geriatr Soc* 1996; 44:1043–1048.
4. Hamel MB, Teno JM, Goldman L, et al. Patient age and decisions to withhold life-sustaining treatments from seriously ill, hospitalized adults. *Ann Intern Med* 1999;130:116–125.
5. Nelson JE, Nierman DM. Special concerns for the very old. In: Curtis JR, Rubenfeld GD, eds. *Managing death in the intensive care unit: the transition from cure to comfort.* New York: Oxford University Press, 2001:349–367.
6. Campion EW, Mulley AG, Goldstein RL, et al. Medical intensive care for the elderly. A study of current use, costs, and outcomes. *JAMA* 1981;246:2052–2056.
7. Boumendil A, Maury E, Reinhard I, et al. Prognosis of patients aged 80 years and over admitted in medical intensive care units. *Intensive Care Med* 2004;30:647–654.
8. Chelluri L, Pinsky MR, Donahoe MP, et al. Long-term outcome of critically ill elderly patients requiring intensive care. *JAMA* 1993; 269:3119–3123.
9. Hamel MB, Davis RB, Teno J, et al. Older age, aggressiveness of care, and survival for seriously ill, hospitalized adults. *Ann Intern Med* 1999;131:721–728.
10. Le GJ, Brun-Buisson C, Trunet P, et al. Influence of age, previous health status, and severity of acute illness on outcome from intensive care. *Crit Care Med* 1982;10:575–577.
11. Fedullo AJ, Swinburne AJ. Relationship of patient age to cost and survival in a medical ICU. *Crit Care Med* 1983;11:155–159.
12. Nicolas F, Le GJ, Alperovitch A, et al. Influence of patients' age on survival, level of therapy and length of stay in intensive care units. *Intensive Care Med* 1987;13:9–13.
13. Sage WM, Hurst CR, Silverman JF, et al. Intensive care for the elderly: outcome of elective and nonelective admissions. *J Am Geriatr Soc* 1987;35:312–318.
14. Chalfin DB, Cohen Il, Lambrinos J. The economics and cost-effectiveness of critical care medicine. *Intensive Care Med* 1995;21: 952–961.
15. Ridley S, Biggam M, Stone P. Cost of intensive therapy. *Anaesthesia* 1991;46:523–530.
16. Wu A, Rubin HR, Rosen MJ. Are elderly people less responsive to intensive care? *J Am Geriatr Soc* 1990;38:621–627.
17. Mahul P, Perrot D, Tempelhoff G, et al. Short and long-term prognosis, functional outcome following ICU for elderly. *Intensive Care Med* 1991;17:7–10.
18. Mayer-Oaks SA, Oye RK, Leake B. Predictors of mortality in older patients following medical intensive care: the importance of functional status. *J Am Geriatr Soc* 1991;39:862–868.
19. Chelluri L, Pinsky MR, Grenvik AN. Outcome of intensive care of the "oldest-old" critically ill patients. *Crit Care Med* 1992;20:757–761.
20. Heuser MD, Case LD, Ettinger WH. Mortality in intensive care patients with respiratory disease. Is age important? *Arch Intern Med* 1992;152:1683–1688.
21. Kass JE, Castriotta RJ, Malakoff F. Intensive care unit outcome in the very elderly. *Crit Care Med* 1992;20:1666–1671.
22. Rockwood K, Noseworthy TW, Gibney RT, et al. One-year outcome of elderly and young patients admitted to intensive care units. *Crit Care Med* 1993;21:687–691.
23. Cohen IL, Lambrinos J. Investigating the impact of age on outcome of mechanical ventilation using a population of 41,848 patients from a statewide database. *Chest* 1995;107:1673–1680.
24. Djaiani G, Ridley S. Outcome of intensive care in the elderly. *Anaesthesia* 1997;52:1130–1136.
25. McLean RF, McIntosh JD, Kung GY, et al. Outcome of respiratory intensive care for the elderly. *Crit Care Med* 1985;13:625–629.
26. Zaren B, Hedstrand U. Quality of life among long-term survivors of intensive care. *Crit Care Med* 1987;15:743–747.
27. Zaren B, Bergstrom R. Survival compared to the general population and changes in health status among intensive care patients. *Acta Anaesthesiol Scand* 1989;33:6–12.
28. Mundt DJ, Gage RW, Lemeshow S, et al. Intensive care unit patient follow-up. Mortality, functional status, and return to work at six months. *Arch Intern Med* 1989;149:68–72.
29. Ridley SA, Wallace PGM. Quality of life after intensive care. *Anaesthesia* 1990;45:808–813.
30. Vasquez-Mata G, Rivera FR, Gonzalez CA, et al. Factors related to quality of life 12 months after discharge from an intensive care unit. *Crit Care Med* 1992;20:1257–1262.
31. Konopad E, Noseworthy TW, Johnston R, et al. Quality of life measures before and one year after admission to an intensive care unit. *Crit Care Med* 1995;23:1653–1659.
32. Lynn J, Harrell FE, Cohn F, et al. Prognoses of seriously ill hospitalized patients on the days before death: implications for patient care and public policy. *New Horiz* 1997;5:56–61.
33. Walter LC, Brand RJ, Counsell SR, et al. Development and validation of a prognostic Index for 1-year mortality in older adults after hospitalization. *JAMA* 2001;285:2987–2994.
34. Knaus WA, Harrell FE, Lynn J, et al. The SUPPORT prognostic model. Objective estimates of survival for seriously ill hospitalized adults. Study to understand prognoses and preferences for outcomes and risks of treatments. *Ann Intern Med* 1995;122: 191–203.
35. Tsevat J, Dawson NV, Wu AW, et al. Health values of hospitalized patients 80 years and older. *JAMA* 1998;279:371–375.
36. Tresch DD, Thakur RK. Cardiopulmonary resuscitation in the elderly. *Emerg Med Clin North Am* 1998;16:649–663.
37. Gulati RS, Bahn GL, Horan MA. CPR of old people. *Lancet* 1983; 2:267–269.
38. Bedell SE, Delbanco TL, Cook EF, et al. Survival after CPR in the hospital. *N Engl J Med* 1983;309:569–575.
39. Taffet GI, Teasdale TA, Luchi RJ. In-hospital CPR. *JAMA* 1988;260: 2069–2072.
40. George AL, Folk BP, Crecelius PL, et al. Pre-arrest morbidity and other correlates of survival after in-hospital CPR. *Am J Med* 1989;87:28–34.
41. Murphy DJ, Murray AM, Robinson BE, et al. Outcomes of CPR in the elderly. *Ann Intern Med* 1989;111:199–205.
42. Peterson MW, Moseley PL, Schwartz DA. Outcome of CPR in a medical intensive care unit. *Chest* 1991;100:168–174.
43. Rosenberg M, Wang C, Hoffman-Wilde S, et al. Results of CPR. *Arch Intern Med* 1993;153:1375.
44. Schneider AP, Nelson DJ, Brown DD. In-hospital cardiopulmonary resuscitation: A 30-year review. *J Am Board Fam Pract* 1993;6:91–101.
45. Schwenzer KJ, Smith WT, Durbin CG Jr. Selective application of CPR improves survival rates. *Anesth Analg* 1993;76:478–484.
46. Tresch DD, Heudebert G, Kutty K, et al. Cardiopulmonary resuscitation in elderly patients hospitalized in the 1990's: a favorable outcome. *J Am Geriatr Soc* 1994;42:137–141.
47. Di Bari M, Chiarlone M, Fumagalli S, et al. CPR of older, inhospital patients: immediate efficacy and long-term outcome. *Crit Care Med* 2000;28:2320–2325.
48. Faber-Langendoen K. Resuscitation of patients with metastatic cancer. *Arch Intern Med* 1991;151:235–239.
49. Vitelli CE, Cooper K, Rogatko A, et al. Cardiopulmonary resuscitation and the patient with cancer. *J Clin Oncol* 1991;9:111–115.
50. Ely EW, Evans GW, Haponik EF. Mechanical ventilation in a cohort of elderly patients admitted to an intensive care unit. *Ann Intern Med* 1999;131:96–104.
51. Nunn JF, Milledge JS, Singaraya J. Survival of patients ventilated in an intensive therapy unit. *Br Med J* 1979;1:1525–1527.
52. Witek TJ, Schachter EN, Dean NL, et al. Mechanically assisted ventilation in a community hospital:immediate outcome, hospital charges, and follow-up of patients. *Arch Intern Med* 1985;145: 235–239.
53. Elpern EH, Larson R, Douglass P, et al. Long-term outcomes for elderly survivors of prolonged ventilator assistance. *Chest* 1989;96: 1120–1124.
54. Tran DD, Groeneveld AB, van dM, et al. Age, chronic disease, sepsis, organ system failure, and mortality in a medical intensive care unit. *Crit Care Med* 1990;18:474–479.

55. O'Donnell A, Bohner B. Outcome in patients requiring prolonged mechanical ventilation: three year experience. *Chest* 1991; 100:29S.

56. Pesau B, Falger S, Berger E, et al. Influence of age on outcome of mechanically ventilated patients in an intensive care unit. *Crit Care Med* 1992;20:489–492.

57. Gracey DR, Naessens JM, Krishan I, et al. Hospital and posthospital survival in patients mechanically ventilated for more than 29 days. *Chest* 1992;101:211–214.

58. Stauffer JL, Fayter NA, Graves B, et al. Survival following mechanical ventilation for acute respiratory failure in adult men. *Chest* 1993;104:1222–1229.

59. Swinburne AJ, Fedullo AJ, Bixby K, et al. Respiratory failure in the elderly. Analysis of outcome after treatment with mechanical ventilation. *Arch Intern Med* 1993;153:1657–1662.

60. Cohen IL, Lambrinos J, Fein IA. Mechanical ventilation for the elderly patient in intensive care. Incremental changes and benefits. *JAMA* 1993;269:1025–1029.

61. Papadakis MA, Lee KK, Browner WS, et al. Prognosis of mechanically ventilated patients. *West J Med* 1993;159:659–664.

62. Dardaine V, Constans T, Lasfargues G, et al. Outcome of elderly patients requiring ventilatory support in intensive care. *Aging* 1995;7:221–227.

63. Steiner T, Mendoza G, De GM, et al. Prognosis of stroke patients requiring mechanical ventilation in a neurological critical care unit. *Stroke* 1997;28:711–715.

64. Kurek CJ, Cohen IL, Lambrinos J, et al. Clinical and economic outcome of patients undergoing tracheostomy for prolonged mechanical ventilation in New York state during 1993: analysis of 6,353 cases under diagnosis-related group 483. *Crit Care Med* 1997;25:983–988.

65. Zilberberg MD, Epstein SK. Acute lung injury in the medical ICU. Comorbid conditions, age, etiology, and hospital outcome. *Am J Respir Crit Care Med* 1998;157:1159–1164.

66. Kurek CJ, Dewar D, Lambrinos J, et al. Clinical and economic outcome of mechanically ventilated patients in New York state during 1993. *Chest* 1998;114:214–222.

67. Ely EW, Evans GW, Haponik EF. Mechanical ventilation in a cohort of elderly patients admitted to an intensive care unit. *Ann Intern Med* 1999;131:96–104.

68. Ely EW, Wheeler A, Thompson B, et al. Recovery rate and prognosis in older persons who develop acute lung injury and the acute respiratory distress syndrome. *Ann Intern Med* 2002;136:25–36.

69. Esteban A, Anzueto I, Alia E, et al. Indications for, complications from, and outcome of mechanical ventilation: effect of age. *Am J Respir Crit Care Med* 2000;161:A385.

70. Ely EW, Wheeler AP, Thompson BT, et al for the Acute Respiratory Distress Syndrome Network. Recovery rate and prognosis in older persons who develop acute lung injury and the acute respiratory distress syndrome. *Ann Intern Med* 2002;136:24–32.

71. Graham C, Ballard C, Sham P. Carers' knowledge of dementia and their expressed concerns. *Int J Geriatr Psychiatry* 1997;12:931–936.

72. Fields SD, MacKenzie CR, Charlson ME, et al. Cognitive impairment. Can it predict the course of hospitalized patients? *J Am Geriatr Soc* 1986;34:579–585.

73. Inouye SK, Bogardus ST, Charpentier PA, et al. A multicomponent intervention to prevent delirium in hospitalized older patients. *N Engl J Med* 1999;340:669–676.

74. Marcantonio ER, Flacker JM, Wright JR, et al. Reducing delirium after hip fracture: a randomized trial. *J Am Geriatr Soc* 2001;49: 516–522.

75. Pisani M, Inouye SK, Mcnicoll L, et al. Screening for pre-existing cognitive impairment in older intensive care unit patients. *J Am Geriatr Soc* 2003;51:689–693.

76. Pisani M, Redlich CA, Mcnicoll L, et al. Underrecognition of pre-existing cognitive impairment by physicians in older ICU patients. *Chest* 2003;124:2267–2274.

77. Inouye SK, Schlesinger MJ, Lyndon TJ. Delirium: a symptom of how hospital care is failing older persons and a window to improve quality of hospital care. *Am J Med* 1999;106(5):565–573.

78. Francis J, Martin D, Kapoor WN. A prospective study of delirium in hospitalized elderly. *JAMA* 1990;263:1097–2101.

79. Inouye SK, Rushing JT, Foreman MD, et al. Does delirium contribute to poor hospital outcomes? A three-site epidemiologic study. *J Gen Intern Med* 1998;13:234–242.

80. Ely EW, Gautam S, Margolin R, et al. The impact of delirium in the intensive care unit on hospital length of stay. *Intensive Care Med* 2001;27:1892–1900.

81. Ely EW, Inouye SK, Bernard GR, et al. Delirium in mechanically ventilated patients:validity and reliability of the confusion assessment method for the intensive care unit (CAM-ICU). *JAMA* 2001;286:2703–2710.

82. Hopkins RO, Weaver LK, Pope DOJF, et al. Neuropsychological sequelae and impaired health status in survivors of severe acute respiratory distress syndrome. *Am J Respir Crit Care Med* 1999;160: 50–56.

83. Jackson JC, Hart RP, Gordon SM, et al. Six-month neuropsychological outcome of medical intensive care unit patients. *Crit Care Med* 2003;31:1226–1234.

84. Elie M, Cole MG, Primeau FJ, et al. Delirium risk factors in elderly hospitalized patients. *J Gen Intern Med* 1998;13(3):204–212.

85. Francis J, Kapoor WN. Delirium in hospitalized elderly. *J Gen Intern Med* 1990;5:65–79.

86. Rogove HJ, Safar P, Sutton-Tyrrell K, et al. Old age does not negate good cerebral outcome after cardiopulmonary resuscitation: analyses from the brain resuscitation clinical trials. The Brain Resuscitation Clinical Trial I and II Study Groups. *Crit Care Med.* 1995 Jan;23(1):18–25.

87. Singer PA, Martin DK, Merrijoy K. Quality end-of-life-care: patients' perspectives. *JAMA* 1999;281:163–168.

88. Phillips RS, Wenger NS, Teno JM, et al. Choices of seriously ill patients about cardiopulmonary resuscitation: correlates and outcomes. Support investigators. The Study to Understand Prognoses and Preferences for Outcome and Risks of Treatments. *Am J Med* 1996;100:128–137.

89. Teno J, Fischer E, Hamel MB, et al. Decision-making and outcomes of prolonged ICU stays in seriously ill patients. *J Am Geriatr Soc* 2000;48:S70–S74.

90. Beach MC, Morrison SR. The effect of do-not-resuscitate orders on physician decision-making. *J Am Geriatr Soc* 2002;50:2057–2061.

91. Fried TR, Bradley EH, Towle VR, et al. Understanding the treatment preferences of seriously ill patients. *N Engl J Med* 2002;346: 1061–1066.

92. Emanuel EJ. Cost saving at the end of life: what do the data show. *JAMA* 1996;275:1907–1914.

93. Chelluri L, Medelshon AB, Belle SH, et al. Hospital costs in patients receiving prolonged mechanical ventilation: does age have an impact? *Crit Care Med* 2003;31:1746–1751.

94. Schneiderman LJ, Jecker NS, Jonsen AR. Medical futility:its meaning and ethical implications. *Ann Intern Med* 1990;112:949–954.

95. Halevy A, Neal RC, Brody BA. The low frequency of futility in an adult intensive care unit setting. *Arch Intern Med* 1996;156: 100–104.

96. Council on Ethical and Judicial Affairs AMA. Medical futility in end-of-life care: report of the council on ethical and judicial affairs. *JAMA* 1999;281:937–941.

97. Prendergast TJ, Luce JM. A national survey of end-of-life care for critically ill patients. *Am J Respir Crit Care Med* 1998;158:1163–1167.

98. Sprung CL, Cohen SL, Sjokvist P, et al. End-of-life practices in European intensive care units. *JAMA* 2003;290:790–797.

99. Kollef MH, Ward S. The influence of access to a private attending physician on the withdrawal of life-sustaining therapies in the intensive care unit. *Crit Care Med* 1999;27:2125–2132.

100. Azoulay E, Pochard F, Chevret S, et al. Meeting the needs of intensive care unit patient families. *Am J Respir Crit Care Med* 2001;163: 135–139.

101. Clarke EB, Curtis JR, Luce JM, et al. Seven end-of-life domains. *Crit Care Med* 2003;31:2255–2262.

102. Goldman L, Caldera DL, Nussbaum SR, et al. Multifactorial index of cardiac risk in noncardiac surgical procedures. *N Engl J Med* 1977;297:845–850.

103. Smetana GW. Preoperative pulmonary evaluation. *N Engl J Med* 1999;340:937–944.

104. Berger DH, Roslyn JJ. Cancer surgery in the elderly. *Clin Geriatr Med* 1997;13:119–141.

105. Fong Y, Blumgart LH, Fortner JG, et al. Pancreatic or liver resection for malignancy is safe and effective for the elderly. *Ann Surg* 1995;122:426–437.

106. Office of Strategic Planning. Medicare and managed care. *HCFA* 1998;2082:59–81.

107. Money SR, Rice K, Crockett D, et al. Risk of respiratory failure after repair of thoracoabdominal aortic aneurysms. *Am J Surg* 1994;168:152–155.

108. Daley J, Khuri SF, Henderson W, et al. Risk adjustment of the postoperative morbidity rate for the comparative assessment of the quality of surgical care: results of the national veterans affairs surgical risk study. *J Am Coll Cardiol* 1997;185:328–340.

109. Wesley Ely, Stephen B. Tatter, L. Douglas Case, et al. Predictors of Successful Extubation in Neurosurgical Patients *Am J Respir Crit Care Med* 2001;163:658–664.

110. Marx GF, Mateo CV, Orkin LR. Computer analysis of postanesthetic deaths. *Anesthesiology* 1973;39:54–58.

111. Djokovic JL, Hedley-Whyte J. Prediction of outcome of surgery and anesthesia in patients over 80. *JAMA* 1979;242:2301–2306.

112. Kroenke K, Lawrence VA, Theroux JF, et al. Operative risk in patients with severe obstructive pulmonary disease. *Arch Intern Med* 1992;152:967–971.

113. Wong D, Weber EC, Schell MJ, et al. Factors associated with postoperative pulmonary complications in patients with severe chronic obstructive pulmonary disease. *Anesth Analg* 1995;80:276–284.

114. Holleman DR, Simel DL. Does the clinical examination predict airflow limitation? *JAMA* 1995;273:313–319.

115. Holleman DR, Simel DL, Goldberg JS. Diagnosis of obstructive airways disease from the clinical examination. *J Gen Intern Med* 1993;8:63–68.

116. Badgett RG, Tanaka DJ, Hunt DK, et al. Can moderate chronic obstructive pulmonary disease be diagnosed by historical and physical findings alone? *Am J Med* 1993;94:188–196.

117. Pickle LW, Mungiole M, Gillum RF. Geographic variation in stroke mortality in blacks and whites in the united states. *Stroke* 1997;28(8):1639–1647.

118. Schapira RM, Schapira MM, Funahashi A, et al. The value of the forced expiratory time in the physical diagnosis of obstructive airways disease. *JAMA* 1993;270:731–736.

119. Dewar DM, Kurek CJ, Lambrinos J, et al. Patterns in costs and outcomes for patients with prolonged mechanical ventilation undergoing tracheostomy: an analysis of discharges under diagnosis-related group 483 in New York State from 1992 to 1996. *Crit Care Med* 2000;27:2640–2647.

120. Gillum, RF. Stroke mortality in blacks. disturbing trends. *Stroke* 1999;30:1711–1715.

121. Matchar D. The value of stroke prevention and treatment. *Neurology* 1998;51:31S–35S.

122. Holland PW. Statistics and causal inference. *J Am Stat Assoc* 1986;81:945–970.

123. Epstein SK, Faling LJ, Daly BD, et al. Predicting complications after pulmonary resection: preoperative exercise testing vs a multifactorial cardiopulmonary risk index. *Chest* 1993;104:694–700.

124. Lawrence VA, Dhanda R, Hilsenbeck SG, et al. Risk of pulmonary complications after elective abdominal surgery. *Chest* 1996;110:744–750.

THE CRITICALLY ILL PATIENT

CHAPTER 20

Nutrition and Ethical Principles in Critical Illness and Injury

Annette Stralovich-Romani

C. Kees Mahutte

John M. Luce

Malnutrition is recognized as a complication of critical illness. The prevention of malnutrition or its detection and subsequent treatment are important goals in the care of ill patients. Critical illness and injury precipitate a hypercatabolic and hypermetabolic response triggered by the release of catecholamines, glucocorticoids, inflammatory cytokines, and other inflammatory products. The metabolic hallmarks of stress and injury include increased energy expenditure, anorexia, impaired immune function, and rapid weight loss associated with significant loss of skeletal muscle mass. Besides impairing wound healing and immune function, malnutrition can have deleterious effects on respiratory function by decreasing respiratory muscle strength and ventilatory drive and by impairing lung defenses.

Nutrition is an integral component of critical care medicine. Identifying patients who will benefit from nutrition intervention will lead to cost-effective and beneficial outcomes. Gaining a better understanding of the metabolic response to stress or injury will allow for the proper determination of nutrient requirements and for the provision of appropriate nutrition support regimens.

Enteral nutrition is the preferred modality of nutrition support because it is cost effective and has beneficial clinical outcomes. Perhaps the most striking clinical benefit of enteral nutrition therapy is preservation of the gastrointestinal (GI) tract. Disruption of the GI barrier is a common occurrence during critical illness and while providing therapies. Early initiation of enteral nutrition will help support the GI tract during critical illness. In addition, the fortification of enteral formulas with specific nutrients that may play a role in the maintenance of GI integrity and immune function is being investigated.

Complications can occur with either enteral or parenteral nutrition (PN). However, with careful monitoring along with new knowledge and technical advances, patient safety and tolerance to nutritional therapy have significantly improved.

FUEL UTILIZATION DURING CRITICAL ILLNESS

Injury caused by burns, trauma, or sepsis evokes increases in both metabolic and catabolic rates. Even in the presence of inadequate intake, these hormone-mediated responses ensure the delivery of abundant glucose, obtained primarily via gluconeogenesis from endogenous proteins, to the sites of injury. Teleologically, one might argue that these metabolic and catabolic responses enhance survival. Both afferent nerve signals and cytokines [interleukin-1 (IL-1), tumor necrosis factor (TNF), and others] originating at the site of injury act on the hypothalamus, which in turn activates the sympathetic nervous system and pituitary gland (1). Consequent increases in norepinephrine, epinephrine, cortisol, glucagon, and insulin ensue. Infusing cortisol, glucagon, and epinephrine into normal subjects elicits the same metabolic stress responses as are seen in critical illness, including the increased levels of insulin (2). The overriding influence of the counterregulatory hormones—cortisol, glucagon, and epinephrine—stimulates gluconeogenesis, glycogenolysis, lipolysis, and proteolysis. As a result, circulating levels of glucose are increased. Substrate cycling (turnover) of carbohydrates, proteins, and fats increase (see Fig. 20-1).

To better understand the changes that occur during the hypermetabolic hypercatabolic state of stress, the hypometabolic catabolic state of nonstressed starvation is discussed first (see Table 20-1).

NONSTRESSED STARVATION

The normal body contains substantial caloric reserves (3). Of these reserves, the oxidative metabolism of fat yields considerably more energy than that of protein or glucose (see Table 20-2).

TABLE 20-1.   Nonstressed Starvation and the Hypermetabolic Hypercatabolic Stress Response

	Starvation	*Stress*
Metabolic rate	↓	↑
Urinary nitrogen losses	↓	↑
Insulin	↓	↑ (resistance)
Counterregulatory hormones[a]	Normal	↑
Ketones	↑	Absent
Glucose	Normal	↑
Gluconeogenesis	Present	↑
Glycogenolysis	↑	↑
Lipolysis	↑	↑
Proteolysis	↓	↑
Primary fuel sources	Fat	Fat

[a] Glucagon, cortisol, catecholamines.

During the initial phase of nonstressed starvation (lasting a few days), glycogen stores are broken down to provide glucose for the brain, erythrocytes, white blood cells, and renal medulla. Glycogen stores are soon depleted because they are less in quantity (containing about 1,000 kcal), and the brain alone requires 100 to 150 g of glucose per day, and in addition, the blood cells require about 40 g per day (3). Insulin levels are low to facilitate mobilization of carbohydrate, fat, and protein for energy. As glycogen is depleted within 48 to 72 hours, fat gradually becomes the major caloric source, providing about 85% of the total required calories from free fatty acids or ketones (produced in the liver). The remaining 15% of calories required by the glucose-dependent tissues (i.e., brain, blood cells, and renal medulla) is obtained from glucose. Most of this glucose is derived from gluconeogenesis of amino acids, and only a small portion of the glucose is derived from gluconeogenesis of glycerol. Within a few days, the brain adapts to the utilization of ketone bodies, which thereafter may supply 50% to 80% of the brain's energy needs. Brain utilization of ketones spares the breakdown of proteins that would otherwise be required for gluconeogenesis. In addition, the metabolic rate may also decrease by 20% to 40% below basal levels. Thus, with prolonged fasting, urinary nitrogen excretion (indicating protein

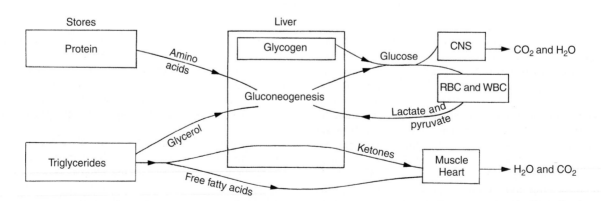

FIGURE 20-1.   Major metabolic pathways. During stress, amino acids are used to produce glucose and fats are used for energy, but the elevated glucose level suppresses ketone production. During nonstressed starvation, ketones are present and supply a substantial portion of the brain's energy.

TABLE 20-2. Normal Caloric Stores in a 70-kg Man

Fuel	Kg	Kcal/g[a]	Calories (kcal)
Fat	15	9.3	140,000
Muscle protein	6	4.4	26,000
Glycogen	0.26	4.2	1,000
Total			167,000

[a] Energy from the body's oxidative metabolism of fat, protein, and carbohydrates (3.7 kcal per g for glucose).

breakdown), which increases from about 10 g per day in the equilibrium state prior to the fast state to about 12 g per day in the initial days, may decrease to about 3 g per day. Despite these adaptive processes and total potential energy stores in a 70-kg man of approximately 170,000 kcal (Table 20-2), death typically occurs in about 2 months.

GLUCOSE METABOLISM DURING STRESS

During the stressed state of critical illness, carbohydrate metabolism is characterized by hyperglycemia, which in turn induces a relative hyperinsulinemia. However, because of the predominance of the counterregulatory hormones (i.e., glucagon, cortisol, and catecholamines), the glucose levels are higher than expected for a given insulin level, leading to the so-called insulin resistance of critical illness. The high glucose levels fuel the cells involved in the reparative processes. These cells are the white blood cells, macrophages, and fibroblasts, all of which require glucose to generate energy via the glycolytic pathway. Because the hyperglycemia of critical illness may therefore be beneficial, it is usually recommended that glucose should not be tightly controlled with insulin, even though there is some evidence that insulin infusion can decrease protein catabolism (4). However, more work is being done to determine whether maintenance of glucose levels in a more normal range may be benefited using insulin infusions.

During very severe stresses, such as those induced by burns, glucose utilization and turnover increase (from normal value of less than 2 mg/kg/minute) and, maximally, may reach 5 to 7 mg/kg/minute (5). Because glycogen stores are rapidly depleted, these extra quantities of glucose are primarily obtained from gluconeogenesis, which occurs in the liver (typically more than 75%) and kidney (less than 25%). The major gluconeogenic precursors are lactate, pyruvate, glycerol, and some amino acids, such as alanine and glutamine. Lactate and pyruvate, resulting from glycolysis of glucose by the red blood and phagocytic cells, are used as substrates for gluconeogenesis in the liver. The newly produced glucose is then again transferred to the peripheral tissues where it is needed and where it is incompletely oxidized via glycolysis to lactate (Cori cycle). Increased rates of lactate cycling via the Cori cycle (see Fig. 20-2) occur in trauma, sepsis, and burns (6). Glycerol, derived from fat, may also be metabolized to glucose. During nonstressed starvation, glycerol accounts for only a small portion of total glucose production (about 3%); during sepsis, the amount of glucose produced from glycerol may reach 20% (7). However, most of the glucose derived from gluconeogenesis originates from degradation of muscle protein. Alanine is the major amino acid precursor in this pathway (see Fig. 20-3). The alanine used for gluconeogenesis is derived from two sources: direct release

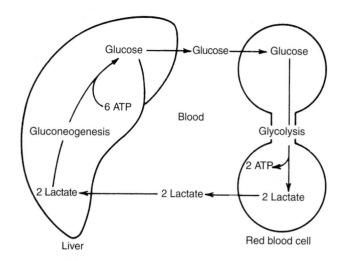

FIGURE 20-2. The Cori cycle. Glucose carbons shuttle potential energy between the liver and anaerobically metabolizing cells. Energy is ultimately derived from lipid. (From Devlin T, ed. *Textbook of Biochemistry.* New York: John Wiley & Sons, 1982, with permission.)

of alanine from muscle and conversion of glutamine (released from muscle) to alanine in the GI tract. Alanine and pyruvate (from glycolysis and protein breakdown) are then converted to glucose via the glucose–alanine cycle. In the stressed patient, the exogenous infusion of glucose (up to 6 mg/kg/minute) only partially suppresses gluconeogenesis, and a portion of the infused glucose is metabolized to glycogen and fat (8). Glucose infusions exceeding 6 mg/kg/minute result in a respiratory quotient (RQ) above 1, indicating net lipogenesis (9). Because these amounts of glucose (6 mg/kg/minute) also do not suppress protein breakdown, glucose alone cannot meet the nutritional requirements in critically ill patients. The overriding stimulation for glucose production appears to be derived from several factors: a decreased level of pyruvate dehydrogenase activity (10), an increase in the glucagon-to-insulin ratio, and an elevation of plasma catecholamine levels.

In summary, during stress, hyperglycemia satisfies the increased peripheral glucose demands. The hyperglycemia is the result of incomplete glucose oxidation (i.e., glycolysis in phagocytic cells and insulin resistance in other tissues) and increased glucose synthesis. The latter uses amino acid, pyruvate, and lactate substrates.

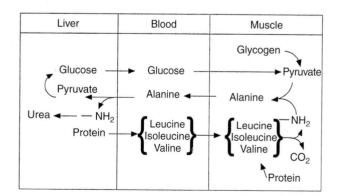

FIGURE 20-3. The glucose–alanine cycle. (From Felig P, Wahren J. Amino acid metabolism in exercising man. *J Clin Invest* 1971;50: 2703–2714, with permission.)

FAT METABOLISM DURING STRESS

Fat becomes the preferred oxidative fuel in the hypermetabolic patient (1,11). This shift from glucose to fat oxidation decreases the muscle proteolysis that would otherwise occur. In contrast to the situation during nonstressed starvation, the increased turnover of fat persists even when exogenous glucose is infused (7,11). Despite this increase in lipolysis, the concentration of free fatty acids is generally not significantly increased, whereas the triglyceride and glycerol concentrations are increased (1,11). Oxidation of free fatty acids may provide 70% to 90% of the total energy needs. However, in septic or injured patients, the elevated glucose levels suppress the conversion of free fatty acids to ketones in proportion to the severity of the insult (12). Thus, in contrast to prolonged nonstressed starvation, during the stressed state, ketone production is inadequate to meet the energy needs of the brain. Therefore, the brain's energy requirements (about 100 to 150 g of glucose per day) must be satisfied via gluconeogenesis fueled (in part) by protein degradation (it takes about 200 g of protein to make 100 g of glucose).

In summary, in the stressed patient, fat becomes the preferred oxidative fuel. Ketone production is decreased and is insufficient to meet the brain's energy demands (necessitating proteolysis to provide glucose).

PROTEIN METABOLISM DURING STRESS

Under normal equilibrium conditions, protein degradation is balanced by protein synthesis. After a few days of starvation in a normal man, the initial catabolic response diminishes and protein sparing occurs. In contrast, with burns, trauma, or sepsis, protein catabolism far exceeds its synthesis. In addition, in contrast to nonstressed starvation, during stress the administration of glucose alone does not suppress the proteolysis that occurs (8). Similarly, administration of fat alone does not suppress proteolysis. Protein sparing is optimal when either a combination of carbohydrate and protein (13) or a combination of fat and protein (14) is administered. Protein requirements range from 1 to 1.5 g/kg/day (15), and excessive protein administration (more than 2 g/kg/day) neither prevents endogenous protein catabolism nor leads to enhanced protein synthesis. During the stress response, only about 20% of the muscle protein that is broken down is used directly for energy generation. The remainder

enters the liver and is used for gluconeogenesis or for synthesis of acute-phase reactant proteins (i.e., C-reactive protein, fibrinogen, and α_1-antitrypsin). As mentioned, glucose is required by the brain and phagocytic cells involved in the reparative processes. The synthesis of acute-phase reactant proteins enhances immune function, coagulation, and antiprotease activity and thereby may enhance survival. The muscle proteolysis occurs because of an increase in stress hormones (i.e., catecholamines, glucagon, and cortisol) as well as cytokines, including IL-1 (16). In the liver, the amino acids not used directly in gluconeogenesis or in acute-phase reactant protein production are deaminated to yield pyruvate (used in gluconeogenesis) and an amino group. The latter is eventually excreted as urea, resulting in increased urinary nitrogen excretion. In the critically ill patient, muscle mass and protein losses may be substantial (see Fig. 20-4). The following example appreciates the magnitude of these losses: 30 g of muscle mass contains 6.25 g of protein, which when fully catabolized leads to 1 g of urinary nitrogen being excreted. Daily urinary nitrogen excretion may range from 20 to 40 g with burns and from 20 to 30 g with trauma or sepsis. Therefore, a loss of 30 g of urinary nitrogen each day corresponds to a loss of 0.9 kg of muscle per day. Such a loss will lead to severe life-threatening protein malnutrition within 1 to 2 weeks.

In summary, during critical illness, increased proteolysis of skeletal muscle occurs. The resultant amino acids are used to produce glucose (via gluconeogenesis) and acute-phase reactant proteins. Massive protein losses (measured by urinary nitrogen excretion) may be incurred rapidly, with catastrophic consequences.

NUTRITIONAL ASSESSMENT

Malnutrition is recognized as a major contributor to the development of morbidity and mortality in hospitalized patients (17). Many studies of nutritional status in hospitalized patients based on anthropometric data have indicated an incidence rate of malnutrition to be 30% to 40% (18). The incidence of nutritional depletion on admission, however, is steadily increasing. Because nutritional status also tends to decline with length of hospital stay, it is imperative to intervene before nutritional depletion becomes more significant. Early identification and intervention of

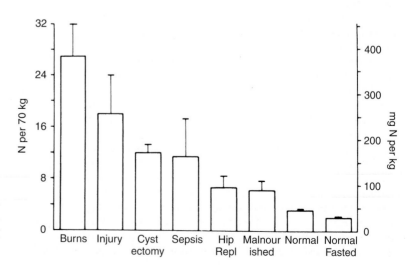

FIGURE 20-4.   Total nitrogen excretion during 5% dextrose infusion in injured, septic, burned, or malnourished patients and normal subjects. Mean + SD. (From Elwyn DH. Protein metabolism and requirements in the critically ill patient. *Crit Care Clin* 1987;3:57–69, with permission.)

patients who are already nutritionally compromised on admission and/or those patients who are at nutritional risk can lead to cost-effective and beneficial outcomes.

The evaluation of nutritional status is a vital step in formulating nutritional care plans for patients. The nutritional assessment process is used to identify those patients with either pre-existing malnutrition or risk for nutritional compromise. One of the greatest challenges for clinicians, however, is to assess body composition and function because there is no gold standard for identifying malnutrition. No single parameter has proven to be useful in all patients. An ideal test for nutritional assessment should be highly sensitive and specific, be unaffected by factors unrelated to nutrition, and correlate with response to nutritional repletion (19). Unfortunately, most markers of malnutrition lack specificity and sensitivity; therefore, until improved methods of identifying malnutrition are developed, it is necessary to perform a comprehensive assessment that includes carefully selected objective parameters, nutritionally focused physical exam, and other subjective parameters. However, in daily clinical practice, the nutritional assessment process must center around assessment parameters that are clinically relevant, easy to obtain, and cost effective (20).

When evaluating nutritional status, it is important to obtain subjective data from the medical history that may bear relevance to the patient's nutritional well-being. For example, acute or chronic illnesses, medications (e.g., immunosuppresive agents and corticosteroids), pyschosocial history, diagnostic tests and procedures, surgeries, or other treatment modalities (e.g., chemotherapy and radiation therapy) may be factors that have a significant impact on nutritional status (21,22). A thorough nutritional history should also be completed and should include weight and appetite changes, diet information, bowel habits, chewing and swallowing abilities, and activity level (23). Another widely accepted nutritional assessment tool is the subjective global assessment (SGA). The SGA relies on history of weight and dietary change, persistent GI symptoms, functional capacity, effects of disease on nutritional requirements, and physical appearance (20).

Careful observation of physical appearance adds a dimension to the evaluation of nutritional adequacy. Severe wasting of lean body mass and subcutaneous fat stores are signs of frank malnutrition. The physical exam should also focus on edema, dermatitis, and overt signs of vitamin and mineral deficiencies (e.g., alopecia, cheilosis, glossitis, stomatitis, bleeding gums, bruising, visual changes, and rickets) (24,25).

Anthropometry can be used to obtain objective parameters for assessment of nutritional status. Body weight is one of the best general parameters for establishing the diagnosis of malnutrition; however, it provides only a crude evaluation of overall fat and muscle stores. *Body mass index* [weight in kilograms divided by height in meters squared (kg per m²)] is often used to help determine nutritional status. The normal range for this index is 20 to 25. Values below 18 signify nutritional depletion. Values above 25 and 30 are defined as overweight and obese, respectively. Usual body weight, rather than ideal body weight, is a much more useful nutritional assessment parameter in patients. Loss of 5% of body weight in 1 month or loss of more than 10% of body weight in the 6 months preceding admission most certainly signifies nutritional depletion. When assessing the weight status of a critically ill patient, caution must be exercised about the kind of weight being used, for weights generally are obscured by fluid shifts and, therefore, are unreliable. Dry weights are more ideal for determining nutritional status, determining nutrient requirements, and monitoring response to nutritional therapy.

Skinfold measurements, although rarely used in the clinical setting, are indirect methods of measuring somatic protein and subcutaneous fat. These measurements have limited utility in the critical care setting due to edema/fluid shifts. Skinfold measurements tend to have more merit in the outpatient arena when nutritional status is being serially evaluated over time or in the pediatric population to assess growth.

One of the more recent techniques for analysis of body composition is bioelectric impedance (BIA). BIA is based on the principle that lean tissue has a higher electric conductivity and a lower impedance relative to water because of its greater electrolyte content (21,26). However, because BIA is considered to be unreliable in the presence of fever, edema, obesity, and electrolyte abnormalities, it is unlikely to be a useful assessment tool in the intensive care setting.

Various serum protein levels have been used in the assessment of nutritional status. Albumin, transferrin, thyroxine-binding prealbumin, and retinol-binding protein are most commonly used in the clinical setting (see Table 20-3). Serum albumin is

TABLE 20-3. Serum Proteins for Nutritional Assessment

Serum Protein	Half-life	Normal Range	Comments
Albumin	20 d	3.5–5.0 g/dL	Large body pool; reliable indicator of morbidity and mortality; reflects chronic vs. acute protein depletion; responds slowly to changes in nutritional status; decreased levels with fluid overload, malabsorptive states, stress (sepsis, burns, trauma, postoperative states); disease process (liver failure, congestive heart failure); increased levels with anabolic agents, dehydration, and infusion of albumin, fresh frozen plasma, and whole blood
Transferrin	8–10 d	200–400 mg/dL	Smaller body pool; sensitive to changes in nutritional status; calculated from total iron binding capacity; decreased with chronic infection, stress, uremia, iron overdose, overhydration, liver failure; increased levels with pregnancy, iron deficiency, hypoxia, hepatitis, dehydration, estrogens
Prealbumin (transthyretin)	2–3 d	15–40 mg/dL	Rapid turnover rate; small body pool; responds quickly with changes in nutritional status; decreased levels with stress, inflammation, surgery, liver disease; increased levels with renal dysfunction
Retinol-binding protein	8–10 h	2.7–7.6 mg/dL	Highly sensitive to changes in nutritional status; decreased levels (same as prealbumin) as well as vitamin A deficiency; increased levels with renal dysfunction and vitamin A supplementation

best evaluated at admission because levels rarely show nutritionally relevant changes during hospitalization because of its long half-life (18 to 20 days). The advantages of albumin as an assessment parameter are that it is an inexpensive laboratory measurement, it is useful with long-term assessments, and it is a valuable prognostic indicator of morbidity and mortality. Serum albumin levels dramatically decrease, however, with metabolic stress/injury because of a combination of factors including down-regulation of the genes for albumin synthesis by TNF and IL-1, increased degradation, increased transcapillary losses, and specific disease state (liver failure). Albumin levels may change quickly as a result of nonnutritional factors and respond slowly even with adequate nutrition support. In fact, plasma albumin levels will not increase in stressed patients until the inflammatory response is remitted. Therefore, little credence should be given to albumin being a marker of nutritional status or being a response to nutritional therapy during a period of metabolic stress (20,23,27,28). Because of their shorter half-lives and smaller protein pools (Table 20-3), transferrin, prealbumin, and retinol-binding protein have been touted as better markers of status. However, like albumin, these constitutive proteins decrease independently of nutritional status during critical illness because of the preferential production of acute-phase reactants over the synthesis of visceral proteins. It should not be assumed, therefore, that decreased levels of serum proteins are caused solely by malnutrition. Normal patterns of hepatic protein synthesis and degradation are altered during critical illness, making evaluation difficult. It is advised to track the trend in visceral protein levels, particularly prealbumin, rather than focusing on isolated values as a method to monitor the response to the nutritional therapy and the overall improvement in the clinical condition of the patient.

NUTRITIONAL REQUIREMENTS

ENERGY REQUIREMENTS

The amount of energy required is a function of resting needs (those required to do daily metabolic work), with adjustments added for activity, specific dynamic action of food, healing, repair of nutritional deficits, painful stimuli, and any catabolic insult such as trauma, sepsis, burns, neurologic injury, and surgery. Several methods exist to determine energy requirements such as predictive equations, nomograms, and indirect calorimetry.

Predictive Equations

Predictive equations are most often estimated using the Harris–Benedict equation (see Table 20-4), which represents resting energy expenditure (REE), and is then multiplied by stress factors ranging from 1.2 to 2.0 depending on the clinical condition of the patient. The utility of this formula in critically ill patients is limited because this equation was developed from data on normal volunteers. Ireton-Jones et al. developed a predictive equation to estimate energy expenditure in both ventilator-dependent and spontaneously breathing hospitalized patients on the basis of statistical analysis of measurements using indirect calorimetry (see Table 20-5) (29).

TABLE 20-4. Harris–Benedict Equation for Estimating Energy Requirement

Men: Resting energy expenditure (REE) = $66.5 + 13.75 \times (W) + 5 \times (H) - 6.76 \times (A)$

Women: Resting energy expenditure (REE) = $655 + 9.56 \times (W) + 1.85 \times (H) - 4.68 (A)$

W = weight (kg)
H = height (cm)
A = age (yr)

Indirect Calorimetry

A more accurate method to calculate energy expenditure, especially in the complex and rapidly changing setting of critical illness is indirect calorimetry. This method can be carried out at the bedside using portable machines that are costly and that require trained personnel to operate. The premise of indirect calorimetry is that it calculates energy expenditure by measurement of respiratory gas exchange, specifically the measurement of oxygen consumption (Vo_2), carbon dioxide production (Vco_2), and minute ventilation (VE). Caloric needs are quantified on the basis of the measurements of Vo_2 and Vco_2 and the application of the Weir equation: (29–31).

Energy expenditure = $[(Vo_2)(3.941) + (Vco_2)(1.11)] \times 1,440$

When measured energy expenditure is obtained from indirect calorimetry, some clinicians add a factor of 10% to 20% to account for 24-hour variability (32). Studies suggest that a 30-minute measurement of a critically ill patient is sufficient to reflect the energy expenditure in a 24-hour period. Besides determining energy expenditure, RQ can also be obtained, which is helpful in guiding caloric and carbohydrate therapy (RQ = Vco_2/Vo_2). RQ values from carbohydrate, fat, and protein are 1.0, 0.7, and 0.8, respectively. An RQ exceeding 1.0 suggests either excessive caloric and or carbohydrate overfeeding, which can result in increased CO_2 production, increased work of breathing, and unwanted net fat synthesis (29). The other valuable information obtained from the indirect calorimetry is that the Vco_2 can be used to calculate dead space in mechanically ventilated patients. The one major limitation to using indirect calorimetry is that the measurement becomes unreliable when the oxygen setting (Fio_2) on the ventilator is greater than 60%. Chest tubes with air leaks, tracheotomy tubes with incompetent or nonexistent tracheal cuffs, or patients receiving inconsistent inspired oxygen make the measurement of energy expenditure unreliable as well.

TABLE 20-5. Ireton–Jones Predictive Equation for Energy Expenditure in Ventilated Patients

Energy expenditure = $1,784 - 11(A) + 5(W) + 244(G) + 239(T) + 804(B)$

A = age (yr)
W = weight (kg)
G = gender (female = 0; male = 1)
T = diagnosis of trauma (absent = 0; present = 1)
B = diagnosis of burn (absent = 0; present = 1)

Fick Equation

When high ventilator settings preclude indirect calorimetry, the cardiovascular Fick equation is an option for determining energy requirements, provided the patient has a pulmonary artery catheter (see Table 20-6).

PROTEIN REQUIREMENTS

The goal of protein provision is to minimize the degree of net nitrogen loss. Because protein reserves do not exist in the body, protein must be continually replenished. Under normal circumstances, the recommended daily intake of protein is approximately 0.8 g of protein per kg body weight (see Table 20-7). In critical illness, the proper provision of protein is crucial as it is the most important macronutrient with stress and/or injury (Table 20-7). Protein requirements are high with trauma, sepsis, neurologic injury (e.g., subarachnoid hemorrhage), and the demands for healing of burns, necrotizing fasciitis, and other types of large wounds. Additionally, with the use of continuous renal replacement therapy the protein requirement is significantly increased (33). In some disease states such as renal failure and hepatic encephalopathy, protein requirements may be reduced (Table 20-7).

Nitrogen Balance

Because protein metabolism changes during the various phases of critical illness, injury, and recovery, assessing protein requirements for patients can pose quite a challenge. Nitrogen balance, when correctly measured and calculated, remains the best available marker of the effects of acute nutrition intervention. In fact, nitrogen balance is the single nutritional parameter associated most consistently with improved outcomes. Nitrogen balance determines the amount of protein required to maintain nitrogen equilibrium by assessing urinary nitrogen losses (34,35). Urinary nitrogen losses following injury and illness tend to parallel the increased energy expenditure with increased degree of stress. The magnitude of nitrogen loss varies with the severity of disease (36). Protein requirements and efficacy of nutrition therapies may be determined from the nitrogen balance calculation. Nitrogen balance is equal to nitrogen intake minus urinary nitrogen output plus obligatory losses from skin, stool, and respiration, ranging from 2 to 4 grams per day.

$$\text{Nitrogen balance (g)} = (\text{Protein intake}/6.25) -$$
$$(\text{Urinary urea nitrogen} + 2 \text{ to } 4)$$

When there are excessive losses of nitrogen from severe diarrhea, fistula drainage, burn exudate, ostomy output, wounds, or pleural drainage, total nitrogen content should be determined when practical.

TABLE 20-6. The Fick Equation for Determining Energy Expenditure

Resting Energy Expenditure (REE) = $CO \times Hgb \times (SaO_2 - SmvO_2)$ $\times 105$

  CO = cardiac output (L/min)
  Hgb = hemoglobin (g/dL)
  SaO_2 = arterial oxygenation saturation percentage
  $SmvO_2$ = mixed venous oxygenation percentage

TABLE 20-7. Estimating Protein Requirements

	Normal Renal Function
Maintenance	0.8–1.2 g of protein/kg/d
Moderate stress	1.3–1.5 g of protein/kg/d
Severe stress	1.5–2.0 g of protein/kg/d
	Renal Failure
Nondialyzed	0.8–1.2 g of protein/kg/d
Hemodialyzed (may be adjusted based on frequency of dialysis)	1.0–1.4 g of protein/kg/d
CAPD/CAVHD/CVVHD	1.3–1.7 g of protein/kg/d
Hepatic failure	Begin at 1.0 g of protein/kg/d, increase as tolerated to 1.5–2.0 g of protein/kg/d
Hepatic failure with encephalopathy	0.6–0.8 g of protein/kg/d (no <40 g/d)

CAPD/CAVHD/CVVHD, continuous ambulatory peritoneal dialysis/continuous arteriovenous hemodialysis/continuous venovenous hemodialysis.

A positive nitrogen balance correlates with net protein synthesis (anabolic state) and suggests adequacy of nutritional support. A negative nitrogen balance, on the other hand, indicates that the rate of protein breakdown exceeds the rate of protein synthesis (catabolic state) and, therefore, will require adjustments in the nutritional support regimen (34). Positive or even neutral nitrogen balance may be difficult to achieve in critically ill patients because of the effects of catabolic hormones, medications, bed rest, fever, and infection. The goal of nutrition support, therefore, is to offset the degree of catabolism rather than to achieve positive balance. Once the source of stress is resolved, an anabolic state can be attainable.

A nitrogen balance study should only be completed after the patient has been on a relatively constant protein and energy intake for 3 days, thus allowing the urea cycle and gluconeogenic enzymes to adjust to protein intake. Urine should be kept on ice during the collection and analyzed within 4 hours to prevent loss of urea due to bacterial conversion to ammonia.

The major limitation of using a standard nitrogen balance study in critically ill patients is that a creatinine clearance >50 mL per minute is required for accurate interpretation (25). When renal function is impaired, nitrogen balance can be calculated using urea kinetic modeling (6). An equation is now available to calculate nitrogen balance for patients on continuous renal replacement therapy. Nitrogen balance studies are usually invalid with hyperammonemic states such as liver failure or valproic acid administration because of decreased urea production.

GOALS OF NUTRITION SUPPORT

Nutrition support is paramount in maintaining the patient's nutritional status during a period of critical illness. Preservation and restoration of lean body mass is the primary objective of nutrition therapy (27). Additionally, specialized nutrition support to provide substrates (macro- and micronutrients) for improving immune function, facilitating wound and tissue repair, and supporting hepatic protein synthesis remain major goals for the management of the critically ill and injured patient (35). Of course, the overall goal of nutrition therapy is to reduce morbidity and mortality and to optimize clinical outcomes to minimize cost and the length of stay in the hospital.

NUTRITIONAL SUPPORT OF VENTILATOR-DEPENDENT PATIENTS

Patients requiring ventilatory support need adequate nutrition to maintain the integrity of their respiratory systems. Ventilator-dependent patients are prone to respiratory infections, especially when nutritional depletion is aggravated by hypercatabolic states such as sepsis, burns, or trauma (37). Catabolism of the respiratory musculature, edema formation from hypoalbuminemia, compromised immune function, decreased surfactant production, prolonged intubation, and decreased repair of epithelial surfaces are the deleterious effects of malnutrition on respiratory function (38).

Electrolyte abnormalities, particularly hypophosphatemia, can have an impact on respiratory function as well. Low serum phosphorous levels can lend to respiratory muscle weakness. Additionally, hypophosphatemia can result in decreased levels of 2,3-diphosphoglycerate in red blood cells, which can lead to increased oxyhemoglobin affinity and decreased oxygen delivery to tissues (37).

When designing the nutrition support prescription for ventilator-dependent patients, it is important to examine the proportion of carbohydrate, fat, and protein. Although there are no definitive recommendations, a well-balanced fuel mix comprised of 30% to 40% of total calories as fat, 40% to 50% of total calories as carbohydrate, and 20% to 25% of total calories as protein is advised. The effect of protein and nitrogen intake on ventilatory drive is controversial. Adequate protein provision is essential for the repletion of lean body mass. One of the major goals of nutritional therapy is to prevent hypercapnia associated with overfeeding. Excessive caloric or carbohydrate administration may cause increased CO_2 production. The substitution of fat as a metabolic fuel may be beneficial when carbohydrate limits have been reached (29). However, increased CO_2 production is primarily related to the total calories administered rather than to the specific carbohydrate:fat calorie ratio (39). Ongoing nutritional assessments and evaluations of clinical status are necessary, with adjustments in total caloric intake and manipulation of nutrient substrate mixtures, as needed, to improve nutritional status and to facilitate weaning from mechanical ventilation.

ROLE OF THE GUT

Besides its role in digestion and absorption, the GI tract has the distinct property of maintaining barrier function and normal bacterial flora of the intestine. GI tissues require direct contact with nutrients to support cell replication and to undergo the numerous metabolic and immunologic functions required for successful adaptation to stress (40). There are nonspecific defense mechanisms (i.e., peristalsis, mucus, gastric acid, bile salts, desquamation, and microflora) that work in concert with immunologic defenses to maintain the function of the gut barrier. However, the single most important influence on intestinal

structure and function are luminal nutrients (40–42). It has been found in human studies that a 10% reduction in mucosal thickness can occur after 1 to 2 weeks of PN (43).

Tissue injury, shock, and other insults increase the inflammatory response, which is followed by immunodepression, which can result in infectious complications and late multiple organ dysfunction (44). Although bacterial translocation was initially considered to be the driving force in this process, the neutrophil [polymorphonuclear (PMN) cell] became suspect in the organ damage (44). The GI tract can prime circulating neutrophils soon after an injury is sustained. Experimentally, lack of enteral feeding leads to an upregulation of adhesion molecules within the small intestine. These primed neutrophils lead to an augmented inflammatory response at extraintestinal sites if subsequent insults are suffered by animals (44).

An integral component of mucosal immunity, besides the epithelial cells that line the GI tract, is the presence of gut-associated lymphoid tissue (GALT). It is estimated that 25% of the intestinal mucosa is lymphoid tissue and that 70% to 80% of all immunologic-secreting cells are located within the intestine. Interestingly, this makes the digestive tract one of the largest immune organs within the body (41). Secretory IgA (sIgA) is the prominent immunoglobulin in the intestine, and it is believed to inhibit bacterial colonization by curtailing adherence of pathogenic microorganisms to the epithelium. Furthermore, sIgA provides protection from antigens that have invaded the enterocytes (42,45).

Alteration of intestinal structure and function may lead to barrier dysfunction of the gut. Impaired immunity, malabsorption, motility disorders, and bacterial translocation are all contributing factors to the breakdown of the gut barrier during critical illness (42).

Intestinal injury or atrophy can potentially lead to a quantitative reduction in GALT, in addition to a decreased production of secretory IgA, both of which can have deleterious immunologic effects (42,45). The malabsorption that typically occurs in critically ill patients can result from bowel wall edema, mucosal atrophy, and impaired mesenteric blood flow. Furthermore, reduced intestinal secretions, causing abdominal distention and dysmotility, and narcotic-induced ileus contribute to altered GI motility in critical illness.

Failure of the intestine to exclude toxic substances, particularly bacteria and their products, may result in bacterial translocation (42). The term *bacterial translocation* implies the migration of gut bacteria or bacterial by-products from the bowel lumen to the bloodstream or lymphatic system (36). Maintenance of the epithelial lining of the GI tract is of utmost importance in preventing gut barrier dysfunction. The physiochemical presence of nutrients in the intestinal lumen is vital in preserving the integrity of mucosal immune function. Absence of luminal nutrient stimulation, therefore, may lead to gut atrophy, which could result in bacterial translocation. Although bacterial translocation has been implicated in the pathogenesis of multisystem organ failure on the basis of animal models in critical illness, there is lack of evidence for bacterial translocation in humans. It is believed, however, that the integrity of intestinal immunity, particularly during a period of physiologic stress, is helpful in preventing infectious complications and may avert the development of multisystem organ failure in the critically ill patients.

For a number of years now, it was thought that an infusion of low volume enteral feeding (i.e., 10 mL per hour) would be sufficient to maintain GI integrity during a period of critical illness. Studies now show that at least 60% of the caloric goal in stressed patients as opposed to 25% in nonstressed patients must be met to achieve the therapeutic benefits of enteral alimentation (46).

GUT FUELS

Over the past few decades, much attention has focused on the use of specific nutrients and growth factors in maintaining GI integrity, improving immune function, and preventing the profound lean tissue dissolution associated with critical illness. Glutamine, fiber, arginine, peptides, omega-3 fatty acids, and antioxidants have all been touted to have salutary effects on intestinal integrity and immunity and possibly alter the metabolic response to stress or injury.

Glutamine is the most abundant amino acid in the plasma. Normally considered to be a nonessential amino acid, recent studies have shown that glutamine is conditionally essential in critical illness (47). During catabolic states, glutamine is preferentially consumed and oxidized by intestinal mucosa in place of glucose (47). Glutamine plays a major role in maintaining intestinal metabolism, structure and function, decreasing mucosal injury, and preventing bacterial translocation. Supplemental glutamine may also preserve gut glutathione levels during ischemia/reperfusion, which may lessen the associated intestinal injury (42).

Recent research has shown that dietary fiber has diverse functions in both the upper and lower GI tract (see Table 20-8). Dietary fiber is classified as either insoluble or soluble on the basis of chemical structure. Besides the functions of fiber listed in Table 20-8, the most pronounced effect of fiber is the colonic fermentation of dietary residue to short-chain fatty acids (i.e., acetate, butyrate, and propionate) (48). Short-chain fatty acids are rapidly absorbed by the intestinal mucosa and are readily metabolized by the intestinal epithelium and the liver. The most desirable effects of the short-chain fatty acids, however, are the trophic effect they exert on the entire intestinal tract and the unfavorable acidic environment they create for bacteria, like *Clostridium difficile*, by their presence in the colon (48,49).

The use of peptide-based diets is beneficial in the critically ill patient with impaired GI absorption. Compared with amino acid diets, peptide diets have been shown to decrease gut permeability by maintaining better intestinal blood flow and protecting intestinal integrity, as well as by stimulating greater release of gut hormones and growth factors. Peptides also

TABLE 20-8. Functions of Fiber

Function	Soluble	Insoluble
Increased water-holding capacity (increased stool weight)	Yes	Yes
Delayed gastric emptying	Yes	No
Hypocholesterolemic effects	Yes	No
Decreased rate of glucose absorption	Yes	No
Short-chain fatty acid production (bacterial fermentation)	Yes	No
Protection against bacterial translocation in gut	Yes	Yes

attenuate hypoalbuminemic diarrhea by excessive protein loss and increasing absorption of protein precursors (50,51).

Arginine is another specific nutrient that has had purported immune-enhancing and wound-healing properties (35). Omega-3 fatty acids may enhance the immune system and have been shown to have anti-inflammatory properties. There are some studies showing the potential benefit of omega-3 fatty acids and antioxidants in inflammatory processes such as acute respiratory distress syndrome (ARDS) (52). At this time, however, there are no specific recommendations for supplementation. Finally, a number of anabolic agents have been investigated for their potential to attenuate the catabolic response, to promote wound healing, and to support the growth and integrity of the GI tract (35).

NUTRITION SUPPORT MODALITIES

ENTERAL NUTRITION

Because of the development of more sophisticated enteral products and feeding techniques, along with all the known clinical benefits of enteral feeding, enteral nutrition is the preferred modality of nutrition support in not only the critically ill but also in all hospitalized patients. Enteral nutrition minimizes many of the inimical responses of the GI tract to critical illness or injury and is favored over PN (42). Enteral feeding is preferred over PN not only for its ease of preparation and administration, lower cost, nitrogen-sparing effect, and decreased weight loss but also, more importantly, because it improves host defenses, promotes blood flow to the gut, maintains a more physiologic state of the GI tract, and reduces infectious complications.

Newer Clinical Applications for Enteral Nutrition

Technological advances in enteral feeding have significantly influenced the practice of enteral nutrition support. Improvements in placement procedures, enteral feeding devices, and nutritional products have allowed enteral nutrition to be provided to patients who previously would not have been candidates for enteral alimentation [e.g., inflammatory bowel disease (IBD), hyperemesis gravidarum, acute pancreatitis, short bowel syndrome, and bone marrow transplantation]. The use of enteral feeding in fistula management is becoming more widespread. The ability to enterally feed is contingent upon the site and extent of usable intestine for feeding. To avoid reflux, it is necessary to administer the feeding 40-cm distal to the fistula. Spontaneous closure rates comparable to total parenteral nutrition (TPN) have been reported (47).

In short bowel syndrome, enteral feeding is used in conjunction with PN. Minimal infusion of enteral nutrition has been shown to foster intestinal adaptation/rehabilitation. Utilization of alternative substrates (e.g., glutamine, fiber, and growth hormone) may be important contributors for successful adaptation. A newer alternative that is becoming the new gold standard for providing nutrition support to the patient with acute pancreatitis has been jejunal feedings placed either nasojejunally or with an operative jejunostomy. Because the cephalic and gastric phases of digestion are bypassed and because there are fewer cholecystokinin (CCK) receptors farther down the GI tract, there is decreased pancreatic stimulation allowing for the safe and efficacious administration of enteral nutrition (53,54). Fewer septic complications with enteral feeding compared to TPN have been reported (55).

Another area in which the efficacy of enteral feeding warrants in-depth investigation is in patients undergoing bone marrow transplantation. Restoration of the GI mucosa following chemotherapy and radiation therapy; prevention of bacterial translocation, especially in an immunocompromised patient; maintenance of normal immune responses; smoother transition to oral feeding; and cost could conceivably be beneficial in this patient population.

Timing of Enteral Nutrition Support

Timing may be crucial when it comes to instituting enteral alimentation in critically ill or injured patients. Changes in gut integrity occur very early, within hours of an acute injury. The timing of initiation of enteral tube feeding significantly affects the degree to which provision of enteral nutrients protects or maintains gut integrity and protects against adverse patient outcome. Preferably, enteral feeding tubes should be placed within 48 hours of admission to the intensive care unit (ICU). Administration of enteral nutrition into the small bowel 8 to 12 hours following surgery is being practiced widely, and with good success, because peristalsis is often well maintained in the small bowel postoperatively. Bowel sounds should be the parameter to indicate not the feasibility of enteral alimentation but rather to indicate the adequacy of gastric emptying. Although gastric and colonic motility are impaired in most critically ill patients, small bowel motility and absorption are usually intact.

The most important features associated with the early administration of enteral nutrition appear to be the minimization of gut atrophy, decreased incidence of sepsis, enhanced immunocompetence, and blunted hypermetabolic response to stress (42). A number of studies have looked at early enteral feeding, within 24 to 36 hours of injury, compared with late feeding, provided 48 hours after the injury. Out of 19 prospective, controlled trials of early versus delayed enteral nutrition therapy, 16 of those studies showed improved outcome. Decreased infectious complications, septic morbidity and mortality, and a reduction in the length of hospital stay and cost were seen (56). The role of pharmacomodulation of the gut has also received increased attention. Pathologic conditions and unavoidable iatrogenic disorders that affect gut function may be managed with drug therapy (e.g., octreotide, propofol, 5-hydroxytryptamine-3, erythromycin, and naloxone) so that the simplest level of enteral feeding may be used (57).

Tube Types and Location

GASTRIC VERSUS SMALL BOWEL FEEDING. The administration of enteral nutrition is generally accomplished by using nasoenteric feeding tubes inserted into the stomach, duodenum, or jejunum. Nasoenteric feeding tubes are the most frequently used because of the ease of placement and the decreased cost and risk to the patient in comparison to a tube requiring surgical insertion (58). Using small bore feeding tubes over the traditional nasogastric tubes (salem sumps) is preferred because there is less risk of tracheoesophageal fistula and aspiration, and they are more comfortable for the patient. The downside to using the

small feeding tubes is that they are prone to collapse and clogging, making it difficult to check for feeding residuals.

In critically ill patients, the best method of delivery remains controversial. There are several studies suggesting that gastric feedings are safe in ICU patients (59,60). Additionally, there are a number of studies showing that transpyloric feedings are better tolerated and have fewer infectious complications due to aspiration than gastric feedings do (61,62). Altered GI motility, disease process, and other clinical conditions render candidacy for small bowel feedings in the critically ill patient (see Table 20-9).

Many bedside placement techniques for passage of weighted tubes beyond the pylorus in patients in the ICU are available and are usually successful. The right lateral decubitus position with auscultation can be used to track the tube into the small intestine (63). However, if the aforementioned method is unsuccessful, then endoscopically or fluoroscopically guided tube placement may be indicated. Prokinetic drugs can also help facilitate tube positioning. Upon placement of the feeding tube, radiographic confirmation is necessary before initiating the enteral feeding regimen.

METHODS OF DELIVERY. Enteral nutrition can be delivered by either bolus, intermittent, or continuous feeding. Bolus feeding is the rapid infusion of a large volume of enteral formula over a short period (64). Frequent GI complications (e.g., diarrhea, nausea, vomiting, aspiration, and distention) are associated with this method of administration. Intermittent feeding using either gravity drip or an infusion pump involves the delivery of a moderate to large volume of enteral formula over a defined period, usually from 1 to 16 hours (64). Continuous tube feeding is the infusion of a small amount of enteral formula over 24 hours using an infusion pump (64). In critically ill patients and with small bowel feedings, the continuous delivery method is essential. Continuous feedings are better tolerated than bolus or intermittent feedings are and are associated with reduced incidence of high gastric residuals, gastroesophageal reflux, and aspiration.

Formula Composition

There are numerous commercially available enteral products that differ in composition and proportion of nutrients as well as cost. All formulas contain the macronutrients, carbohydrate, fat, protein, and water, and the micronutrients, vitamins, minerals, trace elements, and electrolytes (see Table 20-10). Polymeric formulas contain intact nutrients and require normal digestion and

TABLE 20-9. Candidates for Small Bowel Feeding

Altered gastrointestinal motility
Gastroparesis
Gastric ileus
Delayed gastric emptying
Narcotics
Intravenous fat
Propofol
Elevated intracranial pressure
Acute pancreatitis (jejunal feeding)
Absent gag reflex and cough
Early postoperative feeding (within 8–12 h postop)
Noninvasive positive pressure ventilation [Bi-level positive airway pressure (BiPAP)]

TABLE 20-10. Classification of Enteral Formulas

Category	Subcategory	Comments
Polymeric	Blended	Real food; requires normal digestion and absorption; lactose and lactose free; isotonic; nutritionally complete
	Standard	Intact nutrients; lactose free; low residue; isotonic; nutritionally complete; requires normal digestion and absorption
	High nitrogen	Intact nutrients; lactose free; isotonic protein >15% of total kcal; nutritionally complete; requires normal digestion and absorption
	Fiber-enriched	Intact nutrients; lactose free; isotonic; soluble and insoluble fiber; regulation of bowel function; nutritionally complete; requires normal digestion and absorption
	Calorically dense	Intact nutrients, 1.5–2.0 kcal/mL; high osmolality; use with fluid restriction; lactose free; nutritionally complete; requires normal digestion and absorption
	Disease specific	Intact nutrients; protein, fat, and carbohydrate source varies depending on disease state formula designed for; electrolyte content and osmolality vary; require normal digestion and absorption; expensive; efficacy controversial
Oligomeric (partially hydrolyzed)		Hydrolyzed protein; ditripeptides, free amino acids; fat semielemental content varies (3%–40% of total kcal); lactose free; osmolality varies (250–700 mOsm/kg); nutritionally complete; digestion required; limited absorptive surface of GI tract
Monomeric (elemental/chemically-defined)		Free amino acids; lactose free; fat varies (1%–15% of total kcal); high osmolality; may include glutamine; nutritionally complete; minimal digestion required; limited absorptive surface of GI tract
Modular		Individual nutrient (carbohydrate, fat, and protein) modules; used to modify preexisting commercial formula to increase nutrient density or to make unique formula; requires normal digestion and absorption

absorption. Lactose-free mixtures are the basic feeding formulation as a majority of patients have genetic or acquired lactase deficiency (63). Osmolality of these formulas can be isotonic or hypertonic (300 to 800 mOsm per kg of water). Caloric density varies from 1.0 to 2.0 kcal per mL, with 40% to 55% of total calories from carbohydrate, 12% to 20% of total calories from protein, and 30% to 50% of total calories from fat. Fats are provided as long-chain triglycerides (LCTs) and medium-chain triglycerides (MCTs).

Oligomeric and monomeric formulas are classified as elemental and semielemental/peptide-based formulas. They contain one or more partially digested macronutrients and are reserved for patients with compromised GI function (e.g., critical illness, pancreatic or bile salt deficiencies, intestinal atrophy, short bowel syndrome, and IBD) (62). Caloric density is usually 1.0 kcal per mL. The elemental diets have a much higher osmolality than the semielemental diets do. Protein is supplied as crystalline amino acids (monomeric/elemental) or as hydrolyzed whey, casein, or lactalbumin (oligomeric/semielemental). These formulas are considered low fat and may contain a high proportion of fat in the form of MCT (62). The efficacy of elemental diets has been controversial for several years.

Modular formulas are composed of individual nutrient modules (i.e., fat, protein, and carbohydrate) that produce a unique formula customized to meet the specific needs of the patient. Typically, modular components are used to modify a preexisting commercial formula to add caloric and/or protein density.

Widespread use of enteral feeding and an expanding knowledge of specific disease processes has led to an explosion in the development of disease-specific formulas (63). These formulas have been designed for specific organ failure, metabolic dysfuntion, or immunomodulation. Little data exists to suggest the impact on patient outcome from use of other specialty formulas based on specific disease processes or single organ dysfunction. Although sound physiologic principles support the composition and design of certain specialty formulas for specific

patient populations with liver disease, diabetes, renal failure, pulmonary disease, and stress, increased expense and limited data to support their efficacy and impact on patient outcome preclude their use (65). Detailed formula descriptions, clinical indications, and possible benefits are beyond the scope of this chapter (66).

Formula Selection

Enteral formula selection should be based on the patient's digestive and absorptive capacity, organ function, specific nutrient needs, tolerances, and allergies, and should take into account the formula composition and total calories. Attention must also be given to fluid requirements, vitamin and mineral needs, and osmolality. The quantity of water in enteral formulas is often described as water content or moisture content. Most enteral formulas contain water in the general range of 700 to 900 mL per 1,000 mL of enteral formula. The general rule of thumb is to provide 30 mL water per kg body weight, or as clinical status permits. When provided in sufficient volume, most nutritionally complete products contain adequate vitamins and minerals to meet all of the US recommended dietary intake (RDI). If the volume of enteral formula given is inadequate to provide the RDI, a daily multivitamin and mineral supplement is warranted unless contraindicated because of disease states that may reduce requirements of some micronutrients.

The osmolality of enteral formulas can directly affect a patient's GI tolerance to the formula. However, both isotonic formulas (270 to 320 mOsm per kg) and hypertonic formulas (>400 mOsm per kg) can be initiated at full strength.

Initiation and advancement of enteral feedings will vary with the method of administration and the osmolality of the formula. Bolus feedings are generally administered over several minutes and are best tolerated when given at <60 mL per minute (e.g., 240 mL of formula every 3 hours for at least 3 minutes) (67). Intermittent feedings are generally better received if a maximum of 200 to 300 mL of formula is delivered over a 30- to 60-minute period every 4 to 6 hours. Continuous isotonic feedings are introduced at 20 to 30 mL per hour and advanced in 15- to 20-mL increments every 8 hours until the goal flow rate is attained. Hypertonic continuous feedings start at 10 to 15 mL per hour and advance in 10- to 15-mL increments every 8 hours until the final flow rate is achieved. In patients who are critically ill, who have not been fed for an extended period of time, and who are receiving calorie-dense or high-osmolality enteral formulas, conservative initiation and advancement rates are strongly advised (e.g., 10 mL increments every 12 to 24 hours) (67).

Complications

Complications associated with enteral feeding may be avoided and managed with appropriate monitoring. The major goal of monitoring is to minimize the complications of enteral therapy and to maintain the patency of the small bore feeding tube. An assessment of GI tolerance (i.e, nausea, vomiting, abdominal discomfort/distention, and stool pattern) is mandatory when a patient is on enteral nutrition support. Hydration status and laboratory data must also be evaluated when a patient is being enterally fed. Preventive measures should be taken to minimize the risk of aspiration. Keeping the head of the bed elevated at a 30-degree to 45-degree angle and checking for tube feeding residuals are recommended to lessen the potential for aspiration (67). With continuous feeding, residuals should be checked every 4 hours and should not exceed 200 mL. If the patient has a cuffed tracheostomy, the cuff can be deflated 2 hours after bolus feedings; for continuous feeds, the cuff may be deflated only when necessary to prevent tracheal complications (68). Routine flushing of feeding tubes with 30 to 60 mL of water every 4 to 6 hours will help extend the life span of the small tubes.

Enteral nutrition is a safe means of delivering nutritional support. However, there are complications that do arise with this modality of feeding. There are three types of complications: mechanical, GI, and metabolic. Mechanical complications of nasoenteric tube feedings include tube obstruction, displacement, or dislodgement; nasopharyngeal irritation; and gastric rupture. Obstruction or clogging of the tube occurs most frequently because of inadequate crushing of medications and owing to formula residue adhering to the lumen of the tube (68). Giving liquid medications (e.g., elixirs and suspensions) rather than pills or syrups may help avoid clogging of tubes. Flushing with water, as previously described, will help maintain patency of feeding tubes. Following proper procedures for feeding tube placement and verifying tube position will help avoid the complication of tube displacement. By using small soft tubes, lubricating tubes for insertion, and maintaining good hygiene of the mouth and nares, greater patient comfort will ensue.

The most common complications of tube feedings are GI, including diarrhea, nausea, vomiting, constipation, delayed gastric emptying, and GI bleeding (69). Diarrhea is the most common cause of GI intolerance. The major causes of formula-related diarrhea are rapid infusion rate, formula characteristics (i.e., hypertonic, low fiber/residue, and high fat), and bacterial contamination (67). Medications (i.e., sorbitol-containing elixirs, antibiotics, laxatives, and magnesium and phosphorous supplements), pancreatic insufficiency, fecal impaction, and pathogenic

bacteria (*C. difficile*) can all be non–formula-related causes of diarrhea in the tube-fed patient (67). The type of tube feeding formula is rarely the source of diarrhea, and it is not necessary to stop the feeding until the cause is identified (36). Treatment of diarrhea is contingent on the etiology. Antimotility agents (e.g., lomotil, immodium, paregoric, and deodorized tincture of opium) can be used in the treatment of diarrhea provided stool cultures are negative for an infectious etiology (67).

High gastric residuals (i.e., >200 mL) from delayed emptying can result from high fat and fiber formulas, rapid infusion rate, high osmolality formulas, disease state (diabetic gastroparesis), elevated intracranial pressure, sepsis, and medications including narcotics. As previously discussed, checking feeding residuals is an essential component of the monitoring process. If patients have persistently high residuals, giving prokinetic drugs or placing the feeding tube in the small bowel should help alleviate the problem. When checking for residuals during small bowel feedings, there, essentially, should be no residuals obtained. If residuals are obtained, then chances are that the feeding tube has relocated to the stomach, and verification of tube placement is warranted.

Constipation can result from low fiber/residue formulas, inadequate water/fluid intake, inactivity, decreased bowel motility, and medications such as phosphate binders, narcotics, and calcium-channel antagonists. Neuromuscular blocking agents do not paralyze gut smooth muscle but may reduce bowel motility via anticholinergic actions (67,69). Adequate hydration, fiber-enriched formulas, stool softeners, and bowel motility agents are helpful in improving constipation (67,69). If there is narcotic-induced constipation or ileus and if all other bowel motility agents have failed, the use of oral naloxone via the feeding tube can promote defecation. Monitoring the stool pattern of the patient is also important for prevention of fecal impaction.

Metabolic complications that occur during enteral nutrition therapy are similar to those developed during PN but are generally less severe (70). The metabolic disturbances most frequently seen include hyperglycemia, dehydration, and electrolyte imbalances such as hyper–hypophosphatemia, hyper–hyponatremia, and hyper–hypokalemia. Hyperglycemia is common in patients who are diabetic, who have poor glucose utilization due to insulin resistance from stress (i.e., trauma and sepsis), or who are on diabetogenic medications such as corticosteroids (70). Because hyperglycemia and insulin resistance are common in critically ill patients, urine and blood glucose should be monitored at periodic intervals in all patients who receive enteral feeding. Tight glycemic control is the goal of blood glucose management in the ICU. The aim must be to achieve blood glucose levels in the range of 80 to 110 mg per dL. In a single-center unblinded study, intensive insulin administration was reported to reduce morbidity and mortality in some critically ill patients (71). On subcutaneous administration, insulin is poorly absorbed in critically ill patients because of circulatory problems; therefore, an insulin infusion is required for the treatment of hyperglycemia.

Repletion of malnourished patients can result in the intracellular uptake of phosphorus, potassium, and magnesium as anabolism is stimulated, causing decreased serum levels of these electrolytes (67). These electrolytes should be closely monitored for refeeding shifts and replaced as needed. Thiamine supplementation is also needed in the malnourished patient (67). For a comprehensive list of the complications associated with enteral nutrition therapy, along with prevention and treatment strategies, the reader is referred elsewhere (72).

PARENTERAL NUTRITION

PN is the intravenous administration of a hypertonic solution of carbohydrate, fat, protein, electrolytes, vitamins, minerals, and fluid. Although enteral nutrition support is the preferred modality of nutritional therapy, PN is an important technique for nutrient provision in patients who have absolute gut failure such as short bowel syndrome, small bowel obstruction, and fistulas not amenable to enteral feeding. In addition, PN should be initiated in any critically ill patient who cannot tolerate full enteral nutrition support within 5 to 7 days. Guidelines for indications and appropriateness of use of PN have been established by the American Society for Parenteral and Enteral Nutrition (73).

The administration of PN is dependent on the osmolarity of the nutrient solution, anticipated duration of therapy, nutrient requirements, and the need for fluid restriction. The dextrose concentration, however, is the limiting factor for the route of venous access. A central line is necessary when infusing dextrose concentrations >10%, whereas PN solutions with dextrose concentrations <10% can be administered peripherally. Because of the large fluid load generally needed to adequately meet a patient's nutrient goals, peripheral parenteral nutrition (PPN) is not usually feasible in the critical care setting.

Formula Composition

Carbohydrate is the primary energy source in a PN solution. Dextrose monohydrate is the carbohydrate source, yielding 3.4 calories per gram and ranging in concentration from 5% to 70%. The most frequently used dextrose concentrations for critically ill patients are 20% and 25%. The quantity of carbohydrate, however, is based on the patient's caloric requirement, optimal fuel balance, and glucose oxidation rate (i.e., hepatic oxidative capacity). Administration of not >4 to 6 mg dextrose/kg/minute per 24-hour period is recommended for optimal oxidation and prevention of fat synthesis (lipogenesis). Excessive carbohydrate provision is also associated with hepatic dysfunction and increased carbon dioxide production.

Crystalline amino acids are the form in which protein is currently added to the PN admixture and are classified as either standard or modified preparations (74). The standard amino acid solutions contain a balance of nonessential and essential amino acids tailored to the normal serum amino acid profile. Concentrations range from 3% to 15% and yield 4.0 calories per gram.

The modified amino acid formulas contain a blend of amino acids designed to meet disease-specific or age-specific requirements (74). Standard amino acid solutions are glutamine free. Recent studies have shown that glutamine-enriched PN solutions sustain better gut mass than do PN alone; however, PN preparations with glutamine stimulate the gut less effectively than do enteral formulations. In the future, the use of intravenous dipeptides as the source of nitrogen in PN solutions may increase. Preliminary data has indicated that these agents have the same capacity to spare nitrogen and support serum protein synthesis as free amino acids in catabolic patients. Additionally,

the dipeptides have the advantage of being more soluble and stable in aqueous solutions than amino acids do (75). Further studies are required, however, before recommending their use in the clinical setting.

Intravenous fat is an aqueous dispersion containing soybean or safflower oil, egg yolk phospholipid (an emulsifier), and glycerin to achieve isotonicity. Long chain fatty acid emulsions are currently the only commercially available intravenous (IV) fat. They are available as 10%, 20%, or 30% emulsions. Maintenance of essential fatty acid (EFA) requirements can be met by providing 4% to 10% of the total calories as fat (2% to 4% as linoleic acid). The 10% lipid emulsion provides 1.1 kcal per mL; 20% provides 2.0 kcal per mL; 30% provides 3.0 kcal per mL. IV fat is contraindicated in patients with the following: disturbances in normal fat metabolism (i.e, pathologic hyperlipidemia), triglceride levels at upper limit of normal laboratory values (more than 400 to 500 mg per dL), lipoid nephrosis when accompanied by hyperlipidemia, and severe egg allergy because egg yolk phospholipids are used in emulsification. IV fat infusions in patients with pancreatitis of etiologies other than hypertriglyceridemia are not contraindicated. The recommended infusion rate varies depending on the lipid concentrations. A minimum of 8 hours for the 10% emulsion and a minimum of 12 hours for the 20% emulsion are suggested. Propofol is present in 10% IV fat providing 1.1 kcal per mL. Attention must be given to those patients who are on TPN with lipids and on propofol. Because of the dose of propofol that is being administered, occasionally, IV fat will need to be discontinued to avoid the excessive provision of fat and/or total calories. Propofol infusion can be associated with hypertriglyceridemia, so serum triglycerides need to be closely monitored.

Electrolyte requirements in patients receiving PN are patient specific and are influenced by nutritional status. Organ function, acid–base balance, medications, and GI losses will also influence the electrolyte adjustments that will be needed in the PN solution to maintain electrolyte homeostasis (74). In stable patients, acid–base balance can, for the most part, be maintained by adding equal amounts of chloride and acetate (i.e., 1:1 ratio). However, in patients with acid–base disturbances, the acetate, which is metabolized to bicarbonate, and the chloride will need to be adjusted in an effort to help correct the abnormality. For example, in patients with a significant metabolic alkalosis, the acetate should be minimized and the chloride maximized. Alternately, in patients with severe metabolic acidosis, the chloride would be minimized and the acetate maximized. Vitamins and trace elements are added to PN solutions in doses consistent with the American Medical Association Nutrition Advisory Group's recommendations (74) (see Table 20-11). Iron is absent in the multi–trace-element preparation because of the fear of anaphylaxis, but iron can be given as iron dextran either in the PN formula or intramuscularly. Copper and manganese are excreted via biliary excretion. Requirements for both are diminished with cholestatic liver failure to avoid potential toxicities from the hepatic deposition and elevated central nervous system (CNS) levels of these trace elements. Consequently, supplementation of copper and manganese should be discontinued if baseline total bilirubin is three times the upper limit of normal or if total bilirubin triples from baseline value. This can be achieved by deleting the multi–trace-elements from the PN solution and by separately adding back zinc, chromium, and selenium.

TABLE 20-11. Suggested Daily Vitamin and Mineral Intake for Parenteral Nutrition

Vitamin A	3,300 IU
Vitamin D	200 IU
Vitamin E	100 mg
Folic acid	400 μg
Niacin	40 mg
Riboflavin	3.6 mg
Thiamine	3.0 mg
Pyridoxine (vitamin B$_6$)	4.0 mg
Vitamin B$_{12}$	5.0 μg
Pantothenic acid	15.0 mg
Biotin	60 μg
Zinc	2.5–4.0 mg
Copper	0.5–1.5 mg
Chromium	10.0–15.0 μg
Manganese	0.15–0.8 mg

Initiation and Advancement

PN therapy should be initiated at a slow rate (e.g., 30 to 40 mL per hour) using the final concentration planned for therapy and advanced as glucose tolerance permits until the nutrient needs of a patient are met. In critically ill patients, advancement of PN should be conservative (e.g., increasing 20 mL every 24 hours until the goal rate is attained). The slow advancement in rate will help metabolic tolerance in the setting of metabolic disturbances such as hyperglycemia and hypertriglyceridemia. Because dextrose concentration is limited with PPN (5% or 10% dextrose), it may be initiated at the same rate as peripheral IV fluids.

Monitoring

Monitoring guidelines for PN are essential for the successful administration and tolerance of PN support. Blood glucose monitoring via finger sticks every 4 to 6 hours (more frequently in the ICU) is indicated until the infusion rate has stabilized. Serum glucose should be tightly controlled between 80 and 120 mg per dL, as previously mentioned with enteral nutrition, in order to reduce morbidity and mortality among critically ill patients (71). Serum triglycerides should be checked approximately 6 hours after the completion of the IV fat infusion to assess the patient's lipid clearing capacity, especially in the face of hyperglycemia, steroid therapy, and propofol administration. Serum triglyceride levels should be ≤500 mg per dL. Monitoring electrolytes to ensure adequate hydration, renal function, and need for supplementation or restriction is mandatory. Finally, liver function should be periodically monitored to detect hepatic dysfunction related to PN therapy.

Complications

There are several complications that may occur when using PN support including mechanical, metabolic, infectious, and hepatic complications. Pneumothorax is the most common mechanical complication associated with PN. Others include thrombus, catheter occlusion, and air embolus. The infectious complications seen with PN are typically catheter related. Of the metabolic complications, hyperglycemia is the most prevalent.

Risk factors for hyperglycemia include metabolic stress, medications, obesity, diabetes, and excess calories and/or carbohydrate (76). Insulin administration may be warranted to lower blood glucose levels, especially in the critically ill patient. Malnourished patients are prone to refeeding shifts (as discussed in the enteral section of this chapter) with PN therapy. For an extensive list of the metabolic complications of PN and suggestions for prevention and treatment, the reader is referred to a major text on PN (77).

Hepatobiliary abnormalities have been identified in patients on TPN who have no underlying liver disease. Elevated transaminases, alkaline phosphatase, and bilirubin concentrations may occur days to weeks after initiation of parenteral nutrition (76). Enzyme levels may return to normal while a patient is on PN but almost always normalize when PN is discontinued (76). Steatosis (fatty liver) is the most frequent hepatic derangement that occurs with PN. High glucose infusions, exceeding 4 to 6 mg dextrose/kg/minute, are the primary etiologic agent in the production of fatty liver (78). The excessive provision of IV fat can also result in fatty infiltration of the liver. Other proposed etiologies of steatosis are toxins and specific nutritional deficiencies, such as carnitine, EFA, and protein malnutrition, which cause decreased apoprotein synthesis, resulting in impaired hepatic triglyceride transport (78,79).

The possible causes of cholestasis include lack of enteral stimulation, bacterial sepsis, endogenous recycling of lithocholic acid, and molybdenum deficiency (78–80). Gallbladder stasis (biliary sludging) is felt to be the primary cause of PN-associated biliary disease. Stimulating gallbladder contractility with enteral feedings usually reverses this process. Several recommendations exist for the management and prevention of PN-induced hepatic dysfunction, including use of the GI tract whenever possible, avoidance of overfeeding, provision for a well-balanced fuel mix, cycling of the PN regimen, consideration of carnitine and glutamine supplementation, and workup of alternative causes such as hepatitis, biliary obstruction, hepatotoxic drugs, and sepsis (79).

CONCLUSIONS

Nutrition is of vital importance in maintaining nutritional status during a period of critical illness. Appropriate delivery of nutrition support in critical illness is contingent on a thorough understanding of the metabolic response to stress and injury. Stress metabolism, driven by the counterregulatory hormones, is characterized by increased energy expenditure and profound protein catabolism that results in rapid deterioration of nutritional status. The loss of body protein can lead to delayed wound healing and tissue repair, immunosuppression, and loss of muscle strength: an effect that can impede weaning from mechanical ventilation. Because many of the routine nutritional assessment parameters are invalid with critical illness, assessment of nutritional status is difficult. Individualized and ongoing nutritional assessment is imperative to provide optimal nutrition therapy to our critically ill patients. The accurate determination of energy and protein requirements is paramount consideration in delivering proper nutrition support. Measurement of energy expenditure using indirect calorimetry and nitrogen balance studies are recommended in some patients because they can guide nutrition and metabolic management of critically ill patients.

Enteral nutrition therapy is the preferred modality of nutrition support because of the significant benefits on the GI tract, particularly during a period of critical illness or injury. Alimentation via the enteral route preserves gut barrier integrity, physiologic function and cell mass, and prevents bacterial translocation. Initiation of early postoperative or early injury feeding can maintain intestinal mass and barrier function, decrease infection rates, improve immune function and wound healing, blunt the hypermetabolic response to stress, and improve patient outcome. Although enteral nourishment is the optimal route of nutrient administration, at times, it is not medically feasible or well tolerated. Under these circumstances, TPN is indicated; however, every effort should be made to switch to enteral feeding in critically ill patients when possible.

Tight glycemic control (blood glucose kept below 110 mg per dL) may become the standard of care in critically ill patients if there is clear evidence that morbidity and mortality are substantially reduced.

Evidence-based clinical practice changes related to the care of critically ill patients have significantly improved outcomes. More controlled clinical trials of specific nutritional strategies are needed in critically ill patients.

ETHICAL PRINCIPLES

Medical ethics is a set of moral principles that govern the behavior of physicians and other health professionals. As discussed by Beauchamp and Childress, one principle of medical ethics is autonomy—respect for the patient's capacity of self-determination and exercise of personal, informed choice (81). Another principle is nonmaleficence—the obligation not to harm intentionally. A third principle is beneficence—the provision of benefit, which generally is defined as something that promotes well-being. A fourth is distributive justice—the fair, equitable, and appropriate distribution of medical resources in society.

The first three ethical principles outlined in the preceding paragraph are the foundation of the fiduciary relationship that characterizes the practice of medicine. Under the unwritten terms of this relationship, physicians are expected to serve the best interests of their patients, particularly as the patients define these interests (82,83). The fiduciary relationship is based on trust. Patients, who are relatively helpless because of their underlying illnesses and limited familiarity with various treatments, rely on physicians, who are relatively powerful because of their concurrent health and superior knowledge of medicine, to care for them.

MEDICAL DECISION MAKING

Some previously competent patients remain so throughout a critical illness and can participate in medical decisions. However, when patients are incompetent to begin with or are unable to communicate because they are comatose or sedated, their surrogates may become involved in the decision-making process. The proper role for surrogates is to represent patients' interests and previously expressed wishes; surrogates are less helpful in decision making when they represent their own interests or speak only from their own points of view. When family members disagree among themselves about patients' interests and wishes, they should be asked to designate spokespersons

who can represent the group if such spokespersons have not already been selected by the patients. Physicians who work with surrogates of this sort can reach decisions more rapidly than with entire families.

Ideal surrogates are those who have been designated by patients before or during their critical illness to make medical decisions in the event of incapacity. In California and some other states, such surrogates may be granted what is called a "durable power of attorney for health care" (84). Proxy directives of this sort are legally binding so long as patient interests are being protected. They are more helpful than living wills and other instructional directives, most of which are either too broadly or too narrowly drawn.

When surrogates are not available, critical care physicians must rely on other sources of information in determining their patients' wishes. Among these sources are the patients' primary physicians if they have already discussed issues such as resuscitation with the patients. These physicians should be called on to articulate their patients' wishes even if they are not supervising their care in the ICU. Critical care nurses have frequently explored these issues with patients at the bedside while the patients were lucid, and they too should be consulted. So should clergy members who either knew the patients before hospitalization or have come to know them in the hospital.

When surrogates are not available and other sources of information are inadequate, physicians have two options. One is to ask the courts to appoint conservators to help preserve the autonomy of their patients. This approach is cumbersome and time consuming, and conservators usually prefer that physicians make medical decisions anyway. Alternatively, and especially when urgent decisions must be made, physicians may decide what is in their patients' best interests and use beneficence to justify this strategy (85).

Although decisions based on what physicians consider as their patients' best interests may be ethically acceptable, it must be stressed that the principles of beneficence—or medical paternalism, as some would have it—and autonomy frequently conflict in the ICU. This seems inevitable, given the realities of critical care practice, but physicians still should remind themselves of the great personal authority they exercise. Whenever appropriate, they should review their decisions either with colleagues or with members of biomedical ethics committees. Such committees also may be helpful in resolving conflicts between physicians and patients or their surrogates (86,87).

INFORMED CONSENT

The concept of informed consent is contained within the ethical principle of autonomy. This concept may be defined as the voluntary acceptance of physician recommendations by competent patients or surrogates who have been provided with sufficient truthful information regarding risks, benefits, and alternatives and who adequately indicate their comprehension of this information (81). Consent may be implied rather than informed in emergency situations wherein physicians are obligated to provide medically necessary treatment when patients or surrogates have not expressed their wishes or cannot do so. The rationale for treatment in such situations is that patients or surrogates would consent if they could and that harm would result from delaying care.

Informed consent is called for especially when patients are given innovative treatments or are recruited for research. Physicians frequently are tempted to try new therapies in critically ill patients either on a one-time basis or as part of ongoing trials. This is ethically supportable only after consent has been obtained from patients or surrogates or, when consent cannot be obtained, when the treatments are known to be safe and of great potential value. In keeping with the fiduciary relationship, physician obligation is to the present-day patients; such patients should not be experimented on solely because future patients might benefit from what has happened to them. As part of this obligation, physicians should clarify the differences between research and treatment lest a "therapeutic misconception," in which patients or surrogates erroneously assume that research is being done to benefit them personally, occur (88).

FOREGOING LIFE-SUSTAINING THERAPY

Although the fiduciary relationship remains vital to medical practice in the ICU, interpretation of the phrase "best interests of their patients" on the part of physicians has changed over time. ICUs proliferated in the United States and other developed countries during and after the 1950s alongside the advances in scientific knowledge, improvements in artificial ventilation, the introduction of cardiac monitoring, and the need for prolonged support following complex surgeries. For most of their history, ICUs have reported death rates of from 10% to 20%, depending on the types of patients treated therein (89). Today, approximately one fifth of all people who die in the United States do so in the ICU or shortly after discharge (90).

Until recently, most of the patients who died in the ICU did so despite full life support, including attempted cardiopulmonary resuscitation (CPR). The wishes of patients and their surrogates about support were rarely solicited, in our experience, and do-not-resuscitate (DNR) orders were seldom used to limit treatment. This practice has been consonant with the belief, held by health professionals and the public alike, that the ICU and its technologies have the obligation to preserve life whenever possible regardless of the human and economic costs.

In recent years, however, the obligation of the ICU has been challenged, just as its expenses have been scrutinized. For example, clinical research has revealed that many patients, including those with severe respiratory failure and such underlying conditions as advanced hematologic malignancies, rarely leave the ICU alive or do so only after prolonged pain and suffering (91). Furthermore, these and other survivors of critical illness frequently die shortly after being transferred out of the ICU, thereby minimizing its apparent benefits (92). As the clinical limitations of intensive care have become recognized, physicians and hospital administrators have questioned whether the economic resources used to finance ICUs should be used for other, more beneficial medical purposes, especially in our era of capitation and managed care. And although patients and their surrogates seldom pay the ICU bill directly, they nevertheless have come to question the value of intensive care in all instances and to seek ways to refuse it if they so desire.

The right of patients and their surrogates to refuse treatment and have it withdrawn, over the objections of physicians and hospitals if necessary, was first legally affirmed on a state level in the cases of Karen Ann Quinlan in 1976 and Joseph Barber in

1983. In the case of Nancy Cruzan in 1990, the US Supreme Court reaffirmed this right on the part of patients who can participate in medical decisions but allowed states to require evidence of patients' wishes regarding life support if the patients are incapable of decision making. The federal Patient Self-Determination Act of 1991 was passed to encourage the expression of patients' wishes by requiring that health care facilities should ask admitted patients if they have advance directives and help them prepare such directives if they do not (93).

Although the Patient Self-Determination Act and the legal cases that preceded it support patient and surrogate autonomy, more recent cases have involved physicians and hospitals that seek to restrain autonomy. For example in the case of Catherine Gilgunn, the Massachusetts General Hospital and several of its physicians were sued for writing a DNR order for and removing mechanical ventilation from Mrs. Gilgunn over the objections of her daughter. In 1995, a Suffolk County Superior Court jury absolved the physicians and hospital of liability, apparently because they believed that further treatment was futile despite the possibility that Mrs. Gilgunn might have wanted to be kept alive (93). The outcome in this case suggests that some juries are willing to overlook the wishes of patients or their surrogates when the juries believe that physicians and hospitals choose to discontinue treatment they consider nonbeneficial, presumably because such discontinuation is within the medical standard of care.

In parallel with these legal cases from Quinlan to Gilgunn, presidential commissions, individual authors, institutional ethics committees, and professional societies have supported patient and surrogate autonomy while also spelling out circumstances in which futile care should be foregone (94–99). At the same time, the advent of medical cost consciousness related to managed care has restrained the application of therapies that merely prolong death with little hope of long-term cure (100). The legal, ethical, and economic consensus that has resulted from these developments has in turn reinforced a trend toward the limitation of ineffective treatments that is currently reflected in the changing nature of death in the ICU. Whereas critically ill patients previously died despite full support and attempted CPR, such patients are more likely to die today during the withholding and withdrawal of life support with DNR orders in place. Thus, physicians with the implicit or explicit approval of the hospitals in which they practice have increasingly become involved in managing death in the ICU, just as they manage cardiovascular decompensation and respiratory failure.

HOW DEATHS ARE MANAGED

The first major observational study of how critically ill patients die was conducted over the academic year 1987 to 1988 in two medical–surgical ICUs at hospitals affiliated with the University of California, San Francisco (UCSF) (101). During the 1-year period, 228 (13%) of the 1,719 patients admitted to the ICUs died. Of the 224 patients who died, 114 (51%) did so after a decision had been made to limit treatment; 22 patients had life support, including CPR, withheld, and 92 had life support withdrawn. Of the 114 patients who were not supported, 89 died in the ICU and 15 died after they were transferred to other areas of the hospitals with the provision that they would not be readmitted to the ICU if they decompensated. None of the

114 patients received attempted CPR, and DNR orders were written for 109 of them.

Over the academic year 1992 to 1993, 5 years after the first study, a similar investigation was conducted in the same medical–surgical ICUs affiliated with UCSF (102). During this second period, 200 (13%) of the 1,711 patients admitted to the ICUs died, the same proportion as previously. A decision was made to withhold or withdraw life support from 179 (90%) of the 200 patients who died, compared with 51% of patients in the first study. Life support was withheld from 27 of the 179 patients and withdrawn from 140 of them in the second study; 12 patients had only CPR withheld. Of the 179 patients, 162 died in the ICU and 17 died after transfer. None of the 179 patients received attempted CPR, and most had DNR orders.

To determine the generalizability of these observations, the directors of all American postgraduate training programs in critical care medicine were contacted and asked to categorize prospectively all patients who died in their ICUs over a 6-month period in 1994 and 1995 into one of five mutually exclusive categories. The national survey of end-of-life care that resulted from this effort involved 131 ICUs from 110 institutions in 38 states (103). A total of 74,502 patients were admitted to these ICUs during the 6-month study period, 6,300 of whom died (9% mortality in the units). Of the 6,300 patients who died, 1,544 (20%) did so despite full ICU support including attempted CPR, 1,430 (24%) did so after receiving full support but not attempted CPR, 794 (14%) had life support withheld, 2,139 (36%) had life support withdrawn, and 393 (6%) were brain dead. Thus, of the 5,910 patients who died in the ICU who were not brain dead, 4,366 (74%) received less than full support. This percentage probably would have been higher if patients who died shortly after being transferred out of the ICU with no provision for readmission had been included.

One striking finding of the national survey was the wide variation in end-of-life care: The range of proportions of death preceded by failed CPR, DNR status, and withholding or withdrawal of life support was 4% to 79%, 0% to 83%, 0% to 67%, and 0% to 79%, respectively. This variation could not be explained by the types of ICUs (i.e., medical, surgical, medical–surgical, neurosciences, and others), hospital types (i.e., university, community, public, veterans, and others), or the geographic regions of the hospitals. However, a pattern was observed in the two states with strict legal standards for care limitation by surrogates. Thus, ICUs in New York and Missouri had lower proportions of deaths preceded by withdrawal of support than did the entire mid-Atlantic and Midwest regions in which these states are located.

Although the national survey did not demonstrate changes in ICU deaths over time, it did suggest that limits to life support have become so commonplace in the United States as to represent a *de facto* standard of end-of-life care for critically ill patients. This suggestion is reinforced by other studies that document changes in terminal care management at other institutions and in other countries (104–109). Nevertheless, the extreme variation in the categories of ICU death in all these studies underscores the absence of a true consensual approach to end-of-life care. A first step in creating consensus would be for all hospitals to track their own end-of-life practices. The second step would be for critical care specialists to develop guidelines for limiting treatment, as is presently being done.

FUTURE MANAGEMENT OF DEATH

It is likely that critical care specialists will care for most, if not all, ICU patients in the future not only in other countries, as has been the practice for many years, but also in the United States. Kollef in 1996 and Kollef and Ward in 1999 have reported that American intensive care specialists are more likely to limit treatment when appropriate, and other studies have demonstrated that "closed" units in which such specialists direct care are associated with better risk-adjusted mortality, shorter length of stay, and more appropriate use of resources (110–112). Given that death has been and remains commonplace in ICUs (the mortality rate was 9% in the national end-of-life care study), the specialists who will care for critically ill patients in the future must become specialists in the management of death in the ICU if they have not already become proficient in this area.

To help manage death, intensive care specialists must learn how death is managed in ICUs and whether it is managed well. The Study to Understand Prognoses and Preferences for Outcomes and Risks of Treatment (SUPPORT) suggested that physicians do not communicate adequately with patients and surrogates and that patients suffer greatly as they die, at least in the ICUs that were studied (113). Further research is needed to determine whether the SUPPORT findings are generalizable, and if they are not, what measures are useful in improving the quality of death. From such research should come quality indicators for end-of-life care in the ICU, practice guidelines to accompany current recommendations about compassionate care, and clinical tools such as preprinted physician order forms for withdrawing life support (114–116). A recent article from the ethics committee of the Society of Critical Care Medicine provides excellent guidelines for the pharmacologic and clinical management of withdrawal of life support in critically ill patients (117).

In addition to research, critical care specialists require clinical training in death management. In particular, better education in how to prognosticate for ICU patients and how to access and use the large data sets that increasingly make prognostication a scientific process are called for. Training also is needed in communication and conflict resolution, skills that commonly are called for with our patients and their surrogates. Finally, a curriculum in death management for intensive care specialists that befits the changing nature of death in the ICU should be developed.

REFERENCES

1. Goldstein SA, Elwyn DH. The effects of injury and sepsis on fuel utilization. *Annu Rev Nutr* 1989;9:445–473.
2. Bessey PQ, Watters J, Aoki TT, et al. Combined hormone infusion stimulates the metabolic response to injury. *Ann Surg* 1984;200: 264–281.
3. Cahill GF Jr. Starvation in man. *N Engl J Med* 1970;282:668–675.
4. Woolfson AMJ, Heatly RV, Allison SP. Insulin to inhibit protein catabolism after injury. *N Engl J Med* 1979;300:14–17.
5. Wolfe RR, Herndon DN, Jahoor F, et al. Effect of severe burn injury on substrate cycling by glucose and fatty acids. *N Engl J Med* 1987;317:403–408.
6. Clowes GHA, Randall HT, Cha JC. Amino acid and energy metabolism in septic and traumatized patients. *J Parenter Enteral Nutr* 1980;4:195–205.
7. Jeevanadam M, Grote-Holman AE, Chikenji T, et al. Effects of glucose on fuel utilization and turnover in normal and injured man. *Crit Care Med* 1990;18:125–135.

8. Long CL, Kinney JM, Geiger JW. Nonsuppressibility of gluconeogenesis by glucose in septic patients. *Metabolism* 1976;25:193–201.

9. Burke JF, Wolfe RR, Mullany CJ, et al. Glucose requirements following burn injury: parameters of optimal glucose infusion and possible hepatic and respiratory abnormalities following excessive glucose intake. *Ann Surg* 1979;190:274–285.

10. Vary TC, Siegel JH, Nakatani T, et al. Regulation of glucose metabolism by altered pyruvate dehydrogenase activity in sepsis. *J Parenter Enteral Nutr* 1986;10:351–355.

11. Nordenstrom J, Carpentier YA, Askanazi IE, et al. Free fatty acid mobilization and oxidation during total parenteral nutrition in trauma and infection. *Ann Surg* 1983;198:725–735.

12. Birkhahn RH, Long CL, Fitkin DL, et al. A comparison of the effects of skeletal trauma and surgery on ketosis of starvation in man. *J Trauma* 1981;21:513–518.

13. Elwyn DH, Gump FE, Iles M, et al. Protein and energy sparing of glucose added in hypocaloric amounts to peripheral infusions of amino acids. *Metabolism* 1978;27:325–331.

14. Yamazaki K, Maiz A, Sobrado J, et al. Hypocaloric lipid emulsions and amino acid metabolism in injured rats. *J Parenter Enteral Nutr* 1984;8:360–366.

15. Shaw JHF, Wildbore M, Wolfe RR. An integrated analysis of glucose, fat, and protein metabolism in severely traumatized patients: studies in the basal state and the response to total parenteral nutrition. *Ann Surg* 1987;209:66–72.

16. Baracos V, Rodemann HP, Dinarello CA, et al. Stimulation of muscle protein degradation and prostaglandin E_2 release by leukocyte pyrogen (interleukin-1). *N Engl J Med* 1983;308:553–558.

17. Mullen JL, Buzby GP, Matthews DC, et al. Reduction of operative morbidity and mortality by combined pre-operative nutrition support. *Ann Surg* 1980;192:604–613.

18. McWhirter JP, Pennington CR. The incidence and recognition of malnutrition in hospital. *Br Med J* 1994;308:945–948.

19. Buzby GP, Mullen JL. Nutritional assessment. In: Rombeau J, Caldwell MD, eds. *Clinical nutrition,* Vol. 1. Philadelphia: WB Saunders, 1984:127–148.

20. Shronts EP, Fish JA, Pesce-Hammond K. Nutritional assessment. In: Souba WW, Kohn-Keeth C, Mueller C, et al, eds. *The ASPEN nutrition support practice manual.* Silver Spring: ASPEN, 1998.

21. ASPEN. Standards for nutrition support: hospitalized patients. *Nutr Clin Pract* 1995;10(6):208–218.

22. Ireton-Jones CS, Hasse JM. Comprehensive nutritional assessment: The dietitians contribution to the team effort. *Nutrition* 1992;8(2):75–81.

23. Hopkins B. Assessment of nutritional status. In: Gottshclich MM, Matarese LE, Shronts EP, eds. *Nutrition support dietetics core curriculum,* 2nd ed. Silver Spring: ASPEN, 1993.

24. Lang CE, Shutte CV. Nutrition assessment: adult patient. In: Lang CE, ed. *Nutrition support in critical care.* Rockville: Aspen Publishers, 1982:61–91.

25. Grant A, DeHoog S, eds. Biochemical assessment. In: *Nutritional assessment and support.* Seattle: Grant &DeHoog, 1985:35–73.

26. Lipman TO. Nutritional assessment. *Curr Opin Gastroenterol* 1991; 7:271–276.

27. Sax HC, Souba WW. Nutritional goals and macronutrient requirements. In: Souba WW, Kohn-Keeth C, Mueller C, et al, eds. *The ASPEN nutrition support practice manual.* Silver Spring: ASPEN, 1998.

28. Mueller C. True or false: serum hepatic protein concentrations measure nutritional staus. *Support Line* 2004;26(1):8–16.

29. Ireton-Jones CS, Borman KR, Turner WW. Nutrition considerations in the management of ventilator-dependent patients. *Nutr Clin Pract* 1993;8:60–64.

30. McClave SA, Snider HL. Use of indirect calorimetry in clinical nutrition. *Nutr Clin Pract* 1992;7:208–221.

31. Feurer I, Mullen JL. Bedside measurement of resting energy expenditure and respiratory quotient via indirect calorimetry. *Nutr Clin Pract* 1986;1:43–49.

32. Porter C, Cohen N. Indirect calorimetry in critically ill patients: role of the clinical dietitian in interpreting results. *J Am Diet Assoc* 1996;96:49–57.

33. Scheinkestel CD, Adams F, Mahony L, et al. Impact of increasing parenteral protein loads on amino acid levels and balance in critically ill anuric patients on continuous renal replacement therapy. *Nutrition* 2003;19:733–740.

34. Konstantinides FN. Nitrogen balance studies in clinical nutrition. *Nutr Clin Pract* 1992;7:231–238.

35. Barton RG. Nutrition support in critical illness. *Nutr Clin Pract* 1994;9:127–139.

36. Trujillo EB, Robinson MK, Jacobs DO. Critical illness. In: Souba WW, Kohn-Keeth C, Mueller C, et al, eds. *The ASPEN nutrition support practice manual.* Silver Spring: ASPEN, 1998.

37. Spector N. Nutritional support of the ventilator-dependent patient. *Nurs Clin North Am* 1989;24(2):407–413.

38. Schwartz DB. Pulmonary failure. In: Gottschlich MM, Matarese LE, Shronts EP, eds. *Nutrition support core curriculum,* 2nd ed. Silver Spring: ASPEN, 1993.

39. Talpers SS, Romberger DJ, Bunce SB, et al. Nutritionally associated increased carbon dioxide production: excess total calories vs. high proportion of carbohydrate calories. *Chest* 1992;102:551–555.

40. Lord LM, Sax HC. The role of the gut in critical illness. *AACN Clin Issues* 1994;9(4):450–458.

41. Langkamp-Henken B, Glezer JA, Kudsk KA. Immunologic structure and function of the gastrointestinal tract. *Nutr Clin Pract* 1992;7:100–108.

42. Thompson JS. The intestinal response to critical illness. *Am J Gastroenterol* 1995;90(2):190–200.

43. Guedon C, Schmitz J, Lerebours E, et al. Decreased brush border hydrolase activities without gross morphologic changes in human intestinal mucosa after prolonged total parenteral nutrition in adults. *Gastroenterology* 1986;90:373–378.

44. Kudsk KA. Parenteral vs. enteral nutrition. In: Shikora SA, Martindale RG, Schwaitzberg SD, eds. *Nutritional considerations in the intensive care unit.* Dubuque: Kendall /Hunt Publishing Company, 2002:119–130.

45. Albanese CT, Smith SD, Watkins S, et al. Effect of secretory IgA on transepithelial passage of bacteria across the intact ileum in vitro. *J Am Coll Surg* 1994;179:679–688.

46. Sax HC, Illig KA, Ryan CK, et al. Low-dose enteral feeding is beneficial during total parenteral nutrition. *Am J Surg* 1996;171:587–590.

47. Stralovich A. Gastrointestinal and pancreatic disease. In Gottschlich MM, Matarese LE, Shronts EP, eds. *Nutrition support core curriculum,* 2nd ed. Silver Spring: ASPEN, 1993.

48. Palacio JC, Rombeau JL. Dietray fiber: a brief review and potential application to enteral nutrition. *Nutr Clin Pract* 1990;5:99–106.

49. Rombeau JL, Kripke SA. Metabolic and intestinal effects of short-chain fatty acids. *J Parenter Enteral Nutr* 1990;14(5 Suppl): 181S–185S.

50. Brinson RB, Hanumanthu SK, Pitts WM. A reappraisal of the peptide-based enteral formulas: clinical applications. *Nutr Clin Pract* 1989;4:211–217.

51. Zaloga GP. Physiological effects of peptide-based enteral formulas. *Nutr Clin Pract* 1990;5:231–237.

52. Gadek JE, DeMichele SJ, Karlstad MD, et al. Effect of enteral feeding with eicosapentaenoic acid, γ-linoleic acid, and antioxidants in patients with acute respiratory distress syndrome. *Crit Care Med* 1999;17:300–402.

53. Kaushik N, O'Keefe JD. Severe acute pancreatitis: nutritional management in the ICU. *Nutr Clin Pract* 2004;19:25–30.

54. Olah A, Pardavi G, Belagyi T, et al. Early nasojejunal feeding in acute pancreatitis is associated with a lower complication rate. *Nutrition* 2002;18:259–262.

55. McClave SA, Greene LM, Snider HL, et al. Comparison of the safety of early enteral versus parenteral nutrition in mild acute pancreatitis. *J Parenter Enteral Nutr* 1997;21:14–20.

56. Zaloga GP. Early enteral nutritional support improves outcome. Hypothesis or fact? *Crit Care Med* 1999;27:259–261.

57. Bloss CS. Pharmacomodulation of the gut: implications for the enterally fed patient. *Nutr Clin Pract* 1998;13:201–214.

58. Schwartz DB. Enteral therapy. In: Lang CE, ed. *Nutrition support in critcal care.* Rockville: ASPEN publishers, 1982:93–111.

59. Klodell CT, Carroll M, Carrillo EH, et al. Routine intragastric feeding following traumatic brain injury is safe and well tolerated. *Am J Surg* 2000;179:168–171.

60. Spain DA, DeWeese RC, Reynolds MA, et al. Transpyloric passage of feeding tubes in patients with head injuries does not decrease complications. *J Trauma* 1995;39:1100–1102.

61. Heyland DK, Drover JW, MacDonald S, et al. Effect of postpyloric feeding on gastroesophageal regurgitation and pulmonary

microaspiration; Results of a randomized controlled trial. *Crit Care Med* 2001;29:1495–1501.

62. Montecalvo MA, Steger KA, Farber HW, et al, The Critical Care Research Team. Nutritional outcome and pneumonia in critical care patients randomized to gastric versus jejunal tube feedings. *Crit Care Med* 1992;20:1377–1387.

63. American Gastroenterological Association Patient Care Committee. American Gastroenterological Association technical review on tube feeding for enteral nutrition. *Gastroenterology* 1995;108(4):1282–1301.

64. DeLegge MH, Rhodes BM. Continuous versus intermittent feedings: slow and steady or fast and furious? *Support Line* 1998;20(5):11–15.

65. Krystofiak Russell M, Charney P. Is there a role for specialized enteral nutrition in the intensive care unit? *Nutr Clin Pract* 2002;17:156–168.

66. Evans MA, Shronts EP. Intestinal fuels: glutamine, short-chain fatty acids, and dietary fiber. *J Am Diet Assoc* 1992;92:1239–1246, 1249.

67. Lord L, Trumbore L, Zaloga G. Enteral nutrition implementation and management. In: Souba WW, Kohn-Keeth C, Mueller C, et al eds. *The ASPEN nutrition support practice manual*. Silver Spring: ASPEN, 1998.

68. Breach CL, Saldanha LG. Tube feeding complications, part II: mechanical. *Nutr Support Services* 1988;8(5):28–32.

69. Breach CL, Saldanha LG. Tube feeding complications, part I: gastrointestinal. *Nutritional Support Services* 1988;8(30):15–19.

70. Breach CL, Saldanha LG. Tube feeding complications, part III: metabolic. *Nutr Support Services* 1988;8(6):16–19.

71. Van Den Berghe G, Wouters P, Weekers F, et al. Intensive insulin therapy in critically ill patients. *N Engl J Med.* 2001;345(19):1359–1367.

72. Ideno KT. Enteral nutrition. In: Gottschlich MM, Matarese LE, Shronts EP, eds. *Nutrition support dietetics core curriculum*, 2nd ed. Silver Spring: ASPEN, 1993.

73. ASPEN Board of Directors. Guidelines for the use of parenteral and enteral nutrition in adult and pediatric patients. *J Parenter Enteral Nutr* 1993;17(Suppl):1SA–52SA.

74. Strausberg KM. Parenteral nutrition admixture. In: Souba WW, Kohn-Keeth C, Mueller C, et al, eds. *The ASPEN nutrition support Practice Manual*. Silver Spring: ASPEN, 1998.

75. Vazquez JA, Hannelore D, Adibi SA. Dipeptides in parenteral nutrition: from basic science to clinial applications. *Nutr Clin Pract* 1993;8:95–105.

76. Skipper A, Millikan KW. Parenteral nutrition implementation and management. In: Souba WW, Kohn-Keeth C, Mueller C, et al, eds. *The ASPEN nutrition support practice manual*. Silver Spring: ASPEN, 1998.

77. Rombeau JL, Rolandelli RR, eds. *Parenteral nutrition*. Philadelphia: WB Saunders, 1998.

78. Fisher RL. Hepatobiliary abnormalities associated with total parenteral nutrition. *Gastroenterol Clin North Am* 1989;18(3):645–661.

79. Sax HC, Bower RH. Hepatic complications of total parenteral nutrition. *J Parenter Enteral Nutr* 1988;12(6):615–618.

80. Freund HR. Abnormalities of liver function and hepatic damage associated with total parenteral nutrition. *Nutrition* 1991;7(1):1–5.

81. Beauchamp TL, Childress JF. *Principles of biomedical ethics*, 4th ed. New York: Oxford University Press, 1994.

82. Luce JM. Ethical principles in critical care. *JAMA* 1990;213:696–700.

83. Luce JM. Conflicts over ethical principles in the intensive care unit. *Crit Care Med* 1992;20:313–315.

84. Steinbrook R, Lo B. Decision making for incompetent patients by designated proxy. *N Engl J Med* 1984;310:1598–1601.

85. Luce JM. Three patients who asked that life support be withheld or withdrawn in the surgical intensive care unit. *Crit Care Med* 2002;30:775–780.

86. Schneiderman LJ, Gilmer T, Teetzel HD, et al. Effect of ethics consultations on nonbeneficial life-sustaining treatments in the intensive care unit: a randomized controlled trial. *JAMA* 2003;290:1166–1172.

87. Brennan TA. Ethics committees and decisions to limit care in the experience at the Massachusetts General Hospital. *JAMA* 1988;260:803–807.

88. Miller FG, Rosenstein DL. The therapeutic orientation to clinical trials. *N Engl J Med* 2003;348:1383–1386.

89. Thibault GE, Mulley AG, Barnett GO, et al. Medical intensive care: indications, interventions, and outcomes. *N Engl J Med* 1980;302:938–942.

90. Angus D, Barnato AE, Linde-Zwirble WT, et al, on behalf of The Robert Wood Johnson Foundation ICU End-of-Life Peer Group. Use of intensive care at the end of life in the United States: an epidemiologic study. *Crit Care Med* 2004;32:638–643.

91. Rubenfeld GD, Crawford SW. Withdrawing life support from mechanically ventilated recipients of bone marrow transplants: a case for evidence-based guidelines. *Ann Intern Med* 1996;125:625–633.

92. Seneff MG, Wagner DP, Wagner RP, et al. Hospital and 1-year survival of patients admitted to intensive care units with acute exacerbation of chronic obstructive pulmonary disease. *JAMA* 1995;274:1852–1857.

93. Luce JM. Withholding and withdrawal of life support from critically ill patients. *West J Med* 1997;167:411–416.

94. President's Commission for the Study of Ethical Problems in Medicine and Biomedical and Behavioral Research. *Deciding to forego life-sustaining treatment: a report on the ethical, medical, and legal issues in treatment decisions*. Washington: Government Printing Office, 1983.

95. Ruark JE, Raffin TA. Stanford University Medical Center Committee on Ethics. Initiating and withdrawing life support: principles and practice in adult medicine. *N Engl J Med* 1988;318:25–30.

96. Council on Ethical and Judicial Affairs, American Medical Association. Decisions near the end of life. *JAMA* 1992;267:2229–2233.

97. American Thoracic Society. Withholding and withdrawing life-sustaining therapy. *Am Rev Respir Dis* 1991;144:726–731.

98. Task Force on Ethics of the Society of Critical Care Medicine. Consensus report on the ethics of foregoing life-sustaining treatments in the critically ill. *Crit Care Med* 1990;18:1435–1439.

99. Council on Ethical and Judicial Affairs, American Medical Association. Medical futility in end-of-life care: report of the Council on Ethical and Judicial Affairs. *JAMA* 1999;281:937–941.

100. Cher DJ, Lenert LA. Method of Medicare reimbursement and the rate of potentially ineffective care of critically ill patients. *JAMA* 1997;278:1001–1007.

101. Smedira NG, Evans BH, Grais LS, et al. Withholding and withdrawal of life support from the critically ill. *N Engl J Med* 1990;322:309–315.

102. Prendergast TJ, Luce JM. Increasing incidence of withholding and withdrawal of life support from the critically ill. *Am J Respir Crit Care Med* 1997;155:15–20.

103. Prendergast TJ, Claessens MT, Luce JM. A national survey of end-of-life care for critically ill patients. *Am J Respir Crit Care Med* 1998;158:1163–1167.

104. Eidelman LA, Jakobson KJ, Pizov R, et al. Foregoing life-sustaining treatment in an Israeli ICU. *Intensive Care Med* 1998;24:162–166.

105. Keenan SP, Busche KD, Chen LM, et al. A retrospective review of a large cohort of patients undergoing the process of withholding and withdrawal of life support. *Crit Care Med* 1997;25:1324–1331.

106. Turner JS, Michell WL, Morgan CJ, et al. Limitation of life support: frequency and practice in a London and a Cape Town intensive care unit. *Intensive Care Med* 1996;22:1020–1025.

107. Ferrand E, Robert R, Ingrand P, et al, for the French LATAREA group. Withholding and withdrawal of life support in intensive-care units in France: a prospective survey. *Lancet* 2001;357:9–13.

108. Buckley TA, Joynt GM, Tan PYH, et al. Limitation of life support: frequency and practice in a Hong Kong intensive care unit. *Crit Care Med* 2004;32:415–420.

109. Vincent JL, Parquier JN, Preiser JC, et al. Terminal events in the intensive care unit: review of 258 fatal cases in one year. *Crit Care Med* 1989;17:530–533.

110. Kollef MH. Private attending physician status and the withdrawal of life-sustaining interventions in a medical intensive care unit population. *Crit Care Med* 1996;24:968–975.

111. Kollef MH, Ward S. The influence of access to a private attending physician on the withdrawal of life-sustaining therapies in the intensive care unit. *Crit Care Med* 1999;27:2125–2132.

112. Carson SS, Stocking C, Podsadecki T, et al. Effects of organizational change in the medical intensive care unit of a teaching hospital: a

comparison of 'open' and 'closed' formats. *JAMA* 1996;276: 322–328.

113. Desbiens NA, Wu AW, Broste SK, et al. Pain and satisfaction with pain control in seriously ill hospitalized adults: findings from the SUPPORT research investigations. *Crit Care Med* 1996;24: 1953–1961.

114. Clarke EB, Curtis RJ, Luce JM, et al., for the Robert Wood Johnson Foundation Critical Care End-of-Life Peer Workgroup Members. Quality indicators for end-of-life care in the intensive care unit. *Crit Care Med* 2003;31:2255–2262.

115. Brody H, Campbell ML, Faber-Langendoen K, et al. Withdrawing intensive life-sustaining treatment—recommendations for

compassionate clinical management. *N Engl J Med* 1997;336: 652–657.

116. Treece PD, Engelberg RA, Crowley L, et al. Evaluation of a standardized order form for the withdrawal of life support in the intensive care unit. *Crit Care Med* 2004;32:1141–1148.

117. Truog RD, Cist EFM, Brackett SE, et al. Recommendations for end-of-life care in the intensive care unit: the ethics committee of the Society of Critical Care Medicine. *Crit Care Med* 2001;29: 2332–2348.

118. Olree K, Vitello J, Sullivan J, et al. Enteral formulations. In: Souba WW, Kohn-Keeth C, Mueller C, et al, eds. *The ASPEN nutrition support practice manual*. Silver Spring: ASPEN, 1998.

CHAPTER 21

General Principles of Managing a Patient with Respiratory Failure

Rachel H. Dotson

Brian M. Daniel

James A. Frank

ASSESSMENT OF SEVERE RESPIRATORY DYSFUNCTION

CLINICAL EVALUATION

Acute respiratory failure may evolve slowly, over a period of days, or may develop rapidly, within minutes to hours. The clinical manifestations are protean and depend upon the nature of the underlying disease process. In most cases, the symptomatic hallmark of severe respiratory dysfunction is dyspnea.

However, despite the frequent presence of this symptom, dyspnea remains poorly defined, difficult to quantify, and correlates poorly with the degree of respiratory failure (1). Dyspnea is a subjective manifestation, and many factors influence the manner in which it is perceived by the patient. For instance, the sensation of breathlessness may be more intense when it develops acutely. Conversely, patients with disorders resulting in chronic dyspnea may complain of only minor changes from their baseline level of symptoms despite major worsening of gas exchange. Furthermore, dyspnea can be blunted by progressive hypoxemia, hypercarbia, or both, misleading the clinician to underestimate the degree of respiratory impairment that is present. In the setting of sedative–hypnotic or narcotic drug overdoses, patients may not be sufficiently alert to be aware of their respiratory dysfunction or convey their symptoms to others. In patients with neuromuscular disease who have diminished ventilatory drive or cannot exercise due to generalized weakness, significant respiratory muscle impairment may go unrecognized. Also, near-fatal asthma exacerbations have been associated with decreased chemosensitivity to hypoxia and diminished sensation of dyspnea (2).

Although associated symptoms such as cough, sputum production, and chest pain are important for diagnosis and management, they are less helpful than dyspnea as an indicator of respiratory dysfunction. Progressive hypoxemia or hypercapnia may manifest as headache, visual disturbances, memory loss, confusion, hallucinations, or transient loss of consciousness. However, these symptoms are neither specific nor universally present.

The physical examination provides important and objective information in patients with respiratory failure. Early therapeutic interventions can be implemented on the basis of initial exam findings even before a specific diagnosis is made. An assessment of the patient's vital signs, to include oxygen saturation by pulse oximetry, is a crucial first step in evaluating the overall stability of the patient. The respiratory rate (RR), although influenced by a variety of factors, can gauge the severity of respiratory distress and can be used to monitor the response to therapy. As described for the symptom of dyspnea, tachypnea may not be present in patients whose ventilatory drive is blunted. Pulse oximetry is a valuable, noninvasive method for determining oxygen saturation. It should be emphasized that the oxyhemoglobin saturation may be within normal limits in the setting of hypercapnic ventilatory failure. Patients with significant levels of carboxyhemoglobin due to smoke inhalation will also have "normal" oxygen saturation by pulse oximetry; true oxyhemoglobin determination in this setting requires direct measurement by cooximetry. Finally, measurements of oxygen saturation may be inaccurate when perfusion is poor because of local vasoconstriction or low cardiac output states (3). Therefore, in order to best evaluate any patient with severe respiratory dysfunction, direct arterial blood gas sampling is recommended.

An assessment of the patient's general appearance and mental status is of paramount importance when determining the severity of illness. Decreased alertness, diaphoresis, accessory muscle use, and a compromised ability to speak complete sentences constitute evidence of significant distress and may herald imminent respiratory failure. Retraction of the sternum and supraclavicular, suprasternal, and intercostal spaces can be observed when resistance to lung inflation increases, generally because of airway obstruction or infiltrative processes. These findings have been observed to correlate with the severity of airway obstruction in asthma and pneumonia (4,5). An inability to phonate or stridorous breathing raises concern for severe upper airway obstruction.

A directed exam, with particular attention to the cardiopulmonary system, may disclose the etiology and severity of the patient's respiratory failure. The pulmonary findings associated with specific processes are described in Chapter 4, The

Respiratory History and Physical Examination, but several points are worth emphasizing. For example, although wheezing is a characteristic feature of airway obstruction, the absence of wheezing in a patient with dyspnea and obstructive lung disease may be even more alarming. In these cases, airflow may be so diminished that the turbulence required for wheezing is not produced. The presence of a pulsus paradoxus (exaggerated respiratory variation in systemic blood pressure because of large swings in pleural pressure) also correlates with severe airway obstruction (6,7). Unilateral absence of breath sounds in a patient with respiratory distress may be the result of a pneumothorax or obstruction of a main bronchus by a mucous plug, tumor, or foreign body. Physical findings suggestive of a pneumothorax are particularly important to recognize in mechanically ventilated patients because of the heightened risk of tension pneumothorax. Other physical findings pertinent to respiratory failure include subcutaneous emphysema and a systolic "crunch" (the Hamman sign) indicating pneumomediastinum with or without pneumothorax, digital clubbing, cyanosis, abdominal paradox (inward motion of the abdomen during inhalation), flaring of the nasal ala, and neuromuscular abnormalities. Patients should also be examined carefully for evidence of heart failure, although in critically ill patients, the exam findings may not suggest left ventricular failure even when present (8). Right ventricular failure may be the consequence of a chronic pulmonary process complicated by long-standing hypoxemia or acute right ventricular strain secondary to pulmonary embolism. The practitioner must reassess the patient periodically for changes in the exam, be aware that the potential for rapid deterioration exists, and be prepared to respond appropriately.

GENERAL LABORATORY EVALUATION

Although hematologic and serum chemistry studies are considered routine in clinical practice, their utility is rather limited in patients with respiratory failure. However, some helpful information may be provided, such as clues to the acuity or chronicity of the disease process. For example, an elevated hematocrit implies the presence of chronic hypoxemia causing secondary polycythemia. Hypercapnia may be inferred to be chronic if the plasma bicarbonate (HCO_3^-) concentration is increased. Renal compensation for respiratory acidosis develops over a period of days; hence, a rise in HCO_3^- concentration does not occur as a result of acute respiratory failure of short duration (9).

Electrolyte abnormalities can be directly associated with respiratory dysfunction. Hypokalemia and hypophosphatemia may cause respiratory muscle weakness, which can be the primary cause of respiratory failure or may complicate preexisting lung disease (10,11). These abnormalities can also cause difficulty in weaning a patient from mechanical ventilation.

Drug toxicities can cause a spectrum of acute respiratory problems, including pulmonary edema, bronchospasm, and alveolar hemorrhage (12); therefore, a urine drug screen should be considered in all patients with respiratory failure. Overdoses of opiates, benzodiazepines, and barbiturates can induce central hypoventilation, and salicylates can cause central hyperventilation. Salicylates and certain ingestions, such as methanol and ethylene glycol, can cause anion gap metabolic acidosis and tachypnea. Therefore, a salicylate level and measured serum osmolality should be obtained when suggested by the history or the presence of an anion gap metabolic acidosis.

Additional laboratory studies, such as tests to exclude hypothyroidism, vasculitis, or other etiologies of respiratory failure, should be considered when indicated by the patient's history and exam findings. Although the chest radiograph cannot quantify the severity of the respiratory disorder, it is valuable in determining the etiology and is an essential component of the initial evaluation. Figure 21-1 depicts a chest radiograph from a patient with pneumonia and acute respiratory distress syndrome (ARDS). Likewise, the electrocardiogram can detect arrhythmias, myocardial ischemia or infarction, cardiac chamber enlargement, pericarditis, and pericardial effusion.

ARTERIAL BLOOD GASES

The single most useful test in evaluating the critically ill patient with respiratory dysfunction is the measurement of arterial blood gas tensions of oxygen and carbon dioxide (i.e., PaO_2 and $PaCO_2$) and pH. These indices can be used to infer the pathophysiology of the underlying disease process and guide the general approach to treatment.

Hypoxemia

Clinically significant reductions in PaO_2 are most commonly the consequence of ventilation–perfusion $(\dot{V}/\dot{Q})$ mismatch, right-to-left intrapulmonary or intracardiac shunt, or alveolar hypoventilation. Other causes include primary oxygen diffusion defects at the level of the alveolus and low tensions of inhaled oxygen at high altitude. The alveolar–arterial oxygen gradient $(PAO_2 - PaO_2)$ is a measure of pulmonary gas exchange and can help identify the physiologic basis for inadequate oxygenation. For example, a normal $PAO_2 - PaO_2$ is expected when alveolar hypoventilation or high altitude is the sole cause of hypoxemia because the lungs are functionally normal and gas transfer across the alveolar membrane is intact. In contrast, hypoxemia

due to $(\dot{V}/\dot{Q})$ mismatch or anatomic right-to-left shunt is associated with an elevated $PAO_2 - PaO_2$, reflecting abnormalities in oxygen transfer across the alveolar capillary. A defect in the diffusion of oxygen across the alveolar–capillary barrier is not a common cause of hypoxemia but may be seen in *Pneumocystis* pneumonia.

The partial pressure of oxygen in the alveolus (PAO_2) is calculated using the alveolar gas equation:

$$PAO_2 = FIO_2 (P_{atm} - PH_2O) - PaCO_2/R$$

where R is the respiratory quotient (VCO_2/VO_2), FIO_2 is the fraction of inspired oxygen, P_{atm} is the barometric pressure, and PH_2O is the partial pressure of water vapor in fully saturated air at body temperature. At sea level, $P_{atm} = 760$ mm Hg and $PH_2O = 47$ mm Hg. If the patient is breathing 100% oxygen, the respiratory quotient should not be included in the equation. The measured PaO_2 is subtracted from the calculated PAO_2, and the difference is the $PAO_2 - PaO_2$:

$$PAO_2 - PaO_2 \text{ gradient} = PAO_2 - PaO_2$$

The $PAO_2 - PaO_2$ gradient is influenced by age and FIO_2. In young patients breathing room air, the difference should not be greater that 10 mm Hg, but the normal range increases with age (13). The normal $PAO_2 - PaO_2$ gradient can be estimated by the following equation:

$$\text{Normal } PAO_2 - PaO_2 \text{ gradient} = (Age/4) + 4$$

With an increased FIO_2 sufficient to result in a PAO_2 of 200 or greater, the $PAO_2 - PaO_2$ should not exceed 40 mm Hg.

By observing the response to the administration of 100% oxygen, it is possible to distinguish ventilation–perfusion mismatch from pure shunt. Normally, the PaO_2 increases to a greater extent if the hypoxemia is caused primarily by mismatch, whereas with shunt, the increase may be markedly reduced depending on the magnitude of shunt flow (see Fig. 21-2).

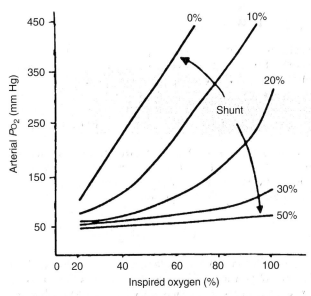

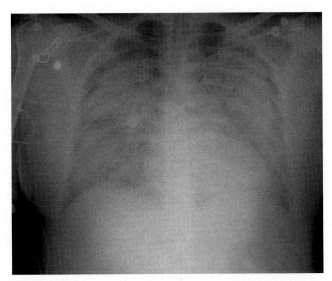

FIGURE 21-1. This chest radiograph shows bilateral diffuse pulmonary infiltrates characteristic of the acute respiratory distress syndrome (ARDS).

FIGURE 21-2. The relationship between inspired oxygen concentration and arterial PO_2 for lungs with varying degrees of shunt. The increase in PO_2 is small for lungs with large shunts. (From Dantzker DR. Gas exchange in ARDS. *Clin Chest Med* 1982;3:57–62, with permission.)

Hypercapnia

Pa_{CO_2} is directly proportional to carbon dioxide production ($\dot{V}_{CO_2}$) and inversely related to alveolar ventilation ($\dot{V}_A$):

$$Pa_{CO_2} \propto \frac{\dot{V}_{CO_2}}{\dot{V}_A}$$

In order to adequately eliminate carbon dioxide and maintain a normal Pa_{CO_2}, alveolar ventilation must adjust according to the level of carbon dioxide production. The amount of alveolar ventilation actually effective in removing carbon dioxide is influenced by the degree of wasted ventilation present. The following equation accounts for wasted ventilation and estimates the *effective* alveolar ventilation ($\dot{V}_A$):

$$\dot{V}_A = (V_T - V_D) \times F$$

where V_T is tidal volume in liters, V_D is wasted or dead-space volume in liters, and F is the RR in breaths per minute. From the above equations, it is evident that the variables determining the Pa_{CO_2} are $\dot{V}_{CO_2}$, V_T, V_D, and F. The product of V_T and F is the total minute ventilation ($\dot{V}_E$) in liters per minute:

$$\dot{V}_E = V_T \times F$$

Thus, increased carbon dioxide production, decreased $\dot{V}_E$, increased wasted ventilation, or a combination of the three mechanisms can set the stage for hypercapnia. Alveolar hypoventilation, whether absolute or relative, must be present for hypercapnia to develop.

Hypercapnia can cause cerebral vasodilation, decreased cardiac contractility, decreased systemic vascular resistance, and depressed consciousness (14). These effects more commonly occur in acute hypercapnia because patients with chronic hypercapnia are generally metabolically compensated. Most adverse consequences associated with hypercapnia result from acidosis or hypoxemia, which often accompany significant elevations of Pa_{CO_2}.

Acid–Base Disturbances

Recognizing and understanding acid–base disturbances in severely ill patients can have major diagnostic and therapeutic implications. A methodic approach to the analysis of acid–base disorders safeguards against misinterpretation of the data. A comprehensive discussion of acid–base disorders is beyond the scope of this section; however, major terms and concepts will be reviewed.

First, an arterial blood gas and serum electrolyte panel must be obtained simultaneously. The relationship between pH, Pa_{CO_2}, and HCO_3^- is depicted by a modified version of the Henderson–Hasselbalch equation:

$$[H^+] = 24 \times \frac{Pa_{CO_2}}{[HCO_3^-]}$$

This equation clearly illustrates that $[H^+]$ (and thus pH) is determined by the ratio of Pa_{CO_2} to HCO_3^- concentration. Also, internal consistency of the laboratory data can be verified using this equation. The Pa_{CO_2} and serum HCO_3^- concentration are used to calculate $[H^+]$, which can predict the pH on the basis of the following relationship: every 1 nEq per L change in H^+

concentration corresponds with a reciprocal change in pH of 0.01 (15). This rule holds true for pH values in the physiologic range 7.1 to 7.5. For example, the concentration of H^+ at pH 7.4 is 40 nEq per L and increases to 50 nEq per L at pH 7.30. Any discrepancy between the calculated H^+ concentration and pH measured directly by arterial blood gas sampling suggests the presence of laboratory error (16). Once internal consistency has been confirmed, the primary disorder(s) can be identified. Table 21-1 lists the equations used to evaluate disorders of acid–base balance.

SIMPLE AND MIXED ACID–BASE DISTURBANCES. Arterial pH is determined by the overall balance between carbon dioxide and HCO_3^- concentration. Therefore, acidemia (pH <7.35) or alkalemia (pH >7.45) can result from simple respiratory, simple metabolic, or mixed acid–base disturbances. In the setting of acidemia, the primary acidosis is respiratory if the Pa_{CO_2} is elevated or metabolic if the Pa_{CO_2} is low. Conversely, when alkalemia is present, a low Pa_{CO_2} is indicative of primary respiratory alkalosis, whereas a normal or elevated HCO_3^- concentration is consistent with primary metabolic alkalosis.

Respiratory and metabolic compensatory responses aim to reverse abnormalities in blood pH. Although compensation can bring the pH toward the normal range, complete normalization of the pH does not result from compensation alone. The rules of compensation listed in Table 21-1 were derived from experimental data (15), which demonstrated that the degree of respiratory or metabolic compensation is predictable. Discrepancies between the calculated and expected compensatory changes in Pa_{CO_2} or HCO_3^- concentration suggest the presence of a concomitant primary acid–base disorder. For example, the presence of an anion gap metabolic acidosis and a coexisting primary respiratory alkalosis raises the possibility of sepsis or salicylate toxicity.

ANION, DELTA, AND OSMOLAR GAPS. The anion gap should be calculated routinely and, if elevated, determination

TABLE 21-1. Equations for Acid–Base Disorders

Rules of Compensation

Acute respiratory acidosis	For every 10 mm Hg rise in P_{CO_2}, HCO_3^- concentration increases 1 mEq/L
Chronic respiratory acidosis	For every 10 mm Hg rise in P_{CO_2}, HCO_3^- concentration increases 3.5 mEq/L
Acute respiratory alkalosis	For every 10 mm Hg decline in P_{CO_2}, HCO_3^- concentration decreases 2 mEq/L
Chronic respiratory alkalosis	For every 10 mm Hg decline in P_{CO_2}, HCO_3^- concentration decreases 4 mEq/L
Metabolic acidosis	$P_{CO_2} = 1.5\,[HCO_3^-] + 8 \pm 2$
Metabolic alkalosis	$P_{CO_2} = 0.9\,[HCO_3^-] + 9 \pm 2$
Anion gap	$Na^+ - Cl^- - HCO_3^-$
Delta gap	(calculated anion gap – normal anion gap)
	(measured HCO_3^- concentration – normal HCO_3^- concentration)
Osmolar gap	Measured osmolarity – calculated osmolarity
Calculated osmolarity	$2[Na^+]$ + glucose/18 + BUN/2.8 + [ethanol]/4.6

P_{CO_2}, partial pressure of carbon dioxide; BUN, blood urea nitrogen.

of the delta gap may reveal a coexisting acid–base disturbance in addition to the anion gap metabolic acidosis. The ratio of the increase in anion concentration and decrease in HCO_3^- concentration is normally between 1 and 1.6. A ratio less than 1 is indicative of a lower than expected HCO_3^- concentration (Table 21-1). This suggests that, in addition to the anion gap metabolic acidosis, a primary non–anion gap metabolic acidosis is present. A primary metabolic alkalosis can result in a ratio greater than 2 because the HCO_3^- concentration is higher than what is predicted by the magnitude of the anion gap.

The osmolar gap detects unmeasured solute and is associated with toxin ingestion. Methanol, ethanol, ethylene glycol, and isopropyl alcohol can result in an elevated osmolar gap. Methanol and ethylene glycol are also causes of increased anion gap acidosis.

ADVERSE EFFECTS OF ACID–BASE DISTURBANCES. Numerous deleterious sequelae can occur secondary to acidemia and alkalemia, particularly when the degree of the disturbance is more profound. In general, acidemia and alkalemia are considered severe when blood pH is less than 7.20 and greater than 7.60, respectively (17,18). Serious consequences of acidemia include obtundation, coma, arrhythmias, and decreased cardiac contractility, cardiac output, and blood pressure (17). Alkalemia may predispose patients to arrhythmias, decreased cardiac output, and reduced seizure threshold (19). Therefore, in addition to treatment of the underlying disease process, severe perturbations in acid–base homeostasis may necessitate interventions directed at improving the pH itself.

MEASUREMENT OF LUNG FUNCTION

In select clinical settings, bedside measurements of vital capacity (VC), maximal inspiratory pressure (MIP), and peak expiratory flow rate (PEFR) are practical lung function studies that can provide useful information and can potentially impact a patient's treatment strategy. Gathering meaningful and interpretable data from these studies requires that the patient be able to cooperate and perform the necessary maneuvers satisfactorily. The VC and MIP (also referred to as PImax) are helpful in patients with progressive neuromuscular disease, whereas the PEFR can help gauge the severity of airway obstruction and guide the management of patients presenting with asthma exacerbations.

The VC is the maximal volume of air that can be exhaled after full inspiration and reflects the patient's ventilatory capability. Because it is influenced by the respiratory muscles, the chest wall, the elastic properties of the lung, and the caliber of the airways, it cannot be used to diagnose abnormalities specifically. Nonetheless, the VC is valuable in the assessment and monitoring of patients with respiratory compromise secondary to neuromuscular disorders. The practitioner should note that the VC may not be significantly reduced until respiratory muscle strength has fallen below 50% of normal (20). A normal VC is 65 mL per kg, and a VC approaching 30 mL per kg is associated with impaired cough and accumulation of secretions (21). Patients with a VC <20 mL per kg should be monitored in the intensive care unit (ICU) and considered for elective intubation (22).

The MIP (PImax) is the negative airway pressure generated by a maximal inspiratory effort against an occluded airway. It is particularly important in the assessment of neuromuscular disease and can facilitate early recognition of respiratory muscle weakness. In a retrospective study by Lawn et al., a 30% decrease in MIP, maximal expiratory pressure (MEP), or VC correlated with progression to respiratory failure requiring intubation in patients with neuromuscular weakness from Guillain–Barré syndrome (23). The MIP and VC are also useful measurements while weaning patients from mechanical ventilation.

The PEFR provides an objective measure of airflow obstruction and is recommended for the management of asthma. PEFR monitoring has the advantage of being both simple and inexpensive; however, the test is highly effort dependent, and artificially low values may occur with submaximal effort. A PEFR less than 50% of the predicted or the patient's personal best value indicates severe obstruction (24). Serial measurements can assess responsiveness to treatment. This test is of limited value in patients with obvious respiratory distress.

The FEV_1 is helpful in diagnosing and assessing the severity of obstructive lung disease in the outpatient setting. However, this measurement may not be possible in the acutely ill patient because of marked tachypnea, and the maneuver may even transiently worsen airway obstruction. Currently, there is no convincing data to support the routine use of FEV_1 in the management of acute exacerbations of chronic obstructive pulmonary disease (COPD) and is therefore not recommended.

TREATMENT MODALITIES

SUPPLEMENTAL OXYGEN

The administration of supplemental oxygen is frequently necessary in patients with any cardiorespiratory disorder resulting in arterial hypoxemia. Treating hypoxemia with external oxygen delivery devices may obviate the need for endotracheal intubation; however, for hypoxemic patients requiring an F_{IO_2} of 0.6 or greater or for those who could potentially suffer serious consequences, it is not prudent to rely on external devices should there be interruption of oxygen delivery due to accidental device malpositioning.

Various external oxygen delivery systems are available, and the selection of a particular device should be based on the patient's degree of hypoxemia, ventilatory pattern, need for precise control of F_{IO_2}, and comfort. Oxygen delivery systems are either low or high flow. Low-flow systems supply oxygen at flow rates lower than the patient's ventilatory requirement and depend on the inspiration of ambient air to meet the patient's demand. The F_{IO_2} actually delivered to the trachea depends upon the oxygen flow rate and the amount of room air entrained. The entrainment of room air is determined by the patient's $\dot{V}_E$. Therefore, in patients with abnormal ventilatory patterns, the inhaled oxygen concentration may be neither controlled nor adequate. In contrast to low-flow devices, most high-flow systems provide the entire inspiratory volume and, therefore, a constant and predictable F_{IO_2} (25). High oxygen concentrations can be delivered with either high-flow or low-flow oxygen.

Low-flow oxygen can be administered by nasal cannulae, simple face masks, or face masks with reservoir bags. Nasal prongs are comfortable and simple to use. In the setting of a normal ventilatory pattern, the F_{IO_2} can be estimated to rise by 0.04 for every 1 L per minute of oxygen supplied. A humidifier can alleviate patient discomfort when flow rates of 4 L per minute or higher dry the nasal mucosa. Simple face masks provide an FIO_2 of 0.4 to 0.5 with oxygen flow rates of 5 to 8 L per minute. Nonrebreathing face masks use reservoir bags to provide an FIO_2 approaching 1.0 at flow rates of 6 to 10 L per minute, although the precise FIO_2 delivered cannot be guaranteed. Proper use of these masks require that the reservoir bag remain partially inflated throughout inspiration (26).

Because the oxygen concentration can be reliably prescribed independent of the $\dot{V}E$, high-flow devices are preferred in some patients. Examples include chronically hypercapnic patients, in whom excessive supplemental oxygen may worsen alveolar hypoventilation, and hypoxemic patients with abnormal breathing patterns who require high oxygen concentrations. The Venturi (jet-mixing) face mask uses a calibrated valve in the delivery line to provide fixed oxygen concentrations of 24%, 28%, 35%, or 40% (27). The mask is supplied by high-flow 100% oxygen, and room air is entrained through the valve by the Venturi effect. However, at an FIO_2 greater than 0.35, precise FIO_2 delivery is less reliable as flow rates often cannot meet the inspiratory demands of patients in respiratory distress (28). Nonetheless, more precise control of FIO_2 can be achieved using Venturi masks, and they are therefore recommended for hypoxemic patients with COPD and carbon dioxide retention. Other high flow devices include reservoir nebulizers with aerosol masks, T-tube adapters, tracheostomy collars, and face tents.

NONINVASIVE POSITIVE PRESSURE VENTILATION FOR ACUTE RESPIRATORY FAILURE

Rationale for Noninvasive Positive Pressure Ventilation in the Acute Setting

Noninvasive positive pressure ventilation (NPPV) is an effective means of providing ventilatory assistance without the use of an endotracheal or tracheotomy tube. Although invasive mechanical ventilation can be lifesaving and, in many cases, should be regarded as the primary intervention for respiratory failure, several disadvantages to this method are well recognized. The potential for NPPV to reduce the morbidity and costs associated with conventional mechanical ventilation led investigators to examine the role of NPPV in acute respiratory failure. A large body of evidence now supports the use of NPPV in select patient populations with acute respiratory failure as it can avoid some of the drawbacks associated with endotracheal intubation. NPPV can be delivered as continuous positive airway pressure (CPAP), in which a constant airway pressure is maintained and no additional assistance is provided during inhalation. NPPV may also be delivered with different inspiratory and expiratory pressures such that the airway pressure is greatest during inhalation. This provides assistance to the muscles of respiration (see Fig. 21-3).

The advantages of NPPV over conventional mechanical ventilation have generated interest in its application in the acute setting. In addition to overcoming some of the risks introduced by endotracheal intubation, such as injury to the upper airway, sinusitis, and nosocomial pneumonia, NPPV does not require the use of sedation and can be continued outside the ICU. Complications of NPPV are typically minor and include facial or nasal bridge ulceration, gastric distension, nasal congestion, sinus pain, and eye irritation. More serious complications, such as aspiration pneumonia, hypotension, and pneumothorax, are

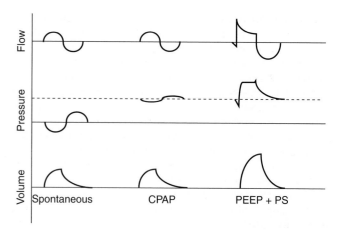

FIGURE 21-3. Airflow, pressure at the airway opening, and VT during various forms of noninvasive ventilation. During spontaneous breathing without any ventilatory assistance, airway pressures oscillate around zero and reflect similar changes in pleural pressures. Delivery of continuous positive airway pressure (CPAP) of 5 cm H_2O via a nasal or face mask results in an increase in airway pressure such that inspiratory and expiratory swings oscillate around 5 cm H_2O. During invasive or noninvasive pressure support ventilation (PSV), inspiratory and expiratory pressures are set by the clinician. In this example, the settings are 10 cm H_2O inspiratory pressure and 5 cm H_2O expiratory pressure. A similar mode of noninvasive ventilation is bilevel positive airway pressure (BiPAP) ventilation.

less common, having been reported in less than 5% of patients (29). Such adverse effects can be minimized by ensuring a properly fitted mask, taking necessary precautions in patients who are at risk of aspiration, adjusting the settings to prevent barotrauma, and selecting patients for NPPV judiciously.

Patient Selection for Noninvasive Positive Pressure Ventilation

Successful NPPV is highly dependent on appropriate patient selection. Prospective, randomized controlled trials have concluded that in certain clinical conditions, a trial of NPPV is justified in the early management of acute respiratory failure; however, not all patients are suitable candidates for noninvasive ventilatory support. Patients must be able to cooperate sufficiently, synchronize breathing with the ventilator, and adequately protect their airway. The potential for reversibility of the underlying process must be considered, and those with contraindications to NPPV should be excluded (see Table 21-2).

TABLE 21-2.   Contraindications to Noninvasive Ventilation

Cardiac or respiratory arrest
Nonrespiratory organ failure
Severe encephalopathy (e.g., glasgow coma scale <10)
Severe upper gastrointestinal bleeding
Hemodynamic instability or unstable cardiac arrhythmias
Facial surgery, trauma, or deformity
Inability to cooperate or protect the airway
Inability to clear respiratory secretions
High risk for aspiration

From International Consensus Conferences in Intensive Care Medicine. Noninvasive positive pressure ventilation in acute respiratory failure. *Am J Respir Crit Care Med* 2001;163:288, with permission.

The decision to institute NPPV must also be based on the current evidence supporting its application for the diagnosis at hand.

Several randomized controlled trials have demonstrated the benefits of NPPV in patients with acute exacerbations of COPD. In these studies, bilevel continuous positive airway pressure (BiPAP) was most commonly used. In this modality, an inspiratory and a lower expiratory pressure are set separately. Decreased mortality, decreased need for endotracheal intubation, fewer infectious complications (primarily nosocomial pneumonia), and decreased length of ICU and hospital stay have been reported (30–33), validating the use of NPPV as a primary intervention in appropriate hypercapnic patients in respiratory failure. Studies have attempted to identify the predictors of success and failure in patients with acute COPD exacerbations managed with NPPV. Improvements in arterial pH and $PaCO_2$ measured 1 to 2 hours after initiating NPPV have been associated with success (34,35). A recent systematic review by Keenan et al. concluded that patients with severe exacerbations of COPD, rather than those with mild exacerbations, benefit from NPPV (36). In a retrospective multivariate analysis, Ambrosino et al. observed that the level of acidemia before starting NPPV was predictive of treatment response (35). A mean baseline pH of 7.28 was associated with treatment success, whereas a mean pH of 7.22 correlated with treatment failure. These findings suggest that although patients with COPD and severe respiratory failure are likely to derive the greatest benefit from NPPV, clinicians must be able to recognize when the severity of illness is so far advanced as to preclude NPPV. In these instances, endotracheal intubation is indicated.

There is considerable evidence that CPAP is efficacious in the management of acute cardiogenic pulmonary edema. In this modality, the airway pressure is maintained at a constant level during inspiration and exhalation. Randomized prospective trials have shown that as compared to supplemental oxygen alone CPAP can significantly improve gas exchange and decrease the need for endotracheal intubation (37,38). Beneficial effects on complication rates or mortality have not been observed. Concerns about the safety of BiPAP in cardiac patients were raised following a controlled trial by Mehta et al., in which randomized patients with acute cardiogenic pulmonary edema received CPAP or BiPAP (39). Although BiPAP improved ventilation more rapidly than CPAP, the study was terminated prematurely because of a higher frequency of acute myocardial infarction in patients receiving BiPAP. Although more patients in the BiPAP group presented with chest pain or left bundle branch block, these baseline differences between the two groups did not reach statistical significance. Recently, Nava et al. conducted a multicenter, prospective trial randomizing patients with acute cardiogenic pulmonary edema receiving standard medical therapy to either supplemental oxygen or NPPV delivered as pressure support (PS) plus positive end-expiratory pressure (PEEP) via face mask (40). This mode of NPPV avoids some of the potential problems of ventilator cycling associated with certain BiPAP devices. In this study, NPPV resulted in more rapid improvement in gas exchange and dyspnea, without changes in duration of hospital stay or mortality. Intubation rates were not decreased except in the subgroup of patients with hypercapnia. Importantly, no differences in adverse events, including acute myocardial infarction, were noted. Further studies are needed to establish the role of BiPAP in acute cardiogenic pulmonary edema.

Recent studies have also examined the use of NPPV in patients with hypoxemic respiratory failure from causes other than cardiogenic pulmonary edema. Although the general use of NPPV for this population has not been fully supported by the literature, certain subgroups of patients may benefit from NPPV. For example, immunocompromised patients with respiratory failure may benefit from NPPV by avoiding the infectious complications of endotracheal intubation and mechanical ventilation. Randomized controlled studies have demonstrated favorable effects in patients with respiratory failure following solid organ transplants (41) and with immunocompromised states and pulmonary infiltrates (42).

Potential Mechanisms of Action

The mechanisms by which NPPV improves gas exchange and symptoms have been studied in patients with acute exacerbations of COPD, and these involve augmenting alveolar ventilation and mitigating work of breathing. Diaz et al. found that gas exchange abnormalities improved with NPPV, primarily by increased alveolar ventilation, without any observed significant changes in ventilation–perfusion mismatching (43). The concept that NPPV reduces inspiratory muscle effort was suggested by one study which found that, in patients with acute exacerbations of COPD, NPPV resulted in decreased indices of inspiratory muscle activity, including transdiaphragmatic pressure and the pressure–time product for the diaphragm (44). NPPV may also decrease work of breathing by overcoming intrinsic PEEP, which commonly complicates obstructive airway disease. For patients with hypoxemic respiratory failure, additional mechanisms for improved oxygenation include increased lung volume and avoidance of the infectious complications of invasive ventilation.

AIRWAY MANAGEMENT

Unambiguous indications for endotracheal intubation that apply to all situations are difficult to define. The decision to proceed to endotracheal intubation is often based on subjective findings and the patient's clinical course. The potential for reversibility of the underlying disorder must be considered when one is determining the appropriateness of endotracheal intubation. Table 21-3 lists the most common indications for endotracheal intubation and mechanical ventilation.

TABLE 21-3. Indications for Endotracheal Intubation and Mechanical Ventilation

Hypoxemia despite supplemental oxygen administration (PaO_2 <60 mm Hg)
Alveolar hypoventilation and hypercapnic respiratory acidosis (pH <7.25)
Altered mental status and inability to protect the airway
Hemodynamic instability, shock, or cardiopulmonary arrest
Flow-limiting obstruction of the upper airway
Requirement of heavy sedation or general anesthesia for completion of a procedure such as endoscopy
Copious secretions with the inability to cough and clear the airway
Postoperative patients in whom maintenance of adequate gas exchange requires excessive energy expenditure (e.g., following cardiac, thoracic, or upper abdominal surgery)
Major trauma

Endotracheal Intubation

Endotracheal tubes may be passed through either the mouth or the nose. The oral route has the advantage of accepting a large diameter tube and is easier to use under emergency circumstances. Because direct laryngoscopy is required, sedation and, often, muscle-relaxing agents are needed. For anatomically challenging intubations, a fiber optic laryngoscope or bronchoscope via the oral route can facilitate endotracheal tube placement. Topical anesthesia is usually necessary for bronchoscope-guided intubation, but, typically, only small doses of systemic agents are required. Intubation should be performed by a physician experienced with the procedure who is familiar with the necessary pharmacologic agents, such as intravenous anesthetics and muscle-relaxing agents.

Nasal endotracheal tubes have certain advantages over oral tubes: they are generally more comfortable for the patient, oral hygiene can be better maintained, and the tube is less likely to become dislodged (45). Nonemergent nasal tube placement in a spontaneously ventilating patient may be accomplished without direct visualization of the vocal cords. As with oral endotracheal tubes, fiber optic bronchoscopy can help guide nasotracheal intubation in difficult cases, such as when the neck is immobilized. However, nasotracheal intubation increases the risk of sinusitis (45). The small diameter of the tube, which can be further narrowed by compression or kinking within the nose or nasopharynx, can hinder suctioning and preclude bronchoscopy. Although there is currently no consensus on which route is best (46), oral tubes are most often used.

Immediately after the tube is placed, the chest must be observed for excursion and auscultated for the presence of bilateral breath sounds. Unilateral breath sounds imply a mainstem intubation. Because of the relatively obtuse angle of the right main bronchus, positioning of the tip of the tube in the right main airway is quite common (see Fig. 21-4). The absence of breath sounds and audible sounds over the midepigastrium or gastric distension indicate esophageal tube placement. Exhaled carbon dioxide detection is a sensitive technique used to verify tube placement within the trachea. If the tube appears to be properly placed, it should be taped securely and the position confirmed by a chest radiograph.

Endotracheal tubes are fitted with high-volume, low-pressure cuffs that occlude the trachea around the tube, enabling positive pressure ventilation and minimizing aspiration of oropharyngeal contents. Care should be taken to avoid overinflation of the cuff (>20 mm Hg), which can cause pressure necrosis of the adjacent tracheal mucosa and increase the risk of developing tracheal stenosis or a tracheoesophageal fistula (47).

Tracheotomy

Tracheotomy is generally recommended for patients requiring prolonged (more than 2 to 3 weeks) ventilatory support as endotracheal tubes can lead to infectious complications and localized tissue damage. Additionally, tracheotomy can facilitate suctioning, may be more comfortable for the patient, and potentially permits oral intake and speech. This procedure can be performed at the bedside percutaneously or in the operating room under direct visualization. The percutaneous technique may be associated with fewer complications than traditional tracheotomy; however, practices vary with each institution (48–51). The optimal timing of tracheotomy has not yet been defined. Given that strong evidence arguing for or against early versus late tracheotomy is lacking, a reasonable approach is to begin planning for tracheotomy within the first week after intubation in patients who will likely require mechanical ventilation for more than 2 weeks (52). Earlier placement is appropriate in patients with irreversible etiologies of respiratory failure.

Airway Care

Because endotracheal and tracheotomy tubes bypass the normal humidifying mechanisms in the upper airway, all inspired gas must be fully humidified. Removal of pulmonary secretions using a suction catheter should be done at regular intervals as determined by the volume of secretions present. Sterile technique must be used for suctioning. Likewise, all gas delivery circuits in direct communication with the airway should be sterile when connected. Replacement of ventilator circuit tubing and inline suction catheters is commonly done on a weekly basis; however, randomized controlled studies demonstrate no increase in nosocomial pneumonia or in duration of mechanical ventilation when these are not changed routinely (53–55).

It is important to realize that once an endotracheal tube is in place, complete responsibility for the airway rests on the individuals caring for the patient. The patient can no longer humidify inspired air, cough effectively, or defend the lower airways against airborne microorganisms. Perhaps more important, the intubated patient cannot call for help or unblock the tube should it become obstructed. For these reasons, in addition to the gravity of the illness for which the airway tube was inserted, virtually all patients with an artificial airway should be managed in a critical care unit.

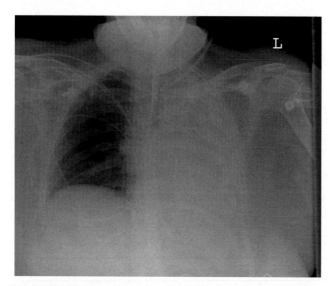

FIGURE 21-4.   This chest radiograph shows an endotracheal tube inserted into the right mainstem bronchus and total left-sided atelectasis.

MECHANICAL VENTILATION

Patients who have severe derangement of gas exchange not corrected with less invasive measures may be temporarily supported with mechanical ventilation until the underlying disease process has resolved. Less commonly, the need for mechanical ventilation may be long term, as in patients with chronic, progressive neuromuscular disease. This section discusses the indications for intubation and mechanical ventilation, reviews the basic features of mechanical ventilators, and describes the most commonly used modes of mechanical ventilation. Strategies of mechanical ventilation in certain clinical situations are reviewed.

Indications for Mechanical Ventilation

Typical indications for mechanical ventilation are listed in Table 21-3; however, there is no substitute for skilled clinical assessment of disease severity, response to therapy, and the potential role of less invasive supportive measures. The most common clinical situations in which mechanical ventilation is necessary include alveolar hypoventilation with severe respiratory acidosis (Chapter 22, Acute Hypercapnic Respiratory Failure: Neuromuscular and Obstructive Diseases) and hypoxemia due to intrapulmonary shunting of blood wherein noninvasive modalities cannot provide a sufficiently high F_{IO_2} (Chapter 23, Acute Hypoxemic Respiratory Failure: Pulmonary Edema and Acute Lung Injury).

Features of Mechanical Ventilators

Modern mechanical ventilators are equipped with several important features to provide support in a variety of respiratory disorders. The most essential feature is the capacity to deliver a wide range of V_T with an adjustable frequency and an accurate, adjustable F_{IO_2}. Ventilator-delivered breaths are provided spontaneously at a predetermined rate or in response to a patient's inspiratory effort. Controls to adjust inspiratory flow rate and the waveform, inspiratory to expiratory time ratio, and inspiratory pressure limit are also necessary. Alarms to alert the clinician to low exhaled V_T, high and low inspiratory pressure, and reduction in F_{IO_2} are provided. Temperature and humidity of inspired gas are controlled. A flow-limiting valve in the expiratory limb of the ventilator circuit allows titration of end-expiratory pressure. In addition to pressure-sensing capability, most ventilators monitor airflow to allow for BiPAP or CPAP in spontaneously breathing patients.

Commonly Used Modes of Mechanical Ventilation

Modes of positive pressure ventilation are described by the relationships among the various types of breaths and by the controlled and independent variables during the inspiratory phase of ventilation. Each mode of ventilation is distinguished by how it initiates a breath (trigger), how it sustains a breath (limit), and how it terminates a breath (cycle). Modes of ventilation can also be distinguished by whether the patient's breath is mandatory, spontaneous, or a combination of the two.

The most basic feature used to categorize modes of mechanical ventilation is the mechanism determining the transition from the inspiratory phase to the expiratory phase. Specifically, the inspiratory phase may be limited by a preset volume or by a preset MIP. The major disadvantage of conventional pressure-targeted ventilation is that a V_T and, therefore, $\dot{V}_E$ cannot be guaranteed. For this reason, volume-cycled modes of ventilation are most commonly used (56).

VOLUME-CYCLED VENTILATION. The oldest and most basic of volume-targeted modes is controlled mechanical ventilation (CMV). During CMV, the ventilator, regardless of patient effort, delivers a preset number of breaths of a specified V_T. Ventilators are designed to provide an assist mode in which the patient's inspiratory effort triggers the machine to deliver a predetermined V_T breath. More precisely, these two modalities are combined as assist-controlled (AC) ventilation; the ventilator delivers a breath with every inspiratory effort and a preset minimum number of breaths if the patient's RR falls below the set rate. Because V_T and RR are set, minimum $\dot{V}_E$ is predetermined.

The disadvantages of volume-targeted AC ventilation include the potential for hyperinflation and resultant lung injury when the RR is high and when insufficient time is allowed for exhalation. This is referred to as "breath stacking," which results in high alveolar pressure and intrinsic PEEP (dynamic hyperinflation) and increases the risk of pneumothorax, pneumomediastinum, and hypotension from decreased cardiac output. Additionally, patients are more likely to develop a respiratory alkalosis because every inspiratory effort results in the delivery of a full-size breath.

In the late 1970s, an alternative mode of volume-cycled ventilation was introduced with the goal of minimizing the risk of hyperinflation and respiratory alkalosis—*intermittent mandatory ventilation* (IMV). IMV combines machine mandatory breaths with spontaneous breaths (see Fig. 21-5). Similar to AC, a preset number of breaths of a set V_T are delivered to the patient each minute. The difference from AC is that the patient may take additional, *unassisted* breaths. The inspired air for these additional breaths comes from a reservoir in parallel with the primary ventilator circuit. In general, the set rate should account for 80% of the patient's minute volume. Essentially, all ventilators in use today provide *"synchronized" intermittent mandatory ventilation* (SIMV) where the ventilator attempts to deliver the machine

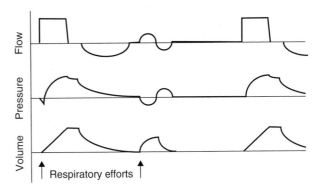

FIGURE 21-5. Airflow, pressure at the airway opening, and tidal volume (V_T) during synchronized intermittent mandatory ventilation (SIMV) without pressure support (PS). Breaths are triggered by patient efforts or by elapsed time on the basis of the rate set by the clinician. Note that up to three styles of breaths are delivered with SIMV. Clinically, SIMV is combined with PS ventilation such that the patient's spontaneous breaths (the middle breath in the figure) are supported to a preset inspiratory pressure.

breaths in response to the patient's intrinsic respiratory efforts. SIMV is usually combined with pressure support ventilation, which is designed to assist inspiratory effort during the spontaneous breaths (57). In selected patients, SIMV with PS may be more comfortable and efficient compared with IMV or AC (58).

The main disadvantage of SIMV is that the clinician may overestimate the amount of support the patient is receiving, resulting in an unrecognized high work of breathing. This may lead to respiratory muscle fatigue. Note that patients may be less likely to develop respiratory alkalosis during SIMV, in part because ventilation is ineffective during the pressure supported breaths (inadequate V_T), and the work of breathing is actually increased (increased V_{CO_2}) compared to AC (59). Therefore, SIMV has no advantage over AC in many patients with low lung compliance and a high work of breathing (60).

PRESSURE-TARGETED VENTILATION. Pressure-targeted ventilation differs from volume-targeted ventilation in that pressure and time rather than volume determine the transition from inspiration to exhalation. Pressure assist-controlled ventilation (PCV) is analogous to volume assist-controlled ventilation, except the controlled variable is pressure (and time) rather than volume. An advantage of this mode is that patients are often more comfortable because the inspiratory flow rate varies with the patient's demand. Another advantage is that mean airway pressure tends to be higher for a given peak pressure setting. This is advantageous in many patients with hypoxemia because the higher mean airway pressure results in larger lung volume for gas exchange. The major disadvantage of PCV is that alveolar $\dot{V}_E$ can be varied. The clinician sets the frequency, MIP, end-expiratory pressure, and the inspiration to exhalation (I:E) ratio. *Inverse ratio ventilation* (IRV), used in patients with very low thoracic compliance and severe refractory hypoxemia, is PCV with an increased inspiratory time such that I:E is 2:1 rather than the more physiologic 1:2 or lower. IRV can also be administered by adding an inspiratory pause to volume-targeted ventilation. This mode theoretically results in higher mean airway pressures allowing a greater percentage of alveoli to open and participate in gas exchange while avoiding high peak airway pressures in select patients with a low thoracic compliance due to ARDS (61). IRV is uncomfortable for the patient and requires the use of heavy sedation and frequently requires muscle relaxation. Higher mean airway pressures also reduce right ventricular filling and cardiac output in many patients.

PRESSURE-REGULATED–VOLUME-CONTROLLED VENTILATION. Pressure-regulated–volume-controlled ventilation (PRVC) is a newer mode of ventilation where the clinician sets a minimum V_T, RR, and inspiratory time. The ventilator delivers the set V_T at the lowest possible pressure within the inspiratory time. The amount of support provided by the ventilator can be varied; if the patient can generate the target tidal volume spontaneously, the ventilator will provide no assistance. PRVC produces lower peak inspiratory pressures (PIPs), and it may decrease the risk of barotrauma-associated complications in neonates (62,63). However, definitive data are not yet available.

PRESSURE SUPPORT VENTILATION. Pressure support ventilation (PSV) is a pressure-targeted mode much like PCV, except that a change in airflow rather than a preset inspiratory time

terminates the breath. During this mode of ventilation, spontaneous inspiratory efforts are rewarded with high airflow until a preset inspiratory pressure above PEEP is reached, usually in the range of 5 to 20 cm H_2O. When the airflow required to maintain this pressure decreases by a predetermined percentage of the initial flow rate, inspiratory support from the ventilator stops and passive exhalation begins (Fig. 21-5). This mode of ventilation can be used alone in a spontaneously breathing patient or in combination with SIMV to provide additional inspiratory support to the patient's spontaneous breaths. PSV is commonly used to wean patients from mechanical ventilation, as discussed later in this chapter. The main advantage of PSV is that the patient has more control over inspiratory time and V_T, resulting in a more physiologic respiratory cycle (64). As with any pressure-targeted mode, the $\dot{V}_E$ cannot be guaranteed when using PSV.

Positive End-Expiratory Pressure

PEEP is an adjunct to any mode of mechanical ventilation. By increasing distending pressure across the walls of the airways and alveoli, PEEP increases the volume of gas in the lung at end exhalation (functional residual capacity). This counteracts the alveolar collapse or microatelectasis characteristic of conditions producing pulmonary edema and low respiratory system compliance such as ARDS. Also termed *alveolar recruitment*, the result is decreased intrapulmonary shunting of blood and improved PaO_2, often allowing the use of lower FiO_2.

The benefits of applied PEEP in patients with respiratory failure due to obstructive airway disease are less clear. These patients commonly develop *intrinsic* PEEP or *auto*-PEEP as a result of small airway obstruction and gas trapping, a condition made worse by insufficient expiratory time. Applied PEEP may actually contribute to this phenomenon. Prospective studies in this patient group have found that applied PEEP raises already high airway and alveolar pressures and may contribute to hyperinflation (65,66). Available data from the few published prospective trials, however, are inconsistent (67). MacIntyre et al. found that PEEP applied to a level of 85% of measured intrinsic PEEP in COPD patients resulted in decreased work of breathing and lower intrinsic PEEP (68). The proposed mechanisms of action for the decrease in the work of breathing associated with the application of PEEP in patients with obstructive airways disease are an overall lower lung volume and greater ease in triggering the ventilator.

HEMODYNAMIC EFFECTS OF POSITIVE END-EXPIRATORY PRESSURE. During positive pressure ventilation, mean airway pressure is dependent on the compliance of the respiratory system, the set level of PEEP, and the peak airway pressure multiplied by the inspiratory time. In most patients, PEEP is the greatest single contributor to a change in mean airway pressure and, therefore, intrathoracic pressure.

Because intrathoracic pressure is increased, PEEP can have hemodynamic consequences; however, the effect in a given patient is unpredictable. This uncertainty results from only partial and varying transmission of applied PEEP to pleural pressure and from differing effects of the pressure change on the right and left heart. In general, the proportion of PEEP that is transmitted to the pleural space is proportional to lung compliance. For example, less of the total PEEP is transmitted to the pleural space in patients with low lung compliance (ARDS) than in patients with high lung compliance (COPD). However, it should be kept in mind that the set levels of PEEP might be much higher in patients with low lung compliance. Decreased chest wall compliance results in greater increases in pleural pressure for a given PEEP level if lung compliance is constant.

Increased intrathoracic pressure from PEEP decreases venous return to the right heart and may compromise cardiac output, particularly in patients with poor right ventricular function or volume depletion (69–71). PEEP also decreases cardiac output by increasing right ventricular afterload while preventing a compensatory increase in preload (72,73). The decrease in cardiac output may actually decrease oxygen delivery to tissues despite an increased PaO_2. Conversely, increased intrathoracic pressure can augment left ventricular emptying in systole and decrease left ventricular afterload, resulting in increased cardiac output in some patients (71).

Determination of the optimal level of PEEP can be difficult. However, levels in the range of 5 to 20 cm H_2O are commonly used. Benefits to oxygenation provided by increased PEEP must be balanced against a decrease in cardiac output and in the effect of PEEP on dynamic airway pressure.

Mechanical Ventilation Strategies

"Conventional" mechanical ventilation refers to the traditional standard ventilator settings targeted at maintaining normal blood pH and arterial blood gases. Table 21-4 shows typical

TABLE 21-4. Commonly Used Initial Ventilator Settings

Volume-cycled Ventilation	
Parameter	*Initial Setting*
Tidal volume	6–10 mL/kg
Respiratory rate	10–20 breaths/min
FIO_2	1.0
PEEP	5–10 cm H_2O
Waveform	Decelerating[b]
Inspiratory flow	60–100 L/min[b]
PIP limit[a]	45–50 cm H_2O
Pressure support (SIMV mode)	5–20 cm H_2O

Pressure-cycled Ventilation	
Parameter	*Initial Setting*
Respiratory rate	10–20 breaths/min
FIO_2	1.0
PIP	25–35 cm H_2O
PEEP	5–10 cm H_2O
I:E	1:2

FIO_2, fraction of inspired oxygen; PEEP, positive end-expiratory pressure; PIP, peak inspiratory pressure; SIMV, synchronized intermittent mandatory ventilation; I:E, inspiratory to expiratory time ratio.

[a]Alarm setting. Other available alarms include low inspiratory pressure (ventilator disconnected from patient), low VE (inadequate spontaneous tidal volume or RR), low exhaled tidal volume (air leak in circuit), and apnea alarm.

[b]Using a square waveform or increasing the inspiratory flow rate results in an effective decrease in inspiratory time (decreased I:E) and usually a higher PIP. Expiratory time is increased.

initial ventilator settings targeted at this goal. An emerging strategy for mechanical ventilation is *protective ventilation*. For patients with obstructive lung disease, this refers to the prevention of high airway pressures and hyperinflation with its associated complications (74). In this context, protective ventilation would include ventilation with low PEEP, lower VTs, and longer exhalation times (e.g., square inspiratory airflow waveform and increased inspiratory flow rate). Although hyperinflation is minimized with this strategy, alveolar ventilation is also decreased. The result is increased $PaCO_2$, a concept known as *permissive hypercapnia* (75). In the subset of patients with severe obstructive lung disease, a protective ventilation strategy may result in fewer ventilator-related complications and may reduce mortality (74,76). However, the resultant hypercapnia can contribute to patient agitation, resulting in the need for more sedation. The associated acidosis may also require treatment with sodium bicarbonate or another buffering agent.

Acute lung injury and ARDS are characterized by proteinaceous pulmonary edema, regional atelectasis, increased shunt fraction, and hypoxemia. Overdistension of relatively normal lung regions, the cyclic collapse and reexpansion of lung regions, and shear forces from the movement of fluid and air through small airways may contribute to further lung injury in these patients (77). A strategy of protective ventilation aimed at minimizing excessive end-inspiratory airway pressures and lung volumes while avoiding low end-expiratory lung volumes through the application of PEEP reduces mortality in patients with acute lung injury and ARDS (78). Optimal ventilation with a lung protective strategy is discussed in Chapter 23, Acute Hypoxemic Respiratory Failure: Pulmonary Edema and Acute Lung Injury.

WEANING FROM MECHANICAL VENTILATION

Discontinuation of mechanical ventilation can be a rapid process, such as following a surgical procedure; however, in many cases, the complexity or severity of the patient's clinical condition necessitates more cautious withdrawal of ventilatory support. This process is commonly referred to as *weaning*. In a literal sense, most patients with respiratory failure do not require "weaning," the gradual withdrawal of ventilator support, but instead require only periodic "readiness testing" to determine when the patient has improved sufficiently to once again breathe spontaneously. This section discusses the various methods used to discontinue mechanical ventilation.

Weaning Criteria

Mechanically ventilated patients should be evaluated frequently to determine whether their clinical condition has sufficiently improved to enable discontinuation from the ventilator. Although the potential complications and costs associated with mechanical ventilation argue for expeditious withdrawal from the ventilator, caution must be taken to avoid premature extubation of patients who still require ventilatory support. For these reasons, clinical criteria and objective indices are used to identify readiness for spontaneous breathing trials (SBTs) and to predict success or failure of extubation (see Table 21-5).

Of the criteria most commonly used for weaning, perhaps the most reliable is the rapid shallow breathing index (RSBI)

TABLE 21-5.   Guidelines for Identifying Candidates for Weaning and Discontinuation of Mechanical Ventilation

General

Resolution of the underlying disorder

Appropriate mental status, wakefulness, and strength to cooperate with weaning

Hemodynamic stability and discontinuation of minimal vasopressors

Adequate nutritional status and repletion of electrolytes (e.g., potassium, calcium, magnesium, and phosphorus)

Absence of upper airway obstruction or edema

Absence of copious secretions

| | *Minimal Weaning Criteria* | |
	Minimum	*Normal (Not Ventilated)*
F_{IO_2}	<0.6	0.21
Vital capacity	>10 mL/kg	60–80 mL/kg
Tidal volume (V_T)	>325 mL	450 mL
Minute ventilation ($\dot{V}_E$)	<10 L/min	6 L/min
MIP	<−20 cm H_2O	<−100 cm H_2O
Respiratory rate/V_T (RSBI)	<105	<30

F_{IO_2}, fraction of inspired oxygen; MIP, maximal inspiratory pressure; RSBI, rapid shallow breathing index.

(79,81). RSBI, as described by Yang and Tobin in 1991, is the RR divided by the V_T in liters while the patient breathes spontaneously on CPAP or a low level of PS. A threshold value of 105 breaths × L per minute measured at the end of an SBT was found to be most predictive (positive predictive value 78% and negative predictive value 95%). Subsequent studies have confirmed an acceptable positive predictive value of the RSBI, although the negative predictive value has been lower in some studies (80,82).

Of the parameters listed in Table 21-5, the V_T and RR should be measured during spontaneous breathing, whether they are used independently or to calculate the RSBI. The remaining indices can be measured during ventilator-supported breaths. It is important to recognize that although several studies demonstrate the predictive potential of these criteria, they are not absolute. Rather, they serve to *guide* the clinician when deciding whether to proceed with an initial SBT or weaning protocol. Some patients, despite meeting established weaning criteria, will require reintubation and reinstitution of mechanical ventilation. Likewise, some patients not meeting criteria can be successfully liberated from the ventilator. Therefore, a patient should prove himself or herself ventilator dependent by direct testing rather than through the use of bedside criteria alone.

WHAT IS A SPONTANEOUS BREATHING TRIAL? When a patient recovering from respiratory failure is deemed a candidate for extubation on the basis of the clinical assessment and objective indices listed in Table 21-5, a trial of spontaneous breathing should be attempted. This is accomplished by either setting the ventilator to a low-level CPAP of 5 cm H_2O with PS of 0 to 7 cm H_2O or connecting the endotracheal tube to a T-piece for 30 minutes to 2 hours. Although the ideal duration of

the SBT is not known, evidence supports the hypothesis that 30-minute trials are as predictive as 2-hour trials (83). If the patient tolerates this SBT, mechanical ventilation can be safely discontinued (84). Criteria commonly used to define SBT failure involve observation of the patient's hemodynamics, RR, oxygenation, and comfort level. In the subset of patients who fail this initial trial, gradual withdrawal of ventilator support may be necessary; however, repeated daily SBTs appear to be the most efficient strategy to assess readiness for liberation from the ventilator for most patients.

Weaning Techniques

Following an unsuccessful SBT, adequate ventilator support should be reinstituted and the reasons for SBT failure must be addressed. When it is appropriate to attempt withdrawal of mechanical ventilation, a weaning strategy should be implemented. Three basic weaning techniques are commonly used in clinical practice today: SBTs, PS ventilation weaning, and IMV weaning. Studies have compared these strategies and have shown that there are clinically important differences among them. Each technique is described followed by a discussion of these differences.

SPONTANEOUS BREATHING TRIALS. In patients who have failed an initial SBT, sequential SBTs are both effective and efficient when used as a method for weaning. SBTs can be conducted with a T-tube circuit, a low level of CPAP, or a low level of PS. T-piece weaning involves attaching the endotracheal tube to a T-piece such that one of the two remaining limbs of the T is connected to the ventilator, which supplies humidified oxygen. The third limb is left open to allow for exhalation. For patients with a high probability of weaning success, the trial may be as short as 30 minutes; for most patients, trials of 2 or more hours duration are frequently used. While T-piece trials can be performed once daily or repeated several times in a day, a randomized trial including medical and surgical patients showed that more than one 2-hour weaning trial per day resulted in neither more rapid weaning nor a higher rate of weaning success compared to a single daily trial (85).

The primary disadvantage of this method of weaning is that apnea, low $\dot{V}_E$, and airway pressure alarms are disabled. Consequently, close visual monitoring is required. An important advantage of T-piece weaning is that it provides a fairly accurate approximation of postextubation breathing. This may result in more rapid recognition of patients able to tolerate discontinuation of mechanical ventilation and faster weaning compared to IMV or PS weaning protocols (85,86).

As an alternative to a T-tube circuit, low level CPAP or PS can be used for both the initial SBT and weaning. These modalities do not require removing the patient from the ventilator, allowing alarms to remain active. Additionally, approximation of postextubation breathing may be superior to T-piece. This is because during T-piece weaning (airway pressure near 0 cm H_2O) the patient may have to assume an increased inspiratory load resulting from resistance in the ventilator tubing and endotracheal tube and potentially increased intrinsic PEEP (in patients with obstructive airways disease) (87,88). Differences between CPAP, PS, and T-piece may not be clinically important (89); however, CPAP with or without PS can be continued noninvasively after extubation.

PRESSURE SUPPORT WEANING. When weaning with PS, the ventilator is changed to a PS mode, usually 5 to 20 cm H_2O, and the level of support is decreased as rapidly as is tolerated by the patient until a minimal level is reached. Generally, decrements of 2 to 5 cm H_2O are attempted in one or two daily adjustments. When the patient tolerates a PS level of 5 to 7 cm H_2O, the decision to discontinue mechanical ventilation can be made on the basis of clinical criteria such as RSBI, arterial or mixed venous blood gases, patient comfort, and the overall clinical trajectory (90,91).

A disadvantage to PS weaning is the tendency to overestimate the amount of work the patient is doing. The amount of PS needed to overcome resistance in the ventilator circuit and other contributions to inspiratory load may indeed be <5 cm H_2O. Therefore, the level of ventilatory assistance received while on PS may occasionally exceed the patient's reserve, resulting in failure of extubation despite acceptable indices on a low level of PS. For this reason, some clinicians will occasionally order a trial of spontaneous ventilation without PS prior to discontinuing mechanical ventilation even for patients receiving PS as low as 5 cm H_2O.

The main potential advantages of PS weaning include a shorter duration of weaning and increased patient comfort compared to IMV because the patient determines the RR and breath size (86,92). However, one study found no difference in patient comfort when PS was compared with SIMV weaning (93). Again, because the patient remains connected to the ventilator, all monitors and alarms remain active during PS weaning.

INTERMITTENT MANDATORY VENTILATION WEANING. IMV has been discussed in detail earlier in this chapter. Its use in weaning from mechanical ventilation is straightforward: the number of machine breaths is gradually decreased by one or more per day until the patient tolerates only 4 to 5 assisted breaths per minute for several hours. One disadvantage of this method of weaning is that the work of breathing required for the unassisted breaths can be high. This is largely due to the resistance to airflow in the ventilator circuit. This additional work of breathing may not be appreciated by the clinician and patient fatigue may ensue. For this reason, IMV weaning is often combined with a low level of PS (5 cm H_2O) such that the unassisted breaths are augmented by PS ventilation (58); however, this variable level of ventilatory support does not necessarily decrease work of breathing, partly because the muscles of respiration contract to the same degree regardless of the level of extrinsic support when the amount of assistance is varied (93,94).

Comparison of Weaning Techniques

In one prospective study, more than 40% of the time that patients remained on mechanical ventilation was attributable to weaning (57). Therefore, an ideal weaning strategy would enable a safe and effective discontinuation of mechanical ventilation in the minimal amount of time required to do so. Two prospective, randomized studies comparing the three weaning techniques in medical and surgical patients failing initial attempts at spontaneous breathing have shown that IMV weaning is up to three times slower than either SBTs via T-piece or PS weaning without a difference in eventual success rates (85,86). This results in fewer days of assisted ventilation in patients weaned with T-piece or PS (85,86). There was no significant difference in weaning time between PS weaning and IMV weaning, although there

was a trend toward a shorter duration of weaning with PS weaning. Differences between SBTs with T-piece and PS are subtle; therefore, it is important to consider the exact protocols used in these studies when comparing these strategies. On the basis of current data, it is reasonable to consider all three weaning techniques as equal with respect to eventual weaning success, but SBTs with T-piece or PS result in more rapid liberation from mechanical ventilation than PS or IMV weaning do, in part because the patient's ability to tolerate spontaneous breathing is recognized earlier.

Weaning Protocols

On the basis of the results of prospective, randomized trials, the use of respiratory therapist–directed or nurse-directed weaning protocols has become widely accepted. This type of protocol requires daily evaluation of readiness for weaning based on the criteria listed in Table 21-5. If minimum criteria are met, the patient is given an SBT (generally, CPAP 5 cm H_2O or T-piece). The physician makes the final decision whether to proceed with extubation if the patient tolerates the trial. Studies have shown that protocol-directed weaning under the direction of nurses and respiratory therapists may result in more rapid liberation from mechanical ventilation without an increase in reintubation rates (95,96). However, one recent study reported that protocol-driven weaning does not necessarily accelerate weaning in an academic ICU with a dedicated ICU team of physicians (97).

Noninvasive Positive Pressure Ventilation and Weaning

NPPV is emerging as a method for weaning, primarily in patients with COPD (98). In two recent controlled trials, patients failing SBTs who were randomized to receive extubation with NPPV support had a shorter duration of mechanical ventilation and ICU stay, as well as reduced complication and mortality rates when compared to those weaned via conventional techniques. One of these investigations was limited to patients with COPD (99), while in the other, patients with COPD constituted most of the patients studied (100). Another trial involving patients intubated for acute-on-chronic respiratory failure who had failed T-piece trials demonstrated a shorter duration of invasive mechanical ventilation in the patients extubated with NPPV when compared to controls weaned by standard methods (101). However, there were no differences in length of ICU or hospital stay and in complication rates or survival, and the overall duration of ventilatory support was longer in the NPPV group. Further studies are necessary to establish protocols for NPPV weaning and to identify other groups of patients likely to benefit from this technique.

NPPV has also been used to prevent reintubation in patients with respiratory distress postextubation. To date, randomized, controlled studies have failed to show benefit from NPPV in this setting (102,103).

EMERGENCIES IN THE VENTILATED PATIENT

Mechanically ventilated patients are subject to many potentially disastrous events, which may be related to the patient's underlying disease process, artificial airway, or malfunctioning of the ventilator. Because some complications are life threatening and can be rapidly fatal, clinicians caring for critically ill patients must be proficient in the assessment and management of these situations.

CLINICAL EVALUATION

The development of respiratory distress in the mechanically ventilated patient is commonly encountered in the ICU. The patient may appear agitated or have physical signs of distress, including tachypnea, diaphoresis, accessory muscle use, or hemodynamic changes. The first priority of the practitioner is to ensure that the patient is receiving adequate oxygenation and ventilation. An assessment of vital signs and physical examination should be performed expeditiously. The patient should be disconnected from the ventilator and manual ventilation should be initiated using an anesthesia bag with 100% oxygen (104). If the patient improves following removal from the ventilator, then the problem is with the ventilator itself. However, if distress continues, then the endotracheal tube and the patient must be thoroughly evaluated. The endotracheal tube should be checked for proper placement and then inspected for external compression such as kinking between the ventilator tubing connection and the nose, mouth, or hypopharynx. If there is no evidence of endotracheal tube migration or compression, the next step is to pass a suction catheter through the tube to check its patency and to remove mucous plugs or blood clots if present. Failure of these maneuvers to resolve the problem suggests that the problem is within the thorax and that the evaluation should center on the patient.

Although the physical examination is more limited in the mechanically ventilated patient, even a rapid cardiopulmonary exam can provide important diagnostic information. Tracheal obstruction manifests as no or markedly reduced entry of air into the lungs. Obstruction of a main bronchus impedes entry of air into the lung distal to the obstruction. Observation of the chest wall may reveal a rocking motion of the chest during inspiration with poor expansion of the affected side and overinflation of the unobstructed side. Peripheral airway obstruction may be suspected from the patient's history and from the presence of wheezing, although with severe bronchoconstriction, severely limited air movement may preclude the development of wheezing. A tension pneumothorax is a life-threatening complication that manifests as difficulty with ventilation, diminished or absent breath sounds, hyperresonance to percussion, contralateral tracheal deviation, hypotension, tachycardia, and elevated jugular venous pressure. In an emergency situation, time does not permit confirmation of the diagnosis via chest roentgenogram, and a presumption of pneumothorax must be acted upon.

HIGH AIRWAY PRESSURE EMERGENCIES

Sounding of the high pressure alarm can signal the presence of a new complication or progression of the underlying disease in patients with or without obvious signs of clinical distress. An understanding of how changes in inspiratory pressures reflect changes in respiratory mechanics can help narrow the differential diagnosis. The peak airway pressure measured at end inspiration is the pressure needed to overcome airway resistance *and* the elastance of the chest wall and lungs (105). By occluding outflow of the ventilator circuit during end inspiration, airflow ceases, and the measured pressure simply represents the elastic

properties of the chest wall and lungs. This is referred to as the *plateau pressure.*

Thus, the difference between the peak airway and plateau pressures is the pressure required to overcome airway resistance (see Fig. 21-6). When the high pressure alarm sounds, comparing the plateau pressure to the rise in end-inspiratory peak pressure can often distinguish whether high pressures are the result of increased airway resistance or decreased compliance. When the peak pressure increases without a concomitant increase in plateau, increased airway resistance, due to biting or mucous plugging of the endotracheal tube, tracheal obstruction, or acute bronchospasm should be suspected. A rise in both peak and plateau pressures indicates decreased compliance of the lungs, such as in pneumothorax (see Fig. 21-7), acute pulmonary edema, progression of pneumonia or ARDS, mainstem intubation, or dynamic hyperinflation. If hyperinflation is suspected, intrinsic PEEP should be measured directly. Although inadequate sedation can explain agitation and elevated pressures, other etiologies must first be excluded.

NORMAL OR LOW AIRWAY PRESSURE EMERGENCIES

When inadequate ventilation is noted and the high pressure limit is not being exceeded, the possible problems to consider are leaks in the ventilator tubing or around the cuff of the artificial airway, ventilator malfunction, bronchopleural fistula, or tracheoesophageal fistula. Again, the first step is to disconnect the ventilator and begin manual ventilation using an FIO_2 of 1.0. At the same time, the position of the tube and the inflation of the cuff should be checked. If the external pilot balloon is deflated, more air should be added. Leaks around the cuff may be indicated by air escaping from the mouth with each ventilator inflation. The leaks may be caused by breaks in the cuff itself or in the

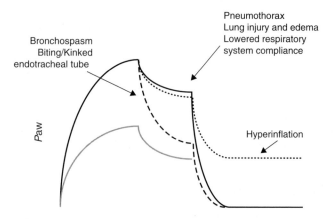

FIGURE 21-6. Peak, plateau, and total end-expiratory pressure to differentiate changes in resistance and compliance. The highest pressure prior to the downward inflection of the curves is the peak pressure, which reflects both airway resistance and respiratory compliance. If airflow is stopped at end inspiration, the airway pressure will decrease to reflect only the respiratory compliance. If airflow is stopped at end exhalation and the airway pressure is allowed to equilibrate, total end-expiratory pressure may be measured. The gray line represents the normal lung on mechanical ventilation. The solid black line represents a change in respiratory compliance, without a change in airway resistance. The dashed black line represents a change in airway resistance without a change in respiratory compliance, and the dotted black line represents hyperinflation and increased total end-expiratory pressure from incomplete exhalation. Although not shown here, hyperinflation is usually accompanied by an increase in airway resistance as well.

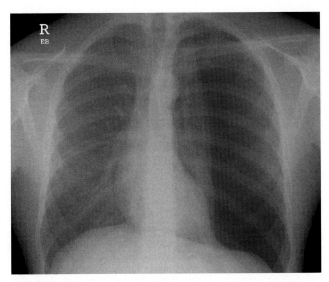

FIGURE 21-7. Anterior–posterior chest radiograph showing a large left pneumothorax in a patient who was being mechanically ventilated for the acute respiratory distress syndrome (ARDS).

external pilot balloon. Occasionally, an endotracheal tube may have migrated too high in the airway with the cuff at the level of the vocal cords or higher, causing air to leak around the cuff. For this reason, visual inspection of the mouth and pharynx is warranted. If the cuff itself is leaking, the tube must be replaced. With some types of tubes, the outer balloon may be replaced without changing the tube. Leaks may also be caused by enlargement of the trachea at the site of the cuff because of the pressure on the tracheal wall. If this is the origin of the leak, adding air to the cuff within the trachea may solve the problem. If air is added, care should be taken, in general, to not exceed a measured intracuff pressure of 20 to 25 mm Hg, especially in patients with systemic hypotension, because this may compromise tracheal perfusion and lead to necrosis (47).

Tracheal dilation is often the precursor of a much more serious problem—formation of a tracheoesophageal fistula. This can usually be prevented by maintaining the intracuff pressures <20 to 25 mm Hg (47). When a fistula does develop, however, it is often catastrophic. Patients with fistulas can sometimes be managed temporarily by placing the tube at a lower level in the trachea with the cuff below the fistula. Definitive management is surgical correction of the fistula.

HYPOXEMIA

Worsening oxygenation is a common emergency and should first be managed by promptly adjusting the inspired FIO_2 (or PEEP) to maintain an oxygen saturation of at least 92%. The most common mechanisms of hypoxemia in the mechanically ventilated patient are $\dot{V}/\dot{Q}$ mismatching and shunt. Although progression of the underlying disease process is frequently the cause, numerous complications can arise in the intubated patient, often as a direct consequence of mechanical ventilation. Ventilator-associated pneumonia, aspiration, atelectasis due to mucous plugging, mainstem intubation, and pneumothorax are frequent. Cardiogenic pulmonary edema can result from volume overload due to intravenous medications, renal failure, or aggressive volume repletion in hypotensive patients. Critically

ill patients are at high risk for pulmonary embolism, and this should always be considered even when deep venous thrombosis prophylaxis has been administered (106). Patients with femoral vein catheters are at particular risk of deep venous thrombosis (107). Leaks or obstruction in the endotracheal tube or malfunctioning of the ventilator circuit can impair oxygenation as well (108). As mentioned previously, pulse oximetry can be inaccurate in certain settings, and arterial blood gas sampling should confirm the presence of hypoxia.

RESPIRATORY MONITORING

In addition to monitoring arterial oxygenation with pulse oximetry and arterial blood gases, several other parameters may be monitored clinically to assess gas exchange in patients with respiratory failure. These other measured variables include exhaled carbon dioxide, the pulmonary dead-space fraction, and respiratory compliance.

CAPNOGRAPHY

The measurement of exhaled carbon dioxide (capnography) can be a useful adjunct to respiratory monitoring. For example, exhaled end-tidal carbon dioxide can be used as a surrogate of alveolar and arterial carbon dioxide. However, exhaled end-tidal carbon dioxide ($PETCO_2$) is always an underestimation of true alveolar $PACO_2$ due to gas mixing in the large airways. For this reason, trends in exhaled PCO_2 over time may be of more value than the actual measurement. When interpreted in conjunction with a measured arterial PCO_2, $PETCO_2$ is also a measure of ventilation–perfusion matching in the lung.

PULMONARY DEAD-SPACE FRACTION

Physiologic dead space is the functionally ineffective part of the tidal volume (VD/VT) and is generally calculated using a modified version of the Bohr equation: $VD/VT = (PaCO_2 - PECO_2)/PaCO_2$ where $PECO_2$ is the partial pressure of carbon dioxide in the exhaled breath collected over several minutes. The VD/VT is normally one third of the VT depending on posture and varies with age and body size. The pulmonary dead-space fraction is elevated in patients with cardiopulmonary disease states, including COPD, pulmonary embolus, and ARDS. Early elevation of VD/VT has been found to be a powerful predictor of poor outcome in patients with ARDS (109).

RESPIRATORY SYSTEM COMPLIANCE

Total respiratory compliance is the sum of lung and chest wall compliance. Dynamic compliance includes the combined effects of airway resistance and the sum of the elastic recoil of the lung and the chest wall. Clinically, dynamic compliance is determined in mechanically ventilated patients as the quotient of tidal volume divided by the ventilator driving pressure (peak airway pressure – end-expiratory pressure). Static compliance includes only the elastic recoil of the lungs and chest wall. Static compliance is calculated as the total volume divided by the plateau airway pressure minus the level of positive end-expiratory pressure. A decrease in dynamic compliance without a change in static compliance indicates airway narrowing due to a partially occluded endotracheal tube or bronchoconstriction.

In the setting of acute respiratory failure, an increase in static compliance suggests parenchymal lung disease such as pulmonary edema, atelectasis, dynamic hyperinflation, or pneumothorax. Because high airway pressures have been associated with ventilator-associated lung injury and worse outcome in lung injury patients, ventilator management strategies for patients with acute lung injury have in part been based on the assessment of respiratory compliance (78).

REFERENCES

1. Wasserman K. Exercise testing in the dyspneic patient. The chairman's postconference reflections. *Am Rev Resp Dis* 1984;129 (Suppl):1–2.
2. Kikuchi Y, Okabe S, Tamura G, et al. Chemosensitivity and perception of dyspnea in patients with a history of near-fatal asthma. *N Engl J Med* 1994;330:1329–1334.
3. Barker SJ, Tremper KK, Gamel DM. A clinical comparison of transcutaneous PO2 and pulse oximetry in the operating room. *Anesth Analg* 1986;65:805–808.
4. McFadden ER, Kiser R, De Groot WJ. Acute bronchial asthma: relations between clinical and physiologic manifestations. *N Engl J Med* 1973;288:221–225.
5. Leventhal JM. Clinical predictors of pneumonia as a guide to ordering chest roentgenograms. *Clin Pediatr* 1982;21:730–734.
6. Rebuck AS, Pengelly LD. Development of pulsus paradoxus in the presence of airways obstruction. *N Engl J Med* 1973;288:66–69.
7. Knowles GK, Clark TJ. Pulsus paradoxus as a valuable sign indicating severity of asthma. *Lancet* 1973;2:1356–1359.
8. Connors AF Jr, McCaffree DR, Gray BA. Evaluation of right-heart catheterization in the critically ill patient without acute myocardial infarction. *N Engl J Med* 1983;308:263–267.
9. Brackett NC Jr, Wingo CF, Muren O, et al. Acid-base response to chronic hypercapnia in man. *N Engl J Med* 1969;280:124–130.
10. Sperelakis N. Pathophysiology of skeletal muscle and effect of some hormones. In: Roussos C, Macklem PT, eds. *The thorax.* New York: Marcel Dekker, 1985:115–140.
11. Newman JH, Neff Ta, Zipporin P. Acute respiratory failure associated with hypophosphatemia. *N Engl J Med* 1977;296:1101–1103.
12. Parsons PE. Respiratory failure as a result of drugs, overdoses, and poisonings. *Clin Chest Med* 1994;15:93–102.
13. Mellemgaard K. The alveolar-arterial oxygen difference: its size and components in normal man. *Acta Physiol Scand* 1967;67:10–20.
14. Weinberger SE, Schwartzstein RM, Weiss JW. Hypercapnia. *N Engl J Med* 1989;321:1223–1231.
15. Narins RG, Emmett M. Simple and mixed acid-base disorders: a practical approach. *Medicine* 1980;59:161–187.
16. Fall PJ. A stepwise approach to acid-base disorders. *Postgrad Med* 2000;107:249–250, 253–254, 257–258.
17. Adrogue HJ, Madias NE. Management of life-threatening acid-base disorders. *N Engl J Med* 1998;338:26–34.
18. Adrogue HJ, Madias NE. Management of life-threatening acid-base disorders. *N Engl J Med* 1998;338:107–111.
19. Kilburn KH. Shock, seizures and coma with alkalosis during mechanical ventilation. *Ann Intern Med* 1966;66:977–984.
20. Rochester DF, Esau SA. Assessment of ventilatory function in patients with neuromuscular disease. *Clin Chest Med* 1994;15:751–763.
21. Bella I, Chad DA. Neuromuscular disorders and acute respiratory failure. *Neurol Clin* 1998;16:391–417.
22. Rabinstein AA, Wijdicks EF. Warning signs of imminent respiratory failure in neurological patients. *Semin Neurol* 2003;23:97–104.
23. Lawn ND, Fletcher DD, Henderson RD, et al. Anticipating mechanical ventilation in Guillain-Barre syndrome. *Arch Neurol* 2001;58:893–898.
24. Guidelines for the diagnosis and management of asthma. NIH Publication No. 97-4051, 1997.
25. O'Connor BS, Vender JS. Oxygen therapy. *Crit Care Clin* 1995;11:67–78.
26. Fulmer JD, Snider GL. American college of chest physicians (ACCP)—National Heart, Lung, and Blood Institute (NHLBI) conference on oxygen therapy. *Arch Intern Med* 1984;144:1645–1655.
27. O'Donohue WJ Jr, Baker JP. Controlled low-flow oxygen in the management of acute respiratory failure. *Chest* 1973;63:818–821.
28. Kallstrom TJ, American Association for Respiratory Care. AARC clinical practice guideline: oxygen therapy for adults in the acute care facility—2002 revision and update. *Respir Care* 2002;47:717–720.
29. Liesching T, Kwok H, Hill NS. Acute applications of noninvasive positive pressure ventilation. *Chest* 2003;124:699–713.
30. Bott J, Carroll MP, Conway JH, et al. Randomised controlled trial of nasal ventilation in acute ventilatory failure due to chronic obstructive airways disease. *Lancet* 1993;341:1555–1557.
31. Brochard L, Mancebo J, Wysocki M, et al. Noninvasive ventilation for acute exacerbations of chronic obstructive pulmonary disease. *N Engl J Med* 1995;333:817–822.
32. Plant PK, Owen JL, Elliot MW. Early use of non-invasive ventilation for acute exacerbations of chronic obstructive pulmonary disease on general respiratory wards: a multicentre randomised controlled trial. *Lancet* 2000;355:1931–1935.
33. Celikel T, Sungur M, Ceyhan B, et al. Comparison of noninvasive positive pressure ventilation with standard medical therapy in hypercapnic acute respiratory failure. *Chest* 1998;114:1636–1642.
34. Soo Hoo GW, Santiago S, Williams AJ. Nasal mechanical ventilation for hypercapnic respiratory failure in chronic obstructive pulmonary disease: determinants of success and failure. *Crit Care Med* 1994;22:1253–1261.
35. Ambrosino N, Foglio K, Rubini F, et al. Non-invasive mechanical ventilation in acute respiratory failure due to chronic obstructive pulmonary disease: correlates for success. *Thorax* 1995;50:755–757.
36. Keenan SP, Sinuff T, Cook DJ, et al. Which patients with acute exacerbation of chronic obstructive pulmonary disease benefit from noninvasive positive pressure ventilation? *Ann Intern Med* 2003;138:861–870.
37. Bersten AD, Holt AW, Vedig AE, et al. Treatment of severe cardiogenic pulmonary edema with continuous positive airway pressure delivered by face mask. *N Engl J Med* 1991;325:1825–1830.
38. Lin M, Yang Y, Chiang H, et al. Reappraisal of continuous positive airway pressure therapy in acute cardiogenic pulmonary edema. *Chest* 1995;107:1379–1386.
39. Mehta S, Jay G, Woolard R, et al. Randomized, prospective trial of bilevel versus continuous positive airway pressure in acute pulmonary edema. *Crit Care Med* 1997;25:620–628.
40. Nava S, Carbone G, DiBattista N, et al. Noninvasive ventilation in cardiogenic pulmonary edema. *Am J Respir Crit Care Med* 2003;168:1432–1437.
41. Antonelli M, Conti G, Bufi M, et al. Noninvasive ventilation for the treatment of acute respiratory failure in patients undergoing solid organ transplantation. *JAMA* 2000;283:235–241.
42. Hilbert G, Gruson D, Vargas F, et al. Noninvasive ventilation in immunosuppressed patients with pulmonary infiltrates, fever, and acute respiratory failure. *N Engl J Med* 2001;344:481–487.
43. Diaz O, Iglesia R, Ferrer M, et al. Effects of noninvasive ventilation on pulmonary gas exchange and hemodynamics during acute hypercapnic exacerbations of chronic obstructive pulmonary disease. *Am J Respir Crit Care Med* 1997;156:1840–1845.
44. Brochard L, Isabey D, Piquet J, et al. Reversal of acute exacerbations of chronic obstructive lung disease by inspiratory assistance with a face mask. *N Engl J Med* 1990;323:1523–1530.
45. Bach A, Boehrer H, Schmidt H, et al. Nosocomial sinusitis in ventilated patients. Nasotracheal versus orotracheal intubation. *Anaesthesia* 1992;47:335–339.
46. Depoix JP, Malbezin S, Videcoq M, et al. Oral intubation v. nasal intubation in adult cardiac surgery. *Br J Anaesth* 1987;59:167–169.
47. Stauffer J, Silvestri R. Complications of endotracheal intubation, tracheostomy and artificial airways. *Respir Care* 1982;27:417–434.
48. Stoeckli SJ, Breitbach T, Schmid S. A clinical and histologic comparison of percutaneous dilational versus conventional surgical tracheostomy. *Laryngoscope* 1997;107:1643–1646.
49. Petros S, Engelmann L. Percutaneous dilatational tracheostomy in a medical ICU. *Int Care Med* 1997;23:630–634.
50. Van Natta TL, Morris JA Jr, Eddy VA, et al. Elective bedside surgery in critically injured patients is safe and cost-effective. *Ann Surg* 1998;227:24–26, 618–624.
51. van Heurn LW, Goei R, de Ploeg I, et al. Late complications of percutaneous dilatational tracheotomy. *Chest* 1996;110:1572–1576.

52. Heffner JE. Tracheotomy application and timing. *Clin Chest Med* 2003;24:389–398.
53. Kollef MH, Shapiro SD, Fraser VJ, et al. Mechanical ventilation with or without 7-day circuit changes. A randomized controlled trial. *Ann Intern Med* 1995;123:168–174.
54. Kollef MH, Prentice D, Shapiro SD, et al. Mechanical ventilation with or without daily changes of in-line suction catheters. *Am J Respir Crit Care Med* 1997;156:466–472.
55. Fink JB, Krause SA, Barrett L, et al. Extending ventilator circuit change interval beyond 2 days reduces the likelihood of ventilator-associated pneumonia. *Chest* 1998;113:405–411.
56. Esteban A, Anzueto A, Frutos F, et al. Characteristics and outcomes in adult patients receiving mechanical ventilation: a 28-day international study. *JAMA* 2002;287:345–355.
57. Esteban A, Alia I, Ibanez J, et al., The Spanish Lung Failure Collaborative Group. Modes of mechanical ventilation and weaning. A national survey of Spanish hospitals. *Chest* 1994;106:1188–1193.
58. Shelledy DC, Rau JL, Thomas-Goodfellow L. A comparison of the effects of assist-control, SIMV, and SIMV with pressure support on ventilation, oxygen consumption, and ventilatory equivalent. *Heart Lung* 1995;24:67–75.
59. Hudson LD, Hurlow RS, Craig KC, et al. Does intermittent mandatory ventilation correct respiratory alkalosis in patients receiving assisted mechanical ventilation? *Am Rev Respir Dis* 1985;132:1071–1074.
60. Leung P, Jubran A, Tobin MJ. Comparison of assisted ventilator modes on triggering, patient effort, and dyspnea. *Am J Respir Crit Care Med* 1997;155:1940–1948.
61. Armstrong BW Jr, MacIntyre NR. Pressure-controlled, inverse ratio ventilation that avoids air trapping in the adult respiratory distress syndrome. *Crit Care Med* 1995;23:279–285.
62. Alvarez A, Subirana M, Benito S. Decelerating flow ventilation effects in acute respiratory failure. *J Crit Care* 1998;13:21–25.
63. Piotrowski A, Sobala W, Kawczynski P. Patient-initiated, pressure-regulated, volume-controlled ventilation compared with intermittent mandatory ventilation in neonates: a prospective, randomised study. *Int Care Med* 1997;23:975–981.
64. Dekel B, Segal E, Perel A. Pressure support ventilation. *Arch Intern Med* 1996;156:369–373.
65. Tuxen DV. Detrimental effects of positive end-expiratory pressure during controlled mechanical ventilation of patients with severe airflow obstruction. *Am Rev Respir Dis* 1989;140:5–9.
66. Ranieri VM, Giuliani R, Cinnella G, et al. Physiologic effects of positive end-expiratory pressure in patients with chronic obstructive pulmonary disease during acute ventilatory failure and controlled mechanical ventilation. *Am Rev Respir Dis* 1993;147:5–13.
67. Guerin C, LeMasson S, de Varax R, et al. Small airway closure and positive end-expiratory pressure in mechanically ventilated patients with chronic obstructive pulmonary disease. *Am J Respir Crit Care Med* 1997;155:1949–1956.
68. MacIntyre NR, Cheng KC, McConnell R. Applied PEEP during pressure support reduces the inspiratory threshold load of intrinsic PEEP. *Chest* 1997;111:188–193.
69. Huemer G, Kolev N, Kurz A, et al. Influence of positive end-expiratory pressure on right and left ventricular performance assessed by Doppler two-dimensional echocardiography. *Chest* 1994;106:67–73.
70. Cheatham ML, Nelson LD, Chang MC, et al. Right ventricular end-diastolic volume index as a predictor of preload status in patients on positive end-expiratory pressure. *Crit Care Med* 1998;26:1801–1806.
71. Schuster S, Erbel R, Weilemann LS, et al. Hemodynamics during PEEP ventilation in patients with severe left ventricular failure studied by transesophageal echocardiography. *Chest* 1990;97:1181–1189.
72. Jardin F, Brun-Ney D, Hardy A, et al. Combined thermodilution and two-dimensional echocardiographic evaluation of right ventricular function during respiratory support with PEEP. *Chest* 1991;99:162–168.
73. Dhainaut JF, Bricard C, Monsallier FJ, et al. Left ventricular contractility using isovolumic phase indices during PEEP in ARDS patients. *Crit Care Med* 1982;10:631–635.
74. Tuxen DV, Williams TJ, Scheinkestel CD, et al. Use of a measurement of pulmonary hyperinflation to control the level of

75. Darioli R, Perret C. Mechanical controlled hypoventilation in status asthmaticus. *Am Rev Respir Dis* 1984;129:385–387.
76. Williams TJ, Tuxen DV, Scheinkestel CD, et al. Risk factors for morbidity in mechanically ventilated patients with acute severe asthma. *Am Rev Respir Dis* 1992;146:607–615.
77. Frank JA, Imai Y, Slutsky A. Pathogenesis of ventilator-induced lung injury. In: Matthay MA, ed. *Acute respiratory distress syndrome*. New York: Marcel Dekker, 2003:201–244.
78. The Acute Respiratory Distress Syndrome Network. Ventilation with lower tidal volumes as compared with traditional tidal volumes for acute lung injury and the acute respiratory distress syndrome. *N Engl J Med* 2000;342(18):1301–1308.
79. Yang KL, Tobin MJ. A prospective study of indexes predicting the outcome of trials of weaning from mechanical ventilation. *N Engl J Med* 1991;324:1445–1450.
80. Epstein SK. Etiology of extubation failure and the predictive value of the rapid shallow breathing index. *Am J Respir Crit Care Med* 1995;152:545–549.
81. Vassilakopoulos S, Zakynthinos S, Roussos C. The tension-time index and the frequency-tidal volume ratio are the major pathophysiologic determinants of weaning failure and success. *Am J Respir Crit Care Med* 1998;158:378–385.
82. Chatilia W, Jacob B, Guaglionone D, et al. The unassisted respiratory rate-tidal volume ratio accurately predicts weaning outcome. *Am J Med* 1996;101:61–67.
83. Esteban I, Alia I, Tobin MJ et al. Spanish Lung Failure Collaborative Group. Effect of spontaneous breathing trial duration on outcome of attempts to discontinue mechanical ventilation. *Am J Respir Crit Care Med* 1999;159:512–518.
84. Esteban A, Alia I, Gordo F, et al., The Spanish Lung Failure Collaborative Group. Extubation outcome after spontaneous breathing trials with T-tube or pressure support ventilation. *Am J Respir Crit Care Med* 1997;156:459–465 [Published erratum appears in *Am J Respir Crit Care Med* 1997;156(6):2028].
85. Esteban A, Frutos F, Tobin MJ, et al., Spanish Lung Failure Collaborative Group. A comparison of four methods of weaning patients from mechanical ventilation. *N Engl J Med* 1995;332:345–350.
86. Brochard L, Rauss A, Benito S, et al. Comparison of three methods of gradual withdrawal from ventilatory support during weaning from mechanical ventilation. *Am J Respir Crit Care Med* 1994;150:896–903.
87. Petrof J, Legare M, Goldberg P, et al. Continuous positive airway pressure reduces work of breathing and dyspnea during weaning from mechanical ventilation in severe chronic obstructive pulmonary disease. *Am Rev Respir Dis* 1990;141:281–289.
88. Appendini L, Purro A, Patessio A, et al. Partitioning of inspiratory muscle workload and pressure assistance in ventilator-dependent COPD patients. *Am J Respir Crit Care Med* 1996;154:1301–1309.
89. Baily R, Jones RM, Kelleher AA. The role of continuous positive airway pressure during weaning from mechanical ventilation in cardiac surgical patients. *Anesthesia* 1995;50:677–681.
90. Jubran A, Mathru M, Dries D, et al. Continuous recordings of mixed venous oxygen saturation during weaning from mechanical ventilation and the ramifications thereof. *Am J Respir Crit Care Med* 1998;158:1763–1769.
91. Bouley H, Froman R, Shah H. The experience of dyspnea during weaning. *Heart Lung* 1992;21:471–476.
92. MacIntyre NR. Respiratory function during pressure support ventilation. *Chest* 1986;89:677–683.
93. Knebel R, Janson-Bjerklie SL, Malley JD, et al. Comparison of breathing comfort during weaning with two ventilatory modes. *Am J Respir Crit Care Med* 1994;149:14–18.
94. Sassoon S, Del Rosario N, Fei R, et al. Influence of pressure- and flow-triggered synchronous intermittent mandatory ventilation on inspiratory muscle work. *Crit Care Med* 1994;22:1933–1941.
95. Kollef H, Shapiro SD, Silver P, et al. A randomized, controlled trial of protocol-directed versus physician-directed weaning from mechanical ventilation. *Crit Care Med* 1997;25:567–574.
96. Ely W, Baker AM, Dunagan DP, et al. Effect on the duration of mechanical ventilation of identifying patients capable of breathing spontaneously. *N Engl J Med* 1996;335:1864–1869.

97. Krishnan J, Moore D, Robeson C, et al. A prospective, controlled trial of a protocol-based strategy to discontinue mechanical ventilation. *Am J Respir Crit Care Med* 2004;169:673–678.

98. International Consensus Conferences in Intensive Care Medicine. Noninvasive positive pressure ventilation in acute respiratory failure. *Am J Respir Crit Care Med* 2001;163:283–291.

99. Nava S, Ambrosino N, Clini E, et al. Noninvasive mechanical ventilation in the weaning of patients with respiratory failure due to chronic obstructive pulmonary disease: a randomized controlled trial. *Ann Intern Med* 1998;128:721–728.

100. Ferrer M, Esquinas A, Arancibia F, et al. Noninvasive ventilation during persistent weaning failure: a randomized controlled trial. *Am J Respir Crit Care Med* 2003;168:70–76.

101. Girault C, Daudenthun I, Chevron V, et al. Noninvasive ventilation as a systematic extubation and weaning technique in acute-on-chronic respiratory failure: a prospective randomized controlled study. *Am J Respir Crit Care Med* 1999;160:86–92.

102. Keenan SP, Powers C, McCormack DG, et al. Noninvasive positive pressure ventilation for postextubation respiratory distress: a randomized controlled trial. *JAMA* 2002;287:3238–3244.

103. Jiang J-S, Kao S-J, Wang S-N. Effect of early application of biphasic positive airway pressure on the outcome of extubation in ventilator weaning. *Respirology* 1999;4:161–165.

104. Tobin MJ. What should the clinician do when a patient "fights the ventilator"? *Respir Care* 1991;36:395–406.

105. Kirby RR, Banner MJ, Downs JB. *Clinical applications of ventilatory support.* New York: Churchill Livingstone, 1990:320–323.

106. Hirsh DR, Ingenito EP, Goldhaber SZ. Prevalence of deep venous thrombosis among patients in medical intensive care. *JAMA* 1995;274:335–337.

107. Merrer J, De Jonghe B, Golliot F, et al., French Catheter Study Group in Intensive Care. Complications of femoral and subclavian venous catheterization in critically ill patients: a randomized controlled trial. *JAMA* 2001;286(6):700–707.

108. Glauser FL, Polatty RC, Sessler CN. Worsening oxygenation in the mechanically ventilated patient. *Am Rev Respir Dis* 1988;138:458–465.

109. Nuckton TJ, Alonso JA, Kallet RH, et al. Pulmonary dead-space fraction as a risk factor for death in the acute respiratory distress syndrome. *N Engl J Med* 2002;346(17):1281–1286.

CHAPTER **22**

Acute Hypercapnic Respiratory Failure: Neuromuscular and Obstructive Diseases

Kamran Atabai
Michael A. Matthay
Carolyn S. Calfee

**NEUROMUSCULAR ETIOLOGIES
OF RESPIRATORY FAILURE**

DRUG OVERDOSES

**CHEST WALL ABNORMALITIES AS A CAUSE
OF ACUTE RESPIRATORY FAILURE**

UPPER-AIRWAY OBSTRUCTION

CHRONIC OBSTRUCTIVE AIRWAYS DISEASE

RESPIRATORY FAILURE IN ASTHMA

This chapter considers the causes of acute respiratory failure that are primarily associated with inadequate alveolar ventilation, which often results in hypercapnia and acute respiratory acidosis. These patients usually have abnormal oxygenation because of ventilation and perfusion mismatch in the lung, but the primary cause of respiratory failure is usually inadequate alveolar ventilation from (a) inadequate central ventilatory drive, (b) insufficient neuromuscular transmission of the respiratory drive, or (c) airway obstruction.

NEUROMUSCULAR ETIOLOGIES
OF RESPIRATORY FAILURE

There are numerous causes of acute respiratory failure from neuromuscular disorders, including the Guillain-Barré syndrome, myasthenia gravis, botulism, poliomyelitis, heavy-metal

intoxication, organophosphate poisoning, and, rarely, administration of aminoglycoside antibiotics. Severe electrolyte disorders such as hypokalemia and hypophosphatemia may also be associated with muscle weakness sufficient to cause or potentiate acute respiratory failure. Respiratory failure also may be worsened by the use of neuromuscular blocking agents in critically ill patients (1). In addition, a variety of congenital and acquired neuromuscular diseases may be associated with progressive respiratory failure. Acute respiratory failure may also follow injury to the spinal cord if the lesion is at a high enough level to affect the function of the phrenic nerve (2). This section focuses on the management of Guillain-Barré syndrome, myasthenia gravis, and diaphragmatic paralysis; the other types of neuromuscular diseases that cause respiratory failure should be managed similarly.

Acute respiratory failure is the most life-threatening complication of the Guillain-Barré syndrome. As in other causes of respiratory failure due to neuromuscular disease, inadequate respiratory muscle strength leads to alveolar hypoventilation, low tidal volume breathing, and diffuse atelectasis. In most large series, approximately 20% to 37% of patients with Guillain-Barré syndrome require mechanical ventilation (3–5). The average duration of mechanical ventilation is 4 to 6 weeks, but the range is quite variable (7 to 93 days in one series) (4–6). Characteristically, patients who require mechanical ventilation have a forced vital capacity (VC) <4 to 5 mL per kg body weight, are progressively unable to handle oral secretions, have a poor cough, and develop hypoventilation. Although this form of acute respiratory failure can be classified primarily as hypercapnic respiratory failure, it is frequently accompanied by a widened alveolar–arterial oxygen gradient secondary to atelectasis and pneumonia (5,7).

Patients who develop Guillain-Barré syndrome should be closely monitored with frequent measurements of VC and arterial blood gases and with careful clinical evaluation of their ability to cough and protect their airway. Initial monitoring in a critical care unit is usually desirable so that immediate ventilatory support can be provided if the patient's respiratory status deteriorates.

Treatment for Guillain-Barré syndrome has traditionally been primarily supportive with mechanical ventilation, intravenous fluids, and nutritional support. In addition, the use of prophylactic subcutaneous heparin is recommended (5). Careful attention to psychosocial issues is very important in managing Guillain-Barré patients in the intensive care unit (ICU) (7,8). In recent years, therapies addressing the underlying autoimmune mechanism of the disease have been employed as well. A prospective controlled study of 245 patients reported that plasmapheresis was superior to conventional, supportive therapy in hastening recovery of muscle strength (9). When plasmapheresis was started before the initiation of mechanical ventilation, the median time on the ventilator was reduced from 23 days to 9 days. The benefit of plasmapheresis in shortening the duration of mechanical ventilation was less clear-cut in patients intubated before plasmapheresis was started. Presumably, the process of plasmapheresis removes from the plasma a circulating factor important in the pathogenesis of acute paralysis. Intravenous immunoglobulin therapy provides a less cumbersome, more accessible alternative to plasmapheresis. Although the possibility of a higher relapse rate has been raised (10), studies suggest that intravenous immunoglobulin may be the better therapy for the subset of patients with GM1 or GM1b antibodies, who tend to have a more rapidly progressive and severe neuropathy (11). A recent randomized trial of 150 patients comparing plasmapheresis and intravenous immunoglobulin found that at 4 weeks the intravenous immunoglobulin group showed more improvement in functional class (53% versus 34%) with shorter time of improvement (27 versus 41 days), less need for intubation (27% versus 41%), and less time on mechanical ventilation (15 versus 22 days) (12). On the other hand, a trial comparing intravenous immunoglobulin, plasmapheresis, or plasmapheresis followed by intravenous immunoglobulin found that at 4 weeks there was no significant difference between the three study arms in ventilatory dependence, disability grade improvement, or time required for independent walking (13). Several smaller studies have reported favorable results with combined treatment modalities such as selective immunoglobulin adsorption followed by extracorporeal elimination or intravenous immunoglobulin combined with high-dose methylprednisolone (10). However, the use of corticosteroid therapy alone is not beneficial (14).

Myasthenia gravis may result in acute respiratory failure at any time in the clinical course of the disease. Some patients initially present with acute respiratory failure, whereas others develop respiratory failure later in their illness, commonly after thymectomy. Frequent monitoring of the VC is useful but should not substitute clinical evaluation of the patient's degree of weakness, ability to protect his or her airway, and measurement of arterial blood gases. In trying to assess the need for postoperative mechanical ventilation in patients undergoing thymectomy, investigators in one study found that four risk factors were particularly helpful in predicting the need for mechanical ventilation: (a) duration of myasthenia gravis, (b) history of chronic respiratory disease, (c) pyridostigmine dosage more than 750 mg per day, and (d) a preoperative VC of <2.9 L (15).

Management of patients with myasthenia gravis who require mechanical ventilation is primarily supportive unless the respiratory failure is complicated by secondary pneumonia. Treatment with anticholinesterase agents is useful for improving muscle strength. Corticosteroids and plasmapheresis have both been effective in treating acute exacerbations in many patients with myasthenia gravis (16–18). In the only trial comparing intravenous immunoglobulin therapy with plasmapheresis for the treatment of acute myasthenia gravis exacerbations, there were no significant differences in the improvement of the myasthenic muscle score at day 15 between the two groups, although the response to intravenous immunoglobulin was slower than that to therapeutic plasmapheresis (19).

Unilateral or bilateral impairment of diaphragmatic function may also lead to acute respiratory failure (20). The diaphragm is the principal muscle of inspiration and is almost totally responsible for inspiration during quiet breathing. Weakness or paralysis of both hemidiaphragms is most frequently caused by chronic neuromuscular disease, but it may also occur as an isolated abnormality or following spinal cord trauma. In addition, the phrenic nerves may be interrupted inadvertently during surgical procedures in the neck or thorax such as coronary artery bypass grafting (21). Clinically, paradoxical (inward) movement of the abdominal wall during spontaneous inspiration in the supine posture may be overlooked, and it may be necessary to use fluoroscopy or ultrasound to demonstrate paradoxical movement of the diaphragm with spontaneous inspiration (the so-called "sniff test"). Additional evaluation with transdiaphragmatic pressure measurements and phrenic nerve conduction studies may be necessary to confirm the diagnosis (22). Ventilatory support by pacing the diaphragm has been used in a number of patients with trauma or infarction of the cervical cord above C2 when the lower motor neurons of the phrenic nerve were clearly viable (22).

DRUG OVERDOSES

Drug overdoses are a common cause of acute respiratory failure, usually through direct depression of respiratory drive. Most patients who require intubation and mechanical ventilation from drug overdoses do not develop primary pulmonary complications other than hypoventilation, which gradually resolves as the drug is removed from circulation or is metabolized. Acute respiratory failure secondary to parenchymal lung disease does occur in some patients following drug overdose and may become the primary clinical problem in the management of the patient (23). Certain drugs, including heroin and tricyclic antidepressants, have been specifically implicated as causative agents of acute lung injury, presumably through a direct toxic effect on the lung parenchyma. In patients overdosed on these drugs, pulmonary edema may occur from an increase in lung vascular permeability resulting in protein-rich edema fluid collecting in the interstitium and air spaces of the lung even in the absence of elevated pulmonary microvascular pressures. In many of these cases, the lung injury is further complicated by gastric aspiration, leading to diffuse and severe lung injury with secondary parenchymal and/or pleural space infections (24).

Heroin is one of the most common drugs implicated in acute respiratory failure and causes both direct suppression of central respiratory drive and intrinsic lung damage. Heroin and other narcotics can also cause noncardiogenic pulmonary edema, though the pathophysiology of this process is not well understood. Potential mechanisms include a direct toxic effect, an acute hypoxic insult to the alveolar–capillary membrane, an allergic/hypersensitivity response, or a neurogenic response to a central nervous system (CNS) insult. In addition, heroin overdose is complicated by gastric aspiration in up to 50% of cases (25).

Tricyclic antidepressants (tricyclics) are another common cause of drug overdose and can cause severe pulmonary complications. Tricyclics can induce both cardiogenic and noncardiogenic pulmonary edema, as well as aspiration-induced lung injury (25). In one large series examining 82 consecutive patients with tricyclic overdose, 80% of the patients had a widened alveolar–arterial oxygen gradient at initial presentation, 75% required mechanical ventilation for an average of 46 hours, and 25% had evidence of aspiration of activated charcoal. Forty percent of these patients developed abnormal chest radiographs within 48 hours. The severity of the chest radiograph abnormalities correlated with the mean blood levels of tricyclics (23).

Both chronic and acute ingestions of salicylates can cause noncardiogenic pulmonary edema resulting in acute respiratory failure (26). In addition, aspirin-sensitive asthmatics may suffer acute respiratory failure and death from aggravated bronchospasm secondary to aspirin ingestion (27).

The management of a patient with a drug overdose begins with the collection of clues about the specific drug and dose ingested. In general, the patient's history may not be reliable, so medication containers and samples of drugs or substances, if they can be obtained, are helpful in the emergency department. Traditionally, initial treatment of the drug overdose patient in the emergency room included careful consideration of whether removal of any unabsorbed drug with induced emesis or gastric lavage was indicated; however, neither of these interventions was supported by strong clinical evidence (28,29). In a patient with a protected airway, activated charcoal can be used to bind and prevent absorption of some drugs that remain in the intestinal tract (30). Further discussion of these issues is available in recent reviews (31,32). The decision to intubate and ventilate patients after a drug overdose is based on the clinical evaluation of the patient including mental status, hemodynamic stability, and ability to protect the airway. As a general rule, it is preferable to intubate patients with known drug overdoses who have a decrease in mental status, even if their arterial blood gases remain acceptable. Thus, in summary, the definitive management of drug-induced respiratory failure is primarily supportive, with meticulous attention to secondary infectious complications, and often requires mechanical ventilation.

CHEST WALL ABNORMALITIES AS A CAUSE OF ACUTE RESPIRATORY FAILURE

Traumatic injury to the chest wall with subsequent rib fractures is the most frequent cause of acute respiratory failure in this category. This type of injury is usually associated with pain that prevents full lung inflation and results in atelectasis and, occasionally, alveolar hypoventilation. If multiple ribs are fractured in multiple locations, lung inflation may be further limited because of the loss of normal chest wall rigidity and subsequent paradoxical motion of the involved area (flail chest). Underlying injury to the lung may also contribute to abnormalities of gas exchange. Some patients can be managed without intubation and mechanical ventilation if their chest wall injury and associated pulmonary dysfunction, as indicated by arterial blood gas tensions, are not overly severe (Chapter 21, General Principles of Managing a Patient with Respiratory Failure). The primary indications for endotracheal intubation and mechanical ventilation in this setting are deteriorating gas exchange, particularly hypoxemia, and a requirement for large doses of narcotic agents to control pain (33).

Chronic deformities of the chest wall or severe pleural disease may also be complicated by acute respiratory failure, although in these situations the pathophysiologic alterations are more complex than in acute injuries to the chest wall (34). Several such "mechanical" causes of respiratory failure are listed in Table 22-1, including scoliosis, severe obesity, fibrothorax, thoracoplasty, and ankylosing spondylitis. Acute respiratory failure in this setting may be exacerbated by (a) ventilation–perfusion mismatching due to premature airway closure when lung volumes are reduced by a deformed thoracic cage, (b) inadequate cough, and/or (c) chronic alveolar hypoventilation and hypoxemia, which in turn may lead to pulmonary hypertension. The pulmonary hypertension may also be related to mechanical compression of portions of the pulmonary circulation because some data suggest a relationship between pulmonary arterial pressures and the angle of spinal deformity in patients with scoliosis (34).

Other important mechanical causes of acute respiratory failure include tension pneumothorax, severe ascites, and metabolic disorders such as hypothyroidism. In addition, chest wall, pleural, or other mechanical abnormalities may contribute to respiratory failure in patients who have a primary pulmonary etiology for their respiratory distress. For example, patients with acute exacerbations of chronic obstructive pulmonary disease (COPD) may have their respiratory failure worsened by ascites, obesity, or hypothyroidism. Similarly, patients with primary chest wall or pleural disease may develop secondary parenchymal processes such as pneumonia or pulmonary edema that, in the presence of an underlying chest wall abnormality, lead to acute respiratory failure.

TABLE 22-1. Clinical Description of Respiratory Failure in Derangements of the Thorax

Category	Respiratory Failure		Clinical Course	Secretions, Atelectasis, and Pneumonia[a]
	Incidence	Severity[a]		
Mechanical				
Scoliosis	Common	+++	Slow	NL+
Obesity–hypoventilation	Common	+++	Periodic	NL or ↑
Fibrothorax	Common	+++	Slow	NL
Thoracoplasty	Common	+++	Slow	NL or ↑
Ankylosing spondylitis	Rare	+	Slow	NL
Neuromuscular				
Postpoliomyelitis	Common	+++	Slow	↑
Amyotrophic lateral sclerosis	Common	+++	Fast	↑
Muscular dystrophies	Common	+	Slow	↑
Spinal cord injury	Common	++	Slow	↑
Multiple sclerosis	Uncommon	+	Slow	↑
Myasthenia gravis	Common	+++	Periodic	↑

[a] +, dyspnea on exertion; ++, dyspnea, mild hypoxemia, and hypercapnia only; +++, severe hypoventilation; NL, normal lungs; ↑, increased incidence.

From Bergofsky EH. Respiratory failure in disorders of the thoracic cage. *Am Rev Respir Dis* 1979;119: 643–649, with permission.

Treatment for acute respiratory failure in patients with chest wall abnormalities described in Table 22-1 must be directed toward reversing hypoxemia and improving alveolar ventilation. There is some evidence that positive-pressure breathing devices or incentive spirometry may be useful in improving lung inflation and oxygenation. In many cases, acute respiratory failure occurs because of the development of an associated lung infection (34). Endotracheal intubation and mechanical ventilation may be necessary to reverse acute deteriorations in blood gases as well as to help clear pulmonary secretions. Mechanical ventilation may also be necessary in patients with the obesity hypoventilation syndrome in whom central respiratory drive is inadequate to maintain ventilation.

UPPER-AIRWAY OBSTRUCTION

Acute upper-airway obstruction can cause respiratory failure in a few minutes. In children, croup and epiglottitis are the most common causes of upper-airway obstruction. Acute epiglottitis also occurs in adults, though aspiration of food, liquid, or foreign bodies is a more common scenario. In addition, upper-airway obstruction may be the result of obstructing tumors, angioedema, closed-space infection in the head or neck, or oropharyngeal bleeding. In some massively obese patients, obstruction of the upper airway may occur when the patient is supine.

Management of acute upper-airway obstruction requires an understanding of the pathogenesis of the disorder. In patients who have severe carbon dioxide retention or apnea, emergency endotracheal intubation must be carried out. If oral intubation is not possible, an emergency cricothyroidotomy or tracheostomy should be performed. In patients with progressive upper-airway obstruction, as may occur in acute epiglottitis, a number of studies have shown that early intubation in a controlled setting in the presence of a skilled anesthesiologist is the best treatment. In some patients with tumors causing upper-airway obstruction, temporizing measures such as treatment with helium–oxygen mixtures have been reported to forestall intubation so that the patient may receive radiation therapy, chemotherapy, and corticosteroids to reduce the size of the tumor (35). Pulmonary edema may complicate upper-airway obstruction in both children and adults through a mechanism that has been recently elucidated (36). In an analysis of three cases of severe postobstructive pulmonary edema, the ratio of pulmonary edema protein to plasma total protein was on average 0.42, suggesting a hydrostatic mechanism for edema fluid formation (37).

CHRONIC OBSTRUCTIVE AIRWAYS DISEASE

Chronic obstructive airways disease is generally regarded as an inexorably, albeit slowly, progressive disorder (38,39). As the airways obstruction progresses, patients become more vulnerable to what in persons with normal lungs would be minor insults. Although acute respiratory failure may be a consequence of severe progressive airways obstruction, first episodes are generally precipitated by some complicating disorder. Most commonly, the precipitating problem is a lower respiratory tract infection, either bronchitis or pneumonia (40,41). The inflammation resulting from the infection, together with increased mucous production, causes further airways narrowing. If pneumonia is present, the alveolar filling causes shunting of blood and worsens lung mechanics. As a result, a vicious cycle may be initiated in which the acute disease process superimposed on chronic airways disease further increases the airway's resistance, worsens gas exchange with increases in arterial carbon dioxide tension ($PaCO_2$) and decreases in arterial oxygen tension (PaO_2), and increases work of breathing.

Acute respiratory failure in the setting of COPD is primarily hypercapnic but may also be hypoxemic. Hypoxemia is caused by mismatching of ventilation and perfusion, a consequence of obstructed airways and, in some cases in which infection is the precipitant, alveolar filling as mentioned above (42). The mechanisms of impaired carbon dioxide elimination are more complex but also relate in part to mismatching of ventilation and perfusion (43). Unless there is severe airways obstruction, reductions in ventilation to some alveoli can be offset by increased ventilation to other alveoli. However, with increasing airways obstruction, this compensatory mechanism is not sufficient to cope with the overall reduction in alveolar ventilation. In addition, because of the increased work of breathing in the presence of hypoxia, the respiratory muscles may become fatigued and may be unable to maintain the necessary level of minute ventilation (43), resulting in increased carbon dioxide production (44). There may also be a decrease in central ventilatory drive, partly genetic and partly acquired (45–47). Finally, either hypercarbia or hypoxemia (or both) may depress central respiratory drive, thus leading to further hypoventilation.

As the abnormalities of gas exchange become more severe, the function of other organs, especially the heart and CNS, may be affected. Cardiac manifestations may include arrhythmias, ischemia, heart failure, or myocardial infarction. Neurologic effects may include alterations in behavior, reduction in level of consciousness, coma, seizures, or myoclonus. Obviously, either cardiovascular or neurologic effects could have a major adverse influence on the course of respiratory failure and could further perpetuate the progressive downward spiral.

The symptoms associated with respiratory failure in patients with chronic airways obstruction usually represent an exacerbation of the patient's baseline symptoms. Most patients with airways obstruction have cough and sputum production. Acute lower respiratory tract infections generally increase these symptoms and are often associated with an increase in the volume of sputum. However, as airways obstruction increases, the ability to clear mucus from the lungs may decrease. Thus, a report of a decrease in sputum production associated with other symptoms may actually be indicative of worsening clinical status.

In some patients, cardiovascular complaints like palpitations, orthopnea, paroxysmal nocturnal dyspnea, ankle swelling, and chest pain may predominate. Complaints related to neurologic dysfunction may also be prominent. Headache, visual problems, sleep disturbances, memory loss, and behavioral alterations may be reported. In some patients, these may be of sufficient severity to obscure the respiratory symptoms.

Findings on physical examination may be quite helpful and may provide an important context in which to evaluate the more objective measurements, such as blood gas tensions. To start with, the general appearance of the patient is very important. A patient who appears reasonably well and is alert and able to cooperate with therapy obviously represents a different management problem than the patient who is confused, combative, stuporous, or comatose, though the patients may have the same blood gas values. Alterations in behavior or level of consciousness may not be caused by the abnormal blood gas tensions *per se* but could be related to drugs or other factors; however, the implications for treatment are the same. The physical examination should be targeted to detect disorders that may have precipitated the acute deterioration. At least in the acute setting, the degree of pulsus paradoxus correlates with the severity of airways obstruction. Chest examination may or may not be helpful. Most patients with acute exacerbations of chronic airways obstruction have supraclavicular and intercostal retractions. The chest is usually hyperinflated and tympanitic with very limited diaphragmatic excursion. Breath sounds commonly are diminished. Wheezing may or may not be heard.

The chest film may simply show the classic changes of longstanding obstructive lung disease (see Fig. 22-1). However, there may also be evidence for pneumonia, left ventricular failure, or pneumothorax that was not evident on physical examination. The electrocardiogram is less often helpful but may show right atrial or right ventricular enlargement, an arrhythmia, or evidence of left ventricular disease. Routine blood studies may provide evidence of other processes, but except for the hematocrit and plasma electrolytes, these do not relate to lung disease. Patients who have been hypoxemic for long periods of time, unless other factors supervene, will have secondary polycythemia (48).

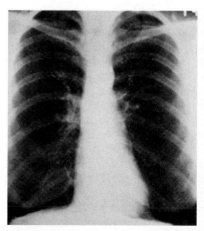
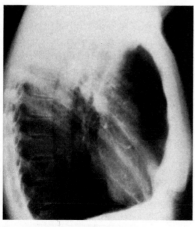

A   B

FIGURE 22-1. Posteroanterior (**A**) and lateral (**B**) chest roentgenograms of a 62-year-old woman with advanced COPD, mainly emphysema, showing low, flattened diaphragms, large retrosternal airspace, vertically oriented heart, and hyperlucency of peripheral lung fields. (From Hinshaw HC, Murray JF. Chronic bronchitis and emphysema. In: Hinshaw HC, Murray JF, eds. *Diseases of the chest* Philadelphia: WB Saunders, 1980:578, with permission.)

Of all the assessments that can be made, measurements of arterial PaO_2, $PaCO_2$, and pH are the most important. Serial blood gases are much more helpful than a single determination and can indicate success or failure of initial therapy. Blood gas values taken together with the general status of the patient often determine the necessary intensity of supportive measures, particularly whether endotracheal intubation and mechanical ventilation will be necessary. Nearly all patients with chronic airways obstruction have some degree of chronic hypoxemia, and some have carbon dioxide retention when they are at their functional baseline. For this reason, a single measurement of $PaCO_2$ without a prior baseline value may be very difficult to interpret; hence, the clinical context should be considered. An elevated plasma bicarbonate concentration is an indication that an elevated $PaCO_2$ has been present for a sufficiently long period to allow metabolic compensation.

Effective management of acute respiratory failure in patients with chronic airways obstruction requires a critical care unit. The approach to treatment should always be directed to providing supportive care while treating the specific processes, such as lower respiratory tract infection that precipitated the acute deterioration.

The major supportive intervention necessary in this setting is provision of supplemental oxygen. Because mismatching of ventilation and perfusion is the pathophysiologic mechanism by which hypoxemia develops, sufficient increases in PaO_2 are easily achieved by administration of low concentrations of oxygen. In patients with an acute decompensation, though, administration of oxygen may lead to further hypercapnia. This change may be due, in part, to a decrease in ventilatory drive from the loss of hypoxic stimulus, although some studies have suggested that an increase in alveolar dead space associated with oxygen therapy may be primarily responsible (49). This concern, however, should not deter oxygen administration. The basic principle should be to administer the lowest amount of oxygen necessary to increase the PaO_2 to approximately 60 mm Hg. Nasal prongs or cannulae with flows of 1 to 2 L per minute are usually sufficient, though occasionally higher flows are needed (see Fig. 22-2). The fraction of inspired oxygen (FIO_2) delivered by devices such as nasal prongs varies considerably depending on the patient's minute ventilation. Although this variability does not usually present a problem, more precise control of the FIO_2 can be provided by a mask that uses a Venturi device to deliver a high flow of oxygen while entraining sufficient room air to produce the desired FIO_2. The disadvantages of the Venturi delivery device are that the inspired gas is usually poorly humidified and that the mask interferes with talking and eating.

Regardless of the oxygen delivery system, arterial blood gas tension must be measured soon after oxygen therapy is begun. The goal, as stated, is to increase the PaO_2 to 60 mm Hg (i.e., 90% oxyhemoglobin saturation) without undue effects on $PaCO_2$. Blood gas measurements should be made thereafter as frequently as the clinical circumstances dictate. In this situation, because of the concern of the interactions of PaO_2 and $PaCO_2$, noninvasive monitoring of oxyhemoglobin saturation alone is usually not sufficient, though it may complement direct measurements of PaO_2 and $PaCO_2$.

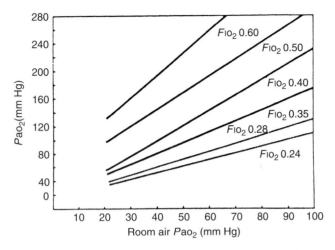

FIGURE 22-2. The relationship of PaO_2 to FIO_2 administered to patients with COPD. Each line gives the expected arterial oxygen tension for the FIO_2 administered. These lines were obtained in a study of patients with acute respiratory failure and stable patients with COPD. (From Bone RC. Treatment of respiratory failure due to advanced chronic obstructive lung disease. *Arch Intern Med* 1980;140:1019, with permission.)

In most patients, provision of supplemental oxygen is the only supportive therapy needed. In some, however, endotracheal intubation and mechanical ventilation are required. Precise criteria for intubation and mechanical ventilation are difficult to define and commonly involve subjective as well as objective assessments. Hypoxemia *per se* is usually not an indication for intubation because of the relative ease with which PaO_2 can be increased with supplemental oxygen provided by external devices. The major indication for ventilatory assistance is a poorly compensated acute respiratory acidosis. This situation may be apparent at the time of initial evaluation and dictate prompt institution of mechanical ventilation, but, frequently, the need for ventilatory assistance is indicated by the patient's failure to improve or by the worsening of the patient's condition with conservative management. This determination should be made through careful monitoring of the response to oxygen administration as well as an assessment of other variables such as respiratory distress, fatigue, mental status, and ability to cooperate with conservative management.

In appropriately selected patients, noninvasive ventilation may reverse the acute respiratory decompensation and allow the patient to avoid endotracheal intubation (50,51). Noninvasive positive-pressure ventilation utilizes a face mask, mouthpiece, or nasal mask to deliver oxygen from a positive-pressure ventilator. In contrast to continuous positive airway pressure (CPAP), different levels of pressure support are set for inspiration and expiration, and a backup rate may be set if desired. Noninvasive ventilation has been shown in multiple randomized controlled trials to decrease mortality and the need for endotracheal intubation when compared with usual medical care in acute exacerbations of COPD (52–56). Further confirmation of these findings has been provided by recent systematic reviews, one of which found that the number of patients needed to be treated with noninvasive ventilation to save one life (commonly referred to as the number needed to treat) was 10, suggesting that noninvasive ventilation is an exceptionally potent intervention (57–59).

Appropriate patient selection for noninvasive ventilation is of paramount importance. Some studies have suggested that patients with a pH of less than 7.3 on initial presentation derive the greatest benefit from noninvasive ventilation, though this cutoff has not been borne out in all reviews (58,59). At the other end of the spectrum, patients with imminent respiratory arrest (or cardiovascular collapse) are poor candidates for noninvasive ventilation. Likewise, patients who are unable to protect their airway, especially patients with altered mental status, should not be considered candidates for noninvasive ventilation. Patients being treated with noninvasive ventilation should be closely monitored, particularly at the onset of therapy. Response to noninvasive ventilation after 1 hour, as measured by salutary changes in arterial blood gas values, should be considered predictive of the likelihood of success of the modality (60,61). A more extensive discussion of this subject can be found in Chapter 21, General Principles of Managing a Patient with Respiratory Failure.

When endotracheal intubation is necessary, mechanical ventilation should be tailored to the individual patient with the goal of resting the respiratory muscles (62). Regardless of the mode of ventilation chosen, the inspiratory volume or pressure delivered by the ventilator should be titrated to achieve maximal synchrony with the awake patient while minimizing the amount of work done by the respiratory muscles. Careful evaluation of the patient and ventilator waveforms is critical in order to recognize wasted efforts made by the patient attempting and failing to trigger the ventilator. Ideally, the respiratory rate should be relatively slow, providing sufficient time for full exhalation so as to avoid stacking breaths with a consequent further increase in functional residual capacity (FRC). Because tachypnea is common in these patients, sedation is often required to enable an optimal ventilatory pattern and to avoid the dynamic hyperinflation that can develop in patients with severe airways obstruction. A long inspiratory time also is desirable to improve the distribution of inspired gas. As a general rule, positive end-expiratory pressure (PEEP) should not be used. The effect of PEEP would be to further increase the already greatly enlarged FRC and cause further overdistention of the lungs. In patients with airways obstruction, an auto-PEEP effect may occur as airways close or as the next breath is delivered before full exhalation (43); if this complication occurs, the judicious use of exogenous PEEP may be required to stent the airways open and allow the trapped air to escape. Alternatively, the patient may need to be momentarily disconnected from the ventilator circuit to allow full exhalation. In mechanically ventilated patients, the overadministration of oxygen is no longer of concern, and the F_{IO_2} should be sufficient to maintain a Pa_{O_2} over 60 mm Hg.

Within 10 to 20 minutes of beginning mechanical ventilation, arterial blood gases should be measured. Because many patients with acute respiratory failure and chronic airways obstruction have had carbon dioxide retention for days, months, or years, metabolic compensation has occurred. This compensation generally is insufficient in the setting of an acute deterioration but is appropriate for the baseline Pa_{CO_2}. When mechanical ventilation is applied, the Pa_{CO_2} generally can be decreased very quickly and, if it is reduced well below the patient's baseline to a normal value of 40 mm Hg, the patient will be left with an uncompensated, sometimes profound, metabolic alkalosis. Alkalemia has a number of potential adverse effects including depressed cardiac output, increased risk of both supraventricular and ventricular arrhythmias, depressed level of consciousness, and seizures (63). For this reason, the adequacy of mechanical ventilation should be determined not by Pa_{CO_2} but by pH. The Pa_{CO_2} should be maintained at a level that keeps the pH no higher than 7.45 to 7.50, and preferably close to a pH of 7.40. Also, because of chronic increases in Pa_{CO_2}, patients are commonly deficient in potassium and chloride. A reduction in plasma bicarbonate concentration does not occur until sufficient chloride has been given (64).

In addition to the supportive ventilatory care described above, treatment of the airways obstruction and the precipitating disorder must be prompt and vigorous. Although there is controversy concerning the use of bronchodilators in patients with chronic airways obstruction, it should always be assumed that there is a reversible component to the obstruction. Inhaled β-adrenergic agonists such as albuterol, metaproterenol, or terbutaline should be used at intervals of 2 to 4 hours at the beginning of treatment, and the frequency of dosage should be decreased if adverse reactions are encountered. These medications can be administered directly via a nebulizer driven by a compressed gas source or through a mechanical ventilator. With either of these devices, the amount of drug actually delivered is difficult to quantify; thus, the dose given should be limited mainly by side effects. Inhaled ipratropium has also been shown to be an effective bronchodilator and may reduce the volume of secretions (65). Metered-dose inhalation is a simpler and usually equally effective route for delivery of these agents in nonintubated patients. Intravenous aminophylline may also be of benefit and should not be forgotten as a therapeutic option, though the data on this topic are somewhat conflicting. Theophylline has been shown to increase respiratory muscle strength, but in one study the dose needed to achieve this effect yielded toxic serum concentrations (66). Another study suggested that theophylline was of minimal benefit in treating acute respiratory failure in COPD patients already treated with β-agonists, antibiotics, and corticosteroids (67).

The benefits of systemic corticosteroids in COPD exacerbations are not as well established as for acute asthmatic attacks (68,69). A recent double-blind randomized controlled trial compared high-dose systemic corticosteroids (given as either 2- or 8-week regimens) to placebo in 271 patients hospitalized for COPD exacerbations. All patients received a 1-week course of antibiotics as well as inhaled corticosteroids, β-agonists, and ipratropium for the follow-up duration (6 months). The patients in the oral corticosteroid treatment arms had significantly shorter hospital stays, significantly less treatment failures at 1 and 3 months, and a small improvement in forced expiratory volume in 1 second (FEV_1). There was no advantage to the longer course of systemic corticosteroids. At 6 months, the three arms had no significant differences in rates of death, intubation, readmission, or treatment intensification (70).

Antimicrobial drugs are of obvious value if bacterial bronchitis or pneumonia accompany obstructive lung disease (71), though many exacerbations of COPD are likely triggered by viral infections (72). The routine use of antibiotics in COPD exacerbations not associated with a clear infection also appears to be beneficial (73). The choice of agents should be guided initially by the results of sputum Gram stains. If Gram stains and cultures do not provide guidance, empiric therapy with trimethoprim–sulfamethoxazole or doxycycline may be used.

Once the above therapies have been employed and the patient has begun to improve, the optimal timing of discontinuation of mechanical ventilation should be addressed. Weaning patients with chronic airways obstruction from mechanical ventilation can present a difficult problem. Implicit in the decision to intubate and ventilate is the assumption that there is a reversible factor contributing to the acute deterioration and that treatment will restore the patient to baseline status. Given this assumption, weaning efforts should begin as soon as the reversible component has improved. In the case of left ventricular failure, for example, this improvement may occur quite rapidly in response to diuresis. On the other hand, if pneumonia has caused the acute deterioration, improvement may be slow.

A number of criteria have been developed as predictors of successful extubation (62). Unfortunately, these criteria are rarely applicable to patients with chronic airways obstruction who may not have been able to perform at the levels indicated by the criteria for many years. For this reason, assessment of ability to be weaned in this setting is more subjective (62,74). Measurements such as VC and maximal inspiratory pressure (MIP) can be made, but low values should not be assumed to predict failure. The patient should be alert and psychologically prepared for weaning. Serum electrolyte concentrations, especially potassium, phosphate, calcium, and magnesium, should be optimized, and the patient should be hemodynamically stable.

In general, before considering extubation, the PaO_2, $PaCO_2$, and pH should be maintained at their baseline values, if known. Thus, patients may be mildly hypoxemic, hypercapnic, and acidemic. All intubated patients should be evaluated for the appropriateness of a spontaneous breathing trial on a daily basis (75). Such a trial can be performed using either a T-piece or a low level of CPAP. If the patient ventilates adequately during a spontaneous breathing trial for 30 minutes to 2 hours without deterioration in arterial blood gas values, hemodynamics, or other subjective or objective measures of stability, the endotracheal tube can usually be removed. Longer periods of spontaneous breathing (especially through a small endotracheal tube <7 mm in diameter) may cause respiratory muscle fatigue because of the high resistance of the tube.

If patients fail a spontaneous breathing trial, ventilatory support should be gradually decreased (i.e., "weaned"). The specific technique of weaning is somewhat controversial, with many clinicians favoring a spontaneous breathing trial with a T-piece or with CPAP and others favoring the use of intermittent mandatory ventilation (IMV) with progressively decreasing ventilatory rates. Though historically different approaches to weaning from mechanical ventilation have been considered equally effective (62,74), there is increasing evidence that spontaneous breathing trials with low-level pressure support or T-piece trials are a more rapid method of weaning than the use of IMV (76–79). In addition, noninvasive ventilation is proving to be a safe and effective technique for extubating patients with chronic lung disease who have failed spontaneous breathing trials but otherwise seem appropriate for extubation (80–83). A more comprehensive discussion of weaning techniques can be found in Chapter 21, General Principles of Managing a Patient with Respiratory Failure.

In managing patients with acute respiratory failure and chronic airways obstruction, important and difficult ethical issues may be raised. As stated previously, undertaking mechanical ventilatory support assumes that the respiratory failure has a reversible component, which may not be the case. In patients with chronic lung disease, acute respiratory failure may simply represent the end stage of an inexorably progressive disease. Providing mechanical ventilation for a patient whose respiratory failure has no reversible component usually means that the patient will not be able to be weaned successfully. Under ideal circumstances, the patient and his or her physician would have had the opportunity to discuss the outlook for the illness prior to acute deterioration, and the patient can make an informed decision about the use of mechanical ventilation. Such a patient may decide that ventilation should be undertaken on the chance that there is a reversible component. If facilities are available, the patient may also choose chronic ventilatory support. Patients who are being ventilated mechanically may also elect to have this support discontinued. In the face of previously reviewed difficulties in predicting weanability, abrupt discontinuation of support may not mean death. If mechanical ventilation is not undertaken or is discontinued, vigorous treatment can still be provided, but particular attention should be paid to the patient's comfort (Chapter 21, General Principles of Managing a Patient with Respiratory Failure).

RESPIRATORY FAILURE IN ASTHMA

Asthma prevalence and mortality has been on the rise in the United States and worldwide (84,85). Most deaths occur in asthmatics from status asthmaticus. Acute airways obstruction in asthma results in increased resistance to airflow during both inspiration and expiration, leading to air trapping and overinflation (86). Because the airflow obstruction is not uniform, the distribution of inspired air is uneven, causing mismatching of ventilation and perfusion and, therefore, hypoxemia and an increase in wasted ventilation (42,87). The hyperinflation serves to maintain airway patency, but as FRC increases and approaches the predicted normal total lung capacity (TLC), a greater change in transpulmonary pressure is required to produce an adequate tidal volume. This cycle, together with the rise in airways resistance, markedly increases the work of breathing. Moreover, increases in wasted ventilation and in carbon dioxide production require greater minute ventilation, which can be achieved only by imposing an additional workload on the respiratory muscles. Because of the hyperinflation, the intercostal, accessory, and diaphragmatic muscles are forced to work at a considerable mechanical disadvantage (88). At some point, if the airways obstruction is not corrected, the system fails, and carbon dioxide retention occurs. In addition, as the oxygen demands of the respiratory muscles begin to outstrip the supply of oxygen, anaerobic metabolism results with subsequent metabolic (lactic) acidosis. Because there is no possibility for respiratory compensation, the pH rapidly decreases. Metabolic acidosis in this setting must be dealt with promptly or rapid deterioration will occur.

Assessment of the severity of an asthmatic episode is of utmost importance in determining the approach toward management of the patient. Although the vast majority of asthma attacks are treated entirely on an outpatient basis, it is essential that both the patient and medical personnel be aware of when more intensive treatment is needed. Although several groups of investigators have attempted to identify factors predictive of the need for hospitalization in asthmatic patients (89), the utility and accuracy of numerical indices derived from such data have been questioned (90,91). Both objective and subjective individualized patient assessments should be used to judge the severity of an asthmatic episode. Factors that should be taken into account in such evaluations are listed in Table 22-2.

The patient's past and recent medical history can be useful in assessing the severity of a given asthmatic episode and may provide information that influences the interpretation of more objective physiologic data. Patients who have a history of having severe attacks tend to continue to have the same. Thus, information from the patient or from the medical record that he or she has previously required hospitalization increases concern for the current episode. The duration of the current attack is also important because the mechanism of airway obstruction changes as the attack persists. Early obstruction is caused mainly by smooth muscle spasm, whereas later mucous plugging and edema play a larger role. Spasm can resolve within minutes, but days may be required to improve the obstruction caused by edema and plugging.

Patients with acute asthmatic episodes are nearly always tachypneic and tachycardic, though neither of these signs correlates well with the degree of airway obstruction. The amount of pulsus paradoxus does, however, increase with greater degrees of obstruction (92) and can be used both to indicate severity and to judge response to therapy. The intensity of wheezing cannot be used to infer the amount of airways obstruction, although prolongation of the expiratory phase varies roughly with obstruction. The absence of wheezing in a patient who by all other indicators has an asthma exacerbation is an ominous finding, indicating that airflow is so reduced that there is no sufficient turbulence to cause wheezing. Unilateral

TABLE 22-2. Important Factors in Assessing Severity of Acute Asthma

1. History of prior hospitalization for asthma
2. History of prior or current corticosteroid therapy
3. Patient's subjective sense of severity of attack
4. Failure to respond to usual treatment (i.e., persistent wheezing despite bronchodilator therapy)
5. Duration of attack
6. Patient is too distressed to talk
7. Silent chest (i.e., minimal breath sounds)
8. Disturbances in mental status
9. Systemic hypertension and tachycardia >110/min
10. Cardiac arrhythmias
11. Cyanosis
12. Prominent accessory muscle use
13. Pulsus paradoxus >10 mm Hg
14. Mediastinal emphysema, pneumothorax
15. FEV_1 <1.0 L
16. Acute respiratory acidosis or arterial PaO_2 <60 on room air

FEV_1, forced expiratory volume in 1 second; PaO_2, arterial oxygen tension.

absence of wheezing may be the result of a pneumothorax or mucous plug in a large airway and is usually indicative of a serious clinical problem. Although not specific, abnormalities in mental status are important in patients with severe airways obstruction as they may indicate hypoxemia or hypercarbia and may interfere with patient cooperation.

Although an understanding of the alterations in pulmonary function is necessary to conceptualize the pathophysiology of asthma, in acute exacerbations the only measurements that can be made routinely are the FEV_1, peak flow, and forced VC. Of these, the peak flow is the most easily obtained because it does not require a full forced exhalation, but rather a short forced puff similar to a cough after a full inhalation. Severe obstruction is indicated by a peak flow of <100 L per minute. This has been shown to correspond to an FEV_1 of <0.7 L (93). The FEV_1 is more difficult to measure because it requires a full inspiration followed by a full forced exhalation, maneuvers that a severe asthmatic may not be able to perform because of dyspnea and that, in some patients, actually worsen the obstruction (94). Nevertheless, the FEV_1 is the most direct measurement of airflow and correlates well with clinical outcomes. Nowak et al. found that an FEV_1 of <1 L or 20% of the predicted value was associated with a poor bronchodilator response, the need for hospitalization, and the likelihood of relapse (93). Similar findings were reported by Kelsen et al. (89). Several investigators have related the FEV_1 to PaO_2 and $PaCO_2$ and have demonstrated that, in acute asthma, carbon dioxide retention begins to occur at an FEV_1 of approximately 0.75 L or 25% of the predicted value (95,96).

The arterial blood gas values are of paramount importance in the management of asthma and must be carefully interpreted. An increase in $PaCO_2$ is a direct consequence of the airways obstruction, which limits ventilatory capability in the face of increased carbon dioxide production. Because mild degrees of acute airways obstruction are usually associated with hyperventilation and a lower than normal $PaCO_2$, the finding of a "normal" value should be viewed with concern. Although there is a tendency for the PaO_2 to decrease with decreasing values of FEV_1, the relationship is not as predictable as with $PaCO_2$ (97). Nearly all patients with airways obstruction have some degree of arterial hypoxemia. Values of <50 mm Hg are distinctly unusual, however, and suggest that factors in addition to airways obstruction are playing a role. Acute hypoventilation results in a reduction in arterial pH of about 0.008 pH unit for every 1 mm Hg increase in $PaCO_2$; thus, an increase in $PaCO_2$ from 40 to 60 mm Hg would result in a pH of 7.25. A reduction in pH that is in excess of that predicted by the change in $PaCO_2$ indicates the presence of a metabolic as well as respiratory acidosis. As discussed previously, in this setting, metabolic acidosis is caused by an imbalance between the supply and consumption of oxygen by the respiratory muscles along with, perhaps, a reduction in clearance of lactate from blood. The finding of metabolic acidosis in a patient with severe asthma is perhaps the single most ominous finding of all (98).

Chest radiographs should be obtained routinely in patients with severe asthma. The most common finding is hyperinflation, but, occasionally, pneumonia, pneumomediastinum, pneumothorax, or atelectasis from mucous plugging of larger airways may be found. Electrocardiograms should also be obtained, especially in older patients. The common abnormalities include P pulmonale, right ventricular strain, and right axis deviation, all of which may be reversible. Much less commonly, changes indicative of ischemia or arrhythmias may be encountered (99).

The treatment modalities employed in severe asthma are directed toward both support of the patient and reversal of the airways obstruction. Supplemental oxygen is an essential supportive measure that should be instituted in all patients with acute airways obstruction. Because there is no concern of depression of ventilatory drive by oxygen in most patients with asthma, the choice of an oxygen delivery system should mainly be made on the basis of patient comfort. For example, face masks that fit tightly may not be tolerated, and humidification of the inspired gas mixture, although desirable, may stimulate more bronchoconstriction. Normal saline is less likely to produce this effect than distilled water is. In addition, heated humidification is preferable.

It can be difficult to determine when to institute mechanical ventilation in severe asthma. There are no uniformly applicable criteria that can guide the decision and, as in all patients approaching the need for mechanical ventilation, both subjective and objective criteria should be used (100). Generally, mechanical ventilation should not be undertaken before the patient has been given maximal bronchodilator therapy, even though marked abnormalities of gas exchange may be present. Exceptions to this generalization include the presence of significant mental status changes, life-threatening cardiac arrhythmias, electrocardiographic evidence of myocardial ischemia, or a history of previous severe asthmatic episodes requiring mechanical ventilation (100).

Patients who continue to deteriorate in the face of aggressive, in-hospital management generally require mechanical ventilation. This development is often foreshadowed by increasing respiratory acidosis, at times accompanied by metabolic acidosis. Hypoxemia by itself is rarely an indication for mechanical ventilation because it can be managed effectively with supplemental oxygen. Placement of an endotracheal tube should be done semielectively rather than waiting until the patient is in extremis. Because there are irritant receptors in the larynx and trachea, the process of endotracheal intubation may provoke increased bronchoconstriction. This response is mediated by the parasympathetic nervous system and may be reduced by premedication with atropine or topical lidocaine. In most patients, orotracheal intubation with sedation and paralysis is necessary.

Once control of the airway is achieved, sedation is generally necessary. Mechanical ventilation should be provided with a volume-cycled ventilator. At least early in the course, the ventilatory mode should be assist-control ventilation rather than IMV to allow more complete resting of the respiratory muscles. Tidal volume should usually be in the range of 5 to 6 mL per kg body weight so as to avoid hyperinflation to the extent possible. Because the FRC is markedly increased, PEEP, which further increases the FRC, should be avoided unless it is necessary to overcome the auto-PEEP phenomenon, as described in the section on chronic obstructive airways disease above.

Appropriate adjustment of the ratio of inspiration to expiration is the most difficult aspect of mechanical ventilation in the setting of severe airways obstruction. An interplay of four factors is involved: (a) marked slowing of the expiratory flow because of the airways obstruction, (b) dyspnea and tachypnea, (c) the need for a minute ventilation that will reduce the $PaCO_2$,

and (d) the desirability of a slow inspiratory time to minimize peak airway pressures and to enable optimal distribution of the inspired gas. Expiratory time should be maximized by setting a low tidal volume, respiratory rate, and I:E ratio with or without increasing inspiratory flow rates. In addition, peak and plateau pressures should be minimized, with most experts recommending that plateau pressures be kept <30 cm H_2O. This strategy minimizes dynamic hyperinflation (also known as auto-PEEP), which can lead to cardiovascular collapse and/or barotrauma if allowed to spiral out of control. Deep sedation with or without paralysis may, at times, be necessary to enact this ventilatory strategy, although the serious risk of myopathy associated with paralytic agents should be kept in mind, particularly in asthmatics who are on high-dose corticosteroids. If paralytics are required, pancuronium or vecuronium should be favored, as curare, succinylcholine, and atracurium cause release of histamine. In addition, hypercapnia should be tolerated as long as the pH remains compatible with life and the $PaCO_2$ does not rise above 90 mm Hg (101–103).

One study reported excellent results with controlled hypoventilation using hyperoxic mixtures in mechanically ventilated patients (104). Peak airway pressures were maintained at <50 cm H_2O; the patients were hypercapnic but well oxygenated. Mortality rates with this strategy compared favorably with those reported in other studies (see Table 22-3).

With mechanical ventilation, PaO_2 and $PaCO_2$ generally can be brought into the normal range quite promptly; however, weaning cannot begin until the airways obstruction remits. Although criteria for weanability in asthma have not been well defined by the literature, reasonable markers of readiness would include a reduction in peak inspiratory pressure, a spontaneous maximum inspiratory force of at least −30 cm H_2O, and a VC of at least 15 mL per kg body weight. Once these measures are achieved, weaning can usually be proceeded using spontaneous breathing trials with a T-piece or CPAP or IMV with a progressively decreasing frequency of mechanical breaths.

In addition to the ventilatory support discussed above, patients with asthma exacerbations should of course receive adjunctive pharmacologic therapy with bronchodilators and corticosteroids. The principles for the use of bronchodilator

TABLE 22-3. Prognosis in Patients Requiring Mechanical Ventilation in Status Asthmaticus

Study	Year	Episodes (n)	Deaths (n)	Mortality (%)
Riding and Ambiavagar	1967	26	4	15
Iisalo et al.	1969	29	4	14
Lissac et al.	1971	19	4	21
Sheehy et al.	1972	22	2	9
Scoggin et al.	1977	21	8	38
Cornil et al.	1977	58	6	10
Westerman et al.	1979	42	4	9.5
Webb et al.	1979	20	7	35
Picado et al.	1983	26	6	23
Darioli et al.	1983	34	0	0

From Darioli R, Perret C. Mechanical controlled hypoventilation in status asthmaticus. *Am Rev Respir Dis* 1994;129:385–387, with permission.

agents apply equally in mild, moderate, and severe asthma. In spite of the poor early response to bronchodilators in patients with severe asthma, these agents together with corticosteroids remain the cornerstone of treatment. β-Adrenergic agonists may be administered orally, by inhalation, subcutaneously, or intravenously, though evidence suggests that the inhaled route yields a more favorable side-effect profile (105,106). Frequently, the use of a metered-dose inhaler is not adequate to deliver the aerosol because of the limitation of inspiratory flow. Placing a spacer or reservoir between the inhaler and the mouth may enable more effective use of the metered-dose inhaler. Alternatively, nebulized therapy is an effective option.

Aerosolized agents have an onset of action within minutes, and the effect of a single dose peaks at 30 to 60 minutes. The duration of effect is 4 to 6 hours following a single dose. In treating severe episodes of asthma, inhalation of a β_2-selective agent should be given nearly continuously during the first hour unless toxicity develops, as indicated by cardiac arrhythmia or intolerable tremor. During the next several hours, inhalation can be given at hourly intervals with close monitoring for toxicity. As the airways obstruction improves, the dosing interval can be increased to 4 to 6 hours, and metered-dose inhalers can be used. In asthmatics who require endotracheal intubation and mechanical ventilation, the drug can be delivered using an in-line nebulizer in the inspiratory limb of the ventilator circuit. Longer-acting β-adrenergic agonists such as salmeterol may also be effective, although the delay in the onset of their action may limit their utility in the acute setting (107).

The use of theophylline was discussed in the preceding section on COPD and acute respiratory failure. In severe asthma, both theophylline and β-adrenergic agonists can be given in doses as guided by blood concentrations (theophylline) or toxicity (β-adrenergic agents and theophylline). In at least two studies, this approach provided more effective bronchodilation than when either agent was given alone in maximal doses; although in a third trial, inhaled isoproterenol proved to have as much effect alone as when combined with aminophylline (108). More recent studies, however, suggest that the addition of theophylline to maximal corticosteroids and β-adrenergic therapy appears to be of marginal benefit in most patients (109). It should be also noted that the factors that tend to alter the pharmacokinetics of theophylline (e.g., pneumonia, heart failure, and severe airways obstruction) are more likely to be present in severe asthma than in milder forms of the same. Further, in patients with severe asthma and multiple coexisting medical conditions, it may be difficult to determine if an untoward event such as an arrhythmia or seizure is truly due to theophylline. For these reasons, the use of theophylline in severe asthma must be monitored closely using measurements of serum drug levels.

Treatment with corticosteroids is essential in severe asthma. In patients who do not respond promptly to initial bronchodilator therapy, treatment with a systemic, generally intravenous, corticosteroid should be instituted (110). This decision does not obligate the patient to a long course of corticosteroids nor will it cause him or her to be steroid dependent. Because the peak effect occurs no sooner than 4 to 6 hours after intravenous administration, it is best to give the initial dose early in the course of treatment and reevaluate the need for continuation at a later time. There appears to be a dose–response relationship between increasing doses of methylprednisolone (15, 40, and 125 mg, all

given three times a day) and FEV_1 in acute severe asthma (111). Given that the adverse effects of even high doses of corticosteroids are minimal if the duration of administration is short, it is probably better to err on the side of giving too much of the drug than too little. On the basis of the scant data that are available, a dose of methylprednisolone in the range of 60 to 120 mg given intravenously at 6- to 8-hour intervals for 48 to 72 hours represents a reasonable initial approach to corticosteroid administration in patients with severe asthma. Higher doses should be used in patients who have been taking chronic corticosteroids or who are taking other drugs such as barbiturates, phenytoin, or rifampin that accelerate the metabolism of corticosteroids (112). The dose can be reduced rapidly to tapering doses given orally or discontinued altogether in patients who respond promptly.

Aerosolized corticosteroids, although effective in maintenance therapy, have no demonstrated role in the management of a severe attack. However, patients who have asthma and are being mechanically ventilated for other reasons can be given agents such as beclomethasone via the endotracheal tube.

Because both airway smooth muscle and mucociliary function are modulated by the parasympathetic nervous system, with stimulation causing both bronchoconstriction and an increase in mucous production, it seems logical that antimuscarinic agents such as atropine might be of benefit in asthma. Although the benefit of adding anticholinergic therapy to maximal β-agonist therapy has not been well studied in critically ill patients, clinical trials comparing combination therapy to β-agonist treatment alone have produced conflicting results. A pooled analysis of three double-blind, randomized control trials involving a total of 1,064 patients treated in the emergency room showed that the combination treatment group had a small improvement in FEV_1 and required hospitalization less frequently (113). A more recent meta-analysis also demonstrated improvement in lung function and a decrease in the rate of hospitalization admission (114).

Antimicrobial agents are of questionable value in the routine management of acute asthmatic episodes in the absence of documented pneumonia or bacterial bronchitis (112). Other strategies that are used in severe asthma exacerbations and that are supported by some clinical data include the use of Heliox or intravenous magnesium sulfate (115). First introduced into the medical armamentarium in the 1930s, Heliox is a mixture of helium and oxygen (usually 80:20, 70:30, or 60:40) that in theory improves laminar flow in obstructed airways. Small, largely uncontrolled trials have demonstrated a reduction in the $PaCO_2$ and a decrease in the alveolar–arterial gradient of intubated asthmatic patients with the addition of Heliox; however, no large-scale randomized trials have been performed in this area (116,117). A recent systematic review evaluating all the published controlled trials of Heliox in acute asthma found little evidence of improvement in spirometric outcomes; however, intubated patients were excluded from this review (118). In general, mucolytic agents are of little use in severe asthma. General anesthesia with inhalational agents has been used in the treatment of refractory asthma for a number of years. Halothane was frequently used in the past because of its inherent bronchodilating effect (119), though isofluorane has now replaced halothane when an inhalational anesthetic is used. These inhalational agents can antagonize the effects of acetylcholine and histamine on smooth muscle as well as reduce antigen-induced bronchospasm in dogs. In addition to the pharmacologic effects of the anesthetic agent, general anesthesia may allow more effective mechanical ventilation, although this objective can also be achieved in the vast majority of instances by proper use of sedatives and muscle relaxants in patients who are already being ventilated mechanically.

REFERENCES

1. Segredo V, Caldwell JE, Matthay MA, et al. Persistent paralysis in critically ill patients after long-term administration of vecuronium. *N Engl J Med* 1992;327(8):524–528.
2. Luce JM. Medical management of spinal cord injury. *Crit Care Med* 1985;13(2):126–131.
3. Govoni V, Granieri E. Epidemiology of the Guillain-Barre syndrome. *Curr Opin Neurol* 2001;14(5):605–613.
4. Gracey DR, McMichan JC, Divertie MB, et al. Respiratory failure in Guillain-Barre syndrome: a 6-year experience. *Mayo Clin Proc* 1982;57(12):742–746.
5. Moore P, James O. Guillain-Barre Syndrome: incidence, management and outcome of major complications. *Crit Care Med* 1981;9(7): 549–555.
6. Melillo EM, Sethi JM, Mohsenin V. Guillain-Barre syndrome: rehabilitation outcome and recent developments. *Yale J Biol Med* 1998;71(5):383–389.
7. Eisendrath SJ, Matthay MA, Dunkel JA, et al. Guillain-Barre syndrome: psychosocial aspects of management. *Psychosomatics* 1983;24(5):465–475.
8. Henschel EO. The Guillain-Barre syndrome, a personal experience. *Anesthesiology* 1977;47(2):228–231.
9. Group G-BSS. Plasmapheresis and acute Guillain-Barre syndrome. The Guillain-Barre syndrome Study Group. *Neurology* 1985;35(8): 1096–1104.
10. Sater RA, Rostami A. Treatment of Guillain-Barre syndrome with intravenous immunoglobulin. *Neurology* 1998;51(6 Suppl 5): S9-15.
11. Yuki N, Ang CW, Koga M, et al. Clinical features and response to treatment in Guillain-Barre syndrome associated with antibodies to GM1b ganglioside. *Ann Neurol* 2000;47(3):314–321.
12. van der Meche FG, Schmitz PI, Dutch Guillain-Barre Study Group. A randomized trial comparing intravenous immune globulin and plasma exchange in Guillain-Barre syndrome. *N Engl J Med* 1992; 326(17):1123–1129.
13. Plasma Exchange/Sandoglobulin Guillain-Barre Syndrome Trial Group. Randomised trial of plasma exchange, intravenous immunoglobulin, and combined treatments in Guillain-Barre syndrome. *Lancet* 1997;349(9047):225–230.
14. Guillain-Barre Syndrome Steroid Trial Group. Double-blind trial of intravenous methylprednisolone in Guillain-Barre syndrome. *Lancet* 1993;341(8845):586–590.
15. Leventhal SR, Orkin FK, Hirsh RA. Prediction of the need for postoperative mechanical ventilation in myasthenia gravis. *Anesthesiology* 1980;53(1):26–30.
16. Gajdos P, Chevret S, Toyka K. Plasma exchange for myasthenia gravis. *Cochrane Database Syst Rev* 2002; Issue 4:CD002275.
17. Grob D. Acute neuromuscular disorders. *Med Clin North Am* 1981; 65(1):189–207.
18. Dau PC, Lindstrom JM, Cassel CK, et al. inventors. Plasmapheresis and immunosuppressive drug therapy in myasthenia gravis. *N Engl J Med* 1977;297(21):1134–1140.
19. Gajdos P, Chevret S, Clair B, et al. Myasthenia Gravis Clinical Study Group. Clinical trial of plasma exchange and high-dose intravenous immunoglobulin in myasthenia gravis. *Ann Neurol* 1997;41(6):789–796.
20. Mickell JJ, Oh KS, Siewers RD, et al. Clinical implications of postoperative unilateral phrenic nerve paralysis. *J Thorac Cardiovasc Surg* 1978;76(3):297–304.
21. Wilcox P, Baile EM, Hards J, et al. Phrenic nerve function and its relationship to atelectasis after coronary artery bypass surgery. *Chest* 1988;93(4):693–698.
22. Glenn WW, Hogan JF, Loke JS, et al. Ventilatory support by pacing of the conditioned diaphragm in quadriplegia. *N Engl J Med* 1984; 310(18):1150–1155.
23. Roy TM, Ossorio MA, Cipolla LM, et al. Pulmonary complications after tricyclic antidepressant overdose. *Chest* 1989;96(4): 852–856.
24. Bynum LJ, Pierce AK. Pulmonary aspiration of gastric contents. *Am Rev Respir Dis* 1976;114(6):1129–1136.
25. Rosenow EC 3rd, Limper AH. Drug-induced pulmonary disease. *Semin Respir Infect* 1995;10(2):86–95.
26. Heffner JE, Sahn SA. Salicylate-induced pulmonary edema. Clinical features and prognosis. *Ann Intern Med* 1981;95(4):405–409.
27. Picado C, Castillo JA, Montserrat JM, et al. Aspirin-intolerance as a precipitating factor of life-threatening attacks of asthma requiring mechanical ventilation. *Eur Respir J* 1989;2:127–129.
28. Krenzelok EP, McGuigan M, Lheur P. Position statement: ipecac syrup. American Academy of Clinical Toxicology; European Association of Poisons Centres and Clinical Toxicologists. *J Toxicol Clin Toxicol* 1997;35(7):699–709.
29. Vale JA, American Academy of Clinical Toxicology; European Association of Poisons Centres and Clinical Toxicologists. Position statement: gastric lavage. *J Toxicol Clin Toxicol* 1997;35(7): 711–719.
30. American Academy of Clinical Toxicology; European Association of Poisons Centres and Clinical Toxicologists. Position statement and practice guidelines on the use of multi-dose activated charcoal in the treatment of acute poisoning. *J Toxicol Clin Toxicol* 1999;37(6):731–751.
31. Mokhlesi B, Leiken JB, Murray P, et al. Adult toxicology in critical care: part I: general approach to the intoxicated patient. *Chest* 2003;123:577–592.
32. Mokhlesi B, Leikin JB, Murray P, et al. Adult toxicology in critical care: part II: specific poisonings. *Chest* 2003;123:897–922.
33. Mayberry JC, Trunkey DD. The fractured rib in chest wall trauma. *Chest Surg Clin North Am* 1997;7(2):239–261.
34. Bergofsky EH. Respiratory failure in disorders of the thoracic cage. *Am Rev Respir Dis* 1979;119(4):643–669.
35. Curtis JL, Mahlmeister M, Fink JB, et al. Helium-oxygen gas therapy. Use and availability for the emergency treatment of inoperable airway obstruction. *Chest* 1986;90(3):455–457.
36. Tami TA, Chu F, Wildes TO, et al. Pulmonary edema and acute upper airway obstruction. *Laryngoscope* 1986;96:506–509.
37. Kallet RH, Daniel BM, Gropper M, et al. Acute pulmonary edema following upper airway obstruction: case reports and brief review. *Respir Care* 1998;43:476–480.
38. Barnes PJ. Chronic obstructive pulmonary disease. *N Engl J Med* 2000;343(4):269–280.
39. Burrows B, Earle RH. Course and prognosis of chronic obstructive lung disease. A prospective study of 200 patients. *N Engl J Med* 1969;280(8):397–404.
40. Gump DW, Phillips CA, Forsyth BR, et al. Role of infection in chronic bronchitis. *Am Rev Respir Dis* 1976;113(4):465–474.
41. Sethi S, Murphy TF. Chronic obstructive pulmonary disease. *N Engl J Med* 2000;343(26):1969–1970; author reply 1970–1.
42. Wagner PD, Dantzker DR, Dueck R, et al. Ventilation-perfusion inequality in chronic obstructive pulmonary disease. *J Clin Invest* 1977;59(2):203–216.
43. Roussos C, Moxham J. Respiratory muscle fatigue. In: Macklem PT, ed. *The thorax*. New York: Marcel Dekker, 1985:829–870.
44. Roussos C. Ventilatory failure and respiratory muscle. In: Macklem PT, ed. *The thorax*. New York: Marcel Dekker, 1985:1253–1279.
45. Anthonisen NR, Cherniak RM. Ventilatory control in lung disease. In: Macklem PT, ed. *The thorax*. New York: Marcel Dekker, 1985:965–987.
46. Mountain R, Zwillich C, Weil J. Hypoventilation in obstructive lung disease. The role of familial factors. *N Engl J Med* 1978;298(10): 521–525.
47. Brodovsky D, Macdonell JA, Cherniack RM. The respiratory response to carbon dioxide in health and in emphysema. *J Clin Invest* 1960;39(5):724–729.
48. Murray J. Classification of polycythemic disorders with comments on the diagnostic value of arterial blood oxygen analysis. *Ann Intern Med* 1966;64:892–903.
49. Aubier M, Murciano D, Fournier M, et al. Central respiratory drive in acute respiratory failure of patients with chronic obstructive pulmonary disease. *Am Rev Respir Dis* 1980;122(2):191–199.
50. Conti G, Antonelli M, Navalesi P, et al. Noninvasive vs. conventional mechanical ventilation in patients with chronic obstructive

pulmonary disease after failure of medical treatment in the ward: a randomized trial. *Intensive Care Med* 2002;28(12):1701–1707.

51. Antonelli M, Conti G, Rocco M, et al. A comparison of noninvasive positive-pressure ventilation and conventional mechanical ventilation in patients with acute respiratory failure. *N Engl J Med* 1998;339(7):429–435.

52. Bott J, Carroll MP, Conway JH, et al. Randomised controlled trial of nasal ventilation in acute ventilatory failure due to chronic obstructive airways disease. *Lancet* 1993;341(8860):1555–1557.

53. Brochard L, Mancebo J, Wysocki M, et al. Noninvasive ventilation for acute exacerbations of chronic obstructive pulmonary disease. *N Engl J Med* 1995;333(13):817–822.

54. Kramer N, Meyer TJ, Meharg J, et al. Randomized, prospective trial of noninvasive positive pressure ventilation in acute respiratory failure. *Am J Respir Crit Care Med* 1995;151(6):1799–1806.

55. Plant PK, Owen JL, Elliott MW. Early use of non-invasive ventilation for acute exacerbations of chronic obstructive pulmonary disease on general respiratory wards: a multicentre randomised controlled trial. *Lancet* 2000;355(9219):1931–1935.

56. Avdeev SN, Tret'iakov AV, Grigor'iants RA, et al. Study of the use of noninvasive ventilation of the lungs in acute respiratory insufficiency due exacerbation of chronic obstructive pulmonary disease. *Anesteziol Reanimatol* 1998;(3):45–51.

57. Lightowler JV, Wedzicha JA, Elliott MW, et al. Non-invasive positive pressure ventilation to treat respiratory failure resulting from exacerbations of chronic obstructive pulmonary disease: Cochrane systematic review and meta-analysis. *Br Med J* 2003; 326(7382):185.

58. Keenan SP, Sinuff T, Cook DJ, et al. Which patients with acute exacerbation of chronic obstructive pulmonary disease benefit from noninvasive positive-pressure ventilation? A systematic review of the literature. *Ann Intern Med* 2003;138(11):861–870.

59. Ram F, Picot J, Lightowler J, et al. Non-invasive positive pressure ventilation for treatment of respiratory failure due to exacerbations of chronic obstructive pulmonary disease. *Cochrane Database Syst Rev* 2004;1:CD004104.

60. Poponick JM, Renston JP, Bennett RP, et al. Use of a ventilatory support system (BiPAP) for acute respiratory failure in the emergency department. *Chest* 1999;116(1):166–171.

61. Anton A, Guell R, Gomez J, et al. Predicting the result of noninvasive ventilation in severe acute exacerbations of patients with chronic airflow limitation. *Chest* 2000;117(3):828–833.

62. Tobin MJ. Advances in mechanical ventilation. *N Engl J Med* 2001;344:1986–1996.

63. Kilburn KH. Shock, seizures, and coma with alkalosis during mechanical ventilation. *Ann Intern Med* 1966;65(5):977–984.

64. Kassirer JP, Berkman PM, Lawrenz DR, et al. The critical role of chloride in the correction of hypokalemic alkalosis in man. *Am J Med* 1965;38:172–189.

65. Ferguson GT, Cherniack RM. Management of chronic obstructive pulmonary disease. *N Engl J Med* 1993;328(14):1017–1022.

66. Dimarco AF, Nochomovitz M, DiMarco MS, et al. Comparative effects of aminophylline on diaphragm and cardiac contractility. *Am Rev Respir Dis* 1985;132(4):800–805.

67. Rice KL, Leatherman JW, Duane PG, et al. Aminophylline for acute exacerbations of chronic obstructive pulmonary disease. A controlled trial. *Ann Intern Med* 1987;107(3):305–309.

68. Singh JM, Palda VA, Stanbrook MB, et al. Corticosteroid therapy for patients with acute exacerbations of chronic obstructive pulmonary disease: a systematic review. *Arch Intern Med* 2002; 162(22):2527–2536.

69. Albert RK, Martin TR, Lewis SW. Controlled clinical trial of methylprednisolone in patients with chronic bronchitis and acute respiratory insufficiency. *Ann Intern Med* 1980;92(6):753–758.

70. Niewoehner DE, Erbland ML, Deupree RH, et al. Department of Veterans Affairs Cooperative Study Group. Effect of systemic glucocorticoids on exacerbations of chronic obstructive pulmonary disease. *N Engl J Med* 1999;340(25):1941–1947.

71. Towes GB. Use of antibiotics in patients with chronic obstructive pulmonary disease. *Semin Respir Med* 1986;165–170.

72. Seemungal TA, Wedzicha JA. Viral infections in obstructive airway diseases. *Curr Opin Pulm Med* 2003;9(2):111–116.

73. Saint S, Bent S, Vittinghoff E, et al. Antibiotics in chronic obstructive pulmonary disease exacerbations. A meta-analysis. *JAMA* 1995;273(12):957–960.

74. Weinberger SE, Weiss JW. Weaning from ventilatory support. *N Engl J Med* 1995;332(6):388–389.

75. Ely EW, Baker AM, Dunagan DP, et al. Effect on the duration of mechanical ventilation of identifying patients capable of breathing spontaneously. *N Engl J Med* 1996;335(25):1864–1869.

76. Brochard L, Rauss A, Benito S, et al. Comparison of three methods of gradual withdrawal from ventilatory support during weaning from mechanical ventilation. *Am J Respir Crit Care Med* 1994;150(4):896–903.

77. Esteban A, Frutos F, Tobin MJ, et al. Spanish Lung Failure Collaborative Group. A comparison of four methods of weaning patients from mechanical ventilation. *N Engl J Med* 1995;332(6):345–350.

78. Esteban A, Alia I, Gordo F, et al. The Spanish Lung Failure Collaborative Group. Extubation outcome after spontaneous breathing trials with T-tube or pressure support ventilation. *Am J Respir Crit Care Med* 1997;156(2 Pt 1):459–465.

79. MacIntyre NR, Cook DJ, Ely EW Jr, et al. Evidence-based guidelines for weaning and discontinuing ventilatory support: a collective task force facilitated by the American College of Chest Physicians; the American Association for Respiratory Care; and the American College of Critical Care Medicine. *Chest* 2001;120 (6 Suppl):375S–395S.

80. Ferrer M, Esquinas A, Arancibia F, et al. Noninvasive ventilation during persistent weaning failure: a randomized controlled trial. *Am J Respir Crit Care Med* 2003;168(1):70–76.

81. Girault C, Daudenthun I, Chevron V, et al. Noninvasive ventilation as a systematic extubation and weaning technique in acute-on-chronic respiratory failure: a prospective, randomized controlled study. *Am J Respir Crit Care Med* 1999;160(1):86–92.

82. Nava S, Ambrosino N, Clini E, et al. Noninvasive mechanical ventilation in the weaning of patients with respiratory failure due to chronic obstructive pulmonary disease. A randomized, controlled trial. *Ann Intern Med* 1998;128(9):721–728.

83. Burns K, Adhikari N, Meade M. Noninvasive positive pressure ventilation as a weaning strategy for intubated adults with respiratory failure. *Cochrane Database Syst Rev* 2003;4:CD004127.

84. Beasley R. The burden of asthma with specific reference to the United States. *J Allergy Clin Immunol* 2002;109(5) Suppl:S482–S489.

85. Grant EN, Wagner R, Weiss KB. Observations on emerging patterns of asthma in our society. *J Allergy Clin Immunol* 1999;104 (2 Pt 2):S1–S9.

86. Woolcock AJ, Read J. Lung volumes in exacerbations of asthma. *Am J Med* 1966;41(2):259–273.

87. Rubinfeld AR, Wagner PD, West JB. Gas exchange during acute experimental canine asthma. *Am Rev Respir Dis* 1978;118(3):525–536.

88. Martin J, Powell E, Shore S, et al. The role of respiratory muscles in the hyperinflation of bronchial asthma. *Am Rev Respir Dis* 1980;121(3):441–447.

89. Kelsen SG, Kelsen DP, Fleeger BF, et al. Emergency room assessment and treatment of patients with acute asthma. Adequacy of the conventional approach. *Am J Med* 1978;64(4):622–628.

90. Centor RM, Yarbrough B, Wood JP. Inability to predict relapse in acute asthma. *N Engl J Med* 1984;310(9):577–580.

91. Rose CC, Murphy JG, Schwartz JS. Performance of an index predicting the response of patients with acute bronchial asthma to intensive emergency department treatment. *N Engl J Med* 1984;310(9):573–577.

92. Rebuck AS, Pengelly LD. Development of pulsus paradoxus in the presence of airways obstruction. *N Engl J Med* 1973;288(2):66–69.

93. Nowak RM, Pensler MI, Sarkar DD, et al. Comparison of peak expiratory flow and FEV1 admission criteria for acute bronchial asthma. *Ann Emerg Med* 1982;11(2):64–69.

94. Nadel JA, Tierney DF. Effect of a previous deep inspiration on airway resistance in man. *J Appl Physiol* 1961;16:717–719.

95. Tai E, Read J. Blood-gas tensions in bronchial asthma. *Lancet* 1967;1(7491):644–646.

96. Rees HA, Millar JS, Donald KW. A study of the clinical course and arterial blood gas tensions of patients in status asthmaticus. *Q J Med* 1968;37(148):541–561.

97. Fanta CH, Rossing TH, McFadden ER Jr. Emergency room of treatment of asthma. Relationships among therapeutic combinations, severity of obstruction and time course of response. *Am J Med* 1982;72:416–422.

98. Appel D, Rubenstein R, Schrager K, et al. Lactic acidosis in severe asthma. *Am J Med* 1983;75(4):580–584.

99. Molfino NA, Nannini LJ, Martelli AN, et al. Respiratory arrest in near-fatal asthma. *N Engl J Med* 1991;324:285–288.

100. FitzGerald JM, Hargreave FE. The assessment and management of acute life-threatening asthma. *Chest* 1989;95(4):888–894.

101. Tuxen DV. Permissive hypercapnic ventilation. *Am J Respir Crit Care Med* 1994;150(3):870–874.

102. Feihl F, Perret C. Permissive hypercapnia. How permissive should we be? *Am J Respir Crit Care Med* 1994;150(6 Pt 1):1722–1737.

103. Bellomo R, McLaughlin P, Tai E, et al. Asthma requiring mechanical ventilation. A low morbidity approach. *Chest* 1994;105(3):891–896.

104. Darioli R, Perret C. Mechanical controlled hypoventilation in status asthmaticus. *Am Rev Respir Dis* 1984;129(3):385–387.

105. Wolfe JD, Tashkin DP, Calvarese B, et al. Bronchodilator effects of terbutaline and aminophylline alone and in combination in asthmatic patients. *N Engl J Med* 1978;298(7):363–367.

106. Larsson S, Svedmyr N. Bronchodilating effect and side effects of beta2- adrenoceptor stimulants by different modes of administration (tablets, metered aerosol, and combinations thereof). A study with salbutamol in asthmatics. *Am Rev Respir Dis* 1977;116(5):861–869.

107. Pearlman DS, Chervinsky P, LaForce C, et al. A comparison of salmeterol with albuterol in the treatment of mild-to-moderate asthma. *N Engl J Med* 1992;327:1420–1425.

108. Rossing TH, Fanta CH, McFadden ER Jr. A controlled trial of the use of single versus combined-drug therapy in the treatment of acute episodes of asthma. *Am Rev Respir Dis* 1981;123(2):190–194.

109. Weinberger M, Hendeles L. Theophylline in asthma. *N Engl J Med* 1996;334:1380–1388.

110. King TE, Chang SW. Corticosteroids therapy in the management of asthma. *Semin Respir Med* 1987;387–399.

111. Haskell RJ, Wong BM, Hansen JE. A double-blind, randomized clinical trial of methylprednisolone in status asthmaticus. *Arch Intern Med* 1983;143(7):1324–1327.

112. Cook JL. Infection in asthma. *Semin Respir Med* 1987.

113. Lanes SF, Garrett JE, Wentworth CE III, et al. The effect of adding ipratropium bromide to salbutamol in the treatment of acute asthma: a pooled analysis of three trials. *Chest* 1998;114:365–372.

114. Rodrigo G, Rodrigo C, Burschtin O. A meta-analysis of the effects of ipratropium bromide in adults with acute asthma. *Am J Med* 1999;107(4):363–370.

115. Rodrigo G, Rodrigo C, Burschtin O. Efficacy of magnesium sulfate in acute adult asthma: a meta-analysis of randomized trials. *Am J Emerg Med* 2000;18(2):216–221.

116. Gluck EH, Onorato DJ, Castriotta R. Helium-oxygen mixtures in intubated patients with status asthmaticus and respiratory acidosis. *Chest* 1990;98(3):693–698.

117. Schaeffer EM, Pohlman A, Morgan S, et al. Oxygenation in status asthmaticus improves during ventilation with helium-oxygen. *Crit Care Med* 1999;27(12):2666–2670.

118. Rodrigo G, Pollack C, Rodrigo C, et al. Heliox for nonintubated acute asthma patients. *Cochrane Database Syst Rev* 2003;4:CD002884.

119. O'Rourke PP, Crone RK. Halothane in status asthmaticus. *Crit Care Med* 1982;10:341–343.

CHAPTER 23

Acute Hypoxemic Respiratory Failure: Pulmonary Edema and Acute Lung Injury

Lorraine B. Ware

Michael A. Matthay

PHYSIOLOGIC AND STRUCTURAL ASPECTS OF FLUID EXCHANGE IN THE LUNG

HIGH-PRESSURE (CARDIOGENIC) PULMONARY EDEMA

IMPLICATIONS FOR TREATMENT OF HIGH-PRESSURE (CARDIOGENIC) PULMONARY EDEMA

INCREASED-PERMEABILITY PULMONARY EDEMA (ACUTE LUNG INJURY AND ACUTE RESPIRATORY DISTRESS SYNDROME)

IMPLICATIONS FOR TREATMENT OF INCREASED-PERMEABILITY EDEMA AND ACUTE RESPIRATORY DISTRESS SYNDROME

This chapter considers the causes of acute respiratory failure that are primarily associated with severe hypoxemia. In most of these patients, the defect in oxygenation is due to filling of the distal air spaces of the lung with edema fluid, blood, or purulent exudate. Microatelectasis and obstruction of the pulmonary capillary bed may also contribute to the hypoxemia. The physiologic basis for the hypoxemia includes both ventilation–perfusion mismatch as well as frank right-to-left intrapulmonary shunting through poorly oxygenated, fluid-filled, or collapsed alveoli. Although alveolar filling may be caused by a variety of disorders, this chapter focuses on pulmonary edema, the most common cause of acute hypoxemic respiratory failure. Two types of pulmonary edema occur in humans: (a) high-pressure edema (usually cardiogenic) and (b) edema secondary to increased permeability of the lung microvascular endothelium and/or the alveolar epithelium (noncardiogenic). The correct diagnosis and appropriate treatment of both kinds of pulmonary edema require a good understanding of the normal

physiology of fluid exchange in the microcirculation of the lung. In addition, familiarity with the structures that surround the fluid-exchanging vessels is essential to understanding how and where edema fluid accumulates in the lung.

This discussion of pulmonary edema is divided into three sections. The first part briefly reviews transvascular fluid and protein movement in the normal lung. This section also considers the influence of the lung structure on the distribution and removal of normal and excessive quantities of fluid. The second part of the chapter describes the interstitial and alveolar phases of high-pressure (cardiogenic) pulmonary edema. The chapter concludes with experimental and clinical examples to illustrate the fundamental physiologic abnormalities that characterize increased-permeability edema. This final section also briefly reviews the common clinical disorders that have been associated with increased-permeability edema, also called acute lung injury or the acute respiratory distress syndrome (ALI/ARDS). Principles of therapy for ALI/ARDS are considered in this chapter, although the general principles for the treatment of acute respiratory failure with mechanical ventilation are discussed in Chapter 21, General Principles of Managing a Patient with Respiratory Failure, and hemodynamic assessment and management are considered in detail in Chapter 24, Thoracic Trauma, Surgery, and Perioperative Management.

PHYSIOLOGIC AND STRUCTURAL ASPECTS OF FLUID EXCHANGE IN THE LUNG

In the normal lung, as in all other organs, there is a net outward movement of fluid from the vascular to the interstitial space. This fluid is removed by lymphatics, which under normal conditions prevent excess fluid from accumulating in the interstitial space of the lung (1). The factors that determine the quantity of fluid that leaves the vascular space are included in the Starling equation for filtration of fluid across a semipermeable membrane (2). A simplified version of the equation is

$$\dot{Q} = K\left[(Pmv - Ppmv) - (\pi mv - \pi pmv)\right]$$

where $\dot{Q}$ is the net transvascular flow of fluid, K quantitatively describes the permeability of the membrane, Pmv is the hydrostatic pressure in the lumen of the microvessels, and $Ppmv$ is the hydrostatic pressure in the perimicrovascular interstitial space. The term πmv is the plasma protein osmotic pressure in the circulation and πpmv is the protein osmotic pressure in the perimicrovascular compartment. This equation is applicable to the microcirculation of the lung because normal pulmonary capillary permeability allows some water and solutes (electrolytes) to leave the circulation but restricts the movement of larger molecules such as plasma proteins. Thus, the net transvascular filtration of fluid ($\dot{Q}$) into the interstitium of the lung depends on the net difference between hydrostatic and protein osmotic pressures, as well as on the permeability of the capillary membrane.

Most evidence suggests that under normal circumstances the $Ppmv$ is close to alveolar pressure, which is approximately zero, or to atmospheric pressure (3). Thus, the main hydrostatic force for fluid filtration in the lung is the Pmv. The absolute value for hydrostatic pressure in the lung microcirculation increases from the top to the bottom of the lung (4). Hydrostatic pressure in the microvessels also varies along the length of the pre- and postcapillary vessels, depending on the resistance of the vessels (5). Hydrostatic pressure also depends on whether the vessel is in a zone 1, 2, or 3 condition. Clinically, it has generally been assumed that the average value for Pmv in the lung is roughly equal to left atrial pressure. However, some investigators have estimated that Pmv is probably closer to the sum of left atrial pressure and about 50% of the difference between mean pulmonary artery pressure and left atrial pressure (6). Thus, pulmonary artery wedge pressure measurements of left atrial pressure remain the most reliable clinical indicator of hydrostatic pressure in the microcirculation of the lung, but the precapillary or pulmonary arterial pressure may also contribute to fluid filtration under some conditions (7).

πmv is higher than πpmv and this gradient is maintained because the normal permeability of the capillary endothelial junctions allows only a small quantity of protein to flow out of the circulation into the interstitial space of the lung. Thus, the sum of protein osmotic pressures normally favors fluid absorption into the circulation and thereby partially offsets the net hydrostatic force that causes fluid to leave the vascular space. In Table 23-1, we have estimated a value for each of the Starling forces and have then calculated a value for net fluid filtration ($\dot{Q}$) that is consistent with experimental studies of transvascular fluid movement in the normal lung (8).

Most of the available evidence indicates that the primary site for fluid exchange in the lung is in the microcirculation of the alveolar vessels. Anatomically, the microvessels in humans have no media or adventitia, and thus, their walls are thinner than those of larger vessels (9). However, a number of experimental studies have shown that some liquid probably also leaks from small arterioles and venules that are located at the corners of alveolar wall junctions (10,11). Figure 23-1 shows an alveolar vessel (capillary) in the lung, surrounded by an interstitial space. In the normal lung, fluid and protein leakage is believed to occur through small gaps between these capillary endothelial cells (12,13).

Fluid that is filtered into the alveolar interstitial space normally does not enter the alveoli because the alveolar epithelium is composed of very tight junctions (Fig. 23-1) that prevent fluid and protein from entering the alveolar air spaces (13–15). Rather, once the filtered fluid enters the alveolar interstitial space, it moves proximally toward the peribronchial and perivascular space in the extraalveolar interstitium (16). Because interstitial pressure in the extraalveolar space is negative relative to the alveolar interstitial space, the loose connective tissue space acts as a sump to drain fluid from the alveolar wall interstitium (17–19). Under ordinary conditions, the lymphatics remove all the filtered fluid from the interstitium and return it to the systemic circulation (see Fig. 23-2). It has been estimated that about 10 to 20 mL of fluid per hour is filtered in the lung and removed by the lymphatics in normal humans (20).

Because surface tension in the normal alveolus is low, it is thought that surface tension has a minimal effect on interstitial pressure around alveolar vessels and, thus, has little effect on normal fluid balance in the lung. However, if surface tension

---

TABLE 23-1.   Starling Equation

$$\dot{Q} = K[(Pmv - Ppmv) - (\pi mv - \pi pmv)]$$

Transvascular fluid flow = permeability fluid flux × [hydrostatic pressure − protein osmotic pressure]. Then, substituting estimated values for the variables under normal conditions:

$$\dot{Q} = K[(10 - 0) - (25 - 19)]$$
$$\dot{Q} = K[10 - 6] = K \times 4$$

1. Net calculated transvascular fluid flow ($\dot{Q}$) is positive from the capillary lumen into the perimicrovascular interstitial space.
2. Note that the protein osmotic pressure gradient normally opposes fluid filtration out of the vessels. If the gradient were abolished, i.e., if protein osmotic pressure were assumed to be equal on both sides of the capillary, then the calculated transvascular fluid flow would more than double.
3. Also, if permeability (K) increases, there are two apparent effects: (a) transvascular fluid flux increases, even at normal hydrostatic pressures, and (b) the protein osmotic pressure difference across the capillary membrane decreases as proteins leak into the interstitium, further increasing transvascular fluid flux.

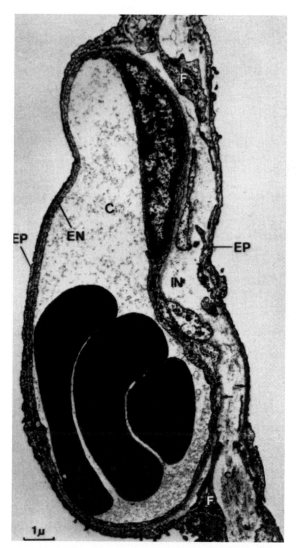

FIGURE 23-1. Electron micrograph of an alveolar capillary (*C*) cross section from human lung. Blood cells are suspended in the interalveolar septum between two alveolar spaces. The alveolar epithelium (*EP*) is the barrier that separates the air spaces from the interstitium (*IN*). The endothelium (*EN*) separates the vascular space from the interstitium. Fluid and protein exchange probably occurs through small gaps between the endothelial cells in the alveolar capillaries. Connective tissue fibers are found in the interstitium, where the basal laminae (*arrows*) of the epithelium and endothelium are separated. *F* indicates a fibroblast cell. (From Fishman AP, Renkin E. *Pulmonary edema*. Bethesda: American Physiological Society, 1979: 4, with permission.)

were high, then *P*pmv could become more negative and thereby increase the transvascular pressure gradient for movement of fluid from the alveolar vessels or the extraalveolar corner vessels into the interstitial space (Table 23-1). A deficiency of surfactant could raise surface tension and possibly favor the development of pulmonary edema (21,22). Clinically, abnormal or inactivated surfactant may contribute to the extent of pulmonary edema in some patients (23). For example, patients with ALI/ARDS have been reported to have both deficiency and inactivity of alveolar surfactant (24).

In summary, there is a constant flow of fluid through the interstitium of the lungs. Small amounts of fluid leak from the alveolar and some extra-alveolar vessels into the perimicrovascular interstitial space. This fluid does not enter the alveolar

space because of the high resistance of the normally tight alveolar epithelium. The filtered fluid moves to the extra-alveolar interstitial space, where lymphatics remove it from the lung.

For experimental purposes, lung lymph of some species (e.g., sheep, goats, or dogs) can be collected to study the normal physiology of fluid and protein balance in the lung as well as to learn how the lung responds to pathologic conditions (8,16). The quantity of lung lymph flow can be used to estimate the quantity of fluid leaving the vascular space in the lung; the protein concentration of the lymph can be measured to determine the amount of protein leaving the microcirculation and, thereby, to evaluate the permeability of the pulmonary microvascular barrier (25). A number of investigators have studied lung lymph flow in animal models in an effort to better understand the pathogenesis of the various kinds of pulmonary edema (26–28).

As stated, pulmonary edema is caused by high pressure, increased permeability, or both. In the next section, high-pressure edema is examined, with an emphasis on correlating the clinical features with the physiologic abnormalities.

HIGH-PRESSURE (CARDIOGENIC) PULMONARY EDEMA

According to the Starling equation, when hydrostatic pressure increases in the microcirculation, the rate of transvascular fluid filtration increases. The clinical counterpart of this physiologic principle occurs in humans when there is a rise in left atrial pressure, usually as a result of left ventricular failure. This increased left atrial pressure is transmitted to the microcirculation of the lung, resulting in an increase in transvascular fluid flow into the interstitium of the lung. With a small increase in left atrial pressure (to 14 to 20 mm Hg), most patients experience only a mild degree of dyspnea. The chest radiograph usually demonstrates prominent interlobular septae (Kerley B lines) consistent with pulmonary edema confined to the interstitium (see Fig. 23-3). Histologically, mild elevations of left atrial pressure lead to interstitial edema in the alveolar septa and in the extraalveolar spaces in the loose connective tissue around the bronchovascular sheath. Figure 23-4 illustrates the prominent perivascular fluid cuffs in this phase of interstitial pulmonary edema.

As left atrial pressure acutely rises above 25 to 30 mm Hg, the capacity of the interstitial space in the lung and the pumping ability of the lymphatics to clear fluid are usually exceeded, and the edema fluid breaks through the alveolar epithelium and begins to flood the alveolar air spaces (1). The development of arterial hypoxemia has been shown experimentally to correlate with alveolar flooding (29).

High-pressure cardiogenic edema has been well studied in experimental animals by using samples of lung lymph to quantify the amount of fluid leaving the vascular space and the protein content of that fluid (8,16). As left atrial pressure is increased by placing an inflatable balloon in the left atrium, lung lymph flow rises and the concentration of protein declines (see Fig. 23-5). This indicates, as the Starling equation predicts, that transvascular flow of water and solutes into the interstitium of the lung is increasing. Because the permeability of the capillary endothelium remains normal, the fluid leaving the circulation has a low protein content, resulting in a fall in the lymph:plasma protein ratio.

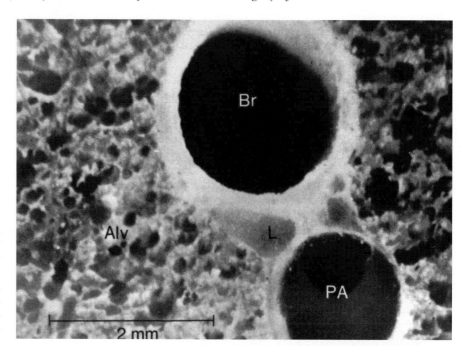

FIGURE 23-2. A photomicrograph from a sheep lung frozen at normal inflation pressure. The bronchus (*Br*), lymphatic (*L*), and partially blood-filled pulmonary artery (*PA*) are surrounded by loose connective tissue. This is the extraalveolar interstitial space. The alveolar ducts and alveoli (*Alv*) surround the bronchovascular sheath. The lymphatics drain fluid that is filtered from the capillaries and return this fluid to the systemic circulation.

During the early, interstitial phase of high-pressure pulmonary edema, the lung has at least three safety factors that function to protect against alveolar flooding. The first safety factor is an increase in lung lymph flow, clearing some of the edema fluid from the interstitium. The second factor is a fall in the concentration of protein in the perimicrovascular interstitial space because of an increase in water and solutes entering the interstitial space surrounding the alveolar vessels. This decrease in perimicrovascular protein concentration leads to an increase in the protein osmotic pressure difference between the plasma and the interstitial fluid (πmv – πpmv). This results in

an increased protein osmotic force that absorbs fluid back into the circulation. It has been estimated that this increased protein osmotic pressure difference offsets about 50% of the rise in transvascular fluid filtration that can occur from a rise in hydrostatic pressure alone (16). In fact, patients with low plasma protein concentrations are likely to develop clinical pulmonary edema at lower levels of left atrial pressure elevation than those with normal plasma protein concentrations (30). The third safety factor against alveolar flooding is the capacity of the interstitial space in the lung to accommodate approximately 500 mL of edema fluid in the bronchovascular cuffs (Fig. 23-4) (16).

When the capacity of the interstitial space is exceeded, the interstitial edema fluid moves through the visceral pleura and causes pleural effusions (31,32). These effusions are primarily related to the elevation of left atrial pressure and to the magnitude of pulmonary edema, as demonstrated by studies in patients with congestive heart failure (32,33) or by experimental studies of hydrostatic pulmonary edema (34) or increased-permeability pulmonary edema (35).

When the capacity of the interstitial space is exceeded, the edema fluid also breaks through the alveolar epithelium and fills the air spaces by bulk flow. Samples of edema fluid in experimental animals have demonstrated that the initial sample of high-pressure, cardiogenic pulmonary edema flow is low in protein content relative to the plasma protein (25). Sampling of undiluted alveolar fluid using a tracheal suction catheter wedged in a distal airway is a useful diagnostic test to separate patients with high-pressure pulmonary edema from those with an increased-permeability edema. Patients with high-pressure edema have an alveolar fluid:plasma protein ratio of less than 65%, whereas patients with increased permeability have an alveolar fluid:plasma protein ratio of 75% or greater, provided the edema fluid is sampled before alveolar fluid reabsorption has begun (36–39).

Both *in vivo* and *in vitro* work have shown that resolution or clearance of edema from the air spaces of the lung depends on active sodium transport across the alveolar epithelial barrier. The primary site of sodium reabsorption is through epithelial

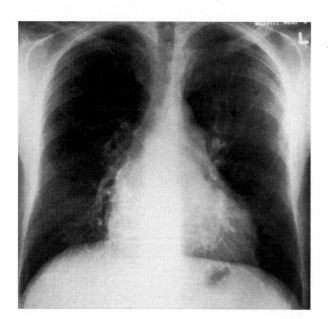

FIGURE 23-3. A posteroanterior chest radiograph from a patient with interstitial pulmonary edema secondary to left ventricular heart failure. Pulmonary capillary wedge pressure was measured at 20 mm Hg. Note the prominent vascular markings in the left upper lobe and the Kerley B lines in the right lower lobe that indicate fluid-filled interlobular septae.

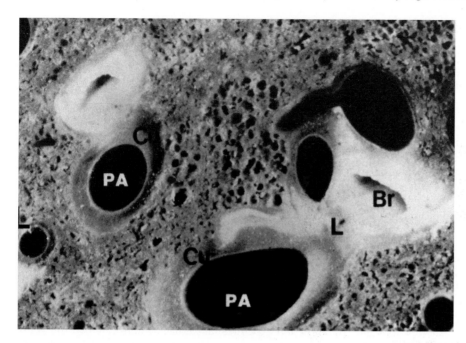

FIGURE 23-4. Photograph of a frozen sheep lung. In this experimental study, left atrial pressure was elevated to 20 cm H₂O for 4 hours. The result is interstitial pulmonary edema with perivascular fluid cuffs (*Cu*) around pulmonary arteries (*PA*) and small airways (*Br*). There are some lymphatics (*L*) visible in the fluid cuffs also.

sodium channels located on the apical membrane of alveolar epithelial type II cells (40–42). Sodium is then actively extruded into the interstitial space via the Na, K-ATPase located on the basolateral membrane of type II cells. Water flows passively, predominantly through water channels, the aquaporins, found on alveolar epithelial type I cells (43,44). Alveolar

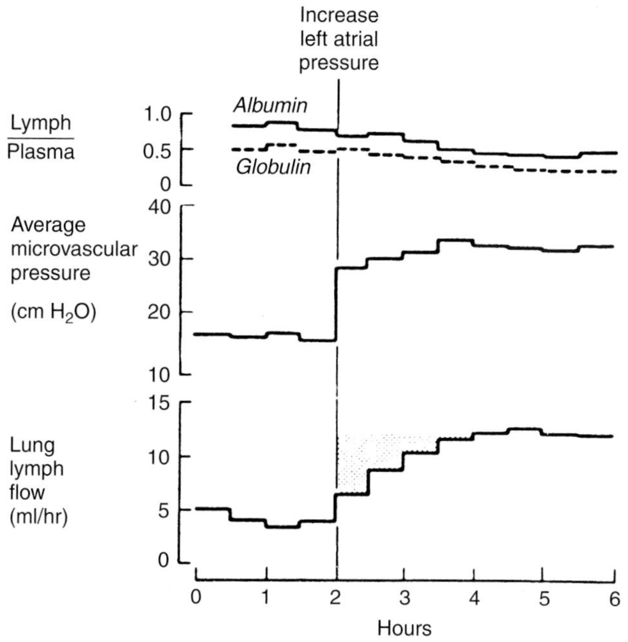

FIGURE 23-5. The time course of a sheep experiment in which left atrial pressure was elevated after a 2-hour stable baseline period. Note that with left atrial hypertension, the lung lymph flow rises sharply and the lymph:plasma protein concentrations fall. This is typical of high-pressure pulmonary edema. (From Erdmann AJ III, Vaughn TR, Brigham KL, et al. Effect of increased vascular pressure on lung fluid balance in unanesthetized sheep. *Circ Res* 1975;37:271–284, The American Heart Association, Inc., with permission.)

fluid is removed even in the face of a rising alveolar edema protein concentration in excess of the plasma protein concentration (45–48). Interestingly, in experimental studies in a variety of species including humans, β-adrenergic agonist therapy is found to increase sodium transport, resulting in a marked increase in the clearance of alveolar liquid (49–56).

Clinically, high-pressure cardiogenic edema is the most common form of pulmonary edema. Measurement of elevated pulmonary arterial wedge pressures with a pulmonary artery catheter helps to confirm that the pulmonary edema is due to high pressure when the etiology of the pulmonary edema cannot be established on clinical grounds alone (57–59). The use of noninvasive techniques such as two-dimensional echocardiography to measure left ventricular contractility and ejection fraction is also extremely helpful. The underlying cause is usually left ventricular failure from ischemic heart disease, aortic or mitral valve disease, diastolic dysfunction, or a cardiomyopathy. Occasionally, patients with normal cardiac function develop high-pressure pulmonary edema from volume overload. In addition, some noncardiogenic causes of pulmonary edema may be complicated by an element of high pressure in the pulmonary circulation (60).

IMPLICATIONS FOR TREATMENT OF HIGH-PRESSURE (CARDIOGENIC) PULMONARY EDEMA

Effective therapy for high-pressure pulmonary edema depends on lowering left atrial pressure and, thus, decreasing the driving force (Pmv − Ppmv) responsible for increased filtration of fluid into the extravascular space. A reduction in left atrial filling pressure (preload) can be accomplished by decreasing venous filling of the heart. Osler's classic method for treatment of cardiogenic pulmonary edema is based on this principle of decreasing venous return to the heart by making the patient sit in the upright position and using rotating tourniquets on the extremities to impede blood return to the heart (61).

For more than 50 years, morphine sulfate has been known to be effective in treating cardiogenic pulmonary edema. Part of the beneficial effect of morphine depends on a reduction in preload to the heart because of systemic venodilation (62). Venodilators such as sublingual, topical, or intravenous nitroglycerin are also effective in reducing venous return and left ventricular preload (63). More potent agents such as sodium nitroprusside can rapidly decrease venous return (64). Nitroprusside also reduces systemic blood pressure, reducing the afterload (resistance) on the left ventricle, which may result in better cardiac function with a subsequent lowering of left atrial filling pressures, particularly if cardiac insufficiency is complicated by systemic hypertension (65). Potent diuretics such as furosemide are a mainstay of therapy, and they lower left atrial filling pressure by decreasing systemic venous tone (when given intravenously) and by inducing diuresis of the expanded extracellular volume (63,66). Newer vasodilating agents are under investigation, including endothelin receptor antagonists and nesiritide (brain natriuretic peptide) (67). Nesiritide is an endogenous neurohormone that functions as both an arterial and venous vasodilator. Initial clinical trials with intravenous nesiritide in acutely decompensated congestive heart failure have been encouraging, but more extensive clinical trials are needed to better define its role (68).

Finally, agents that improve myocardial contractility can lower cardiac filling pressures. Acutely, this can be accomplished with inotropic vasopressors such as dopamine or dobutamine given in low doses (69,70). Phosphodiesterase inhibitors such as milrinone have both vasodilating and inotropic properties. Milrinone may be useful in selected patients, but caution is warranted because it may produce significant tachycardia and ventricular arrhythmias (67). In patients with chronic congestive heart failure and pulmonary congestion, digitalis augments myocardial contractility and thereby decreases left atrial and left ventricular filling pressures (71).

Patients with acute cardiogenic pulmonary edema and severe respiratory distress often generate very negative pleural pressures in an effort to maintain adequate alveolar ventilation. These negative pleural pressures may increase left ventricular transmural pressure and thus increase left ventricular afterload (72). Patients with acute pulmonary edema also are more susceptible to respiratory muscle fatigue (73,74). It is not surprising, therefore, that some patients with acute cardiogenic pulmonary edema develop refractory hypoxemia and hypercapnia even with adequate supplemental oxygen and appropriate pharmacologic therapy. These more seriously ill patients usually require endotracheal intubation and positive-pressure mechanical ventilation to achieve adequate arterial oxygenation and adequate alveolar ventilation, although recently, some patients have been treated successfully with noninvasive positive-pressure ventilation (see Chapter 21, General Principles of Managing a Patient with Respiratory Failure). Institution of positive-pressure ventilation in patients with acute cardiogenic pulmonary edema usually results in prompt improvement in oxygenation and sometimes in cardiac output as well. The improved oxygenation is due to better lung inflation with improved matching of ventilation and perfusion. An improvement in left ventricular function may occur because of at least four possible factors: (a) improved arterial oxygen saturation and hence better myocardial oxygen supply, (b) reduction in the extreme pleural pressure swings that present with spontaneous ventilation and hence reduction in afterload on the left ventricle, (c) less workload on the failing heart because the work of breathing (and the oxygen needed to perform it) has been assumed by a mechanical ventilator, and (d) reduction in atrial filling pressure (preload) because positive-pressure ventilation decreases venous return to the heart.

INCREASED-PERMEABILITY PULMONARY EDEMA (ACUTE LUNG INJURY AND ACUTE RESPIRATORY DISTRESS SYNDROME)

The Starling equation predicts that a change in permeability of the microvascular membrane (K) will result in a marked increase in the amount of fluid and protein leaving the vascular space. Pulmonary edema of this type should have a high protein content because a more permeable vascular membrane does not have a normal capacity to restrict the outward movement of larger molecules such as plasma proteins. Results of clinical and experimental studies demonstrate that this is exactly what happens in most types of noncardiogenic pulmonary edema (26,27,47,75,76).

Increased-permeability pulmonary edema usually develops in the setting of an ALI. The ALI syndrome of poor oxygenation, dense pulmonary infiltrates, and decreased lung compliance was first described by Petty and Ashbaugh in 1971 and was termed the adult respiratory distress syndrome (77). A more specific definition that requires quantitative scoring of the physiologic and radiographic abnormalities to determine whether the ALI is mild, moderate, or severe ARDS was proposed in 1988 (78). This lung injury score also takes into account the presence or absence of nonpulmonary organ failure and the associated clinical disorder because prognosis depends on these factors as well as on the extent of ALI (79,80). In 1994, American–European Consensus Conference proposed a simplified definition for what is now termed the acute (rather than adult) respiratory distress syndrome (81). Using this definition, ARDS is defined as the acute onset of bilateral infiltrates indistinguishable from cardiogenic pulmonary edema, with a ratio of arterial oxygen to fraction of inspired oxygen (Po_2:Fio_2 ratio) of <200 and no clinical evidence of left atrial hypertension. A less severe form of ARDS, termed ALI, was defined similarly to ARDS but with a Po_2:Fio_2 ratio of <300. These new consensus definitions for ALI and ARDS are widely used and have improved standardization of clinical trials. However, they fail to take into account the underlying cause of ALI and the presence or absence of multiorgan failure, both of which can influence outcome (82–86).

The list of clinical disorders associated with the development of ALI/ARDS is impressively long (see Table 23-2) (87–89). The ALI can occur via either the blood (i.e., sepsis or fat embolism) or the airways (i.e., liquid aspiration or pulmonary infections). In some clinical disorders, such as drug overdose or acute pancreatitis, the route of lung injury is not known. Because of this heterogeneity of causes and clinical manifestations of ALI/ARDS and the lack of standardized definitions prior to 1994, the incidence of ALI/ARDS has been difficult to quantify. A recent epidemiologic study from 20 hospitals in the National Institutes of

TABLE 23-2. Clinical Disorders Associated with Adult Respiratory Distress Syndrome (ARDS)

Sepsis
Trauma
    Fat emboli
    Lung contusion
    Nonthoracic trauma
Liquid aspiration
    Gastric contents
    Fresh and salt water (drowning)
    Hydrocarbon fluids
Drug-associated disorders
    Heroin
    Methadone
    Propoxyphene
    Barbiturates
    Colchicine
    Ethchlorvynol
    Aspirin
    Hydrochlorothiazide
Inhaled toxins
    Smoke
    Oxygen (high concentration)
    Corrosive chemicals
    (e.g., NO_2, Cl_2, NH_3, and phosgene)
Shock of any etiology
Hematologic disorders
    Massive blood transfusion
    Disseminated intravascular coagulation
Metabolic
    Acute pancreatitis
    Uremia
Miscellaneous
    Lymphangiography
    Reexpansion pulmonary edema
    Increased intracranial pressure
    Postcardiopulmonary bypass
    Eclampsia
    Air emboli
    Amniotic fluid embolism
    Ascent to high altitude
Primary pneumonias
    Viral
    Bacterial
    Mycobacterium
    Tuberculosis
    Fungal
    Pneumocystis carinii

Health (NIH) ARDS Network utilizing the American–European Consensus Conference definitions of ALI and ARDS estimated a yearly incidence of ALI/ARDS in the United States to be 64.2 cases per 100,000 population, higher than the previously estimated value (90).

Mortality in ALI/ARDS has been exceedingly high, from 50% to 70%, partly because of associated multiorgan failure as well as uncontrolled or recurrent infection (79,82,83,86). Two recent studies suggest that mortality from ALI/ARDS may be declining (91,92). The reasons for this decline are unclear but are perhaps related to better supportive care of critically ill patients or better management of sepsis. Although the lung appears to be the primary target organ for failure in ALI/ARDS, a number of studies have shown that mortality in ALI/ARDS is closely related to multiorgan failure, uncontrolled infection, and chronic medical diseases such as liver failure that are associated with ALI/ARDS (78–80,93). In fact, mortality seems to be directly caused by respiratory failure alone in <20% of ARDS cases, although most patients die with severe respiratory failure (79). Sepsis appears to be the most important cause of both early and late mortality (79,93).

The principal clinical manifestations of ALI/ARDS are similar, regardless of what the associated clinical condition may be. The typical findings are (a) severe hypoxemia that is unresponsive to low-flow oxygen and due to intrapulmonary right-to-left shunting of blood through fluid-filled and atelectatic alveoli (94); (b) bilateral, fluffy infiltrates on the chest radiograph, indistinguishable from cardiogenic pulmonary edema (see Fig. 23-6); and (c) a decrease in the static lung compliance. Clinically, this change in the mechanical properties of the lungs is manifested by the high ventilatory pressures that are required to deliver an adequate tidal volume. Pulmonary dead-space fraction is also increased and higher levels correlate with worse outcomes (95).

In the acute phase of increased-permeability pulmonary edema and respiratory failure, the densities on the chest radiograph result from a combination of interstitial and alveolar edema and a variable degree of atelectasis. Typically, the lung volumes are reduced because of a change in the mechanical properties of the lung. A reduction in vital capacity and functional residual capacity and an increase in lung compliance occur for three main reasons: (a) edema fluid in the air spaces displaces air, decreasing gas volumes; (b) edema in peribronchovascular interstitial spaces causes airways to narrow down or close, which results in atelectasis (Fig. 23-4); and (c) there may be a reduction in surfactant (secondary to alveolar epithelial injury), which could increase surface tension and thereby decrease lung compliance (23,24,96).

Histologically, in this acute phase of lung injury, there is widespread interstitial and alveolar edema, with an abundance of polymorphonuclear leukocytes, erythrocytes, macrophages, cell debris, plasma proteins, and strands of fibrin. Electron microscopy studies have shown injury to the capillary endothelium and denuding of the alveolar epithelium (see Fig. 23-7) (21). If the patient survives the acute phase of the lung injury, the pulmonary edema may resolve and the patient may completely recover normal lung function over a few months (97,98).

However, some patients with ALI/ARDS progress to a subacute phase over 7 to 14 days, during which time they still require mechanical ventilation with high airway pressures and high fractions of inspired oxygen and may have worsening pulmonary hypertension (see Fig. 23-8) (99). These patients develop fibrosis and capillary obliteration in the lungs, a condition which is termed *fibrosing alveolitis* (21,100). It is not clear why in some patients the injured lungs are successfully repaired and they recover, whereas progressive fibrosis and even bullae develop in the lungs of others (see Fig. 23-9). The development of fibrosis and the resultant reduced lung compliance predispose patients to develop barotrauma, which may manifest as pneumothoraces, pneumomediastinum, and subcutaneous emphysema (see Fig. 23-10) (101,102). However, barotrauma may also occur early and is associated with higher levels of positive endexpiratory pressure (PEEP) (103). The role of secondary lung injury from oxygen toxicity has been difficult to quantify experimentally or even to estimate clinically (100,104,105).

Numerous experimental and clinical studies have been done during the last 15 years to determine the mechanisms of ALI in noncardiogenic pulmonary edema. Because many disorders are associated with ARDS, the cause of the increased-permeability

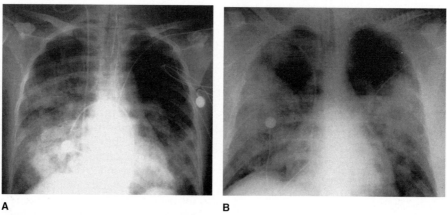

A   **B**

FIGURE 23-6. **A:** Anteroposterior chest radiograph from a 40-year-old man with acute respiratory failure from gastric aspiration. Note that the endotracheal tube is in good position. The pulmonary artery line, inserted through the right internal jugular vein, passes through the superior vena cava, right atrium, right ventricle, and main pulmonary artery and terminates in a branch of pulmonary artery in the right lower lobe. The wedge pressure was 2 mm Hg. The radiographic pattern indicates a typical location for pulmonary aspiration into dependent segments of the left lower lobe, right lower lobe, and right upper lobe. Before tracheal intubation, this patient's PaO_2 was 55 mm Hg on an FIO_2 of 0.9. The fluffy bilateral infiltrates progressed to involve all lung zones within 3 days. However, the patient ultimately recovered after 2 weeks of treatment with antibiotics and mechanical ventilation with positive end-expiratory pressure (PEEP). **B:** Anteroposterior chest radiograph from a 55-year-old man who developed noncardiogenic pulmonary edema from gram-negative sepsis. The pulmonary artery line was inserted through the right subclavian vein and terminated in a posterior branch (visible on a lateral chest film) of the right pulmonary artery. The cardiac silhouette appears slightly enlarged, but the wedge pressure was 4 mm Hg and the cardiac output was high (consistent with sepsis). The PaO_2 was 45 mm Hg on an FIO_2 of 0.90 prior to ventilation with positive pressure. The patient's acute respiratory failure and sepsis were successfully treated and the FIO_2 was lowered to 0.50 with 15 cm H_2O of PEEP within 2 days. Subsequently, the patient did not improve, and he ultimately developed recurrent sepsis and died with severe adult respiratory distress syndrome (ARDS).

edema may depend on the specific associated etiology. For example, neutrophils have been implicated as a major factor in lung injury from sepsis and microembolism (106,107). Complement activation in sepsis may play a role in activating white blood cells (WBC) to release toxic enzymes (e.g., proteases) that could increase endothelial permeability in the lung (108). One study showed that neutrophil elastolytic activity in air spaces is very high in 50% of ARDS patients (109). However, some investigators have shown that neither WBC nor complement is necessary for some kinds of permeability pulmonary edema (110,111). Also, other investigators have implicated the fibrinogen and coagulation system in the pathogenesis of ALI (112–114). The possible role of proinflammatory cytokines, such as tumor necrosis factor, interleukin-1, or interleukin-8, in mediating pulmonary and systemic lung injury from sepsis has been studied in experimental and clinical studies (107,115,116). Recently, the role of oxidants in mediating ALI has also been explored. There are several reviews that summarize much of the progress that has been made in unraveling the mechanisms of ALI (87,117,118). Further research in the next few years will probably result in more specific information about the basic causes of ALI.

The process by which basic pathogenetic research can be translated to clinical therapies is well illustrated by the concept of ventilator-induced lung injury (119). Experimental studies have demonstrated that mechanical ventilation at high volumes and pressures injures the lung (120) causing increased-permeability pulmonary edema in the uninjured lung (121,122) and enhanced edema formation in the injured lung (123,124). These deleterious effects were initially thought to be due to

capillary stress failure from alveolar overdistension. Recently, however, cyclic opening and closing of atelectatic alveoli during mechanical ventilation has been recognized as causing lung injury independent of alveolar overdistension. Alveolar overdistension coupled with the repeated collapse and reopening of alveoli can actually initiate a proinflammatory cytokine cascade, a phenomenon that has been observed both experimentally (125) and clinically (126). The experimental description of ventilator-induced lung injury has led directly to clinical trials of protective ventilatory strategies designed to prevent alveolar overdistension and alveolar collapse and to prevent the superimposition of ventilator-associated lung injury on pre-existing ALI or ARDS and has fundamentally altered the treatment of patients with ALI/ARDS. Strategies for mechanical ventilation in ALI/ARDS are further discussed under the section "Implications for Treatment of Increased-Permeability Edema and Acute Respiratory Distress Syndrome."

An in-depth discussion of each of the associated causes of ALI/ARDS is not possible in this chapter. However, two of the most common clinical disorders associated with the development of ARDS, gastric aspiration and sepsis, are considered below.

The acute respiratory failure that can follow gastric aspiration is a good example of ALI/ARDS resulting from direct injury to the alveolar epithelium and air spaces of the lung (Fig. 23-6A). Aspiration of gastric contents injures the lung if the pH is <2.5, even if the volume of aspirated fluid is as small as 50 mL (127). The aspirated, acidic fluid acutely causes an increase in the permeability of the alveolar epithelium and a rapid development of pulmonary edema (128).

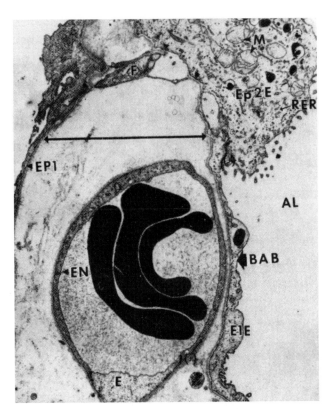

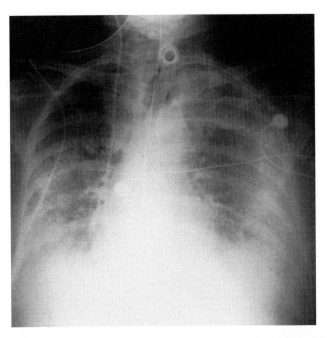

FIGURE 23-7. Electron micrograph of an alveolar capillary in the interalveolar septum between alveolar spaces (*AL*) from a patient with adult respiratory distress syndrome (ARDS). The interstitial space is widened by edema fluid (*arrows*), and the capillary endothelium has normal areas (*EN*) and swollen, abnormal areas (*E*). Some of the alveolar epithelium is normal (*EP1*), whereas other type 1 and 2 cells are swollen (*E1E* and *Ep2E*). The damaged type 2 cell shows degenerative features with swollen mitochondria (*M*) and degranulating rough endoplasmic reticulum (*RER*). There is a fibrocyte (*F*) that anchors the epithelial basement membrane. (From Fishman AP, Renkin E. *Pulmonary edema.* Bethesda: American Physiological Society, 1979:103, with permission.)

FIGURE 23-8. Anteroposterior chest radiograph of a 42-year-old woman being ventilated through a cuffed tracheostomy tube. Her respiratory failure had begun 3 weeks previously when she developed adult respiratory distress syndrome (ARDS) from severe acute pancreatitis. Note the diffuse ground-glass appearance of the lung fields. At this point in her clinical course, she had noncompliant lungs that required very high airway pressures to provide an adequate tidal volume. She died of persistent respiratory failure 1 week after this chest radiograph was taken. Postmortem examination of the lungs revealed extensive interstitial fibrosis and hyaline membranes.

The severe hypoxemia that occurs after massive gastric aspiration has been attributed to a combination of pulmonary edema and the atelectasis resulting from alterations of surfactant activity and subsequent closure of small airways (129). In fact, mortality in patients with ALI/ARDS secondary to gastric aspiration can be predicted in part by the severity of the arterial hypoxemia in relation to the alveolar oxygen tension (the $Pa_{O_2}:PA_{O_2}$ ratio). If the $Pa_{O_2}:PA_{O_2}$ ratio is < 0.50 immediately after gastric aspiration, the mortality rate is 50% as compared with 14% in patients with a ratio of > 0.50 (130). The ultimate outcome in patients with ALI/ARDS from gastric aspiration is also influenced by the delayed development of secondary bacterial lung infections with aerobic and anaerobic bacteria (131).

Whereas massive gastric aspiration is a good illustration of acute respiratory failure from direct injury to the alveolar epithelium, systemic sepsis is an example of ALI/ARDS that develops from injury to the endothelium of the pulmonary microcirculation (Fig. 23-6B). Clinical studies have shown that ALI develops in about 60% of patients with sepsis syndrome, and about 25% to 35% of these patients develop severe ALI/ARDS (132,133). The mortality from ARDS secondary to sepsis ranges from 60% to 90% (133).

Studies in experimental animals have provided important information about the early phase of ALI from sepsis. Brigham

et al. (26,134,135) demonstrated that when sheep are given either *Pseudomonas* organisms or *Escherichia coli* endotoxin intravenously, lung lymph flow increases markedly. In these studies, the increase in lymph flow is associated with a high lymph:plasma protein ratio and a dramatic rise in lymph protein transport (see Fig. 23-11). The increased lung lymph flow cannot be accounted for exclusively by a change in hydrostatic or protein osmotic pressures in the microcirculation of the lung and, therefore, must be due partly to an increase in lung vascular permeability. Histologic examination of the sheep lungs in this early phase shows interstitial edema with perivascular fluid cuffs, as seen in the interstitial phase of high-pressure pulmonary edema (Fig. 23-4). In the next phase of pulmonary edema, the edema fluid floods into the air spaces, although recent experimental studies have shown that the alveolar epithelium is more resistant than the lung endothelium to the injurious effects of *E. coli* endotoxin (26,134,135).

Clinically, the early phase of increased-permeability pulmonary edema from sepsis with interstitial edema is often not recognized (12). This is partly due to the lack of sensitive clinical indicators of a mild increase in extravascular lung water. The chest radiograph, for example, may not show edema until there is a 30% increase in lung water content (136,137). Also, major arterial blood gas abnormalities do not usually develop until edema fluid enters the air spaces, when there is a dramatic decrease in arterial oxygenation secondary to both ventilation–perfusion mismatch and right-to-left shunting of blood through fluid-filled alveoli (29,94).

Clinical studies of patients with increased-permeability pulmonary edema from sepsis have shown that the pulmonary

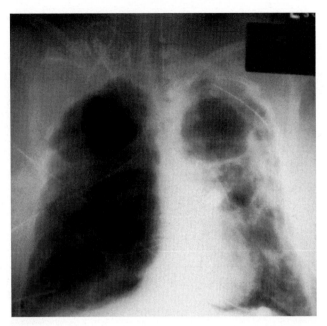

FIGURE 23-9. Anteroposterior chest radiograph of a 36-year-old woman who had developed adult respiratory distress syndrome (ARDS) from gram-negative sepsis 6 weeks prior to this chest film. Her clinical course was characterized by persistent respiratory failure and ventilator dependence. Her chest radiograph initially showed noncardiogenic pulmonary edema with fluffy infiltrates (as in Fig. 23-6B). About 2 weeks following the development of ARDS from sepsis, her chest radiograph showed a diffuse ground-glass appearance (as in Fig. 23-6) and her lungs became very noncompliant. Finally, 5 weeks following the onset of ARDS, she developed bilateral bullae in the upper and lower lung zones and required multiple chest tubes to drain recurrent pneumothoraces. She died 2 days after this chest film was taken. At postmortem examination, her lungs showed large bullae with extensive loss of lung tissue. She had no prior history of smoking and her chest film was normal prior to the onset of sepsis and ARDS.

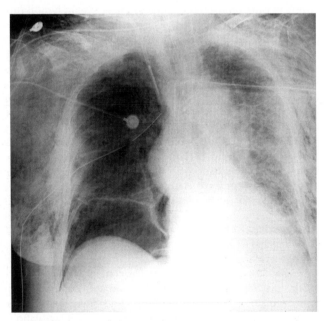

FIGURE 23-10. Anteroposterior chest radiograph of a 42-year-old woman who developed severe adult respiratory distress syndrome (ARDS) from aspiration of gastric contents. This radiograph was taken 10 days into her course. Note the severe barotrauma with bilateral chest tubes, pneumomediastinum, and severe subcutaneous emphysema.

edema fluid has a high protein concentration (75% to 100%) compared to the plasma protein level (36,37,47,76,138). In addition, measurements of cardiac filling pressures with a pulmonary artery catheter usually demonstrate normal or even low pressures (75). Both these findings further support the concept that pulmonary edema from sepsis occurs because of an increase in permeability of the vascular endothelium and perhaps the alveolar epithelium as well.

IMPLICATIONS FOR TREATMENT OF INCREASED-PERMEABILITY EDEMA AND ACUTE RESPIRATORY DISTRESS SYNDROME

Ideal treatment for patients with increased-permeability edema would be an agent that could restore the abnormal vascular permeability of the pulmonary microcirculation and the alveolar epithelium to its normal state. This would prevent additional leakage of protein-rich fluid into the interstitium and alveoli of the lung. Unfortunately, no such agent is available at present. Although corticosteroids and antioxidant agents have been shown experimentally to modestly ameliorate ALI if they are given before or immediately after the injury occurs, clinical studies have demonstrated no benefit of glucocorticoids or antioxidants for treatment of sepsis-induced ARDS (139).

At present, the best therapeutic approach for ARDS is to identify and treat, if possible, the precipitating cause of the acute respiratory failure. The most treatable causes of ARDS are sepsis, respiratory infections, and shock. In many cases, such as smoke inhalation, trauma, and gastric aspiration, the injury has already occurred when the patient is first seen. In other cases, such as acute pancreatitis or viral pneumonia, the cause of the ARDS cannot be easily controlled. Supportive care for patients with ALI/ARDS is also critically important and should include adequate nutrition, identification, treatment and prevention of nosocomial infection, and prevention of thromboemboli and gastrointestinal bleeding (139,140).

The diagnosis of noncardiogenic pulmonary edema may need to be confirmed by measuring the vascular filling pressures in the pulmonary circulation to be certain that the pulmonary edema is not of cardiogenic origin (58). A pulmonary arterial catheter can be passed percutaneously into the pulmonary artery via the internal jugular, subclavian, femoral, or antecubital vein. The pulmonary artery wedge pressure usually reflects the left atrial filling pressure. Normal or low pressures (<12 mm Hg) indicate that the pulmonary edema is from a noncardiogenic cause. Occasionally, patients with pulmonary edema primarily due to increased permeability also have an element of fluid overload with mildly elevated wedge pressures (140). As the Starling equation predicts, an increase in hydrostatic pressure (Pmv) in the face of increased vascular permeability (K) will result in an exponential rise in transvascular fluid flux (20,140–142). These patients may benefit from treatment (such as diuretics) that decreases left atrial filling pressures to a normal range.

Because most patients with ARDS have severe pulmonary edema and poorly compliant lungs, they usually experience respiratory muscle fatigue from the hypoxemia and the increased work of breathing. Mechanical ventilation with positive pressure is usually necessary to improve oxygenation

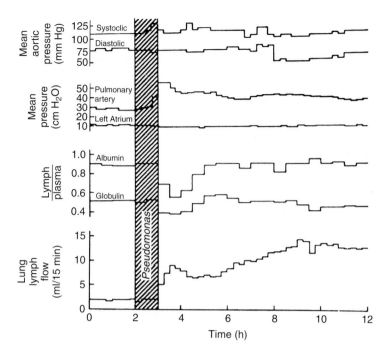

FIGURE 23-11. Effects of infusion of *Pseudomonas aeruginosa* on lung vascular pressures, lymph flow, and lymph:plasma protein concentration in an unanesthetized sheep. Note that the lymph flow rises steeply several hours after the infusion of *Pseudomonas* organism, indicating that the capillary leak of protein-rich fluid occurs a few hours after the septic insult. (From Brigham KL, Woolverton WC, Blake LH, et al. Increased sheep lung vascular permeability caused by Pseudomonas bacteria. *J Clin Invest* 1974;54:792–804, with copyright permission of the American Society for Clinical Investigation.)

and stabilize alveolar ventilation in patients with ARDS. The appropriate mode of mechanical ventilation for patients with ALI/ARDS has been controversial since the syndrome was first described. In the past, high tidal volumes of 12 to 15 mL per kg were routinely advocated to maintain normal levels of alveolar ventilation in the setting of decreased lung compliance. However, experimental evidence has been accumulating to suggest that ventilation with high tidal volumes and pressures may be injurious to the lung and may worsen or prolong a preexisting lung injury (123,143,144). For this reason, several clinical trials of low tidal volume ventilation for ALI/ARDS have recently been completed. Although initial small trials were discouraging (145–147), a recently completed NIH-sponsored multicenter trial in 861 patients of 6 mL per kg versus 12 mL per kg tidal volume showed a 20% reduction in ALI/ARDS mortality with the low tidal volume approach (148). Because ventilation with low tidal volumes may cause alveolar hypoventilation and respiratory acidosis, patients must be carefully monitored and profound acidosis should be treated with bicarbonate administration. The ARDS Network low tidal volume ventilator protocol is summarized in Table 23-3.

PEEP has been known to improve oxygenation in ALI/ARDS since the syndrome was first described. PEEP in the range of 5 to 15 cm H_2O improves oxygenation by inflating poorly ventilated alveoli and thereby decreasing the amount of venous admixture (or intrapulmonary shunting) in the lung (140). PEEP is also thought to prevent the repetitive end-expiratory collapse of alveoli, which may contribute to ventilator-induced lung injury. The addition of PEEP usually permits the fraction of inspired oxygen to be lowered, also reducing the risk of superimposed oxygen toxicity to the lungs. However, the optimal level of PEEP has been debated. Although some investigators have attempted to maximize alveolar recruitment in individual patients by adjusting the level of PEEP on the basis of static pressure–volume curves measured after the administration of neuromuscular blocking agents (143), the implementation of

this approach in a large clinical trial has not been feasible. The ARDS Network protocol for low tidal volume mechanical ventilation (Table 23-3) includes a set of allowable PEEP and FIO_2 combinations. Use of higher levels of PEEP is not recommended because a recently completed ARDS Network trial of increased PEEP levels compared with those in the original trial showed no benefit (149).

PEEP does not, however, alter the course of the primary lung injury. It does not, for example, reduce extravascular lung water content in pulmonary edema (150,151). High levels of PEEP (>10 cm H_2O) usually cause a reduction in cardiac output (140). This reduction in cardiac output may result in an even higher arterial PaO_2. This improved oxygenation with a declining cardiac output results from either decreased blood flow to poorly ventilated lung regions or a longer time for oxygen diffusion in edematous lung units when pulmonary blood flow is reduced. Clinically, a reduction in cardiac output from PEEP may interfere with overall oxygen transport even if the arterial oxygen tension is adequate. Careful monitoring of the effects of PEEP on cardiac output and perfusion to vital organs (e.g., brain and kidney) may be helpful in patients with ALI/ARDS and a low-output syndrome (140).

In addition to low tidal volume ventilation, a number of other novel ventilator strategies are being investigated. Prone positioning of the ARDS patient, although cumbersome, may temporarily improve oxygenation. However, in a randomized multicenter trial, prone positioning did not improve mortality in patients with ARDS (152). High-frequency ventilation (153) and partial liquid ventilation (154) have also been studied, but there has yet to be a demonstration of benefit in a large multicenter trial. Although often used in neonates and children, extracorporeal membrane oxygenation has not been found to be beneficial in adults with ARDS (155).

In the future, other modalities of therapy for ALI/ARDS may be helpful, including surfactant replacement (156), monoclonal antibody treatment for sepsis (157), and modulation of pulmonary vascular tone. However, recent experience with

TABLE 23-3. National Institutes of Health (NIH) Adult Respiratory Distress Syndrome (ARDS) Network Lower Tidal Volume Ventilation for Acute Lung Injury/Acute Respiratory Distress Syndrome (ALI/ARDS) Protocol Summary [a]

Ventilator Mode	Volume Assist-Control
Tidal volume	≤6 mL/kg PBW
Plateau pressure	≤30 cm H$_2$O
Ventilation set rate/pH goal	6–35, adjusted to achieve arterial pH ≥7.30 if possible
Inspiratory flow, I:E	Adjust flow to achieve I:E = 1:1–1:3
Oxygenation goal	55 mm Hg ≤PaO$_2$ ≤80 mm Hg or 88% ≤SaO$_2$ ≤95%

Allowable FIO$_2$/PEEP Combinations

FIO$_2$	0.3	0.4	0.4	0.5	0.5	0.6	0.7	0.7	0.7	0.8	0.9	0.9	0.9	1.0
PEEP cm H$_2$O	5	5	8	8	10	10	10	12	14	14	14	16	18	18, 22, 24

(Further increases in PEEP to 34 cm H$_2$O allowed but not required)

Weaning	Attempt to wean by pressure Support when FIO$_2$/PEEP ≤0.40/8

PBW, predicted body weight; I:E, ratio of the duration of inspiration to the duration expiration; PaO$_2$, partial pressure of oxygen in arterial blood; SaO$_2$, oxyhemoglobin saturation by pulse oximetry; FIO$_2$, fraction of inspired oxygen; PEEP, positive end-expiratory pressure.

Male PBW = 50 + 2.3 [height (inches) − 60] or
50 + 0.91 [height (cm) − 152.4]

Female PBW = 45.5 + 2.3 [height (inches) − 60] or
45.5 + 0.91 [height (cm) − 152.4]

[a] More details available at *www.ardsnet.org*.
From *www.ardsnet.org*, with permission.

these approaches has not been encouraging (158–160). Manipulation of cytokine balance and antioxidant therapy may also have a role in the future, but clinical studies are lacking. It is also possible that efforts directed at accelerating recovery from ALI may offer more long-term promise for effective therapy (161–165).

In summary, progress continues to be made in understanding both the pathogenesis and treatment of acute hypoxemic respiratory failure. New treatments have been developed for both cardiogenic pulmonary edema and noncardiogenic pulmonary edema. The establishment of the NIH ARDS Network for clinical trials has been particularly important in improving both the quantity and quality of large multicenter clinical trials in patients with ALI/ARDS. The advent of new research tools such as genetic analysis, genomics, and proteomics, along with a continued effort to move therapies from bench to bedside (166), should ultimately lead to further improvements in outcomes from acute hypoxemic respiratory failure.

REFERENCES

1. Staub NC. Pulmonary edema. *Physiol Rev* 1974;54:678–811.
2. Starling EH. On the absorption of fluids from the connective tissue spaces. *J Physiol* 1986;19:312–326.
3. Staub NC. The pathogenesis of pulmonary edema. *Prog Cardiovasc Dis* 1980;23:53–80.
4. Blake LH, Staub NC. Pulmonary vascular transport in sheep. A mathematical model. *Microvasc Res* 1976;12:197–220.
5. Bhattacharya J, Staub NC. Direct measurement of microvascular pressure in the isolated, perfused dog lung. *Microvasc Res* 1979;17(Part 2):586.
6. Gaar KA, Taylor AE, Owens LJ. Pulmonary capillary pressure and filtration coefficient in the isolated perfused lung. *Am J Physiol* 1967;213:910–914.
7. Brigham KL. Mechanisms of acute lung injury. *Clin Chest Med* 1982;3:9–24.
8. Erdmann JA, Vaughn TRJ, Brigham KL, et al. Effect of increased vascular pressure on lung fluid balance in unanesthetized sheep. *Circ Res* 1975;37:271–284.
9. Reid I, Meyrick B. Microcirculation: definition and organization at tissue level. *Ann NY Acad Sci* 1982;384:3–20.
10. Albert RK, Lakshminarayan S, Kirk W, et al. Lung inflation can cause pulmonary edema in zone I of in situ dog lungs. *J Appl Physiol* 1980;49:815–819.
11. Bo G, Hauge A, Nicolayson G. Alveolar pressure and lung volume as determinants of net transvascular fluid filtration. *J Appl Physiol* 1977;42:476–482.
12. Schneeberger-Keeley EE, Karnovscy MJ. The ultrastructural basis of alveolar capillary membrane permeability to peroxidase used as a tracer. *J Cell Biol* 1968;37:781–793.
13. Gorin AB, Stewart PA. Differential permeability of endothelial and epithelial barriers to albumin flux. *J Appl Physiol* 1979;47:1315–1324.
14. Gee MH, Havil AM. The relationship between pulmonary perivascular cuff fluid and lung lymph in dogs with edema. *Microvasc Res* 1978;19:209–216.
15. Taylor AE, Gaar KAJ. Estimation of equivalent pore radii of pulmonary capillary and alveolar membranes. *Am J Physiol* 1970;218:1133–1140.
16. Howell JBL, Permutt S, Proctor DF, et al. Effect of inflation of the lung on different parts of the pulmonary vascular bed. *J Appl Physiol* 1961;16:71.
17. Gee MH, William DO. Effect of lung inflation on perivascular cuff fluid volume in isolated dog lung lobes. *Microvasc Res* 1979;17:192–201.
18. Goshy M, Lai-Fook SJ, Hyatt RE. Perivascular pressure measurements by wick-catheter technique in isolated dog lobes. *J Appl Physiol* 1979;46:950–955.

19. Staub NC. Pulmonary edema. Physiologic approaches to management. *Chest* 1978;74:559–564.
20. Albert RK, Lakshminarayan S, Hildebrandt J, et al. Increased surface tension favors pulmonary edema formation in anesthetized dogs' lungs. *J Clin Invest* 1979;63:1015.
21. Gregory TJ, Longmore WJ, Moxley MA, et al. Surfactant chemical composition and biophysical activity in acute respiratory distress syndrome. *J Clin Invest* 1991;88:1976–1981.
22. Raj U. Alveolar liquid pressure measured by micropuncture in isolated lungs of mature and immature fetal rabbits. *J Clin Invest* 1987;79:1579–1588.
23. Vreim CE, Snashall PD, Demling RH, et al. Lung lymph and free interstitial fluid protein composition in sheep with edema. *Am J Physiol* 1976;230:1650–1653.
24. Hallman M, Spragg R, Harrell JH, et al. Evidence of lung surfactant abnormality in respiratory failure. A study of bronchoalveolar lavage phospholipids, surface activity, phospholipase activity, and plasma myoinositol. *J Clin Invest* 1982;70:673–683.
25. Brigham KL, Woolverton WC, Blake LH, et al. Increased sheep lung vascular permeability caused by Pseudomonas bacteremia. *J Clin Invest* 1974;54:792–804.
26. Ohkuda K, Nakahara K, Weidner WJ, et al. Lung fluid exchange after uneven pulmonary artery obstruction in sheep. *Circ Res* 1978;43:152–161.
27. Jayr C, Matthay MA. Alveolar and lung liquid clearance in the absence of pulmonary blood flow in sheep. *J Appl Physiol* 1991;71:1679–1687.
28. Bongard F, Matthay MA, Mackeasie RC, et al. Morphologic and physiologic correlates of increased extravascular lung water. *Surgery* 1984;96:395–403.
29. DaLuz PL, Shubia H, Weil MH. Pulmonary edema related to changes in colloid osmotic and pulmonary artery pressure in patients after acute myocardial infarction. *Circulation* 1975;51:350–357.
30. Aberle DR, Wiener-Kronish JP, Webb WR, et al. Hydrostatic versus increased permeability pulmonary edema: diagnosis based on radiographic criteria in critically ill patients. *Radiology* 1988;168:73–79.
31. Wiener-Kronish JP, Matthay MA. Pleural effusions associated with hydrostatic and increased permeability pulmonary edema. *Chest* 1988;93:852–858.
32. Wiener-Kronish JP, Matthay MA, Collen PE, et al. Relationship of pulmonary hemodynamics to pleural effusions in patients with heart failure. *Am Rev Respir Dis* 1988;132:1253–1256.
33. Wiener-Kronish JP, Goldstein R, Matthay RA, et al. Chronic pulmonary arterial and right atrial hypertension are not associated with pleural effusions. *Chest* 1987;92:967–970.
34. Broaddus VC, Wiener-Kronish JP, Staub NC. Removal of pleural liquid and protein by lymphatics in awake sheep. *J Appl Physiol* 1990;64:384–390.
35. Wiener-Kronish JP, Broaddus VC, Albertine K, et al. Relationship of pleural effusions to increased permeability pulmonary edema in anesthetized sheep. *J Clin Invest* 1988;82:1422–1429.
36. Fein A, Grossman RF, Jones JG, et al. The value of edema protein measurements in patients with pulmonary edema. *Am J Med* 1979;67:32–39.
37. Matthay MA, Eschenbacher WC, Goetzl EJ. Elevated concentrations of leukotriene D4 in pulmonary edema fluid of patients with adult respiratory distress syndrome. *J Clin Immunol* 1984;4:479–483.
38. Matthay MA, Landolt CC, Staub NC. Differential liquid and protein clearance from the alveoli of anesthetized sheep. *J Appl Physiol* 1982;53:96–104.
39. Verghese GM, Ware LB, Matthay BA, et al. Alveolar epithelial fluid transport and the resolution of clinically severe hydrostatic pulmonary edema. *J Appl Physiol* 1999;87:1301–1312.
40. Basset G, Crone C, Saumon G. Significance of active ion transport in transalveolar water absorption: a study on isolated rat lung. *J Physiol* 1987;384:311–324.
41. Goodman BE, Fleisher RS, Crandall ED. Evidence for active sodium transport by cultured monolayers of pulmonary alveolar epithelial cells. *Am J Physiol* 1982;245:C78–C83.
42. Matalon S, Benos DJ, Jackson RM. Biophysical and molecular properties of amiloride-inhibitable sodium channels in alveolar epithelial cells. *Am J Physiol* 1996;271:L1–L22.
43. Dobbs LG, Gonzalez R, Matthay MA, et al. Highly water-permeable type I alveolar epithelial cells confer high water permeability between the airspace and vasculature in rat lung. *Proc Natl Acad Sci USA* 1998;95:2991–2996.
44. Matthay MA, Folkesson HG, Verkman AS. Salt and water transport across alveolar and distal airway epithelia in the adult lung. *Am J Physiol* 1996;270:L487–L503.
45. Matthay MA, Berthiaume Y, Staub NC. Long-term clearance of liquid and protein from the lungs of unanesthetized sheep. *J Appl Physiol* 1985;59:928–934.
46. Goodman BE, Brown JE, Crandall EP. Regulation of transport across pulmonary alveolar epithelial cell monolayers. *J Appl Physiol* 1984;57:703–710.
47. Matthay MA, Wiener-Kronish JP. Intact epithelial barrier function is critical for the resolution of alveolar edema in humans. *Am Rev Respir Dis* 1990;142:1250–1257.
48. Effros RM, Hacker A, Silverman P, et al. Protein concentrations have little effect on reabsorption of fluid from isolated rat lungs. *J Appl Physiol* 1991;70:416–422.
49. Berthiaume Y, Staub NC, Matthay MA. Beta-adrenergic agonists increase lung liquid clearance in anesthetized sheep. *J Clin Invest* 1987;79:335–343.
50. Berthiaume Y, Broaddus VC, Gropper MA, et al. Alveolar liquid and protein clearance from normal dog lungs. *J Appl Physiol* 1988;65:585–593.
51. Garat C, Carter E, Matthay M. New in situ mouse model to quantify alveolar epithelial fluid clearance. *J Appl Physiol* 1998;84:1763–1767.
52. Crandall ED, Heming TA, Palombo RL, et al. Effects of terbutaline on sodium transport in isolated perfused rat lung. *J Appl Physiol* 1986;60:289–294.
53. Maron MB. Dose-response relationship between plasma epinephrine concentration and alveolar liquid clearance in dogs. *J Appl Physiol* 1998;85:1702–1707.
54. Jayr C, Garat C, Meignan M, et al. Alveolar liquid and protein clearance in anesthetized, ventilated rats. *J Appl Physiol* 1994;76:2636–2642.
55. Sakuma T, Folkesson HG, Suzuki S, et al. Beta-adrenergic agonist stimulated alveolar fluid clearance in ex vivo human and rat lungs. *Am J Respir Crit Care Med* 1997;155:506–512.
56. Ware LB, Fang X, Wang Y, et al. Selected contribution: mechanisms that may stimulate the resolution of alveolar edema in the transplanted human lung. *J Appl Physiol* 2002;93:1869–1874.
57. Swan HJC, Ganz W, Forrester J, et al. Catheterization of the heart in man with use of a flow directed balloon-tipped catheter. *N Engl J Med* 1970;283:447–451.
58. Conners AF, McCaffree RD, Gray BA. Evaluation of right heart catheterization in the critically ill patient without acute myocardial infarction. *N Engl J Med* 1983;308:263–267.
59. Matthay MA, Chatterjee K. Bedside catheterization of the pulmonary artery: risks versus benefits. *Ann Intern Med* 1988;109:826–834.
60. Unger KM, Shibel EM, Moser KM. Detection of left ventricular failure in patients with the adult respiratory distress syndrome. *Chest* 1975;67:8–13.
61. Osler W. *The principles and practice of medicine.* New York: D. Appleton and Co., 1927.
62. Lee G, De Maria A, Amsterdam EA, et al. Comparative effects of morphine, meperidine, and pentazocine on cardiocirculatory dynamics in patients with acute myocardial infarction. *Am J Med* 1976;60:949–955.
63. Parmley WW, Chatterjee MB. *Cardiology.* Philadelphia: JB Lippincott and Co, 1988.
64. Packer M. Do vasodilators prolong life in heart failure? *N Engl J Med* 1987;316:1471–1473.
65. Cohn JN. Physiologic basis for vasodilator therapy for heart failure. *Am J Med* 1981;71:135–139.
66. Biddle TL, Ju PN. Effect of furosemide on hemodynamics and lung water in acute pulmonary edema secondary to myocardial infarction. *Am J Cardiol* 1979;43:86–90.
67. Young JB. New therapeutic choices in the management of congestive heart failure. *Rev Cardiovasc Med* 2001;2:S19–S24.
68. de Denus S, Pharand C, Williamson DR. Brain natriuretic peptide in the management of heart failure. *Chest* 2004;125:652–668.

69. Goldstein RA, Passamani ER, Roberts R. A comparison of digoxin and dobutamine in patients with acute infarction and cardiac failure. *N Engl J Med* 1980;303:846–850.

70. Gray R, Shah PK, Singh B, et al. Low cardiac output states after open heart surgery. *Chest* 1981;80:16–22.

71. Arnold SB, Byrd RC, Meister W. Long-term digitalis therapy improves left ventricular function in heart failure. *N Engl J Med* 1980;303:1443–1448.

72. Buda AJ, Pinsky MR, Ingels NBJ, et al. Effect of intrathoracic pressure on left ventricular performance. *N Engl J Med* 1979;301:453–459.

73. Macklem PT. Respiratory muscles: the vital pump. *Chest* 1980;78:753–758.

74. Aubier M, Trippenback T, Roussos C. Respiratory muscle fatigue during cardiogenic shock. *J Appl Physiol* 1981;51:499–508.

75. Anderson RR, Holliday RL, Driedger AA. Documentation of pulmonary capillary permeability in the adult respiratory distress syndrome accompanying human sepsis. *Am Rev Respir Dis* 1979;119:869–877.

76. Ware LB, Matthay MA. Alveolar fluid clearance is impaired in the majority of patients with acute lung injury and the acute respiratory distress syndrome. *Am J Respir Crit Care Med* 2001;163:1376–1383.

77. Petty TL, Ashbaugh DG. The adult respiratory distress syndrome: Clinical features, factors influencing prognosis and principles of management. *Chest* 1971;60:273–279.

78. Murray JF, Matthay MA, Luce JM, et al. An expanded definition of the adult respiratory distress syndrome. *Am Rev Respir Dis* 1988;138:720–723.

79. Montgomery AB, Stager MA, Carrico CJ, et al. Causes of mortality in patients with the adult respiratory distress syndrome. *Am Rev Respir Dis* 1985;132:485–489.

80. Rubin DB, Wiener-Kronish JP, Murray JF, et al. Elevated von Willebrand factor antigen is an early plasma predictor of acute lung injury in nonpulmonary sepsis. *J Clin Invest* 1990;86:474–480.

81. Bernard GR, Artigas A, Brigham KL, et al. The American-European Consensus Conference on ARDS. Definitions, mechanisms, relevant outcomes, and clinical trial coordination. *Am J Respir Crit Care Med* 1994;149:818–824.

82. Doyle RL, Szaflarski N, Modin GW, et al. Identification of patients with acute lung injury. Predictors of mortality. *Am J Respir Crit Care Med* 1995;152:1818–1824.

83. Zilberberg MD, Epstein SK. Acute lung injury in the medical ICU. Comorbid conditions, age, etiology and hospital outcome. *Am J Respir Crit Care Med* 1998;157:1159–1164.

84. Sloane PJ, Gee MH, Gottlieb JE, et al. A multicenter registry of patients with acute respiratory distress syndrome. *Am Rev Respir Dis* 1992;146:419–426.

85. Baumann WR, Jung RC, Koss M, et al. Incidence and mortality of adult respiratory distress syndrome: A prospective analysis from a large metropolitan hospital. *Crit Care Med* 1986;14:1–4.

86. Monchi M, Bellenfant F, Cariou A, et al. Early predictive factors of survival in the acute respiratory distress syndrome. A multivariate analysis. *Am J Respir Crit Care Med* 1998;158:1076–1081.

87. Ware LB, Matthay MA. Medical progress: The acute respiratory distress syndrome. *N Engl J Med* 2000;342:1334–1349.

88. Pepe PE, Potkin RT, Reus DH, et al. Clinical predictors of the adult respiratory distress syndrome. *Am J Surg* 1982;144:124–130.

89. Fowler AA, Hamman RF, Good JT, et al. Adult respiratory distress syndrome: risk with common predispositions. *Ann Intern Med* 1983;98:593–597.

90. Goss CH, Brower RG, Hudson LD, et al., The ARDS Network. Incidence of acute lung injury in the United States. *Crit Care Med* 2003;31:1607–1611.

91. Milberg JA, Davis DR, Steinberg KP, et al. Improved survival of patients with acute respiratory distress syndrome (ARDS): 1983–1993. *JAMA* 1995;273:306–309.

92. Abel SJC, Finney SJ, Brett SJ, et al. Reduced mortality in association with the acute respiratory distress syndrome. *Thorax* 1998;53:292–294.

93. Bell RC, Coalson JJ, Smith JD, et al. Multiple organ system failure and infection in adult respiratory distress syndrome. *Ann Intern Med* 1983;99:293–298.

94. Dantzker DR, Brook CJ, Dehart P, et al. Ventilation-perfusion distributions in adult respiratory distress syndrome. *Am Rev Respir Dis* 1979;120:1039–1052.

95. Nuckton TJ, Alonso JA, Kallet RH, et al. Pulmonary dead-space fraction as a risk factor for death in the acute respiratory distress syndrome. *N Engl J Med* 2002;346:1281–1286.

96. Said SI, Avery ME, Davis RK, et al. Pulmonary surface activity in induced pulmonary edema. *J Clin Invest* 1965;44:458–464.

97. Elliott CG, Morris AH, Cengiz M. Pulmonary function and exercise gas exchange in survivors of adult respiratory distress syndrome. *Am Rev Respir Dis* 1981;123:492–495.

98. Bachofen M, Weibel ER. Alterations of the gas exchange apparatus in adult respiratory insufficiency associated with septicemia. *Am Rev Respir Dis* 1977;116:589–615.

99. Lakshminarayan S, Stanford RE, Petty TL. Prognosis after recovery from adult respiratory distress syndrome. *Am Rev Respir Dis* 1976;113:7–16.

100. Zapol WM, Snider MT. Pulmonary hypertension in severe acute respiratory failure. *N Engl J Med* 1977;296:476–480.

101. Nash G, Blennerhassett JB, Pontoppidan H. Pulmonary lesions associated with oxygen therapy and artificial ventilation. *N Engl J Med* 1981;276:368–374.

102. Gammon RB, Shin MS, Groves RHJ, et al. Clinical risk factors for pulmonary barotrauma: a multivariate analysis. *Am J Respir Crit Care Med* 1995;152:1235–1240.

103. Eisner MD, Thompson BT, Schoenfeld D, et al., the Acute Respiratory Distress Syndrome Network. Airway pressures and early barotrauma in patients with acute lung injury and acute respiratory distress syndrome. *Am J Respir Crit Care Med* 2002;165:978–982.

104. Schnapp LM, Chin DP, Szaflarski N, et al. Frequency and importance of barotrauma in 100 patients with acute lung injury. *Crit Care Med* 1995;23:272–278.

105. Pratt PC, Vollmer RT, Shelburne JD, et al. Pulmonary morphology in a multihospital collaborative extracorporeal membrane oxygenation project. *Am J Pathol* 1979;95:191–214.

106. Witschi HR, Haschek WM, Klein-Szanto AJR, et al. Potentiation of diffuse lung damage by oxygen: determining variables. *Am Rev Respir Dis* 1981;123:98.

107. Rinaldo J. Mediation of ARDS by leukocytes. *Chest* 1986;89:590–593.

108. Pittet JF, MacKersie RC, Martin TR, et al. Biological markers of acute lung injury: prognostic and pathogenetic significance. *Am J Respir Crit Care Med* 1997;155:1187–1205.

109. Stevens JH, O'Hanley P, Shapiro JM, et al. Effects of anti-C5a antibodies on the adult respiratory distress syndrome in septic primates. *J Clin Invest* 1986;77:1812–1816.

110. Lee CT, Fein AM, Lipmann M, et al. Elastolytic activity in pulmonary lavage fluid from patients with adult respiratory distress syndrome. *N Engl J Med* 1981;304:192–196.

111. Maunder RJ, Hackman RC, Riff E, et al. Occurrence of the adult respiratory distress syndrome in neutropenic patients. *Am Rev Respir Dis* 1986;133:313–316.

112. Rinaldo JE, Borovetz H. Deterioration of oxygenation and abnormal lung microvascular permeability during resolution of leukopenia in patients with diffuse lung injury. *Am Rev Respir Dis* 1985;131:579–583.

113. Haynes JB, Hyers TM, Giclas PC, et al. Elevated fibrinogen degradation products in the adult respiratory distress syndrome. *Am Rev Respir Dis* 1980;122:841–847.

114. Idell S. Coagulation, fibrinolysis, and fibrin deposition in acute lung injury. *Crit Care Med* 2003;31:S213–S220.

115. Tracey KJ, Fong Y, Hesse DG, et al. Anti-cachectin/TNF monoclonal antibodies prevent septic shock during lethal bacteremia. *Nature* 1987;330:662–664.

116. Malik AB, Vander Zee H. Mechanism of pulmonary edema induced by microembolism in dogs. *Circ Res* 1978;42:72–79.

117. Miller EJ, Cohen AB, Nagao S, et al. Elevated levels of NAP-1/interleukin-8 are present in the airspaces of patients with adult respiratory distress syndrome and are associated with increased mortality. *Am Rev Respir Dis* 1992;146:427–432.

118. Sethi JM, Waxman AB. Mediators of acute lung injury: a review. *Clin Pulm Med* 2001;8:214–225.

119. Matthay M, Bhattacharya S, Gaver D, et al. Ventilator-induced lung injury: in vivo and in vitro mechanisms. *Am J Physiol Lung Cell Mol Physiol* 2002;283:L678–L682.

120. Webb HH, Tierney DF. Experimental pulmonary edema due to intermittent positive pressure ventilation with high inflation pressures. Protection by positive end expiratory pressure. *Am Rev Respir Dis* 1974;110:556–565.

121. Dreyfuss D, Soler P, Basset G, et al. High inflation pressure pulmonary edema. Respective effects of high airway pressure, high tidal volume, and positive end-expiratory pressure. *Am Rev Respir Dis* 1988;137:1159–1164.

122. Parker JC, Townsley MI, Rippe B, et al. Increased microvascular permeability in dog lungs due to high peak airway pressure. *J Appl Physiol* 1984;57:1809–1816.

123. Corbridge TC, Wood LDH, Crawford GP, et al. Adverse effects of large tidal volumes and low PEEP in canine acid aspiration. *Am Rev Respir Dis* 1990;142:311–315.

124. Frank J, Gutierrez J, Jones K, et al. Low tidal volume reduces epithelial and endothelial injury in acid-injured rat lungs. *Am J Respir Crit Care Med* 2002;165:242–249.

125. Slutsky AS, Tremblay LN. Multiple system organ failure: is mechanical ventilation a contributing factor. *Am J Respir Crit Care Med* 1998;157:1721–1725.

126. Ranieri VM, Suter PM, Tortorella C, et al. Effect of mechanical ventilation on inflammatory mediators in patients with acute respiratory distress syndrome. *JAMA* 1999;282:54–61.

127. Luce JM, Montgomery BA, Marks JD, et al. Ineffectiveness of high-dose methylprednisolone in preventing parenchymal lung injury and improving mortality in patients with septic shock. *Am Rev Respir Dis* 1988;136:62–68.

128. Cameron JL, Zuidema GD. Aspiration pneumonia. Magnitude and frequency of the problem. *JAMA* 1972;219:1194–1196.

129. Jones JG, Grossman RF, Beny M, et al. Alveolar-capillary membrane permeability. *Am Rev Respir Dis* 1979;120:339–410.

130. Wynne JW, Modell JH. Respiratory aspiration of stomach contents. *Ann Intern Med* 1977;87:466–474.

131. Bynum LJ, Pierce AK. Pulmonary aspiration of gastric contents. *Am Rev Respir Dis* 1976;114:1129–1136.

132. Bartlett JG, Gorback SL, Finegold SM. The bacteriology of aspiration pneumonia. *Am J Med* 1974;56:202–208.

133. Kaplan RL, Sahn SA, Petty TL. Incidence and outcome of the respiratory distress syndrome in Gram-negative sepsis. *Arch Intern Med* 1979;139:867–869.

134. Hechtman HB, Lonergan EA, Shepro D. Platelet and leukocyte lung interactions in patients with respiratory failure. *Surgery* 1978;83:155–163.

135. Brigham KL, Bowers RE, Haynes J. Increased lung vascular permeability caused by E. Coli endotoxin. *Circ Res* 1979;45:292–297.

136. Wiener-Kronish JP, Albertine KH, Matthay MA. Differential responses of the endothelial and epithelial barriers of the lung in sheep to Escherichia coli endotoxin. *J Clin Invest* 1991;88:864–875.

137. Staub NC. Conference report on a workshop on the measurement of lung water. *Crit Care Med* 1980;8:752–759.

138. Pistolesi M, Guintini C. Assessment of extravascular lung water. *Radiol Clin North Am* 1978;16:551–574.

139. Brower RG, Ware LB, Berthiaume Y, et al. Treatment of ARDS. *Chest* 2001;120:1347–1367.

140. Saint S, Matthay MA. Risk reduction in the intensive care unit. *Am J Med* 1998;105:515–523.

141. Broaddus VC, Berthiaume Y, Biondi J, et al. A. Management of pulmonary hemodynamics in patients with the adult respiratory distress syndrome. *J Intensive Care Med* 1987;2:190–213.

142. Ohkuda K, Nakahara K, Binder A, et al. Venous air emboli in sheep: reversible increase in lung microvascular permeability. *J Appl Physiol* 1981;51:887–894.

143. Amato MB, Barbas CS, Medeiros DM, et al. Effect of a protective-ventilation strategy on mortality in the acute respiratory distress syndrome. *N Engl J Med* 1998;338:347–354.

144. Tremblay L, Valenza F, Ribeiro SP, et al. Injurious ventilatory strategies increase cytokines and c-fos mRNA expression in an isolated rat lung model. *J Clin Invest* 1997;99:944–952.

145. Dreyfuss D, Basset G, Soler P, et al. Intermittent positive-pressure hyperventilation with high inflation pressures produces pulmonary microvascular injury in rats. *Am Rev Respir Dis* 1985;132:880–884.

146. Stewart TE, Meade MO, Cook DJ, et al. Evaluation of a ventilation strategy to prevent barotrauma in patients at high risk for acute respiratory distress syndrome. *N Engl J Med* 1998;338:355–361.

147. Brochard L, Roudot-Thoraval F, Roupie E, et al. Tidal volume reduction for prevention of ventilator-induced lung injury in acute respiratory distress syndrome. *Am J Respir Crit Care Med* 1998;158:1831–1838.

148. The Acute Respiratory Distress Syndrome Network. Ventilation with lower tidal volumes as compared with traditional tidal volumes for acute lung injury and the acute respiratory distress syndrome. *N Engl J Med* 2000; 342:1301–1308.

149. The Acute Respiratory Distress Syndrome Network. A trial of mechanical ventilation with higher versus lower positive end-expiratory pressures in patients with acute lung injury and acute respiratory distress syndrome. *N Engl J Med* 2004;351:327–336.

150. Prewitt RM, McCarthy J, Wood LDH. Treatment of acute low pressure pulmonary edema in dogs. *J Clin Invest* 1981;67:409–418.

151. Demling RH, Staub NC, Edmunds LHJ. Effect of end-expiratory airway pressure on accumulation of extravascular lung water. *J Appl Physiol* 1975;38:907–912.

152. Gattinoni L, Tognoni G, Pesenti A, et al. Effect of prone positioning on the survival of patients with acute respiratory failure. *N Engl J Med* 2001;345:568–573.

153. Derdak S, Mehta S, Stewart T, et al. The multicenter oscillatory ventilation for acute respiratory distress syndrome trial (MOAT) study investigators: high-frequency oscillatory ventilation for acute respiratory distress syndrome in adults: a randomized controlled trial. *Am J Respir Crit Care Med* 2002;166:801–808.

154. Kaisers U, Kelly KP, Busch T. Liquid ventilation. *Br J Anaesth* 2003;91:143–151.

155. Kopp R, Kuhlen R, Max M, et al. Evidence-based medicine in the therapy of the acute respiratory distress syndrome. *Intensive Care Med* 2002;28:244–255.

156. Merritt TA, Hallman M, Bloom BT, et al. Prophylactic treatment of very premature infants with human surfactant. *N Engl J Med* 1986;315:785–789.

157. Baumgartner JD, McCutchan JA, Melle GV, et al. Prevention of Gram-negative shock and death in surgical patients by antibody to core glycolipid. *Lancet* 1985;2:59–63.

158. Rossaint R, Falke KJ, Lopez F, et al. Inhaled nitric oxide for the adult respiratory distress syndrome. *N Engl J Med* 1993;328:399–405.

159. Anzueto A, Baughman RP, Guntupalli KK, et al. Aerosolized surfactant in adults with sepsis-induced acute respiratory distress syndrome. *N Engl J Med* 1996;334:1417–1421.

160. Dellinger RP, Zimmerman JL, Taylor RW. Effects of inhaled nitric oxide in patients with acute respiratory distress syndrome: Results of a randomized phase II trial. *Crit Care Med* 1998;26:15–23.

161. Payen D, Vallet B, The Genoa Group. Results of the French prospective multicentric randomized double-blind placebo-controlled trial on inhaled nitric oxide in ARDS. *Intensive Care Med* 1999;25:S166.

162. Matthay MA. Function of the alveolar epithelial barrier under pathological conditions. *Chest* 1994;105:67S–74S.

163. Bitterman PB. Pathogenesis of fibrosis in acute lung injury. *Am J Med* 1992;92:39S–43S.

164. Wortel CH, Doerschuk CM. Neutrophils and neutrophil-endothelial cell adhesion in adult respiratory distress syndrome. *New Horiz* 1993;1:631–637.

165. Berthiaume Y, Lesur O, Dagenais A. Treatment of adult respiratory distress syndrome: plea for rescue therapy of the alveolar epithelium. *Thorax* 1999;54:150–160.

166. Matthay MA, Zimmerman GA, Esmon C, et al. Future research directions in acute lung injury: summary of a National Heart, Lung and Blood Institute working group. *Am J Respir Crit Care Med* 2003; 167:1027–1035.

CHAPTER 24

Thoracic Trauma, Surgery, and Perioperative Management

Michael W. Owens

Shawn A. Milligan

Jane M. Eggerstedt

The introduction of modern, safe anesthesia and improved operative techniques has dramatically reduced the incidence of complications of surgery. In spite of these vast improvements, pulmonary complications remain a significant cause of morbidity and increased health care expenditure. Prediction of the probability of developing postoperative complications is important clinically and has been the subject of debate for most of the 20th century. Several preoperative tests and composite classification systems have been devised, but the perfect preoperative indicator of operative morbidity remains elusive.

CARDIOPULMONARY EFFECTS OF ANESTHESIA

RESPIRATORY EFFECTS

Virtually every aspect of general anesthesia contributes negatively to pulmonary physiology. Most anesthetic agents depress the central ventilatory response to hypercapnia and hypoxemia and cause a decrease in tidal volume. There is also an increase in dead space because of the decreased minute ventilation (1). Other significant effects on the respiratory system include a reduction in muscle tone and an upward movement of the diaphragm, causing a decrease in functional residual capacity (FRC) by about 15% to 20% (2).

Intraoperative atelectasis develops in the dependent lung zones in approximately 90% of patients receiving general anesthesia. Typically, about 10% of the lung develops atelectasis; however, this can be much more extensive in some patients. Atelectasis leads to intrapulmonary shunting and hypoxemia.

Induction of general anesthesia produces a loss of tone in the inspiratory muscles and diaphragm. This changes the shape of the chest wall and diaphragm, resulting in compression of lung tissue. This mechanism probably explains the rapid onset of atelectasis with induction of general anesthesia (3). Areas of the lung with low ventilation–perfusion ($\dot{V}/\dot{Q}$) ratios are at risk for absorptive atelectasis. In these low $\dot{V}/\dot{Q}$ areas, gas leaves the alveolus faster than it can enter, resulting in alveolar collapse (3). As oxygen is more soluble than nitrogen, the use of high oxygen levels promotes the development of absorptive atelectasis. Mucous plugging is an exacerbating factor. Lastly, atelectasis occurs because of loss of surfactant.

A fractional inspired oxygen concentration (FIO_2) of 1.0 is frequently used to preoxygenate patients prior to intubation and immediately prior to extubation. The risk of atelectasis during these procedures must be balanced by the risk of hypoxia with lower concentrations of oxygen. Using a lower FIO_2 can also lessen the development of atelectasis during surgery. Alveolar recruitment methods using positive end-expiratory pressure (PEEP) and/or vital capacity (VC) maneuvers are modern strategies used to decrease atelectasis and improve oxygenation during general anesthesia (4,5).

Endotracheal intubation in patients with asthma may provoke clinically significant bronchospasm. Pretreatment with inhaled albuterol will blunt this response; however, intravenous (IV) lidocaine is not effective (6). The type of induction agent is important, with propofol resulting in a lower respiratory resistance than etiomidate or thiopental (7). The choice of inhaled anesthetic is also important in asthmatics. Halothane and isoflurane are known to decrease bronchial smooth muscle tone and airway resistance (8). More recently, sevoflurane has been shown to have more bronchodilator effects than halothane, isoflurane, or thiopental–nitrous oxide anesthesia (9). Some studies have suggested an increased incidence of postoperative respiratory complications in patients who have had a recent upper respiratory infection. Elective surgery should be postponed for a few weeks after a viral respiratory infection (10,11).

CARDIOVASCULAR EFFECTS

All inhalational anesthetic agents are myocardial depressants. Halothane has a marked depressant effect and also causes a reduction in heart rate. Isoflurane causes minimal myocardial depression but has a marked vasodilator effect that results in tachycardia. The effects of enflurane on myocardial contractility and heart rate are intermediate between those of halothane and isoflurane (12). Nitrous oxide tends to cause less myocardial depression and also has intrinsic sympathomimetic effects.

Among the IV induction agents, barbiturates are more potent myocardial depressants compared with the narcotic agents. Morphine sulfate can cause histamine release, resulting in bronchospasm and hypotension. The newer sedative agents fentanyl, sufentanil, and alfentanil are preferred agents in patients with underlying heart disease. Ketamine and etomidate also have fewer adverse hemodynamic consequences (13).

GENERAL VERSUS REGIONAL ANESTHESIA

Epidural anesthesia has been advocated as an alternative in high-risk patients with underlying lung or heart disease. However, epidural anesthesia inhibits intercostal and abdominal muscle function and may contribute to a postoperative reduction in VC and FRC (14). Epidural anesthetics exert a negligible effect on central ventilatory drive.

The hemodynamic effects of regional anesthesia are more pronounced. Vasodilatation occurs as a result of sympathetic blockade and may result in significant hypotension (13,15). In addition, all the local anesthetic agents used in regional anesthesia can cause a dose-dependent myocardial depression.

A recent review of more than 10,000 patients undergoing various types of surgery examined the outcomes of patients treated with regional (i.e., epidural or spinal) versus general anesthesia (16). Regional anesthesia was associated with a 59% decrease in respiratory depression, a 55% decrease in pulmonary embolism, and a 40% decrease in postoperative pneumonia. The use of regional anesthesia resulted in a 30% reduction in mortality rate at 30 days. The regional anesthesia was found to be beneficial regardless of whether it was used alone or in combination with general anesthesia (16). A lower incidence of postoperative respiratory failure with regional anesthesia was also found in the Veterans Affairs multifactorial risk index study (odds ratio 1.91 for general anesthesia and 1.00 for spinal or epidural anesthesia) (17). However, in the Veterans Affairs study, the site and type of surgery were more robust predictors of postoperative respiratory failure than was the type of anesthesia. In summary, modern anesthetic practice uses combined general and regional anesthesia in addition to advanced postoperative analgesic techniques (18). Future studies will determine whether these combined techniques lead to lower incidences of complications.

POSTOPERATIVE ANALGESIA

Thoracic and abdominal surgery commonly disrupts the normal breathing pattern in the postoperative period. This is a multifactorial process because of surgical disruption of muscles, pain, and reflex inhibition of phrenic and other motor neurons due to visceral stimulation (14). These factors contribute to decreases in lung volume, atelectasis, and potentially more serious postoperative complications such as pneumonia and respiratory failure.

It has been suggested that patients who are pain free will have an earlier recovery of their pulmonary function and a decreased incidence of postoperative complications. Epidural administration of local anesthetics and narcotic agents has been studied extensively (19–21). A recent meta-analysis compared the benefits of various postoperative analgesic techniques (22). Epidural administration of opioids resulted in less atelectasis compared with systemic opioids. Epidural local anesthetics significantly reduced the incidence of pulmonary infection and other pulmonary complications as compared with systemic opioids. Unfortunately, none of the analgesic techniques yielded a significant improvement in pulmonary function.

Intercostal nerve blockade, infiltration of the wound, and intrapleural administration of local anesthetics are other regional analgesic techniques (22–24). Some evidence suggests that intercostal nerve blockade may decrease the incidence of respiratory complications in patients undergoing upper abdominal surgery. Review of all such studies in the meta-analysis demonstrated that the use of intercostal nerve block did not improve analgesia or other outcome measures as compared with systemic opioids (22). However, intercostal nerve blockade may be a useful option for patients in whom epidural analgesia cannot be achieved or is otherwise contraindicated (23).

Intrapleural infusion of local anesthetics is very successful in providing postoperative analgesia after cholecystectomy and thoracotomy. However, it has been difficult to demonstrate improvements in pulmonary function (22). Furthermore, in thoracotomy patients, this technique requires intermittent clamping of the chest tube to retain the local anesthetic. It is often unsafe to clamp tubes in the early postoperative period. To circumvent this problem, the catheter can be tunneled in the extrapleural paravertebral space (25). In a small study using this new method, there were significant improvements in thoracotomy pain, VC, and atelectasis in the group receiving local anesthetic via the catheter compared with systemic analgesia (25). In summary, modern postoperative analgesia usually involves a combination of regional analgesic techniques combined with systemic nonsteroidal and narcotic analgesics.

SURGICAL INCISION SITE AND DIAPHRAGMATIC FUNCTION

In the normal awake subject, the diaphragm is the predominant inspiratory muscle. The intercostal and other accessory muscles assume a more central role during the first few days after surgery. This results in rapid, shallow breathing with small tidal volumes (26). Upper abdominal surgery results in a higher incidence of diaphragmatic dysfunction compared to lower abdominal incisions (27). Reflex inhibition of diaphragmatic motor activity resulting from the handling of abdominal viscera and the parietal peritoneum is one of the proposed mechanisms of diaphragmatic dysfunction (28).

Recently, a large prospective study on 994 patients was carried out to assess the role of the surgical incision site in perioperative hypoxemia. The results showed that hypoxemia [arterial oxygen saturation (SaO_2) below 90%] during the early postoperative period was closely related to operative site. Patients who had thoracoabdominal incisions had a 52% incidence of hypoxemia compared to a 38% incidence in those who underwent abdominal surgery. Only 7% of the patients who underwent elective superficial plastic surgery developed

significant hypoxemia (29). In another study, subcostal incisions were reported to be associated with a lower rate of postoperative pulmonary complications (POPCs) than midline incisions were (30). Transverse abdominal incisions are associated with the lowest pulmonary complication rate.

Laparoscopic surgery has been promoted as an alternative to conventional laparotomy because of shorter hospital stay, decreased postoperative pain, and early ambulation. There is some evidence that laparoscopic surgery may result in lower incidence of postoperative respiratory complications (31–33). Video-assisted thoracoscopic surgery (VATS) is also known to cause lesser postoperative pain and impairment of pulmonary function compared to standard thoracotomy techniques (34–36).

POSTOPERATIVE PULMONARY COMPLICATIONS

Estimates of POPCs have varied depending on the patient population studied, the procedure performed, and the criteria used to define a POPC. The overall incidence of POPC in the general population is approximately 5% but is below 1% for nonabdominal, nonthoracic procedures (37). Patients undergoing major vascular, upper abdominal, and thoracic surgery are at higher risk and constitute a special group, and POPCs are reported to occur in up to 50% of these patients (38–42).

Most pulmonary abnormalities after surgery are minor and self-limited. These include minor postoperative atelectasis, bronchospasm, hypoxemia, dyspnea, and cough. Major complications include postoperative pneumonia, lobar atelectasis, aspiration, and ventilatory failure and are infrequent. Death and prolonged ventilator dependence are rare even among patients with severe chronic obstructive pulmonary disease (COPD) (42,43). Obese patients are at risk for respiratory failure from obstructive sleep apnea (OSA). In the postoperative period, residual anesthetic effects and the use of narcotic analgesics are predisposing factors for OSA (44).

POSTOPERATIVE ATELECTASIS AND HYPOXEMIA

The major cause of postoperative hypoxemia is the formation of atelectasis, resulting in areas of low $\dot{V}/\dot{Q}$ ratio. Other causes include hypoventilation, pulmonary edema, thromboembolism, and bronchial obstruction by retained secretions (see Table 24-1). Residual anesthesia, pain, and immobilization also contribute to hypoxemia (2).

The anesthetic and surgical factors outlined above result in a decreased FRC. In individuals with no underlying lung disease,

TABLE 24-1.   Common Mechanisms of Postoperative Hypoxemia

Atelectasis
Microatelectasis
Segmental or lobar atelectasis
Hypoventilation
Residual anesthetic
Narcotic analgesics
Pain with splinting
Pulmonary edema
Venous thromboembolism
Bronchial mucous plugging

arterial partial pressure of oxygen (PaO_2) may decrease to 80% of baseline value. The forced expiratory volume in 1 second (FEV_1) and forced vital capacity (FVC) also decrease to approximately two-thirds of the preoperative levels after low-risk lower abdominal surgery (45). These decrements in lung function are more severe after upper abdominal surgery (46). In up to 33% of patients, atelectasis can persist up to the third or fourth postoperative day. The extent of atelectasis has a direct correlation with the severity of postoperative hypoxemia and with the decrease in FEV_1 and FVC.

The volume of the lung at which small dependent airways begin to collapse is called the *closing volume*. In normal healthy patients, the closing volume is less than FRC so that the airways remain open during tidal breathing. The closing volume begins to increase with age and approaches the FRC in patients more than 65 years old. Patients with COPD, obesity, or a history of smoking have higher closing volumes. Even a small decrease in the FRC in these patients leads to dependent airway closure, placing them at very high risk for the formation of atelectasis (2,47). Patients given 100% oxygen during surgery and the immediate postoperative period tend to have a higher incidence of atelectasis, probably because of resorption of oxygen in areas of decreased ventilation, as noted above (48,49).

Atelectasis in the dorsal and basal lung regions has been demonstrated by computerized tomography (CT) scan in virtually 100% of patients undergoing abdominal surgery (50). These regions are generally well perfused, and blood shunts through the airless lung units. In most patients, atelectasis is asymptomatic and resolves spontaneously. However, among high-risk patient groups, atelectasis may be persistent, and pneumonia can result from retained secretions in collapsed lung units (45).

PREVENTION AND TREATMENT OF ATELECTASIS

The primary physiologic alteration in postoperative atelectasis is a reduction in FRC; therefore, the main therapeutic objective is to restore FRC to preoperative levels. Repositioning the patient in bed every 2 hours and early mobilization should be routine practice in every postoperative patient. Respiratory techniques that produce a sustained maximal inspiration are most efficacious in reversing atelectasis. Incentive spirometry (IS) is generally the first modality employed in patients who are mentally alert and without excessive secretions. The goal of the IS effort is to inflate the lung to near total lung capacity for 5 to 10 seconds. The patient should perform 8 to 10 IS maneuvers every 1 to 2 hours while awake (50). Volume and flow type IS are available; however, the goal with both is to achieve a large inspired volume. The advantage of IS includes ease of use, low cost, and the ability of the patient to monitor their progress. IS can be combined with breath stacking to further increase lung volumes by 15% to 20%.

The technique of blow bottles is an expiratory method. It is useful only to the extent that the patient must inspire before the forceful expiratory maneuver (50). Intermittent positive-pressure breathing is not more effective than IS and is associated with more complications. Because of cost and potential barotrauma, it is no longer recommended for postoperative atelectasis.

When heavy secretions coexist with the atelectasis, methods to mobilize the sputum are useful. Simple coughing is effective in patients who are not debilitated and have good

pain control. Debilitated or oversedated patients may benefit from suctioning and/or percussion with postural drainage during the cough maneuver (50). These techniques may induce transient oxygen desaturation; therefore, oximetry monitoring should be considered. If the atelectasis is refractory to these maneuvers, fiber-optic bronchoscopy is useful in removing mucous plugs.

Continuous positive airway pressure (CPAP) with a nasal or full-face mask increases end-expiratory pressure and is useful to inflate the lung and to reverse atelectasis. It can be used for 2- to 4-hour intervals with time off as tolerated. CPAP should be considered when atelectasis and hypoxemia prove refractory to more conservative methods or in patients who are unable to perform these techniques (18,50). Patients should be monitored for gastric distension, which may induce aspiration. Other complications include hypoventilation, barotrauma, conjunctivitis, skin breakdown at the mask site, and patient intolerance to CPAP.

Noninvasive mask ventilation with bilevel positive airway pressure (BiPAP) utilizes a higher inspiratory pressure to promote an increased inspiratory volume in combination with a lower end-expiratory pressure to recruit atelectatic lung. The use of BiPAP in the intensive care unit (ICU) may be used to treat postoperative patients with incipient respiratory failure in an attempt to avoid reintubation (51). It is also useful to treat atelectasis but is generally recommended when more conservative techniques have failed.

Morbidly obese patients are at increased risk of decreased FRC, hypoxemia, and atelectasis in the postoperative period (52). In the postoperative period, obese patients have a larger percentage of atelectatic lung and a longer duration of atelectasis than those with normal weight. CPAP, BiPAP, and the reverse Trendelenburg position are useful in treating hypoxemia associated with morbid obesity (3,52).

It has been difficult to demonstrate which of these respiratory interventions is superior for the management of postoperative atelectasis. This is due to multiple factors including the heterogeneity of respiratory therapy methods used, types of surgery, outcome measures, and use of control groups (18,50). For example, a recent meta-analysis has demonstrated that postoperative complications following upper abdominal surgery are significantly less in patients receiving IS or deep-breathing exercises compared with those not receiving any therapy (53). There was no significant difference in complications when various respiratory therapy measures were compared with each other. However, the primary consideration is that the use of some type of lung-expansion method is superior to not using any method regardless of the type of surgery (50,53). Furthermore, these methods are more efficacious when the patient is instructed about the use of these methods prior to surgery (18). In summary, the present state of knowledge suggests that a stepwise approach utilizing an increase in intensity of therapy based on the severity of illness can be employed.

PREOPERATIVE PULMONARY FUNCTION TESTING

Pulmonary function testing (PFT) has three purposes in the preoperative evaluation of patients. Patients who will undergo lung resection should have a preoperative PFT done to determine their ability to tolerate the procedure. Secondly, lung function testing is useful in the diagnosis of obstructive or restrictive disease in patients with dyspnea. Lastly, spirometry can assist in achieving optimal presurgical bronchodilation in patients with diseases such as asthma. It should be emphasized that patients with COPD have an increased risk of postoperative complications such as pneumonia and respiratory failure (18). However, lung function testing and arterial blood gas analysis have not been clearly demonstrated to serve as an independent risk factor for predicting postoperative complications (14,18,54). For example, in a case–control study of pulmonary complications following abdominal surgery, abnormal findings on lung exam or chest radiograph were important for predicting complications (55). The degree of obstructive impairment on spirometry was not a predictive factor (55). In summary, lung function tests should be ordered for specific reasons, as outlined above, with the understanding that uniform testing of all preoperative patients is costly and without proven benefit.

SMOKING IN THE PREOPERATIVE PERIOD

Cigarette smoking has been identified as a risk factor for POPC in several studies (56–61). In a series of upper abdominal and thoracic surgery patients, the incidence of POPC in current smokers was almost twice that of past smokers and five times that of subjects who had never smoked (59). Two recent studies in patients undergoing lung resection demonstrated that patients who continued to smoke within 1 month of surgery had higher rates of postoperative complications (56,57).

In an effort to reduce the risk of postoperative complications, many physicians recommend smoking cessation prior to surgery. However, there is sometimes a paradoxical increase in complications in those who discontinue cigarettes immediately prior to surgery. In a study of 200 consecutive patients undergoing coronary artery bypass surgery, the risk for postoperative complications was reported to be four times higher in those who stopped smoking within 8 weeks prior to surgery compared with those who had given up smoking for more than 8 weeks prior to surgery (60). In another study, patients who were able to reduce their cigarette smoking prior to surgery had a seven times higher risk of developing postoperative complications compared with smokers who were unable to reduce their cigarette consumption (59). It appears that patients should give up smoking at least 8 weeks prior to surgery for the most beneficial outcome. Short-term preoperative smoking cessation may be beneficial by causing a reduction in blood carbon monoxide levels; however, heavy smokers may experience a nicotine withdrawal in the perioperative period that can have harmful effects (58–61).

PERIOPERATIVE ASPIRATION

Clinically significant aspiration of gastric contents is an uncommon but feared perioperative complication. Initially described by Mendelson in obstetric patients, the syndrome has been reported in patients undergoing all types of surgery (62). Modern anesthetic techniques and mandatory overnight preoperative fasting have decreased the incidence of aspiration. The incidence of aspiration in the surgical population has varied from study to study, varying from 0.2 to 2 per 10,000 cases, with an associated mortality rate of 2 to 3 per 100,000 anesthetic

cases. A decrease in mortality has been seen over the past two decades (63,64).

It is estimated that the minimum amount of gastric contents needed to cause significant changes is about 0.4 mL per kg. The cutoff for gastric pH below which aspiration pneumonitis can occur is approximately 2.5 to 3.5 (62,65).

Risk factors for aspiration include the extremes of age (i.e., the very young and the elderly), pregnancy, obesity, intestinal obstruction, esophageal disorders, decreased gastric motility, depressed levels of consciousness, emergency surgery, and recent oral intake. The only factors that have been independently associated with aspiration are emergency surgery and poor preoperative physical status. In one large study, all the deaths attributed to aspiration occurred in patients with American Society of Anesthesiologists (ASA) class 4 or higher preoperative risk category (64). The periods of an operation when aspiration is most likely to occur are during laryngoscopy and tracheal extubation (62,64).

Signs and symptoms of aspiration of gastric contents include cough, hypoxemia, and wheezing. Complications include pneumonitis, respiratory failure requiring mechanical ventilation, and death. Fortunately, the incidence of serious complications is very low. Patients who do not develop any symptoms within 2 hours of a witnessed aspiration are very unlikely to develop complications and can be safely monitored in a non-ICU setting. Those who develop respiratory symptoms or a new infiltrate on chest radiograph within 2 hours of a witnessed aspiration have a high incidence of respiratory complications and should be closely monitored.

A number of pharmacologic agents including antacids, H_2 blockers, prokinetic agents, antimuscarinic agents, and proton pump inhibitors have been used preoperatively to reduce the incidence of complications. The goal has been to keep the gastric pH above 2.5 and the volume of gastric aspirate prior to induction below 25 mL. Cricoid pressure is also a very effective measure to reduce the incidence of aspiration during endotracheal intubation (65). H_2 blockers and proton pump inhibitors are effective in increasing gastric pH but do not decrease gastric volume. Pirenzepine, which is an antimuscarinic agent, has been shown to decrease gastric volume (66–71). In obstetric and pediatric cases, preoperative use of H_2 antagonists or prokinetic agents is commonly practiced. Whether such treatment should be offered to all patients undergoing surgery is controversial.

Treatment of aspiration pneumonitis is mainly supportive and includes the current procedural terminology (CPT) measures outlined above. As much of the aspirated material as possible should be coughed up and/or suctioned. Bronchoscopic removal is possible in some cases but is not routinely helpful. Steroids do not help after aspiration occurs. Antibiotics are useful only for secondary infections.

POSTOPERATIVE PNEUMONIA

The surgical patient is at risk for various nosocomial infections including urinary tract infections, surgical wound infections, and pneumonia. Pneumonia is the leading fatal postoperative nosocomial infection. Malnutrition and poor general medical condition constitute important risk factors for postoperative pneumonia in addition to other risk factors for POPC outlined in Table 24-2.

TABLE 24-2. Risk Factors for Postoperative Pulmonary Complications

Age >70
Past or current smoking
Major surgery
   Upper gastrointestinal incisions
   Thoracic and thoracoabdominal operations
Emergency surgery
Coronary artery bypass grafting in COPD
Prolonged operations (>120 min)
General anesthesia involving muscle relaxants
Chronic obstructive lung disease
MI within past year
Chronic heart failure
Malnutrition

COPD, chronic obstructive pulmonary disease; MI, myocardial infarction.

TABLE 24-3. Preparing for Elective Surgery in Patients with Moderate to Severe Chronic Obstructive Pulmonary Disease

Clinical evaluation including a full medical history and examination.
Evaluation of severity of respiratory symptoms like cough, wheezing, etc. Surgery should be postponed in patients who have a URI or active symptoms.
Objective assessment of the severity of obstruction with ABG, spirometry/PFTs; treat reversible component with steroids prior to surgery if possible.
Detailed medication review. Discontinue β-blockers; these can worsen bronchospasm even if used as eye drops.
Physical therapy consultation for instruction in postural drainage, deep breathing, incentive spirometry, etc. CPT should start preoperatively and should continue till patient is ambulatory.
Prescribe bronchodilator therapy in the perioperative period for patients who have evidence of bronchospasm.
Theophylline may improve pulmonary function; however, data is insufficient to recommend routine use of aminophylline infusions during the perioperative period.
Steroid-dependent patients should receive stress-dose steroids in the perioperative period.
DVT prophylaxis should be practiced in all patients.

URI, upper respiratory infection; ABG, artery bypass grafting; PFT, pulmonary function testing; CPT, current procedural terminology; DVT, deep venous thrombosis.

In one study of surgical patients, the incidence of postoperative pneumonia was 50% in malnourished patients versus 15% for patients with normal nutritional status (72,73). The organisms responsible for postoperative pneumonia are different from those of community-acquired pneumonia. A large proportion of postoperative pneumonias are caused by gram-negative organisms, including *Pseudomonas*, *Klebsiella*, *Escherichia coli*, *Proteus*, and *Enterobacter* species (74). *Staphylococcus aureus* is also an important and frequent cause of ventilator-associated pneumonia.

Postoperative pneumonia is associated with 50% mortality rate, increasing to 80% in pneumonias caused by *Pseudomonas* species. Diagnosis of postoperative pneumonia requires a high index of clinical suspicion. Sputum Gram stains and tracheal aspirates are often nonspecific and the positive predictive value of a positive isolate is low. Invasive diagnostic methods like bronchoalveolar lavage (BAL) and/or protected specimen brushing (PSB) with quantitative cultures may be helpful for accurate diagnosis, but often these studies are not available, and empirical antibiotic therapy is prescribed. The antibiotic regimen used should provide broad-spectrum coverage, including antipseudomonal coverage in severely ill patients because hospital-acquired pneumonia is polymicrobial in up to 40% of the cases. However, a recent study suggests that the choice of antibiotic regimen had little impact on mortality (75). Those who have pneumonia secondary to aspiration should also be treated for anaerobic and staphylococcal infection. Staphylococcal coverage should be considered in patients with diabetes, renal failure, head trauma, and coma (76).

SURGICAL CONSIDERATIONS IN A PATIENT WITH CHRONIC OBSTRUCTIVE PULMONARY DISEASE

Patients with severe COPD have an increased risk of complications after major surgery. A decreased FEV_1 has been identified as an independent risk factor for POPC. Kroenke et al. studied a group of patients with severe COPD who underwent major abdominal and thoracic surgery excluding lung resection surgery (42). POPC occurred in 29% of 107 patients.

The incidence of complications was strongly associated with ASA class and the type and duration of surgery. Most of the patients did not experience a life-threatening complication. There were six deaths for the entire group, most of which occurred in the patients undergoing coronary artery bypass grafting (CABG). Three of these were due to cardiac causes and three were due to multiple causes, but respiratory failure was a contributing factor. Hence, the overall mortality rate was 6% and the mortality rate attributable to COPD was 3%. The mortality rate in non-CABG patients was only 1.3%, suggesting that patients undergoing operations not involving lung resection should not be denied an operation because of the severity of their lung disease. Patients who have severe COPD have a tendency for a worse outcome in CABG operations secondary to coexisting heart disease and other medical illnesses (42,43,77). Perioperative management of the patient with COPD is outlined in Table 24-3.

SURGICAL CONSIDERATIONS IN THE ASTHMATIC PATIENT

In a recent prospective study of 706 asthmatic patients undergoing surgery, the risk for perioperative bronchospasm was 2% (78). Although refractory bronchospasm leading to respiratory failure is rare (78,79), those patients who have been recently hospitalized for asthma or have required an emergency room or office visit within 30 days preceding surgery are at much greater risk of developing a significant exacerbation in the perioperative period (78). Operations associated with a higher incidence of bronchospasm include bronchoscopy and oropharyngeal instrumentation such as gastroscopy and ears, nose, and throat (ENT) surgery. Mediastinoscopy can also provoke bronchospasm by reflex mechanisms.

Elective surgery should be postponed for a few weeks in patients with a recent asthma attack. All bronchodilators used preoperatively should be continued during the postoperative period. Intravenous aminophylline can be used in patients who are unable to take their oral medication, although inhaled bronchodilators are more efficacious. Inhaled steroids should be continued. Patients who are on systemic steroid medication should be given stress-dose steroids in the perioperative period to prevent adrenal insufficiency. Humidified air and oxygen should be used in the perioperative period. Regional anesthesia may be an option for patients who have significant bronchospasm despite optimal medical therapy.

EVALUATION OF SUITABILITY FOR LUNG RESECTION

Although spirometry has not been shown to be a good predictor of pulmonary complications in patients undergoing nonresectional thoracic or abdominal surgery, it has a definite role in evaluating patients for lung resection. The predicted postoperative FEV_1 has been shown to correlate significantly with postoperative complications (80).

While evaluating fitness for lung resection, the possibility of a pneumonectomy should always be considered. Patients who are deemed to be unfit for a pneumonectomy should be offered less aggressive surgical options such as VATS or nonsurgical therapy rather than open thoracotomy.

In the past, patients were excluded from surgery if they did not meet the fitness criteria outlined in Table 24-4 (80–85). There are varying recommendations about the lowest acceptable value of the postoperative percent-predicted FEV_1 and diffusing capacity of carbon monoxide (D_{LCO}) by different authors. Markos et al. found a mortality rate of 50% if the predicted postoperative FEV_1 was <40%. Predicted postoperative D_{LCO} below 40% of the predicted value was associated with a 33% mortality rate (86).

PREDICTING POSTOPERATIVE PULMONARY FUNCTION AND COMPLICATIONS

Ventilation and Perfusion Lung Scanning

The contribution of each lung to pulmonary function can be assessed by quantitative ventilation and perfusion lung scans. After IV injection of technitium 99m–labeled macroaggregates of albumin, images are obtained with a gamma camera linked to a computer. The counts are then recorded over each hemithorax from an anterior and posterior view, and the sum of these is divided by the total counts from both lungs to

TABLE 24-4. Contraindications to Lung Resection

Hypercarbia >45 mm Hg at rest or exercise.
FEV_1 <2 L, FVC below 2 L, and MVV <50% of the
  predicted value for patients undergoing pneumonectomy.
FEV_1 <1.5 L in those in whom a lobectomy is required.
Predicted postoperative FEV_1 <800 mL determined
  preoperatively by spirometry and quantitative perfusion scans.

FEV_1, forced expiratory volume in 1 second; FVC, forced vital capacity; MVV, maximal voluntary ventilation.

determine the contribution of each lung to overall perfusion. Standard oblique views can also be obtained to assess the contribution of each lobe to lung perfusion. Predicted postoperative FEV_1 is then measured as follows:

Predicted postoperative FEV_1
  = Preoperative FEV_1 × (1 − fractional contribution
    of the affected lung or lobe)

Calculation of predicted postoperative FEV_1 can also be performed by using preoperative PFT data and the number of bronchopulmonary segments to be removed (84). If it is assumed that each of the 19 bronchopulmonary segments contributes equally to ventilatory function, each segment would account for 5.26% of pulmonary function. Hence, a right pneumonectomy is assumed to cause a loss of 55% of pulmonary function, whereas a left pneumonectomy would cause a loss of approximately 45% of lung function. On the basis of these assumptions, the predicted postoperative function can be calculated by the formula:

$$\text{Predicted postoperative } FEV_1 = \text{preoperative } FEV_1 \times [1 - (S \times 5.26/100)]$$

where S = the number of segments to be resected

Exercise Testing

Several studies have evaluated the usefulness of preoperative exercise testing for predicting the incidence of postoperative complications (87–94). Whether or not exercise testing is superior to measurement of predicted postoperative lung function is controversial. There are studies to support both approaches, but neither method has been shown to be superior. Exercise testing is attractive because exercise capacity is not dependent on lung function alone. It also measures hemodynamic performance and peripheral tissue oxygen utilization.

The exercise protocol used by most centers involves a graded increase in workload using a bicycle ergometer. Gas exchange is monitored and analyzed along with electrocardiogram (ECG) monitoring, pulse oximetry, and frequent blood pressure monitoring. Some centers routinely use invasive blood pressure monitoring devices. Exercise is stopped when the patient develops limiting symptoms. The data is analyzed, and the maximum oxygen consumption (V_{O_2}max) is then calculated.

Most studies have reported a strong correlation between decreased exercise capacity and the frequency of cardiopulmonary complications. However, the threshold V_{O_2}max for identifying high-risk patients has been difficult to define. In the study by Smith et al., patients who achieved a V_{O_2}max above 20 mL/kg/minute had only a 10% incidence of postoperative complications, whereas all the patients with a V_{O_2}max below 15 mL/kg/minute suffered postoperative complications (88). In another study by Morice et al., two out of the six patients with a V_{O_2}max above 15 mL/kg/minute had postoperative complications after lung resection. Patients who had a V_{O_2}max below 15 mL/kg/minute were not offered lung resection in that study (90). Most centers offer lung resection to patients if their V_{O_2}max is above 15 mL/kg/minute and if there are no other contraindications to surgery. The V_{O_2}max has not been shown to correlate with spirometric measurements of pulmonary function (88).

Predicted postoperative maximal oxygen consumption (Vo_2max-ppo) can be estimated with the use of preoperative pulmonary perfusion scans and exercise testing in a manner similar to the prediction of postoperative FEV_1 and $DLco$. A Vo_2max-ppo below 10 mL/kg/minute was associated with a 100% mortality rate in a study by Bolliger et al. (89). In another study, eight out of nine patients who had a Vo_2max below 60% of the predicted value suffered POPC, including three deaths (93).

The ability of the patient to climb stairs is also a good predictor of postoperative complications after high-risk surgery, such as thoracotomy, sternotomy, and upper abdominal laparotomy (92). The inability to climb two flights of stairs had a positive predictive value of 82% for postoperative complications. There also appears to be a correlation between the $DLco$ measurement at rest and during exercise (i.e., at 70% of the patient's maximal workload) and the incidence of postoperative complications. If the $DLco$ at 70% of maximal workload was less than 10% more than the $DLco$ at rest, there was a 100% complication rate, compared with a 10% rate in patients in whom the differences were more than or equal to 10% (95).

Invasive cardiopulmonary exercise testing has also been employed to determine lung resectability. In a study by Olsen et al., patients who tolerated lung resection poorly were found to have a lower cardiac index, oxygen delivery, and oxygen consumption compared with patients who tolerated resection well (96). A pulmonary vascular resistance (PVR) >190 dynes second per cms has been proposed as a contraindication to lung resection by Fee et al. (94). However, in the study by Olsen et al., PVR was not significantly different between the patients who tolerated lung resection and those who were classified as being intolerant (96).

Epstein et al. have devised a cardiopulmonary risk index (CPRI) by combining a modified Goldman index and six factors that have been shown to be associated with increased POPC (see Table 24-5). These risk factors include obesity, cigarette smoking, productive cough within 5 days prior to surgery, diffuse ronchi or wheezing on physical examination, FEV_1/FVC <70%, and a arterial partial pressure of carbon dioxide ($Paco_2$) >45 mm Hg. The total possible score for the pulmonary index is six. The Goldman index was modified using an echocardiographic or radionuclide estimation of cardiac ejection fraction, and points were assigned for each of the four classes described by Goldman. The combined CPRI had a total possible score of 10. In a series of 42 patients undergoing

lung resection, Epstein et al. observed that a CPRI score of >4 was associated with a 73% incidence of postoperative cardiopulmonary complications versus 11% when the score was <4. The CPRI was shown to have a sensitivity of 73%, a specificity of 89%, a positive predictive value of 79%, and a negative predictive value of 98%. The predictive value of CPRI is improved if it is combined with exercise testing using cycle ergometry (97,98). In a recent prospective study of 180 patients undergoing lung resection, the CPRI had an overall sensitivity of 23% and a specificity of 80% for predicting postoperative complications. In patients undergoing pneumonectomy, the sensitivity was improved to 44% and the specificity was 100% (99). The CPRI cannot be recommended as a screening test for all patients undergoing lung resection. It may be of value for the evaluation of elderly lung resection candidates who are likely to have a high prevalence of cardiac or pulmonary diseases.

CARDIAC CONSIDERATIONS FOR LUNG RESECTION AND GENERAL SURGERY

A large number of patients with COPD also have cardiovascular disease that contributes significantly to postoperative morbidity and mortality. Goldman et al. devised a multifactorial cardiac risk index to predict operative morbidity in unselected patients more than 40 years old (100) (see Table 24-6). This "Goldman Index" was based on a prospective study of 1,001

TABLE 24-5. Cardiopulmonary Risk Index

Variable	Points
Obesity (BMI >27 kg/m²)	1
Cigarette smoking (within 8 wk of surgery)	1
Productive cough within 5 d	1
Diffuse wheezing or ronchi within 5 d of surgery	1
FEV_1/FVC <70%	1
$Paco_2$ >45 mm Hg	1
Total	6

BMI, body mass index; FEV_1, forced expiratory volume in 1 second; FVC, forced vital capacity; $Paco_2$, arterial partial pressure of carbon dioxide.

TABLE 24-6. Goldman Multifactorial Risk Index

	Points
History	
Age >70	5
MI within 6 mo	10
Physical	
JVD or S3 gallop[a]	11
Significant valvular aortic stenosis	3
Electrocardiogram	
Rhythm other than sinus or PACs on preoperative ECG	7
More than five PVCs per minute at any time prior to surgery	7
Poor General Medical Status	3
Po_2 <60 mm Hg or Pco_2 <50 mm Hg	
K^+ <3.0 or HCO3$^-$ <20 mEq/L	
BUN >50 or creatinine >3 mg/dL	
Abnormal SGOT, chronic liver disease	
Bedridden due to noncardiac disease	
Operation	
Intrathoracic, intraperitoneal, or aortic surgery	3
Emergency surgery	4
Total Points	53

Class 1 = 0–5 points, Class 2 = 6–12 points, Class 3 = 13–25 points, Class 4 = >26 points.[b]

MI, myocardial infarction; JVD, jugular venous distension; PAC, premature atrial contraction; ECG, electrocardiogram; PVC, premature ventricular contraction; Po_2, partial pressure of oxygen; Pco_2, partial pressure of carbon dioxide; BUN, blood urea nitrogen; SGOT, serum glutamic-oxaloacetic transaminase.

[a]In cardiopulmonary risk index (CPRI) described by Epstein et al., left ventricular ejection fraction (LVEF) <40% was also included.
[b]In CPRI, Goldman class 1 = 1 point, Class 2 = 2 points, Class 3 = 3 points, and class 4 = 4 points.

consecutive patients undergoing noncardiac surgery. The study identified nine risk factors that were associated with increased cardiac complications. Scores were assigned to each risk factor after multivariate analyses. The patients were assigned four risk categories according to their total score. This index provides clinicians with a simple way of assessing and modifying cardiac risk. It has been found to be reproducible and has been validated in several studies.

Lee et al. have developed a Revised Cardiac Risk Index, which utilizes six factors to assess the risk of complications in patients undergoing major noncardiac surgery (101). The predictors were preoperative creatinine >2.0 mg per dL, preoperative insulin therapy, history of cerebrovascular disease, history of ischemic heart disease, history of congestive heart failure (CHF), and higher-risk surgery. If three or more factors were present, then the major cardiac complication rate was 9%.

Age alone does not appear to be an independent risk factor for cardiac complications in major noncardiac surgery (102).

SURGICAL RISK IN PATIENTS WITH ANGINA

The Goldman index does not address surgical risk in patients with angina pectoris. Patients with stable angina as their only risk factor are at low cardiac risk during noncardiac surgery. Patients with unstable angina are at significantly increased risk, and coronary revascularization should be considered prior to major surgery. For patients with myocardial infarction (MI) within the past 6 months, it is best to delay elective surgery. However, operations can be safely performed within 4 to 6 weeks after an MI if a delay is potentially dangerous. Patients who undergo successful revascularization following an MI can also undergo surgery 4 to 6 weeks after their MI.

It has been shown that in the perioperative period, β-blockers significantly reduce the risk of MI and cardiac death, so perioperative β-blockers should be considered unless they are contraindicated (103). Additionally, perioperative clonidine reduces cardiac ischemic episodes in patients with known or suspected coronary artery disease (104).

CHEST TRAUMA

In spite of the implementation of a standardized assessment and management program for care of trauma patients, development of designated regional trauma centers, intensive training of paramedical personnel, and advances in the fields of trauma surgery and critical care medicine, trauma remains one of the five most common causes of death in the United States (105). Nearly 150,000 deaths occur in the United States yearly from trauma, and twice as many patients are left permanently disabled each year.

Injuries to the chest occur in approximately 60% of all victims with multisystem injuries and very often represent the most life-threatening component of the injury complex. For this reason, physicians caring for these patients should be trained in standardized advanced trauma life support (ATLS) assessment and procedures (106). Application of ATLS principles couples the initiation of the ABCs (Airway, Breathing, and Circulation) of general resuscitation with the rapid initial assessment of the trauma patient or primary survey (see Table 24-7). The purpose

TABLE 24-7. Initial Survey of Thoracic Injuries

Primary Survey—Assessment of IImmediately Life-Threatening Injuries
  Airway obstruction
  Tension pneumothorax
  Open pneumothorax
  Massive hemothorax
  Flail chest
  Cardiac tamponade

Secondary Survey—Assessment of Potentially Life-Threatening Injuries
  Simple pneumothorax
  Hemothorax
  Pulmonary contusion
  Traumatic aortic rupture
  Tracheobronchial disruption
  Esophageal disruption
  Traumatic diaphragmatic injury
  Blunt cardiac injury
  Penetrating wounds traversing the mediastinum

of the primary survey is rapid identification and treatment of immediately life-threatening injuries. Most of these injuries involve structures located within the chest cavity. Following stabilization of these injuries, a secondary survey is performed. This is a full examination of the patient, assessing injuries in all systems and identifying specifically those that are deemed potentially life threatening. Use of these ATLS management methods has greatly decreased morbidity and mortality in victims of trauma.

DIAGNOSTIC AND THERAPEUTIC MODALITIES

Radiologic Studies

In all patients with polytrauma, chest radiography (CXR) is a vital diagnostic tool. This study should be done early in the course of the patient's care, after general resuscitation measures and the primary survey are completed. Most CXRs obtained in this early care setting are portable anterior/posterior views and are taken with the patient in a supine position. Patient position combined with body habitus and the presence of emergency transport equipment (e.g., cervical collar) may limit the clinician's ability to interpret this initial film, and this should be taken into account when evaluating abnormalities. Evaluation of the initial CXR should be done in a systematic manner (e.g., bony skeleton, soft tissues, pleural spaces, lungs, mediastinum, and diaphragm) so that no abnormality is overlooked. Repeat CXRs should be done following procedures such as endotracheal intubation, central venous line placement, or chest tube insertion, or if technical aspects of the initial film prevent adequate interpretation.

Thoracic Bony Skeleton

Detection of rib fractures is important in that it may be associated with other significant injuries within the chest. It also indicates the need for pain control to help prevent secondary complications such as atelectasis and pneumonia. If clinical examination leads to the suspicion that a rib fracture is present, the patient should be treated for it even without radiologic confirmation because rib fractures are not always evident on the chest film. The single best and most cost-effective test for detection of rib fractures is an upright posterior/anterior chest radiograph in full inspiration. In most chest trauma cases, this will be a repeat film and not the initial CXR that is performed and will only be done after more critical studies and therapeutic procedures are completed. Occasionally, more specific views may be indicated for fractures of ribs 1 to 3 and 9 to 12 because fractures in these areas have a greater chance of association with significant underlying injuries (107,108). These additional films should only be obtained after full stabilization of the patient (109). When looking for rib fractures, the clinician should look particularly in the area of the anterior and posterior axillary lines because it is in these areas of curvature that most rib fractures occur with anterior chest compression injuries.

Sternal fractures are uncommon and their detection is difficult. The best radiologic study for evaluation is a lateral CXR using a horizontal beam. The presence of a sternal fracture is often associated with more significant soft tissue injury beneath, particularly cardiac or pulmonary contusion. The clinician should be alert to the possibility of these injuries.

Because a significant amount of force is required for fracture of the scapula, the clinician should always be suspicious of more severe damage to vital intrathoracic structures if it is seen. A large percentage of scapular fractures are missed on initial evaluation of the CXR. More sensitive studies such as CT scan may be needed for diagnosis. Vertebral fractures often produce a paravertebral hematoma, a finding that commonly obscures the normal intrathoracic vascular structures and widens the mediastinal shadow on initial CXR. This may lead many clinicians to suspect a major vascular injury. If suspected from the initial CXR, a repeat CXR that is overpenetrated can often be useful in determining the existence of vertebral injuries (110). If vertebral injury is noted or suspected, more sensitive diagnostic studies such as CT scan would be indicated.

Computerized Tomography and Magnetic Resonance Imaging

CT scan of the chest is a much more sensitive study for identifying intrathoracic injuries than the supine anteroposterior CXR, but it requires patient transport, is more time consuming and costly, and requires more expertise for appropriate interpretation. If deemed necessary for evaluation of the chest in a trauma patient, this study should never be done until the secondary survey is completed. Information obtained from a chest CT study in this initial phase of patient care infrequently alters management. In specific instances, a CT scan may provide valuable information that is not noted on the admission CXR (e.g., a small pneumothorax in a patient requiring positive-pressure ventilation) (110). In some centers, CT scan is used prior to aortography to evaluate the patient with a widened mediastinal shadow and possible aortic transection. Some believe that this is a very valuable diagnostic step because absence of a mediastinal hematoma eliminates the need for aortography (111–113). Others believe that a CT study for aortic transection is excessively time consuming and has an unacceptably high false-negative rate (114). Until these controversies are sorted out, it is safe to say that at most medical facilities any suspicion of aortic transection should be immediately studied with the single most definitive test for this problem, aortography. Use of CT scan may prove to be more valuable later in the course of the trauma patient's care to evaluate abnormalities such as retained hemothorax, loculated empyema, pulmonary contusion, and intrapulmonary hematoma (114).

Magnetic Resonance Imaging (MRI) also provides more detail than plain radiographs but, like CT scan, is virtually never indicated in the acute trauma setting for evaluation of the chest (110). It may prove helpful in a limited number of cases later in the course of the trauma patient's management for identification of residual abnormalities within the chest.

Ultrasound/Echocardiography/Aortography

Transthoracic ultrasound has become a mainstay for assessment of the pericardial space in the setting of acute chest trauma. A good view of the pericardial space can be obtained using the subxiphoid view, thus allowing rapid diagnosis of intrapericardial fluid (113). This technology can be done rapidly and reliably by physicians with limited training. Several series have shown that this study has excellent sensitivity at centers in which it is used regularly.

More recently, ultrasound has been described as a tool for detection of pneumothorax and hemothorax. Several busy trauma centers have extended their standard focused abdominal sonography for trauma (FAST) scan protocols to include evaluation of the thoraces for pneumothorax in acute trauma victims. This technology may prove to be a useful extension of the physical examination in the trauma setting because of its accuracy, portability, and ability to provide diagnostic data instantly. In addition, mastery of this technology appears relatively easy for surgeons and other physicians caring for the injured. Limitations of this technology, however, do exist in the assessment of various other thoracic injuries, such as those of the thoracic skeleton and mediastinal structures. Thus at present, thoracic ultrasound can be considered an adjunct to standard CXR (115,116).

Transesophageal echocardiography (TEE) has been used successfully for the diagnosis of acute dissection of the ascending aorta, but its value in the diagnosis of traumatic aortic transection has been questionable (113). Some centers report a significant number of false-negative studies. Also, this study requires specially trained personnel and is time consuming. TEE is not presently a valuable diagnostic tool for diagnosis in acute chest trauma.

Aortography has long been considered the gold standard for diagnosis of acute aortic transection and remains so in the opinion of many. Except for this and for diagnosis of trauma to the brachiocephalic vessels, arteriography has very little value in acute chest trauma.

Bronchoscopy

Flexible fiber-optic bronchoscopy can be a very valuable diagnostic tool in chest trauma. The clinician should have a low threshold for its use in chest trauma patients presenting with any of the signs of major tracheobronchial injury (117) or airway foreign bodies (114). The procedure can be done in the emergency department, the operating room, or the ICU and is particularly easy in patients who have already been endotracheally intubated for airway control. One *caveat* that should not be overlooked in the intubated patient is the fact that the entire airway of a patient suspected of having a tracheobronchial injury should be visualized, not merely the portion distal to the endotracheal tube (118). This may require a coordinated effort by several personnel so that airway control is maintained. The endotracheal tube can be backed out over the fiber-optic bronchoscope up to the level of the vocal cords while the upper portion of the trachea is viewed, and the endotracheal tube can then be safely reinserted over the bronchoscope.

Rigid bronchoscopy may be required in the chest trauma patient presenting with massive hemoptysis and in some cases of tracheobronchial injury (117). This procedure must be done in the operating room and is performed for localization of the source of bleeding prior to thoracotomy.

Tube Thoracostomy

Chest tube insertion is the most frequent therapeutic procedure performed for blunt and penetrating chest trauma and is a mainstay in the management of pneumothorax and hemothorax. Adequate chest tube size and proper intrathoracic placement are two important features in successful evacuation of a fluid collection within the chest cavity. A list of the indications for tube thoracostomy in the setting of chest trauma is given in Table 24-8. Though a common therapeutic procedure in chest trauma, it is associated with a complication rate of >30% in some series. It goes without saying that proper technique is mandatory when inserting a chest tube (119). Additionally, a number of studies suggest that administration of prophylactic antibiotics in the setting of tube thoracostomy placement for chest trauma reduces the incidence of infectious complications (120,121).

Thoracoscopy

Over the past decade, video-assisted technology has been found increasingly applicable in patients suffering from chest trauma. It has been used as a diagnostic tool to identify and primarily control sources of bleeding within the chest in hemodynamically stable patients (122). Even when the site of bleeding cannot be readily controlled with these minimally invasive methods, limited thoracotomy plus thoracoscopic visualization can be used to approach the bleeding site (123,124). Thoracoscopic methods have also been used for identification and repair of diaphragmatic injuries (124). This minimally invasive technology is most commonly used later in the course of the trauma patient's care for evacuation of retained hemothoraces (125–127) and in select patients who develop an empyema after chest injury. One important management point to be observed is patient respiratory stability during a thoracoscopic procedure. Patients undergoing video-assisted thoracoscopic procedures must be able to tolerate single-lung ventilation while positioned in a lateral decubitus position on the operating table. This places the ventilated lung in a dependent position and may not be tolerated well by patients whose ventilatory status is marginal (122). Also, for this procedure, exchange of a standard endotracheal tube for a double-lumen tube is commonly required. This maneuver alone may be risky in marginally stable patients. Trauma patients who are difficult to oxygenate and/or ventilate because of massive pulmonary contusion, adult respiratory distress syndrome (ARDS), pulmonary edema, or other conditions are not likely to tolerate the positioning and ventilatory settings required to perform a thorough thoracoscopic examination of the chest.

Thoracotomy

Thoracotomy is indicated in a small percentage of chest trauma patients in whom the injury is not adequately managed by other means such as tube thoracostomy (128). Large hemothorax and persistent hemorrhage are two common indications for exploration of the chest (see Table 24-9).

Indications for thoracotomy in the emergency department are few. The best survival data for emergency department thoracotomy is found in patients who have sustained penetrating trauma to the chest and have vital signs detected at the scene of the injury but experience loss of vital signs en route to the hospital or in the emergency department (129). Those who have sustained blunt chest injury and have no vital signs at the scene have been shown to derive virtually no benefit from thoracotomy in the emergency department and are not considered candidates for this procedure. It should be emphasized that emergency department thoracotomy should only be performed by qualified physicians with appropriate surgical training.

INJURIES TO THE CHEST WALL

Sternal Fractures

Motor vehicle crashes and, more recently, the mandatory use of seat belts have increased the incidence of sternal fracture. The classic scenario is that of a patient whose anterior chest wall strikes the steering wheel. Less common mechanisms are direct blows to the sternum or hyperflexion of the thoracic spine. These fractures are most common in women, patients over the age of 50, and those using shoulder restraints (130). The signs

TABLE 24-8.   Indications for Tube Thoracostomy in Thoracic Trauma

---

Simple pneumothorax associated with any chest trauma
Tension pneumothorax
Pneumothorax increasing in size
Pneumothorax in any unstable patient
Bilateral pneumothorax
Hemothorax or hemopneumothorax
Pneumothorax in an intubated, ventilated patient (including those about to undergo general anesthesia)
Open pneumothorax ("sucking" chest wound) in association with application of sterile occlusive dressing over the chest wall defect

---

TABLE 24-9.   Indications for Thoracotomy in Thoracic Trauma

Operating Room Thoracotomy
  Initial evacuation of 1,500 mL of blood or more from
    thoracostomy tube
  Persistent hemorrhage (>250 mL/hr for 2–4 hr)
  Failure of tube thoracostomy with enlarging hemothorax
  Hemodynamic instability despite adequate resuscitation
Emergency Department Thoracotomy
  Penetrating injury with trauma arrest en route to or in the
    emergency department

---

and symptoms are anterior chest pain, overlying tenderness, ecchymosis, crepitus, swelling, and/or deformity. Although some sternal fractures are evident on plain CXR, a lateral film of the sternum is the best diagnostic tool. The upper and mid-portions of the sternum are most prone to fracture.

Treatment is initially directed toward associated injuries, reported in approximately 50% of patients, with rib fractures, long bone fractures, and head injury reported in 40%, 25%, and 18%, respectively (131,132). There is considerable controversy about whether sternal fractures are a hallmark for underlying cardiac injuries. ECG and radionuclide abnormalities have been demonstrated in >50% of the patients who present with sternal fracture, but the incidence of blunt cardiac injury does not seem to exceed that of the multiply injured population (133–138). Certainly, the possibility of blunt cardiac injury should receive consideration and investigation in patients with sternal fracture and with a history of high-energy mechanism of injury and in those with hemodynamic instability. Therapy of sternal fracture is nearly always limited to pain relief and avoidance of excessive motion. Only patients with grossly displaced sternal fragments and severe pain need operative fixation (see Fig. 24-1). Patients with isolated sternal fracture can often be managed on an outpatient basis.

Rib Fractures

The most commonly encountered bony injury to the chest is a rib fracture, although the exact incidence is unknown. This diagnosis should be suspected in any patient with a blunt mechanism of injury who complains of chest pain and tenderness, particularly if there is an overlying abrasion or contusion.

Motor vehicle crashes account for most rib fractures; the incidence is not significantly reduced by using seat belts (139). Penetrating trauma to the chest is not a common cause of rib fracture. In the conscious patient, careful physical examination will detect most rib fractures; however, Trunkey noted that 50% of rib fractures are not readily apparent on the initial anteroposterior chest films routinely obtained in trauma patients (140,141). In unconscious and severely injured patients, rib fractures are more difficult to detect. Rib detail films may aid in confirming a clinical suspicion on the basis of mechanism of injury and physical examination.

The treatment of rib fractures is primarily directed at pain relief, maintenance of effective pulmonary function, and prevention of complications. The optimal method of accomplishing these goals is dependent on a variety of factors that include the severity of injury to the chest, overall injury severity, patient factors such as age and medical condition, and the clinical modalities that are available within the treatment facility.

Patients who have one or two rib fractures, are in good medical condition, and have no other major injuries or complications can often be managed as outpatients with oral analgesics. The use of rib belts for additional analgesia remains controversial. There is at least one clinical study that indicates that rib belts relieve pain without significantly impairing chest wall mechanics (142). However, in general, rib belts are disfavored because of the concept that restricted chest wall motion leads to atelectasis and other complications such as pneumonia. There is no major support in the literature for these ideas as they specifically relate to rib belts, and further study is needed. If a patient is to be treated as an outpatient, adequate pain relief and education on cough, deep breathing,

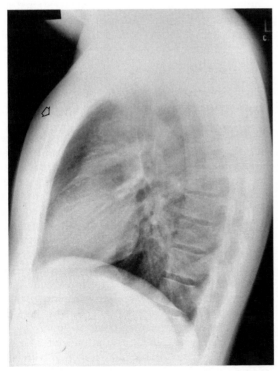
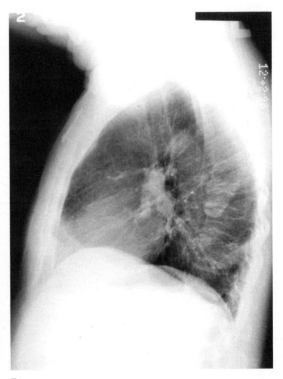

A
B

FIGURE 24-1. **A, B:** Sternal dislocation. This sternal dislocation required repair because of nonunion and chronic pain.

and general pulmonary toilet are essential. The patient should also clearly understand the signs and symptoms that would necessitate a return to the hospital (i.e., dyspnea, tachypnea, persistent pain, fever, and yellow sputum).

Three or more rib fractures or flail segments are indications of a greater overall injury severity, both inside and outside the chest cavity (143). Of particular note is that pneumothorax, hemothorax, and lung parenchymal and intraabdominal injuries are more common. These patients should be treated initially in the hospital. Also, individuals who are elderly or pediatric, multiply injured, medically complicated, in a questionable state of health, or have inadequate pain control with oral analgesics should be hospitalized. Complications occur in one-third of these patients. Predicting the need for ICU care and mechanical ventilation is challenging, and outpatient management is risky (144,145). The respiratory therapy service should be involved with the patient and physician to establish an individualized program for maintaining pulmonary toilet and function. Pain management also must be individualized. There is no consensus on the best modality, although success has been reported with oral and IV narcotics, patient-controlled analgesia (PCA), intrapleural catheters, and intermittent and continuous epidural catheters. For nonintubated patients with mid–to-lower chest wall injuries involving multiple ribs, there is some evidence that continuous epidural management is superior to PCA and intrapleural catheters in maintaining tidal volume, VC and maximum inspiratory pressure, and pain relief (146,147).

Special consideration should be given to patients with fractures of the first and second ribs. A fracture at this level indicates a high level of kinetic injury and is associated with a higher incidence of injury to the aorta and great vessels, as well as intraabdominal and intracranial structures. Investigations of these areas should be undertaken on a selective basis. Many of these patients will require inpatient observation to rule out other injuries.

In summary, rib fractures are a common sequela of trauma. Although patients with simple fractures can be treated as outpatients, multiple rib fractures are predictors of severe injury and patients with these fractures often require hospitalization, not only for the treatment of pain and maintenance of adequate pulmonary function but also for the treatment of complications of nonchest injuries. Previous research indicates that 50% of these patients will require operative or ICU care (148).

Flail Chest

Flail chest is a multiple injury pattern of the chest wall that results in paradoxical motion of the hemithorax with breathing. The injured segment moves inward during inspiration and outward during expiration. Usually, flail chest results from the fractures of three or more ribs in two locations, typically posteriorly and laterally or anteriorly and laterally, but it may also result from a combination of fractures of the ribs and costal cartilages and/or sternum (see Fig. 24-2). Flail chest may not be diagnosed initially in patients who arrive at the hospital intubated by prehospital personnel and may only be suspected after chest radiographs or during weaning from the ventilator. Flail chest is diagnosed by physical examination and may be confirmed radiographically.

As with rib fracture alone, treatment of flail chest is supportive. Pulmonary function abnormalities seen in flail chest

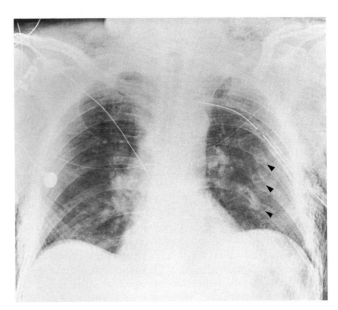

FIGURE 24-2.   Multiple rib fractures. Multiple rib fractures with subcutaneous emphysema can be seen. Greater than three rib fractures correlates with an increased overall injury severity score. Outpatient treatment is inadvisable.

include decreases in the VC, total static lung compliance, maximum inspiratory force, and arterial oxygenation and increases in airway resistance and the work of breathing. This pathophysiology is related to pain, splinting, and abnormal chest wall mechanics, and in many cases, underlying pulmonary contusion.

Management concepts have changed through the years. Until the 1950s, emphasis was placed on external stabilization of the chest wall using a variety of operative and nonoperative techniques. In 1956, Avery et al. advocated internal stabilization of the chest wall with volume-control ventilators (149). More recently, Richardson et al. and Sheckford et al. have demonstrated that adequate analgesia and aggressive pulmonary toilet reduce morbidity and hospital stay without need for mechanical ventilation (145,150).

Even with these measures, a significant number of patients will require ventilator assistance. Factors associated with a greater need for mechanical ventilation are the overall injury severity, particularly injuries to the head, multiple long bone fractures, and truncal injuries requiring operation; blood transfusions in the first 24 hours; and shock on admission (151). Also affecting outcome adversely are age above 50, bilateral flail segments, the presence of a hemothorax and/or pneumothorax requiring a chest tube, and underlying pulmonary contusion. Patients involved in a motorcycle accident, pedestrians hit by automobiles, and fall victims also have a poorer prognosis (152).

Intubation is recommended for individuals with tachypnea (respiratory rate >40 breaths per minute), tidal volumes <10 mL per kg, hypoxemia (PaO_2 <60 mm Hg on an FIO_2 of >50%), and/or hypercapnia ($PaCO_2$ >50 mm Hg in patients with no history of COPD), and in patients whose associated injuries necessitate intubation. Extubation criteria are similar to those used in other ventilated patients. Adequate unassisted tidal volume and respiratory rates of 30 breaths per minute or less suggest that the chest wall has stabilized sufficiently to allow extubation.

In rare circumstances, patients require operative stabilization of the chest wall. Although criteria are not strictly established, paradoxical motion of the chest wall that prevents weaning from the ventilator and severe chest wall deformity with >5 cm depression are accepted indications. Patients who are ventilated principally for severe pulmonary contusion have not been shown to benefit from chest wall stabilization. Patients who require thoracotomy for other traumatic indications (e.g., persistent air leak, diaphragmatic rupture, retained hemothorax, etc.) should also receive chest wall stabilization. Thomas et al. showed shortened duration of mechanical ventilation, improved pain control, and improved anatomic healing with early stabilization (153).

Long-term pulmonary disability exists in approximately 60% of patients recovering from a flail chest. All of the following complications have been documented: chest wall pain and deformity, dyspnea on exertion varying from months to lifetime, decreased minute ventilation, and mild restrictive pulmonary disease (154,155). Despite modern improvements in care, the mortality rate remains high (10% to 35%). Death is principally due to associated injuries and sepsis (152,156).

Pneumothorax

Pneumothorax is a common sequela of both blunt and penetrating chest trauma. The three types of pneumothorax seen in trauma victims are simple, open, and tension.

Simple pneumothorax most commonly occurs when air escapes from the visceral pleural surface of the lung. As the space within the thorax fills with air, the lung parenchyma collapses. If the lung injury is small, it may be rapidly sealed by platelets in the low-pressure setting of the lung. Mechanisms of lung injury include penetrating objects and missiles, iatrogenic causes such as central lines and bronchoscopic biopsy, and rib fractures. Blunt rupture of blebs and lung parenchyma may occur with high kinetic energy transmission across the chest wall, such as in motor vehicle crashes and falls. Patients complain of shortness of breath and have decreased breath sounds and tympany to percussion in the affected hemithorax.

In the setting of trauma, it is neither necessary nor advisable to await a chest radiograph prior to instituting therapy. Initial treatment can be with a large-bore needle in the second intercostal space or a chest tube. If needle decompression is elected, chest tube placement should follow expeditiously. Except in iatrogenic trauma, use of needle-catheter drainage system is not recommended because of the high incidence of reaccumulation and concomitant presence of blood within the chest cavity. Chest tubes for trauma should be placed in the fourth or fifth intercostal space laterally and be directed posteriorly. Because up to 25% of patients have pleural symphysis, chest tube placement should always be performed by or with the supervision of an experienced physician. A 32F to 40F size tube will prevent inadequate evacuation of air and blood secondary to clots within the tube. Careful attention should be directed to ascertaining that all the holes in the chest tube are within the thoracic cavity. Sturdy stitches (usually size 0, no. 1, or no. 2) should secure the tube to the skin and underlying fascia. Chest tubes should be placed on suction of approximately 20 cm H_2O. A CXR should be obtained after the tube is placed to assess the expansion of the lung and chest tube position.

A question often asked is whether a trauma patient can be treated for pneumothorax without a chest tube. There is little scientific data on this matter. In general, most experienced physicians would recommend this therapy only under the following circumstances: (a) the pneumothorax is unilateral and small (<20% of the volume of the hemithorax), (b) there is no associated hemothorax or detectable air leak, (c) there are no other major injuries, (d) the patient can understand worsening signs and symptoms and ask for assistance, (e) there is no requirement for positive-pressure ventilation or anesthetic, (f) the patient requires no further transfer by ground or air, (g) an individual who can urgently place a chest tube on the patient is present in the hospital, and (h) the patient is largely asymptomatic. When in doubt, the placement of a chest tube is the safer option. If management without a chest tube is elected, a second CXR should be obtained within 4 to 6 hours to be certain that the pneumothorax is not increasing in size. Any worsening of symptoms should result in prompt insertion of a chest tube.

An open pneumothorax occurs when there is an opening in the chest wall that exceeds two-thirds of the diameter of the trachea. This creates a "sucking wound" that allows ingress and egress of air and blood. In the prehospital setting, the wound should be covered with occlusive gauze and taped on three sides only. A completely occlusive dressing taped on four sides may convert the open pneumothorax to a tension pneumothorax. In the emergency room setting, a chest tube should be expeditiously placed and a fully occlusive bandage applied after the placement. The chest tube should not be introduced through the area of injury. Most of these wounds should proceed to the operating room for debridement and closure. Smaller wounds can be successfully managed in the emergency room setting. A CXR should be obtained after chest tube placement to check for adequate expansion of the lung, evacuation of air and blood, location of the tube, and concomitant injuries to other organs within the thorax.

A tension pneumothorax occurs when air escapes from the lungs and/or mediastinal structures or, less commonly, enters from outside and fills the hemithorax. Not only does the lung collapse but also a continued accumulation of air will shift the mediastinum to the opposite hemithorax. If untreated, it will kink the vena cava and impede venous return to the heart. If the preload to the heart becomes sufficiently reduced, hypotension and cardiac arrest will occur. Tension pneumothorax should be suspected in any patient presenting with blunt or penetrating chest injury plus hypotension. Common presenting findings include absent breath sounds, tympany to percussion, deviation of the trachea, neck vein distension, pulsus paradoxus, and/or worsening tachycardia, but these symptoms may be absent or difficult to detect. Additionally, the symptoms may mimic pericardial tamponade. If a tension pneumothorax is suspected, the patient should undergo an immediate large-bore–needle decompression in the second intercostal space followed by prompt chest tube placement. One should never wait for a CXR when there is high clinical suspicion of tension pneumothorax.

Hemothorax

Hemothorax simply means blood within the pleural cavity. It is seen with both penetrating and blunt trauma. In penetrating trauma, there is nearly always associated trauma to the chest wall, lungs, great vessels, heart, or intra-abdominal contents such as spleen or liver, with an associated diaphragmatic injury. Blunt trauma produces hemothorax via injuries to the chest wall, particularly rib fractures with associated intercostal artery bleeding, lacerations to the lung due to rib punctures and/or shear forces on the pulmonary parenchyma, and tearing of adhesions between the visceral and parietal pleura. Great vessel injury is also seen with blunt injuries, particularly aortic injury.

Patients with isolated hemothorax and blood loss of <250 mL will present with few symptoms. Generally, these hemothoraces are detected by blunting of the costophrenic angle on chest film. Patients with a greater blood loss present with all or a combination of the following signs and symptoms: chest pain, tachypnea, tachycardia, decreased or absent breath sounds, dullness to percussion, pallor, hypotension, and cardiovascular collapse. Shift of the mediastinum is also possible with hemothorax but is less common than with tension pneumothorax (see Fig. 24-3).

Initial treatment for hemothorax is with a tube thoracostomy. Thoracentesis is not indicated. Eighty-five percent of patients with hemothorax can be successfully managed with chest tube alone. Large size tubes, such as a 36F or 40F, placed in the fifth intercostal space and directed posteriorly will most effectively evacuate blood and are less likely to clot. If a large hemothorax is suspected, it may be beneficial to use an evacuation device with autotransfusion capability. The amount of blood collected should be serially monitored.

If >800 mL of blood is collected with insertion of the chest tube, it is defined as a massive hemothorax. Only 10% to 15% of patients requiring a chest tube progress to operative intervention, but this is a high-risk group. Early surgical consultation is mandatory. Criteria for operative intervention varies somewhat from surgeon to surgeon, but nearly all surgeons will operate if the chest tube output within the first hour after injury exceeds 1.5 liters or is >250 mL per hour thereafter.

Approximately 5% of patients presenting with hemothorax will develop the complication of a clotted hemothorax. Small, clotted hemothoraces that do not become infected will resolve on their own without significant pulmonary sequela. If chest tubes do not successfully drain large blood clots within the chest cavity, the patient may develop an empyema or have trapping and fibrosis of a significant portion of the lung. Research by Coselli et al. recommends that a clotted hemothorax be operatively evacuated if a lung volume loss of 25% or greater is detected on chest film or if signs of infection, such as fever and leukocytosis, develop (157). Timing of evacuation of a clotted hemothorax remains controversial. Generally, if a decision is made prior to 1 week, many patients can undergo an evacuation using the video-assisted thoracoscope (158). After 1 week, the patient is more likely to need a formal thoracotomy, resulting in increased morbidity and prolongation of the hospital stay (159,160).

INJURIES TO THE PULMONARY PARENCHYMA

Pulmonary Contusion

Pulmonary contusion is a common finding after trauma, seen in about 20% of adult patients with multiple injuries (161). Pulmonary contusion is more common in children because of increased compliance of the chest wall (162). Motor vehicle accidents, falls, and penetrating injuries are the most common causes for pulmonary contusion in civilian settings. In a military setting, pulmonary contusions often result from high velocity missiles and blast injuries from explosives.

There are three basic components in the pathophysiology of pulmonary contusion:

1. *The spalling effect:* This describes the shearing or burst effect that occurs at a gas/liquid interface with the dissipation of an applied force. In the lung, for example, the impact of the pulmonary parenchyma against the chest wall leads to a disruption of alveoli.

2. *The inertial effect:* The low density alveolar tissues are stripped from the hilum as they accelerate at different rates.

3. *The implosion effect:* Gas bubbles rebound and overexpand after the shock wave passes.

Injury to the lung results from the actual transmission of mechanical forces from the chest wall, increased tissue pressure and tearing of tissues, direct laceration of the lung by ribs or penetrating objects, bleeding into uninvolved lungs, increased mucous production with decreased clearance, and decreased production of surfactant leading to alveolar collapse (163). On the microscopic level, animal models reveal interstitial hemorrhage initially, followed by edema within 1 to 2 hours of injury. In 24 hours, this progresses to alveoli filled with protein, red cells, inflammatory cells, fibrin deposits, and loss of architecture. At 48 hours, these processes are worsened, and cellular debris, granules from type II alveolar cells, macrophages, and neutrophils are also present. Lymphatics are dilated and are filled with protein, and edema is massive. Healing with minimal scarring is present at 7 to 10 days (164,165).

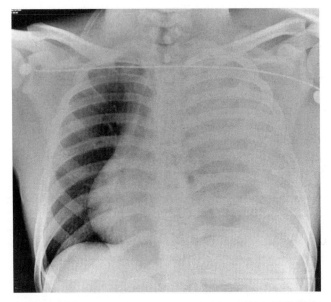

FIGURE 24-3. Hemothorax. This patient has a massive left hemothorax with mediastinal shift. A missile can be seen in the left hemothorax. Chest tube placement, volume resuscitation, and prompt surgical consultation are needed.

This pathology is manifested clinically as hypoxemia, hypercarbia, and increased work of breathing. Ventilation–perfusion mismatch, intrapulmonary shunt, increased lung water, and loss of compliance can lead to respiratory failure. CXR anomalies may not be present until 4 to 6 hours after the injury and may underestimate the degree of damage (166,167) (see Fig. 24-4). CT scan of the lungs reveals the presence and extent of injury earlier and more accurately. Wagner and Jamieson have demonstrated that consolidation of 28% or more of the airspaces was 100% predictive of the need for mechanical ventilation. Chest CT scan, however, is not always practical in the multiply injured patient (167). Clinical decisions based on the mechanism of injury and examination of the patient may be required.

Treatment is primarily supportive. Supplemental oxygen, including mechanical ventilation, is the mainstay of therapy. The mode of ventilation must be tailored to the patient, but protective strategies that avoid overdistension of the uninvolved lung are recommended. Patients with severe unilateral disease and significant $\dot{V}/\dot{Q}$ mismatch and intrapulmonary shunting may benefit from dual lung ventilation and/or nitric oxide therapy (168). Extracorporeal membrane oxygenation is not usually practical as significant bleeding may occur within the lung or from associated injuries. In extreme cases, lobectomy may be necessary. Excellent pulmonary toilet is also needed. In addition to cough, deep breathing, and postural drainage, pain management is required to optimize patient effort. Intravenous bolus or patient-controlled intrapleural and epidural analgesia all have a potential role in pain management. Except in the smallest of contusions, patients should be initially cared for with continuous cardiovascular monitoring and pulse oximetry in an ICU.

Several controversies exist in the management of pulmonary contusion. The controversy that is most often investigated is fluid resuscitation. Overzealous fluid administration has been shown to be deleterious in animal models. However, in humans, there is no evidence that volume restriction or use of diuretic therapy has a positive impact on outcome (169). The current recommendation is that fluids be given on the basis of the need for adequate hydration and perfusion of vital organs.

Fluid restriction and diuretics should only be used in patients with volume overload. A second controversy regarding fluids is the use of colloid instead of crystalloid to avoid increased lung water, pulmonary edema, and the potential sequelae of these factors in lung injury. There is no strong evidence to support the use of colloids over crystalloids in resuscitation of patients with pulmonary contusion (169–172). Controversy also exists about the use of corticosteroids in pulmonary contusion. Animal models have shown both diminution of hypoxemia and decrease in lesion size (173). In humans, Svennevig et al. showed a decrease in PVR with high-dose steroids but no change in clinical outcomes (174). Currently, the use of steroids is not recommended.

Generally, the pulmonary derangements associated with pulmonary contusion will resolve in less than a week, but problems with systemic immune response, ARDS, and secondary nosocomial pneumonia are not uncommon. Morbidity and mortality are related to injury severity scores, the severity of lung injury, and the development of complications. Long-term morbidity for recovered patients includes the possibility of decreased FRC and oxygenation, disabling dyspnea, and pulmonary fibrosis (175).

Pulmonary Hematoma

Pulmonary hematoma is a discrete collection of blood contained within the pulmonary parenchyma. This rather uncommon finding usually follows pulmonary contusion and laceration from blunt or penetrating injury (114). On initial radiologic studies, pulmonary hematoma is masked by the manifestations of the pulmonary contusion. It is usually later in the patient's course, after clearing of the acute pulmonary injury, that it becomes visible, often seen as a discrete density or mass within the lung tissue. Occasionally, if the original pulmonary parenchymal injury involved small airway structures in addition to pulmonary vessels, the loculation may have an air-fluid level or may present as a posttraumatic pneumatocele. Spontaneous resolution of these posttraumatic collections generally takes about 5 to 6 weeks, and unless infection or air

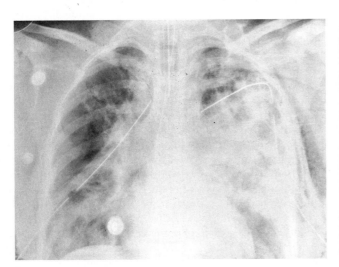

A

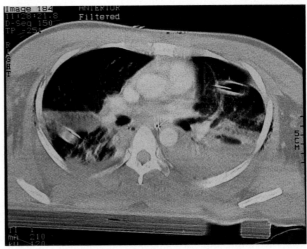

B

FIGURE 24-4. **A, B:** Pulmonary contusion. Chest radiograph and computerized tomography (CT) scan of a patient with blunt chest injury. Pulmonary contusions are often more evident on CT scans than on plain films.

leak develop, or evidence of continued hemorrhage exists, observation is continued and management is nonoperative. In cases where resolution has not occurred within 5 to 6 weeks, further investigation is warranted (176). Ideally, prior available CXRs would be helpful in revealing an abnormality that existed prior to the injury. Additional studies helpful in differentiating a persistent hematoma from some other type of lung lesion are CT scan and MRI (177). These have been used by some centers to follow residual posttraumatic masses and avoid surgical intervention. More commonly, when resolution of the mass lesion has not occurred in the anticipated period, surgical excision of the lesion is performed.

Pulmonary Laceration and Air Embolization

Pulmonary laceration occurs more often after penetrating trauma but is also associated with blunt injury. In blunt trauma cases, it may result from direct penetration by fractured ribs or may occur from shear forces exerted upon the lung tissue during severe chest compression followed by sudden decompression (178). In these situations, both intrapulmonary vessels and airways can be torn, resulting in hemothorax, pneumothorax, or a combination of the two. Because perfusion pressure within the lungs is low and the injured vessel's caliber is small, bleeding is generally selfcontained. Radiologic identification of a pulmonary laceration on plain CXR is often difficult because its presence may be masked by the picture of contusion. CT scan is a much more exacting study for the delineation of pulmonary lacerations (178). Surgical intervention is required in about 5% of patients for either persistent bleeding or unresolved air leak.

Although most pulmonary lacerations are successfully treated with tube thoracostomy or with a thoracoscopic or surgical procedure, a few sustain potentially lethal air embolization. Left-sided air embolization is by far the more dangerous and potentially lethal form. Lung injuries involving adjacent bronchi and pulmonary venous structures can cause a bronchopulmonary venous fistula, setting the stage for air entry into the left heart and systemic arterial circulation. While air can travel to any end organ, the greatest risk for morbidity and mortality occurs with embolization to the coronary or cerebral circulation. Less than 1 mL of air in a critical vessel like the left anterior descending coronary artery is enough to cause ventricular fibrillation and death. With regard to the cerebral circulation, symptoms of air embolization include dizziness, headache, and visual disturbance. Clinical manifestations can occur suddenly and include loss of consciousness, focal seizures or convulsions, and a variety of neurologic deficits. Air may be visible in the retinal vessels on ophthalmologic examination.

Right-sided air embolization is most common in relation to accidental infusion from IV therapy. In cases of lung or chest wall trauma, air can enter via injured bronchial or intercostal veins or via the superior vena cava or its major tributaries. In most cases, a moderately large amount of right-sided air can be tolerated, although rapid infusion can affect the ability of the patient to tolerate air in the right-sided circulation. Large amounts of right-sided air (5 to 8 mL per kg) can be fatal. A secondary complication of right-sided air embolization is paradoxical embolization. Patients having any type of potential right-to-left shunt are at risk for this complication. This includes

patients with a patent foramen ovale (15% to 25% of the population) or other types of congenital intracardiac defects and those who develop an intrapulmonary right-to-left shunt within injured lung tissue as a result of the trauma they experience. In paradoxical embolization, air can traverse the intracardiac defect or intrapulmonary shunt, enter the left side of the heart, and then travel to critical coronary or cerebral arteries. These patients are subject to the same risks as those patients who have primary systemic arterial air embolization (179).

It must be remembered that iatrogenic air embolization can easily occur in the trauma setting. Significant amounts of air can be infused into the systemic veins during hasty initiation of fluid resuscitation therapy. More importantly, vigorous positive-pressure ventilation in patients with lung contusion or laceration may increase the likelihood of air embolization by forcing air through lacerated bronchial structures into adjacent injured pulmonary vessels. If clinical findings suggest systemic air embolism, the single best diagnostic study is TEE (180). The diagnosis can be made quickly and accurately because air bubbles are easily visible in the cardiac chambers. At times, the diagnosis is made when thoracotomy is performed.

Treatment of systemic air embolism includes maintenance of adequate intravascular volume, appropriate use of cardiotonic agents to sustain adequate systemic blood pressure, and judicious management of mechanical ventilation. Use of low tidal volume, decreased PEEP, and in some cases, high-frequency jet ventilation may greatly reduce the detrimental hemodynamic consequences associated with systemic air embolization (180). Using TEE for continuous observation of cardiac function while adjusting pharmacologic agents or ventilatory modes can be very useful.

INJURIES TO THE DIAPHRAGM

Traumatic rupture of the diaphragm is seen with increasing frequency. Ten percent to 15% of patients with lower chest/upper abdomen–penetrating trauma and up to 5% of hospitalized victims of motor vehicle crashes will have a diaphragmatic injury (181–183).

The diagnosis of a ruptured hemidiaphragm is not always easy, particularly if there is no radiologic abnormality on chest film and if the patient has no obvious need for thoracic or abdominal operation. The diagnosis is most frequently made on the left side, but that does not necessarily mean that it is more frequent on the left side. Most commonly, symptoms are due to associated injuries of the chest or abdominal cavity. Patients may present with dyspnea, orthopnea, and chest or abdominal pain. If gastric dilatation with obstruction occurs, the patient may have severe respiratory distress with ipsilateral lung collapse and symptoms that mimic tension pneumothorax. Patients may also be entirely asymptomatic. Physical signs of rupture include absence of breath sounds over the left hemithorax, displacement of the cardiac dullness to the right, presence of bowel sounds in the left chest, diminished left chest wall excursion, and cardiac and respiratory dysfunction. In the classic case of diaphragmatic rupture, the diagnosis can be made by a CXR, which shows an elevated left diaphragm and coiling of the nasogastric tube in the left chest. One may also see the curvilinear shadows of other abdominal viscera such as colon or small bowel in the thorax. The accuracy of the

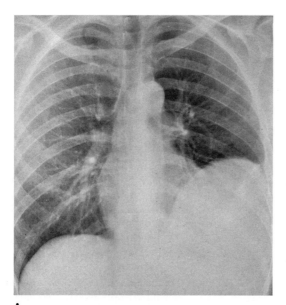

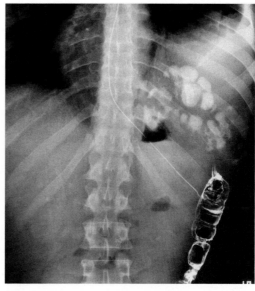

A   B

FIGURE 24-5. **A, B:** Diaphragmatic rupture. This patient has an elevated left hemidiaphragm after receiving blunt chest trauma. Diaphragmatic rupture should always be ruled out in such cases. The injury was not diagnosed in the acute setting but was later discovered when the patient underwent a barium enema.

CXR in the diagnosis of diaphragmatic rupture has been quoted to be from 13% to 94% (184) (see Fig. 24-5). Although it is impossible to know the accuracy of chest film, it is obvious that the potential for missed injury is significant. Therefore, a high index of suspicion should prompt further testing. Additional studies that have proved useful in making the diagnosis include upper gastrointestinal contrast studies, barium enema, ultrasonography, CT scans, radioisotopic scintigraphy, MRI, fluoroscopy, thoracoscopy, laparoscopy, and diagnostic peritoneal lavage (DPL). Generally, DPL is used to diagnose injury in penetrating wounds, and the positive red cell count is dropped to 20,000 instead of 100,000. None of the modalities are foolproof. In general, one should consult with the radiologists and surgeons in their own hospital to determine the modality with which they are experiencing the most success in making an accurate diagnosis. The estimated incidence of missed injury is 12% to 60% (185–188).

Discovery of a diaphragmatic injury should prompt expeditious surgical consultation. Most surgeons will approach acute ruptures via a celiotomy. If there has been a significant delay of months to years in the diagnosis, most will approach the herniation through the chest. There is, however, disagreement about the best approach.

Morbidity and mortality are most often due to associated injuries. Mortality rates vary in the literature from 4.3% to 41%, with blunt injuries causing a higher mortality. Morbidity associated with diaphragmatic injury and repair includes atelectasis, pneumonia, respiratory failure, systemic sepsis, failed repair, empyema, diaphragmatic paresis or paralysis, strangulation of visceral structures within the herniation, and lung and liver abscesses. The overall incidence of complications is 40% to 60%. Diaphragmatic injury is rarely an isolated event. Prevention of morbidity and mortality demands careful attention to the overall condition of the patient and care of associated injuries in addition to prompt and proper repair.

INJURIES TO THE MEDIASTINUM

Esophageal Injury

The course of the esophagus includes the neck, thorax, and abdomen. This discussion will be principally confined to injuries below the neck.

The exact incidence of trauma to the esophagus is unknown. The most common causes are penetrating wounds to the back, neck, and chest and iatrogenic instrumentation. Blunt trauma rarely produces esophageal injury; the overall incidence is <0.1% in motor vehicle crashes. Accidental insufflation of pressurized air through the mouth during resuscitation is another rare mechanism of injury. Because of the close anatomic relationship of the esophagus and trachea, both penetrating and blunt injuries may have associated tracheal injury.

Following injury to the esophagus, air and secretions escape into the mediastinum and cause extensive chemical and bacterial mediastinal contamination. Symptoms at presentation range from none to critical sepsis, depending on the size and layer of penetration of the wound, associated injuries, and the time frame of development. The most common symptom is pain in the chest or epigastrium. Other potential signs and symptoms include fever, hoarseness, dysphagia, subcutaneous emphysema, mediastinal crunch, splinting of the chest wall, respiratory distress, and shock. Abdominal pain and rigidity usually herald perforation at the esophagogastric junction rather than in the chest.

Diagnosis can be suspected by history, physical examination, and CXR. Typical radiographic findings are mediastinal emphysema, hydrothorax, pneumothorax, and/or widening of the mediastinum (see Fig. 24-6). There may be increased space between the vertebral bodies and the trachea. In rare cases, the chest film may be without anomaly, or anomalies may be attributable to concomitant injuries. For this reason,

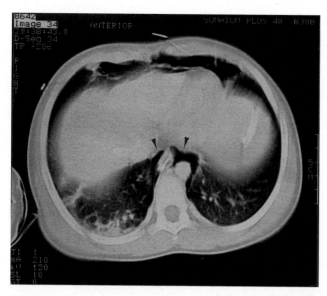

FIGURE 24-6. Pneumomediastinum and pneumopericardium. The computerized tomography (CT) scan demonstrates obvious air in the mediastinum and pericardium in a patient who suffered blunt chest trauma. Air in these locations can be easily missed on chest radiographs. Its presence should alert the physician to the possibility of esophageal and/or tracheobronchial injury and warrants further study of these structures.

esophagrams should be performed on patients with transthoracic missile injuries near the mediastinum and stab wounds. In rare cases, esophagrams may be falsely negative. In patients in whom there is a high index of suspicion with a negative esophagram or in those whose condition does not technically permit esophagography, esophageal endoscopy is an accurate diagnostic alternative.

As soon as the diagnosis is suspected, treatment should begin. The general recommendations for any esophageal perforation are suspension of all oral intake, placement of a nasogastric tube with continuous suction, and antibiotic administration. Antibiotics should cover mouth flora (gram positives and anaerobes) and possible gram-negative contaminants from penetrating wounds. If hydrothorax or pneumothorax is present, a chest tube is inserted. Surgical consultation should be made at the earliest possible juncture as the morbidity and mortality associated with this injury increases with time to operation. Mortality rate ranges from 9% to 25% in various series (189).

Tracheal and Bronchial Disruption

Traumatic disruption of the tracheobronchial tree is an uncommon but potentially life-threatening injury resulting from either blunt or penetrating trauma. In civilian populations, it is most commonly associated with blunt injury, occurring in <3% of cases (117,190). Although infrequent, this injury is highly lethal because nearly 80% of patients sustaining it expire before they reach a hospital. Factors believed to contribute to this high mortality rate include anatomic location and degree of injury, severity of associated injuries, and asphyxia (191). Of the patients who reach the hospital alive, present data shows that roughly 10% do not survive. This number has greatly decreased over the past 50 years, dropping from about 36%, and can be attributed to improvement of prehospital care and transport, advancements in perioperative

and intraoperative management, and rapidity of diagnosis and treatment (190,192,193).

In cases of penetrating injury, the nature of the disruption depends upon the trajectory and force of the penetrating weapon or object. Much more controversy exists about the exact nature of the injury mechanism in cases resulting from blunt trauma. A number of theories have been described. Rapid deceleration is one proposed mechanism in which a shearing effect takes place at the point between the fixed airway structures in the mediastinum and the relatively more mobile portions in the pleural spaces. A second theory suggests that injury occurs with anteroposterior compression of the airway structures between sternum and vertebral column, with simultaneous lateral "splaying" of the major bronchi from the trachea. The third theory describes a barotrauma or "blowout" type of injury that occurs in cases where compressive thoracic trauma immediately follows deep inspiration and closure of the glottis (190,192,194). More than 80% of these injuries occur within 2.5 cm of the carina (191). Injuries in this region vary from simple linear lacerations to complex stellate disruptions (117,194) or even complete transection. Distal (lobar or segmental) bronchial injuries occur even more uncommonly and are usually associated with extensive pulmonary parenchymal damage.

Disruption of the tracheobronchial tree can produce a constellation of early manifestations, some of which can be extremely subtle. Tracheobronchial injuries are most obvious when they communicate with the pleural space and produce findings that include a large pneumothorax, extensive and progressive subcutaneous and mediastinal emphysema with dyspnea and hypoxemia, persistent pneumothorax or air leak in spite of functioning thoracostomy tube, or failure of the affected lung to reexpand with appropriate thoracostomy drainage (117,191). Hemoptysis occurs in about 20% of cases (191). Whereas airway injuries communicating with the pleural space are rather obvious, injuries that are contained by surrounding peribronchial tissues and pleura often present with more subtle findings. Patients may present with a small initial leak of air into the pleural space or, more commonly, into the mediastinal tissues. Shortly after the leak occurs, the injury site is sealed by the surrounding tissues or clot. Hemoptysis is rare in these cases. Because air dissects predominantly into the peribronchial and mediastinal tissue planes in these cases, subcutaneous emphysema is the most common finding on CXR. Other associated findings may include pneumomediastinum, pneumothorax, and rib fractures. A subtle yet very reliable early finding on plain CXR is emphysema in the deep soft tissues of the neck (191).

Prior to the undertaking of any further diagnostic procedures, establishment of a stable airway and adequate gas exchange is of prime importance. If endotracheal intubation and positive-pressure ventilation are required for management, these must be done with great caution and with attention to the location of the injury. Imprudent placement of an endotracheal tube or vigorous positive-pressure ventilation may worsen the condition of the patient by enlarging a laceration or by reopening one that has been sealed. Positive-pressure ventilation may increase an already existing ventilation–perfusion mismatch because a large percentage of each delivered breath will preferentially exit the injury site, leaving the uninjured lung underventilated. To secure satisfactory airway control in some cases, it may be necessary to direct the endotracheal tube into the uninjured bronchus or to use a double-lumen endotracheal tube (195). In cases where standard techniques of intubation may be difficult or dangerous, it may be prudent to position the endotracheal tube under direct vision by inserting it over a flexible fiber-optic bronchoscope. Also, in cases where the laceration is in the trachea or carina, an alternate mode of mechanical ventilation such as high-frequency ventilation may be useful.

For diagnosis of tracheobronchial injuries, the single best study is bronchoscopy (117,194,196). Although most clinicians prefer the ease and ready availability of flexible fiber-optic bronchoscopy, rigid bronchoscopy is also useful in experienced hands. In cases where the leak is large or patient stability is in question, this procedure should be performed in the operating room so that thoracotomy can be immediately performed if needed. Bronchoscopy is performed to identify the existence, location, and extent of a laceration. It can be done quickly but must include the entire tracheobronchial tree, including the portion proximal to the distal tip of the endotracheal tube. The method for doing this has previously been described. In some cases, repeat bronchoscopy is needed to establish or confirm diagnosis (117). Bronchography is not indicated for patients with acute injuries (191).

After the extent and location of the injury have been identified, it is best to proceed with early surgical repair in most cases. Only a few exceptions allow for nonoperative management of these injuries in the acute setting (191), and these are listed in Table 24-10. When surgical repair is done, the approach to most tracheobronchial injuries is a posterolateral incision through the right thorax at the fourth intercostal space. This allows for access to the entire right mainstem bronchus, the carina, and virtually the entire intrathoracic trachea. Injuries to the left mainstem bronchus distal to the carina are repaired through the left chest (117,194). Whenever possible, the anastomosis is reenforced externally with a pleural or intercostal muscle flap and is then tested for residual leak prior to closure of the chest. Critical care management postoperatively must be directed at avoiding prolonged intubation and positive-pressure ventilation so that disruption of the anastomosis does not occur (117).

When tracheobronchial injury is missed in the acute setting, fibrous scarring occurs at the site over time, usually resulting in stricture formation (118). If left untreated, this complication leads to persistent atelectasis of the lung parenchyma distal to the stricture or recurrent infection secondary to retained secretions in the affected area with the ultimate development of a bronchiectatic picture (194). Complete evaluation of pulmonary anatomy and functional status should be performed before undertaking surgery in these cases because depending on the degree of airway injury and on the amount of damaged distal lung parenchyma, the operative procedure may range from tracheobronchial repair to distal lung resection such as lobectomy

or pneumonectomy. If repair is attempted >6 months after injury, it is unlikely that the patients will have improvement in pulmonary function.

Finally, tracheoesophageal fistulae can result from thoracic trauma but are extremely rare (194). Certainly, a penetrating injury directed toward the posterior mediastinum can result in injury to both structures. In cases of blunt trauma, the tracheobronchial injury likely occurs in one of the ways previously mentioned, and the adjacent esophagus is also ruptured. If an esophageal injury is suspected in association with a tracheobronchial injury, esophagoscopy is warranted in addition to bronchoscopy (197). Once a fistula is discovered, airway protection is of primary importance with placement of an endotracheal tube distal to the injury site so that aspiration of gastric contents can be prevented. Endoscopic examination and barium swallow are indicated, followed by early surgical repair (198). If early operative intervention is done, both structures can be treated with local debridement and primary repair. If surgery is done at a later time, a more complex esophageal repair may be needed.

FAT EMBOLISM SYNDROME

First described by Zenker in 1861, fat embolism syndrome (FES) is still one of the least well-defined entities in trauma. A variety of traumatic and nontraumatic conditions are associated with FES (199) (see Table 24-11). In the trauma patient, FES is most commonly found in patients with fractures of the long bones and pelvis. The clinical prevalence of FES in these patients is 0.25% to 10% (200–202).

TABLE 24-10. Indications for Nonoperative Management of Tracheobronchial Disruption

Tracheobronchial injury involves one-third or less of the circumference of the affected lumen

PLUS

Complete resolution of any accompanying pneumothorax and full reexpansion of the affected lung after tube thoracostomy

PLUS

No residual air leak

TABLE 24-11. Clinical Settings for Fat Embolism

Trauma
  Lower extremity long bone fractures
  Pelvic fractures
  Child abuse with or without fractures
  Blast concussion
  Liver contusion
  Severe burns
  Massive soft tissue injury
Surgery
  Total joint replacement
  Intramedullary nailing of femoral shaft
  Closed femoral osteotomy
  Femoral elongation
  Spinal fusion
  Liposuction
  Bone marrow transplant
  Renal transplant
Nonsurgical
  External cardiac massage
  Lipid emulsions in intravenous feedings
  Intraosseous venography
  Acute pancreatitis
  Carbon tetrachloride poisoning
  Prolonged corticosteroid therapy
  Fatty liver secondary to alcohol
  Acute osteomyelitis
  Bone infarction in sickle cell disease
  Epilepsy
  Diabetes mellitus
  Extracorporeal circulation
  Severe infection, especially clostridial species
  High altitude

The pathophysiology of FES is poorly understood. There are two prevalent hypotheses:

1. The mechanical hypothesis suggests that disruption of intramedullary veins allows fat to gain access to the pulmonary and cardiac circulation. Echocardiography studies performed during intramedullary nailing demonstrate fat emboli to the heart. However, true FES was not demonstrated in most of these patients (203). In addition, fat can be detected in the bronchoalveolar lavage fluid (BALF) of patients with FES (204). However, Aoki et al. demonstrated fat in the BALF of patients who underwent intramedullary nailing and did not clinically progress to FES (205). Thus, a purely mechanical etiology of FES seems unlikely.

2. The physiochemical hypothesis states that fracture sites produce chemical mediators that change intravascular lipid solubility causing coalescence into fat globules and pulmonary embolism. Related is the hypothesis that free fatty acids produce mediators leading to FES (206,207).

FES is a clinical syndrome classically characterized by respiratory insufficiency, thrombocytopenia with petechiae, and deteriorating mental status. Respiratory insufficiency typically presents as tachypnea and hypoxemia. Classic locations of petechiae are the axillae, chest, root of the neck, and conjunctiva. Retinal emboli may also be visible on funduscopic exam. Mental status changes may include restlessness, disorientation, stupor, or coma (208). Tachycardia, fever, and anemia may also develop. Peak incidence of FES is 24 to 48 hours after injury, with a range of 6 to 72 hours. Because trauma patients are prone to a variety of mechanisms producing respiratory insufficiency, the diagnosis of FES relies on the exclusion of other causes and an appropriate clinical setting. FES can coexist with ARDS, pulmonary contusion, and aspiration pneumonitis. No specific laboratory or radiographic test is pathognomic. Yoshida et al. have shown that MRI can be useful in the detection of fat emboli in the cerebrum, cerebellum, and brainstem. However, transport and monitoring of patients, the frequent presence of ferromagnetic materials in fracture patients, expense, and time consumption render MRI impractical (209). Fat globules may be detected in the blood, sputum, BALF, urine, and/or cerebrospinal fluid; however, the diagnosis of fat embolism is based on the history; clinical signs of pulmonary, cerebral, and cutaneous manifestations; and hypoxemia in the absence of other disorders.

Treatment is largely directed at prevention and supportive measures: adequate oxygenation, fracture splinting or fixation, judiciously administered fluids with avoidance of excessive hydration, and avoidance of unnecessary transport of the patient. FES has been treated with a variety of agents, including ethanol, heparin, hypertonic glucose, and corticosteroids. There are no prospective, controlled studies to support any of these interventions. Timing and type of fixation of fractures are currently under scrutiny, but currently it does not appear that the type of fixation plays a major role in the development of FES. In most cases, FES is a self-limited process. Pulmonary function will return to normal if the patient has adequate oxygenation, and severe complications such as ARDS do not develop. Long-term morbidity, when present, is usually in the form of cerebral neurologic deficits (210,211). The mortality rate from complicated FES is 5% to 15%.

REFERENCES

1. Stoelting RK. Inhaled anesthetics. In: *Pharmacology and physiology in anesthetic practice.* Philadelphia: JB Lippincott Co, 1987:35–68.
2. Scweieger I, Gamulin Z, Suter PM. Lung function during anesthesia and respiratory insufficiency in the postoperative period. *Acta Anaesthesiol Scand* 1989;33:527–534.
3. Magnusson L, Spahn DR. New concepts of atelectasis during general anesthesia. *Br J Anesth* 2003;91:61–72.
4. Tusman F, Bohm SH, de Anda GFV, et al. Alveolar recruitment strategy improves arterial oxygenation during general anesthesia. *Br J Anesth* 1999;82:8–13.
5. Magnusson L, Zemgulis V, Tenling A, et al. Use of a vital capacity maneuver to prevent atelectasis after cardiopulmonary bypass—an experimental study. *Anesthesiology* 1998;88:134–142.
6. Maslow AD, Regan MM, Israel E, et al. Inhaled albuterol but not intravenous lidocaine protects against intubation—induced bronchoconstriction in asthma. *Anesthesiology* 2000;93:1198–1204.
7. Eames W, Rooke G, Wu R, et al. Comparison of the effects of etomidate, propofol and thiopental on respiratory resistance after tracheal intubation. *Anesthesiology* 1996;84:1307–1311.
8. Hirshman CA, Edelstein G, Peetz S, et al. Mechanism of action of inhalational anesthesia on airways. *Anesthesiology* 1982;56:107–111.
9. Rooke G, Choi J, Bishop M. The effects of isoflurane, halothane, sevoflurane and thiopental/nitrous oxide on respiratory system resistance after tracheal intubation. *Anesthesiology* 1997;86:1294–1299.
10. Tait AR, Knight PR. Intraoperative respiratory complications in patients with upper respiratory tract infections. *Can J Anesth* 1987;34:300–303.
11. Fennelly ME, Hall GM. Anesthesia and upper respiratory tract infections—a non existent hazard?—editorial. *Br J Anaesth* 1990; 64:535–536.
12. Pavlin EG. Cardiopulmonary pharmacology. In: Miller RD, ed. *Anesthesia*, 3rd ed. New York: Churchill Livingstone, 1990:105–134.
13. Sykes L, Bowe E. Cardiorespiratory effects of anesthesia. *Clin Chest Med* 1993;14:211–226.
14. Warner DO. Preventing postoperative pulmonary complications. *Anesthesiology* 2000;92:1467–1472.
15. Cousins MJ, Bromage PR. Epidural neural blockade. In: *Neural blockade in clinical anesthesia and pain management*, 3rd ed. JB Lippincott Co, 1988.
16. Rodgers A, Walker N, Schug S, et al. Reduction postoperative mortality and morbidity with epidural or spinal anaesthesia: results from an overview of randomized trials. *Br Med J* 2000; 321:1493–1497.
17. Arozullah A, Daley J, Henderson WG, et al. Multifactorial risk index for predicting postoperative respiratory failure in men after major noncardiac surgery. *Ann Surg* 2000;232:242–253.
18. Arozullah A, Conde MV, Lawrence VA. Preoperative evaluation for postoperative pulmonary complications. *Med Clin North Am* 2003;87:153–173.
19. Jayr C, Thomas H, Rey A, et al. Postoperative pulmonary complications: epidural analgesia using bupivacaine and opioids versus parenteral opioids. *Anesthesiology* 1993;78:666–676.
20. Hendloin H, Lahtinen J, Lansimies E, et al. The effect of thoracic epidural analgesia on respiratory function after cholecystectomy. *Acta Anaesthesiol Scand* 1987;31:645–651.
21. Cuschieri RJ, Morran CG, Howie JC, et al. Postoperative pain and pulmonary complications: comparison of three analgesic regimens. *Br J Surg* 1985;72:495–498.
22. Ballantyne JC, Carr CB, De Ferranti S, et al. The comparative effects of postoperative analgesic therapies on pulmonary outcome: cumulative meta-analyses of randomized controlled trials. *Anesth Analg* 1998;86:598–612.
23. Engberg G, Wiklund L. Pulmonary complications after upper abdominal surgery: their prevention with intercostal blocks. *Acta Anaesthesiol Scand* 1988;32:1–9.
24. Kaiser AM, Zollinger A, Lorezi DD, et al. Prospective randomized comparison of extrapleural versus epidural analgesia for postthoracotomy pain. *Ann Thorac Surg* 1998;66:367–372.
25. Bilgin M, Akcali Y, Oguzkaya F. Extrapleural regional versus systemic analgesia for relieving postthoracotomy pain: a clinical study of bupivacaine compared with methamizol. *J Thorac Cardiovasc Surg* 2003;126:1580–1583.

26. Ford GT, Whitelaw WA, Rosenal TW, et al. Diaphragm function after upper abdominal surgery in humans. *Am Rev Respir Dis* 1983;127:431–436.

27. Dureuil B, Cantineau JP, Desmonts JM. Effects of upper or lower abdominal surgery on diaphragmatic function. *Br J Anaesth* 1987;59:1230–1235.

28. Prabhakar NR, Marek W, Loeschcke HH. Altered breathing patterns elicited by stimulation of abdominal visceral afferents. *J Appl Physiol* 1985;58:1755–1760.

29. Xue FS, Li BW, Zhang GS, et al. The influence of surgical sites on early postoperative hypoxemia in adults undergoing elective surgery. *Anesth Analg* 1999;88:213–219.

30. Vaughan RW, Wise L. Choice of abdominal operative incision in the obese patients: a study using blood gas measurements. *Ann Surg* 1975;181:829–835.

31. Frazee R, Roberts J, Okeson G, et al. Open versus laparoscopic cholecystectomy: a comparison of postoperative pulmonary function. *Ann Surg* 1991;213:651–653.

32. Grace PA, Quereshi A, Colenian J, et al. Reduced postoperative hospitalization after laparoscopic cholecystectomy. *Br J Surg* 1991;78:160–162.

33. Meyers WA, Southern Surgeons Club. A prospective analysis of 1518 laparoscopic cholecystectomies. *N Engl J Med* 1991;324:1073–1078.

34. Mack MJ, Aronoff RJ, Acuff TE, et al. Present role of thoracoscopy in the diagnosis and treatment of diseases of the chest. *Ann Thorac Surg* 1992;54:403–409.

35. Landrenau RJ, Hazelrigg SR, Ferson PF, et al. Thoracoscopic resection of 85 pulmonary lesions. *Ann Thorac Surg* 1992;54:415–420.

36. Daniel TM, Kern JA, Tribble CJ, et al. Thoracoscopic surgery for diseases of the lung and pleura. *Ann surg* 1993;217:566–575.

37. Pederson T, Eliasen K, Henriksen E. A prospective study of risk factors and cardiopulmonary complications associated with anaesthesia and surgery: risk indicators of cardiopulmonary morbidity. *Acta Anaesthesiol Scand* 1990;34:144–155.

38. Celli BR, Rodriguez KS, Snider GL. A controlled trial of intermittent positive pressure breathing, incentive spirometry and deep breathing exercises in preventing pulmonary complications after abdominal surgery. *Am Rev Respir Dis* 1984;130:12–15.

39. Svensson L, Hess KR, Coselli JS, et al. A prospective study of respiratory failure after high risk surgery on the thoracoabdominal aorta. *J Vasc Surg* 1991;14:271–282.

40. Vodinh J, Bonnet F, Touboul C, et al. Risk factors for postoperative pulmonary complications after vascular surgery. *Surgery* 1989;105:360–365.

41. Roukema JA, Carol EJ, Prins JG. The prevalence of pulmonary complications after upper abdominal surgery in patients with noncompromised pulmonary status. *Arch Surg* 1988;123:30–34.

42. Kroenke K, Lawrence VA, Theroux JF, et al. Operative risk in patients with severe obstructive pulmonary disease. *Arch Intern Med* 1992;152:967–971.

43. Wong DH, Weber EC, Schell MJ, et al. Factors associated with postoperative pulmonary complications in patients with severe chronic obstructive pulmonary disease. *Anesth Analg* 1995;80:276–284.

44. Meoli AL, Rosen CL, Kristo D, et al. Upper airway management of the adult patient with obstructive sleep apnea in the perioperative period—avoiding complications. *Sleep* 2003;26:1060–1065.

45. Lindberg P, Gunnarsson L, Tokics L, et al. Atelectasis and lung function in the postoperative period. *Acta Anaesthesiol Scand* 1992;36:546–553.

46. Christensen EF, Schultz P, Jensen OV, et al. Postoperative pulmonary complications and lung function in high risk patients: a comparison of three physiotherapy regimens after upper abdominal surgery in general anesthesia. *Acta Anaesthesiol Scand* 1991;35:97–104.

47. Strandberg A, Brismar B, Lundquist H, et al. Constitutional factors promoting development of atelectasis during anaesthesia. *Acta Anaesthesiol Scand* 1987;31:21–24.

48. Rothen HU, Sporre B, Engberg G, et al. Prevention of atelectasis during general anaesthesia. *Lancet* 1995;345:1387–1391.

49. Rothen HU, Sporre B, Engberg G, et al. Influence of gas composition on recurrence of atelectasis after a reexpansion maneuver during general anesthesia. *Anesthesiology* 1995;82:832–842.

50. Strandberg A, Tokics L, Brismar B, et al. Atelectasis during anaesthesia and in the postoperative period. *Acta Anaesthesiol Scand* 1986;30:154–158.

51. Kindgen-Milles D, Buhl R, Gabriel A, et al. Nasal continuous positive airway pressure. A method to avoid endotracheal reintubation in postoperative high-risk patients with severe nonhypercapnic oxygenation failure. *Chest* 2000;117:1106–1111.

52. Eichenberger AS, Proietti S, Wicky S, et al. Morbid obesity and postoperative pulmonary atelectasis: an underestimated problem. *Anesth Analg* 2002;95:1788–1792.

53. Thomas JA, McIntosh JM. Are incentive spirometry, intermittent positive pressure breathing, and deep breathing exercises effective in the prevention of postoperative pulmonary complications after upper abdominal surgery? A systematic overview and meta-analysis. *Phys Ther* 1994;74:3–16.

54. Fisher BW, Majumdar SR, McAlister FA. Predicting pulmonary complications after nonthoracic surgery: a systematic review of blinded studies. *Am J Med* 2002;112:219–225.

55. Lawrence VA, Dhanda R, Hilsenbeck SG, et al. Risk of pulmonary complications after elective abdominal surgery. *Chest* 1996;110:744–750.

56. Vaporciyan AA, Merriman KW, Ece F, et al. Incidence of major pulmonary morbidity after pneumonectomy: association with timing of smoking cessation. *Ann Thorac Surg* 2002;73:420–426.

57. Nakagawa M, Tanaka H, Tsukuma H, et al. Relationship between the duration of the preoperative smoke-free period and the incidence of postoperative pulmonary complications after pulmonary surgery. *Chest* 2001;120:705–710.

58. Brooks-Brunn JA. Predictors of postoperative pulmonary complications following abdominal surgery. *Chest* 1997;111:564–571.

59. Bluman LG, Mosca L, Newman N, et al. Preoperative smoking habits and postoperative pulmonary complications. *Chest* 1998;113(4):883–889.

60. Warner MA, Offord KP, Warner ME, et al. Role of preoperative cessation of smoking and other factors in postoperative pulmonary complications: a blinded prospective study of coronary artery bypass patients. *Mayo Clin Proc* 1989;64:609–616.

61. Pearce AC, Jones RM. Smoking and anesthesia: preoperative abstinence and perioperative morbidity. *Anesthesiology* 1984;61:576–584.

62. Mendelson CL. Aspiration of stomach contents into lungs during obstetric anesthesia. *Am J Obstet Gynecol* 1946;53:196–205.

63. Olsson GL, Hallen B, Hambreas-Jonzon K. Aspiration during anaesthesia: a computer aided study of 185,358 anaesthetics. *Acta Anaesthesiol Scand* 1986;30:84–92.

64. Warner MA, Warner ME, Weber JG. Clinical significance of pulmonary aspiration during the perioperative period. *Anesthesiology* 1993;78:56–62.

65. Sellick BA. Cricoid pressure to control regurgitation of stomach contents during induction of anesthesia. *Lancet* 1961;2:404–406.

66. Orr DA, Bill KM, Gillon KRW, et al. Effects of omeprazole, with and without metclopramide, in elective obstetric anaesthesia. *Anaesthesia* 1993;48:114–119.

67. Manchikanti L, Colliver JA, Marrero TC, et al. Assessment of age related acid aspiration risk factors in pediatric, adult and geriatric patients. *Anesth Analg* 1985;64:11–17.

68. Levack ID, Bowie RA, Braid DP, et al. Comparison of the effects of two dose schedules of oral omeprazole with oral ranitidine on gastric pH and volume in patients undergoing elective surgery. *Br J Anaesth* 1996;76:567–569.

69. Maekawa N, Nishina K, Mikawa K, et al. Comparison of pirenzepine, ranitidine and pirenzepine-ranitidine combination for preoperative gastric fluid acidity and volume in children. *Br J Anaesth* 1998;80:53–57.

70. Salmenpera M, Kortilla K, Kalima T. Reduction of the risk of acid pulmonary aspiration in anesthetized patients after cimetidine premedication. *Acta Anaesthesiol Scand* 1980;24:25–30.

71. Wingtin LNG, Glomaud D, Hardy F, et al. Omeprazole for prophylaxis in elective surgery. *Anaesthesia* 1990;45:436–438.

72. Windsor JA, Hill GL. Risk factors for postoperative pneumonia—the importance of protein depletion. *Ann Surg* 1988;208:209–214.

73. Garibaldi RA, Britt MR, Coleman ML, et al. Risk factors for postoperative pneumonia. *Am J Med* 1981;70:677–680.

74. Montravers P, Veber B, Auboyer C, et al. Diagnostic and therapeutic management of nosocomial pneumonia in surgical patients: results of the Eole study. *Crit Care Med* 2002;30(2):368–375.
75. Dupont H, Montravers P, Gauzit R, et al. Club d'infectiologie en anesthesie-reanimation. Outcome of postoperative pneumonia in the Eole study. *Intensive Care Med* 2003;29(2):179–188.
76. Campbell GD Jr, Neiderman MS, Broughton WA et al., ATS Consensus Committee. Hospital acquired pneumonia in adults: diagnosis, assessment of severity, initial antimicrobial therapy and preventive strategies. *Am J Respir Crit Care Med* 1995;153:1711.
77. Samuels LE, Kaufman MS, Morris RJ, et al. Coronary artery bypass grafting in patients with COPD. *Chest* 1998;113:378–382.
78. Warner DO, Warner MO, Barnes RD, et al. Perioperative respiratory complications in patients with asthma. *Anesthesiology* 1996;85:460–467.
79. Olsson GL. Bronchospasm during anesthesia. A computer aided incidence study of 136,929 patients. *Acta Anaesthesiol Scand* 1987;31:244–252.
80. Zibrak JD, O'Donnell CR, Marton K. Indications for pulmonary function testing. *Ann Intern Med* 1990;112:763–771.
81. Gaensler EA, Cugell DW, Lindgren I, et al. The role of pulmonary insufficiency in mortality and invalidism following surgery for pulmonary tuberculosis. *J Thorac Cardiovasc Surg* 1955;29:163–187.
82. Keagy BA, Schorlemmer GR, Murray GF, et al. Correlation of preoperative pulmonary function testing with clinical course in patients after pneumonectomy. *Ann Thorac Surg* 1983;36:253–257.
83. Milledge JS, Nunn JF. Criteria of fitness for anesthesia in patients with chronic obstructive lung disease. *Br Med J* 1975;3:670–673.
84. Kearney DJ, Lee TH, Reilly JJ, et al. Assessment of operative risk in patients undergoing lung resection-importance of predicted pulmonary function. *Chest* 1994;105:753–759.
85. Olsen GN, Block AJ, Swenson EW, et al. Pulmonary function evaluation of the lung resection candidate: a prospective study. *Am Rev Respir Dis* 1975;111:379–387.
86. Markos J, Mullan BP, Hillman DR, et al. Preoperative assessment as a predictor of mortality and morbidity after lung resection. *Am Rev Respir Dis* 1989;139:901–910.
87. Holden DA, Rice TW, Stelmach K, et al. Exercise testing, 6 minute walk test and stair climb in the evaluation of patients at high risk for pulmonary resection. *Chest* 1992;102:1774–1779.
88. Smith TP, Kinasewitz GT, Tucker WY, et al. Exercise capacity as a predictor of post-thoracotomy morbidity. *Am Rev Respir Dis* 1984;129:730–734.
89. Bolliger CT, Wyser C, Roser H, et al. Lung scanning and exercise testing for the prediction of postoperative performance in lung resection candidates at increased risk for complications. *Chest* 1995;108:341–348.
90. Morice RC, Peters EJ, Ryan MB, et al. Exercise testing in the evaluation of patients at high risk for complications from lung resection. *Chest* 1992;101:356–361.
91. Olsen GN, Bolton JWR, Weiman DS, et al. Stair climbing as an exercise test to predict the postoperative complications of lung resection. *Chest* 1991;99:587–590.
92. Girish M, Trayner E Jr, Dammann O, et al. Symptom-limited stair climbing as a predictor of postoperative cardiopulmonary complications after high-risk surgery. *Chest* 2001;120(4):1147–1151.
93. Bolliger CT, Jordan P, Soler M, et al. Exercise capacity as a predictor of postoperative complications in lung resection candidates. *Am J Respir Crit Care Med* 1995;151:1472–1480.
94. Fee JH, Holmes EC, Gerwirtz HS, et al. Role of pulmonary resistance measurement in preoperative evaluation of candidates for lung resection. *J Thorac Cardiovasc Surg* 1975;75:519–524.
95. Wang JS, Abboud RT, Evans KG, et al. Role of CO diffusing capacity during exercise in the preoperative evaluation for lung resection. *Am J Respir Crit Care Med* 2000;162(4 Pt 1):1435–1444.
96. Olsen GN, Weiman DS, Bolton JWR, et al. Submaximal invasive exercise testing and quantitative lung scanning in the evaluation for tolerance of lung resection. *Chest* 1989;95:267–273.
97. Epstein SK, Faling LJ, Daly BDT, et al. Predicting pulmonary complications after pulmonary resection—preoperative exercise testing vs a multifactorial cardiopulmonary risk index. *Chest* 1993;104:694–700.
98. Epstein SK, Faling J, Daly BDT, et al. Inability to perform bicycle ergometry predicts increased morbidity and mortality after lung resection. *Chest* 1995;107:311–316.
99. Melendez J, Carlon VA. Cardiopulmonary risk index does not predict complications after thoracic surgery. *Chest* 1998;114:69–75.
100. Goldman L, Caldera DL, Nussbaum SR, et al. Multifactorial index of cardiac risk in non cardiac surgical procedures. *N Engl J Med* 1977;297:845–850.
101. Lee TH, Marcantonio ER, Mangione CM, et al. Derivation and prospective validation of a simple index for prediction of cardiac risk of major noncardiac surgery. *Circulation* 1999;100(10):1043–1049.
102. Polanczyk CA, Marcantonio E, Goldman L, et al. Impact of age on perioperative complications and length of stay in patients undergoing noncardiac surgery. *Ann Intern Med* 2001;134(8):637–643.
103. Auerbach AD, Goldman L. Beta-blockers and reduction of cardiac events in noncardiac surgery: scientific review. *JAMA* 2002;287(11):1435–1444.
104. Nishina K, Mikawa K, Uesugi T, et al. Efficacy of clonidine for prevention of perioperative myocardial ischemia: a critical appraisal and meta-analysis of the literature. *Anesthesiology* 2002;96(2):323–329.
105. Tortella BJ, Trunkey DD. Trauma care systems. *Trauma Q* 1984;11:17–24.
106. American College of Surgeons Committee on Trauma. Course overview: the purpose, history and concepts of the ATLS program for doctors. In: *Advanced trauma life support for doctors: instructor course manual.* Chicago: American College of Surgeons, 1997:9–19.
107. Yee ES, Thomas AN, Goodman PC. Isolated first rib fracture: clinical significance after blunt chest trauma. *Ann Thorac Surg* 1981;32:278–283.
108. Phillips EM, Rogers WF, Gaspar MR. First rib fractures: incidence of vascular injury and indications for angiography. *Surgery* 1981;89:42–47.
109. Thompson BM, Finger W, Tonsfeldt D, et al. Rib radiographs for trauma: useful or wasteful? *Ann Emerg Med* 1986;15:261–265.
110. Chan O, Hiorns M. Chest trauma. *Eur J Radiol* 1996;23:23–34.
111. Mirvis SE, Bidwell JK, Buddemeyer EU, et al. Value of chest radiography in excluding traumatic aortic rupture. *Radiology* 1987;163:487–493.
112. Richardson P, Mirvis SE, Scorpio R, et al. Value of CT in determining the need for angiography when findings of mediastinal hemorrhage on chest radiographs are equivocal. *Am J Roentgenol* 1991;156:273–279.
113. Madayag MA, Kirshenbaum KJ, Nadimpalli SR, et al. Thoracic aortic trauma: role of dynamic CT. *Radiology* 1991;179:853–855.
114. Boyd AD, Glassman LR. Trauma to the lung. *Chest Surg Clin North Am* 1997;7:263–284.
115. Dulchavsky SA, Schwarz KL, Kirkpatrick AW, et al. Prospective evaluation of thoracic ultrasound in the detection of pneumothorax. *J Trauma* 2001;50:201.
116. Ma OJ, Mateer JR. Trauma ultrasound examination versus chest radiography in the detection of hemothorax. *Ann Emerg Med* 1997;29:312.
117. Huh J, Milliken JC, Chen JC. Management of tracheobronchial injuries following blunt and penetrating trauma. *Am Surg* 1997;63:896–899.
118. Pembroke AP, Klineberg P, Johnson DC. Traumatic tracheal disruption-diagnostic difficulties. *Anaesth Intensive Care* 1995;23:206–207.
119. Etoch SW, Bar-Natan MF, Miller FB, et al. Tube thoracostomy: factors related to complications. *Arch Surg* 1995;130:521–526.
120. Fallon WF, Wears RL. Prophylactic antibiotics for the prevention of infectious complications including empyema following tube thoracostomy for trauma: results of meta-analysis. *J Trauma* 1992;33:110.
121. Gonzalez RP, Holevar MR. Role of prophylactic antibiotics for tube thoracostomy in chest trauma. *Am Surg* 1998;64:617–621.
122. Graeber GM, Jones DR. The role of thoracoscopy in thoracic trauma. *Ann Thorac Surg* 1993;56:646–648.
123. Abolhoda A, Livingston DH, Donahoo JS, et al. Diagnostic and therapeutic video assisted thoracic surgery (VATS) following chest trauma. *Eur J Cardiothorac Surg* 1997;12:356–360.
124. Wong MS, Tsoi EK, Henderson VJ, et al. Videothoracoscopy: an effective method for evaluating and managing thoracic trauma patients. *Surg Endosc* 1996;10:118–121.

125. Coselli JS, Mattox KL, Beall AC. Reevaluation of early evacuation of clotted hemothorax. *Am J Surg* 1984;148:786–790.

126. Heniford BT, Carrillo EH, Spain DA, et al. The role of thoracoscopy in the management of retained thoracic collections after trauma. *Ann Thorac Surg* 1997;63:940–943.

127. Meyer DM, Jessen ME, Wait MA, et al. Early evacuation of traumatic retained hemothoraces using thoracoscopy: a prospective, randomized trial. *Ann Thorac Surg* 1997;64:1396–1401.

128. Richardson JD. Indications for thoracotomy in thoracic trauma. *Curr Surg* 1985;42(5):361–364.

129. Cogbill TH, Moore EE, Millikan JS, et al. Rationale for selective application of emergency department thoracotomy in trauma. *J Trauma* 1983;23:453–458.

130. Cogbill TH, Landercasper J. Injury to the chest wall. In: Feliciano N, Moore DV, Maddox EE, eds. *Trauma*, 3rd ed. Stanford: Appleton & Lange, 1996.

131. Buckman R, Troskin SZ, Slancbaum L, et al. The significance of stable patients with sternal fracture. *Surg Gynecol Obstet* 1997; 164:261.

132. Wojcik JB, Morgan AS. Sternal fracture the natural history. *Ann Emerg Med* 1998;17:912.

133. Buckman R, Troskin SZ, Slancbaum L, et al. The significance of stable patients with sternal fracture. *Surg Gynecol Obstet* 1997;164:261.

134. Harley DP, Mena I. Cardiac and vascular sequelae of sternal fractures. *J Trauma* 1968;26:553.

135. Brookes JG, Dunn RJ, Rogers IR. Sternal fractures, a retrospective analysis of 272 cases. *J Trauma* 1993;35:46.

136. Hills MW, Delprado AM, Deane SA. Sternal fractures: associated injuries and management. *J Trauma* 1993;35:55.

137. Jackson M, Walker WS. Isolated sternal fractures, a benign injury. *Injury* 1992;23:535.

138. Garzon AA, Seltzer B, Carlson KE. Pathophysiology of crushed chest injury. *Ann Surg* 1968;168:128.

139. Newman RJ, Jones IS. A prospective study of 413 consecutive car occupants with chest injuries. *J Trauma* 1984;24:129.

140. Pate JW. Chest wall injuries. *Surg Clin North Am* 1989;69:59.

141. Trunkey DD. Cervicothoracic trauma. In: Blaisdell FW, Trunkey DD, eds. *Trauma management*, Vol. 3. New York: Thieme Medical Publishers, 1986.

142. Quick G. A randomized clinical trial of rib belts for simple fractures. *Am J Emerg Med* 1990;8:277–281.

143. Lee RB, Bass SM. Three or more rib fractures as an indicator for transfer to a Level I trauma center: a population based study. *J Trauma* 1990;30(6):689–694.

144. Ziegler DW, Agarwahl NN. The morbidity and mortality of rib fractures. *J Trauma* 1994;37:975–979.

145. Richardson JD, Adams L, Flint LM. Selective management of flail chest and pulmonary contusion. *Ann Surg* 1992;196:481.

146. Luchette FA, Radafsharsm SM, Kaiser R, et al. A prospective evaluation of epidural vs intrapleural catheters for analgesia in chest wall trauma. *J Trauma* 1994;39:865–870.

147. Mackersie RC, Karaginnes TG, Hoyt DB, et al. Prospective evaluation of epidural and intravenous administration of fentanyl for pain control and restoration of ventilatory function following multiple rib fractures. *J Trauma* 1991;31:443–451.

148. Ziegler DW, Agarwahl NN. The morbidity and mortality of rib fractures. *J Trauma* 1994;37:975–979.

149. Avery EE, Morch ET, Benson DW. Critically crushed chest. A new method of treatment with continuous mechanical hyperventilation to produce alkalotic apnea in internal pneumatic stabilization. *J Thorac Surg* 1956;32:291.

150. Shacford SR, Virgilio RW, Peters RM. Selective use of ventilatory in flail chest injury. *J Thorac Cardiovasc Surg* 1981;81:194.

151. Freedland M, Wilson RF, Bender JS, et al. The management of flail chest injury: factors effecting outcome. *J Trauma* 1990;30:1460.

152. Voggenreiter G, Newdeck S, Aufmkolh M, et al. Operative chest wall stabilization and flail chest. Outcomes of patients with and without pulmonary contusion. *J Am Coll Surg* 1998;187:130.

153. Thomas AN, Blaisdell FW, Lewis FR Jr, et al. Operative stabilization for flail chest with blunt trauma. *J Thorac Cardiovasc Surg* 1978;75:793.

154. Landercasper J, Cogbill TH, Lindesmith LA. Long term disability after flail chest injury. *J Trauma* 1984;24:410.

155. Beal SL, Oreskovich MR. Long term disability associated with flail chest injury. *Am J Surg* 1985;150:324.

156. Schaal MA, Fischer RP, Perry JF. The unchanged mortality of flail chest injuries. *J Trauma* 1979;19:492.

157. Coselli JS, Mattox KL, Beall AC. Reevaluation of early evacuation of clotted hemothorax. *Am J Surg* 1984;148:786–790.

158. Meyer DM, Jessen ME, Wait MA, et al. Early evacuation of traumatic retained hemothoraces using thoracoscopy: a prospective, randomized trial. *Ann Thorac Surg* 1997;64:1396–1401.

159. Richardson JD, Miller FB. Injuries to the lungs and pleura. In: Feliciano D, Moore EE, Mattox KK, eds. *Trauma*, 3rd ed. Stanford: Appleton & Lange, 1996.

160. Eggerstedt JM. Hemothorax. *eMedicine Journal* [serial online] 2003. Available at: *http://www.emedicine.com/med/topic2915.htm*.

161. Cohn SM. Pulmonary contusion: a review of the clinical entity. *J Trauma* 1997;42:973.

162. Pecklet MH, Newman KD, Eichelberger MR, et al. Thoracic trauma in children, an indicator of increased mortality. *J Pediatr Surg* 1990;25:961.

163. Fulton RL, Peter ET. The progressive nature of pulmonary contusion. *Surgery* 1970;67:499.

164. Casley-Smith JR, Eckert P, Foldia-Borcsok. The fine structure of pulmonary contusion and the effects of various drugs. *Br J Exp Pathol* 1976;57:487.

165. Alfano GS, Hale HW. Pulmonary contusion. *J Trauma* 1965;5:647.

166. Schield HH, Strunk H, Webber W, et al. Pulmonary contusion: CT vs plain radiograms. *J Comput Assist Tomogr* 1979;13:417.

167. Wagner RB, Jamieson PM. Pulmonary contusion: evaluation and classification by computed tomography. *Surg Clin North Am* 1989;69:31.

168. Johannigman JA, Campbell RS, Davis K Jr, et al. Combined differential lung ventilation and inhaled nitric oxide therapy in the management of unilateral pulmonary contusion. *J Trauma* 1977; 42:108.

169. Johnson JA, Cogbill TH, Winga ER. Determinants of outcome after pulmonary contusion. *J Trauma* 1986;26:695.

170. Dodek PM, Rice TW, Bonsignore MR, et al. Effects of plasmapheresis and hypoproteinemia on lung liquid conductance in awake sheep. *Circ Res* 1986;58:269.

171. Bongard FS, Lewis FR. Crystalloid resuscitation of patients with pulmonary contusion. *Am J Surg* 1984;148:145.

172. Hoff SJ, Shotts SD, Eddy VA, et al. Outcome of isolated pulmonary contusion in blunt trauma patients. *Am Surg* 1994; 60:138.

173. Foranz JL, Richardson JD, Grover FL, et al. Effect of methylprednisolone sodium succinate on experimental pulmonary contusion. *J Thorac Cardiovasc Surg* 1974;68:842.

174. Svennevig JL, Bugge-Asperheim B, Vaage J, et al. Corticosteroids in the treatment of blunt injury of the chest. *Br J Accident Surg* 1984;16:80.

175. Kishikawa M, Yoshioka T, Shimazu T, et al. Pulmonary contusion causes long term respiratory dysfunction with decreased functional residual capacity. *J Trauma* 1991;31:1203.

176. Mathai M, Byrd RP Jr, Roy TM. The posttraumatic pulmonary mass. *J Tenn Med Assoc* 1996;89:41–42.

177. Takahashi N, Murakami J, Murayama S, et al. MR evaluation of intrapulmonary hematoma. *J Comput Assist Tomogr* 1995;19: 125–127.

178. Hollister M, Stern EJ, Steinberg KP. Type 2 pulmonary laceration: a marker of blunt high-energy injury to the lung. *Am J Roentgenol* 1995;165:1126.

179. Thomas AN, Stephens BG. Air embolism: a cause of morbidity and death after penetrating chest trauma. *J Trauma* 1974;14:633–638.

180. Saada M, Goarin J-P, Riou B, et al. Systemic gas embolism complicating pulmonary contusion: diagnosis and management using transesophageal echocardiography. *Am J Respir Crit Care Med* 1995;152:812–815.

181. Rodrigus-Morales G, Rodrigus A, Shatney CH. Acute rupture of the diaphragm and blunt trauma: analysis of 60 patients. *J Trauma* 1968;26:438.

182. Voeller GR, Risser JR, Fabian TC, et al. Blunt diaphragm injuries: a five year experience. *Am Surg* 1990;56:28.

183. Brant ML, Luks FI, Spigland NA, et al. Diaphragmatic injury in children. *J Trauma* 1992;32:298.

184. Ascensio JA, Demetriades D, Rodrigus A. Injury to the diaphragm. In: Feliciano D, Moore EE, Maddox KK, eds. *Trauma*, 3rd ed. Stanford: Appleton & Lange, 1996:471.

185. Guth AA, Pachter HL, Kim U. Pitfalls in the diagnosis of blunt diaphragmatic trauma. *Am J Surg* 1995;170:5.

186. Shah R, Sabanathan S, Mearns AJ, et al. Traumatic rupture of the diaphragm. *Ann Thorac Surg* 1995;60:1444.

187. Estrera AS, Platt MR, Mills LJ. Traumatic injuries of the diaphragm. *Chest* 1979;75:306.

188. Puffer P, Gaebler M. Traumatic diaphragmatic rupture in a forensic medicine autopsy symbol. *Beitr Gerichtl Med* 1991;49:149.

189. Symbas PN. Injury to the esophagus, trachea and bronchus. In: Feliciano D, Moore EE, Maddox KK, eds. *Trauma*. Stanford: Appleton & Lange, 1998.

190. Kiser AC, O'Brien SM, Detterbeck FC. Blunt tracheobronchial injuries: treatment and outcomes. *Ann Thorac Surg* 2001;71:2059–2065.

191. Halttunen PE, Kostianen SA, Meurala HG. Bronchial rupture caused by blunt chest trauma. *Scand J Thorac Cardiovasc Surg* 1984; 18:141–144.

192. Kirsch MM, Orringer MB, Behrendt DM, et al. Management of tracheobronchial disruption secondary to nonpenetrating trauma. *Ann Thorac Surg* 1976;22:93–101.

193. Cassada DC, Munyikwa MP, Moniz MP. Acute injuries of the trachea and major bronchi: importance of early diagnosis. *Ann Thorac Surg* 2000;69:1563–1567.

194. Amauchi W, Birolini D, et al. Injuries to the tracheobronchial tree in closed trauma. *Thorax* 1983;38:923–928.

195. Wu M-H, Tseng Y-L, Lin M-Y, et al. Surgical results of 23 patients with tracheobronchial injuries. *Respirology* 1997;2:127–130.

196. Matsumoto K, Noguchi T, Ishikawa R, et al. The surgical treatment of lung lacerations and major bronchial disruptions caused by blunt thoracic trauma. *Surg Today* 1998;28:162–166.

197. Rupprecht H, Rumenapf G, Petermann H, et al. Transthoracic bronchial intubation in a case of main bronchus disruption. *J Trauma* 1996;41:895–898.

198. Feliciano DV. The diagnostic and therapeutic approach to chest trauma. *Semin Thorac Cardiovasc Surg* 1992;4:156–162.

199. Johnson MJ, Lucas GL. Fat embolism syndrome. *Orthopaedics* 1996;19:41.

200. Peltier LF. Fat embolism, a current concept. *Clin Orthop* 1969;66:241.

201. Eddy A, Rice C, Carrico C. Fat embolism syndrome: monitoring and management. *J Crit Illness* 1987;2:24.

202. Muller C, Rahn B, Pfister U, et al. The incidence, pathogenesis, diagnosis and treatment of fat embolism. *Orthop Rev* 1994;23:107.

203. Pell ACH, Christi J, Keating J, et al. The detection of fat embolism by transesophageal echocardiography during reamed intramedullary nailing. *J Bone Joint Surg* 1993;75:921.

204. Chastre J, Fagon JY, Soler P, et al. Bronchoalveolar lavage for rapid diagnosis of fat embolism syndrome in trauma patients. *Ann Intern Med* 1990;113:583.

205. Aoki OBN, Kazui S, Masateru S, et al. Evaluation of potential fat emboli during placement of intramedullary nails after orthopaedic fractures. *Chest* 1998;113:178.

206. Fonte DA, Hausberger FX. Pulmonary free fatty acids in experimental fat embolism. *J Trauma* 1971;11:668.

207. Gossing HR, Pellegrini VD Jr. Fat embolism syndrome: a review of the pathophysiology and physiologic basis of treatment. *Clin Orthop* 1982;165:68.

208. Bulger EM, Smith DG, Maier RV, et al. Fat embolism syndrome: a ten year review. *Arch Surg* 1997;132:435.

209. Yoshida A, Okada Y, Nagata Y, et al. Assessment of cerebral fat embolism by magnetic resonance imaging in the acute stage. *J Trauma* 1996;40:437.

210. Moylan JA, Birnbaum M, Katz A, et al. Fat emboli syndrome. *J Trauma* 1976;16:341.

211. Jacobson DM, Terrance CF, Reinmuth OM. The neurologic manifestations of fat embolisms. *Neurology* 1986;36:847.

CHAPTER 25

Managing the Patient with Shock, Sepsis, and Multiple Organ Failure

Richard H. Savel

Michael A. Matthay

Michael A. Gropper

This chapter initially focuses on (a) the methods available for the diagnosis and monitoring of hemodynamic insufficiency in critically ill patients, (b) the indications for invasive hemodynamic monitoring in critically ill patients, and (c) the basic principles of determining the etiology of shock. The second half of the chapter considers multiple organ failure (MOF) in critically ill patients, with a particular focus on sepsis.

CARDIOVASCULAR MONITORING

In this section, techniques for monitoring the hemodynamic and respiratory status of critically ill patients with respiratory failure are discussed. In the last three decades, many invasive techniques for monitoring the systemic and pulmonary circulation have been developed. However, there has been increasing interest in developing noninvasive methods for monitoring important physiologic variables with the goal of reducing the risk and expense of invasive measurements whenever possible. This is particularly pertinent with the use of pulmonary artery (PA) catheters, which has become increasingly controversial.

SYSTEMIC ARTERIAL CATHETERIZATION

Systemic arterial catheters are widely used in a variety of critically ill patients. They are most useful for monitoring systemic arterial blood pressure in patients who are hemodynamically unstable, including patients with severe, uncontrolled hypertension as well as patients with hypotension and clinical shock. In addition, systemic arterial catheters are useful as a means of obtaining repeated blood samples from patients, thus obviating the need for repeated percutaneous venous or arterial puncture. In general, systemic arterial catheters are well tolerated, although there are a few important concerns about insertion technique and complications that need to be remembered.

Insertion Techniques for Systemic Arterial Catheters

Peripheral arterial cannulation is accomplished most frequently by percutaneous insertion of a no. 18 or no. 20 gauge catheter using sterile technique. The radial artery is usually chosen because of its accessibility and because there is generally good collateral circulation via the ulnar artery. Prior to insertion, the status of this collateral circulation may be assessed with an Allen test. With this test, both the ulnar and radial arteries are occluded by applying pressure at the wrist; after the hand becomes pale and cool, releasing only the ulnar artery occlusion restores adequate circulation within 5 seconds. The femoral, dorsales pedis, and axillary arteries may also be cannulated. Cannulation of the brachial artery should be avoided because of the lack of collateral circulation at that site.

Complications of Systemic Arterial Catheters

Infection and ischemia are the most important major complications that may occur from systemic arterial catheterization. Ischemia may occur secondary to either thrombosis with local occlusion or distal embolization. In one large prospective study, a 4% incidence of catheter-related septicemia and an 18% incidence of local infection (defined by semiquantitative culture of the catheter tip) were found (1). Catheters should be inserted using sterile technique after skin decontamination using chlorhexidine or an iodine-containing solution. Infection may originate in the transducer or fluid-delivery apparatus. One prospective study indicated that catheter-related infection can be decreased markedly if a continuous flush device is located immediately distal to the transducer apparatus rather than close to the insertion site (2). This eliminates a long proximal static fluid column between the transducer and flush intake. With this design and with careful sterile precautions in the blood-sampling stopcock technique, the incidence of catheter-related septicemia reduces to <1%. Arterial lines should not be routinely changed unless there is clinical evidence of infection.

Clinically significant thrombosis or embolism is rare. In more than 12,000 consecutive placements of arterial lines (including radial, axillary, and/or dorsalis pedis arteries), necrosis of the fingers or toes occurred in only 15 patients (0.2%) (3).

Similarly, in another study, only 3 (0.6%) of 531 patients required emergency thrombectomies for distal ischemia (4). The clinical risk factors for acute distal ischemia include systemic hypotension, severe peripheral vascular disease, and the use of vasopressor drugs. Even though clinically important ischemia is rare, reversible subclinical arterial occlusion or reduced flow is common, with up to 24% of arteries still occluded 1 week after catheter removal (5). The risk factors for such occlusion include larger catheter size (no.18 versus no. 20 gauge), smaller wrist size (e.g., in women and children), repeated attempts before successful cannulation, and duration of cannulation (risk increases after 3 to 4 days). Ulnar refill time determined by the Allen test prior to insertion is also of some predictive value.

Once the catheter is placed, distal perfusion should be assessed at least daily by noting any changes in skin color, temperature, or capillary refill time. If the arterial pressure tracing becomes persistently dampened, or if blood-drawing is difficult, thrombus formation on the catheter tip is likely, and removal of the catheter should be considered because the risk of occlusion is high (6).

PULMONARY ARTERY CATHETERIZATION

There are numerous clinical conditions for which PA catheterization has been considered to be a reasonable procedure (7,8). These include shock associated with acute myocardial infarction, sepsis, or major trauma; acute respiratory failure from cardiogenic or noncardiogenic pulmonary edema; and management of patients following cardiac surgery. However, there has been increasing concern that clinicians need to be better informed about the risk and potential benefits of PA catheterization (9–11). The clinical literature contains numerous examples of how incorrect information may be conveyed from pulmonary capillary wedge pressure (PCWP) measurements when physicians and nurses are not sufficiently skilled at interpreting pressure and waveform tracings (12,13). In addition, the use of PA catheters to guide resuscitation has not been shown to improve outcomes (14–16).

Insertion Techniques

The pulmonary circulation can be monitored by percutaneous insertion of a balloon-tipped PA catheter via the subclavian, internal jugular, external jugular, femoral, or antecubital vein. Catheterization can be done at the patient's bedside with only pressure waveform and amplitude and electrocardiographic monitoring. Fluoroscopy is usually not necessary, although the prescribed waveform must be displayed on the bedside monitor. The PA catheter used most frequently has four lumina plus a small thermistor near the tip for thermodilution cardiac output measurements. One lumen is used to inflate the balloon on the tip of the catheter. After the catheter is advanced into the thorax, the balloon is inflated. The flow-directed catheter then usually passes easily from the right atrium, across the tricuspid valve, through the right ventricle, and into the PA (see Fig. 25-1). If the catheter is advanced further with the balloon inflated, it will wedge in the PA and occlude blood flow. The distal lumen, which opens at the tip of the catheter, will then record the downstream vascular pressure, the pulmonary arterial wedge pressure (PAWP) (Fig. 25-1). When the balloon is deflated, the distal lumen records the

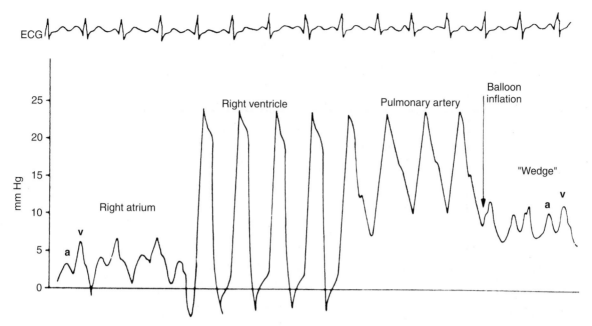

FIGURE 25-1. Representative recording of pressures as a Swan-Ganz catheter is inserted through an internal jugular vein through the right side of the heart into the pulmonary artery. The first recorded waveform is a right atrial tracing with characteristic *a* and *v* waves. In the right ventricle, note that end-diastolic pressure is zero. In the pulmonary artery, a normal pressure waveform is recorded. The catheter is then advanced to the wedge position with the balloon inflated. The wedge pressure tracing shows *a* and *v* waves transmitted from the left atrium. The wedge tracing is not always this clear, but it should not be overly damped. The pressures shown here are normal. [From Matthay MA. Invasive hemodynamic monitoring in critically ill patients. *Clin Chest Med* 1983;4(2):233–249, with permission.]

phasic pulmonary arterial pressure. The proximal lumen, located 30 cm from the tip of the catheter, will then be positioned in the right atrium to measure central venous pressure (CVP) when the tip of the catheter is in the PA. This proximal lumen is also used to inject a bolus of indicator (10 mL of normal saline) to determine cardiac output by thermodilution. The bolus is injected through the lumen in the right atrium so that the thermistor near the tip of the catheter in the PA can sense the change in temperature as the bolus flows into the PA. A small bedside computer then integrates the time–temperature curve and determines cardiac output using the Stewart–Hamilton equation. The fourth lumen, located 31 cm from the tip of the catheter, is used for infusion of intravenous solutions. An introducer sheath that has an additional lumen is also available for the intravenous infusion of fluids.

Obtaining Reliable Pressure Measurements

Once the catheter is in place, the pressure is transmitted via the catheter through the fluid-filled tubing to the diaphragm of a transducer and then converted to an electronic signal. The signal is amplified, the pressure waveform is shown on an oscilloscope, and the pressure is shown on a digital display (Fig. 25-1). Correct pressure measurements depend on accurately calibrated transducers, a fluid-filled catheter system without blood clots or air bubbles, and a monitor that displays the pressure tracing in an appropriate size to demonstrate the waveforms clearly. The pulmonary arterial and wedge pressure tracing in Figure 25-1 fulfills these requirements. Note that there is a single major pulmonary arterial pressure wave

for each spike on the electrocardiogram (ECG). Correct amplitude settings (generally in the range of 0 to 30 or 0 to 60 mm Hg) are needed to display the waveform correctly. In addition, the contour of the tracing is important. Figure 25-2 illustrates the dampening effect of a small air bubble in the catheter system. Another common pitfall is improper location of the zero reference point, particularly because patients are moving from side to side or the head of the bed is raised or lowered. In general, the proper zero reference is the midchest position (phlebostatic axis).

Perhaps the most common source of error in making intrathoracic pressure measurements is failure to take into account the effects of respiration on these pressure measurements (7,8,12,17). Pleural pressure becomes *negative* during inspiration in a spontaneously breathing patient and *positive* during the inspiratory cycle of a mechanically ventilated patient. In Figure 25-3, the recording of PAWP is interrupted by deep troughs in the tracing produced by the patient's spontaneous inspiratory efforts. During these troughs, the pressure reading is zero. Thus, the problem is how to obtain a reliable transmural pressure measurement when the reference pressure (pleural pressure) is changing. To minimize the effects of changing pleural pressure, pulmonary arterial pressures should be measured at *end-expiration* when pleural pressures will be close to zero. In Figure 25-3, end-expiration can be clearly seen in both the pulmonary arterial pressure and the wedge pressure tracing. This approach enables the clinician to consider the measured pressure at end-expiration as a very close approximation of the true transmural pressure. This approach can be complicated if the patient is breathing so rapidly that the end-expiratory phase is very brief (see Figure 25-4).

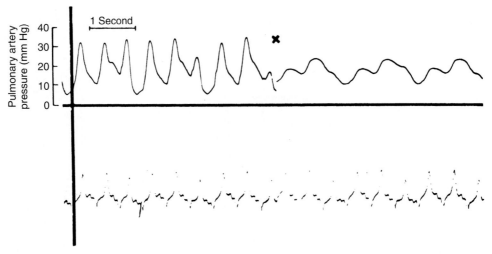

FIGURE 25-2.   Pulmonary artery tracing after introduction of 0.5 mL of air into the connecting tubing at *X*, with the electrocardiogram recorded below. The phasic contour of the pulmonary artery tracing is damped out by the air bubble; the same pattern can be produced by clots in the catheter or on the catheter tip. (From Quinn K, Quebbeman EJ. Pulmonary artery pressure monitoring in the surgical intensive care unit. *Arch Surg* 1981;116:872–876, with permission.)

In most circumstances, the best approach for obtaining a reliable pressure tracing is to obtain a printout of the actual pressure tracing.

Accurate measurements of pulmonary arterial pressures can be particularly difficult in patients with acute, severe airway obstruction. In order to overcome the high airway resistance, patients generate very positive intrathoracic pressures throughout expiration, and this leads to an elevated pulmonary arterial pressure or an elevated wedge pressure. During inspiration, the patient's pleural pressure may be markedly negative, and there will be a wide swing in the pulmonary arterial pressure tracing in the opposite direction. Similar problems occur while measuring pressures in patients on positive end-expiratory pressure (PEEP) (see the section Effect of Positive End-Expiratory Pressure on Wedge Pressure Measurements). There is no reliable method to determine the effect of positive intrathoracic pressure on hemodynamic measurements with the PA catheter. Additional information about cardiac filling may be obtained using transthoracic echocardiography or transesophageal echocardiography (TEE).

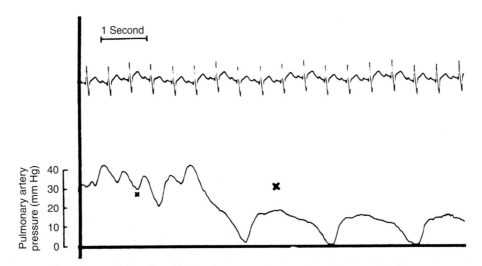

FIGURE 25-3.   Continuous monitoring of the electrocardiogram and the phasic pulmonary artery pressure plus a segment of a pulmonary artery wedge tracing. Note that the troughs in the pulmonary artery and in the wedge tracings occur when the patient takes a spontaneous breath and pleural pressure becomes negative, thus causing a downward deflection in the tracing. The *X* marks indicate end-expiration in the respiratory cycle. At end-expiration, pleural pressure is zero; therefore, the measured intraluminal pressure should be close to the real transmural pressure. Wedge pressure is about 15 mm Hg below the pulmonary artery end-diastolic pressure; the patient had pulmonary hypertension from acute pulmonary embolism, which accounts for the gradient between the end-diastolic and the wedge pressures. (From Quinn K, Quebbeman EJ. Pulmonary artery pressure monitoring in the surgical intensive care unit. *Arch Surg* 1981;116:872–876, with permission.)

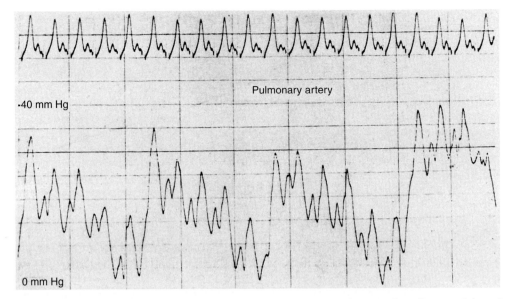

FIGURE 25-4. Example of how rapid, labored respirations can result in rapid oscillations of the pulmonary artery pressure tracing and highly variable pressure measurements. The patient's respiratory rate was 40 breaths per minute and the peak pulmonary artery pressure varied from 35–40 to 18 mm Hg. A brief period of end-expiration could be identified, but the electronic digital readout could not reflect that brief end-expiratory period alone. So the pulmonary artery tracing was recorded on calibrated paper and the pressures read off the paper at the point of end-expiration. [From Matthay MA. Invasive hemodynamic monitoring in critically ill patients. *Clin Chest Med* 1983;4(2):233–249, with permission.]

Relation of Wedge Pressure to Left Arterial Pressure

The PAWP is used widely as an index of left atrial filling pressure. In general, most studies have demonstrated that the correlation between wedge pressure and left atrial pressure in patients is very good (7,8,17). The correlation of left atrial pressure to left ventricular end-diastolic pressure, likewise, is good, provided there is no mitral valve disease. The pulmonary arterial end-diastolic pressure provides an accurate indication of the PAWP except when there is an increase in pulmonary vascular resistance, in which case the end-diastolic pressure will be much higher than the wedge pressure. Pulmonary vascular resistance is elevated in several clinical conditions associated with acute or chronic pulmonary hypertension (see Chapters 10, Lung Transplantation and Lung Volume Reduction Surgery; 11, Pulmonary Thromboembolism and Other Pulmonary Vascular Diseases; 13, Occupational and Environmental Lung Disease; and 22, Acute Hypercapnic Respiratory Failure: Neuromuscular and Obstructive Diseases).

Effect of Positive End-Expiratory Pressure on Wedge Pressure Measurements

Accurate transmural arterial and wedge pressure measurements may be more difficult to obtain in patients on PEEP in excess of 10 cm H_2O. PEEP may interfere with accurate measurements in two ways. First, it may result in an undetermined increase in pleural pressure. Second, the airway pressure generated by PEEP may be transmitted to the pulmonary microcirculation (17). Because PEEP prevents transpulmonary pressure from falling to zero at the end of expiration, the pleural pressure remains positive at the end of expiration; thus, the reference pressure for the pulmonary arterial pressure measurement is not zero. Hence, the recorded intraluminal pressure (i.e., CVP, pulmonary arterial pressure, or wedge pressure) may be higher than the actual transmural pressure. One way to solve this problem is to measure esophageal pressure as an indicator of pleural pressure in order to obtain a more accurate reference pressure. However, reliable esophageal pressure measurements are difficult to obtain, especially in a supine patient in a critical care unit. One partial solution to the problem is to make an estimate of pleural pressure and subtract this value from the measured wedge pressure. In clinical studies in which pleural pressure was measured in patients with acute respiratory distress syndrome (ARDS), pleural pressure did not usually become significantly positive with levels of PEEP below 10 cm H_2O (18,19). For every 5 cm H_2O increase in PEEP levels above 10 cm H_2O, pleural pressure was increased 2 to 3 cm H_2O (18,19).

The other potential difficulty with levels of PEEP above 10 cm H_2O is that if alveolar pressure exceeds the pulmonary arterial pressure, the catheter tip may reflect airway pressure rather than vascular pressures. Theoretically, the wedge pressure will reflect left atrial pressure if the wedged catheter tip is located in a portion of the lung where pulmonary arterial and pulmonary venous pressures exceed the alveolar pressure (zone 3) (7,8,17). If the catheter tip is in an area where alveolar pressure exceeds venous pressure when pulmonary arterial flow is occluded with balloon inflation, the recorded pressure will be airway pressure rather than PA pressure. If the catheter is located in zone 3, the wedged catheter can look through the pulmonary vasculature to sense the left atrial pressure. Thus, to have an accurate indication of left atrial pressure, the PA catheter must be in a zone 3 area.

Usually, the flow-directed PA catheter migrates to zone 3, and the wedge pressure accurately reflects left atrial pressure (7,8). If PEEP is increased, it is possible that the zone 3 area, where the catheter was initially placed, may become a zone 2 area, where alveolar pressure exceeds venous pressure. Although this does not happen very often, it has been shown experimentally that if the tip of the PA catheter is at or below the left atrium, the mean wedge pressure at end-expiration still reflects left atrial pressure, even with levels of PEEP up to 30 cm H_2O (20). Therefore, it is reasonable to confirm the position of the catheter tip with an anteroposterior portable chest roentgenogram and, if necessary, with a lateral chest radiograph (7,8). When a question arises about the location of the catheter tip, there are a few maneuvers that can be done to verify zone 3 conditions (see Table 25-1) (21). For wedge pressure tracings outside zone 3, the wedge contour appears unusually smooth and the PA end-diastolic pressure tends to be lower than the balloon-occlusion pressure. In zones 1 and 2, changes in the wedge pressure tend to follow alveolar rather than left atrial pressure.

Thus, the swings in the wedge pressure during ventilation with positive pressure are unusually wide because only 50% or less of the change in static airway pressure (peak greater than plateau pressure) transmits to the pleural spaces, left atrium, and intrathoracic vessels. For the same reason, a trial of PEEP reduction causes the wedge pressure to fall by an unexpected magnitude (more than 50% of the PEEP decrement) when the catheter tip is in zone 1 or 2 (Table 25-1) (21).

One recent study reported that there is considerable interobserver variability in pressure measurement using pulmonary arterial catheter tracings (22). Nurse–physician differences were not substantially greater than physician–physician differences. Significant differences in measurement were more common in patients whose PAWP had a higher degree of respiratory variation, probably because of disagreement in identifying end-expiration on the tracings (22). The observed differences were likely to be clinically significant and potentially led to inappropriate clinical decisions and clinical interventions.

ECHOCARDIOGRAPHY AND OTHER NONINVASIVE MONITORING TECHNIQUES

Given some recent data showing that invasive hemodynamic monitoring may not necessarily be associated with improved outcomes, many intensivists are using noninvasive techniques to gain similar data (23–26). One of the most common techniques is the use of echocardiography to rapidly assess cardiac function in the critical care setting (27). Though more and more intensivists are leaving their critical care training with some knowledge of echocardiography, accurate interpretation in the critically ill patient can often be quite complex, and the equipment can be rather costly. Other new technologies include the combination of lithium dilution cardiac output and beat-to-beat variability of the arterial line tracing to give a real-time measure of stroke volume (28). Though this technique appears to be valid and accurate, studies will need to be performed to see whether their use is associated with improved outcome. Additional techniques include using gastric or sublingual tonometry to detect early splanchnic hypoperfusion (29,30), as well as esophageal Doppler probes and thoracic electrical bioimpedance to estimate cardiac output (23,31).

PULMONARY ARTERY CATHETERIZATION: CLINICAL INDICATIONS

The most common clinical conditions for which PA catheterization is used in intensive care units (ICUs) include acute pulmonary edema, shock, and hemodynamic management of patients after cardiac surgery (7–9).

ACUTE CARDIOGENIC PULMONARY EDEMA

Patients with acute pulmonary edema in association with systemic hypotension secondary to an acute myocardial infarction present difficult management problems. A number of studies have documented that the hemodynamic profiles of patients within this group may vary considerably. Some patients will have markedly elevated left ventricular end-diastolic pressures in association with a very low cardiac output, whereas others may have a much more moderate elevation in the PAWP and better ventricular function (11,32). Occasionally, patients thought to have left ventricular failure will be found to have noncardiogenic pulmonary edema. Rational decisions about the use of vasopressors, vasodilators, and volume replacement may be better made with knowledge of the left ventricular filling pressure and systemic vascular resistance (SVR) (9,11), providing the measurements are accurate (22).

ACUTE NONCARDIOGENIC PULMONARY EDEMA

There are several reasons why pulmonary arterial catheterization may be indicated in selected patients with suspected noncardiogenic pulmonary edema. First, differentiation of cardiogenic from noncardiogenic pulmonary edema can be difficult both radiographically (33) and clinically. In one study, the clinical diagnosis of noncardiogenic pulmonary edema was substantiated on PA catheterization in only 56% of patients (34). In addition, some patients who have primary lung injury also may have a mild elevation in the PAWP that contributes to the pulmonary edema (35).

In patients with ARDS who have received a PA catheter, it should be removed within 3 to 4 days to reduce the risk of secondary infection and to convert the central line onto a triple-lumen catheter that can be used for the administration of fluids and antibiotics and, if necessary, for hyperalimentation (see Chapter 26, Prevention of Nonpulmonary Complications of Intensive Care). There are some patients with ARDS who

TABLE 25-1. Checklist for Verifying Position of Pulmonary Arterial Catheter

Condition	Zone 3	Zone 1 or Zone 2
Respiratory variation of PW	≤1/2 ΔPalv	>1/2 ΔPalv
PW contour	Cardiac ripple	Unnaturally smooth
Catheter tip location	LA level or below	Above LA level
Decrease PEEP trial	ΔPW ≤1.2 PEEP	ΔPW >1/2 ΔPEEP
Ppad vs. PW	Ppad >PW	Ppad ≤PW

PW, wedge pressure; Palv, static airway pressure; LA, left atrium; PEEP, positive end-expiratory pressure; Ppad, pulmonary artery diastolic pressure.

From Marini JJ. Obtaining meaningful data from the Swan-Ganz catheter. *Respir Care* 1985;30:572, with permission.

are very stable hemodynamically and in whom the oxygenation defect is not very severe. Most of these patients can be managed without pulmonary arterial catheterization (36,37).

SHOCK

One of the original justifications for PA catheterization rests on the evidence that some patients with acute myocardial infarction may have a normal CVP in the presence of an elevated PAWP (38). Also, some patients with an acute myocardial infarction and shock are found to have low left ventricular filling pressures that can be best treated with volume expansion to increase preload. Thus, the argument has been that pulmonary arterial catheterization helps provide information that cannot be obtained by clinical examination alone. In fact, one study confirmed that clinical assessment of hemodynamic variables in patients with shock prior to insertion of a PA catheter was poor (34). In patients with PAWPs >18 mm Hg, the wedge pressure was predicted correctly only 35% of the time. Similarly, in the same group of patients with a measured cardiac index of <2.2 L/minute/m^2, the cardiac index was predicted correctly only 55% of the time. It is important to remember that the PA catheter is a monitor, and not a therapy, and has not been shown to decrease mortality in patients with septic shock.

MANAGEMENT OF PATIENTS AFTER CARDIAC SURGERY

The indications for PA catheterization in patients who have had cardiac surgery are controversial (9). In some institutions, for example, clinicians insert PA catheters in all patients who have undergone cardiac surgery, whereas in other institutions, even cardiac transplant patients do not have routine PA pressure monitoring. Increasing use of intraoperative TEE has led to decreasing utilization of PA catheters in the operating room. However, available data about risks versus benefits of PA catheterization after cardiac surgery support a more selective approach, reserving PA catheterization for patients with a reduced left ventricular ejection fraction (9). Moreover, one study demonstrated that the PAWP was not a reliable indicator of left ventricular preload in the immediate period following coronary artery bypass surgery (39).

HOW TO DETERMINE THE PHYSIOLOGIC BASIS FOR SHOCK

There is no specific blood pressure that defines shock. Shock is present if evidence of multisystem organ hypoperfusion is apparent. Evidence of hypoperfusion obtained during the rapid initial clinical evaluation of a patient in case of suspected shock may include tachycardia, a low mean blood pressure, an altered mental status, and a decreased urine output. There are several causes of shock that need to be differentiated as early as possible in the patient's clinical course.

A systematic approach to determining the etiology of shock is helpful in the initial diagnosis and management of the hypotensive patient. This approach acknowledges that shock is identified in most patients by systemic hypotension and that mean arterial blood pressure is the product of cardiac output

and the SVR (40,41). Accordingly, hypotension may be due to reduced cardiac output or reduced system vascular resistance. Initial examination of the hypotensive patient seeks to determine whether cardiac output, and therefore systemic oxygen delivery, is reduced. High–cardiac-output hypotension is most often signaled by a large pulse pressure, a low diastolic pressure, warm extremities, fever (or hypothermia), and leukocytosis (or leukopenia); these clinical findings strongly suggest a working diagnosis of septic shock, the initial treatment for which is broad-spectrum antimicrobial therapy combined with early and aggressive expansion of the vascular volume (see Table 25-2).

By contrast, a low cardiac output is indicated by a small pulse pressure and cool extremities with poor nail bed capillary refill. In this case, the clinical need is to determine whether the left ventricle is overdistended and is failing. A heart that is too full in a hypotensive patient is signaled by elevated jugular venous pressure (JVP), peripheral edema, crepitations on lung auscultation, a large heart with extra heart sounds (S$_3$ and S$_4$), chest pain, ischemic changes on the ECG, and a chest radiograph showing a large heart with dilated upper-lobe vessels and pulmonary edema. These findings suggest cardiogenic shock, most often due to ischemic heart disease, and are generally absent when the low cardiac output is due to hypovolemia (Table 25-2). Then, clinical examination reveals manifestations of blood loss (i.e., hematemesis, tarry stools, abdominal distension, and reduced hematocrit), trauma, or manifestations of dehydration (i.e., reduced tissue turgor, vomiting or diarrhea, or negative fluid balance). This distinction between cardiogenic and hypovolemic shock allows initial therapy to focus on vasoactive drugs or on volume infusions, respectively (Table 25-2).

Whenever the clinical formulation is not obvious, it is helpful to determine what does not fit (41). Most often, the answer is that the hypotension is due to two or more etiologies of shock: (a) septic shock complicated by myocardial ischemia or hypovolemia, (b) cardiogenic shock complicated by hypovolemia or sepsis, and (c) hypovolemic shock masking as sepsis or ischemic heart disease. It should be remembered that in septic shock, ventricular function is almost always depressed, even when cardiac output is elevated. In these situations, more data is needed and it frequently can be obtained from echocardiography and pulmonary arterial catheterization. Proper interpretation of this data, along with response to initial therapy, frequently confirm that multiple etiologies for shock exist or it leads to a broader differential diagnosis of the etiologies of shock (Table 25-2).

MULTIPLE ORGAN FAILURE

This section considers MOF with a focus on definitions, epidemiology, pathogenesis, management, and prevention (42). One of the earliest descriptions of MOF was written by Baue in 1975:

> The sequence of events often begins with a period of shock or circulatory failure at some point during the initial injury, accompanied sooner or later by failure of ventilation and the need for ventilatory support. This may be followed by renal failure, hepatic failure (jaundice and decreasing albumin levels), gastrointestinal failure (stress ulcers and gastrointestinal bleeding), and metabolic

TABLE 25-2. Characteristics of Septic, Cardiogenic, and Hypovolemic Shock

Abnormalities in Shock	Septic	Cardiogenic	Hypovolemic
Blood pressure	↓	↓	↓
Heart rate	≥	≥	≤
Respiratory rate	≥	≥	≤
Mentation	↓	↓	↓
Urine output	↓	↓	↓
Arterial pH	↓	↓	↓
Pulse pressure	↓	↓	↓
Diastolic pressure	↓↓↓	↓	↓
Extremities/digits	Warm	Cool	Cool
Temperature	≤ or ↓	↔	↔
White cell count	≤ or ↓	↔	↔
Site of infection	+ +	—	—
Is the Heart Too Full?	No	Yes	No
Symptoms/clinical context	Sepsis/liver failure	Ischemia/infarction	Hemorrhage/dehydration
Jugular venous pressure	↓	≥	↓
S₃, S₄, gallop rhythm	—	+ + +	—
Chest radiograph	Normal (early in course)	Large heart (sometimes) ≥ upper lobe flow pulmonary edema	Normal
What Does Not Fit?			
Overlapping etiologies (septic + cardiogenic, septic + hypovolemic, cardiogenic + hypovolemic)			
Short list of other etiologies	High-output hypotension Thyroid storm Arteriovenous fistula Paget disease	High right atrial–pressure hypotension Cardiac tamponade Right ventricular infarction Pulmonary hypertension	Nonresponsive hypovolemia Adrenal insufficiency Anaphylaxis Spinal shock
Obtain more information	Echocardiography, right-heart catheterization		

↓, decrease; ↑, increase; ≥, increased or unchanged; ≤, decreased or unchanged; ↔, unchanged.
From Hall JB, Schmidt GA, Wood LDH, eds. *Principles of critical care.* New York: McGraw-Hill, Inc., 1992:1393–1395, with permission.

failure (decrease in lean body mass and weakness due to progressive catabolism). Our ability to support a single system that has failed, transiently at least, is reasonably good. The support of two or more failed units, however, stresses our knowledge and capability. Survivors of multiple systems failure are infrequent (43).

Since this description, several medical and surgical studies have reported a high mortality rate associated with MOF in critically ill patients. Sepsis syndrome is clearly the most frequently encountered clinical problem associated with the development of MOF (43). Some patients who have MOF, however, do not seem to have a clear-cut infectious etiology. For example, patients who have been treated with interleukin-2 (IL-2) for malignant disorders frequently develop renal failure, gastrointestinal failure, neurologic disturbances, and sometimes even acute respiratory failure. These observations suggest that release of potent endogenous humoral factors during noninfectious disorders (e.g., severe hypovolemic shock) may produce the clinical features of the sepsis syndrome without necessarily being related to the infection. Finally, it is also possible that primary lung injury itself can lead to the development of nonpulmonary organ failure (43). In any case, sepsis often complicates MOF, even if sepsis is not the initial clinical disorder (44,45).

DEFINITION AND EPIDEMIOLOGY

MOF is often a major complication in patients with shock from sepsis, major trauma, severe pancreatitis, drug overdose, or thermal injury (42–47). The extent to which an individual organ is likely to be damaged in these clinical settings depends on numerous factors, including age, preexisting medical illnesses, severity of illness on admission to the ICU, and the specific precipitating event (42,45,46). The clinical features of organ dysfunction in this patient group are also variable and have been defined by different criteria. Specifically, organ dysfunction in critically ill patients ranges in spectrum from minor biochemical abnormalities to irreversible organ failure. Nonetheless, the incidence of renal, gastrointestinal, hepatic, central nervous, and hematologic failure has been studied, especially in patients with acute respiratory failure. The definition and incidence of acute respiratory failure are discussed subsequently after considering criteria for failure of the nonpulmonary organ systems.

Cardiovascular Failure

The incidence of cardiovascular failure among critically ill patients varies from 10% to 23% (42). Although a uniform definition in critically ill patients has yet to be established, most clinicians agree that cardiovascular failure exists when one or more of the following are present: (a) mean arterial pressure ≤60 mm Hg, (b) cardiac index of 2 L/minute/m² or less, and (c) reversible ventricular fibrillation or asystole. This definition could include a patient with an acute myocardial infarction and severe pump failure. It could also include a patient with septic shock who has a high cardiac output, a low SVR, and a low mean arterial blood pressure. Cardiovascular failure, therefore, includes those disturbances that cause a major decrease in myocardial function as well as those clinical disorders associated with abnormalities in the peripheral circulation.

Although human septic shock is usually characterized by elevated cardiac output and reduced SVR, it may also be associated with a decrease in the left ventricular ejection fraction. In addition, studies have shown that septic patients have increased left ventricular ejection fraction, increased end-systolic and end-diastolic volumes, normal or decreased stroke work, and decreased right ventricular ejection fraction. These cardiovascular parameters normalize among patients who survive (48).

The mechanism of myocardial dysfunction during sepsis is not entirely known (48,49). Nonetheless, serum obtained from patients with septic shock has been shown to depress myocardial cell contractility *in vitro*. Moreover, evidence suggests that tumor necrosis factor (TNF), an important humoral mediator of sepsis, is capable of depressing myocardial cell contractility. It is likely that one or more of these myocardial depressants are responsible for the reduction in ejection fraction and for the ventricular volume changes that occur during sepsis.

Given the complexities associated with the diagnosis and management of cardiovascular dysfunction in acutely ill patients, the use of right-heart catheterization has become routine for many physicians caring for ICU patients. However, a recent prospective study suggested that the use of right-heart catheters was associated with an increase in both 30-day mortality [odds ratio (OR) = 1.24; 95% confidence interval (CI) = 1.03 to 1.49] and resource utilization (11).

Two other important features of sepsis syndrome are the abnormal vasodilation of the systemic circulation and the abnormalities of peripheral oxygen uptake. These issues are discussed in the section on pathogenesis.

Renal Failure

Renal dysfunction is a frequent complication in critically patients (40% to 55% incidence) and is manifested by reductions in urine output and by an increase in the serum urea and creatinine levels (42,49). Specifically, renal failure may be defined in this patient group as a serum creatinine value in excess of 2 mg per dL and a urine output <600 mL per 24 hours (45).

The three most important risk factors for the development of renal failure in critically ill patients are hypotension, sepsis, and nephrotoxic drugs (50,51). Acute nonoliguric renal failure, associated primarily with nephrotoxic drugs, has a better prognosis than acute oliguric renal failure that occurs with septic shock or after major cardiovascular surgery. In spite of supportive therapies such as hemodialysis and continuous renal replacement therapy, acute renal failure in the setting of sepsis is strongly associated with mortality.

Gastrointestinal Failure

Alterations in gastrointestinal tract function are estimated to occur in 30% of critically ill patients (42,49). The pathologic basis for gastrointestinal dysfunction appears to be both an alteration in microvascular permeability and mucosal ischemia. For example, TNF infusion into experimental animals causes necrosis of intestinal villi. These morphologic observations suggest a pathologic basis for the functional abnormalities of the gastrointestinal tract that occur in critically ill patients (52).

The clinical features of gastrointestinal tract dysfunction are variable and include hemorrhage, ileus, malabsorption (i.e., inability to tolerate enteral feedings), and occasionally, acalculous cholecystitis or pancreatitis. Among these complications, gastrointestinal bleeding is common but is difficult to quantify. However, gastrointestinal blood loss in excess of 1 g per dL of hemoglobin per 24 hours is generally accepted to be clinically significant (53).

An intact gastrointestinal tract mucosa provides an essential barrier to the entry of bacteria into the systemic circulation. Because mucosal integrity of the gastrointestinal tract is frequently impaired in critically ill patients, bacteria may translocate or migrate from the bowel lumen into the peritoneal cavity, or to regional gastrointestinal lymph nodes, and to the portosystemic circulation. To the extent that this occurs, the process of bacterial translocation may propagate septic shock and result in further organ dysfunction.

Clinical data in support of the central role of the gastrointestinal tract in the pathogenesis of MOF in acutely ill patients is increasing. In this regard, marked alterations in gastrointestinal permeability were demonstrated to occur in a prospectively studied group of ICU patients using monosaccharide and disaccharide probes (54). Perhaps even more significant, however, was the observation that the patients who developed MOF had significantly greater alterations in intestinal permeability upon ICU admission than those who did not ultimately develop MOF. Taken together, these observations suggest that altered gastrointestinal tract function plays an important if not central role in the pathogenesis of MOF in critically ill patients. Early enteral nutrition is an important strategy in the maintenance of gut mucosal integrity.

Hepatic Failure

Fulminant hepatic failure as a feature of organ failure in critically ill patients is uncommon and occurs in <10% of critically ill patients (42,49). By contrast, reversible elevations in serum transaminases and elevations in serum bilirubin or abnormal clotting parameters are common and may be found in as many as 95% of critically ill patients. Criteria for hepatic failure in critically ill patients are in a state of evolution. Nonetheless, elevations in serum bilirubin that exceed 4 to 5 mg per dL, a prothrombin time of more than 1.5 times control, and a serum albumin level below 2 g per dL are indicative of significant hepatic dysfunction (45,55).

As a complication of septic shock or other critical illnesses, hepatic dysfunction is of more than academic interest. The liver is an important reticuloendothelial organ whose function is also altered when the liver is damaged. For example, fibronectin, an opsonin that is important in the maintenance of host defense, is frequently decreased in critically ill patients. Mortality data indicate the importance of intact hepatic function in the outcome of critically ill patients. Mortality rate from septic shock approaches 100% in patients with severe hepatic damage. Also, when hepatic failure occurs in the setting of acute respiratory failure, the prognosis for recovery from the acute lung injury (ALI) is poor (55). Thus, evidence is accumulating to suggest that the various systemic organs are not merely targets of damage during critical illnesses. Rather, once these organs are damaged, their dysfunction has a substantial impact on host defense and on the propagation of the underlying injury.

Central Nervous System Failure

Abnormalities of central nervous system (CNS) function have been frequently described in critically ill patients (46,49,56,57). For example, CNS dysfunction, including disorientation, confusion, agitation, obtundation, and seizures, occurs commonly in septic patients. One study reported a 9% incidence of CNS dysfunction, defined as an inability to follow simple commands, in 106 patients with intra-abdominal sepsis. By contrast, another study, using an altered sensorium as the criteria for CNS dysfunction, reported a 33% incidence of CNS abnormalities in sepsis (42). Delirium in mechanically ventilated patients can lead to increased length of stay and other morbidities (58).

Use of the Glasgow Coma Scale helps to provide a more uniform, standard approach to defining CNS function (56). The Glasgow Coma Scale provides a measurement of visual, motor, and verbal (e.g., orientation) responsiveness (see Table 25-3). The Glasgow Coma Scale can be used in intubated patients, and a score of less than 6 to 8 in critically ill patients is considered abnormal (maximal score = 15). Using these criteria, abnormalities of CNS function have been found to occur in 7% to 30% of critically ill patients. The factors that underlie CNS dysfunction in this patient population are unclear but may include the production of false neurotransmitters, direct microvascular injury, and brain ischemia from global or regional reductions in cerebral blood flow (56,57).

Hematologic Failure

Hematologic abnormalities occur among critically ill patients with a frequency that ranges from 0% to 26% (42,49). There is

TABLE 25-3.   Glasgow Coma Scale

Parameter	Score
EYE OPENING	
Spontaneous	4
To speech	3
To pain	2
None	1
MOTOR RESPONSE	
Obeys verbal commands	6
Responds appropriately to painful stimuli (localizes pain)	5
Withdraws to pain	4
Decorticate posturing	3
Decerebrate posturing	2
No response	1
VERBAL RESPONSES	
Oriented and conversant	5
Disoriented but conversant	4
Inappropriate response	3
Incomprehensible sounds	2
No response	1

little clinical consensus about the definition of hematologic failure in this patient group. Several parameters, including the platelet count, the white blood cell count, fibrinogen levels, and coagulation parameters, have been used to assess the adequacy of the hematologic system in these patients. Despite some differences, most clinical studies employ criteria that include a platelet count ≤50,000 cells per μL, a white blood cell count ≤1,000 cells per μL, and a fibrinogen level <100 mg per dL to define hematologic failure. Obviously, the presence of severe neutropenia decreases host resistance to infection, and thrombocytopenia increases the risk of bleeding and the need for transfusion of blood products. Disseminated intravascular coagulation is sometimes associated with ALI (59).

Acute Respiratory Failure

The incidence of acute respiratory failure in critically ill patients varies considerably depending on the criteria used to define failure of the respiratory system. Although the term ARDS has been very useful for designating the clinical syndrome, a more quantitative definition is needed. A recent American–European Consensus Conference proposed a simplified, uniform definition of ALI and ARDS (60). ALI is defined as a patient with a $PaO_2:FIO_2$ ratio <300, with chest radiographic evidence of bilateral pulmonary infiltrates. Exclusion criteria include the presence of interstitial lung disease or left ventricular failure assessed by history, physical examination, or laboratory criteria. As previously noted, the role of right-heart catheterization in the management of patients with ARDS is controversial and will be the subject of an upcoming National Institutes of Health–sponsored clinical trial.

ARDS is defined with the same criteria as ALI except that the $PaO_2:FIO_2$ ratio is <200. As such, the distinction between ALI and ARDS is based entirely on the severity of the gas exchange alterations. The clinical relevance of this distinction remains to be proven. Nonetheless, the notion that the distinction between ALI and ARDS may not be relevant was underscored by a recent study in which the overall mortality rate in medical patients with ALI was 58% and was identical to the mortality rate in the subset of these patients who had ARDS.

A quantitative scoring system for assessing ALI has also been used to evaluate the severity of lung injury (see Table 25-4) (61). This system is based on the severity of hypoxemia and on the extent of infiltrates on the chest radiograph. If the patient is mechanically ventilated, abnormalities in the compliance of the lungs and the level of PEEP are also scored. Using these criteria, patients can be classified as having mild, moderate, or severe lung injury (61). The pathophysiology and treatment of ALI/ARDS are discussed extensively in Chapter 23, Acute Hypoxemic Respiratory Failure: Pulmonary Edema and Acute Lung Injury.

Special Considerations

Although not unique to any particular organ system, a number of serious problems exist with respect to the MOF syndrome. Because there is a general lack of consensus about the criteria for individual organ system failure, the incidence of organ failure is variable among different study centers and contributes to the confusion in this area. Until uniform criteria

TABLE 25-4. Components of the Acute Lung Injury Score

	Value
CHEST RADIOGRAPH SCORE	
No alveolar consolidation	0
Alveolar consolidation in 1 quadrant	1
Alveolar consolidation in 2 quadrants	2
Alveolar consolidation in 3 quadrants	3
Alveolar consolidation in all 4 quadrants	4
HYPOXEMIA SCORE	
$PaO_2:FIO_2 \geq 300$	0
$PaO_2:FIO_2$ 225–299	1
$PaO_2:FIO_2$ 175–224	2
$PaO_2:FIO_2$ 100–174	3
$PaO_2:FIO_2 < 100$	4
RESPIRATORY SYSTEM COMPLIANCE SCORE (WHEN VENTILATED)	
Compliance ≥ 80 mL/cm H_2O	0
Compliance 60–79 mL/cm H_2O	1
Compliance 40–59 mL/cm H_2O	2
Compliance 20–39 mL/cm H_2O	3
Compliance ≤ 19 mL/cm H_2O	4
POSITIVE END-EXPIRATORY PRESSURE SCORE (WHEN VENTILATED)	
PEEP ≤ 5 cm H_2O	0
PEEP 6–8 cm H_2O	1
PEEP 9–11 cm H_2O	2
PEEP 12–14 cm H_2O	3
PEEP ≥ 15 cm H_2O	4

The final value is obtained by dividing the aggregate sum by the number of components that were used.

SCORE	
No lung injury	0
Mild-to-moderate lung injury	0.1–2.5
Severe lung injury (ARDS)	>2.5

$PaO_2:FIO_2$, ratio of partial pressure of oxygen to fractional inspired oxygen concentration; PEEP, positive end-expiratory pressure; ARDS, acute respiratory distress syndrome.

From Murray JF, Matthay MA, Luce J, et al. An expanded definition of the adult respiratory distress syndrome. *Am Rev Respir Dis* 1988; l38:720, with permission.

are established, the true incidence and natural history of MOF will remain unclear. These problems are further compounded by the lack of uniform diagnostic criteria for the definition of septic shock and ALI. The net effect of this diagnostic imprecision is that patients with dissimilar critical illnesses are often inappropriately grouped together. However, a number of cooperative efforts have been undertaken to reach consensus on this issue and to more precisely define the criteria for organ system failure in this patient group (62).

Despite the current uncertainties, several important issues about MOF among critically ill patients have been resolved. First, the number of involved organ systems impacts significantly on patient mortality (46). Mortality rate ranges from 15% to 30% for a single organ failure and from 45% to 55% for failure of two organ systems. By contrast, mortality rate exceeds 80% when three or more organ systems have failed and reaches 100% if the MOF persists beyond 4 hospital days (46). Second, certain organ systems (e.g., heart, kidney, lung, and liver) are involved more frequently than other organ systems. Third, although individual organs may be preferentially injured in specific situations (e.g., renal failure and respiratory failure in septic shock), MOF may occur after acute cardiorespiratory failure of any etiology. Finally, early detection and treatment of the underlying cause of the MOF may offer the best hope for treatment of this potentially fatal disorder (52,63–65).

PATHOGENESIS

The MOF syndrome occurs in a variety of clinical settings, including infection, severe hypotension, and multiple trauma. Prototypic among the risk factors for MOF is septic shock. Although a scientific consensus has yet to be established, there is evidence to suggest that MOF during sepsis, and perhaps other critical illnesses, is due to widespread organ injury that is caused by activated inflammatory cells and a variety of humoral mediators (49,52,66,67). However, any theory about the pathogenesis of MOF during sepsis or other acute catastrophic illnesses must also take into account the abnormalities in systemic gas exchange that occur in these disorders and those that manifest as an abnormal relationship between oxygen uptake (VO_2) and oxygen delivery (QO_2).

As illustrated in Figure 25-5, whole-body oxygen uptake is normally maintained at a constant level over wide ranges of oxygen delivery (68). This is accomplished by means of local compensatory mechanisms, which include increases in oxygen extraction and increases in recruitable capillary reserves (e.g., the cross-sectional area of perfused capillaries within an individual organ). Once these mechanisms for the preservation of a constant oxygen uptake are exhausted, volume of oxygen uptake, VO_2, falls in a manner that is directly related to the reductions in oxygen delivery. The level of oxygen delivery below which oxygen uptake begins to fall is termed QO_{2c} (i.e., critical threshold for oxygen delivery), and it signifies the level of QO_2 below which oxygen supply–demand imbalances exist (68,69).

In contrast to the situation described above for the normal VO_2–QO_2 relationship, the relationship between VO_2 and QO_2 in critically ill patients is often markedly altered (70,71). For example, in many critically ill patients, VO_2 depends on QO_2 at nearly all levels of oxygen delivery, including levels that would normally be more than adequate to meet tissue metabolic demands. These abnormalities indicate that oxygen supply–demand imbalances exist at all levels of QO_2 in these patients.

In recent years, the concept that the VO_2–DO_2 relationship is altered in the critically ill patient has been challenged. In particular, the fact whether VO_2 is calculated using the Fick equation [VO_2 = cardiac output $\times$ (a–vO_2 content difference)] or measured using a metabolic cart may affect whether an abnormal VO_2–DO_2 relationship is observed in these patients. The explanation for differences in measured versus calculated VO_2–DO_2 is not intuitively obvious. When both VO_2 and DO_2 are calculated, however, it is believed an artifactual mathematical coupling occurs because both VO_2 and DO_2 share the variables of cardiac output and arterial oxygen content. This problem may be avoided by measuring VO_2 directly, using a metabolic cart. However, an abnormal relationship between VO_2 and DO_2 can be observed whether VO_2 is measured using

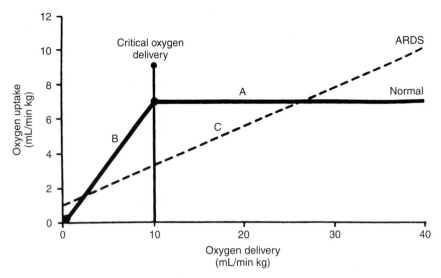

FIGURE 25-5.   Oxygen uptake–oxygen delivery (V_{O_2}–Q_{O_2}) relationships in normal subjects and in patients with acute respiratory distress syndrome (ARDS). V_{O_2} is regulated by whole body metabolic demand and is normally constant over a wide range of Q_{O_2}. This is accomplished by local compensatory mechanisms, including increases in oxygen extraction and increases in the cross-sectional density of perfused capillaries. Once these compensatory mechanisms are exhausted, further reductions in Q_{O_2} are accompanied by reductions in V_{O_2} (line B). The Q_{O_2} below which V_{O_2} begins to decrease is termed the critical threshold for Q_{O_2} ($Q_{O_{2c}}$). In contrast to the normal situation, V_{O_2} is dependent at nearly all levels of Q_{O_2} in ARDS. This finding indicates that an oxygen supply–demand imbalance exists at all levels of Q_{O_2} in ARDS patients. (From Dorinsky PM, Gadek JE. Mechanisms of multiple nonpulmonary organ failure in ARDS. *Chest* 1989;96:885, with permission.)

a metabolic cart or calculated using the Fick equation. As such, criticisms of the method by which V_{O_2} is determined do not negate the concept that V_{O_2}–D_{O_2} relationships can be altered in the setting of sepsis or ALI—a fact that has been well established experimentally. Rather, these observations underscore the notion that whole-body V_{O_2}–D_{O_2} relations in humans may be unreliable and that a better method for assessing oxygenation in individual tissues needs to be established.

There are several mechanisms that may explain both the nonpulmonary organ failure and the V_{O_2}–Q_{O_2} abnormalities that occur in this patient population. These may be divided into two broad categories: (a) altered blood flow distribution and (b) endothelial or parenchymal injury (38).

Altered Blood Flow Distribution

Oxygenated blood that bypasses nutrient capillary beds could alter V_{O_2}–D_{O_2} relationships and cause organ damage. This sequence of events may result from (a) a redistribution of cardiac output to organs with inherently low oxygen extraction fractions (e.g., skeletal muscle), (b) an increase in the fraction of cardiac output that bypasses nutrient capillaries through anatomic, precapillary arteriovenous channels (e.g., shunt flow), (c) local blood flow heterogeneities such that tissue oxygen supply and demand are imbalanced, or (d) a reduction in recruitable capillary reserves that would prevent effective compensation for reductions in oxygen supply (71).

Endothelial or Parenchymal Injury

Endothelial injury may be accompanied by local edema formation, with subsequent increases in diffusion distances for oxygen or reductions in capillary surface area (e.g., reduced

recruitable capillary reserves) or both. Alternatively, direct parenchymal cell injury may impair oxygen use at any level of oxygen delivery by impairing cellular oxidative metabolism.

Possible Mechanisms of Injury

Little direct experimental evidence exists to support the idea that either MOF or the systemic V_{O_2}–Q_{O_2} alterations associated with ARDS, septic shock, and other critical illnesses are caused by primary alterations in the distribution of cardiac output (e.g., increased anatomic shunt flow or increased blood flow to organs with low oxygen extraction). However, there is evidence to indicate that nonpulmonary organs are damaged both structurally and functionally during critical illness, and this damage often includes alterations in individual organ V_{O_2}–Q_{O_2} matching (68–71).

The best studied experimental model for MOF has been septic shock that is produced either by live bacterial organisms or by endotoxin. In this context, structural studies of endothelial monolayers exposed to endotoxin show that these cells undergo contraction, become pyknotic, and finally die. Likewise, it is known that endotoxin or live bacteria can induce the release of various mediators, each of which can cause cell injury (67,72). Considerable experimental evidence indicates that both cyclooxygenase and lipoxygenase products of arachidonic acid metabolism participate in the hemodynamic, pathologic, and metabolic derangements that occur during sepsis. Also, complement is activated in sepsis, and there is some evidence to indicate that the elevated levels of a C5a derivative correlate with the severity of hypotension and metabolic acidosis during sepsis. There has also been considerable interest in the possible role of cytokines (e.g., TNF) in mediating systemic organ injury during sepsis (67,73). In this regard, antibodies to TNF are capable of preventing the development of endotoxin-mediated hypotension, fibrin deposition, and death in animals. Likewise, anti-TNF antibody prevented shock and death in baboons given live *Escherichia coli* organisms but only if the antibody was given 2 hours before the bacteremia (74). However, clinical studies using strategies to neutralize TNF-α in sepsis patients have not been effective (67).

Many studies (but not all) suggest a central role for neutrophils in mediating both the systemic and pulmonary injury from bacteria or endotoxin (52,75). Along this line, monoclonal antibodies to the adherence-promoting leukocyte glycoprotein complex (i.e., CD18) reduce systemic organ injury and improve survival from hemorrhagic shock in many species of animals. Although many schemes have been proposed to explain the mechanism by which neutrophils cause tissue injury, some works suggest that there may be important interactions between elastases and toxic oxygen radicals elaborated by neutrophils (67). Thus, in septic shock, endotoxin and bacteria may directly damage endothelial cells and promote the activation of polymorphonuclear leukocytes and mononuclear cells, as well as mediate the release of numerous proinflammatory agents (e.g., kinins, prostaglandins, complement, and monokines). Acting in concert, these events culminate in widespread organ injury.

Finally, evidence from several sources suggest that there may also be a link between the organ injury that occurs during sepsis and other critical illnesses and the Vo_2–Do_2 alterations that occur in these settings. It has generally been presumed that the mechanism for the altered Vo_2–Do_2 relationships in these disorders involves insufficient delivery of oxygen to metabolically active tissues. However, altered oxygen metabolism, especially during sepsis, cannot be totally accounted for by this proposed mechanism. This may explain the fact that several clinical trials have shown that augmentation of oxygen delivery in the setting of established sepsis or ALI fails to reduce mortality, and in some studies, the mortality actually increased. This apparent clinical paradox may be reconciled by a hypothesis that proposes that both organ injury and Vo_2–Do_2 alterations during sepsis and other critical illnesses are the result of mitochondrial injury. Experimental data in support of this notion is increasing. However, future studies are needed to address more definitively the validity of this compelling hypothesis.

EARLY RECOGNITION AND PREVENTION OF MULTIPLE ORGAN FAILURE

Early Recognition

Several studies have been published that identify patients who are at the highest risk for developing MOF. Patients with multiple trauma and hypotension who require emergency surgery and multiple transfusions are one common group of patients at high risk. Other patients considered to be at high risk for the development of MOF include patients with septic shock, patients with advanced chronic diseases (e.g., chronic liver disease or chronic renal failure) who are hospitalized for cardiac failure or a primary infection, and patients with the acquired immunodeficiency syndrome (AIDS). Finally, patients who are immunosuppressed because of an underlying malignancy or its treatment may be at particularly high risk for MOF, both from the toxic effects of the chemotherapy as well as from the increased susceptibility to septicemia.

Some investigators have evaluated clinical factors as well as easily measurable plasma factors that might predict which patients with nonpulmonary sepsis syndrome would progress to develop ALI. In one study, the possible value of a product of endothelial cells for predicting ALI was studied (45). This study was based on the premise that endothelial cell injury is a ubiquitous early event in the pathogenesis of sepsis. In this regard, several *in vitro* and *in vivo* studies have shown that both pulmonary and systemic endothelial cell injury occur during endotoxemia and septicemia. The investigators measured plasma levels of von Willebrand factor–antigen (VWF–Ag) because VWF–Ag has been shown to be released from endothelial cells *in vitro* when they are injured, and two prior clinical studies demonstrated that plasma VWF–Ag levels are markedly elevated in patients with established acute respiratory failure. In this study, plasma VWF–Ag levels were increased twofold in patients with nonpulmonary sepsis who subsequently developed ALI compared with patients with nonpulmonary sepsis who did not progress to develop ALI. Moreover, of the 15 patients who developed ALI from sepsis, 14 patients died (93% mortality rate). An elevated VWF–Ag level above 450 (percentage of control) was predictive of the development of ALI (87% sensitivity and 77% specificity) and had a positive predictive value of 80% for identifying septic patients who were not likely to survive. Subsequent studies have explored the predictive value of several biologic markers, many of which have some pathogenetic and prognostic value (76,77).

More studies are needed to combine clinical factors and readily measurable plasma factors to identify those patients with sepsis syndrome who have the greatest risk of developing ALI and not surviving. These patients might be reasonable candidates for early treatment with immunotherapy, antiinflammatory agents, and other new treatments that may become available in the future. Unfortunately, a recent study testing administration of human growth hormone to critically ill patients had a deleterious effect on outcome, perhaps because of an adverse effect on host defense against infection (78).

Prevention

There has been a growing interest in various approaches to reduce the risk of MOF, particularly because the outcome is so poor once a patient develops MOF. Although specific treatment approaches have yet to be established, a number of general supportive measures are available. Perhaps the most important supportive measure is prevention of infection. Nosocomial infection can be reduced by good hand washing, removal of unnecessary intravascular and urinary catheters, keeping the head of the bed elevated, and the prevention of skin ulcers. See Chapter 26, Prevention of Nonpulmonary Complications of Intensive Care, for a more complete discussion of these issues.

MANAGEMENT OF THE PATIENT WITH MULTIPLE ORGAN FAILURE

Critically ill patients at risk for developing MOF generally present with one or more of the following clinical problems: shock (i.e., hypovolemic, cardiac, or septic), acute respiratory failure, or major alterations in mental status. These clinical problems initially require a prompt therapeutic response to stabilize the patient. In general, initial management is directed toward maintaining an adequate blood pressure and supporting gas exchange (35). For example, patients who present with hypovolemic shock, either from trauma or from gastrointestinal bleeding, require rapid intravascular volume expansion with blood. Likewise, patients who have severe alterations in mental status with failure to protect the airway and/or progressive respiratory failure require prompt endotracheal intubation and mechanical ventilation. It is important that the physician caring for critically ill patients recognize that the initial priority must be to stabilize the patient's circulatory and respiratory status. The decision, for example, to insert a pulmonary arterial catheter should not take precedence over initial management of the hypotension and respiratory failure (9,35). Once the patient is stabilized and appropriate support has been given to the circulatory and respiratory systems, a careful assessment of the likely cause of the patient's condition should be undertaken.

A logical starting point in the evaluation of critically ill patients is to search for the usual causes of shock, which include sepsis, cardiac failure (especially acute myocardial infarction), gastrointestinal bleeding, acute pancreatitis, drug overdose, and occult bleeding from recent trauma. However, one must always maintain a high index of suspicion for the presence of septicemia. There should be a low threshold for obtaining blood cultures and appropriate cultures of other possible sources of infection. In addition, patients with even presumptive evidence for infection should be promptly placed on broad-spectrum antibiotics. Given these general supportive measures, the remainder of this section is devoted to a discussion of specific issues related to support of the circulatory system.

Guidelines for Fluid and Blood Replacement

With the exception of patients with acute blood loss, for whom there is a need to transfuse blood to maintain the hematocrit between 25% and 30%, most patients also need crystalloid or colloid therapy (35). Most medical and surgical centers favor the use of crystalloid in preference to colloid for volume expansion. This preference is based, in part, on the fact that crystalloid, unlike colloid, can restore both the intravascular and the interstitial component of the extracellular fluid space. Some physicians do administer colloid in an attempt to maintain circulating plasma protein osmotic pressure, but large volumes of colloid are often needed to achieve this objective, and the clearance of infused protein from the intravascular space is usually quite rapid (35). Despite the apparent advantages of crystalloid versus colloid, red blood cells remain the ideal volume expander because they have the advantage of both increasing oxygen transport to the tissues as well as maintaining intravascular volume. However, new evidence suggests that clinical criteria for transfusions in many critically ill patients have been higher than necessary. In one recent study, restrictive red cell transfusion criteria resulted in a better survival (79).

The appropriate guidelines for fluid therapy depend on the cause of the patient's shock. For the patient with an acute myocardial infarction, fluid replacement should be titrated to maintain the PAWP between 15 and 20 mm Hg. By contrast, for patients with hypovolemic shock, traumatic shock, or septic shock, an increase in the CVP or PAWP to 15 to 20 mm Hg may not be optimal. For example, in one study that examined

volume resuscitation in patients with septic shock, the investigators found that increases in PAWP beyond 11 to 12 mm Hg did not result in a higher cardiac output (35).

Ideally, optimal fluid resuscitation in any form of shock should include the restoration of euvolemia. Euvolemia is often difficult to define in critically ill patients. In addition, the adjustment of fluid therapy will depend on the use of vasoactive agents (35). Finally, although invasive hemodynamic monitoring with a pulmonary arterial catheter is frequently used to assist in the management of patients with septic shock, no evidence suggests that this kind of monitoring changes outcome (9,11). Given these uncertainties, the best indices for evaluating fluid replacement therapy are the patient's acid–base status, mental status, skin perfusion, and, perhaps most importantly, urine flow and renal function.

Vasoactive Agents

The most useful vasopressor for treating patients with septic shock may be norepinephrine (80). It is a powerful vasoconstrictor, but it does not appear to have the clinical splanchnic vasoconstriction that is a theoretic concern for this agent. Dopamine can also be used as a vasoconstrictor but tends to cause more tachycardia than norepinephrine. Phenylephrine, a synthetic pure α-agonist, is also commonly used in this setting.

In some patients, septic shock will be unresponsive even to high doses of norepinephrine. In these patients, vasopressin can be added to provide an increase in systemic arterial pressure. Epinephrine is another catecholamine that can be used for blood pressure support in severe septic shock. In doses of >10 μg per minute, epinephrine causes primarily α-stimulation. High doses of any of these potent vasopressors will cause vasoconstriction that may maintain systemic blood pressure, but blood flow to the kidneys, splanchnic bed, muscles, and skin may be markedly reduced.

It is often difficult to determine the level of mean arterial pressure or cardiac output that is optimal in septic shock. In general, it is best to try to adjust the mean arterial pressure and cardiac output to a level that stabilizes the metabolic acidosis associated with sepsis and improves tissue perfusion, particularly as indicated by urine flow. Some patients with severe septic shock will require high doses of dopamine, norepinephrine, and epinephrine to maintain even a barely adequate blood pressure.

Antibiotics

Selection of appropriate antibiotics for patients with septic shock and MOF is important. In general, a careful search for the likely source of sepsis should be undertaken and appropriate broad-spectrum antibiotics should then be administered. The antibiotic spectrum should include gram-negative enteric bacteria as well as β-lactamase producers. Effects of the agents on renal function should be considered and monitored.

Nutritional Support

Nutritional and metabolic support is an essential part of the management of patients with MOF. Hypermetabolism develops early in the syndrome, and severe malnutrition can become a prominent feature within days after the onset of illness.

The characteristics of the hypermetabolic state include (a) increases in resting energy expenditure and oxygen consumption, (b) increased use of carbohydrate, fat, and amino acids as energy substrates, and (c) increased loss of nitrogen in the urine. The hypermetabolic state results in profound protein catabolism, which is associated with a decrease in total-body protein synthesis. The mechanism for the alteration of metabolism observed in patients with MOF appears to be related to the inflammatory mediators and to the hormonal response to injury. Unfortunately, these fundamental alterations in metabolism do not appear to be readily altered by therapy. However, if adequate nutritional support is not provided, then it is likely that organ dysfunction will be accelerated.

The goal of nutritional support in patients with or at risk for MOF is to prevent substrate-limited metabolism and to support, rather than attempt to alter, the hypermetabolism (see Chapter 20, Nutrition and Ethical Principles in Critical Illness and Injury, for a detailed discussion of nutritional support). In general, nutrition should be provided by the enteral route whenever possible. Enteral feedings eliminate cholestasis and reduce the risk of acalculous cholecystitis. Enteral alimentation may also offer some protection against gastrointestinal hemorrhage in mechanically ventilated patients.

Ethical Support

It is important for physicians to assess carefully the likelihood of meaningful recovery in each critically ill patient with MOF. This assessment will depend on the natural history of the patient's underlying disease, as well as on the extent and severity of his or her organ failure. There is a growing awareness among the medical community that reasonable limits should be exercised by physicians and by patients' families in supporting patients with critical illnesses and MOF. Studies have demonstrated that some patient groups have a particularly poor prognosis for recovery. For example, patients with ARDS following bone marrow transplantation have a less than 10% chance for recovery, and patients with a combination of hepatic failure and ALI have a nearly 100% mortality rate. In addition, one study in two ICUs at the University of California Medical Center has shown that withdrawal of life support was the mechanism for death in about 50% of patients in the ICU setting (81). As more information about prognostic indices for specific disease processes become available, it may help guide decisions to discontinue life support in patients who do not have a reasonable chance for meaningful recovery. See Chapter 20, Nutrition and Ethical Principles in Critical Illness and Injury, for more discussion of ethical issues.

EVIDENCE-BASED APPROACH TO SEVERE SEPSIS SYNDROME

PATHOPHYSIOLOGY

The past decade has seen an explosion in the molecular understanding of severe sepsis syndrome (SSS). It has been fairly clear for some time that the primary response in sepsis is an overwhelming inflammatory response to a nidus of infection. In response to endotoxin or exotoxin, tissue macrophages release proinflammatory mediators such as TNF-α or IL-1β. Recent data has revealed, however, that the inflammatory and

coagulation cascades are much more intimately linked than was once thought (82). Endothelial injury appears to be a key step in the pathogenesis of a lack of hemostasis in the coagulation and fibrinolytic cascades. In an intact endothelium, thrombomodulin binds to thrombin, the combination of which then activates protein C. Activated protein C (APC) has anticoagulant properties through its ability to inactivate factors V and VIII. It also has profibrinolytic properties via the inhibition of thrombin-activatable fibrinolysis inhibitor (TAFI) and plasminogen activator inhibitor-1 (PAI-1). Finally, APC is felt to have direct antiinflammatory properties primarily through NF-κB (83).

ACTIVATED PROTEIN C

As a consequence of the great molecular understanding of the sepsis pathway, multiple putative agents were developed to block key steps in the cascade with the hope that these agents would lead to improved outcomes. Some of these agents include recombinant human tissue factor pathway inhibitor, antithrombin III, as well as antibody against TNF-α (84). To date, the only agent that has been proven effective in reducing 28-day mortality in patients with SSS is APC (83). In the trial of 1,690 patients with SSS, mortality rate was reduced from 30.8% to 24.7%, a nearly 20% relative risk reduction. Afterwards, the Food and Drug Administration (FDA) approved the drug for use in patients with SSS and high risk of death, as documented by either an Acute Physiology and Chronic Health Evaluation (APACHE) II score greater than or equal to 25 or two or more organ system dysfunctions (80). Though the drug is somewhat costly compared to other agents used in the critical care setting, analyses reveal that if the drug is used according to the FDA guidelines, it appears to be cost effective (85).

EARLY GOAL-DIRECTED THERAPY

Given the cytopathic hypoxia and abnormal relationship between oxygen delivery and consumption seen in SSS, it was hypothesized that providing supraphysiologic delivery of oxygen to the tissues might lead to improved clinical outcomes. Two well-designed studies were performed in the 1990s, which not only did not show a benefit to this approach but were also actually suggestive of a worse outcome (14,15). This topic was revisited, however, in a recent landmark study by Rivers et al. (86). All the patients with SSS who were entered into the study had the same resuscitative endpoints [CVP between 8 and 12 mm Hg, mean arterial pressure (MAP) $\geq$65 mm Hg, and urine output $\geq$0.5 mL/kg/hour]. How the clinicians reached those endpoints differed depending on the arm of the study. In the control group, it was at the discretion of the clinician as to how to reach the aforementioned goals. In the intervention group, a specific algorithm was used. The first step in the protocol was to measure CVP through a central line and to give fluids (either colloids or crystalloids) until the CVP measured between 8 and 12 mm Hg. Next, vasoactive agents were used if the MAP was outside the target range of between 65 and 90 mm Hg. In this study, a special central line was used that could give a continuous saturation of the central venous blood ($ScvO_2$). Though not fully substantiated by the literature, it was used in this study as a surrogate marker for mixed venous oxygen saturation. If the $ScvO_2$ was less than 70%, the patient was transfused until the hematocrit was greater than or equal to 70%. At this point, if the patient still had an $ScvO_2$ less than 70%, inotropes were started with a goal to increase the $ScvO_2$ greater than 70%. This cycle of fluids, vasoactive agents, blood transfusions, and inotropes was repeated until the goals were met. The patients in the early goal-directed therapy (EGDT) arm had their 28-day mortality rate significantly reduced from 49.2% to 33.3%, and this difference remained significant up to 60 days in the study.

There were concerns that the EGDT group might receive more fluids than the control group. Though the EGDT group received approximately 1.5 L more than the control group during the first 6 hours of the study ($P <0.001$), by 72 hours both groups had received approximately the same volume of fluids. Significantly, more patients in the EGDT group received blood transfusions. The clinical implications of this part of the EGDT trial are somewhat unclear given the results of the Hébert study (79). In the first 6 hours, the intervention arm also had a significantly greater use of inotropes. This data is certainly in concordance with recent evidence of significant cardiogenic dysfunction in early SSS (80). Though the precise role of $ScvO_2$ remains to be proven, this study reinforces the concept that early recognition and aggressive resuscitory efforts in SSS are associated with improved outcomes.

LOW-DOSE STEROIDS IN REFRACTORY SHOCK

As we have described above, SSS is felt to be, at least in part, an overwhelming inflammatory response to an infectious agent. As such, it was felt that the antiinflammatory properties of corticosteroids might have a beneficial effect. Large doses were tried in the past with no evidence of benefit, and it was felt that the concept had been laid to rest. In the mid-1990s, however, the idea was looked at in a slightly different way. The concern was that if too high a dose of steroids is given, the patient may go from being immunomodulated to being immunosuppressed (87,88). This hypothesis led to the study performed by Annane et al. in 2002 (89). They analyzed 300 patients with SSS and randomized them to receive steroids [hydrocortisone 50 mg intravenously every 6 hours and a mineralocorticoid (fludrocortisone) 50 μg orally every day] or placebo for 7 days. They performed an adrenocorticotropic hormone (ACTH)-stimulation test on all patients (measuring baseline serum cortisol, followed by injecting patients with cosyntropin 250 μg, and measuring serum cortisol 30 and 60 minutes later). They defined partial adrenal insufficiency ("nonresponders") as a difference of 9 μg per dL or less between the baseline serum cortisol level and the highest postcosyntropin level. Though the 28-day mortality for all patients was not improved by giving steroids, in the nonresponders, their 28-day mortality rate was reduced from 63% to 53% ($P = 0.04$). Approximately 75% of the patients in this study were nonresponders. In the responder group (without evidence of adrenal insufficiency), the mortality rate increased from 53% to 61% if steroids were given ($P = 0.96$). A current reasonable recommendation is to have a low threshold test for adrenal insufficiency in patients with SSS and to treat with steroids those patients with insufficiency. An alternative recommendation is to start steroids early in patients with SSS and stop them when the patient is found to be free from adrenally insufficient. This requires the

ability to obtain the results of a cosyntropin stimulation test in a timely manner.

GLUCOSE CONTROL IN THE CRITICALLY ILL

Though there has been ample data in the diabetic outpatient that long-term tight glucose control is associated with improved outcomes (90), this issue had not been fully addressed in the critically ill patient. Van den Berghe et al. recently randomized 1,548 patients (primarily patients after heart surgery) to receive either "intensive insulin therapy" with an insulin infusion started if the serum glucose was >110 mg per dL with a serum glucose goal of between 80 and 110 mg per dL, or "conventional therapy" with an insulin infusion being started for blood glucose >215 mg per dL with the goal in this group being between 180 to 200 mg per dL (91). The ICU mortality rate of the patients in the intensive therapy group decreased from 8% to 4.6% ($P <0.04$). For those patients who were in the ICU for more than 5 days, the mortality rate decreased from 20% to 10% ($P = 0.005$). In addition, the patients who received intensive insulin therapy had a statistically decreased rate of septicemia, need for renal replacement therapy, as well as red blood cell transfusions. Interestingly, they also had a lower incidence of critical illness polyneuropathy and were also less likely to require prolonged mechanical ventilation. This dramatic improvement in mortality was seen with tight glucose control in spite of the fact that only 13% of the patients in this study were diabetics. Follow-up data appears to show that it is the tight glucose control *per se* rather than the amount of insulin given that appears to be more important (92). Future studies will need to be performed in specific subgroups (e.g., septic, surgically critically ill, etc.) to enhance the generalizability of this important study.

QUESTIONABLE EFFICACY OF THE PULMONARY ARTERY CATHETER

One of the great controversies that exist in managing patients with hemodynamic insufficiency is the role of the PA catheter. Since its initial publication in 1970, it has been widely used in ICUs without any large randomized controlled trials (RCT) documenting any benefit. Given the fact that two studies, one from 1987 and one from 1990, were unable to document a benefit in patients with acute coronary syndromes, national societies called for either a moratorium on the PA catheter or a large RCT (93–95). The future appeared bleak when, in 1991, the first attempt at a large RCT had to be stopped because of the inability to recruit patients (96).

The next landmark study was by Connors et al. in 1996, which has been discussed previously in this chapter (11). Though it did not meet the criteria of an RCT, it was again unable to document any obvious benefit on the use of the PA catheter, and there was a possibility of increased mortality. This was followed up by a similar study by Polanczyk et al. in 2001 (97). Here again, no obvious benefit could be found, though the use of the catheter was associated with an increased length of stay. As is well described in a recent editorial, there are three reasons why the benefit of using the PA catheter cannot be easily detected (95). Firstly, PA catheters are placed in many ICUs where properly trained intensivists are not present, leading to misinterpretation of the data. The second possibility is that the use of the PA catheter may be a marker of an aggressive style of care that itself may be associated with poor outcomes. Finally, the lack of benefit may be related to adverse outcomes secondary to the placement of the catheter itself (such as arrhythmia or infection).

In early 2003, the Canadian Critical Care Trials Group published the results of a 10-year RCT of 1,994 high-risk patients scheduled for surgery (16). Importantly, 54% of those eligible were randomized into the study. In the patients where a PA catheter was placed, a protocol was used with goals being to normalize oxygen delivery, cardiac index, MAP, heart rate, PCWP, and hematocrit. The primary endpoint, in-hospital mortality rate, was 7.7% in the group without the catheter and 7.8% in the group with PA catheter–guided therapy ($P = 0.93$). This is despite the fact that there was a greater use of inotropes, vasodilators, colloids, and red blood cell transfusions in the PA catheter group. The only significant difference between the two groups was the rate of pulmonary emboli (8 in the catheter group and 0 in the group without catheter, $P = 0.004$). The importance of this study cannot be overemphasized, yet again pointing out the concept of exposure to risk without proven benefit when using the PA catheter in the high-risk surgical patient.

Most recently, in December 2003, Richard et al. published their RCT of the use of the PA catheter in patients with shock, ARDS, or both (98). In this particular trial, the clinicians resuscitated their patients without any particular protocol, more closely mimicking the real-world situation. As in most critical care trials, their primary endpoint was 28-day mortality, of which they could find no difference between the two groups. Though many intensivists still feel that hemodynamic monitoring is important in their patients with hemodynamic instability and insufficiency, it has been extremely difficult for researchers to find a subgroup of patients in whom the placement of the PA catheter has been associated with a clear improvement in outcome.

REFERENCES

1. Band JD, Maki DG. Infections caused by arterial catheters used for hemodynamic monitoring. *Am J Med* 1979;67:735–741.
2. Shinozaki T, Deane RS, Mazuzan JE Jr, et al. Bacterial contamination of arterial lines. A prospective study. *JAMA* 1983;249:223–225.
3. Shapiro BA. Monitoring gas exchange in acute respiratory failure. *Respir Care* 1983;28:605–607.
4. Gardner RM, Schwartz R, Wong HC, et al. Percutaneous indwelling radial-artery catheters for monitoring cardiovascular function. Prospective study of the risk of thrombosis and infection. *N Engl J Med* 1974;290:1227–1231.
5. Bedford RF. Long-term radial artery cannulation: effects on subsequent vessel function. *Crit Care Med* 1978;6:64–67.
6. Davis FM, Stewart JM. Radial artery cannulation. A prospective study in patients undergoing cardiothoracic surgery. *Br J Anaesth* 1980;52:41–47.
7. Wiedemann HP, Matthay MA, Matthay RA. Cardiovascular-pulmonary monitoring in the intensive care unit (Part 2). *Chest* 1984; 85:656–668.
8. Wiedemann HP, Matthay MA, Matthay RA. Cardiovascular-pulmonary monitoring in the intensive care unit (Part 1). *Chest* 1984; 85:537–549.
9. Matthay MA, Chatterjee K. Bedside catheterization of the pulmonary artery: risks compared with benefits. *Ann Intern Med* 1988;109:826–834.
10. Robin ED. The cult of the Swan-Ganz catheter. Overuse and abuse of pulmonary flow catheters. *Ann Intern Med* 1985;103:445–449.
11. Connors AF Jr, Speroff T, Dawson NV et al., SUPPORT Investigators. The effectiveness of right heart catheterization in the initial care of critically ill patients. *JAMA* 1996;276:889–897.
12. Matthay MA. Invasive hemodynamic monitoring in critically ill patients. *Clin Chest Med* 1983;4:233–249.
13. Quinn K, Quebbeman EJ. Pulmonary artery pressure monitoring in the surgical intensive care unit. Benefits vs difficulties. *Arch Surg* 1981;116:872–876.
14. Hayes MA, Timmins AC, Yau EH, et al. Elevation of systemic oxygen delivery in the treatment of critically ill patients. *N Engl J Med* 1994;330:1717–1722.
15. Gattinoni L, Brazzi L, Pelosi P et al. SvO2 Collaborative Group. A trial of goal-oriented hemodynamic therapy in critically ill patients. *N Engl J Med* 1995;333:1025–1032.
16. Sandham JD, Hull RD, Brant RF, et al. A randomized, controlled trial of the use of pulmonary-artery catheters in high-risk surgical patients. *N Engl J Med* 2003;348:5–14.
17. O'Quin R, Marini JJ. Pulmonary artery occlusion pressure: clinical physiology, measurement, and interpretation. *Am Rev Respir Dis* 1983;128:319–326.
18. Dhainaut JF, Devaux JY, Monsallier JF, et al. Mechanisms of decreased left ventricular preload during continuous positive pressure ventilation in ARDS. *Chest* 1986;90:74–80.
19. Jardin F, Farcot JC, Boisante L, et al. Influence of positive end-expiratory pressure on left ventricular performance. *N Engl J Med* 1981;304:387–392.
20. Tooker J, Huseby J, Butler J. The effect of Swan-Ganz catheter height on the wedge pressure-left atrial pressure relationships in edema during positive-pressure ventilation. *Am Rev Respir Dis* 1978;117:721–725.
21. Marini JJ. Obtaining meaningful data from the Swan-Ganz catheter. *Respir Care* 1985;30:572–578.
22. Al-Kharrat T, Zarich S, Amoateng-Adjepong Y, et al. Analysis of observer variability in measurement of pulmonary artery occlusion pressures. *Am J Respir Crit Care Med* 1999;160:415–420.
23. Chaney JC, Derdak S. Minimally invasive hemodynamic monitoring for the intensivist: current and emerging technology. *Crit Care Med* 2002;30:2338–2345.
24. Pinsky MR. Rationale for cardiovascular monitoring. *Curr Opin Crit Care* 2003;9:222–224.
25. Bellomo R, Uchino S. Cardiovascular monitoring tools: use and misuse. *Curr Opin Crit Care* 2003;9:225–229.
26. Boldt J. Clinical review: hemodynamic monitoring in the intensive care unit. *Crit Care* 2002;6:52–59.
27. Brown JM. Use of echocardiography for hemodynamic monitoring. *Crit Care Med* 2002;30:1361–1364.
28. Jonas MM, Tanser SJ. Lithium dilution measurement of cardiac output and arterial pulse waveform analysis: an indicator dilution calibrated beat-by-beat system for continuous estimation of cardiac output. *Curr Opin Crit Care* 2002;8:257–261.
29. Hameed SM, Cohn SM. Gastric tonometry: the role of mucosal pH measurement in the management of trauma. *Chest* 2003;123: 475S–481S.
30. Boswell SA, Scalea TM. Sublingual capnometry: an alternative to gastric tonometry for the management of shock resuscitation. *AACN Clin Issues* 2003;14:176–184.
31. Laupland KB, Bands CJ. Utility of esophageal Doppler as a minimally invasive hemodynamic monitor: a review. *Can J Anaesth* 2002;49:393–401.
32. Chatterjee K, Swan HJ, Kaushik VS, et al. Effects of vasodilator therapy for severe pump failure in acute myocardial infarction on short-term and late prognosis. *Circulation* 1976;53:797–802.
33. Aberle DR, Wiener-Kronish JP, Webb WR, et al. Hydrostatic versus increased permeability pulmonary edema: diagnosis based on radiographic criteria in critically ill patients. *Radiology* 1988; 168:73–79.
34. Connors AF Jr, McCaffree DR, Gray BA. Evaluation of right-heart catheterization in the critically ill patient without acute myocardial infarction. *N Engl J Med* 1983;308:263–267.
35. Matthay MA, Broaddus VC. Fluid and hemodynamic management in acute lung injury. *Semin Respir Med* 1994;15:271–288.
36. Matthay MA, Eschenbacher WL, Goetzl EJ. Elevated concentrations of leukotriene D4 in pulmonary edema fluid of patients with the adult respiratory distress syndrome. *J Clin Immunol* 1984;4:479–483.

37. Rinaldo JE. Indicators of risk, course, and prognosis in adult respiratory distress syndrome. *Am Rev Respir Dis* 1986;133:343–344.

38. Swan HJ, Ganz W, Forrester J, et al. Catheterization of the heart in man with use of a flow-directed balloon-tipped catheter. *N Engl J Med* 1970;283:447–451.

39. Hansen RM, Viquerat CE, Matthay MA, et al. Poor correlation between pulmonary arterial wedge pressure and left ventricular end-diastolic volume after coronary artery bypass graft surgery. *Anesthesiology* 1986;64:764–770.

40. Hall JB, Schmidt GA, Wood LDH, eds. *Principles of critical care.* New York: McGraw-Hill, 1992:1393–1395.

41. Tobin MJ. *Principles and practice of intensive care monitoring.* New York: McGraw-Hill, 1998.

42. Dorinsky PM, Matthay MA. Management of the critically ill patient with multiple organ failure. In: Kelley WN, ed. *Textbook of internal medicine.* Philadelphia: JR Lippincott Co, 1992:1850–1856.

43. Baue AE. Multiple, progressive, or sequential systems failure. A syndrome of the 1970s. *Arch Surg* 1975;110:779–781.

44. Bell RC, Coalson JJ, Smith JD, et al. Multiple organ system failure and infection in adult respiratory distress syndrome. *Ann Intern Med* 1983;99:293–298.

45. Rubin DB, Wiener-Kronish JP, Murray JF, et al. Elevated von Willebrand factor antigen is an early plasma predictor of acute lung injury in nonpulmonary sepsis syndrome. *J Clin Invest* 1990; 86:474–480.

46. Knaus WA, Wagner DP. Multiple systems organ failure: epidemiology and prognosis. *Crit Care Clin* 1989;5:221–232.

47. Montgomery AB, Stager MA, Carrico CJ, et al. Causes of mortality in patients with the adult respiratory distress syndrome. *Am Rev Respir Dis* 1985;132:485–489.

48. Parrillo JE, Parker MM, Natanson C, et al. Septic shock in humans. Advances in the understanding of pathogenesis, cardiovascular dysfunction, and therapy. *Ann Intern Med* 1990;113:227–242.

49. Dorinsky PM, Gadek JE. Mechanisms of multiple nonpulmonary organ failure in ARDS. *Chest* 1989;96:885–892.

50. Kraman S, Khan F, Patel S, et al. Renal failure in the respiratory intensive care unit. *Crit Care Med* 1979;7:263–266.

51. Graber M, Chestnutt M. Acute renal failure and electrolyte disturbances in the intensive care unit. In: Matthay MA, Schwartz DE, eds. *Complications in the intensive care unit.* New York: Chapman & Hall, 1997:228–265.

52. St John RC, Dorinsky PM. Immunologic therapy for ARDS, septic shock, and multiple-organ failure. *Chest* 1993;103:932–943.

53. Harris SK, Bone RC, Ruth WE. Gastrointestinal hemorrhage in patients in a respiratory intensive care unit. *Chest* 1977;72:301–304.

54. Doig CJ, Sutherland LR, Sandham JD, et al. Increased intestinal permeability is associated with the development of multiple organ dysfunction syndrome in critically ill ICU patients. *Am J Respir Crit Care Med* 1998;158:444–451.

55. Schwartz DB, Bone RC, Balk RA, et al. Hepatic dysfunction in the adult respiratory distress syndrome. *Chest* 1989;95:871–875.

56. Prough DS, ed. Neurologic critical care. *Critical care clinics.* Philadelphia: WB Saunders, 1989.

57. Kelly BJ, Nicholau DK. Neurologic complications of intensive care medicine. In: Matthay MA, Schwartz DE, eds. *Complications in the intensive care unit.* New York: Chapman & Hall, 1997:291–316.

58. Ely EW, Gautam S, Margolin R, et al. The impact of delirium in the intensive care unit on hospital length of stay. *Intensive Care Med* 2001;27:1892–1900.

59. Bone RC, Francis PB, Pierce AK. Intravascular coagulation associated with the adult respiratory distress syndrome. *Am J Med* 1976;61:585–589.

60. Artigas A, Bernard GR, Carlet J, et al. The American-European Consensus Conference on ARDS, part 2: ventilatory, pharmacologic, supportive therapy, study design strategies, and issues related to recovery and remodeling. Acute respiratory distress syndrome. *Am J Respir Crit Care Med* 1998;157:1332–1347.

61. Murray JF, Matthay MA, Luce JM, et al. An expanded definition of the adult respiratory distress syndrome. *Am Rev Respir Dis* 1988;138:720–723.

62. Bone RC, Balk RA, Cerra FB et al., the ACCP/SCCM Consensus Conference Committee, American College of Chest Physicians/ Society of Critical Care Medicine. Definitions for sepsis and organ failure and guidelines for the use of innovative therapies in sepsis. *Chest* 1992;101:1644–1655.

63. Macho JR, Luce JM. Rational approach to the management of multiple systems organ failure. *Crit Care Clin* 1989;5:379–392.

64. Pinsky MR, Matuschak GM. Multiple systems organ failure: failure of host defense homeostasis. *Crit Care Clin* 1989;5:199–220.

65. Pinsky MR. Multiple systems organ failure: malignant intravascular inflammation. *Crit Care Clin* 1989;5:195–198.

66. Goris RJ, te Boekhorst TP, Nuytinck JK, et al. Multiple-organ failure. Generalized autodestructive inflammation? *Arch Surg* 1985; 120:1109–1115.

67. Wheeler AP, Bernard GR. Treating patients with severe sepsis. *N Engl J Med* 1999;340:207–214.

68. Cain SM. Acute lung injury. Assessment of tissue oxygenation. *Crit Care Clin* 1986;2:537–550.

69. Cain SM. Oxygen delivery and uptake in dogs during anemic and hypoxic hypoxia. *J Appl Physiol* 1977;42:228–234.

70. Danek SJ, Lynch JP, Weg JG, et al. The dependence of oxygen uptake on oxygen delivery in the adult respiratory distress syndrome. *Am Rev Respir Dis* 1980;122:387–395.

71. Dorinsky PM, Costello JL, Gadek JE. Relationships of oxygen uptake and oxygen delivery in respiratory failure not due to the adult respiratory distress syndrome. *Chest* 1988;93:1013–1019.

72. Baumgartner JD, Glauser MP, McCutchan JA, et al. Prevention of gram-negative shock and death in surgical patients by antibody to endotoxin core glycolipid. *Lancet* 1985;2:59–63.

73. Tracey KJ, Beutler B, Lowry SF, et al. Shock and tissue injury induced by recombinant human cachectin. *Science* 1986;234:470–474.

74. Tracey KJ, Fong Y, Hesse DG, et al. Anti-cachectin/TNF monoclonal antibodies prevent septic shock during lethal bacteraemia. *Nature* 1987;330:662–664.

75. Ware LB, Matthay MA. The acute respiratory distress syndrome. *N Engl J Med* 2000;342:1334–1349.

76. Pittet JF, Mackersie RC, Martin TR, et al. Biological markers of acute lung injury: prognostic and pathogenetic significance. *Am J Respir Crit Care Med* 1997;155:1187–1205.

77. Parsons PE, Moss M. Early detection and markers of sepsis. *Clin Chest Med* 1996;17:199–212.

78. Takala J, Ruokonen E, Webster NR, et al. Increased mortality associated with growth hormone treatment in critically ill adults. *N Engl J Med* 1999;341:785–792.

79. Hébert PC, Wells G, Blajchman MA et al., Transfusion Requirements in Critical Care Investigators, Canadian Critical Care Trials Group. A multicenter, randomized, controlled clinical trial of transfusion requirements in critical care. *N Engl J Med* 1999;340: 409–417.

80. Dellinger RP. Cardiovascular management of septic shock. *Crit Care Med* 2003;31:946–955.

81. Smedira NG, Evans BH, Grais LS, et al. Withholding and withdrawal of life support from the critically ill. *N Engl J Med* 1990; 322:309–315.

82. Matthay MA. Severe sepsis—a new treatment with both anticoagulant and antiinflammatory properties. *N Engl J Med* 2001; 344:759–762.

83. Bernard GR, Vincent JL, Laterre PF, et al. Efficacy and safety of recombinant human activated protein C for severe sepsis. *N Engl J Med* 2001;344:699–709.

84. Angus DC, Crowther MA. Unraveling severe sepsis: why did OPTIMIST fail and what's next? *JAMA* 2003;290:256–258.

85. Angus DC, Linde-Zwirble WT, Clermont G, et al. Cost-effectiveness of drotrecogin alfa (activated) in the treatment of severe sepsis. *Crit Care Med* 2003;31:1–11.

86. Rivers E, Nguyen B, Havstad S, et al. Early goal-directed therapy in the treatment of severe sepsis and septic shock. *N Engl J Med* 2001;345:1368–1377.

87. Lefering R, Neugebauer EA. Steroid controversy in sepsis and septic shock: a meta-analysis. *Crit Care Med* 1995;23:1294–1303.

88. Cronin L, Cook DJ, Carlet J, et al. Corticosteroid treatment for sepsis: a critical appraisal and meta-analysis of the literature. *Crit Care Med* 1995;23:1430–1439.

89. Annane D, Sebille V, Chapentier C, et al. Effect of treatment with low doses of hydrocortisore and fludrocortisore or mortality in patients with septic shock, *JAMA* 2002;288(7):862–871.

90. Spellman CW. Management of diabetes in the real world: tight control of glucose metabolism. *J Am Osteopath Assoc* 2003;103: S8–S13.

91. Van den Berghe G, Wouters P, Weekers F, et al. Intensive insulin therapy in the critically ill patients. *N Engl J Med* 2001;345: 1359–1367.

92. Van den Berghe G, Wouters PJ, Bouillon R, et al. Outcome benefit of intensive insulin therapy in the critically ill: Insulin dose versus glycemic control. *Crit Care Med* 2003;31:359–366.

93. Gore JM, Goldberg RJ, Spodick DH, et al. A community-wide assessment of the use of pulmonary artery catheters in patients with acute myocardial infarction. *Chest* 1987;92:721–727.

94. Zion MM, Balkin J, Rosenmann D et al., SPRINT Study Group. Use of pulmonary artery catheters in patients with acute myocardial infarction. Analysis of experience in 5,841 patients in the SPRINT Registry. *Chest* 1990;98:1331–1335.

95. Parsons PE. Progress in research on pulmonary-artery catheters. *N Engl J Med* 2003;348:66–68.

96. Guyatt G, Ontario Intensive Care Study Group. A randomized control trial of right-heart catheterization in critically ill patients. *J Intensive Care Med* 1991;6:91–95.

97. Polanczyk CA, Rohde LE, Goldman L, et al. Right heart catheterization and cardiac complications in patients undergoing noncardiac surgery: an observational study. *JAMA* 2001;286:309–314.

98. Richard C, Warszawski J, Anguel N, et al. Early use of the pulmonary artery catheter and outcomes in patients with shock and acute respiratory distress syndrome: a randomized controlled trial. *JAMA* 2003;290:2713–2720.

CHAPTER **26**

Prevention of Nonpulmonary Complications of Intensive Care

Mark D. Eisner
Michael A. Matthay
Sanjay Saint

VENOUS THROMBOEMBOLISM
Prevalence and Risk Factors
Prevention
Recommendations

STRESS-RELATED UPPER GASTROINTESTINAL BLEEDING
Risk Factors
Prevention
Recommendations

VASCULAR CATHETER–RELATED INFECTION
Types of Infection
Risk Factors
Prevention
Recommendations

URINARY CATHETER–RELATED INFECTION
Risk Factors
Prevention
Bladder Irrigation
Antimicrobial Agents in the Drainage Bag
Rigorous Meatal Cleaning
Systemic Antibiotic Therapy
Summary of Preventive Methods against Catheter-Related
    Urinary Tract Infection
Recommendations

CONCLUSIONS

ACKNOWLEDGMENT

As previously described in this section of the book, Section IV: The Critically Ill Patient, sophisticated supportive care is provided to critically ill medical and surgical patients in the intensive care unit (ICU) setting. A variety of invasive interventions are performed, such as endotracheal intubation, mechanical ventilation, and central venous catheterization. As a result, patients may develop new medical problems that result from intensive care. ICU-acquired infection, for instance, affects about 20% of critically ill patients and confers excess risk of mortality (1).

This chapter reviews four common life-threatening nonpulmonary complications of intensive care: venous thromboembolism, stress-related gastrointestinal bleeding, vascular

catheter–related infection, and urinary catheter–related infection. For each complication, we review preventive strategies designed to reduce the risk posed to critically ill patients. We provide evidence-based recommendations for preventing these common ICU-related complications.

VENOUS THROMBOEMBOLISM

Hospitalized patients, especially those who are critically ill, are at risk for venous thromboembolism (2–4). Both deep venous thrombosis and pulmonary embolism are difficult to

608

diagnose, presenting with nonspecific clinical manifestations (3,5). Pulmonary embolism, in particular, confers a substantial risk of mortality (10%) (5). Because of the silent and potentially lethal nature of this complication, prevention is of paramount importance (6). Screening high-risk patients is insensitive and impractical and is less cost effective than preventive strategies (7–11).

PREVALENCE AND RISK FACTORS

Critically ill patients often have risk factors for venous thromboembolism (see Table 26-1) (4,12–15). Although ICU patients have heterogeneous illnesses, they often have advanced age, malignancy, or prolonged immobility. Similarly, trauma and postoperative surgical patients are commonly encountered. As a result, the prevalence of venous thromboembolism is substantial in ICU patients (see Table 26-2).

Although fewer studies have examined deep venous thrombosis in critically ill medical patients, numerous studies have documented a high prevalence in general surgical (25%) and trauma (51%) patients (16). In the few studies conducted in medical ICUs, about one third of patients had documented deep venous thrombosis (4,12,13). Compared with medical ward patients, the risk of deep venous thrombosis was about threefold higher among ICU patients (12).

PREVENTION

Because pulmonary embolism is life threatening, prevention of deep venous thrombosis is widely recommended for hospitalized patients (6). Some experts advocate prophylaxis for virtually all hospitalized patients (10). Although few studies have examined critically ill medical patients, the efficacy of venous thromboembolism prophylaxis has been clearly established in general surgical patients (6). A review of 70 randomized controlled clinical trials demonstrated a reduction of deep venous thrombosis from 25% in untreated controls to 7% to 8% in those patients receiving either unfractionated or low molecular weight heparin (16,17). Furthermore, these studies found a 50% reduction in fatal pulmonary embolism with

TABLE 26-1. Risk Factors for Venous Thromboembolism

Risk Factors for Venous Thromboembolism
Age above 40
Previous venous thromboembolism
Malignancy
Obesity
Prolonged immobility or paralysis
Major surgery (e.g., abdomen, pelvis, or lower extremity)
Trauma
Congestive heart failure
Acute myocardial infarction
Stroke
Fracture (e.g., pelvic, hip, or leg)
Estrogen replacement therapy
Hypercoagulable states

From Saint S, Matthay MA. Risk reduction in the intensive care unit. *Am J Med* 1998;105:515–523, with permission.

TABLE 26-2. Prevalence of Venous Thromboembolism in Hospitalized Patients

Patient Group	Deep Venous Thrombosis (%)	Pulmonary Embolism (%)
General surgery	25	1.6
Trauma	51	0.5–2.0
Ischemic stroke	63	0.8
Myocardial infarction	24	N/A
Other medical conditions	9.1–26	N/A
Medical ICU	29–33	N/A

ICU, intensive care unit; N/A, not available.

Data are summarized from the American College of Chest Physicians Consensus Conference (11). Prevalence for medical ICU patients is also derived from Hirsch DR, Ingenito EP, Goldhaber SZ. Prevalence of deep venous thrombosis among patients in medical intensive care. *JAMA* 1995;274:335–337 and Cade JF. High risk of the critically ill for venous thromboembolism. *Crit Care Med* 1982;10:448–450, with permission.

heparin prophylaxis. A more recent meta-analysis found that unfractionated heparin substantially reduced the risk of venous thromboembolism after colorectal surgery [pooled odds ratio (OR), 0.32; 95% confidence interval (CI), 0.20 to 0.53] (18). Similar benefit has been observed after major gynecologic and urologic surgery (14,19). Among general surgery patients, unfractionated and low molecular weight heparin appear to be equally effective (14,18,20,21). Intermittent pneumatic compression also reduces the risk of deep venous thrombosis by about 50% in surgical patients (17,22). In higher-risk surgical procedures, especially orthopedic surgery involving total hip or knee replacement, low molecular weight heparin is more efficacious than low-dose unfractionated heparin (14,17). In postoperative patients, then, venous thromboembolism prophylaxis is clearly warranted.

The optimal duration of heparin therapy for prevention of venous thromboembolism after major surgery remains uncertain. Although most studies have focused on treatment during hospitalization, a recent study of high-risk patients undergoing abdominal or pelvic surgery for cancer found that 4 weeks of enoxaparin prophylaxis reduced the risk of venous thromboembolism by more than 50% compared to 6 to 10 days of treatment (23). Further studies are needed to evaluate longer-term prophylaxis in other surgical patient groups.

Although less extensive, the available evidence supports preventive strategies targeted at venous thromboembolism in critically ill medical patients. The commonly employed prophylactic measures include low-dose unfractionated heparin, low molecular weight heparin, and intermittent pneumatic compression of the lower extremities.

Low-dose unfractionated heparin, usually administered in doses of 5,000 U to 7,500 U every 8 to 12 hours by subcutaneous (SQ) injection, reduces the incidence of deep venous thrombosis in patients with myocardial infarction (24–26) and ischemic stroke (27,28). Fewer trials have assessed efficacy in other medical patients. In a randomized trial enrolling patients with congestive heart failure or respiratory infection, preventive treatment with low-dose unfractionated heparin (5,000 units SQ every 8 hours) reduced the incidence of deep venous thrombosis from 26% to 4% (29). Only one randomized clinical trial examined venous thromboembolism in critically ill ICU patients by comparing low-dose unfractionated heparin (5,000 units SQ every 12 hours) with placebo (12). Investigators found a substantial reduction of deep venous thrombosis in patients receiving heparin (13%) compared with placebo (29%).

Low molecular weight heparin also appears to be effective among medical patients. A randomized controlled trial evaluated the efficacy of enoxaparin in 1,102 hospitalized medical patients, most of whom were not in the ICU (30,31). Low molecular weight heparin reduced the incidence of venous thromboembolism by two thirds.

Nonrandomized studies have also examined the impact of preventive therapy on pulmonary embolism and death. In a retrospective review of patients admitted to a respiratory ICU, low-dose unfractionated heparin was associated with a reduced incidence of pulmonary embolism (32). Among 1,358 general medical ward patients nonrandomly assigned to low-dose unfractionated heparin or no prophylaxis, heparin treatment reduced mortality rate from 10.9% to 7.8% (33). An unblinded multicenter trial enrolling 11,693 subjects hospitalized with infectious diseases found that low-dose heparin reduced the incidence of nonfatal pulmonary embolism (34). There was, however, no significant difference in the risk of fatal pulmonary embolism or death (34). Taken together, the available evidence indicates that low-dose unfractionated heparin reduces the risk of deep venous thrombosis and pulmonary embolism in critically ill medical patients.

Although low molecular weight heparin is more efficacious than unfractionated heparin in orthopedic surgery, trauma, and high-risk general surgery patients (6,35–39), few trials have compared this agent to unfractionated heparin in medical patients. In a randomized controlled trial of 270 hospitalized medical patients, low molecular weight heparin (enoxaparin 60 mg SQ daily) reduced the incidence of deep venous thrombosis threefold compared with placebo (9.1% versus 3.0%) (40). The risk of injection site hematoma, however, was significantly increased in the low molecular weight heparin-treated group (40). Three other randomized controlled trials compared low molecular weight heparin with low-dose unfractionated heparin in hospitalized medical patients (41). A multicenter trial of 442 elderly medical inpatients found no difference in the rate of venous thromboembolism between low molecular weight heparin (enoxaparin 20 mg SQ daily) and low-dose unfractionated heparin (5,000 units SQ twice daily) (4.8% versus 4.6%, respectively) (42). Similarly, a randomized trial of 166 hospitalized medical patients found no difference in the incidence of deep venous thrombosis between treatment with low molecular weight heparin and low-dose unfractionated heparin (41). Another randomized trial conducted among 451 patients with heart failure or severe respiratory disease found similar efficacy for low molecular weight heparin (enoxaparin 40 mg daily) and unfractionated heparin (5,000 units SQ three times daily) (43). On the basis of the available evidence, unfractionated and low molecular weight heparin seem to have similar efficacy among medical patients.

Most patients admitted to the ICU have at least one risk factor for venous thromboembolism (4). Evidence from surgical and medical patients, which has been reviewed above, supports the use of unfractionated heparin or low molecular

weight heparin in critically ill patients. There have been very few trials of heparin for prevention of venous thromboembolism in the ICU (4). More than 20 years ago, Cade found that low-dose unfractionated heparin (5,000 units SQ twice daily) reduced the risk of deep venous thrombosis from 29% to 13% among 119 critically ill patients (12). More recently, Fraisse et al. randomized 223 patients who were mechanically ventilated for chronic obstructive pulmonary disease (COPD) to low molecular weight heparin (nadroparin) versus placebo (44). Nadroparin reduced the risk of deep venous thrombosis by nearly 50%.

Intermittent pneumatic compression has been extensively studied in surgical patients. In patients undergoing a variety of surgical procedures—general, neurologic, orthopedic, cardiac, gynecologic, and urologic surgery—pneumatic compression reduces the risk of venous thromboembolism (16,22,42,45,46). For example, five randomized clinical trials conducted in general surgical patients demonstrated a 60% reduction in the risk of deep venous thrombosis (16). Unfortunately, this strategy has not been adequately evaluated in medical patients or in patients with critical illness (47). Despite the lack of direct evidence, this strategy does seem likely to have some efficacy. In critically ill medical patients with a contraindication to heparin, pneumatic compression may be the preferred preventive strategy.

Bleeding is a potentially important adverse effect of heparin. Evidence from surgical patients, however, indicates that both forms of heparin are relatively safe. No increase in major bleeding due to low-dose unfractionated heparin has been observed in individual trials, but two meta-analyses (16,17) found a statistically significant absolute increase (2%) in minor bleeding episodes (e.g., wound hematomas). Compared with low-dose unfractionated heparin, low molecular weight heparin probably causes less major and minor bleeding (35,48,49). In critically ill medical patients, the benefit of venous thromboembolism prophylaxis appears to outweigh the small excess of minor bleeding episodes.

Another potential risk is heparin-induced thrombocytopenia, an IgG-mediated effect associated with thrombotic complications (49). A recent randomized trial (50) in patients undergoing hip surgery found that low-dose unfractionated heparin had a significantly lower incidence of heparin-induced thrombocytopenia than low molecular weight heparin did (2.7% versus 0%). Other trials have also demonstrated an approximate 3% incidence of heparin-induced thrombocytopenia in patients given low-dose unfractionated heparin (49).

RECOMMENDATIONS

1. Most critically ill patients are at moderate to high risk for venous thromboembolism and should receive prophylaxis.

2. Low-dose unfractionated heparin or low molecular weight heparin are probably both efficacious agents in critically ill medical patients. Although low molecular weight heparin is more effective in critically ill surgical and trauma patients, unfractionated heparin and low molecular weight heparin seem to have similar efficacy in medical patients.

3. Intermittent pneumatic compression has not been studied in critically ill medical patients but may be the preferred strategy in patients at high risk for bleeding.

STRESS-RELATED UPPER GASTROINTESTINAL BLEEDING

Gastrointestinal bleeding is a well-recognized complication in critically ill patients. Most such bleeding results from stress ulceration of gastric or duodenal mucosa (51). Gastrointestinal ulceration during critical illness appears to be distinct in etiology from peptic ulcer disease presenting in ambulatory patients (52,53). In particular, critically ill patients with gastrointestinal ulceration have a lower prevalence of *Helicobacter pylori* infection and nonsteroidal antiinflammatory drug (NSAID) use than ambulatory patients with ulcer bleeding have. Furthermore, hospitalized patients who develop gastrointestinal bleeding have worse outcomes than ambulatory patients, with higher transfusion requirements, rate of rebleeding, and duration of hospital stay (52,53). Mortality, also, is greater among hospitalized patients who develop gastrointestinal bleeding (25% to 50%) compared with ambulatory patients (5% to 10%) (54–58). Because the morbidity and mortality from gastrointestinal hemorrhage in critically ill patients is substantial, many investigators have examined preventive strategies.

In critically ill patients, Cook et al. have proposed the following classification scheme (57). *Overt bleeding* is defined as hematemesis, gross blood or "coffee grounds" material in a nasogastric aspirate, hematochezia, or melena. *Clinically important* bleeding is overt bleeding complicated by any of the following symptoms within 24 hours: a spontaneous decrease in systolic blood pressure by more than 20 mm Hg, an increase in heart rate by at least 20 beats per minute or a decrease in systolic blood pressure by 10 mm Hg when sitting upright, or a decrease in hemoglobin level by more than 2 g per dL.

RISK FACTORS

In modern ICUs, a significant minority (<5%) of critically ill patients develop overt gastrointestinal bleeding (57,59). Patients who bleed, however, have a 12.5% excess mortality rate (59). As a result, investigators have attempted to define patient subgroups at higher risk of gastrointestinal bleeding. In a study of 179 critically ill medical patients, Schuster et al. found that 14% had evidence of either occult or overt bleeding. Mechanical ventilation and the presence of a coagulopathy (defined as a platelet count <50,000 per mm^3 or a prolonged prothrombin or partial thromboplastin time) were independent risk factors for gastrointestinal bleeding (60). This result was confirmed in a larger prospective cohort study of 2,252 critically ill medical and surgical patients (57). Although 30% of patients received prophylaxis, investigators found a 4.2% incidence of overt bleeding and a 1.5% incidence of clinically important bleeding. As before, respiratory failure requiring mechanical ventilation (for more than 48 hours) and coagulopathy was the only independent risk factor for gastrointestinal bleeding (57). Importantly, the presence of coagulopathy or mechanical ventilation identified nearly all patients who developed clinically important bleeding, with only 0.1% of the cases occurring among those patients with neither risk factor. In a subsequent study by the same investigators, renal failure was also identified as a risk factor for clinically important gastrointestinal bleeding in mechanically ventilated patients (61). On the basis of other studies, additional high-risk groups include surgical patients with extensive burns and those with head trauma or multiple traumatic injuries (62).

PREVENTION

Because gastrointestinal bleeding is associated with increased mortality, preventive strategies for critically ill patients have been developed (58). These techniques include prophylaxis with histamine H$_2$-receptor antagonists, sucralfate, antacids, and proton-pump inhibitors (57,63–67). Multiple randomized trials and meta-analyses have addressed the prevention of stress ulceration (68–71). When considering these studies, the impact of prophylaxis on three clinical outcomes must be considered. The first outcome is the rate of clinically important gastrointestinal bleeding—the target of prevention. The second is the incidence of nosocomial pneumonia. Many studies indicate that H$_2$-receptor antagonists and antacids may increase the probability of gastric bacterial colonization and late-onset nosocomial pneumonia (67,72–74). In particular, the risk of nosocomial pneumonia may be highest among patients who are mechanically ventilated for more than 4 days and who are receiving H$_2$-receptor antagonist prophylaxis (73). Sucralfate, primarily a cytoprotective agent, may not have this disadvantage (67,72,75) and may have limited antibacterial activity (68,72,76). Third is the impact of prophylaxis on mortality, which reflects the effects on both gastrointestinal bleeding and nosocomial pneumonia.

Although many randomized controlled trials have been published, the clinical benefit of stress ulcer prophylaxis remains uncertain (68–71,77,78). Cook et al. conducted a meta-analysis that attempted to resolve discrepancies among available studies (see Table 26-3) (69). Compared with placebo, H$_2$-receptor antagonists substantially reduced the incidence of clinically important gastrointestinal bleeding. There was a suggestion, however, that H$_2$-receptor antagonists were associated with a higher

TABLE 26-3. Comparison of Randomized Trials of Stress-Related Upper Gastrointestinal Bleeding

Comparison	Number of Trials	Pooled Odds Ratio (95% Confidence Interval)
H$_2$-RECEPTOR ANTAGONISTS VS CONTROL/PLACEBO		
Clinically important bleeding	10	0.44 (0.22–0.88)
Pneumonia	8	1.25 (0.78–2.00)
Mortality	15	1.15 (0.86–1.53)
SUCRALFATE VS CONTROL/PLACEBO		
Clinically important bleeding	1	1.26 (0.12–12.87)
Pneumonia	2	2.11 (0.82–5.44)
Mortality	4	1.06 (0.67–1.67)
SUCRALFATES VS H$_2$-RECEPTOR ANTAGONISTS		
Clinically important bleeding	4	1.28 (0.27–6.11)
Pneumonia	11	0.78 (0.60–1.01)
Mortality	11	0.83 (0.62–1.09)

From Cook DJ, Reeve BK, Guyatt GH, et al. Stress ulcer prophylaxis in critically ill patients. Resolving discordant meta-analyses. *JAMA* 1996;275:308–314, with permission.

risk of pneumonia and death. A more recent meta-analysis summarized five trials of ranitidine, three of which were included in Cook's earlier meta-analysis; studies of cimetidine were excluded (78). Ranitidine did not reduce the risk of clinically important gastrointestinal bleeding (OR 0.95; 95% CI, 0.37 to 2.43) or increase the risk of pneumonia (OR 1.10; 95% CI, 0.45 to 2.66). Although differential effectiveness of cimetidine and ranitidine could explain the different results of these two meta-analyses, these differences could also be explained by methodologic quality of the original trials.

Fewer trials have compared sucralfate with placebo. Compared with placebo, sucralfate was not effective in reducing clinically important gastrointestinal bleeding in Cook's meta-analysis (69). Also, use of sucralfate may have increased the risk of nosocomial pneumonia. Randomized trials have also compared sucralfate to H_2-receptor antagonists. According to the most recent meta-analysis, there was no significant difference in gastrointestinal bleeding between sucralfate-treated and H_2-receptor antagonist–treated patients (69). However, a more recent randomized trial of 1,200 critically ill mechanically ventilated patients demonstrated that ranitidine reduced the risk of clinically important gastrointestinal bleeding compared to sucralfate [relative risk (RR) 0.44; 95% CI, 0.21 to 0.92] (59). Ranitidine-treated patients had an 18% increased risk of ventilator-associated pneumonia, although the CI did not exclude absence of difference (RR 1.18; 95% CI, 0.92 to 1.51). There was also no difference in mortality between the two treatment groups. Despite the relatively large sample size and excellent methodology, this trial may have been underpowered to detect a clinically important difference in nosocomial pneumonia, as suggested by the wide CI.

Because proton-pump inhibitors are superior for raising gastric pH, they are being widely used as prophylaxis for gastrointestinal bleeding in the ICU. Studies show that omeprazole and other proton-pump inhibitors are effective in raising gastric pH among critically ill patients (79–82). A small randomized controlled trial of 67 high-risk ICU patients compared omeprazole (oral or nasogastric tube) with ranitidine (continuous intravenous infusion). Clinically important gastrointestinal bleeding occurred less commonly in the omeprazole-treated group (6% versus 31%, P <0.05). The study had several methodologic limitations that precluded clear conclusions, including no blinding, the lack of prespecified protocol for evaluating suspected gastrointestinal bleeding, and statistical analysis that did not conform to the intention-to-treat principle. Currently, there are inadequate data to evaluate the safety and efficacy of proton-pump inhibitors for prevention of gastrointestinal bleeding. A major concern is the effect of these medications on the risk of nosocomial pneumonia, given their powerful effect on increasing gastric pH. A final conclusion awaits data from well-designed clinical trials.

On the basis of the available data, the decision to institute preventive therapy for gastrointestinal bleeding is complex (65). Unfortunately, the most effective agents for preventing gastrointestinal bleeding (H_2-receptor antagonists) are also associated with a greater risk of nosocomial pneumonia. Although sucralfate may carry a lower risk of pneumonia, clinical trials have not established its efficacy compared with placebo. Neither agent has an established mortality benefit.

Because the risk of clinically important gastrointestinal bleeding is low (0.1%) in patients without mechanical ventilation or coagulopathy, preventive therapy is usually not indicated. If prophylaxis is selected in higher-risk patients, the choice between H_2-receptor antagonists and sucralfate should depend on the anticipated duration of mechanical ventilation. Nosocomial pneumonia related to H_2-receptor antagonists primarily occurs among patients ventilated for 4 or more days (73). In those patients who may require mechanical ventilation for less than 4 days, H_2-receptor antagonists may be used because they have proven efficacy compared with placebo (unlike sucralfate). Because sucralfate may decrease the risk of nosocomial pneumonia compared to H_2-receptor antagonists, it may be the superior choice when the clinician anticipates more prolonged mechanical ventilation. However, further clinical trials comparing sucralfate versus placebo are required to establish its efficacy. Proton-pump inhibitors, because they have been inadequately studied, cannot be recommended as prophylaxis at this time. One approach (83) to deciding whether prophylaxis is required and what agent to use is outlined in Figure 26-1.

RECOMMENDATIONS

1. In critically ill medical patients without mechanical ventilation or coagulopathy, prophylactic therapy is not indicated. In those patients with either of the risk factors, prophylaxis may be warranted.

2. Prophylaxis with H_2-receptor antagonists prevents clinically important upper gastrointestinal bleeding in critically ill patients, but a mortality benefit has not been shown.

3. If prophylaxis is selected, the choice between H_2-receptor antagonists and sucralfate may depend upon whether a prolonged (i.e., >4 days) intubation is anticipated.

4. The use of proton-pump inhibitors cannot be recommended until data from well-designed clinical trials become available.

VASCULAR CATHETER–RELATED INFECTION

Central venous and pulmonary arterial (PA) catheters provide vascular access and hemodynamic monitoring in critically ill patients (84), but are associated with infectious complications. Each year, more than 200,000 cases of nosocomial bacteremia occur in the United States. Central venous catheters (CVCs) account for most of these episodes. The consequences of catheter-related bacteremia are substantial, resulting in longer hospital stays, increased medical costs, and an excess mortality rate of 10% to 35% (85–89). This section will focus on prevention of *short-term* central venous and pulmonary artery catheter–related infection.

TYPES OF INFECTION

The placement of CVCs can result in three major infectious syndromes (90). The first is local infection at the insertion site, manifested by regional warmth, erythema, swelling, or expression of purulent material. When untreated, this local skin infection can lead to other, more advanced syndromes of catheter infection (90). The second is catheter colonization without evidence of systemic infection. Significant colonization is defined as a semiquantitative roll-plate catheter culture yielding more

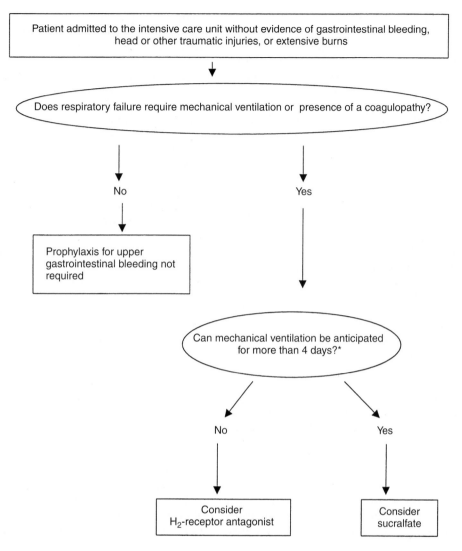

Patient admitted to the intensive care unit without evidence of gastrointestinal bleeding, head or other traumatic injuries, or extensive burns

Does respiratory failure require mechanical ventilation or presence of a coagulopathy?

No

Yes

Prophylaxis for upper gastrointestinal bleeding not required

Can mechanical ventilation be anticipated for more than 4 days?*

No

Yes

Consider H₂-receptor antagonist

Consider sucralfate

*This decision node is based on insufficient and conflicting data.

FIGURE 26-1. Stress-related upper gastrointestinal bleeding prophylaxis algorithm. (From Hiramoto JS, Terdiman JP, Norton JA. Evidence-based analysis: postoperative gastric bleeding: etiology and prevention. *Surg Oncol* 2003;12:9–19, with permission.)

than 15 colony forming units (cfus) of bacterial growth (91) or quantitative catheter culture (sonication method) revealing more than 1,000 cfus (92). On the basis of the landmark study by Maki et al., this semiquantitative culture cutoff identified all cases that subsequently developed bloodstream infection (91). More recent reports indicate that the quantitative culture technique has even higher sensitivity for local and bacteremic catheter infection (84,93–95).

The third infectious syndrome is catheter-related bloodstream infection (CR-BSI), resulting in bacteremia and clinical manifestations of sepsis (90). According to the most recent Infectious Disease Society of America (IDSA) guidelines, CR-BSI is defined as clinical signs and symptoms of bacteremia, such as fevers and chills, without other sources of bacteremia. A central component of the definition is that positive simultaneous blood cultures from the CVC and peripheral vein yield the same organism (96). In addition, there must be either catheter-tip colonization (>15 cfus for semiquantitative culture) with the same

organism (same species and antibiogram) isolated from the blood cultures *or* simultaneous quantitative blood cultures in which the number of cfus isolated from the blood drawn through the CVC was at least fivefold greater than the number isolated from blood drawn percutaneously. Another possible criterion may be differential time to positivity (positive blood culture occurs at least 2 hours earlier from the CVC than from the peripheral blood), which has a sensitivity and specificity of 81% and 92%, respectively, for catheters in place for less than 30 days (positive and negative likelihood ratios were 10.5 and 0.21, respectively) (97).

In recent studies, the incidence of CVC colonization ranged from 13.7% to 71.4% (85). In two recent clinical trials, the rate of colonization was approximately 25 per 100 catheters (92,98). The incidence of CR-BSI is substantially lower, ranging from 2.1% to 11.7% (72). The best estimate is 5 CR-BSI per 100 catheters or 7 CR-BSI per 1,000 catheter days (98). The incidence of catheter-related bacteremia varies substantially by type of ICU, with the lowest rates in cardiothoracic ICUs (2.8 infections per 1,000 catheter days) and the highest in burn units (10 infections per 1,000 catheter days) (99).

The most common organisms causing catheter-related infections are staphylococci (coagulase-negative and *Staphylococcus aureus*), enterococci, gram-negative rods, and *Candida* species. Resistance to antimicrobials has increased over the past decade for many of the common pathogens (99). Among ICU isolates, approximately 25% of enterococci are now resistant to vancomycin, 23% of *Pseudomonas aeruginosa* are quinolone-resistant, and more than 50% of *S. aureus* isolates are resistant to methicillin (99).

RISK FACTORS

There have been numerous attempts to identify the clinical factors associated with a higher risk of CVC-related infection (see Table 26-4). The duration of central venous catheterization is an important risk factor for infection. Hampton and Sheretz (100) pooled data from 25 prospective trials to estimate the risk of local infection associated with different types of catheters. The risk for peripheral venous catheters was 1.3% per day and that for CVCs was 3.3% per day (100). The risk of infection over time, however, is nonlinear, with a markedly increased incidence after 3 days of catheterization (84,92,98, 100). After 7 days of central venous catheterization, the risk of bloodstream infection is increased nearly ninefold (101). Pooling data from four large prospective trials of PA catheter infection (nearly 1,000 catheters), Mermel and Maki found that the cumulative incidence of CR-BSI was very low (<1%) until day 4, when the risk of infection increased exponentially (90). Longer duration of central venous catheterization, then, appears to result in higher risk of infection.

The site of central venous catheterization affects the risk of infection. A recent randomized trial conducted in eight French ICUs found that femoral vein catheterization caused more catheter-related infections (19.8% versus 4.5%, P <0.001) and thrombotic complications (21.5% versus 1.9%, P <0.001) (102). Observational studies of both central venous and pulmonary artery catheters have documented an increased risk of infection for internal jugular vein compared to subclavian vein placement (92,101,103–105). There are several explanations for the increased infection risk with internal jugular vein catheterization, including anatomic proximity to the respiratory tract, presence of facial hair, and difficulty maintaining tight-fitting dressings on the neck (104). Although subclavian catheters have a lower infection risk, mechanical complications (e.g., pneumothorax) are more common than with internal jugular

TABLE 26-4. Risk Factors for Vascular Catheter–Related Infection

Risk Factors

Longer duration of catheterization
Location of catheter
Use of transparent dressing
Lack of systemic antibiotic therapy
Less stringent barrier precautions during placement
Multilumen catheters (controversial)

From Saint S, Matthay MA. Risk reduction in the intensive care unit. *Am J Med* 1998;105:515–523, with permission.

catheters (98,102,106,107). Placement of PA catheters in the operating room, compared with the ICU, conferred increased risk of infection in a prospective, multivariate analysis (103). This increased risk was attributed to less rigorous sterile technique employed by anesthesiologists in the operating room. A similar analysis demonstrated a higher risk of CVC infection with placement outside the ICU (92). Supporting the impact of setting and technique, a prospective randomized trial of maximal barrier precautions versus routine sterile procedure revealed a sixfold lower risk of CVC infection with maximal precautions (90,108). A difficult catheter insertion has also been associated with higher risk of CVC infection, supporting the impact of technique on the rate of catheter infection (74).

The type of dressing may also be important in determining the risk of CVC-related infection. A meta-analysis of seven prospective randomized controlled trials comparing transparent polyurethane dressings with standard gauze dressings found a nearly twofold increased risk of CVC-tip infection with transparent dressings (109). There was a suggestion of increased risk of catheter-related sepsis (RR 1.69; 95% CI, 0.97 to 2.95) and bacteremia (RR 1.63; 95% CI, 0.76 to 3.47). Another more recent trial, however, found no significant difference between transparent or gauze dressing in local or bacteremic infection in 442 patients with PA catheters (110). In addition, a more recent meta-analysis of nine trials found no evidence linking dressing type with the risk of infection (111). In sum, it remains unclear whether dressing type is a risk factor for CVC-related infection.

Many investigators have suggested that multilumen catheters increase the risk of CR-BSI compared with single lumen devices. Several nonrandomized trials (112–114) have found an association between multilumen catheter use and higher risk of infection. However, illness severity confounds this association and complicates interpretation of these studies—patients requiring multilumen catheters may have greater disease severity. Randomized trials have provided conflicting results, with some studies demonstrating an increased risk with multilumen catheters (115,116) and others finding no significant difference in risk of infection (117,118). A recent meta-analysis of 15 randomized controlled trials found that multilumen catheters were associated with a greater risk of CR-BSI (OR 2.15; 95% CI, 1.00 to 4.66) but not with catheter colonization (OR 1.78; 95% CI, 0.92 to 3.47) (119). When higher quality studies were examined, there was no impact of multilumen catheters on the risk of infection. As a practical consideration, many critically ill ICU patients require multilumen catheters to provide adequate medication and nutrition delivery.

PREVENTION

Strict adherence to proper hand washing and aseptic technique during any catheter manipulation are crucial aspects of catheter infection prevention (120,121). We review the other strong evidence-based preventive strategies. A recent Centers for Disease Control and Prevention (CDC) guideline covers additional preventive techniques (122).

Site and Duration of Catheterization

Because the risk of CVC infection increases with time, clinicians should minimize the duration of catheterization. Whenever possible, reducing duration of central venous catheterization to 7 or fewer days is desirable. PA catheterization should not exceed 4 days, after which the risk of infection increases exponentially. Because of the higher risk of infectious and thrombotic complications, the femoral site should be avoided whenever possible. The choice between internal jugular and subclavian vein sites should be based on a clinical assessment that includes balancing the risk of infectious and mechanical complications.

Insertion Site Preparation and Maintenance

Strict adherence to proper hand washing techniques and use of maximal barrier precautions during CVC insertion are critical for infection prevention (122). Maximum sterile barrier precautions should include the use of sterile gloves, long-sleeved gowns, mask, cap, and a full-size drape (122).

Most CVC infections originate from cutaneous site colonization with microorganisms (90,123). Several investigators have examined whether site preparation with antiseptic compounds reduces the rate of CVC colonization. Cleansing the insertion site with povidone–iodine solution moderately reduces the rate of catheter colonization (124,125). The best agent for suppressing cutaneous microorganisms, however, is chlorhexidine gluconate. In a randomized trial of 668 central venous and arterial catheters, Maki et al. found that the incidence of local infection was significantly lower with chlorhexidine (2.3%) than with alcohol (7.1%) or povidone–iodine (9.3%) (124). The investigators observed a suggestion of decreased risk of CR-BSI in the chlorhexidine group, but the CI did not exclude absence of benefit (OR 0.23, 95% CI, 0.03 to 1.8). A more recent randomized trial in critically ill surgical patients also found that an antiseptic solution containing chlorhexidine gluconate decreased the risk of local infection (RR 0.4; 95% CI, 0.1 to 0.9) and catheter-related sepsis (RR 0.4; 95% CI, 0.1 to 1.0) compared with povidone–iodine (126). A meta-analysis of eight studies involving 4,143 catheters found that chlorhexidine reduced the risk of CR-BSI by 50% compared with povidone–iodine (127). On the basis of the available evidence, chlorhexidine should be routinely used for central venous catheterization.

An important component of site maintenance is the dressing system. As discussed above, there is no clear evidence that transparent dressings are associated with a higher risk of infection. Moreover, transparent dressings have significant clinical advantages, such as permitting continuous visual inspection of the catheter site, less frequent dressing changes, and patient bathing without disrupting the dressing. The recent CDC guidelines make no recommendation about dressing type.

Antimicrobial or Antiseptic-Impregnated Catheters

Antiseptic-impregnated catheters have been evaluated as means to prevent CVC infection. In a randomized controlled trial of 158 medical–surgical ICU patients, Maki et al. demonstrated that CVCs impregnated with chlorhexidine and silver sulfadiazine reduced the risk of CVC colonization (RR 0.56; 95% CI, 0.36 to 0.89) and bloodstream infection (RR 0.21; 95% CI, 0.03 to 0.95) when compared with control catheters (98). A recent meta-analysis of 11 randomized trials (2,603 catheters) comparing antiseptic-impregnated CVCs with standard catheters found a decreased risk of colonization (OR 0.44, 95% CI, 0.36 to 0.54) and CR-BSI (OR 0.56, 95% CI, 0.37 to 0.84) in the former (85). Therefore, CVCs impregnated with chlorhexidine

and silver sulfadiazine are effective in reducing catheter colonization and bloodstream infection.

Antibiotic-coated CVCs may even be more effective than antiseptic catheters in preventing CR-BSI (128). A recent randomized trial of minocycline/rifampin (i.e., antibiotic-coated) versus chlorhexidine/silver sulfadiazine (i.e., antiseptic) catheters demonstrated a significant decrease in the incidence of CR-BSI in the group receiving the antibiotic-coated catheter (0.3% versus 3.4%, P <0.002) (101). Compared to the antiseptic catheters, the antibiotic-coated catheters reduced the rate of CR-BSI from 4.1 per 1,000 catheter days to 0.3 per 1,000 catheter days. When deciding which antimicrobial catheter is to be used, it is important to note that minocycline and rifampin are still occasionally used as systemic antimicrobial agents; their use in catheters raises the theoretic concern of emerging antimicrobial resistance.

A formal economic evaluation compared chlorhexidine/silver sulfadiazine catheters to standard catheters, finding that chlorhexidine/silver sulfadiazine catheters led to both clinical and economic advantages in patients who were considered to be at high risk for infection (e.g., the critically ill or immunocompromised patients) who received central venous catheterization for 2 to 10 days. (129) Using a decision modeling approach, Marciante et al. found that minocycline/rifampin catheters were likely to be cost effective compared to chlorhexidine/silver sulfadiazine when used in patients catheterized for 8 or more days (130). Moreover, the antibiotic-coated catheters lead to overall cost savings for patients who are catheterized for 2 weeks or longer. Consequently, antiseptic or antimicrobial-coated catheters should be used in most ICU patients. The recent CDC guidelines recommend using these catheters for adults whose catheter is expected to remain in place for more than 5 days (122).

Scheduled Catheter Replacement

Because the risk of infection increases with duration of catheterization, routine catheter replacement has been advocated by some investigators. Two randomized controlled trials have examined whether scheduled central venous and pulmonary artery catheter replacement reduces infection when compared to catheter replacement for suspected infection or mechanical malfunction (131,132). In both studies, scheduled catheter replacement failed to reduce the incidence of catheter colonization or bloodstream infection. In fact, Cobb et al. (132) found that patients receiving replacement catheters at new insertion sites had no decrease in the risk of infection. These patients did, however, have an increased incidence of mechanical complications. Those patients undergoing routine replacement via guidewire exchange had a trend towards higher risk of bloodstream infection compared with patients who had catheter replacement only when clinically indicated. Therefore, routine replacement of central venous or pulmonary artery catheters appears to increase, rather than decrease, the overall complication rate. CVCs should be replaced only for well-defined clinical indications.

Prophylactic Antibiotics and Heparin

In two prospective multivariate analyses, use of systemic antibiotics was associated with a lower risk of central venous (92) and pulmonary artery catheter colonization (123). The effectiveness of "prophylactic" systemic antibiotics has been mixed, but overall there seems to be no compelling evidence for reduction of CVC infection rates (90,123). Given the problem of emerging antimicrobial resistance, prophylactic antibiotics cannot be recommended.

Catheter-related venous thrombosis may predispose patients to infection. Flushing CVCs with heparin may prevent thrombus formation and, as a result, infection. A recent meta-analysis of 12 randomized controlled trials found that use of heparin, including infusion, SQ administration, or bonding to the catheter, reduced catheter-related deep venous thrombosis (RR 0.43; 95% CI, 0.23 to 0.78), catheter colonization (RR 0.18; 95% CI, 0.06 to 0.6), and bloodstream infection (RR 0.26; 95% CI, 0.07 to 1.03) (133). The complications of heparin-induced thrombocytopenia and bleeding may limit the benefit of this strategy. At present, further evaluation is necessary before heparin flushes can be routinely recommended.

RECOMMENDATIONS

1. Maximal barrier precautions should be used for central venous and pulmonary artery catheter insertion. Strict adherence to proper hand washing should be maintained during all phases of catheter care.

2. The duration of catheterization should be minimized. Whenever possible, pulmonary artery catheter placement should be limited to 4 days.

3. The agent of choice for disinfecting the skin prior to and during catheterization is chlorhexidine gluconate.

4. CVCs impregnated with antiseptic or antibacterial agents should be used in all patients requiring prolonged (i.e., more than 2 days of) central venous catheterization.

5. Central venous and PA catheters should be changed only when clinically indicated. Routine, scheduled catheter replacement should not be employed.

URINARY CATHETER–RELATED INFECTION

Urinary catheters are widely utilized among hospitalized patients, with 25% receiving an indwelling urinary catheter (134). Unfortunately, urinary catheter–related urinary tract infection (UTI) is the most common nosocomial infection seen in medical ICUs, accounting for nearly one third of nosocomial infections (135). The daily incidence of bacteriuria in catheterized patients is approximately 3% to 10% (136). Among patients with bacteriuria, up to 25% will develop symptoms of local UTI and about 1% to 4% will develop bacteremia (136–139). The consequences of nosocomial catheter-related UTI are not benign—these infections increase the risk of mortality by nearly threefold (140). Because urinary catheter–related infection increases the risk of morbidity and mortality, preventive strategies should be employed in ICUs.

RISK FACTORS

The definition of catheter-related UTI varies by investigator, with interchangeable use of the terms bacteriuria and UTI. Low-level growth from a catheterized specimen (i.e., 10^2 cfu per mL) usually progresses to higher-grade bacteriuria

TABLE 26-5. Significant Risk Factors for Developing Urinary Tract Infection in Patients with an Indwelling Urinary Catheter

Risk Factors
Increasing duration of catheterization
Not receiving systemic antibiotic therapy
Female sex
Older age
Azotemia (serum creatinine concentration >2.0 mg/dL)
Diabetes mellitus
Rapidly fatal underlying illness
Nonsurgical disease
Faulty aseptic management of the indwelling catheter
Bacterial colonization of drainage bag

($>10^4$ cfu per mL) within days (141). For patients with indwelling urinary catheters, most experts agree that culturing $\geq 10^2$ cfu per mL of a predominant bacterial pathogen represents catheter-related UTI (142). Several investigators have evaluated risk factors for urinary catheter–related UTI (see Table 26-5). The most consistent risk factor is the duration of indwelling catheterization (137,143–147). The lack of systemic antimicrobial agents has also been found to increase the risk of catheter-related UTI in several studies (143–146,148). Most studies found that women have a higher risk of UTI than men do (137,143,145,146,148). Other possible risk factors include catheter care violations (143,145,149), rapidly fatal underlying illness (143), older age (143,146), diabetes mellitus (145), and azotemia (>2 mg per dL) at the time of catheterization (145).

Unfortunately, risk factors for UTI-related bloodstream infection have been less clearly defined (see Table 26-6). Because fewer than 4% of patients with catheter-related UTI develop catheter-related bacteremia (136,139), most studies had low statistical capacity to examine risk factors. During a prospective 23-month hospital surveillance study, investigators identified 1,233 patients with nosocomial UTI (incidence 3 cases per 100 admissions) (139). Nearly all patients with UTI had an indwelling urinary catheter (86%). Of the patients with UTI, 2.7% developed bloodstream infection. Risk factors for bloodstream infection were UTI due to *Serratia marcescens* (compared with other organisms, RR = 3.5) and male sex (RR = 2.0). No other factors (e.g., age, race, underlying disease, and hospital service) were related to the risk for bacteremia.

A retrospective case-control study compared patients with community-acquired, bacteremic UTI to nonbacteremic UTI (150). Risk factors for bacteremia were old age, noninfectious urinary tract disease (e.g., nephrolithiasis or prostatic

TABLE 26-6. Significant Risk Factors for Developing Bacteremia in Patients with Bacteriuria

Risk Factor
Male sex
Infection with *Serratia marcescens*
Old age
Noninfectious urinary tract disease (e.g., nephrolithiasis or prostatic hypertrophy)
Presence of an indwelling urinary catheter

hypertrophy), and indwelling urinary catheter placement. Clearly, indwelling bladder catheters are the major risk factor for UTI-related bacteremia. Other patient characteristics cannot be used to easily screen for patients at high risk for UTI-related bacteremia.

PREVENTION

Avoiding Indwelling Catheterization

Because most nosocomial UTIs are related to indwelling urinary catheters, the cornerstone of prevention is avoiding unnecessary indwelling catheterization. Although urinary catheters may have important functions in critically ill patients, their use is often inappropriate. A recent prospective study found that medical ICU patients often underwent urinary catheterization for inappropriate indications (in 13% of 135 catheterized medical ICU patients) (151). Even when urinary catheter placement was initially indicated, catheters were often continued for longer than necessary. Of 597 patient-days of continued indwelling bladder catheterization, 41% were judged as being unnecessary (151).

Consequently, urinary catheters should be removed immediately when there are no longer strong clinical indications for continued indwelling catheterization. To this end, an automatic urinary catheter "stop order" or reminder would be useful. This innovative structural intervention, similar to an antibiotic "stop order," (152) would remind physicians that their patient has an indwelling catheter, which in turn could reduce inappropriate catheterization. Indeed, a recent before-and-after crossover study found that a computerized reminder system for urinary catheters may be beneficial (153). Although no change in UTI rates were found in this small study, the computerized urinary catheter reminder system decreased catheterization duration by nearly 3 days ($P = 0.01$) (153).

Intermittent Catheterization

If continued urinary collection is required, options other than indwelling catheterization should be considered. Intermittent catheterization, that is, inserting and removing a sterile urinary catheter several times daily, may reduce the risk of UTI compared with an indwelling catheter. Most observational studies as well as review articles have concluded that long-term intermittent catheterization is associated with a decrease in UTI risk compared with long-term indwelling catheterization (154–158). Therefore, intermittent catheterization appears to be a reasonable alternative to long-term indwelling catheterization.

External (Condom) Catheters

External urine collection systems may be associated with a lower risk of bacteriuria than are indwelling catheters. Although devices have been developed for women, these systems are almost exclusively used in men. The proper role of condom catheters in hospitalized patients remains unclear. One prospective study conducted in a Department of Veterans Affairs (VA) Medical Center demonstrated a low risk of UTI among men wearing condom catheters (approximately 12% per month) (159). The rate was substantially higher, however, in those patients who frequently manipulated their catheters. In two parallel cohort studies in a VA nursing home, the incidence

of symptomatic UTI was about 2.5 times greater in men with a chronic indwelling catheter compared to those wearing a condom catheter (160,161). In contrast, a recent cross-sectional study in Denmark reported that the risk of UTI in hospitalized patients was twofold higher in those wearing condom catheters than in those with indwelling catheters (162). Because most of these studies were conducted in extended care facilities, the effectiveness of condom catheters for preventing UTI in the ICU remains unclear. Until randomized controlled trial data become available, external catheters cannot be recommended for prevention of UTI in the ICU.

Antiinfective Urinary Catheters

Antiinfective agents applied to the surface of urinary catheters, usually silver, appear to be effective in preventing bacteriuria. Most of these data, however, are based on hospitalized patients who are not in the ICU. Although the results reported in eight randomized controlled trials evaluating the silver-coated catheter were mixed, certain types of silver-coated urinary catheters, notably silver alloy catheters, appear to reduce the rate of bacteriuria according to a meta-analysis (OR 0.24; 95% CI, 0.11 to 0.52) (163). Five studies of silver alloy urinary catheters were published after the meta-analysis, which focused mostly on bacteriuria. Two of the studies demonstrated a small benefit of silver alloy catheters (164,165); both studies included patients in an ICU. However, when Karchmer et al. performed subgroup analysis on ICU patients, there was no statistically significant benefit seen in patients given silver alloy catheters (RR 0.94; 95% CI, 0.64–1.38) (164). One study, which included intensive care and neurosurgical patients, did not support the efficacy of silver alloy catheters (166); another study, which only evaluated postoperative urologic patients, found a benefit in those receiving the silver alloy catheter for about 5 days but not in those given the catheter for 14 days (167). In a before-and-after evaluation that focused entirely on ICU patients, Bologna et al. found a significant benefit in the silver alloy catheter group in the unadjusted analyses (37% risk reduction; $P <0.001$) but not in the adjusted analyses (40% risk reduction; $P = 0.13$) (168). Although the evidence is mixed, we recommend silver alloy catheters for patients at highest risk for infection (e.g., immunocompromised) because there are limited alternative preventive strategies currently.

Catheters coated with antibacterial substances other than silver have also been evaluated, but to a much lesser extent compared with silver catheters. A recent randomized study of men undergoing radical prostatectomy found that patients who received antimicrobial-impregnated catheters coated with minocycline and rifampin had significantly lower rates of gram-positive bacteriuria than the control group who were given standard catheters, but similar rates of gram-negative bacteriuria and candiduria were observed in both groups (169). Future studies are needed to evaluate the effectiveness of antimicrobial catheters before they can be recommended for use.

Among critically ill patients, urinary catheterization may often be unavoidable. As a result, strategies to reduce infection in patients with indwelling catheters are essential. The most important infection control advance is the closed catheter drainage system, including the use of sealed urinary catheter junctions (170–173). Proper aseptic technique, including aseptic insertion and maintenance of the catheter and drainage bag, remain essential in preventing catheter-related UTI (142,143,

149,174,175). Ideally, the collection bag should remain below the level of the bladder in order to prevent reflux of urine into the bladder. Finally, glove use and proper hand washing practices are important methods for preventing infection (176,177).

BLADDER IRRIGATION

Investigators have examined bladder irrigation with antiseptic (e.g., povidone—iodine and chlorhexidine) or antibacterial (e.g., neomycin and polymyxin) agents to prevent catheter-associated UTI. When modern closed drainage systems are used, this method has minimal efficacy (178–182). Because of the potential for local toxicity, bladder irrigation cannot be recommended.

ANTIMICROBIAL AGENTS IN THE DRAINAGE BAG

In catheterized patients, UTIs may occur when bacterially colonized urine in a drainage bag refluxes into the patient's bladder. Several studies have evaluated addition of antibacterial agents (e.g., chlorhexidine, hydrogen peroxide, and povidone–iodine) to the drainage bag. Although some studies have suggested a reduction in catheter-related UTI (183–186), well-controlled randomized trials have demonstrated no significant benefit (187–189). Importantly, adding solutions to the drainage bag violates aseptic handling of the closed drainage system.

RIGOROUS MEATAL CLEANING

Bacteria colonizing the urethral meatus may ascend along the urinary catheter's external surface and infect the urinary bladder. Reduction of urethral meatal colonization, then, might decrease the risk of UTI. Despite sound theoretic benefits, two large randomized trials have shown no impact of rigorous meatal cleansing on the risk of UTI (190,191). In one trial, investigators observed an increased prevalence of bacteriuria among patients undergoing meatal cleansing (190). As a result, rigorous meatal cleaning is not recommended.

SYSTEMIC ANTIBIOTIC THERAPY

Because systemic antibiotic therapy has been associated with a lower risk of catheter-related UTI, investigators have studied the use of systemic antimicrobial agents to prevent catheter-related infection (143–145,147). Evaluation of existing data is limited by retrospective study design, different definitions of UTI, and variation of antibiotic usage. Systemic antibiotics appear most useful in patients requiring urinary catheterization for 3 to 14 days (192–197). With shorter catheter duration, the risk of UTI is very low; longer duration is associated with near universal bacteriuria regardless of therapy. However, most experts do not recommend routine prophylactic antibiotics in catheterized patients because of cost, potential adverse effects, and emerging antibacterial resistance (172,198–200). Supporting this contention, studies demonstrate a higher rate of development of resistant organisms among patients receiving antibiotic prophylaxis (192,193,195). Furthermore, most critically ill patients receive antibiotic therapy for other indications (146,148).

Specific subgroups may benefit from prophylactic antibiotics to prevent catheter-related infection, including patients who undergo renal transplantation and transurethral resection of the prostate gland (201–203).

SUMMARY OF PREVENTIVE METHODS AGAINST CATHETER-RELATED URINARY TRACT INFECTION

Urinary catheter–related infection is common, costly, and morbid. Few interventions attenuate the risk of this important complication. Silver alloy urinary catheters may reduce nosocomial UTI among the critically ill patients. It is less clear as to what effect silver alloy urinary catheters will have on outcomes such as urinary catheter-related bacteremia and mortality. At present, using silver alloy catheter in those patients at highest risk for catheter-related UTI (e.g., immunocompromised) seems reasonable. Regardless of which type of urinary catheter is used, two aspects remain critical. First, a urinary collection device should be used only when appropriate and should be discontinued as soon as catheterization is no longer required. Second, aseptic technique should be used at all times during both the insertion and management of the catheter, and the drainage system should be manipulated as infrequently as possible.

RECOMMENDATIONS

1. Avoid using a urinary catheter whenever possible. When catheters are placed, minimize the duration of use.
2. Always insert a catheter aseptically, use a closed drainage system, and properly maintain the catheter during use.
3. Consider using silver alloy–coated catheters in patients at high risk for UTI.
4. For incontinent men, a condom catheter may be preferable if they will not manipulate the device.
5. Bladder irrigation, antibacterial instillation in the drainage bag, and rigorous meatal cleaning should not be used.

CONCLUSIONS

The clinical outcomes of critically ill patients can be improved by reducing common complications of intensive care. In this chapter, we have reviewed the strategies that are most effective in reducing nonpulmonary complications. These complications are associated with longer duration of ICU stay, higher mortality, and increased cost. By rigorously employing these preventive strategies, the outcomes of critical illness will continue to improve.

ACKNOWLEDGMENT

Dr. Eisner was supported by K23 HL04201 from the National Heart, Lung, and Blood Institute. Dr. Saint is supported by a Career Development Award from the Health Services Research & Development Program of the Department of Veterans Affairs and a Patient Safety Developmental Center Grant from the Agency for Healthcare Research and Quality (P20-HS11540).

REFERENCES

1. Vincent JL, Bihari DJ, Suter PM et al., EPIC International Advisory Committee. The prevalence of nosocomial infection in intensive care units in Europe. Results of the European Prevalence of Infection in Intensive Care (EPIC) study. *JAMA* 1995;274:639–644.
2. Carter CJ. The natural history and epidemiology of venous thrombosis. *Prog Cardiovasc Dis* 1994;36:423–438.
3. Alpert JS, Dalen JE. Epidemiology and natural history of venous thromboembolism. *Prog Cardiovasc Dis* 1994;36:417–422.

4. Geerts W, Selby R. Prevention of venous thromboembolism in the ICU. *Chest* 2003;124:357S–363S.
5. Moser KM. Venous thromboembolism. *Am Rev Respir Dis* 1990; 141:235–249.
6. Clagett GP, Anderson FA Jr, Heit J, et al. Prevention of venous thromboembolism. *Chest* 1995;108:312S–334S.
7. Oster G, Tuden RL, Colditz GA. A cost-effectiveness analysis of prophylaxis against deep-vein thrombosis in major orthopedic surgery. *JAMA* 1987;257:203–208.
8. Hull RD, Hirsh J, Sackett DL, et al. Cost-effectiveness of primary and secondary prevention of fatal pulmonary embolism in high-risk surgical patients. *Can Med Assoc J* 1982;127:990–995.
9. Salzman EW, Davies GC. Prophylaxis of venous thromboembolism: analysis of cost effectiveness. *Ann Surg* 1980;191:207–218.
10. Goldhaber SZ, Morpurgo M. Diagnosis, treatment, and prevention of pulmonary embolism. Report of the WHO/International Society and Federation of Cardiology Task Force. *JAMA* 1992; 268:1727–1733.
11. Oster G, Tuden RL, Colditz GA. Prevention of venous thromboembolism after general surgery. Cost-effectiveness analysis of alternative approaches to prophylaxis. *Am J Med* 1987;82:889–899.
12. Cade JF. High risk of the critically ill for venous thromboembolism. *Crit Care Med* 1982;10:448–450.
13. Hirsch DR, Ingenito EP, Goldhaber SZ. Prevalence of deep venous thrombosis among patients in medical intensive care. *JAMA* 1995;274:335–337.
14. Geerts WH, Heit JA, Clagett GP, et al. Prevention of venous thromboembolism. *Chest* 2001;119:132S–175S.
15. Geerts W, Cook D, Selby R, et al. Venous thromboembolism and its prevention in critical care. *J Crit Care* 2002;17:95–104.
16. Clagett GP, Anderson FA Jr, Geerts W, et al. Prevention of venous thromboembolism. *Chest* 1998;114:531S–560S.
17. Collins R, Scrimgeour A, Yusuf S, et al. Reduction in fatal pulmonary embolism and venous thrombosis by perioperative administration of subcutaneous heparin. Overview of results of randomized trials in general, orthopedic, and urologic surgery. *N Engl J Med* 1988;318:1162–1173.
18. Wille-Jorgensen P, Rasmussen M, Andersen B, et al. Heparins and mechanical methods for thromboprophylaxis in colorectal surgery. *Cochrane Database Syst Rev* 2003;4:CD001217.
19. Oates-Whitehead R, D'Angelo A, Mol B. Anticoagulant and aspirin prophylaxis for preventing thromboembolism after major gynaecological surgery. *Cochrane Database Syst Rev* 2003; 4:CD003679.
20. Koch A, Bouges S, Ziegler S, et al. Low molecular weight heparin and unfractionated heparin in thrombosis prophylaxis after major surgical intervention: update of previous meta-analyses. *Br J Surg* 1997;84:750–759.
21. Nurmohamed MT, Rosendaal FR, Buller HR, et al. Low-molecular-weight heparin versus standard heparin in general and orthopaedic surgery: a meta-analysis. *Lancet* 1992;340:152–156.
22. Handoll HH, Farrar MJ, McBirnie J, et al. Heparin, low molecular weight heparin and physical methods for preventing deep vein thrombosis and pulmonary embolism following surgery for hip fractures. *Cochrane Database Syst Rev* 2002;4:CD000305.
23. Bergqvist D, Agnelli G, Cohen AT, et al. Duration of prophylaxis against venous thromboembolism with enoxaparin after surgery for cancer. *N Engl J Med* 2002;346:975–980.
24. Warlow C, Terry G, Kenmure AC, et al. A double-blind trial of low doses of subcutaneous heparin in the prevention of deep-vein thrombosis after myocardial infarction. *Lancet* 1973;2:934–936.
25. Gallus AS, Hirsh J, Tutle RJ, et al. Small subcutaneous doses of heparin in prevention of venous thrombosis. *N Engl J Med* 1973; 288:545–551.
26. Handley AJ. Low-dose heparin after myocardial infarction. *Lancet* 1972;2:623–624.
27. McCarthy ST, Turner JJ, Robertson D, et al. Low-dose heparin as a prophylaxis against deep-vein thrombosis after acute stroke. *Lancet* 1977;2:800–801.
28. Turpie AG, Gent M, Cote R, et al. A low-molecular-weight heparinoid compared with unfractionated heparin in the prevention of deep vein thrombosis in patients with acute ischemic stroke. A randomized, double-blind study. *Ann Intern Med* 1992;117:353–357.
29. Belch JJ, Lowe GD, Ward AG, et al. Prevention of deep vein thrombosis in medical patients by low-dose heparin. *Scott Med J* 1981;26:115–117.
30. Samama MM, Cohen AT, Darmon JY et al., Prophylaxis in Medical Patients with Enoxaparin Study Group. A comparison of enoxaparin with placebo for the prevention of venous thromboembolism in acutely ill medical patients. *N Engl J Med* 1999;341:793–800.
31. Alikhan R, Cohen AT, Combe S, et al. Prevention of venous thromboembolism in medical patients with enoxaparin: a subgroup analysis of the MEDENOX study. *Blood Coagul Fibrinolysis* 2003;14:341–346.
32. Pingleton SK, Bone RC, Pingleton WW, et al. Prevention of pulmonary emboli in a respiratory intensive care unit: efficacy of low-dose heparin. *Chest* 1981;79:647–650.
33. Halkin H, Goldberg J, Modan M, et al. Reduction of mortality in general medical in-patients by low-dose heparin prophylaxis. *Ann Intern Med* 1982;96:561–565.
34. Gardlund B, the Heparin Prophylaxis Study Group. Randomised, controlled trial of low-dose heparin for prevention of fatal pulmonary embolism in patients with infectious diseases. *Lancet* 1996;347:1357–1361.
35. Anderson DR, O'Brien BJ, Levine MN, et al. Efficacy and cost of low-molecular-weight heparin compared with standard heparin for the prevention of deep vein thrombosis after total hip arthroplasty. *Ann Intern Med* 1993;119:1105–1112.
36. Turpie AG, Levine MN, Hirsh J, et al. A randomized controlled trial of a low-molecular-weight heparin (enoxaparin) to prevent deep-vein thrombosis in patients undergoing elective hip surgery. *N Engl J Med* 1986;315:925–929.
37. Levine MN, Hirsh J, Gent M, et al. Prevention of deep vein thrombosis after elective hip surgery. A randomized trial comparing low molecular weight heparin with standard unfractionated heparin. *Ann Intern Med* 1991;114:545–551.
38. Prins MH, Gelsema R, Sing AK, et al. Prophylaxis of deep venous thrombosis with a low-molecular-weight heparin (Kabi 2165/Fragmin) in stroke patients. *Haemostasis* 1989;19:245–250.
39. Turpie AG, Levine MN, Hirsh J, et al. Double-blind randomised trial of Org 10172 low-molecular-weight heparinoid in prevention of deep-vein thrombosis in thrombotic stroke. *Lancet* 1987; 1:523–526.
40. Dahan R, Houlbert D, Caulin C, et al. Prevention of deep vein thrombosis in elderly medical in-patients by a low molecular weight heparin: a randomized double-blind trial. *Haemostasis* 1986;16:159–164.
41. Harenberg J, Kallenbach B, Martin U, et al. Randomized controlled study of heparin and low molecular weight heparin for prevention of deep-vein thrombosis in medical patients. *Thromb Res* 1990;59:639–650.
42. Bergmann JF, Neuhart E, The Enoxaparin in Medicine Study Group. A multicenter randomized double-blind study of enoxaparin compared with unfractionated heparin in the prevention of venous thromboembolic disease in elderly in-patients bedridden for an acute medical illness. *Thromb Haemost* 1996;76:529–534.
43. Kleber FX, Witt C, Vogel G, et al., Randomized comparison of enoxaparin with unfractionated heparin for the prevention of venous thromboembolism in medical patients with heart failure or severe respiratory disease. *Am Heart J* 2003;145:614–621.
44. Fraisse F, Holzapfel L, Couland JM et al. The Association of Non-University Affiliated Intensive Care Specialist Physicians of France. Nadroparin in the prevention of deep vein thrombosis in acute decompensated COPD. *Am J Respir Crit Care Med* 2000;161: 1109–1114.
45. Hull RD, Pineo GF. Intermittent pneumatic compression for the prevention of venous thromboembolism [Editorial; Comment]. *Chest* 1996;109:6–9.
46. Ramos R, Salem BI, De Pawlikowski MP, et al. The efficacy of pneumatic compression stockings in the prevention of pulmonary embolism after cardiac surgery. *Chest* 1996;109:82–85.
47. Mazzone C, Chiodo Grandi F, Sandercock P, et al. Physical methods for preventing deep vein thrombosis in stroke. *Cochrane Database Syst Rev* 2002;1:CD001922.
48. Levine MN, Raskob G, Landefeld S, et al. Hemorrhagic complications of anticoagulant treatment. *Chest* 1995;108:276S–290S.
49. Hirsh J, Raschke R, Warkentin TE, et al. Heparin: mechanism of action, pharmacokinetics, dosing considerations, monitoring, efficacy, and safety. *Chest* 1995;108:258S–275S.
50. Warkentin TE, Levine MN, Hirsh J, et al. Heparin-induced thrombocytopenia in patients treated with low-molecular-weight heparin or unfractionated heparin. *N Engl J Med* 1995;332:1330–1335.

51. Schuster DP. Stress ulcer prophylaxis: in whom? With what? [Editorial; Comment]. *Crit Care Med* 1993;21:4–6.

52. Terdiman JP. Update on upper gastrointestinal bleeding. Basing treatment decisions on patients' risk level. *Postgrad Med* 1998;103: 43–47, 51–52, 58–59.

53. Terdiman JP, Ostroff JW. Gastrointestinal bleeding in the hospitalized patient: a case-control study to assess risk factors, causes, and outcome. *Am J Med* 1998;104:349–354.

54. Zimmerman J, Meroz Y, Siguencia J, et al. Upper gastrointestinal hemorrhage. Comparison of the causes and prognosis in primary and secondary bleeders. *Scand J Gastroenterol* 1994;29:795–798.

55. Loperfido S, Monica F, Maifreni L, et al. Bleeding peptic ulcer occurring in hospitalized patients: analysis of predictive and risk factors and comparison with out-of-hospital onset of hemorrhage. *Dig Dis Sci* 1994;39:698–705.

56. Zimmerman J, Meroz Y, Arnon R, et al. Predictors of mortality in hospitalized patients with secondary upper gastrointestinal haemorrhage. *J Intern Med* 1995;237:331–337.

57. Cook DJ, Fuller HD, Guyatt GH et al. Canadian Critical Care Trials Group. Risk factors for gastrointestinal bleeding in critically ill patients. *N Engl J Med* 1994;330:377–381.

58. Cook DJ, Griffith LE, Walter SD, et al. The attributable mortality and length of intensive care unit stay of clinically important gastrointestinal bleeding in critically ill patients. *Crit Care* 2001;5: 368–375.

59. Cook D, Guyatt G, Marshall J et al. Canadian Critical Care Trials Group. A comparison of sucralfate and ranitidine for the prevention of upper gastrointestinal bleeding in patients requiring mechanical ventilation. *N Engl J Med* 1998;338:791–797.

60. Schuster DP, Rowley H, Feinstein S, et al. Prospective evaluation of the risk of upper gastrointestinal bleeding after admission to a medical intensive care unit. *Am J Med* 1984;76:623–630.

61. Cook D, Heyland D, Griffith L et al. Canadian Critical Care Trials Group. Risk factors for clinically important upper gastrointestinal bleeding in patients requiring mechanical ventilation. *Crit Care Med* 1999;27:2812–2817.

62. Ben Menachem T, McCarthy BD, Fogel R, et al. Prophylaxis for stress-related gastrointestinal hemorrhage: a cost effectiveness analysis. *Crit Care Med* 1996;24:338–345.

63. Yang YX, Lewis JD. Prevention and treatment of stress ulcers in critically ill patients. *Semin Gastrointest Dis* 2003;14:11–19.

64. Hiramoto JS, Terdiman JP, Norton JA. Evidence-based analysis: postoperative gastric bleeding: etiology and prevention. *Surg Oncol* 2003;12:9–19.

65. Steinberg KP. Stress-related mucosal disease in the critically ill patient: risk factors and strategies to prevent stress-related bleeding in the intensive care unit. *Crit Care Med* 2002;30:S362–S364.

66. Cash BD. Evidence-based medicine as it applies to acid suppression in the hospitalized patient. *Crit Care Med* 2002;30:S373–S378.

67. Tryba M, Kulka PJ. Critical care pharmacotherapy. A review. *Drugs* 1993;45:338–352.

68. Cook DJ, Witt LG, Cook RJ, et al. Stress ulcer prophylaxis in the critically ill: a meta-analysis. *Am J Med* 1991;91:519–527. [published erratum appears in *Am J Med* 1991;91(6):670]

69. Cook DJ, Reeve BK, Guyatt GH, et al. Stress ulcer prophylaxis in critically ill patients. Resolving discordant meta-analyses. *JAMA* 1996;275:308–314.

70. Tryba M. Sucralfate versus antacids or H2-antagonists for stress ulcer prophylaxis: a meta-analysis on efficacy and pneumonia rate. *Crit Care Med* 1991;19:942–949.

71. Lacroix J, Infante Rivard C, Jenicek M, et al. Prophylaxis of upper gastrointestinal bleeding in intensive care units: a meta-analysis. *Crit Care Med* 1989;17:862–869.

72. Tryba M. Side effects of stress bleeding prophylaxis. *Am J Med* 1989;86:85–93.

73. Prod'hom G, Leuenberger P, Koerfer J, et al. Nosocomial pneumonia in mechanically ventilated patients receiving antacid, ranitidine, or sucralfate as prophylaxis for stress ulcer. A randomized controlled trial. *Ann Intern Med* 1994;120:653–662.

74. Garvey BM, McCambley JA, Tuxen DV. Effects of gastric alkalization on bacterial colonization in critically ill patients. *Crit Care Med* 1989;17:211–216.

75. McCarthy DM. Sucralfate. *N Engl J Med* 1991;325:1017–1025.

76. Tryba M, Mantey Stiers F. Antibacterial activity of sucralfate in human gastric juice. *Am J Med* 1987;83:125–127.

77. Hanisch EW, Encke A, Naujoks F, et al. A randomized, double-blind trial for stress ulcer prophylaxis shows no evidence of increased pneumonia. *Am J Surg* 1998;176:453–457.

78. Messori A, Trippoli S, Vaiani M, et al. Bleeding and pneumonia in intensive care patients given ranitidine and sucralfate for prevention of stress ulcer: meta-analysis of randomised controlled trials. *BMJ* 2000;321:1103–1106.

79. Lasky MR, Metzler MH, Phillips JO. A prospective study of omeprazole suspension to prevent clinically significant gastrointestinal bleeding from stress ulcers in mechanically ventilated trauma patients. *J Trauma* 1998;44:527–533.

80. Balaban DH, Duckworth CW, Peura DA. Nasogastric omeprazole: effects on gastric pH in critically ill patients. *Am J Gastroenterol* 1997;92:79–83.

81. Phillips JO, Metzler MH, Palmieri MT, et al. A prospective study of simplified omeprazole suspension for the prophylaxis of stress-related mucosal damage. *Crit Care Med* 1996;24:1793–1800.

82. Jung R, MacLaren R. Proton-pump inhibitors for stress ulcer prophylaxis in critically ill patients. *Ann Pharmacother* 2002;36: 1929–1937.

83. Saint S, Matthay MA. Risk reduction in the intensive care unit. *Am J Med* 1998;105:515–523.

84. Raad II, Bodey GP. Infectious complications of indwelling vascular catheters. *Clin Infect Dis* 1992;15:197–208.

85. Veenstra DL, Saint S, Saha S, et al. Efficacy of antiseptic-impregnated central venous catheters in preventing catheter-related bloodstream infection: a meta-analysis. *JAMA* 1999;281:261–267.

86. Corona ML, Peters SG, Narr BJ, et al. Infections related to central venous catheters. *Mayo Clin Proc* 1990;65:979–986.

87. Arnow PM, Quimosing EM, Beach M. Consequences of intravascular catheter sepsis. *Clin Infect Dis* 1993;16:778–784.

88. Pittet D, Tarara D, Wenzel RP. Nosocomial bloodstream infection in critically ill patients. Excess length of stay, extra costs, and attributable mortality. *JAMA* 1994;271:1598–1601.

89. Smith RL, Meixler SM, Simberkoff MS. Excess mortality in critically ill patients with nosocomial bloodstream infections. *Chest* 1991;100:164–167.

90. Mermel LA, Maki DG. Infectious complications of Swan-Ganz pulmonary artery catheters. Pathogenesis, epidemiology, prevention, and management. *Am J Respir Crit Care Med* 1994;149:1020–1036. [published erratum appears in *Am J Respir Crit Care Med* 1994;150(1):290]

91. Maki DG, Weise CE, Sarafin HW. A semiquantitative culture method for identifying intravenous-catheter-related infection. *N Engl J Med* 1977;296:1305–1309.

92. Raad I, Darouiche R, Dupuis J et al., the Texas Medical Center Catheter Study Group. Central venous catheters coated with minocycline and rifampin for the prevention of catheter-related colonization and bloodstream infections. A randomized, double-blind trial. *Ann Intern Med* 1997;127:267–274.

93. Raad II, Hanna HA. Intravascular catheter-related infections: new horizons and recent advances. *Arch Intern Med* 2002;162:871–878.

94. Raad II, Sabbagh MF, Rand KH, et al. Quantitative tip culture methods and the diagnosis of central venous catheter-related infections. *Diagn Microbiol Infect Dis* 1992;15:13–20.

95. Raad II. The pathogenesis and prevention of central venous catheter-related infections. *Middle East J Anesthesiol* 1994;12:381–403.

96. Mermel LA, Farr BM, Sherertz RJ, et al. Guidelines for the management of intravascular catheter-related infections. *Clin Infect Dis* 2001;32:1249–1272.

97. Raad I, Hanna HA, Alakech B, et al. Differential time to positivity: a useful method for diagnosing catheter-related bloodstream infections. *Ann Intern Med* 2004;140:18–25.

98. Maki DG, Stolz SM, Wheeler S, et al. Prevention of central venous catheter-related bloodstream infection by use of an antiseptic-impregnated catheter. A randomized, controlled trial. *Ann Intern Med* 1997;127:257–266.

99. *Am J Infect Control*, National Nosocomial Infections Surveillance (NNIS) system report, data summary from January 1992-April 2000, issued June 2000. 2000;28:429–448.

100. Hampton AA, Sherertz RJ. Vascular-access infections in hospitalized patients. *Surg Clin North Am* 1988;68:57–71.

101. Darouiche RO, Raad II, Heard SO et al. Catheter Study Group. A comparison of two antimicrobial-impregnated central venous catheters. *N Engl J Med* 1999;340:1–8.

102. Merrer J, De Jonghe B, Golliot F, et al. Complications of femoral and subclavian venous catheterization in critically ill patients: a randomized controlled trial. *JAMA* 2001;286:700–707.

103. Mermel LA, McCormick RD, Springman SR, et al. The pathogenesis and epidemiology of catheter-related infection with pulmonary artery Swan-Ganz catheters: a prospective study utilizing molecular subtyping. *Am J Med* 1991;91:197S–205S.

104. Richet H, Hubert B, Nitemberg G, et al. Prospective multicenter study of vascular-catheter-related complications and risk factors for positive central-catheter cultures in intensive care unit patients. *J Clin Microbiol* 1990;28:2520–2525.

105. Gil RT, Kruse JA, Thill Baharozian MC, et al. Triple- vs single-lumen central venous catheters. A prospective study in a critically ill population. *Arch Intern Med* 1989;149:1139–1143.

106. Goetz AM, Wagener MM, Miller JM, et al. Risk of infection due to central venous catheters: effect of site of placement and catheter type. *Infect Control Hosp Epidemiol* 1998;19:842–845.

107. Meredith JW, Young JS, O'Neil EA, et al. Femoral catheters and deep venous thrombosis: a prospective evaluation with venous duplex sonography. *J Trauma* 1993;35:187–190.

108. Raad II, Hohn DC, Gilbreath BJ, et al. Prevention of central venous catheter-related infections by using maximal sterile barrier precautions during insertion. *Infect Control Hosp Epidemiol* 1994;15:231–238.

109. Hoffmann KK, Weber DJ, Samsa GP, et al. Transparent polyurethane film as an intravenous catheter dressing. A meta-analysis of the infection risks. *JAMA* 1992;267:2072–2076.

110. Maki DG, Stolz SS, Wheeler S, et al. A prospective, randomized trial of gauze and two polyurethane dressings for site care of pulmonary artery catheters: implications for catheter management. *Crit Care Med* 1994;22:1729–1737.

111. Gillies D, O'Riordan L, Carr D, et al. Gauze and tape and transparent polyurethane dressings for central venous catheters. *Cochrane Database Syst Rev* 2003;4:CD003827.

112. Pemberton LB, Lyman B, Lander V, et al. Sepsis from triple- vs single-lumen catheters during total parenteral nutrition in surgical or critically ill patients. *Arch Surg* 1986;121:591–594.

113. Yeung C, May J, Hughes R. Infection rate for single lumen v triple lumen subclavian catheters. *Infect Control Hosp Epidemiol* 1988;9:154–158.

114. Hilton E, Haslett TM, Borenstein MT, et al. Central catheter infections: single- versus triple-lumen catheters. Influence of guide wires on infection rates when used for replacement of catheters. *Am J Med* 1988;84:667–672.

115. Clark Christoff N, Watters VA, Sparks W, et al. Use of triple-lumen subclavian catheters for administration of total parenteral nutrition. *JPEN J Parenter Enteral Nutr* 1992;16:403–407.

116. McCarthy MC, Shives JK, Robison RJ, et al. Prospective evaluation of single and triple lumen catheters in total parenteral nutrition. *JPEN J Parenter Enteral Nutr* 1987;11:259–262.

117. Farkas JC, Liu N, Bleriot JP, et al. Single- versus triple-lumen central catheter-related sepsis: a prospective randomized study in a critically ill population. *Am J Med* 1992;93:277–282.

118. Powell C, Fabri PJ, Kudsk KA. Risk of infection accompanying the use of single-lumen vs double-lumen subclavian catheters: a prospective randomized study. *J Parenter Enteral Nutr* 1988;12:127–129.

119. Dezfulian C, Lavelle J, Nallamothu BK, et al. Rates of infection for single-lumen versus multilumen central venous catheters: a meta-analysis. *Crit Care Med* 2003;31:2385–2390.

120. Nystrom B. Impact of handwashing on mortality in intensive care: examination of the evidence. *Infect Control Hosp Epidemiol* 1994;15:435–436.

121. Doebbeling BN, Stanley GL, Sheetz CT, et al. Comparative efficacy of alternative hand-washing agents in reducing nosocomial infections in intensive care units. *N Engl J Med* 1992;327:88–93.

122. O'Grady NP, Alexander M, Dellinger EP, et al. Guidelines for the prevention of intravascular catheter-related infections. Centers for disease control and prevention. *MMWR Recomm Rep* 2002;51:1–29.

123. Rello J, Coll P, Net A, et al. Infection of pulmonary artery catheters. Epidemiologic characteristics and multivariate analysis of risk factors. *Chest* 1993;103:132–136.

124. Maki DG, Ringer M, Alvarado CJ. Prospective randomised trial of povidone-iodine, alcohol, and chlorhexidine for prevention of

125. Levy JH, Nagle DM, Curling PE, et al. Contamination reduction during central venous catheterization. *Crit Care Med* 1988;16:165–167.

126. Mimoz O, Pieroni L, Lawrence C, et al. Prospective, randomized trial of two antiseptic solutions for prevention of central venous or arterial catheter colonization and infection in intensive care unit patients. *Crit Care Med* 1996;24:1818–1823.

127. Chaiyakunapruk N, Veenstra DL, Lipsky BA, et al. Vascular catheter site care: the clinical and economic benefits of chlorhexidine gluconate compared with povidone iodine. *Clin Infect Dis* 2003;37:764–771.

128. Raad I, Darouiche R, Dupuis J et al., the Texas Medical Center Catheter Study Group. Central venous catheters coated with minocycline and rifampin for the prevention of catheter-related colonization and bloodstream infections. A randomized, double-blind trial. *Ann Intern Med* 1997;127:267–274.

129. Veenstra DL, Saint S, Sullivan SD. Cost-effectiveness of antiseptic-impregnated central venous catheters for the prevention of catheter-related bloodstream infection. *JAMA* 1999;282:554–560.

130. Marciante KD, Veenstra DL, Lipsky BA, et al. Which antimicrobial impregnated central venous catheter should we use? Modeling the costs and outcomes of antimicrobial catheter use. *Am J Infect Control* 2003;31:1–8.

131. Eyer S, Brummitt C, Crossley K, et al. Catheter-related sepsis: prospective, randomized study of three methods of long-term catheter maintenance. *Crit Care Med* 1990;18:1073–1079.

132. Cobb DK, High KP, Sawyer RG, et al. A controlled trial of scheduled replacement of central venous and pulmonary-artery catheters. *N Engl J Med* 1992;327:1062–1068.

133. Randolph AG, Cook DJ, Gonzales CA, et al. Benefit of heparin in central venous and pulmonary artery catheters: a meta-analysis of randomized controlled trials. *Chest* 1998;113:165–171.

134. Haley RW, Hooton TM, Culver DH, et al., Nosocomial infections in U.S. hospitals, 1975–1976: estimated frequency by selected characteristics of patients. *Am J Med* 1981;70:947–959.

135. Richards MJ, Edwards JR, Culver DH et al., National Nosocomial Infections Surveillance System. Nosocomial infections in medical intensive care units in the United States. *Crit Care Med* 1999;27:887–892.

136. Saint S. Clinical and economic consequences of nosocomial catheter-related bacteriuria. *Am J Infect Control* 2000;28:68–75.

137. Tambyah PA, Maki DG. Catheter-associated urinary tract infection is rarely symptomatic: a prospective study of 1,497 catheterized patients. *Arch Intern Med* 2000;160:678–682.

138. Bryan CS, Reynolds KL. Hospital-acquired bacteremic urinary tract infection: epidemiology and outcome. *J Urol* 1984;132:494–498.

139. Krieger JN, Kaiser DL, Wenzel RP. Urinary tract etiology of bloodstream infections in hospitalized patients. *J Infect Dis* 1983;148:57–62.

140. Platt R, Polk BF, Murdock B, et al. Mortality associated with nosocomial urinary-tract infection. *N Engl J Med* 1982;307:637–642.

141. Stark RP, Maki DG. Bacteriuria in the catheterized patient. What quantitative level of bacteriuria is relevant? *N Engl J Med* 1984;311:560–564.

142. Stamm WE. Urinary tract infections. In: Brachman PS, ed. *Hospitals infections.* Philadelphia: Lippincott–Raven Publishers, 1998.

143. Garibaldi RA, Burke JP, Dickman ML, et al. Factors predisposing to bacteriuria during indwelling urethral catheterization. *N Engl J Med* 1974;291:215–219.

144. Hustinx WN, Mintjes de Groot AJ, Verkooyen RP, et al. Impact of concurrent antimicrobial therapy on catheter-associated urinary tract infection. *J Hosp Infect* 1991;18:45–56.

145. Platt R, Polk BF, Murdock B, et al. Risk factors for nosocomial urinary tract infection. *Am J Epidemiol* 1986;124:977–985.

146. Riley DK, Classen DC, Stevens LE, et al. A large randomized clinical trial of a silver-impregnated urinary catheter: lack of efficacy and staphylococcal superinfection. *Am J Med* 1995;98:349–356.

147. Shapiro M, Simchen E, Izraeli S, et al. A multivariate analysis of risk factors for acquiring bacteriuria in patients with indwelling urinary catheters for longer than 24 hours. *Infect Control* 1984;5:525–532.

148. Johnson JR, Roberts PL, Olsen RJ, et al. Prevention of catheter-associated urinary tract infection with a silver oxide-coated

urinary catheter: clinical and microbiologic correlates. *J Infect Dis* 1990;162:1145–1150.

149. Maki DG, Tambyah PA. Engineering out the risk for infection with urinary catheters. *Emerg Infect Dis* 2001;7:342–347.

150. Jerkeman M, Braconier JH. Bacteremic and non-bacteremic febrile urinary tract infection—a review of 168 hospital-treated patients. *Infection* 1992;20:143–145.

151. Jain P, Parada JP, David A, et al. Overuse of the indwelling urinary tract catheter in hospitalized medical patients. *Arch Intern Med* 1995;155:1425–1429.

152. Zoebelein E, Levy M, Greenwald RA. The effect of quality assurance review on implementation of an automatic stop-order policy. *Qual Rev Bull* 1982;8:12–17.

153. Cornia PB, Amory JK, Fraser S, et al. Computer-based order entry decreases duration of indwelling urinary catheterization in hospitalized patients. *Am J Med* 2003;114:404–407.

154. Weld KJ, Dmochowski RR. Effect of bladder management on urological complications in spinal cord injured patients. *J Urol* 2000;163:768–772.

155. Bennett CJ, Young MN, Adkins RH, et al. Comparison of bladder management complication outcomes in female spinal cord injury patients. *J Urol* 1995;153:1458–1460.

156. Cardenas DD, Hooton TM. Urinary tract infection in persons with spinal cord injury. *Arch Phys Med Rehabil* 1995;76:272–280.

157. Shekelle PG, Morton SC, Clark KA, et al. Systematic review of risk factors for urinary tract infection in adults with spinal cord dysfunction. *J Spinal Cord Med* 1999;22:258–272.

158. Jamil F. Towards a catheter free status in neurogenic bladder dysfunction: a review of bladder management options in spinal cord injury (SCI). *Spinal Cord* 2001;39:355–361.

159. Hirsh DD, Fainstein V, Musher DM. Do condom catheter collecting systems cause urinary tract infection? *JAMA* 1979;242:340–341.

160. Ouslander JG, Greengold B, Chen S. Complications of chronic indwelling urinary catheters among male nursing home patients: a prospective study. *J Urol* 1987;138:1191–1195.

161. Ouslander JG, Greengold B, Chen S. External catheter use and urinary tract infections among incontinent male nursing home patients. *J Am Geriatr Soc* 1987;35:1063–1070.

162. Zimakoff J, Stickler DJ, Pontoppidan B, et al. Bladder management and urinary tract infections in Danish hospitals, nursing homes, and home care: a national prevalence study. *Infect Control Hosp Epidemiol* 1996;17:215–221.

163. Saint S, Elmore JG, Sullivan SD, et al. The efficacy of silver alloy-coated urinary catheters in preventing urinary tract infection: a meta-analysis. *Am J Med* 1998;105:236–241.

164. Karchmer TB, Giannetta ET, Muto CA, et al. A randomized crossover study of silver-coated urinary catheters in hospitalized patients. *Arch Intern Med* 2000;160:3294–3298.

165. Maki DG, Knasinski V, Halvorson K, et al. A novel silver-hydrogel-impregnated indwelling urinary catheter reduces catheter-related urinary tract infections. A prospective double-blind trial [Abstract]. *Infect Control Hosp Epidemiol* 1998;19:682(A10).

166. Thibon P, Le Coutour X, Leroyer R, et al. Randomized multi-centre trial of the effects of a catheter coated with hydrogel and silver salts on the incidence of hospital-acquired urinary tract infections. *J Hosp Infect* 2000;45:117–124.

167. Verleyen P, De Ridder D, Van Poppel H, et al. Clinical application of the Bardex IC Foley catheter. *Eur Urol* 1999;36:240–246.

168. Bologna RA, Tu LM, Polansky M, et al. Hydrogel/silver ion-coated urinary catheter reduces nosocomial urinary tract infection rates in intensive care unit patients: a multicenter study. *Urology* 1999;54:982–987.

169. Darouiche RO, Smith JA Jr, Hanna H, et al. Efficacy of antimicrobial-impregnated bladder catheters in reducing catheter-associated bacteriuria: a prospective, randomized, multicenter clinical trial. *Urology* 1999;54:976–981.

170. Wolff G, Gradel E, Buchman B. Indwelling catheter and risk of urinary infection: a clinical investigation with a new closed-drainage system. *Urol Res* 1976;4:15–18.

171. Thornton GF, Andriole VT. Bacteriuria during indwelling catheter drainage. II. Effect of a closed sterile drainage system. *JAMA* 1970;214:339–342.

172. Meares EM Jr. Current patterns in nosocomial urinary tract infections. *Urology* 1991;37:9–12.

173. Kunin CM, McCormack RC. Prevention of catheter-induced urinary-tract infections by sterile closed drainage. *N Engl J Med* 1966;274:1155–1161.

174. Wong ES. Guideline for prevention of catheter-associated urinary tract infections. *Am J Infect Control* 1983;11:28–36.

175. Pratt RJ, Pellowe C, Loveday HP et al., Department of Health (England). The epic project: developing national evidence-based guidelines for preventing healthcare associated infections. Phase I: Guidelines for preventing hospital-acquired infections. *J Hosp Infect* 2001;47:S3–S82.

176. Schaberg DR, Haley RW, Highsmith AK, et al. Nosocomial bacteriuria: a prospective study of case clustering and antimicrobial resistance. *Ann Intern Med* 1980;93:420–424.

177. Larson EL. APIC guideline for handwashing and hand antisepsis in health care settings. *Am J Infect Control* 1995;23:251–269.

178. Warren JW, Platt R, Thomas RJ, et al. Antibiotic irrigation and catheter-associated urinary-tract infections. *N Engl J Med* 1978;299:570–573.

179. Kirk D, Dunn M, Bullock DW, et al. Hibitane bladder irrigation in the prevention of catheter-associated urinary infection. *Br J Urol* 1979;51:528–531.

180. Gelman ML. Antibiotic irrigation and catheter-associated urinary tract infections [Editorial]. *Nephron* 1980;25:259.

181. Dudley MN, Barriere SL. Antimicrobial irrigations in the prevention and treatment of catheter-related urinary tract infections. *Am J Hosp Pharm* 1981;38:59–65.

182. Bastable JR, Peel RN, Birch DM, et al. Continuous irrigation of the bladder after prostatectomy: its effect on post-prostatectomy infection. *Br J Urol* 1977;49:689–693.

183. Southampton Infection Control Team. Evaluation of aseptic techniques and chlorhexidine on the rate of catheter-associated urinary-tract infection. *Lancet* 1982;1:89–91.

184. Maizels M, Schaeffer AJ. Decreased incidence of bacteriuria associated with periodic instillations of hydrogen peroxide into the urethral catheter drainage bag. *J Urol* 1980;123:841–845.

185. Sujka SK, Petrelli NJ, Herrera L. Incidence of urinary tract infections in patients requiring long-term catheterization after abdominoperineal resection for rectal carcinoma: does Betadine in the Foley drainage bag make a difference? *Eur J Surg Oncol* 1987;13:341–343.

186. al Juburi AZ, Cicmanec J. New apparatus to reduce urinary drainage associated with urinary tract infections. *Urology* 1989;33:97–101.

187. Sweet DE, Goodpasture HC, Holl K, et al. Evaluation of H_2O_2 prophylaxis of bacteriuria in patients with long-term indwelling Foley catheters: a randomized controlled study. *Infect Control* 1985;6:263–266.

188. Thompson RL, Haley CE, Searcy MA, et al. Catheter-associated bacteriuria. Failure to reduce attack rates using periodic instillations of a disinfectant into urinary drainage systems. *JAMA* 1984;251:747–751.

189. Gillespie WA, Simpson RA, Jones JE, et al. Does the addition of disinfectant to urine drainage bags prevent infection in catheterised patients? *Lancet* 1983;1:1037–1039.

190. Burke JP, Garibaldi RA, Britt MR, et al. Prevention of catheter-associated urinary tract infections. Efficacy of daily meatal care regimens. *Am J Med* 1981;70:655–658.

191. Burke JP, Jacobson JA, Garibaldi RA, et al. Evaluation of daily meatal care with poly-antibiotic ointment in prevention of urinary catheter-associated bacteriuria. *J Urol* 1983;129:331–334.

192. van der Wall E, Verkooyen RP, Mintjes de Groot J, et al. Prophylactic ciprofloxacin for catheter-associated urinary-tract infection. *Lancet* 1992;339:946–951.

193. Verbrugh HA, Mintjes de Groot AJ, Andriesse R, et al. Postoperative prophylaxis with norfloxacin in patients requiring bladder catheters. *Eur J Clin Microbiol Infect Dis* 1988;7:490–494.

194. Vollaard EJ, Clasener HA, Zambon JV, et al. Prevention of catheter-associated gram-negative bacilluria with norfloxacin by selective decontamination of the bowel and high urinary concentration. *J Antimicrob Chemother* 1989;23:915–922.

195. Mountokalakis T, Skounakis M, Tselentis J. Short-term versus prolonged systemic antibiotic prophylaxis in patients treated with indwelling catheters. *J Urol* 1985;134:506–508.

196. Little PJ, Pearson S, Peddie BA, et al. Amoxicillin in the prevention of catheter-induced urinary infection. *J Infect Dis* 1974;129: S241–S242.

197. Britt MR, Garibaldi RA, Miller WA, et al. Antimicrobial prophylaxis for catheter-associated bacteriuria. *Antimicrob Agents Chemother* 1977;11:240–243.

198. Warren JW. Catheter-associated urinary tract infections. *Int J Antimicrob Agents* 2001;17:299–303.

199. Platt R, Polk BF, Murdock B, et al. Prevention of catheter-associated urinary tract infection: a cost-benefit analysis. *Infect Control Hosp Epidemiol* 1989;10:60–64.

200. Stamm WE. Catheter-associated urinary tract infections: epidemiology, pathogenesis, and prevention. *Am J Med* 1991;91:65S–71S.

201. Tolkoff Rubin NE, Cosimi AB, Russell PS, et al. A controlled study of trimethoprim-sulfamethoxazole prophylaxis of urinary tract infection in renal transplant recipients. *Rev Infect Dis* 1982;4: 614–618.

202. Fox BC, Sollinger HW, Belzer FO, et al. A prospective, randomized, double-blind study of trimethoprim-sulfamethoxazole for prophylaxis of infection in renal transplantation: clinical efficacy, absorption of trimethoprim-sulfamethoxazole, effects on the microflora, and the cost-benefit of prophylaxis. *Am J Med* 1990;89:255–274.

203. Amin M. Antibacterial prophylaxis in urology: a review. *Am J Med* 1992;92:114S–117S.

SUBJECT INDEX

Page numbers followed by *f* indicate figures; those followed by *t* indicate tables

A

AA (arachidonic acid), metabolism of, 18
Abdominal muscles, 4, 5
Abdominal surgery, pleural effusions after, 427
ABPA (allergic bronchopulmonary aspergillosis), 138
ABPF (allergic bronchopulmonary fungoses), 138
Abscess
  intraabdominal, pleural effusions with, 426
  lung, 354, 368, 369f, 370f
    pleural effusions with, 186–188
    sputum with, 62
    symptoms of, 60, 62, 63
AC (assist-controlled) ventilation, 525, 527t
Acanthosis nigricans, with lung cancer, 332
Accessory muscles, of inspiration, 4–6
Accolate (zafirlukast), for asthma, 143, 150
ACE (angiotensin-converting enzyme)
  in sarcoidosis, 248
  vasoactive properties of, 17, 18f
Acetaldehyde, inhalation injury due to, 297t
Acetazolamide (Diamox), for central sleep apnea, 467
Acetylcholine, in respiratory muscle function, 6
Acid aerosols, air pollution due to, 311
Acid-base balance, disturbances in, 51
  diagnosis of, 54–56
    metabolic acidosis, 52
    metabolic alkalosis, 53
    mixed, 54
    respiratory acidosis, 51
    respiratory alkalosis, 52
Acid-base abnormalities, in respiratory failure, 520–521
Acid–base analysis, 97
Acid–base balance
  normal, 49–51

Acquired immunodeficiency syndrome (AIDS)
  aspergillosis in, 393
  bacterial infections in, 378f, 404
  bronchoscopy in, 120
  coccidioidomycosis in, 410
  cryptococcosis in, 393, 410
  evaluation in, 405–411
  highly active antiretroviral therapy for, 405
  histoplasmosis in, 387, 389f, 390f, 410
  noninfectious pulmonary complications of, 401t
  open-lung biopsy in, 124
  pneumonia in, 363, 376–378, 379f, 377t, 405, 409f, 410, 410f
  pulmonary effusion lymphoma in, 424
  respiratory infections in, 353
  tuberculosis in, 382, 383, 409, 410
Acquired immunodeficiency syndrome (AIDS), 386, 410
Acrylonitrile, carcinogenicity of, 298t, 309
Actinomycosis, pleural effusions due to, 421
Acute and subacute diseases, 291
Acute interstitial pneumonia, 237
Acute lung injury (ALI), 554, 559, 560t
  clinical course of, 557, 558f, 559f
  clinical disorders associated with, 554, 560t
  clinical manifestations of, 555, 556f
  defined, 554
  diagnosis of, 559
  due to gastric aspiration, 556f
  due to sepsis, 555, 556f, 558f
  early recognition of, 601
  in critically ill patients, 597–598
  mechanism of, 560
  mortality in, 554
  pulmonary edema in, 554, 558f
  scoring system for, 598, 599t
  treatment for, 559
Acute lupus pneumonitis (ALP), 256

Acute rejection, after lung transplantation, 192–193
Acute respiratory distress syndrome (ARDS), 554
  clinical course of, 557, 558f
  clinical disorders associated with, 554, 560t
  clinical manifestations of, 556, 557f
  defined, 554
  diagnosis of, 559
  due to gastric aspiration, 556f, 557
  due to pancreatitis, 557f
  due to sepsis, 556f, 558f
  in critically ill patients, 598–599
  mechanism of lung injury in, 558
  oxygen uptake in, 599, 600f
  pneumonia in, 353, 363t, 374–376, 375f
  pulmonary artery catheterization for, 594
  pulmonary edema in, 554, 557f
  right-to-left shunting in, 47
  surfactant in, 29
  treatment for, 559
ADA (adenosine deaminase)
  in pleural fluid, 116
  in tuberculous pleuritis, 420
Adenocarcinoma, 320, 323–325
Adenoid cystic carcinoma, 327
Adenoma(s)
  alveolar, 327
  bronchial, 326–327
  pleomorphic, 327
Adenosine deaminase (ADA)
  in pleural fluid, 116
  in tuberculous pleuritis, 420
Adenosine triphosphatase (ATPase), in respiratory muscle function, 4–6
Adenosine triphosphate (ATP)
  in exercise, 99, 103
  in respiratory muscle function, 6
Adenovirus, pneumonia due to, 373t

in middle compartment, 432*t*, 436–437, 436*f*
in posterior compartment, 437–438
of vascular origin, 437, 438*f*
Mediastinitis, 439–440
acute, 439
after cardiac surgery, 439
fibrosing, 439
granulomatous, 439–440
lymph node involvement in, 436
Mediastinoscopy, 123
in lung cancer, 337*f*
Mediastinotomy, in lung cancer, 337–338
Mediastinum, 432
computed tomography of, 433
injuries to, 572*t*, 581–583, 582*f*
Medical decision-making, 511
Medihaler-150 (isoproterenol HCl)
for asthma, 142*t*, 145
Mediterranean fever, familial, pleural
effusions with, 425
Medroxyprogesterone (Provera)
for obstructive sleep apnea, 462
for pulmonary lymphangiomyomatosis,
428
Meigs syndrome, 428
Meningeal coccidioidomycosis, 393
Meningitis
coccidioidal, 393
cryptococcal, 393, 410
tuberculous, 384
Meningocele, mediastinal, 438
Meningomyelocele, mediastinal, 438
Mercury, inhalation injury due to, 298
Mesenchymal tumors, mediastinal, 436
Mesodermal tumors, 327–328
Mesothelial cysts, 437
Mesothelioma
localized benign pleural, 424
malignant, 424
asbestos and, 310
Metabolic acidosis, in respiratory failure,
520
Metabolic alkalosis, in respiratory failure,
521
Metabolic complications, of tube feeding,
508
Metabolic equivalents (METs), 99
Metabolic manifestations, of lung cancer,
330–331
Metal fume fever, 298
Metal(s), irritant, 298, 307*t*
Metaproterenol (Alupent, Metaprel)
for asthma, 142*t*, 145, 541
Metastases
evaluation for, 339
in staging of lung cancer, 334, 335*t*, 336*t*
pulmonary, CT of, 78*f*
signs and symptoms of, 329–330
Metastatic lymph node enlargement, 436–437
Metered dose inhalers (MDIs), 133, 152
Methotrexate
for asthma, 154
for Wegener's granulomatosis, 264
pulmonary reaction to, 275
Methylisocyanate, inhalation injury due to,
297*t*
Methylphenidate (Ritalin), for narcolepsy, 456

Methylprednisolone sodium succinate
(Medrol, Solu-Medrol)
for asthma, 144*t*, 153, 545
for COPD, 179
Methylxanthines
for asthma, 143*t*
for COPD, 173
Methysergide, pleural effusions due to, 427
Metronidazole, for amebiasis, 422
Mica-associated lung disease, 306
Microscopic polyangiitis, 266
Midexpiratory flow rate, maximal, 91
Miliary tuberculosis, 374
Minerals, in parenteral nutrition, 509–510, 510*t*
Minute ventilation (VE)
and alveolar ventilation, 46
and work capacity, 103
normal, 6
total, 41, 520
with exercise, 6
MIP (maximal inspiratory pressure), 25–26, 521
Mitomycin C, pulmonary reaction to, 275
Mitral stenosis, pulmonary hypertension
due to, 222–225
Mixed venous saturation, 44*t*, 100–103*t*
Mixed ventilatory dysfunction, pulmonary
function testing with, 107
Mixed-dust pneumoconiosis, 306
MMF (maximal midexpiratory flow rate), 91
MMF (mycophenolate mofetil)
for bronchiolitis obliterans, 194
for lung transplantation, 198, 198*t*
MMO (maxillary mandibular osteotomy),
for obstructive sleep apnea, 463
MMVFs (manmade vitreous fibers)
carcinogenicity of, 307*t*, 309
pneumoconiosis due to, 306
Modafinil, for narcolepsy, 456
Mometasone furoate (Asmanex), for
asthma, 143*t*
Monge disease, 224
Monitoring
airflow, 453
cardiovascular, 589–595
of peak expiratory flow, 133, 137
respiratory, 531–532
of sleep, 448–451, 449*f*, 450*f*, 453–455, 454*t*
Monoclonal anti–T lymphocyte antibodies,
for lung transplantation, 199–201
Montelukast (Singulair), for asthma, 143*t*,
150–152
Moraxella spp, bronchitis due to, 359
Morphine sulfate
cardiovascular effects of, 565
for pulmonary edema, 554
MOTT (mycobacteria other than
tuberculosis), 386–387
Mountain sickness, chronic, 224
Mouth breathing, during exercise, 7
MRI (magnetic resonance imaging), 79–82
of chest trauma, 573
of lung cancer, 336
MS (mainstream smoke), 310
MSDSs (Material Safety Data Sheets), 291
MSLT (multiple sleep latency test), 454
in obstructive sleep apnea syndrome,
456

Mucin-associated antigens, 11
Mucociliary escalator, 19–20
Mucoepidermoid carcinoma, 327
Mucolytic therapy
for COPD, 177
for pneumonia, 381
Mucormycosis, 395
Mucosa, respiratory, metabolic and secretory
functions of, 10, 11
Mucous cells, functional anatomy of, 10
Mucous glands
functional anatomy of, 9
hypertrophy of, 10
in mucociliary escalator, 19, 20*f*
Mucus
formation of, 19
gel layer of, 19–20
sol layer of, 19, 20*f*
Mucus secretion
in chronic bronchitis, 166, 168
in COPD, 168
in idiopathic pulmonary fibrosis, 264
Multibreath nitrogen washout, 94, 97
Multidrug-resistant tuberculosis (MDRTB),
382, 385–387
with HIV infection, 409
Multiple organ failure (MOF), 595–605
cardiovascular failure in, 595–597
CNS failure in, 598
defined, 595
early recognition of, 601
epidemiology of, 596–599
gastrointestinal failure in, 597
hematologic failure in, 598
hepatic failure in, 597–598
management of, 601–605
mortality with, 599
pathogenesis of, 599–601, 600*f*
prevention of, 601
renal failure in, 597
respiratory failure in, 598–599
Multiple sclerosis, respiratory failure with,
538*t*
Multiple sleep latency test (MSLT), 454
in obstructive sleep apnea syndrome, 456
Muromonab-CO3 (Orthoclone OKT3)
for bronchiolitis obliterans, 194
for lung transplantation, 190
Muscle fatigue, functional anatomy of, 6
Muscular dystrophies, respiratory failure
with, 538*t*
Muscular efforts, volume-pressure relations
during, 25–29
Mustard gas, carcinogenicity of, 308*t*, 309
MVV (maximal voluntary ventilation), 92
and work capacity, 92
MWT (maintenance of wakefulness test), 455
Myasthenia gravis
respiratory failure in, 536, 538*t*
with thymoma, 434
Mycobacteria other than tuberculosis
(MOTT), 386–387
Mycobacterium avium complex (MAC),
386, 409
Mycobacterium tuberculosis, 382
Mycobacterial infections, 353, 386–387
with silicosis, 300